ALEXANDER'S
CARE OF THE PATIENT IN SURGERY

ALEXANDER'S
CARE OF THE PATIENT
IN SURGERY

Margaret Huth Meeker, RN, BSN, CNOR
Director of Perioperative Nursing
The Ohio State University Hospitals
Columbus, Ohio

Jane C. Rothrock, RN, DNSc, CNOR
Professor and Program Coordinator, Perioperative Nursing
Delaware County Community College
Media, Pennsylvania

NINTH EDITION

with 2296 illustrations

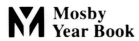 **Mosby
Year Book**

St. Louis   Baltimore   Boston   Chicago   London   Philadelphia   Sydney   Toronto

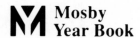
Mosby
Year Book
Dedicated to Publishing Excellence

Editor: Nancy L. Coon
Senior Developmental Editor: Susan R. Epstein
Project Manager: Annette Hall
Design: Susan Lane

NINTH EDITION

Printed in the United States of America

Mosby–Year Book, Inc.
11830 Westline Industrial Drive
St. Louis, Missouri 63146

Library of Congress Cataloging-in-Publication Data

Meeker, Margaret Huth.
    Alexander's care of the patient in surgery/Margaret Huth Meeker,
  Jane C. Rothrock.—9th ed.
      p.   cm.
    Includes bibliographical references.
    Includes index.
    ISBN 0-8016-3387-7
    1. Surgical nursing.   2.   Therapeutics, Surgical.   I.   Title.
    [DNLM: 1.   Nursing Care.   2.   Surgical Nursing.   WY 161 M494a]
  RD99.M387   1991
  610.73′677—dc20
  DNLM/DLC
  for Library of Congress   90-13509
                                                                       CIP

GW/VH/VH   9   8   7   6   5   4   3   2   1

In the Preface to the first edition of *Alexander's Care of the Patient in Surgery,* Edythe Alexander wrote, "From the moment an operation is decided upon, every phase of the handling of the patient, every detail, no matter how small, becomes of greatest importance." The first edition of her book, and all of the subsequent editions, have been committed to attending to the details of perioperative patient care. **Edythe Louise Alexander,** always generous in expressing her appreciation and gratitude to those who contributed to *Alexander's,* died on February 18, 1989. This ninth edition of *Alexander's Care of the Patient in Surgery* is dedicated to her, with our appreciation and gratitude for the earnest, sincere, and far-reaching effort she made on the part of perioperative nurses and their patients. Hers was an effort "of the greatest importance."

Contributors

Kay A. Ball, RN, MSA, CNOR
Laser Program Director
Mt. Carmel Health
Columbus, Ohio

Billie Fernsebner, RN, MSN, CNOR
Perioperative Clinical Nurse Specialist
Massachusetts General Hospital
Boston, Massachusetts

Virginia L. Finnie, RN, BSN, CNOR, CPSN
Plastic Surgery Clinical Specialist
University of Chicago
Section of Plastic and Reconstructive Surgery
Chicago, Illinois

Myrna K. Graves, RN
Assistant Manager, Operating Room
Grant Medical Center
Columbus, Ohio

Brenda S. Gregory, RN, BSN, CNOR
Assistant Manager, Nursing Education, Operating Rooms and
 Post Anesthesia Care Units
The Methodist Hospital
Houston, Texas

Jayne Henry, RN, BSN
Product Manager, Operating Rooms
The Ohio State University Hospitals
Columbus, Ohio

John Lee Hoffer, PhD, MD
Associate Professor in Anesthesiology and Physiology
Northeastern Ohio University School of Medicine;
Medical Director
Aultman Center for One Day Surgery
Canton, Ohio

Patricia P. Kapsar, RN, MBA
Director of Nursing
Bethesda General Hospital
St. Louis, Missouri

Susan V. M. Kleinbeck, RN, MS
Assistant Professor, Nursing
The Wichita State University
Wichita, Kansas

Karen S. McNeely, RN, MS
Nurse Manager, Operating Rooms
The Ohio State University Hospitals
Columbus, Ohio

Patricia Felice Meckes, RN, MN, CNOR
Assistant Director of Education and Training
Kaiser Foundation Hospital
Bellflower, California

Gratia M. Nagle, RN, RNFA, CNOR
Charge Nurse, Urology Service
Paoli Memorial Hospital
Paoli, Pennsylvania

Gwen Lynn Nelson, RN, BSN, CNOR
Staff Development Instructor, Perioperative Services
Pennsylvania Hospital
Philadelphia, Pennsylvania

Lynda R. Petty, RN, BSN
Research Associate—Surgical Oncology
College of Medicine
The Ohio State University
Columbus, Ohio

Merry Anne Pierson, RN, MSN, CNOR
Director, Surgical Services
Westside Hospital, Centennial Medical Center
Nashville, Tennessee

Leslie Eileen Ricker, RN, BSN
Staff Nurse, Ambulatory Operating Rooms
The Ohio State University Hospitals
Columbus, Ohio

Rosemary Ann Roth, RN, MSN, CNOR
Surgical Suite Nursing Director
The Genesee Hospital
Rochester, New York

Cheryl A. Sangermano, RN, BSN, CNOR
Nurse Manager, OR, PACU, Ambulatory Surgery Center
Grant Medical Center
Columbus, Ohio

Patricia C. Seifert, RN, MSN, CNOR
Operating Room Coordinator
Cardiac Surgery
The Arlington Hospital
Arlington, Virginia

Sue Silcox, RN, CNOR
Head Nurse, Otorhinolaryngology Operating Rooms
The Neurosensory Center
The Methodist Hospital
Houston, Texas

Judith J. Stellar, RN, MS, CPNP
Clinical Nurse Specialist, Surgery and Trauma
St. Christopher's Hospital for Children
Philadelphia, Pennsylvania

Elaine Thomson-Keith, RN, BSN, CNOR
Manager, Neurosensory Operating Rooms and Post Anesthesia
 Care Units
The Methodist Hospital
Houston, Texas

Ruth E. Vaiden, RN, CNOR
Director, Surgical Services
Humana Hospital St. Luke's
Richmond, Virginia

Jane Scott Witchey, RN, BSN
Nurse Manager, Orthopedics
The Ohio State University Hospitals
Columbus, Ohio

Anita Lee Malen Wynne, RN, PhD
Associate Professor
University of Portland School of Nursing
Portland, Oregon

Reviewer Panel

Pat Aimino, RN, BSN
Nursing Educator
Education Department
North Colorado Medical Center
Greeley, Colorado

A. E. Lyn Ames, RN, MS, CNOR
AMI Rancho Encino Hospital
Encino, California

Roberta P. Bartee, RN, BS, MS
Former Assistant Professor
Louisiana State University Medical Center
School of Nursing
New Orleans, Louisiana

Carol Baumann, RN, MSN(R), CNOR
Education Coordinator
Missouri Baptist Medical Center
St. Louis, Missouri

Larry Brock
Surgical Technical Instructor
Red River Vocational Tech School
Duncan, Oklahoma

Mary Ann Coble, RN, CNOR
OR Education/Resource
Surgical Services Department
Swedish Hospital Medical Center
Seattle, Washington

Lura B. Dorsey, RN
Sweetwater, Texas

Gerry Downen, RN, BA
Swedish Hospital Medical Center
Seattle, Washington

Linda Edgeton, RN, MSN
RN First Assistant for Klint H. Stander, M.D.
Provo, Utah

Janice Fortune, RN
North Core Team Leader, Main Surgery
Surgical Services Department
Swedish Hospital Medical Center
Seattle, Washington

Mary T. Gilley, RN, BSN, CNOR
Clinical Specialist
Division of Colon/Rectal Surgery
Jewish Hospital at Washington University
St. Louis, Missouri

Pauline Goske, RN, BSN, CNOR
Director of Operative Services
Lyndon Baines Johnson Hospital
Harris County Hospital District
Houston, Texas

Mary E. Grech, RN, MA
Lecturer
University of California–Los Angeles
Los Angeles, California

Betty Haddock, RN
Director of School of Surgical Technology
Presbyterian Hospital
Charlotte, North Carolina

Norma Ester Harnack, RN, BSN, CNOR
Clinical Specialist/Staff Nurse
St. Joseph Hospital–Kirkwood
Kirkwood, Missouri

Linda Herzog, RN, MA, CNOR
Perioperative Nurse Educator
Phoenix Baptist Hospital
Phoenix, Arizona

Edwinia Ion, RN
Cardiovascular Nurse Specialist
Dunn Operating Room
The Methodist Hospital
Houston, Texas

Joan Irving, RN, BSN, CNOR
Supervisor of Education and Resources for Surgical Services
Swedish Hospital Medical Center
Seattle, Washington

Nyla Juhl, RN, PhD
Chair, Family and Community Nursing
University of North Dakota
Grand Forks, North Dakota

Rosemary Kesler, RN, MA, CNOR
Program Director for Surgical Technology
Gateway Community College
Phoenix, Arizona

Barbara Kopec, RN, CNOR
Staff Nurse, Operating Room
Memorial Medical Center
Springfield, Illinois

Debra Lentz, RN, BSN, CNOR
OR Supervisor
St. Joseph Hospital–Kirkwood
Kirkwood, Missouri

Edwina A. McConnell, RN, PhD
Independent Nurse Consultant
Madison, Wisconsin

Margaret McGregor, RN
Director/Instructor
Surgical Technological Program
Simi Valley Adult School
Simi Valley, California

Thomas McLaren, RN, BSN
Director of Nursing for Surgical Services
Baptist Hospital
Pensacola, Florida

Elaine K. Neel, RN, MSN
Perioperative Nursing Instructor
The Methodist Medical Center
Peoria, Illinois

Jane A. Oyler, RN, BSN, CNA, CNOR
Director of Surgical Services
Gettysburg Hospital
Gettysburg, Pennsylvania

Sandra E. Paddock, RN
Clinical Education Charge Nurse
Surgical Services
Swedish Hospital Medical Center
Seattle, Washington

Ann E. Prather, RN, CNOR
Operating Room Nurse Educator
Memorial City Medical Center
Houston, Texas

Rosanne Rapone-Tomich, RN, BSN, CNOR
Supervisor of Education and Resources for Surgical Services
Swedish Hospital Medical Center
Seattle, Washington

Dorothy Ross, RN, MS, CNOR
Head Nurse, Operating Rooms
VA Medical Center
Oklahoma City, Oklahoma

Lexy Rotzell, RN
Operating Room Clinical Educator
Meriter Madison General Hospital
Madison, Wisconsin

Judith Sands, RN
Associate Professor
University of Virginia
School of Nursing
Charlottesville, Virginia

Deborah Sears, RN, CNOR
Quality Assurance Coordinator, Surgery
Laser Safety Officer, Surgery
Bryon Memorial Hospital
Lincoln, Nebraska

Carol A. Stephenson, RN, EdD
Associate Professor
Texas Christian University
Harris College of Nursing
Fort Worth, Texas

Pam Stevenson, RN, BSN
Surgical Services
Swedish Hospital Medical Center
Seattle, Washington

Roger Stone, RN, MS(N), CNOR
Divisional Director of Perioperative Nursing
Cook County Hospital
Chicago, Illinois

Miriam Struzyna, RN, BSN
Surgical First Assistant, Plastic Surgery, for Gilbert Eade, M.D.
Seattle, Washington

Dorothy Thomas, RN, MSN
Instructor, School of Nursing
Missouri Baptist Medical Center
St. Louis, Missouri

Sarah Jane Bradford Tobiason, RN
Assistant Professor of Nursing
Arizona State University
Tempe, Arizona

Susan K. Yakubisin, RN, CNOR
Coordinator Plastics and Assistant Coordinator Ophthalmology
Timpken Mercy Medical Center
Canton, Ohio

Mary Lou Young, RN, BSN
St. Louis, Missouri

Preface

The ninth edition of *Alexander's Care of the Patient in Surgery* has been extensively updated to reflect new concepts in perioperative nursing practice and the increased sophistication and complexity of high-tech surgical procedures. However, the goal of this text remains essentially the same: to provide a comprehensive basic reference that will assist perioperative personnel to more effectively meet the needs of patients during surgical intervention.

The standard in perioperative nursing for nearly 50 years, *Alexander's Care of the Patient in Surgery* is written primarily for professional perioperative nurses, but is also useful for nursing students, surgical technologists, health care industry representatives, medical students, interns, residents, and government officials concerned with health care issues. Nurse practitioners and educators from many geographic areas of the United States have served as contributors to this text, providing a broad range of perioperative experience and procedural information.

This thoroughly revised edition highlights the most current techniques and innovations in surgery. Hundreds of illustrations, including many new photographs and drawings, help familiarize the reader with new methods and equipment. Classic illustrations, particularly of surgical anatomy, have been preserved to enhance the text.

Overall, the text imparts state-of-the-art information that reflects quality contemporary practice and promotes the delivery of comprehensive perioperative patient care.

Part One, "General Considerations," provides information on basic principles and procedures utilized in all surgical suites. Significant revisions in the chapter on "Management of Perioperative Nursing Services" address organization theories and management systems that will assist the nurse manager in more efficiently and effectively managing complex surgical services. The chapter on "Anesthesia" has been expanded to include common problems that can occur during recovery from anesthesia. This vital information will assist the PACU nurse with assessment of patients during the immediate postoperative period and initiation of early intervention therapy. A separate chapter on "Lasers" is new to this edition and details contemporary and future applications of this exciting surgical technology.

The care and procedures involved with nearly 400 general and specialty surgical interventions are included in Part Two. Each chapter provides an overview of pertinent anatomy and details the steps of each procedure. Perioperative nursing considerations have been expanded and are now presented within the nursing process framework. Related NANDA-approved nursing diagnoses and Sample Care Plans for each surgical specialty will assist the nurse in planning, implementing, and evaluating individualized perioperative patient care. Increased emphasis on preoperative and postoperative teaching will assist the reader in preparing patients for surgical intervention and early discharge.

Part Three, "Special Considerations" discusses the unique needs of pediatric, geriatric, and ambulatory surgery patients. The new chapter on "Geriatric Surgery" provides valuable information that will enable the perioperative nurse to more effectively care for members of this fast growing population. The expanded "Ambulatory Surgery" chapter continues to reflect the expectation that these patients will receive the same standard of perioperative care as traditional inpatients. "Pediatric Surgery" highlights special considerations for the child in surgery.

Many expert practitioners have contributed to this ninth edition, and we owe a debt of gratitude to each of them. We also acknowledge the valuable assistance of editors, reviewers, photographers, and illustrators who have contributed their time and expertise to the revision of this text.

Alexander's Care of the Patient in Surgery is written by and for perioperative nurses, and is dedicated to excellence in perioperative nursing practice.

Margaret Huth Meeker
Jane C. Rothrock

Contents

ALEXANDER'S
CARE OF THE PATIENT IN SURGERY

Part One

GENERAL CONSIDERATIONS

1 Concepts basic to perioperative nursing

ANITA LEE MALEN WYNNE

The specialty of perioperative nursing has come of age in both image and practice. In the few years since the last edition of this text was published, perioperative nurses have expanded their practice patterns and responsibilities, continued to enhance their self-concepts, and firmly established perioperative nursing as a professional nursing specialty.

The term *perioperative nursing* is now used in both nursing and medical circles. Perioperative nursing is recognized and practiced in surgical suites and ambulatory surgery centers across the United States. Historically, the term "operating room nursing" was used to describe the care of patients in the immediate preoperative, intraoperative, and postoperative phases of the surgical experience. Such a term, however, had implied geographic limitations; it intimated that nursing care activities were circumscribed to the geographic limits of the surgical suite. The term may have contributed to stereotypic images of a nurse who took care of the operating room and had little interface or nursing responsibility for medicated and anesthetized patients in the surgical suite. In this perspective, nursing practitioners outside the operating room had difficulty ascribing important elements of the nursing process and patient care accountability to the nurse who practiced behind the doors of the surgical suite.

Perioperative nursing includes the preoperative, intraoperative, and postoperative periods of the patient's surgical experience. It connotes, however, the delivery of nursing care through the framework of the nursing process. In such a framework, the perioperative nurse engages in patient assessment; collects, organizes, and prioritizes patient data; develops and implements a plan of nursing care; and evaluates that care in terms of outcomes achieved by the patient. In these activities, the perioperative nurse functions dependently, independently, and interdependently. The perioperative nurse collaborates with other health care professionals, makes appropriate nursing referrals, and delegates and supervises nursing care. When perioperative nursing is practiced in its broadest scope, nursing care may begin in the patient's home, a clinic, a physician's office, the patient care unit, or the holding area. Following the surgical intervention, nursing care may continue in postanesthesia care or in patient evaluation on the patient care unit, in the physician's office, in the patient's home, in a clinic, or through written or telephone patient surveys. Perioperative nursing may be practiced in diverse settings. When perioperative nursing is practiced in the narrower sense, patient care activities may be confined to the common areas of the surgical suite. Assessment and data collection may take place in the holding area; evaluation may take place on discharge from the operating room to the postanesthesia care unit. Despite the way perioperative nursing is operationalized in a health care setting, it is underscored by the nursing process and all the care activities inherent in that process.

CONSIDERATIONS

The various perioperative nursing roles all subsume elements of the behaviors and technical practices that characterize professional nursing. Probably no other area of nursing requires the broad knowledge base, the instant recall of nursing science, the need to be intuitively guided by past nursing experience, the diversity of thought and action, the stamina, and the flexibility needed in perioperative nursing endeavors. Whether a generalist or specialist, the perioperative nurse depends on stored knowledge pertinent to surgical anatomy, physiologic alterations and their consequences for the patient, intraoperative risk factors, potentials for patient injury and the means of preventing them, and psychosocial implications of surgery for the patient and significant others, as well as on clues to needs of the patient or surgical team. This stored knowledge enables the perioperative nurse to initiate nursing actions on a minute's notice. Such excellence in practice is the hallmark of perioperative nursing.

The size of this mental repertoire is staggering and points out the constant discipline, attention, ongoing education, and presence of mind demanded in perioperative nursing. However, the greater the requirements, the more satisfactory and indelible are the joys that come to the perioperative nurse who practices at this level of excellence. The perioperative nurse recognizes self, and is recognized by other members of the health care team, as an integral team member, truly an expert!

Perioperative nursing is a purposeful, dynamic, professional process. Through the process of planning patient care and identifying required nursing interventions and actions, perioperative nurses assure surgical patients of scientific, professional nursing care. Perioperative nurses historically have assumed responsibility for providing a safe, efficient, and caring environment for surgical patients, one in which the surgical team can function smoothly and efficiently to achieve positive patient outcomes. Such mutuality between nursing and other health care disciplines and the role of patient advocacy continues to be part of the essence of perioperative nursing in the 1990s.

This textbook is in part technical. A significant part of perioperative nursing is the delivery of scientifically based care. Understanding the necessity for certain techniques of care; knowing how and when to initiate them; being creative in maintaining a technique when the situation calls for flexibility; and evaluating the safety, cost, and outcomes of the technical aspects of nursing science are all part of professional nursing responsibility. Knowledge of nursing skills, procedures, setups, instruments, and equipment is essential during the implementation phase of nursing care. Without such knowledge, the perioperative nurse is unable to prepare for or anticipate the steps in the surgical procedure, with their concomitant implications for the patient and for the surgical team. Nurses who are well versed in the detailed nursing techniques contained in this text can best foresee the needs of both the patient and the surgical team during care plan implementation. Scientific nursing techniques are at the heart of perioperative nursing. In the many chapters of this text that focus on surgical interventions common to patients in the 1990s, these nursing techniques have clearly and deliberately been incorporated as part of the care plan. Such conceptualization integrates them as important elements of nursing care.

In this chapter, perioperative nursing is considered as an entity. The purpose is to place it in perspective by spelling out the place for and details of some of the behavioral and conceptual components. It sets the scene for the remainder of the text. A fundamental assumption is that perioperative nursing is a blend of the technical and behavioral; it is thinking as well as doing, patient caring and people caring as well as instrument handling.

DESCRIPTION OF PERIOPERATIVE NURSING

Perioperative nursing, a term describing the scope and practice of nursing in surgical settings, has gained wide acceptance. Emanating from the work and influence of the Association of Operating Room Nurses (AORN), the term has helped to define and elucidate the activities of the professional nurse during three patient care phases: preoperative, intraoperative, and postoperative. A model depicting perioperative practice would illustrate a continuum on which the nurse functions, from beginning competency to excellence.

Such a perioperative practice concept brings together both traditional and expanded nursing activities during intraoperative care, preoperative and postoperative patient education, counseling, assessment, planning, and evaluation functions. Perioperative nurses scrub, circulate, assist the surgeon (RN first assistant), manage, teach, and conduct research. Because of an increased concern with containment of costs associated with the delivery of health care services, surgical procedures are now performed not only in traditional hospital operating rooms but also in freestanding surgical centers, ambulatory care or short-stay units, emergency departments, and physicians' offices. In these settings, the professional nurse is a primary care giver. From admission through discharge and home follow-up, the perioperative nurse plays a significant role in overseeing the patient's care. Such practice has helped to popularize and confirm the nature of a broad foundation for perioperative nursing roles. In the 1990s, research should continue to test and validate the contribution of perioperative nursing to patient care outcomes in all settings where it is practiced.

Within such a conceptual framework for the practice of perioperative nursing, a description of a comprehensive combination of head and hand skills emerges. A schema is provided whereby such nursing is viewed in a professional perspective and the nursing process is a pervasive thread.

NURSING PROCESS

Perioperative nursing is a planned process, a series of integrated steps. If viewed only as "setting up cases," perioperative nursing becomes nothing more than rote equipment preparation and paper shuffling. If, rather, it is viewed as *patient care,* it becomes a scientific process and an exciting stimulus for the nurse to perform optimally.

The nursing process is a way of looking at nursing and bringing it into perspective as *a methodical thought process that guides actions,* which contrasts to considering nursing as only a set of cookbook rituals and procedures to be learned. The focus of the nursing process is on the patient, and the nursing interventions prescribed are those that meet patient needs. Because of the setting and the nature of the work, perioperative nursing is particularly vulnerable to being considered only a conglomeration of mechanical techniques and a carrying out of surgeons' orders. By using the nursing process, perioperative nurses can focus on the patient and, at the same time, put skills and know-how in proper perspective in dealing with patients *and* implementing procedures.

Use of the nursing process and nursing care plans has become an integral part of patient care in hospital nursing units. Their use in the perioperative setting has been less evident, in part because the perioperative setting is sufficiently different to require some alterations from the formal processes implemented on other nursing units. Because of

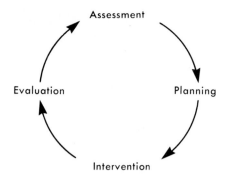

Assessment

Evaluation

Planning

Intervention

Fig. 1-1. Four phases of nursing process.

these differences, including the short time the nurse has contact with the conscious patient and the movement through three different areas in the operative process, the perioperative nurse must adapt the process to the setting.

In its simplest form the nursing process consists of four phases: assessment, planning, intervention, and evaluation (Fig. 1-1). The process is circular and continuous.

Assessment is the collection of relevant data about the patient. Sources of data may be a preoperative interview with the patient and the patient's family by a perioperative or unit nurse; review of the nursing care plans, Kardex, and patient's chart; and consultation with the surgeon and anesthesiologist, unit nurses, or other personnel.

The format this assessment takes may vary from institution to institution but should always include both the physiologic and the psychosocial aspects of the patient. (See Bibliography at the end of the chapter.)

For a perioperative nurse, assessment often means a thoughtful, quick scan of the patient and chart, a review of the surgical procedure, and a mental rehearsal of the resources and knowledge necessary to direct the patient through an operative course. At other times the nurse must thoroughly assess all aspects of the patient and the patient's condition, along with preoperative and postoperative reviews.

In a discussion of assessment, the question of whether perioperative nurses should perform preoperative interviews invariably arises. Preoperative interviews or visits are standard procedure in many institutions. In others these interviews are not done and are not supported by the administration because of such reasons as shortages of time and personnel.

Preoperative visits by perioperative nurses are neither an end in themselves nor a means of "getting nurses in touch with their patients." Also, preoperative patient contact alone does not mean that true perioperative practice exists; the perioperative nurse should beware of this fallacy. However, if planned properly to fill the needs of both patients and nurses, preoperative (and postoperative) interviews can be extremely beneficial (Fig. 1-2).

When thinking about preoperative interviewing and teaching, the nurse should consider the following: Is relevant, concise patient information already being transmitted to the perioperative nursing staff? Is enough infor-

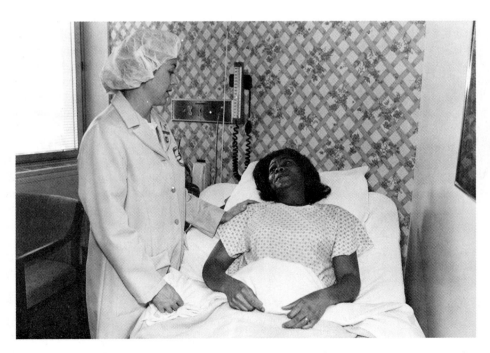

Fig. 1-2. Perioperative nurse interviews surgical patient. Purpose of visit is to assess patient needs, to obtain information about patient and family, and to teach patient regarding common routines, sensations, and nursing care.

mation available to allow perioperative nurses to consider patient care needs when setting up the room (special equipment, supports, instruments, sutures)? Is sufficient time available to initiate a meaningful nurse-patient interaction before induction? Are surgical patients satisfied with their perioperative nursing care (do they express feelings of comfort and satisfaction regarding their care in the surgical setting), and do they have knowledge of the perioperative nurse's role? Is there continuity of care between the operating room and other nursing care units?

Being able to exchange information about their patients in face-to-face meetings (Fig. 1-3) or by telephone or written messages is helpful for unit and perioperative nurses. A thorough assessment, made and recorded by the unit nurses, can accompany patients to the operating room and serve as a guide to perioperative nursing personnel. Often, however, this assessment is not done or the information supplied is not useful to the nurses in the surgical suite. Then the perioperative nurse has the responsibility to do more in-depth preoperative patient assessment.

Individual sessions with patients may be the answer to the issue of preoperative assessment. In some hospitals, group preoperative classes not only help nurses get to know the patients but also permit them to impart information on common routines, reactions, sensations, and nursing procedures that will take place preoperatively, intraoperatively, and postoperatively. The important point is that some form of assessment and teaching should be done.

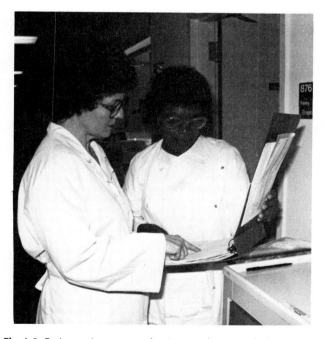

Fig. 1-3. Perioperative nurse and unit nurse discuss and plan patient care and preparation for surgery by sharing findings and relevant data.

How it is accomplished is up to the particular facility and nursing staff.

Assessment, then, is knowing and understanding the patient as a feeling, thinking, and responsible person and as a candidate for a surgical procedure.

Based on the data collected and interpreted during patient assessment, a nursing diagnosis is formulated and pertinent patient information is recorded.

Diagnosis is the process of identifying and classifying the data collected in the assessment in a way that will yield a focus for the planning of nursing care. Nursing diagnoses have been evolving since they were first introduced in the 1950s. They have now reached the stage of development of being identified, named, and classified. The group responsible for delineating the accepted list of nursing diagnoses is the North American Nursing Diagnosis Association (NANDA) (see box, p. 6). References related to these diagnoses are found in the bibliography at the end of the chapter.

Not all patient problems encountered in the perioperative setting can be described by the existing list of accepted nursing diagnoses, but the list is expanding. The perioperative nurse is encouraged to assist in the description and naming of new nursing diagnoses that describe these problems.

Having collected and interpreted the patient data and arrived at appropriate nursing diagnoses, the perioperative nurse is prepared to plan the nursing care for the patient. Viewing the patient as an individual and not as a case allows the nurse to gain more satisfaction because the *person* having the surgery is now considered *as well as* the tools, setups, and environmental controls needed to perform the surgery. If perioperative nursing care fails to put its main emphasis on the human having the operation, it can no longer be labeled professional nursing.

Planning, the second step in the nursing process, means that perioperative nurses use their nursing knowledge and information about the patient to prepare the operating room environment. They check equipment, have unusual and usual supplies ready, and use their knowledge of anatomy to have proper instruments and sutures on hand for the procedure to be performed. They know the usual steps in a procedure and use the surgeon's preference cards and nursing care guides to have the room and equipment completely ready for the patient.

Planning is knowing ahead of time what will happen and being prepared. Planning also means knowing the patient and the patient's unique needs so that alterations in positioning or in the surgical process may be readily made if adaptation to these unique needs is required. Planning requires some knowledge of the patient's feelings about the proposed operation so an extra, needed explanation or a comforting hand grasp can be provided during the critical preinduction period (Fig. 1-4).

Planning involves a broad understanding of operating

NANDA-APPROVED NURSING DIAGNOSES (1990)

Activity intolerance
Altered family processes
Altered growth and development
Altered health maintenance
Altered nutrition: less than body requirements
Altered nutrition: more than body requirements
Altered nutrition: potential for more than body requirements
Altered oral mucous membrane
Altered parenting
Altered protection
Altered patterns of urinary elimination
Altered role performance
Altered sexuality patterns
Altered thought processes
Altered (specify type) tissue perfusion, (cerebral, cardiopulmonary, renal, gastrointestinal, peripheral)
Anticipatory grieving
Anxiety
Bathing/hygiene self-care deficit
Body-image disturbance
Bowel incontinence
Chronic low self-esteem
Chronic pain
Colonic constipation
Constipation
Decisional conflict (specify)
Decreased cardiac output
Defensive coping
Diarrhea
Dressing/grooming self-care deficit
Dysfunctional grieving
Dysreflexia
Effective breastfeeding
Family coping: potential for growth
Fatigue
Fear
Feeding self-care deficit
Fluid volume deficit (1)
Fluid volume deficit (2)
Fluid volume excess
Functional incontinence
Health seeking behaviors (specify) or desire for high-level wellness (specify)
Hopelessness
Hyperthermia
Hypothermia
Impaired adjustment
Impaired gas exchange
Imparied home maintenance management
Impaired physical mobility

Impaired skin integrity
Impaired social interaction
Impaired swallowing
Impaired tissue integrity
Impaired verbal communication
Ineffective airway clearance
Ineffective breastfeeding
Ineffective breathing pattern
Ineffective denial
Ineffective family coping: compromised
Ineffective family coping: disabled
Ineffective individual coping
Ineffective thermoregulation
Knowledge deficit (specify)
Noncompliance (specify)
Pain
Parental role conflict
Perceived constipation
Personal identity disturbance
Post-trauma response
Potential activity intolerance
Potential altered body temperature
Potential fluid volume deficit
Potential for aspiration
Potential for disuse syndrome
Potential for infection
Potential for injury
Potential for poisoning
Potential for suffocating
Potential for trauma
Potential for violence: self-directed or directed at others
Potential impaired skin integrity
Powerlessness
Rape-trauma syndrome
Rape-trauma syndrome: compound reaction
Rape-trauma syndrome: silent reaction
Reflex incontinence
Self-esteem disturbance
Sensory perceptual alterations (specify) (auditory, gustatory, kinesthetic, olfactory, tactile, visual)
Sexual dysfunction
Situational low self-esteem
Sleep pattern disturbance
Social isolation
Spiritual distress (distress of the human spirit)
Stress incontinence
Toileting self-care deficit
Total incontinence
Unilateral neglect
Urge incontinence
Urinary retention

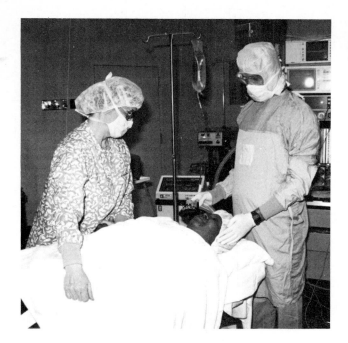

Fig. 1-4. Critical time for each surgical patient is preinduction phase.

room routines and perioperative nursing. It requires participating in continuing education programs (Fig. 1-5), reading journals, and keeping up-to-date in the rapidly advancing world of perioperative nursing. Education is discussed in more detail later in this chapter.

Intervention is performing the nursing care that was planned and responding to changes in routine or to emergencies with calmness and orderly thinking. It is employ-

ing established standards of nursing care and other guidelines developed and maintained by the nursing profession (see Bibliography at end of chapter). Intervention also means being the patient's advocate by carrying out nursing care as part of a team whose individual responsibilities in the operating room are well defined. The role of patient advocate is especially important in the operating room, where patients are usually unconscious and unable to speak for themselves.

Accurate documentation of nursing care is an integral part of all phases of the nursing process, especially intervention. A description of the patient, the nursing care given, and the patient's response to care (outcomes) should be included in the patient's record. The AORN *Standards of Perioperative Nursing Practice* state that documentation of the nursing care given should include more than the technical aspects of care, such as the sponge count or the application of the electrosurgical dispersive pad. Nursing care documentation should be related to nursing diagnoses, with preestablished goals against which the appropriateness of care may be judged.

The form for this documentation may include both standardized interventions and space to write in interventions that are unique to individual patients. Documentation should require little time to complete, be specific to the perioperative setting, and provide continuity across the various areas in surgery from presurgery holding areas to the postanesthesia care units.

Implicit in intervention is teamwork. Nowhere is a smoothly functioning team of more importance to the patient than in the operating room. Respect for others' expertise, the ability to work harmoniously, and the art of

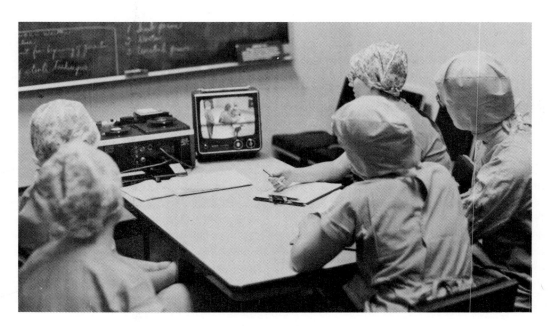

Fig. 1-5. Continuing education is necessary for all perioperative nurses. Self-instruction, use of literature, conferences, and informal discussions are examples.

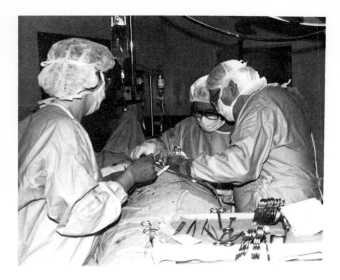

Fig. 1-6. Teamwork in the operating room implies collegial relationships, efficient use of skills and knowledge, and effective, respectful communication among team members (surgeons, anesthesiologists, and perioperative nurses).

Assess	Review medical record, validate important findings, corroborate with patient. Formulate *nursing diagnoses* based on analysis, interpretation, and prioritization of patient information.
Plan	Incorporate information into a plan for the patient's care. Set goals based on identified nursing diagnoses; identify nursing interventions.
Implement	Carry out nursing plan. Gather equipment and supplies; participate in/guide/supervise patient preparation (transfer to OR bed, anesthesia induction, antimicrobial skin preparation, draping, patient positioning, physiologic alterations during surgery), and patient discharge (transfer from OR bed, discharge to postanesthesia or postoperative unit).
Evaluate	Determine whether goals were met; use outcome statements. Incorporate outcomes that have been met and those that are pending in report to nurse in postanesthesia care unit/discharge area.

Fig. 1-7. The nursing process is continuous, leading to a higher level of care.

communicating effectively are necessary ingredients for a well-functioning team (Fig. 1-6).

Evaluation, the fourth phase of the nursing process, is checking, observing, and appraising the results of what was done. Evaluation of perioperative nursing care can be performed through on-the-spot correction of deficiencies and through education to keep personnel up-to-date on new procedures and equipment. It is also accomplished through traditional quality assurance activities, notably monitoring, problem identification, problem solving, and peer review. Resources such as conferences, workshops, textbooks, and journal articles are available to assist in the initiation of these processes.

Hospital quality assurance programs demonstrate many ways of evaluating and improving care, including that given to surgical patients. Quality assurance programs identify problems in patient care, propose solutions, and monitor and evaluate specified actions in solving the problems.

Evaluation must also include reassessment of patients to determine outcomes and reactions to their surgical experiences. Evaluation, then, is a learning process in which both strengths and weaknesses are exposed and examined. The emphasis is always on outcomes.

The nursing process is continuous in that evaluation may lead back to assessment. Changes in patient care patterns may require new assessments and plans. The nursing process is never a dead end; it is continuous and always leads to a higher level of care (Fig. 1-7).

CONTINUING EDUCATION

The pace and complexity of today's health care scene demand constant attention to professional development.

Perioperative nurses who keep abreast of new information and techniques will be assets to the operating room team. A word of caution—only the fittest will survive and thrive as professional nurses.

Who are the fittest? They are those professionals who are tenacious in their search for relevant, practical knowledge that leads to better daily functioning in perioperative clinical practice. This search can be thought of as quality assurance for the perioperative nurse (Fig. 1-8). Quality assurance in health care means monitoring and correction of problems, which lead to predictability of proper outcomes; it can have similar meanings for the perioperative nurse who wishes to be above average, even superior, in practice. Quality assurance also implies assessment of resources and goals, participation in and high regard for continuing education, use of learning props (Fig. 1-5), and evaluation of professional goal achievements, roadblocks, and effectiveness of continuing education programs.

Rigorous professional and personal credentialing is becoming familiar to perioperative nurses and will be the

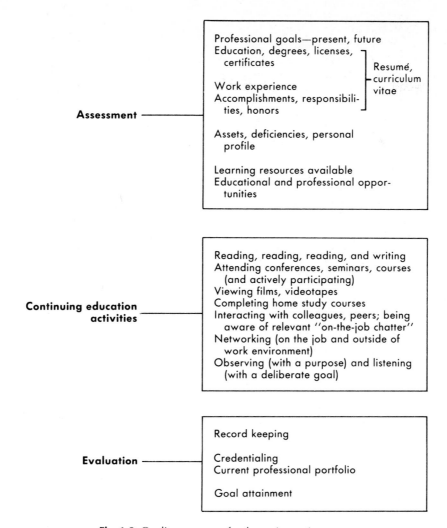

Fig. 1-8. Quality assurance for the perioperative nurse.

accepted process for seeking or changing employment and for remaining professionally viable. Credentialing is verification and evaluation of education and experience according to professional and institutional standards and policies. A standard procedure in medicine, credentialing is fast becoming the modus operandi in other health care professions, including nursing.

Above all, continuing education requires great awareness and curiosity, the acquisition of practical and theoretical knowledge, and a disciplined, habitual reading of literature that pertains to the business and political worlds, the health care marketplace, the profession of nursing, and the specialty of perioperative nursing.

NURSING ROLES IN THE FUTURE

The profession of nursing is in a state of self-evaluation, renewal, and emergence as a strong force in health care. Nurses, as well as many others outside the profession, are questioning the profession's identity, status, and reward system. The triad of nurse-physician-administrator is under scrutiny. New roles, new definitions, and new parameters of practice are being proposed and tested. Regardless of title and function, every nurse working in the operating room is assuming greater responsibility and is becoming a colleague of other health care professionals in patient care.

The role of the perioperative nurse as assistant at surgery is a good example of an evolving new role. In 1984, the AORN approved an official statement on the RN first assistant. This nurse, who must have formal education or documented independent study for role preparation, works collaboratively with the surgeon (and the patient and surgical team) by handling tissue and instruments, providing exposure and hemostasis, and suturing. Many experienced perioperative nurses have obtained additional education to prepare themselves for this role. Performing as an RN first assistant allows the experienced perioperative nurse to advance in clinical knowledge and skill while still remaining directly involved with the provision of perioperative nursing care. This new role, which has gained acceptance, value, and importance in operating rooms across the country, is just one of the ways perioperative nurses are developing themselves to meet the changing needs of health care delivery.

In addition to practitioner–care giver, the roles of the professional nurse also include teacher, advocate, and researcher. The perioperative nurse teaches staff and patients and counsels patients who need assistance in adjusting to a new diagnosis or a changed body image. The nurse monitors the care given to the patient in the operating room and serves as patient advocate to assure a high quality of care. The consistent use of the nursing process is one form of the researcher role. For each patient, data are collected, problems are diagnosed, hypotheses in the form of nursing interventions are written to propose ways to solve the problem, the interventions are tested as they are carried out, and they are judged against expected patient outcomes. Each perioperative nurse has to use this process and document it appropriately to facilitate the development of the science as well as the art of nursing. Perioperative nurses also need to assist nurse researchers to delineate problems in the perioperative setting that need to be studied and to participate in those studies.

Finally, the perioperative nurse works in collaboration with surgeons, anesthesiologists, and other health care providers to plan the best course of action for each patient. To assure the highest quality of care, input from each of the health care disciplines represented in the operating room is crucial. Because the education of the professional nurse has more breadth than that of many other health care providers, the nurse is often in the best position to serve in a leadership role in fostering collegiality and collaboration among a variety of disciplines.

With greater responsibility comes accountability. Perioperative nurses are accountable to their patients and demonstrate it by using standards, recommended practices, and quality assurance activities and by constantly strengthening their professional skills through education.

As perioperative nursing progresses, new roles will emerge. Each of these roles, whether staff nurse, clinician, manager, or researcher, will make use of the nursing process and will demonstrate humanized care for surgical patients and their families. Perhaps a perioperative practitioner's role will include assisting during the operation or greater consultation with patients' families. Perioperative nurses can also be excellent teachers of health promotion, disease prevention, and wellness regimens. Each new function must be tested with time and should be integrated into the profession only if it enhances overall care and wellness of people, especially those who require surgical interventions.

Scrubbing and *circulating* may in the future become obsolete terms; already we know that they define circumscribed functions that are only a part of the perioperative nurse's sphere of responsibility. The future may bring new titles and functions but will never erase the critical function in surgical patient care that every perioperative nurse fulfills.

The future of perioperative nursing is directly related to the sophistication of its practitioners. Sophistication means that perioperative nurses must be superior thinkers *and* doers. If either knowledge *or* practice is neglected, perioperative nursing as a profession will decline and give way to rote tasks.

The nature of nurse-physician working relationships will continue to be scrutinized. This relationship is critical to good patient outcomes but often is contaminated by power struggles and turf battles. Physician-nurse conflicts are not only professional-technical and master-servant in nature but have status and socioeconomic roots as well. That physicians are often in independent practice whereas nurses usually have employee status enlarges the gap between the two groups. However, true peer respect is emerging and must be nurtured, although it is not yet reality in many operating rooms.

Outcomes of operations are directly related to the quality of perioperative nursing care provided, which in turn reflects the aptitudes and motivations of the practitioners. With this perspective, the reader should consider the remainder of this book as one part of a perioperative nurse's knowledge bank. The remaining chapters contain vital information related to the nursing process that is needed to function in a surgical setting.

BIBLIOGRAPHY

AORN policy, plan and priority statement on nursing research, AORN J. 48:436, 1988.

AORN's official statement on R.N. first assistant, AORN J. 41:141, 1984.

AORN standards and recommended practices for perioperative nursing, Denver, 1990, Association of Operating Room Nurses, Inc.

Association of Operating Room Nurses, Inc.: Perioperative nursing credentialing model, AORN J. 43:262, 1986.

Atkinson, L.J., and Kohn, M.L.: Berry and Kohn's introduction to operating room technique, ed. 6, New York, 1986, McGraw-Hill Book Co.

Barrett, N., and Schwartz, M.D.: What patients really want to know, Am. J. Nurs. 81:1642, 1981.

Bower, F.L.: The process of planning nursing care, ed. 3, St. Louis, 1982, The C.V. Mosby Co.

Brennan, P.E.: Preoperative visits: controlling the stress, Today's OR Nurse 4:9, 1982.

Brown, D., and Peake, J.: Presurgical education: establishing a program, AORN J. 39:1163, 1984.

Burden, N.: The ambulatory surgery setting: adding the caring touch, J. Post Anesthesia Nurs. 3:411, 1988.

Cook, T.D.: Major research analysis provides proof: patient education does make a difference, Promoting Health 5:4, 1984.

Cozad, J.: Nursing diagnosis, Point of View 25:16, 1988.

Damron, C., and Stetson, P.: A preoperative teaching program: preparing a child for ambulatory surgery, AORN J. 41:352, 1985.

Davis, N.: Charting a course for the R.N. first assistant, AORN J. 32:1032, 1980.

Defining a first assistant credential, OR Manager 4:9, 1988.

Griffith, J.W., and Christensen, P.J.: Nursing process: application of theories, frameworks, and models, St. Louis, 1982, The C.V. Mosby Co.

Griffith, N.L.: A review of the literature: the patient and the perioperative period, Point of View 22:14, 1985.

Jordan, C.H.: If we teach holistic care, can we exclude perioperative nursing? AORN J. 32:797, 1980.

Kathol, D.K.: Anxiety in surgical patients' families, AORN J. 40:131, 1984.

Kim, M.J., McFarland, G.K., and McLane, A.M., editors: Classification of nursing diagnosis: proceedings of the fifth national conference, St. Louis, 1984, The C.V. Mosby Co.

Kim, M.J., McFarland, G.K., and McLane, A.M., editors: Pocket guide to nursing diagnosis, St. Louis, 1984, The C.V. Mosby Co.

Kneedler, J.A.: Perioperative nursing research: intraoperative chemical and physical hazards to personnel, AORN J. 49:829, 1989.

Kneedler, J.A.: Perioperative nursing research: potential intraoperative biological hazards to personnel, AORN J. 49:1066, 1989.

Kneedler, J.A., and Dodge, G.H.: Perioperative patient care: the nursing perspective, Boston, 1987, Blackwell Scientific Publications.

Koehler, J.S.: Perioperative nursing can be cost effective, AORN J. 32:1068, 1980.

Leske, J.S., and McKnight, E.A.: First assistants: planning and implementing a course, AORN J. 42:185, 1985.

Lierman, J.: Perioperative assessments: can we afford to do without them? AORN J. 47:586, 1988.

Lindeman, C.A., and Van Aernam, B.: Nursing intervention with the presurgical patient: the effects of structured and unstructured preoperative teaching, Nurs. Res. 20:319, 1971.

McHugh, N.G., Christman, N.J., and Johnson, J.E.: Preparatory information: what helps and why, Am. J. Nurs. 82:780, 1982.

Malen A.L.: Perioperative nursing diagnosis: what, why and how, AORN J. 44:829, 1986.

Novak D., and others: The OR nurse universe study, AORN J. 48:26, 1988.

Patterson, P.: Time for a first assistant credential? OR Manager 4:6, 1988.

Pesetski, J.D.: A practical guide for perioperative practice, AORN J. 32:1049, 1980.

Phippen, M.: Perioperative nursing: implementing change, AORN J. 39:601, 1984.

Porter-O'Grady, T.: Credentialing, privileging, and nursing bylaws: assuring accountability, J. Nurs. Admin. 15:32, 1985.

Reeder, J.M.: Perioperative nursing competencies: the process and study. AORN J. 48:215, 1986.

Rothrock, J.C.: A college without walls: learning first assistant skills, AORN J. 45:1150, 1987.

Rothrock, J.C.: Perioperative care planning, St. Louis, 1990, The C.V. Mosby Co.

Rothrock, J.C.: Perioperative nursing research: preoperative psychoeducational interventions, AORN J. 49:597, 1989.

Rothrock, J.C.: The RN first assistant: an expanded perioperative nursing role, Philadelphia, 1987, J.B. Lippincott Co.

Santore, A.M.: The expanding role of the OR nurse, Today's OR Nurse 2:69, 1982.

Schur, V., and others: Documenting perioperative care, Today's OR Nurse 8:24, 1986.

Stone, L.A. and others: Nursing care documentation: creating a perioperative nursing record, AORN J. 49:808, 1989.

2 Management of perioperative nursing services

PATRICIA P. KAPSAR

Professional nursing standards comprise the framework within which perioperative nursing services are provided. Consumers rightfully expect to receive cost-effective care that is consistent with those standards of practice and provided by qualified practitioners. With rapidly changing technology, shrinking financial resources because of federally mandated reimbursement programs (such as the prospective payment systems for both inpatients and outpatients), and even more stringent reimbursement policies of the private sector, perioperative nursing personnel are obligated to implement new approaches in the provision of patient care. They must continually develop essential knowledge and skills associated with new concepts. Management practices that are consistent with the needs of a rapidly changing health care environment should assure that the department provides quality care for the surgical patient.

The management of perioperative nursing services should be consistent with that of the nursing department and the hospital. Professional management guidelines allow for the establishment and maintenance of good interdepartmental and intradepartmental relationships.

The purpose of this chapter is to highlight key aspects of managing perioperative nursing services. It introduces the concepts of management strategies that can stimulate perioperative nursing managers to pursue further knowledge related to effective management.

PHILOSOPHY, PURPOSE, AND OBJECTIVES OF PERIOPERATIVE NURSING
Philosophy

A written statement of perioperative nursing philosophy describes values and beliefs that pertain to nursing practice in the surgical services department and serves as the basis for choosing the means to accomplish objectives. It formalizes nurses' visions of what practice is believed to be. Philosophy statements are value statements about people as patients or employees, about work that will be performed by nurses for patients, about nursing as a profession, about education as it pertains to nurses' competence, and about the setting in which nursing services are provided. The philosophy of perioperative nursing should blend with those of the hospital and the department of nursing, the general and specialty surgical programs, and appropriate educational and research programs.

One philosophy of perioperative nursing service may be summarized as follows:

1. Perioperative nursing is a dynamic, behavioral, and technical process directed toward provision of quality patient care during surgical intervention.
2. Perioperative nursing service comprises distinct functions concerned with a safe physical environment and protection of patients, with continuous awareness of the dignity of humans and their physical and spiritual needs.
3. Perioperative nursing service promotes the knowledge and skills of its personnel to facilitate implementation of scientific and technological advances in health care.
4. Perioperative nursing service frequently adjusts its organization and functions in accordance with current health and educational programs.

The philosophy defined by the professional perioperative nursing staff should be consistent with that of the department of nursing.

Purpose

Every nursing department exists for a reason. The reason for existence is the purpose or mission of the department. Just as the nursing department has a purpose, so should surgical services. This purpose should be based on the philosophy, written in realistic terms and developed or revised with the participation of the perioperative nursing personnel who are governed by it. They should know and understand it. A meaningful statement of purpose indicates the relationships between the perioperative nursing personnel and patients, other personnel, the nursing department, and the hospital.

A statement of purpose of perioperative nursing might include the following:

1. To plan and provide perioperative nursing care that is consistent with standards for professional nursing practice as defined by the professional nurses of the staff and by the *Standards of Perioperative Nursing Practice*

2. To collaborate and cooperate with other members of the health care team in meeting the emergency, restorative, and preventive health needs of patients in a safe, comfortable, and therapeutic environment

Objectives

The objectives of perioperative nursing should be practical, specific, and measurable for the persons performing nursing functions. They should be detailed statements supporting the defined philosophy and employing the nursing process. Well-stated objectives serve as criteria by which personnel can measure achievement of purpose. Effective objectives are developed and changed in accordance with overall institutional policy through the cooperative efforts of the director, supervisors, and other staff members. In the absence of unified objectives, difficulties frequently arise in the delegation, coordination, and establishment of standards.

In developing objectives the professional nursing staff should consider the following factors:

1. Overall objectives of the department of nursing should be the core around which the perioperative nursing staff members work.
2. Objectives should be written in terms of the process to be used or the results to be achieved. The objectives should clearly reflect the overall functions of the personnel concerned, the limits of authority, and the managerial and training functions of the various staff members.
3. Objectives should provide for assignment of duties to permit staff members to perform at the highest potential and provide a means for them to broaden their knowledge base.
4. Objectives should be reasonable, attainable, behavioral, and measurable in the light of existing and foreseeable conditions, such as availability of trained personnel and facilities, operating time scheduled, and operational costs.
5. Overlapping objectives within the institution should promote cooperation among group members and coordination among departments. From the institutional aspects of perioperative nursing, the housekeeping department has similar objectives concerning the prevention and control of infection.
6. Objectives should be written for, freely available to, and understood by all personnel. A positive attitude on the part of the director, supervisors, head nurses, and staff members is essential to the fulfillment of objectives. The nursing staff should be encouraged through daily conferences and training programs to help set measurable goals to meet the objectives.
7. Objectives should be reviewed and revised periodically.

Following are sample objectives for perioperative nursing:

1. Quality intraoperative nursing care that is professionally planned, implemented, and evaluated will be administered in an efficient, cost-effective manner.
2. Knowledgeable and skilled nursing personnel will be provided to meet the patient's individual needs during surgical intervention.
3. A safe and therapeutic environment will be provided for patients and personnel.
4. Proper equipment and supplies will be provided for all operative procedures.
5. Perioperative nursing standards will be evaluated and revised in accordance with current nursing practice.
6. Educational opportunities that encourage individual motivation and growth will be provided for personnel.

ORGANIZATION DESIGN

An *organization* may be defined as a framework within which people in various groups perform certain jobs for the accomplishment of a purpose under authority and leadership. Organization theory is based largely on the systematic investigation of the different concepts of how organizations work. Although the literature on organization design reveals varying terminology, the formal elements consist of structure and systems that involve measurement of the work of the organization and selection, development, and rewarding of the people within the organization.

Organization theories

Two major schools of thought that have had a major impact on health care organizations are classical theory and the human relations theory. Both theories are very prescriptive in nature and espouse "one best way" of achieving organization coordination. The principles of these schools are division of labor, chain of command (scalar principle), hierarchical structure, and span of control. Hospitals in the past were relatively stable, static organizations with emphasis placed upon the internal structure and little regard for the external environment. The traditional theories were successfully used in this type of closed system organization.

With rapid sociotechnological changes, however, organizations, and especially health care institutions, realized that they could not survive without considering the external environment. From this awareness the systems school has evolved. General systems theory addresses not only how the organization functions but also how it interacts with its environment. Systems theorists purport that there are two views of systems: closed and open. Closed systems operate independently of their environment

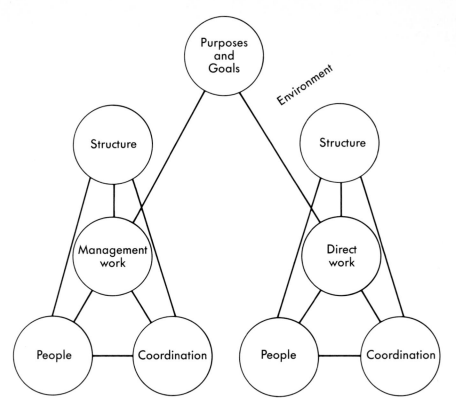

Fig. 2-1. Contingency model for organization and management. (From Charns, M.P., and Schaefer, M.J.: Health care organizations: a model for management, © 1983, p. 1. Reprinted by permission of Prentice-Hall, Inc., Englewood Cliffs, N.J.)

whereas open systems must take into account how well the organization accommodates to the outside world. Hospitals can no longer be viable without considering how they impact on the external environment and, equally critical, how the external environment affects them. To meet the demands of this open system approach, a contingency theory for organizations and management is evolving.

Contingency theory is based upon both classical and human relations theories in addition to sociotechnical and cognitive theories. The contingency school is based upon the premise that an organization's relationship to its total environment (external as well as internal) "depends upon the situation." This view requires the organizational structure as well as its managers to be more adaptable, flexible, and ingenious in the decision-making process.

Although several models of contingency theory can be found in the literature, the Charns-Schaefer model is particularly suited to health care (Charns and Schaefer, 1983). It is based on the premise that organizations are open systems that exist and interact with their environments, they exist to do work, and the requirements for the organization depend upon the characteristics of that work. The model makes a distinction between management work and direct (clinical) work and reflects the relationships among people, structure, and coordination to each type of

work as determined by the purposes and goals of the organization and its external environment. The model offers no prescriptions for management activities but rather presents a framework for analyzing the highly complex nature of health care organizations and, as a direct result of that analysis, assists managers in making informed decisions (Fig. 2-1).

Organization structure

Organizations are structured (or restructured) to improve their effectiveness, efficiency, adaptability and survival. Theoretically, an organization can be structured in many ways, but in practice only a few basic forms are found. The functional form is probably the one most frequently seen in health care organizations. In this form, work is divided into departments specialized by functional area. For example, nursing, dietary, radiology, and clinical laboratories are departments of a hospital that are divided by a specific function. The divisional design is often found in health care organizations that have high technological complexity and in which semiautonomous units can be defined. An example is the large academic medical center. The current trend is to divide the units into product lines rather than the traditional medical specialties. The matrix organization is characterized by a dual authority system.

In this design, functional and product line (or program) managers report to a common superior, with both managers exercising authority over workers within the matrix. This design violates the classical theorists' "unity of command" and scalar principles. However, it is being used by organizations that have organized around product lines as a response to third-party payers that demand better control and accountability for program costs. The major advantages of this form include the potential for having the highest degree of adaptability to changes in environment. The disadvantages are the costs and efforts expended in getting people acclimated to the continual process of change. Because of difficulty in implementation of the matrix, a parallel design modification may be utilized. In this structure, routine activities are handled functionally whereas the parallel structure is used for complex problem solving and strategic planning. Choice of structure will be determined by size, complexity, and the political environment of the specific institution. Whichever is chosen, the structure must be flexible, dynamic, and capable of growing with the institution.

Perioperative nursing managers must be knowledgeable about organization and management theories in order to remain effective in the current environment. Although they may not be actively involved in the organizational design, their subunit of surgical services can be structured to best meet the needs of the department. The scope of this chapter cannot provide an in-depth examination of these theories, but professional managers are obligated to their patients, their profession, their staffs, and themselves to explore further the concepts presented here.

ELEMENTS OF PROFESSIONAL MANAGEMENT

The effective practice of management is based upon cognitive skills, strongly aided by human and technological skills. "Skill" indicates both knowledge and the ability to translate that knowledge into action. A body of knowledge, based upon theoretical concepts, forms the foundation for the practice of management. The distinction between professional and nonprofessional managers is their cognitive skill in using theoretical concepts as a basis for action. Emphasis has been placed on the prescriptive processes of management, but the ability of the manager to recognize the uniqueness of the specific department is what enables the manager to identify, analyze, and resolve problems. Although definitions of management may vary widely, it is, in a universal perspective, decision making related to the achievement of the stated departmental goals and objectives.

Management systems

Management involves achieving the organization's stated goals. The work of Burns and Stalker (1961) suggests that the type of management within an organization fits into a bipolar systems form. At the extremities are the mechanistic and organic forms of management systems. In between are intermediate stages that can be applied, depending upon the stability and complexity of the organization.

A *mechanistic* management system is usually applied where conditions are stable and the work is routine. The characteristics of this system are the classical theorists' model of specialization; hierarchic structure of control, authority, and communication; rigid policies and procedures; and close supervision of the work to be done.

The *organic* form is appropriate in an unstable environment where new problems surface frequently and requirements that cannot be anticipated or foreseen cannot be resolved by the functional approach. This form is characterized by continual redefinition of the individual tasks and their relationship to the entire institution; a network structure of control, authority, and communication; and a decentralized approach to decision making.

Because, in reality, an organization applies a management form that is somewhere in the intermediate stages of this view of management systems, the characteristics that are relevant to perioperative nursing management should be explored further.

Specialization means learning one thing in depth. Perioperative nurses achieve excellence of performance through intensive education in their particular specialties. Because of the increased technological demands of perioperative nursing, some degree of specialization is almost a prerequisite to effective performance. The size of the department and the resources available are factors to consider in determining the degree of specialization within the department. Professional nursing shortages cause the manager to evaluate the degree of specialization appropriate to maintain safe provision of nursing care.

Hierarchic structure—a reflection of the chain of command from top down—continues to be used in most health care institutions. An *organization chart*—a map used to represent the organization's structure—generally uses a line-staff model in this structure. The term *line responsibility* stems from the chain of command that is transferred from the top executive officer down the line through various levels in the hierarchy to the point where the basic activities of the organization are carried out. Line functions consist of the action-producing duties on the job. In perioperative nursing practice, line would be represented by the director of the department at the top of the chart flowing downward through the head nurses, team leaders, staff nurses, and the nursing support personnel. The term *staff responsibility* denotes a function that may be advisory in nature or provide a service or counsel to the line. An example of this might be the human resources personnel within the hospital. Clarifying the position of all staff advisors is extremely important; if staff and line do not clearly understand their roles in the organization, conflict may develop. Departments that tend toward the organic form of management use the line-staff function less often.

Centralization or decentralization is a choice to be made within the management system. A growing trend is to place decision making lower in the organization. Factors leading to this trend are the increase in technology, which dilutes the expert power of management, and findings from the behavioral sciences that taking responsibility is often associated with increased work motivation. Factors influencing centralization are the size of the units, capital costs of consolidating expensive equipment in one area, operational costs (locating specialized services in one unit rather than in several functional areas), and the use of mechanized administrative tools such as computers. The advantages of decentralization are quicker decisions, administrative development, reduced levels of organization, and the freeing of supervisors to concentrate on broader responsibilities. Decentralization provides flexibility and better communication within the group involved. It can be extremely effective when the majority of the group are professionals. Placing the decision-making process at the staff nurse level provides a climate for "buying into" the system and thus increasing its effectiveness.

The systems approach to management attempts to look at the organization as a unified, purposeful system composed of interrelated parts. It gives managers a way of viewing an organization as a whole and as a part of the larger, external environment. Consequently, managers can see that the activity of any part of the organization affects the activity of every other part. Systems theory has its own vocabulary. Some of these words are:

- Subsystems: The parts that make up the whole
- Synergy: The whole is greater than the sum of its parts
- System boundary: The demarcation of the system and its environment; closed system boundaries are rigid, open ones are flexible
- Flow: Information, materials, and energy (including humans) flow into the system as inputs, undergo transformation within the system, and exit as outputs
- Feedback: The key to systems control

Systems theory incorporates concepts from all earlier management schools of thought and permeates current management thinking. The contingency theory of management uses the same "it depends" approach to problem solving as organization theory.

Management functions

Regardless of the form of management system adopted by the department, looking at the process of management is necessary. The process is comprised of a series of separate parts, or functions. The major functions of management are planning, organizing, directing, and controlling. The organizational structure determines the emphasis placed on each function, but the manager should be familiar with each one.

Planning is the process of formulating in advance the direction a department intends to follow in fulfilling its stated objectives. It is largely conceptual, but evidence that it occurred is visible. Planning includes the prior determination of who is to do a task and when and where it is to be done. Within this management function, proper selection and training of a staff take place.

Organizing involves arranging the various components of any unified effort—the people, tasks, and materials necessary for putting plans into operation. The purpose of the organizing function is to correlate these elements to orient them toward executing plans and meeting objectives. For managers to fulfill the function of organizing, six essential steps in the process must be considered: (1) establishment of objectives, (2) identification of tasks, (3) logical grouping of tasks, (4) assignment of employees, (5) delineation of authority and responsibility, and (6) establishment of authority and responsibility relationships. Organizing enables a manager to develop order, promote cooperation among personnel, and foster productivity.

Directing is the complex managerial function concerned with the supervision of employees as they perform their assignments. Directing is doing things through others. A manager is actively involved with the human factor in the directing process. To accomplish the department's objectives, the nursing manager must deal with conflict and motivate and discipline staff. These tasks require good communication skills, assertive behavior, and positive motivation.

Controlling is seeing that plans that have been developed are carried through to completion. The basic steps in this management function are (1) setting standards, (2) measuring performance against these standards, (3) reporting the results, and (4) taking corrective action.

Coordination

Another function of management that merits separate consideration is coordination. *Coordination* is the conscious activity of integrating the different work efforts so they function harmoniously to attain the department's objectives (Fig. 2-2).

Several formal approaches to coordination are possible. The approach selected varies with the characteristics of the work to be performed. Six major approaches are: (1) use of standards and policies, (2) skill standardization, (3) outcome standards, (4) direct supervision, (5) peer review, and (6) group coordination. These approaches are divided into two categories: programming methods and feedback methods.

Programming methods are used when the work is well

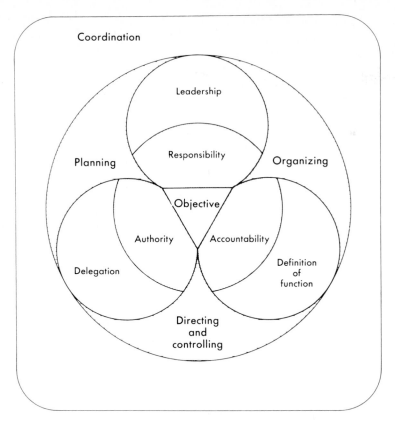

Fig. 2-2. Management functions. (From Arndt, C., and Huckabay, L.M.D.: Nursing administration: theory for practice with a systems approach, ed. 2, St. Louis, 1980, The C.V. Mosby Co.)

understood and has a high degree of certainty related to its outcome (programmable). The standardization of the performance of work is a programmable method of co-ordination. It is done through (1) use of standards, policies, procedures, protocols, and regulations; (2) use of job or position descriptions so that required skills are standardized; and (3) standardization of output so that the results of the activities are clearly specified. In perioperative nursing practice, many areas are coordinated through these approaches. Among them are standards of nursing practice, administrative and departmental policies and procedures, and position descriptions, which are discussed in more detail later in this chapter.

Feedback methods are used in more complex situations in which the work is less certain and deviations from the desired outcome are likely. They are (1) direct supervision, (2) mutual adjustment, which can be a result of exchange of information between peers through a review process, and (3) group coordination in the form of meetings, committees, conferences, or task forces. Feedback approaches are much more time-consuming but are necessary for effective coordination. Because of the need to avoid the pitfalls of nonproductive time spent in group activities in

the current cost-reduction and cost-containment environment, committees and meetings are addressed separately.

Committees

Horizontal coordination of activities occurs between departments and other professional groups within the hospital hierarchy.

The *committee* structure of the hospital and department should not perform functions that, dependent upon the organization structure, should be performed by established departments for which individuals can be held accountable.

Committee action has advantages and disadvantages. Advantages of committees are that they (1) disseminate information and ideas, (2) provide for integration of ideas, (3) deter hasty decision making, (4) provide for coordinated action by individuals having line and staff responsibilities, and (5) broaden individual viewpoints pertaining to a specific problem or plan. The disadvantages of committee action are (1) difficulty in achieving control of action, (2) time consumed to achieve general agreement of the group, (3) difficulty in getting members to attend, especially when emergency decision making is needed,

(4) difficulty in appraising results because of diffusion of responsibilities within the group, and (5) potential for decreased quality of decisions because compromises may be necessary for consensus.

Within a department in the hospital, committees—administrative, advisory, judicial, executive, and others—combine a number of functions and characteristics. Organizationally, a committee may have line or staff responsibility. A line or staff committee may be delegated decision making or enforcement responsibilities established by the governing board. For example, the director of surgical services, as a member of the nursing service steering (executive) committee, has a staff responsibility for decision-making in accordance with the established functions of the committee. The director, because of line responsibility, may become a staff advisor as a member of the surgical committee.

A formal or standing committee has a permanent place in the organizational structure of the hospital and department. The informal, temporary, or special ad hoc committee does not have a permanent place in the organizational chart. It is appointed to collect and analyze data and make recommendations. When those tasks are completed, the ad hoc committee is discharged. In developing or revising a committee structure, the following factors should be considered: (1) establishment and statement of the purposes of each committee, (2) determination of the rules and regulations pertaining to selection and tenure of members and their responsibilities for providing effective functioning, and (3) approval of the committee structure by the governing board.

The operating room committee (surgical committee) is a standing committee in most organizational structures and serves in a staff capacity. It recommends policies and procedures affecting the therapeutic aspects of patient care. The committee should consist of representatives from the surgery department, anesthesia department, hospital administration, perioperative nursing department, and other departments as appropriate to the individual facility.

Perioperative nursing personnel should participate as members of committees to improve perioperative nursing practices and their own knowledge and skills. They should also serve as representatives on nursing and hospital committees.

Meetings

The three major types of meetings are informational, advisory, and problem solving. Before a meeting is scheduled, several decisions must be made regarding (1) the purpose of the meeting, (2) who should attend (always considering their responsibility and authority), (3) who should conduct the meeting, and (4) how it should be conducted.

PERIOPERATIVE NURSING PRACTICE STANDARDS

The perioperative nurse manager is responsible for identifying, interpreting, and implementing contemporary professional standards. The provision of perioperative nursing services should be based on these standards. The Association of Operating Room Nurses (AORN) has established standards for perioperative nursing practice that can serve as guidelines for measuring the quality of patient care. They are sound principles that are broad in scope, attainable, definitive, and relevant for perioperative nurses. The standards represent a comprehensive approach to meeting the health care needs of surgical patients.

Nursing care standards encompass three parameters: structure, process, and outcome. Structure standards describe organizational characteristics, administrative and fiscal accountabilities, personnel qualifications, and facilities and environmental requirements. The *AORN Standards of Administrative Nursing Practice: OR* provides structure standards and guidance for professionals in management roles (see box at right).

Process standards relate to nursing activities, interventions, and interactions and are used to evaluate the extent to which nursing objectives have been met. An example of process standards is *Standards of Perioperative Nursing Practice,* which has been jointly published by the AORN and the American Nurses' Association (ANA). These standards pertain to nursing during the perioperative period and are based on the nursing process.

Outcome standards identify patients' observable physiologic and psychologic responses to nursing interventions. Patient outcomes are probably the most valid indicator of the quality of care. *Patient Outcome Standards for Perioperative Nursing,* published by the AORN, provides guidelines for judging patient responses. The common goal of all three categories of standards is quality care for the surgical patient. They should be used in conjunction with the AORN recommended practices, which are optimum goals that perioperative nursing personnel should strive to achieve.

POLICIES AND PROCEDURES

The governing board of the institution delegates to the medical board the responsibility for the medical treatment of patients and to the hospital personnel, through the executive administrative staff, clearly defined functions and lines of authority concerned with meeting patients' needs.

A *policy* may be defined as a written statement that explains how goals will be achieved and outlines the general course and scope of activities permissible for goal achievement. A *procedure* may be defined as a guide to action that enumerates the chronologic sequence of steps needed to accomplish a task.

Text continued on p. 25.

STANDARDS OF ADMINISTRATIVE NURSING PRACTICE: OR

The Association of Operating Room Nurses believes that professions must regulate themselves and demonstrate accountability to the consumer and other health care professionals. As a professional association, AORN is committed to the development of mechanisms that establish accountability and measure the quality and effectiveness of health care.

Standards are an effective tool for identifying activities that are appropriate in the development of a contemporary health care system. Implementation of professional standards creates an environment that is beneficial to the consumers of health care and to the professionals rendering care. Standards are established through the collaboration of experts in the field of practice, consumers, and other health care professionals.

These administrative standards should be used in conjunction with the Standards of Perioperative Nursing Practice and the recommended technical and aseptic practices established by AORN. The Standards of Perioperative Nursing Practice are based on the nursing process and encompass nursing activities of preoperative assessment and preparation, intraoperative intervention, and postoperative evaluation. The recommended technical and aseptic practices are based on principles of microbiology and research and are directed toward providing a safe operating room environment for the patient.

The Standards of Administrative Nursing Practice: Operating Room were developed to guide professionals in administrative roles and to provide a model for evaluating practice. The standards are broad in scope, definitive, relevant, attainable, and subject to ongoing evaluation and revision.

These standards have been developed by the Standards of Administrative Nursing Practice: Operating Room Committee and are intended to assist agencies in establishing administrative practice in their settings. Compliance with these standards is voluntary.

Standard I. A Philosophy, Purpose, and Objectives Shall be Formulated to Guide Operating Room Services.
Criteria
1. The philosophy, purpose, and objectives are based on those of the agency and nursing department.
2. The philosophy explains the beliefs of the operating room personnel and determines how operating room personnel will accomplish the purpose.
3. The purpose is a statement that describes the reason for operating room services, and is based on the philosophy.
4. The objectives are realistic and are used to measure the accomplishment of the purpose.
5. Operating room personnel share in the formulation, implementation, and periodic review and revision of the philosophy, purpose, and objectives.
6. The philosophy, purpose, and objectives are distributed and interpreted to the agency administration and medical staff.

Interpretive Statement
Realistic, easily understood, and functional statements of philosophy, purpose, and objectives serve as guidelines for operating room services.

Standard II. An Organizational Plan for the Operating Room Shall be Developed and Communicated.
Criteria
1. The plan reflects the philosophy, purpose, and objectives of operating room services.
2. The plan identifies the lines of formal authority, responsibility, accountability, and communication within the operating room.
3. The plan describes the relationship of the operating room to administration, medical staff, and other departments.
4. The plan depicts relationships between people and/or functions.
5. The plan is a tool for developing descriptions of functions within the operating room.

Continued.

STANDARDS OF ADMINISTRATIVE NURSING PRACTICE: OR—cont'd

Interpretive Statement

The organizational plan is an arrangement of functions and resources that contribute to the achievement of the objectives of the operating room.

Standard III. A Registered Nurse Shall be Authorized with Administrative Accountability and Responsibility for the Operating Room Services.
Criteria

1. The registered nurse administrator has experience and expertise in perioperative nursing practice. Perioperative nursing is professional operating room nursing during preoperative, intraoperative, and postoperative phases of the patient's surgical experience.
2. The registered nurse administrator is prepared in management and leadership skills through education and experience.
   a. Management skills include but are not limited to the ability to plan, organize, direct, control, and evaluate.
   b. Leadership skills include but are not limited to flexibility, effective communication, and the ability to establish a climate to facilitate group effort.
3. The registered nurse administrator maintains competencies in management practices through participation in continuing education offerings.
4. The administrative responsibilities must be delegated to another registered nurse in the registered nurse administrator's absence.

Interpretive Statement

The registered nurse administrator is responsible for the interpretation, direction, and evaluation of nursing practice and the coordination of operating room services through the use of clinical, management, and leadership skills. Registered nurses with these skills must be the managers of operating room suites. They must have the authority to negotiate with other health care disciplines on policy matters.

Standard IV. The Registered Nurse Administrator Shall be Accountable and Responsible for Developing Mechanisms that Assure Optimal Patient Care.
Criteria

1. The registered nurse administrator has responsibility for the identification, interpretation, and implementation of the standards of nursing care.
2. The registered nurse administrator has responsibility for
   a. fiscal management
   b. policy development, implementation, and revisions
   c. integration and coordination of the activities of other health care disciplines in the operating room
   d. management of human, material, and environmental services.
3. The registered nurse administrator interacts with other departments and serves on hospital committees.

Interpretive Statement

The registered nurse administrator is accountable and responsible for the integrated management of multifaceted services. Operating room services require management of human resources, fiscal resources, facilities, and material. Optimal patient care is assured through collaboration, communication, coordination, and effective interdepartmental relationships.

Standard V. The Operating Room Management Team Shall Develop and Manage the Budget for Operating Room Services.
Criteria

1. The budget is developed.
   a. Assessment factors include but are not limited to
   historical data
   changes in patient population
   changes in services offered
   changes in composition of medical staff
   changes in delivery of health care services
   changes in nursing practice
   impact of regulatory agencies.
   b. Fiscal impact of trends is forecast.
   c. The budget is submitted and appropriate approval obtained.

STANDARDS OF ADMINISTRATIVE NURSING PRACTICE: OR—cont'd

2. The budget is implemented.
   a. An action plan is developed, which should include but is not limited to setting priorities and schedules for the procurement of human resources, equipment, and supplies.
   b. The budget is communicated to operating room personnel, medical staff, and supportive service departments.
3. The budget is monitored and investigated for variances, and corrective action is taken as necessary.
   a. Periodic review of comparative data, including human resources, equipment, and supply costs related to revenue, is carried out.
   b. Results of the periodic review are shared with staff for their contributions to corrective action.
   c. Corrective action is taken.

Interpretive Statement
Fiscal management is a major administrative nursing responsibility in the operating room. Budget preparation, implementation, and monitoring are paramount to sound fiscal management of the unit. Fiscal management assures the consumer of management's commitment to a balance between cost and quality.

The operating room management team must be aware of current and future technological changes that will have a fiscal impact. Input must be obtained from the agency administration, medical staff, operating room personnel, and supporting departments about trends that could affect the preparation or implementation of the budget for the operating room.

Standard VI. The Operating Room Service Shall have Written Standards of Nursing Practice.
Criteria
1. The standards are based on accepted standards of nursing practice.
2. Operating room nursing personnel share in the formulation of the standards of nursing practice and interpretation to other disciplines.
3. The standards are implemented, periodically reviewed, and revised to reflect change in nursing practice.

Interpretive Statement
The standards provide guidelines for measuring the quality of patient care. They are a means of establishing accountability for care.

Standard VII. The Operating Room Services Shall have Written Policies and Procedures that Serve as Operational Guidelines.
Criteria
1. Policies and procedures are written, dated, and enforceable.
2. Operating room personnel share in formulation of policies and procedures and yearly review and revision.
3. Obsolete policies and procedures are removed from the manual. One copy is filed for reference.
4. Policies and procedures for the operating room shall include but are not limited to
   a. operative and special consents
   b. fire and disaster plans
   c. environmental control
   d. visitor and traffic control
   e. safety regulations
   f. infection control
   g. care and disposition of surgical specimens, cultures, and foreign bodies
   h. care of special equipment including preventive maintenance contracts and records where necessary
   i. emergency actions, such as cardiopulmonary resuscitation
   j. orientation of all personnel entering the operating room.
5. Policies and procedures are approved and interpreted to all appropriate persons.
6. All deviations from established policy shall be documented as directed by the agency.
7. Policy and procedure manuals available to operating room personnel should include but are not limited to
   a. operating room policy manual
   b. operating room procedure manual
   c. personnel policies
   d. agency policies and rules and regulations
   e. anesthesia policies
   f. medical staff rules and regulations.

Continued.

STANDARDS OF ADMINISTRATIVE NURSING PRACTICE: OR—cont'd

Interpretive Statement

The registered nurse administrator is accountable and responsible for assuring there are clear, concise, and current written policies and procedures. They are used to standardize practices, assist staff, and minimize risk factors.

Standard VIII. The Operating Room Management Team Shall be Responsible for Establishing Staffing Requirements, Selecting Personnel, and Planning for Appropriate Utilization of Human Resources.

Criteria

1. Staffing requirements and patterns are determined by
   a. philosophy, purpose, and objectives
   b. complexity of consumer acuity
   c. scope of services
   d. fiscal resources.
2. Selection of personnel is determined by
   a. philosophy and objectives guiding the quality of care to be delivered
   b. hiring policies of the agency and department
   c. job requirements
   d. vacancies
   e. qualifications
   f. availability.
3. The utilization of human resources is consistent with needs of the consumer, the nature of support functions, and agency requirements.
   a. Clinical assignments are based on consumer needs and the competence of the categories of human resources.
   b. Use of personnel is based on identified levels of competency.

Interpretive Statement

Staffing is an administrative function. Staffing patterns, selection, and utilization have a direct bearing on the well-being of the consumer, the effectiveness and efficiency of the agency, and the cost of health care. Staffing depends on the size of the agency and the scope of its services.

Standard IX. Staff Development Programs Shall be Provided for Operating Room Personnel.

Criteria

1. Orientation programs are established and required for all personnel. Content includes but is not limited to
   a. philosophy, mission, and role of the agency
   b. philosophy, purpose, and objectives of operating room services
   c. policies and procedures of agency and operating room
   d. job descriptions and performance standards
   e. skills assessment.
2. Technical and professional programs and experiences are scheduled based on
   a. identified learning needs of the personnel
   b. need to communicate agency and OR directives, policies, and procedures
   c. need to maintain and promote clinical and management competencies.
3. There should be planned learning experiences designed to promote clinical competence.
4. Involvement in career development activities is encouraged and facilitated.
5. Involvement in professional activities is encouraged. This includes but is not limited to
   a. participation in professional organizations
   b. reading professional journals
   c. participation in educational programs and meetings
   d. collegial interchange.

Interpretive Statement

Orientation programs assist employees to adjust to the organization, environment, and duties. Staff development programs enhance performance and foster professional and personal growth. Basic or advanced technical and professional programs are designed to develop job knowledge, skills, and attitudes as they affect direct patient care.

STANDARDS OF ADMINISTRATIVE NURSING PRACTICE: OR—cont'd

Standard X. A Safe Operating Room Environment Shall be Established, Controlled, and Consistently Monitored.
Criteria
1. Technical and aseptic practice guidelines are established, maintained, and periodically reviewed and revised in accordance with AORN recommended practices of technical and aseptic practice for the operating room.
2. Electrical safety is maintained, consistent with accepted agency, regional, and national standards.
3. Occupational safety for personnel is maintained by
   a. safety programs and surveillance
   b. infection control program and surveillance
   c. radiation monitoring and protection
   d. minimizing exposure to toxic substances, infectious wastes, and other hazards
   e. employee health programs.
4. Physical facilities are maintained by
   a. temperature control within acceptable ranges
   b. humidity control within acceptable ranges
   c. adequate air circulation and filtration system
   d. proper maintenance of air filtering system
   e. fire alert systems
   f. constantly monitored gas systems
   g. constantly monitored vacuum system
   h. automatic auxiliary power system
   i. electrical safety monitors.
5. Guidelines and regulations not limited to the following are used in determining and monitoring operating room safety
   a. governing boards
   b. licensing agencies
   c. National Fire Protection Association
   d. Joint Commission on Accreditation of Hospitals
   e. Occupational Safety and Health Administration
   f. US Department of Health and Human Services
   g. Environmental Protection Agency
   h. American National Standards Institute
   i. manufacturers' equipment manuals.

Interpretive Statement
A safe, comfortable, therapeutic operating room environment is maintained for patients and health care providers.

Standard XI. The Operating Room Management Team Shall Promote the Discovery and Integration of New Knowledge by Encouraging Development of and Use of Nursing Research.
Criteria
1. Operating room nursing management recognizes its professional responsibility to expand the knowledge base in perioperative nursing.
2. Operating room nursing management affirms the value of nursing research by encouraging staff to initiate, promote, and support nursing research projects.
3. Research studies are conducted in accordance with the American Nurses' Association ethical standards of nursing research.
4. Operating room nursing management facilitates the application of research findings to perioperative nursing practice, education, and administration.

Interpretive Statement
Research is increasingly important in perioperative nursing. Continual development of a scientific body of knowledge is fundamental to improving practice and the quality of service offered to clients.

Standard XII. The Operating Room Staff Shall Maintain Appropriate Documentation Related to OR Activities.
Criteria
1. Perioperative nursing care is documented on the patient record as outlined in *Recommended Practices for Documentation of Perioperative Nursing Care.*
2. An operative record is maintained for each patient that includes but is not limited to
   a. patient's name
   b. patient's agency number
   c. date and times
   d. surgeon(s)
   e. anesthetist
   f. assistant(s) to surgeon
   g. scrub person and circulating nurse
   h. preoperative and postoperative diagnosis
   i. operative procedure
   j. wound status
   k. implants
   l. specimen and disposition
   m. complications.

Continued.

STANDARDS OF ADMINISTRATIVE NURSING PRACTICE: OR—cont'd

3. Records are maintained to provide statistical data that include but are not limited to
   a. the numbers, types, and duration of operative procedures
   b. utilization of operating room, manpower, supplies, and equipment
   c. environmental controls
   d. infection control.
4. The operating room administration and medical record department maintain and control records for the length of time required by the agency and legal statute.
5. Minutes of meetings are maintained.
6. Current personnel performance records are maintained.
7. Confidentiality of records is established by the agency and legal statute.

Interpretive Statement
The responsibility of the operating room management team includes the assurance of appropriate documentation of activities. A record of perioperative care, which becomes a part of the patient's permanent record, is documented. Records maintained for statistical data are used to determine increases or decreases in specialty activity for future budget and special agency requirements. Personnel records are maintained for current employees that include staff development activities and pertinent chronological entries regarding the individual's achievement of established performance standards.

Standard XIII. The Operating Room Management Team Shall Recognize a Professional Responsibility to Promote, Provide, and Participate in a Learning Environment for Students in Health Care Disciplines.
Criteria
1. A written agreement is made, as appropriate, with each educational provider seeking to use the agency or staff.
2. There is ongoing collaboration with faculty and the learner to facilitate the achievement of educational objectives.
3. The safety and welfare of the consumer must be maintained while providing a controlled learning experience for students.

Interpretive Statement
The operating room offers health care students a clinical laboratory where they can experience a variety of activities not performed elsewhere. This experience is essential to their understanding the trauma of surgery, the care required to ensure the safety of the anesthetized patient, the necessity for proper patient preparation, interdisciplinary team functioning, stress management, and the application of medical-surgical asepsis. Use of the operating room for these student experiences must be controlled. This experience will broaden the competencies of the beginning health care practitioner, promoting higher quality patient care.

Standard XIV. There Shall be a Quality Assurance Program for Operating Room Services.
Criteria
1. An ongoing review process of nursing practice in the operating room is established and documented. The goal of this review is to assure optimal achievable care for the consumer.
2. Continued competence in meeting performance standards is assured by ongoing personnel performance appraisal.
3. The safety and cost effectiveness of purchased goods and services are assured by ongoing multidisciplinary product evaluation.
4. A safe, comfortable, and therapeutic environment is assured the consumer and personnel through
   a. adherence to guidelines and regulations established for operating room safety
   b. ongoing monitoring of the facility.
5. The optimal use of human, facility, and fiscal resources is assured through periodic evaluation of
   a. staffing patterns
   b. scheduling methodology
   c. case load distribution
   d. provisions for emergency care
   e. facilities utilization
   f. budget review.
6. The plan of action is developed, implemented, and monitored.
7. The quality assurance program for the operating room interfaces with and supports the agency's quality assurance program.

STANDARDS OF ADMINISTRATIVE NURSING PRACTICE: OR—cont'd

8. A confidentiality policy guides how quality assurance information is reported and stored and which qualified individuals will have access to it.

Interpretive Statement

The quality assurance program in the operating room is flexible and encourages innovative approaches to patient care. The activity begins with the identification of real or potential problems. The identification may be accomplished through many activities, such as audit procedures, peer review, committee meetings, staff meetings, review of incident reports, and patient or staff surveys or comments. The problems are resolved through a plan of action. This plan of action includes an assessment of the problems through data collection, comparison of findings to acceptable standards, and recommended changes. Following the assessment, problems are ranked according to their impact on patient care. Once implemented, the change is closely monitored through a review process. A positive outcome is permanently incorporated into standard operating procedures. Negative outcomes warrant identifying and selecting other alternatives to correct the problem.

Medical staff policies

Policies pertaining to dependent functions of the medical staff are formulated by a representative committee and are recommended to the administrative staff for approval by the governing board. Many policies and rules relate to the interdependent functions of medicine and nursing. The medical, hospital, and nursing administrative staffs have joint responsibilities in formulating overall policies related to therapeutic aspects of patient care.

Administrative policies and procedures

The objectives of administrative policies and procedures are to protect patients and personnel from injury and to meet state and national safety codes; local, state, and federal laws; and the *Standards for Hospital Accreditation of the Joint Commission on Accreditation of Healthcare Organizations*. The laws concerning negligence, legal obligations, and grounds for liability vary from state to state. The policies should interpret existing laws that affect the hospital, patient, and personnel.

Nursing administrative manual

The nursing administrative manual should include the philosophy and objectives of nursing, the qualitative nursing standards to meet patient care needs, procedures for the control of equipment and supplies, budgetary information (costs and expenditures), organizational chart, committee structure of the department and related departments, and personnel policies. In some hospitals the personnel policies, including position descriptions, master staffing plan, and performance appraisal format, are given in a separate personnel policies manual.

The staff development and in-service education manual should include the purpose, content, methods of instruction, hours, and length of the program for orientation of various categories of personnel, on-the-job training, and leadership staff development.

Surgical services policies and procedures

Written policies and procedures must be available to all personnel who provide patient care in the surgical setting. This information should be maintained in a readily accessible manual to facilitate uniform interpretation and administration of policies and procedures. The manual should be reviewed annually and revised as often as needed to meet the changing standards of practice. Policies and procedures affecting perioperative personnel should be formulated by representatives of the groups concerned with the delivery of patient care in this area.

A perioperative nursing policy and procedure committee comprised of nursing personnel from all levels and specialties is an effective vehicle for drafting realistic new or revised policies and procedures. Participation of staff members in policy and procedure development increases their knowledge of the subject matter and generates a sense of ownership of the drafts. These effects usually result in meaningful interpretation of the approved policy or procedure to peers and successful implementation.

The surgical committee recommends policies and procedures relating to therapeutic aspects of patient care.

The surgical services policy and procedure manual should address but not be limited to the following:

1. Safety of patients and personnel
   a. Fire and disaster plans
   b. Safety regulations

    c. Infection control requirements

    d. Incident reports

    e. Emergency actions, such as cardiopulmonary resuscitation

    f. Handling of nuclear materials

2. Admission of patients

    a. Identification of patient

    b. Laboratory tests and other diagnostic procedures

    c. Consent for surgical procedures

3. Records

    a. Operative record

    b. Anesthesia record

    c. Tissue examination request form

4. Surgical and aseptic techniques

5. Care and handling of instruments and equipment

6. Sponge, sharp, and instrument counts

7. Administration of narcotics

8. Care and disposition of surgical specimens

9. Postmortem care

10. Environmental controls

11. Visitor and traffic control

12. Surgical staff privileges

13. Orientation of personnel

14. Quality assurance and risk management program

15. Personnel policies

    a. Dress code

    b. Attendance

    c. Vacation

    d. Performance appraisals

    e. Promotion

    f. Sick leave and leave of absence

16. Public relations

Most surgical departments have separate procedure manuals or cards that enumerate surgeons' preferences for instruments, sutures, supplies, and equipment for each type of operation.

Scheduling policies and procedures

Clearly defined scheduling policies and procedures promote effective and economical services to patients and provide all surgeons with an equitable opportunity to use the facilities. The most common methods of surgical scheduling are block and open. *Block scheduling* is the allocation of a specific block of time (number of operating room hours per room per day) to a surgical service or an individual surgeon based on defined needs. Allocations are reserved for the respective service or surgeon until a set number of hours (usually 24 to 72) before the day of surgery. After that time, any unscheduled time may be scheduled by another service or surgeon. An advantage of block scheduling is that the assigned service or surgeon is assured scheduling time on a consistent day. A disadvantage is that a surgeon without allocated time may not be able to schedule an elective patient at the desired time. Utilization of block times must be monitored regularly, and allocations evaluated and reassigned as indicated.

In contrast, *open scheduling* is handled on a first-come, first-served basis. Every service or surgeon has access to any unscheduled time on any day of the week. In some facilities open scheduling is perceived as more flexible in meeting the varying needs of a surgeon. However, a disadvantage of this method is that services having a high volume of strictly elective surgery, such as plastic surgery or oral surgery, may schedule months in advance and usurp many hours of prime available time.

The most effective scheduling systems appear to be a mix of block and open scheduling. Factors affecting scheduling include the following:

1. Scheduling of procedures should be under the control of one scheduler.

2. Room and time availability must be clearly indicated.

3. Specific facts must be obtained:

    a. Patient's name and age

    b. Surgeon's name

    c. Admission type (inpatient, morning admission, or ambulatory surgery)

    d. Type and classification (elective or urgent) of procedure

    e. Estimated operative time

    f. Potential blood replacement requirements (transfusion or cell salvage)

    g. Type of anesthesia

    h. Special instrumentation and equipment requirements

    i. Date and time requested

A system of measurements and controls should be initiated to enhance the daily effectiveness of the scheduling policies. Data should be collected at periodic intervals for (1) the variations of actual numbers of procedures per week from predicted scheduling policies, (2) the range of total hours of actual operating room time used, showing the minimum and maximum hours used each week, (3) the average setup time and the average terminal cleanup time, and (4) the unused available time resulting from variations in the schedule or noncompliance with protocols.

Collection and analysis of data help management personnel determine methods for decreasing excessive expenditures for staffing and equipment that result when staffing is based on the maximum for the existing caseload rather than on the expected demand for services. This becomes a real challenge for the nurse manager as the competitive environment demands convenience and availability. Flexible staffing patterns are needed to meet this demand.

DEVELOPING POSITION DESCRIPTIONS FOR PERIOPERATIVE NURSING
Terminology

In preparation for position analysis and the resultant position description, the staff should know common definitions and understand the terminology.

A *task,* or duty, is a unit of work or human effort exerted to achieve a specific purpose. Examples are checking identification bands on patients, checking patient charts to ensure the safety of each patient, and assembling surgical instruments in a metal sterilizer tray. When a sufficient number of similar tasks have developed, a position is created for one person.

A *function* is a group of closely related tasks (duties) that logically fall into a unified unit of work for the accomplishment of a responsibility delegated to a staff member or a department. An example is to plan, organize, and control the staffing pattern to ensure effective use of personnel in meeting the nursing care needs of a group of patients. This function comprises several tasks performed by the administrative supervisor or head nurse.

A *position* is a collection of tasks and responsibilities rendered by one staff member who is delegated to perform specific functions.

Position analysis is the study of a position to determine the knowledge, skills, aptitude, and personal characteristics needed to perform the responsibilities successfully. Ultimately, the position analysis determines minimum position requirements and sets standards for such factors as education, experience, and individual specifications. An effective position analysis program depends on several important factors, as follows:

1. The individual who performs the position analysis should have the ability to get along with people and be able to express ideas effectively and analytically.

2. The program must be planned in detail, as much as is possible.
3. The program must be approved and supported by the administration.
4. The personnel concerned must understand the purpose and mechanics of the program.
5. The supervisory staff must review the collected data.
6. The analyst must observe and interview the personnel, write the first draft, review it with the supervisory staff, and then revise the draft until it is accepted by the department head.

The *position specification* clearly and specifically sets forth the qualifications required for a position. It includes the level of education; the amount of previous experience in similar work; special training, knowledge, and skills required; physical requirements; and legal requirements such as licensure. It ultimately determines the pay range and classification of a position.

A *position description* is a written statement of the requirements, major duties and responsibilities, and organizational relationships of a given position.

Position relationships refer to the interrelatedness of staff members within and outside the department who have similar duties or joint responsibilities to achieve specific objectives.

Position descriptions

Position descriptions should be current, accurate, and realistic. The title of the position indicates the major responsibilities and sets the position apart from others. The position description should be a complete but not detailed summary of primary duties (Fig. 2-3). Duties should be arranged in a logical order and stated concisely in action terms. Position descriptions help prevent overlapping of duties and subsequent conflict and frustration. They play

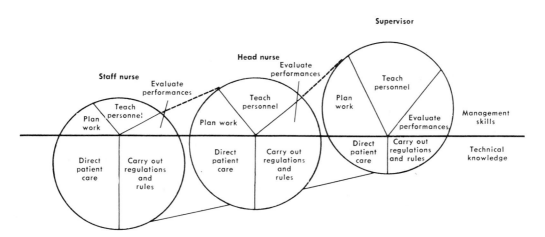

Fig. 2-3. Allocation of functions and responsibilities of staff nurse, head nurse, and supervisor in relation to planning of work, teaching, direct patient care, and rules and regulations.

an important part in performance appraisals and in decisions concerning promotions and salary rates.

The professional nurse, regardless of position in the nursing service hierarchy, performs clinical, managerial, and operational nursing duties. In the upward progression of the hierarchy, clinical leadership duties increase and operational (performance) duties decrease. The functions of the administrative supervisor involve almost entirely clinical leadership duties. Many perioperative nursing departments have implemented a manager/coordinator program to coordinate nonnursing functions.

The number and type of positions required to meet perioperative patient care needs depend on the extent and complexity of the surgical services offered to patients.

FISCAL RESPONSIBILITIES OF MANAGEMENT

Never has containing costs while striving to improve the quality of and access to health care been more critical. Consumer expectations, increased costs of technology, and competition among health care organizations have created an untenable position for hospitals as they strive to implement cost-containment measures in the face of shrinking reimbursements. Sound business management techniques, both operationally and strategically, must be developed, but the greater challenge is to balance the issues of cost, quality, and access.

Impact of reimbursement changes

In the face of rising costs since the inception of Medicare in the mid-1960s, the federal government reacted by creating the prospective payment system in the early eighties. The system, based upon diagnosis-related groups (DRGs), intended to reimburse for a specific diagnosis that required similar treatment and consumed a similar amount of resources as measured by cost and length of stay. The initial system was intended for inpatients, but within a few years a prospective payment system based upon categories of outpatient surgical procedures was added to the plan. Commercial insurers in the private sector followed very rapidly; managed care plans such as preferred provider organizations, health maintenance organizations, and other alternative delivery systems followed suit. Where once billed charges were a good indicator of revenues, hospitals have had to learn to deal with either discounting, per capita, or per diem reimbursement programs. One result has been that organizational performance must be measured and monitored by every department in the institution.

Effectiveness and efficiency

Organizational performance means performance in two areas: effectiveness and efficiency. *Effectiveness* is the degree to which goals and objectives are successfully met. *Efficiency* is related to the cost of producing those services. Efficiency and productivity are closely related. Efficiency examines the cost per unit (procedure) of the services, whereas productivity is the ratio of the final product (volume of procedures) to the resources that were used to achieve the product. The difficulty for perioperative nurse managers, not uncommon to all of nursing, is measuring the final product. One of the major emphases of the manager in a turbulent environment is to monitor organizational performance.

Productivity must be critically analyzed to determine the bottom line for fiscal resources. Staffing patterns must be carefully scrutinized to determine if all positions are essential. A benefit-cost or cost effectiveness analysis may be required to provide documentation for support of positions that may be subject to cutbacks. Preoperative patient teaching can be adversely affected because of the shortened period between a patient's arrival to the hospital or ambulatory surgery unit and the time of surgery. Innovative methods for providing outpatient preoperative education have been developed to provide quality care during relatively brief perioperative experiences.

Operating room use must be carefully assessed and revised as needed to eliminate gaps in the surgical schedule. With the rapid shift of patients from inpatient surgery to ambulatory surgery and to admission on the morning of surgery, managers through their staff must ensure greater efficiency in the provision of perioperative nursing care without a reduction in quality.

The budget-curbing effect of the reimbursement changes has had a significant impact on management of surgical services materials. Competitive bids on equipment and supplies greatly influence purchasing decisions. No longer can purchasing a more expensive item be justified if a less expensive one is acceptable and does not jeopardize patient care. Inventory levels must be evaluated and par levels adjusted to just-in-time inventories to reduce overhead as much as possible. Frequent in-service education programs on cost-effectiveness can increase personnel awareness of costs and may help motivate staff members to monitor the use of supplies and equipment. The various infection-control practices must be validated by research and not ritualism. Departmental budgets must be fiscally responsive to the financial resources of the institution.

Budget process

Budget management is a key responsibility of the perioperative nurse manager. To be responsible and accountable for controlling costs, managers must be actively involved in the preparation of the departmental budget.

The objectives of budgeting are to present a written quantitative expression of the policies and plans of the department, to provide a basis for evaluation of financial performance compared to those plans, to supply a tool for controlling costs, and to create cost awareness. Departmental budgets are developed according to cost centers to which expenses are allocated. The two main types of budgets are operating and capital equipment. The operating budget encompasses all revenue and expenses generated by the respective cost center. Operating expenses are divided into direct (for example, salaries, supplies, and repairs) and indirect (overhead, usually based on square footage occupied by the department). The capital equipment budget identifies major purchases with an expected life span, above a baseline cost.

To develop an accurate, realistic budget, the operating room manager should use the following process:

1. Develop departmental goals and objectives for the budget year, using the hospital operational goals and objectives as a framework.
2. Establish a timetable for the completion of each aspect of budget development.
3. Consult with surgeons in each surgical specialty to identify any anticipated new or revised procedures that might have budgetary implications, such as new instruments or equipment or additional staff requirements.
4. Consult with head nurses and staff members to determine need for duplication or replacement of instruments and equipment.
5. Review historical, statistical, and financial data for the previous year to identify trends.
6. Prepare budget figures for operating expenses based on the previous year's expenses, projected units of service, staffing objectives, new or different supplies needed, new practices recommended for implementation, and projected inflation rates as applicable.
7. Forecast revenue based on current charge structure adjusted for appropriate reimbursements.
8. Prepare capital equipment budget. Categorize each item as new or replacement, and provide thorough justification for every item requested. Establish priorities and estimated times of purchase.
9. Present proposed budget to appropriate administrator or budget committee. Highlight key areas that may have a positive budgetary impact.
10. Receive approval of budget as proposed or adjusted.

Following the approval of the budget, the manager should communicate it to surgical services staff, medical staff, and support services as appropriate. Ongoing monitoring of the budget is essential. Variances should be investigated and corrective action taken as necessary.

AUTOMATED INFORMATION SYSTEMS APPLICATIONS FOR PERIOPERATIVE NURSING

Pressures for more efficient management of fiscal, material, and human resources have stimulated many surgical services managers to pursue automated information systems for diverse management functions. Prompt access to accurate data is essential to maintain and improve the management and functioning of a surgical suite. A well-designed management information system can efficiently synthesize large volumes of data into meaningful reports. Ad hoc reporting capabilities are a vital component that can enhance the surgical services manager's decision making.

In many hospitals, integrated surgical services management information systems are entered on a mainframe computer. This linkage to other systems in the hospital reduces data redundancy and paper flow. The availability of programmers and sufficient room on the mainframe to accommodate extensive surgical services applications is a critical factor in determining whether to pursue this route or to purchase a microcomputer and appropriate software for use in the surgical services department.

The commercial development of surgical services management information systems has skyrocketed during the past few years and yielded a wide variety of software systems. Available and potential applications include the following:

1. Scheduling of patients and surgical procedures
2. Recording of patient information (surgical services log)
3. Production of management reports, such as procedural hours, room use, volume and productivity statistics, and procedure-specific costs
4. Preparation of surgeons' preference cards
5. Inventory control
6. Capturing of patient charges
7. Equipment usage
8. Revenue by surgical service
9. Tracking of wound classifications for infection control purposes
10. Registry of implants
11. Staffing
12. Case cart ordering
13. Nursing care plans
14. Intraoperative documentation
15. Quality assurance measures

Weekly, monthly, year-to-date, and ad hoc reports are possible with most systems.

When a management information system is chosen, the software must be adaptable to the specific needs of the surgical services manager and have the capacity for future enhancement to meet changing needs. A detailed user's manual should accompany the software and enable the user to adapt quickly to the system.

QUALITY ASSURANCE

Trends in health care reimbursement have mandated increased control of costs, decreased lengths of stay for hospitalized patients, and shifting of many procedures from an inpatient to an outpatient basis. These trends emphasize the need for continued quality in the provision of patient care. The Joint Commission on Accreditation of Healthcare Organizations has taken a strong position on the need for monitoring and evaluating the quality and appropriateness of care and for resolving any identified problems.

The surgical services quality assurance program should be based on the established standards of care. The intent of each standard should be reflected in realistic, measurable criteria. Specific indicators should be identified that reflect important aspects of care directly related to a specific standard. Thresholds should be established that identify the level of acceptability of variance for each indicator. Numerous measurement methods may be used to assess the attainment of standards or the degree of difference between actual practice and the standards. Methods may include retrospective review, review of incident reports, utilization review, patient surveys, and peer review. Emphasis has evolved from process auditing to the current emphasis on outcome or end results in terms of patient health and satisfaction.

A problem-focused approach facilitates measurement of perioperative patient care. When problems are identified, they must be resolved through a systematic plan of action. Following assessment of the problems, they should be given priority according to impact on patient care, and solutions should be identified and implemented. Ongoing monitoring and a scheduled, documented follow-up indicate if the solutions were successful. If not, alternative approaches must be taken and evaluated.

Staff involvement in the development and implementation of a surgical services quality assurance program can strengthen their commitment to meeting standards and enhance program effectiveness. Staff members must be informed of how quality assurance findings will be used, which can be accomplished through periodic educational programs on quality assurance activities. Documentation of quality assurance activities is channeled through the appropriate reporting mechanisms to the hospitalwide quality assurance committee.

RISK MANAGEMENT

Although risk management has been used in industry for many years, in health care organizations it has emerged only this past decade. Risk management is a set of activities that identifies, evaluates, and addresses potential and actual uncertainties of economic loss. The goals are to prevent harm to patients, visitors, and staff and to minimize financial loss once an exposure to risk has occurred. Risk management programs must be individualized to the institution based on size, claims history, organizational structure, and the political environment of the institution.

The methodology for identifying risks and selecting the best method for treating the risk follows the same form as that of quality assurance. In fact, the two have many over-

laps: quality assurance is dedicated to patient care and risk management to economic loss, but the quality assurance activity of utilization review can affect the institution's financial resources if reimbursement is dependent upon compliance with precertification and second opinion requirements. Because of the many overlaps, the Joint Commission has set standards that require operational linkages between the two functions. Otherwise, duplication and fragmentation would result in excessive costs. As with quality assurance, a systematic method for documentation must reflect the effectiveness of the risk management program and demonstrate that the program is evaluated and modified on an ongoing basis.

ISSUES FOR THE FUTURE

The perioperative nurse manager will be faced with many continued challenges for the future. As nurses leave institutional settings for alternative practice arenas, a major concern will be recruitment and retention of a competent nursing staff. New practice models will have to be developed to address this concern. A redefinition of *minimal standard of care*—defined as the minimum amount of nursing intervention each patient requires—for each individual practice setting will be based upon the resources of the institution. The balance must be to retain a high quality, but nursing standards cannot be so high as to be unrealistic. Traditional practices must be validated by research. Perioperative nurse managers will have to examine past practices and determine what actions will best meet the purposes and objectives of the department for the future. The challenge will be to track the critical elements within each specific nursing action that make a difference in providing care and direct the limited resources into those elements that do make a difference. Failure to meet the challenge will result in managers who simply observe rather than influence the future.

REFERENCES

Burns, T., and Stalker, G.: The management of innovation, London, 1961, Tavistok.

Charns, M., and Shaefer, M.: Health care organizations, Englewood Cliffs, N.J., 1983, Prentice-Hall, Inc.

BIBLIOGRAPHY

Arndt, C. and Huckabay, L.: Nursing administration: theory for practice with a systems approach, ed. 2, St. Louis, 1980, The C.V. Mosby Co.

Association of Operating Room Nurses: AORN standards and recommended practices for perioperative nursing. Denver, 1990, The Association.

Balzer, M.D.: Computerized systems for the OR, AORN J. 43:187, 1986.

Bartolo, D.M., and Heffelfinger, W.: Establishing operating room rates based on costs of surgical procedures, Perioper. Nurs. Q. 1:17, 1985.

Byars., L., and Rue, L.: Human resource management, ed. 2, Homewood, Ill., 1987, Richard D. Irwin, Inc.

Covvey, H.D., Craven, N.H., and McAlister, N.H.: Concepts and issues in health care computing, St. Louis, 1985, The C.V. Mosby Co.

Creighton, H.: Law every nurse should know, ed. 5, Philadelphia, 1986, W.B. Saunders Co.

Decker, C.M.: Quality assurance: accent on monitoring, Nurs. Manage. 16:20, 1985.

Groah, L.K.: Preparing the OR budget, AORN J. 41:547, 1985.

Hackay, B.A., and others: Maximizing resources: efficient scheduling of the OR, AORN J. 39:1174, 1984.

Hejna, W., and Gutmann, C.: Management of surgical facilities, Rockville, Md., 1984, Aspen Publishers, Inc.

Issac, E.K.: Financial planning, AORN J. 42:708, 1985.

Joint Commission on Accreditation of Healthcare Organizations: Accreditation manual for hospitals, Chicago, 1990, The Commission.

Kneedler, J.A., and Dodge, G.H.: Perioperative patient care, ed. 2, Boston, 1987, Blackwell Scientific Publications.

Koontz, H., and Fulmer, R.: Business, ed. 4, Homewood, Ill., 1984, Richard D. Irwin, Inc.

Long, B.C., and Phipps, W.J., editors: Essentials of medical-surgical nursing, St. Louis, 1985, The C.V. Mosby Co.

Lucas, Henry: Information systems concepts for management, ed. 3, St. Louis, 1986, McGraw-Hill Book Co.

Mackie, R.J., Peddie, R., and Pendleton, R.: Quality assurance: a design for perioperative nurses, AORN J. 42:58, 1985.

Monagle, R.: Risk management, Rockville, Md., 1985, Aspen Publishers, Inc.

Nelson, C., and Goldstein, A.: Health care quality, Health Care Management Review 14:2, Spring 1989.

Schulz, R., and Johnson, A.: Management of hospitals, ed. 2, St. Louis, 1983, McGraw Hill Book Co.

Shortell, S., and Kaluzny, A.: Healthcare management, ed. 2, New York, 1988, John Wiley and Sons.

Stoner, J.A.: Management, ed. 2, Englewood Cliffs, N.J., 1982, Prentice-Hall.

3 Design of the surgical suite

MERRY ANNE PIERSON

Increased federal restraints on building and renovation programs, mandates of the prospective payment system, decreased use of inpatient facilities, and greater competition among health care providers are forcing health care administrators to assume an expanded role in the planning and construction of new or revamped facilities. Control of costs has never been more important. Health systems agencies exercise stringent controls to prevent the duplication of services while ensuring the availability of appropriate facilities to meet consumers' health care needs.

The early involvement of nurses and physicians in planning new buildings or renovation yields the most functional facilities for the provision of efficient, high-quality patient care. Surgeons and perioperative nurses can provide knowledgeable, progressive advice on surgical suite design. From practical experience they know which aspects of the current suite have been functional and which have not. They can be invaluable in the planning and design process.

The purpose of this chapter is to outline an approach to thoughtful analysis of planning and design. It includes consideration of systems analysis, suite and operating room configuration, environmental control, and safety. The result must be a surgical suite that functions effectively and facilitates provision of safe, contemporary patient care.

APPROACH TO THE ANALYSIS

The request for an analysis by perioperative nursing personnel is usually initiated by the architect through the hospital and nursing administrators. However, the nursing division may be consulted only after the fact, for example, after plans have been drawn by the architect and approved by the hospital administration or renovation and building committees. This timing is unwise. Perioperative nursing management must be involved in the planning from inception. Few surgeons or administrators are familiar with all aspects of the daily process by which the surgical suite functions. Initiative, assertion of the right to advise, and well-defined proposals promptly submitted are necessary if a functional, technologically efficient, and cost-effective new surgical suite is to meet patient and nursing care needs.

The analysis should begin with consideration of the demands on the surgical suite: Is any major demographic shift within the community anticipated? Is the local health systems agency considering restrictions on specific functions and services, such as open heart surgery? What new surgical technology is expected during the next 10 to 15 years? What services will decrease with the advent of new technology? How will the institution's strategic plan affect surgical suite requirements? Will certain services require additional surgical beds to accommodate growth? Will additional surgical specialties be added? What changes can be anticipated in relation to the provision of inpatient versus outpatient surgery? What are the deficits of the current suite? What does a utilization analysis reveal about the volume of surgeries performed, the hours required to accommodate those procedures, and the unique space and equipment needs for specialty procedures? What level of trauma service is provided? After considering this information, perioperative nursing managers can determine the surgical suite requirements for the anticipated type and number of surgical procedures.

The second consideration is the materials-handling systems in use. If a renovation of existing facilities is planned and the central supply area will be unchanged, the flow and work patterns of personnel may be dictated in part by the way materials enter and leave the suite. An analysis of instrument processing, sterilization systems, the type of materials used (reusable, disposable), storage of supplies and equipment, decontamination methods, and delivery systems (cartage, mechanical, manual) should be included.

The third consideration is the needs of the persons involved: patients, nursing personnel, surgeons, anesthesiologists, and ancillary staff. Lack of in-depth analysis of the characteristics of surgical personnel, human activity patterns, and time-efficiency data has resulted in dissatisfaction with new or renovated facilities. In-depth consideration of the intraoperative needs of the pathology and radiology departments as well as other support staff is necessary. Analysis depends in part on the organization of perioperative nursing personnel. If personnel are assigned to specific surgical services in which duties and responsibilities are fairly constant and well defined, suggestions should come up the line through each specialty nurse manager to the administrative supervisor and then to the director of surgical services. Studies should be made of the activity patterns of each specialty team. Inefficient movements result in slower case turnover and increased costs.

OPERATING ROOM SYSTEMS

Once the general requirements for the performance of surgery in the community and the hospital have been considered, the analysis may be carried into more detail and specificity by reducing the surgical suite activities into four major systems: surgical support systems (design and function of the physical environment); traffic and commerce systems (movement of patients, personnel, and materials into, within, and out of the suite); communications systems; and administrative systems. These systems are discussed in the remainder of this chapter.

Surgical support systems
Surgical suite design

Suite design is dictated in part by the number of operating rooms required. In hospitals with 100 or fewer beds, many functions (sterilization, storage, delivery) can be carried on within the same area of the surgical suite. Single-corridor or L-shaped designs are applicable for two or three operating rooms and support areas. In hospitals with a capacity of 500 to 600 beds, 12 to 15 operating rooms will be required, and double-corridor, U- or T-shaped suites are more suitable. In larger hospitals all of

these designs have been used, as well as cluster, circular, and rectangular patterns with either central core and radial distribution or a peripheral corridor plan. Although the peripheral corridor scheme tends to be more expensive because of excessive corridor space, it is one of the most common designs utilized. The large passageway becomes a storage area for movable equipment. Two designs are illustrated (Figs. 3-1 and 3-2). The peripheral corridor design incorporates the operating rooms surrounding a central supply area with a patient/staff corridor around the perimeter. The basic modular design usually has four operating rooms with a system of peripheral patient/staff corridors and a central supporting core. This modular approach is the most flexible because identical modules can be added with little disruption.

In both designs the flow of supplies is from the clean core area through the operating rooms to the peripheral corridor. Soiled materials should not reenter the clean core area. Soiled linen and trash collection areas should be separated from personnel and patient traffic areas, if possible, for infection control purposes. If instruments and other supplies are partially or totally reprocessed within the surgical suite, a unidirectional traffic pattern should ensure movement of items from the decontamination area to processing and storage. Work areas for each task should be clearly identified to eliminate crossover or mixing of soiled and cleaned instruments or supplies. When planning a remote central processing system for operating room instruments and supplies, keeping fragile instruments and high-cost, low-volume items within the surgical suite may

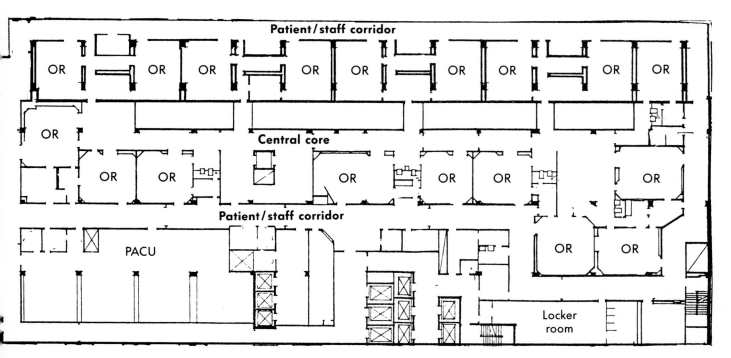

Fig. 3-1. Peripheral corridor design. (Courtesy of The Ohio State University Hospitals, Columbus, Ohio.)

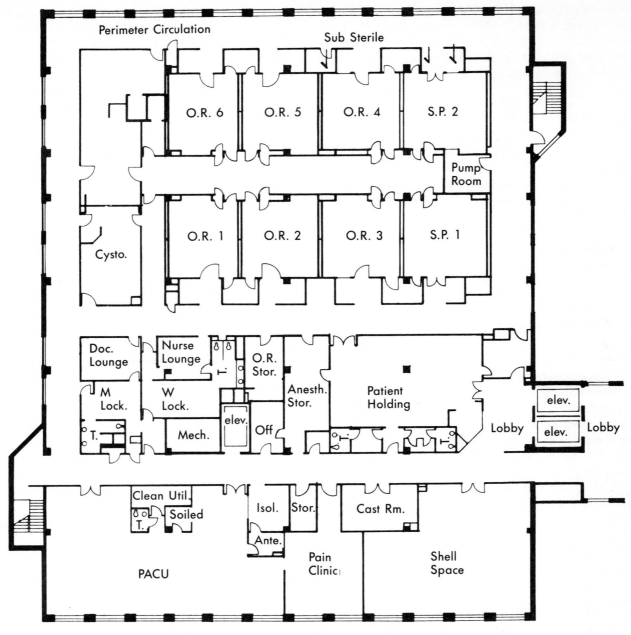

Fig. 3-2. Modular design within a peripheral corridor. (Modified from Ellerbe Becket, Architects and Engineers, New York, N.Y., 1989.)

be wise. To facilitate appropriate processing of these items, a decontamination area and a processing area must be located in the suite.

Three basic faults frequently found in newly constructed surgical suites are poorly designed traffic patterns, inefficient materials handling, and insufficient, poorly organized storage space. A common misconception among hospital and operating room designers is that a large central processing and supply area negates the need for storage within the surgical suite. A continual lament of many surgical suite managers is the lack of storage space. A

quick perusal of any suite reveals various pieces of equipment that must be kept within the department. With continuing technologic advances in surgery, an increased volume of equipment can be anticipated. In addition, backup supplies and instruments must be available in the suite for unanticipated needs that arise in even the best planned system of surgical supplies management. These supplies and equipment should be stored as close as possible to the point of use to facilitate quick retrieval. Specialty service carts containing unique and frequently needed specialty items provide a convenient, easily accessible mode of storage. In-depth analysis of operating room functioning and thoughtful planning can eliminate or reduce the problems that frequently occur in newly constructed surgical suites.

A preoperative patient holding area should be provided in the design of a new or renovated suite. It should be near the main entrance of the suite and have a quiet, restful atmosphere. Here patient identification and planned procedure are verified, the patient may receive preoperative medications and the incisional site may be shaved, if required. Intravenous therapy is initiated, and the chart is checked to ascertain that all requested diagnostic tests have been completed and results recorded. The proximity of the holding area enables the perioperative nurse to perform an immediate preoperative assessment of the patient and alter the plan of intraoperative care if warranted. The surgeon and anesthesiologist may also visit the patient in the patient holding area. Use of a holding area is psychologically advantageous to the patient and reduces preparation time in the operating room.

Outpatient surgery facilities

Large-volume outpatient surgery facilities are becoming common because of escalating costs of inpatient hospital care, validated safety of ambulatory surgery, and the convenience to patients and their families. Careful consideration of present and future community needs and the direction of hospital growth must be made before planning such a facility. Outpatient surgery services have been integrated into major operating room facilities or have been built as separate, economically self-sustaining units. The advantages of the integrated suite are the consolidation of staff, equipment, and supplies; the delivery of quality care by a knowledgeable staff; the convenience to the surgeon of being able to go from surgical outpatients to inpatients without changing clothes and violating traffic flow; and the use of outpatient operating rooms for inpatient surgery or vice versa when those rooms are not being used for the designated type of surgery. Ambulatory surgery is discussed in detail in Chapter 28.

Outpatient surgery facilities require special considerations because most patients are fully awake on entering the operating room. Traffic design is highly important; the most successful facilities have a one-way traffic pattern. The outer clerical and waiting area should be attractively furnished and have a warm, friendly atmosphere that provides a sense of security. A designated area where families may wait is essential and should be equipped with telephones, television, and reading space. A patient preparation room should be provided in a clean area. This room should have privacy and should permit changing of clothes, skin washing, and access to toilet facilities. Entrance to the operating room should be direct and protective, so that the previous patient is not seen. After the operation, the patient is taken to the postanesthesia care area or observation room. When ready for discharge, the

patient dresses and leaves the facility without retracing any steps. Double-doored lockers that open on one side in the admission dressing room and on the other in the discharge dressing room facilitate one-way traffic flow. Special attention must be given to the psychologic aspects of surgical care by consideration of color, excessive noise, privacy, music, and conduct of perioperative nursing personnel.

Operating room design

Operating rooms have been built in a myriad of shapes, but the rectangle or square remains the most practical and flexible and the least expensive. Ovoid and multifaceted rooms have not offered significant advantages over simpler designs that lend themselves to modular and prefabricated construction techniques.

The ideal size of an operating room is controversial. A 400-square-foot area is satisfactory except when procedures require extensive peripheral equipment such as a cardiopulmonary bypass machine and lasers. Open heart and complex neurosurgical procedures may require as much as 600 square feet of usable space. Conversely, endoscopy, cystoscopy, and some outpatient diagnostic rooms may require only 200 square feet. Thus a modular unit system can be devised that will accommodate each need by halving or doubling the basic unit for special applications. State and local building codes may affect architectural plans by specifying minimum square footage requirements.

The interior of the operating room has specific requirements for environmental control. Ceilings and walls should be nonporous, smooth, easy to clean, waterproof, and fire resistant. Soundproofing is desirable. Ceiling heights should be approximately 10 feet to accommodate ceiling-mounted surgical lighting fixtures. Where possible, a 4-foot space between the ceiling and the next floor should be allowed to facilitate maintenance. Room lighting should be flush-mounted in the ceiling and should have prismatic lenses and fixtures solidly grounded for elimination of transient radio frequency interference.

High-impact vinyl materials and flexible wall coverings, together with new adhesives, permit completely sealed wall, ceiling, and floor joints so that the surfaces may be washed effectively with microbicidal cleaning solutions. Tile walls are not desirable because most grout lines are porous and can harbor microorganisms.

All cabinets, view boxes, and receptacles should be recessed. Wall-mounted shelves and cabinets and free-standing storage cabinets are being used less and less because of the difficulty of cleaning and maintaining supplies. The trend is toward use of a cart system in which mobile units may be easily supplied and cleaned on a consistent basis.

No windows should be installed in the operating rooms because of the critical need for precise illumination during surgery and energy-saving requirements. However, personnel should have access to natural light in corridors or lounges. Several authors have reported that persons confined in an artificially lighted environment for an extended time experience psychologic and physiologic changes that may result in decreased vitality and attentiveness (Keep, 1980; Hardy, 1978).

Floor coverings have the same requirements as the wall surfaces but in addition must be highly wear resistant. Conductive flooring is not required where flammable anesthetic gases are prohibited. Slip-proof surfaces should be used for floors at scrub sinks for safety purposes.

Sliding doors should be used in the operating room to eliminate the air turbulence caused by swinging doors. A marked increase in microbial counts is noted when swinging doors are opened or closed. Doors should be made of the surface-sliding type, if possible, so that all surfaces may be washed. Fire regulations require that the doors be capable of being swung open if necessary. All door frames should be at least 5 feet wide to allow equipment access.

Color requirements of the ceiling, walls, doors, and floors are few. Obviously, the chosen hue must be generally acceptable. The traditional cool white or green is being replaced in most new surgical suites with warmer colors for a more cheerful atmosphere. Similar colors or the same colors throughout give a sense of increased space.

Certain surgical specialties require consideration of special needs. For example, flush-mounted, snap-lock water connections for the heart-lung machine, x-ray facilities, space for neurocryosurgery, and special outlets for air-powered or water cooled equipment may be required. Numerous specialties use fiberoptics, lasers, or special built-in television or cine cameras. Each service should be consulted for any anticipated specific needs that require preparation, operation, or maintenance by nursing personnel.

Environmental conditions

Appropriate environmental design aids in the control of surgical infections. Temperature should be maintained between 20° and 24° C (68° and 75° F) to reduce metabolic demands on patients, and humidity at a minimum of 50% to reduce bacterial growth and suppress static electricity (DHEW, 1978). Each operating room should have individual controls for adjusting the temperature of the room as needed, for example, when increased warmth is required for severely compromised patients during operative procedures. New operating rooms should have at least 25 room air exchanges per hour, five of which should be fresh air. High-efficiency particulate air (HEPA) filters are now used in many conventional operating room ventilation systems. Dispersion of inlet air should come from vents in the central portion of the ceiling, and return air exhaust ducts should be located near the floor on opposite walls. Air should move down and through the room, with a minimum of draft, to the floor for exhaust. Slightly less air is

exhausted than is introduced to create positive pressure within the room. Positive pressure is created to prevent potentially contaminated air from entering the operating room from adjacent areas. This objective mandates keeping the doors to the operating room closed at all times other than patient and personnel entry and exit. Without the use of HEPA filters, conventional operating room air may contain as many as 10 to 15 bacteria per cubic foot and as many as 250,000 particles per cubic foot. The level of airborne bacterial contamination increases as the number of personnel in the operating room increases.

High-flow unidirectional ventilation

The use of laminar airflow systems in the operating room has been a source of controversy since its implementation by the aerospace industry in the early 1960s. Laminar airflow is described as the flowing of air at a uniform velocity along parallel flow lines within a confined area. The term *laminar flow system* is actually a misnomer when applied to operating rooms because of the air turbulence created by the operating room team and objects in the room. A more accurate description is *high-flow unidirectional ventilation system.* When designing a clean air system, properly planning the use of the surgical area is essential so that airflow turbulence is reduced and does not occur over the operative site. A volume of 500 to 600 room air changes per hour may be achieved through an entire wall or ceiling covered with HEPA filters. When the filters are not plugged or damaged, they filter out all particles down to 0.3 microns, or macrovirus size. Although a definitive relationship between airborne contamination and surgical infections is not universally agreed on, clean air systems do reduce bacterial contamination of the surgical wound at the time of operation. Wound infections are directly related to the type and number of organisms that are deposited in the wound and the host's ability to combat infection. Airborne contamination plays a more important role when a prosthesis is implanted into a surgical wound than when no foreign body is implanted.

In summary, high-flow unidirectional ventilation systems provide a cleaner operating room environment and may reduce the potential for infection in certain procedures in which prosthetic materials are employed. Of far greater importance in the control of wound infections are meticulous surgical technique, strict maintenance of sterile technique, preoperative elimination of clinical and subclinical infection in the patient, containment of the surgical team through the use of barrier gowns and proper operating room attire, reduction of activity within the operating room, and control of traffic into and out of the room.

Operating room lighting

Lighting is an important aspect of the operating room environment. An effective lighting system should provide ambient room lighting that complements the operating task (spot) light. General room illumination should be a minimum of 200 foot-candles uniformly distributed, with provision for reducing the level. To minimize eye fatigue, the ratio of task light intensity to general room lighting should range from 3:1 to 5:1. These light levels should also be maintained in the adjacent corridor and scrub rooms to facilitate more rapid visual accommodation as the surgical team approaches the surgical field.

Of the variety of surgical task lights available today, most are designed for use by all surgical specialties. Because different surgeons may perform various procedures in the same operating room, each surgeon should review the specifications of a lighting system to see if individual requirements are met. The Illuminating Engineering Society recommends that a surgical lighting system provide a minimum of 2500 foot-candles at the center of a 10-inch circle on the illuminated surgical field that is 42 inches from the lower edge of the lamp cover or reflector. At the periphery of the circle, 500 foot-candles is desirable.

Diverse surgical exposures require that the main beam of light be capable of coming from a variety of directions. Gimbal-mounted lights appear to have more versatility and mobility than do track-mounted lights. Movement of track-mounted lights may shower dust on the surgical field, because the tracks are difficult to clean thoroughly. The scrub nurse or surgeon can control the direction of many surgical lights by use of a sterile handle, but this procedure is subject to criticism because of the questionable maintenance of sterility of the handle.

Shadow reduction is an important consideration when choosing a surgical light. Theoretically, the shadowing effect can be minimized by providing a sufficiently diffuse number of light sources to bypass the heads and hands of the surgical team. Surgical lights produce heat at the source and at the point where the light strikes. Some lighting systems reduce the heat problem through multilayer reflectors or glass lenses.

Perception of the color of tissue is determined by the character of the tissue as well as the light reflected from it. Although no tests have documented the color of light that is best for surgery, most surgeons prefer light at about 5000 K, which is approximately the color of noon sunlight. Other factors to consider when evaluating a surgical light are mobility, stability, and memory.

An increasing number of surgeons are employing fiberoptic headlights to enhance surgical task lighting, especially in small or deep incisions.

Safety design

Safety design incorporates features that prevent or control the potential of infection, flame, explosion, and electrical hazards. Well-devised traffic patterns, materials-handling systems, and disposal systems; strict adherence to aseptic technique; containment of shedding through proper attire; positive-pressure and well-dispersed clean ventilation; and high-flow unidirectional ventilation systems for special applications all contribute to a safe surgical environment. Flame and explosion hazards have decreased significantly in recent years as a result of the use of nonflammable anesthetics and skin prepping agents. Electrical hazards continue to be a problem.

Currently, problems revolve about the grounding systems and the increasing use of electronic monitoring. If a voltage exists between any two electrical conductors touching the patient, an electrical current flows that can lead to ventricular fibrillation and sudden death. Although isolated power systems are no longer required in nonflammable anesthetizing locations by the National Fire Protection Association, some operating rooms have these systems referenced to a common ground. The maximum point-to-point resistance of the systems should be less than 50 milliohms. Each isolated power system must have a continually operating line isolation monitor that indicates possible leakage or fault currents (Spooner, 1983). Most monitors have a green signal lamp that remains lighted when the system is isolated from ground. A red signal lamp and an audible warning signal are energized when a ground fault is detected.

The static electricity hazard is greatly reduced with control of the humidity at a minimum of 50% and the use of nonflammable anesthetics. The extensive use of electronic monitoring for cardiac patients has led to wider application of its use in all surgical specialties. The electrocardiogram is electively monitored in most operations. Electronic measurement of vascular pressures requires the use of voltage in most pressure transducers. Damaged transducers can cause current flow in the patient and result in disaster. Thus special attention must be directed to rooms that will require special engineering to yield a safe environment for the surgical patient.

Traffic and commerce

Traffic patterns for patients and personnel must be designated, dependent on the entrances and exits to the suite. When renovation of existing facilities is planned, central supply and storage areas should be brought as close to the point of utilization as possible. When new wings, buildings, or hospital complexes are being considered, traffic patterns and materials-handling and storage systems may be optimally designed around the requirements of the surgical suite.

Traffic-control design should address movement into and out of the suite, as well as movement within the suite. A three-zone concept clearly designates one area from another. The three zones are the unrestricted area, the semirestricted area, and the restricted area. Individuals in street clothes are permitted in the *unrestricted* area. This zone permits limited access for communication with department personnel, hospital personnel, and patients' families. The unrestricted area may have an intermingling of inside and outside traffic, mixing individuals in street clothes with personnel in scrub attire. The locker rooms, surgical scheduling office, operating room supervisor's office, and postanesthesia care areas where families are present are examples of an unrestricted zone. Scrub attire and caps are required of all persons entering the *semirestricted* zone. This zone includes most peripheral support areas of the suite, instrument processing and storage areas, and corridors to restricted zones. Barriers or points of demarcation are often present in areas where semirestricted and unrestricted zones meet. Scrub attire, caps, and masks are required in the *restricted* zone, which is limited to inside traffic. This area includes operating rooms, substerile rooms, scrub rooms, clean cores, and any other areas in which sterile procedures are carried out. The operating room control office may be in any of the three zones but should be adjacent to the locker rooms to aid in monitoring personnel traffic into and out of the restricted area. This point is often used for transmitting messages and information between operating room personnel and outside areas.

Patients should be transported into, through, and out of the surgical suite by the most direct route that prevents cross-contamination and protects them from potentially upsetting sights and sounds. Patients are transported from their rooms on stretchers or beds and may be transferred to a clean or "inside" stretcher on entry into the restricted area. Several problems are inherent with this transfer. The safe transfer of certain patients, such as one immobilized by traction, would be impossible. A logistical problem occurs when several patients arrive at the transfer point at the same time. When a patient is being transported out of the suite immediately after surgery, the additional movement could be painful or hazardous. Keen assessment of the patient and good judgment must determine if the transfer can be safely and expeditiously accomplished. A meaningful decrease in environmental contamination has not been documented with the transfer process. A scheduled program of frequent cleaning of floors and of stretcher wheels and frames should diminish any threat of environmental contamination from "outside" stretchers.

Commerce in the surgical suite refers to the movement of reusable and disposable supplies, equipment, laundry, and trash. The location of the instrument and supplies processing area must be determined before any other planning for a new or renovated surgical suite takes place. Transfer of processing to a central area outside the surgical suite is occurring more frequently in hospital design. Studying the patterns of instruments and supplies usage at the outset is essential.

Remote processing of instruments can be extremely costly. Depending on the location and staffing of the processing area and the delivery system used, the instrument inventory in most instances needs to be tripled when processing is remote. The inefficiencies of a remote processing system include delayed response when unanticipated instruments are needed, potential contamination of sterile sets during transport if not properly contained, distribution of instruments to incorrect areas of the hospital, and damage or loss of delicate or highly specialized instruments. The original concept of central processing suggested that all surgical instruments be removed from the surgical suite. However, many hospitals that have instituted this process have revised the system and by necessity have returned certain types of instruments to be processed and stored within the surgical suite.

An efficient materials-handling system is critical to effective use of the surgical suite. Materials-handling systems are often difficult to integrate into the desired traffic pattern. Three options are available: a horizontal system in which all materials handling is on the same floor, a stacked or vertical system in which materials travel by elevator or dumbwaiter, and a combination of the two. The decision as to which system to use may be determined by vertical versus horizontal construction costs, the degree of automation of the materials delivery system that is employed, and the cost of storage of disposables as opposed to reusable items. Conveyor systems can be time-saving and cost-effective, even though mechanical problems may occur.

At the onset of planning, the operating room manager should carefully evaluate the travel time required for automated materials transport from the central processing area to the operating room. In many suites where this factor was not considered during initial design, the time required to send an item from the central processing area to the operating room is at least 15 minutes. In these situations, additional supplies and instruments must be maintained in the operating room to meet unanticipated needs. Contrary to architects' claims, numerous hospitals have found that the capital cost and high operational expenses of an automated transport system more than offset any predicted cost savings.

Traffic patterns for clean and sterile supplies and equipment should be separated by space or time from those employed for soiled items and waste. External packing containers must be removed before materials are transported to the semirestricted area of the surgical suite. Sterile and clean supplies should be delivered to and transported within the surgical suite in containers or vehicles that protect the integrity of the items. Soiled materials and equipment should be handled according to the AORN recommended practices for operating room sanitation (AORN, 1990).

The proximity of ancillary services within the hospital to the surgical suite can have a significant impact on the amount of time a patient is in the operating room. Such services include those of the x-ray and pathology departments, the various laboratories, and the blood bank. Careful planning of physical facilities should expedite movement between the surgical suite and these areas.

Communications system

The third system to consider in design is the communications system. The increased capabilities and sophistication of solid-state electronics have generated expanded communications systems for hospital use. A surgical suite installation might include the telephone system; interdepartmental and intradepartmental intercom with privacy and announcing features; television for surveillance, communication, and education; emergency call and code systems; music system; clock system; and staff management system.

An analysis of the number of telephone lines required to the control desk and to the surgical suite administrative offices is necessary. A reliable intercom system is required between each operating room and the control desk and from there to the blood bank, operating room director's office, postanesthesia care unit, intensive care unit, and surgical pathology, x-ray, and central supply departments. A two-way audiovisual system between the surgical pathology department and the operating room facilitates the surgeon's direct communication with the pathologist. A similar hookup between the operating room and the x-ray department permits viewing x-ray films on an operating room television screen. In large suites the staff management component of a diversified communications system may consist of a staff registry using a visual display, a pocket paging system, television surveillance, or an audible call system.

Many surgical suites are now being designed to facilitate the use of computers in monitoring patients, obtaining diagnostic data and calculations, documenting intraoperative care, scheduling surgery, billing, and ordering supplies. Hospital designers plan for computer terminals to be directly accessible in each operating room in some new surgical suites.

Pneumatic tube systems have been of value as an accessory supply and communications network. They are excellent for rapid transport of diagnostic reports, forms and correspondence, small supplies and instruments furnished by central supply or the materials management department, and laboratory specimens. The potential for environmental contamination exists if laboratory specimens are not contained or handled properly. A pneumatic tube system that runs vertically and horizontally is the fastest, lowest-cost automated materials-handling device available for hospitals.

Administration

The last major system in the delineation of surgical suite activities—administration—is discussed in Chapter 2.

SUMMARY

An approach to analysis of the requirements of a surgical suite in terms of systems, materials, and human needs has been outlined. Specificity of design can be determined with consideration of the four major operating room systems: (1) surgical support systems, (2) traffic and commerce, (3) communications, and (4) administration. Specific suite design depends on the number of operating rooms involved. Single-corridor and L-shaped configurations are most applicable to suites with two or three operating rooms, whereas the double-corridor T and U shapes are more appropriate for suites with 12 to 15 operating rooms. The peripheral corridor modular design has become popular in large suites. The principal faults found in newly constructed surgical suites have been poorly designed traffic patterns, insufficient storage areas, and inefficient materials-handling systems. The rectangular or square operating room has been found most useful; an average unit size of 400 square feet is required. Specialty rooms may require half to twice the unit size. Uniform size and shape aid in cost-effective construction. All interior surfaces must be washable. Conventional tile walls are not recommended. Doors should be of the sliding type, and floors need not be conductive if flammable gases are not used. The unique needs of specialty operating rooms are emphasized. Environmental design includes consideration of highly filtered center ceiling air distribution with at least 25 room air changes per hour. Relative humidity should be closely controlled at a minimum of 50% with the temperature between 20° and 24° C (68° and 75° F). The effectiveness of high-flow unidirectional ventilation systems in the prevention of surgical wound infections has not been proved. Gimbal-mounted surgical lights are suggested, as is appropriate room illumination to prevent sharp contrast of lighting zones. Safety design has been emphasized to reduce the potential of electrical hazards to the patient.

The most important concepts in renovating or designing a surgical suite are infection control, safety, flexibility and efficiency of operation, capability of expansion, and accessibility to ancillary hospital services. Perioperative nursing management, the architect, surgeons, anesthesiologists, and administrators should all be part of the team that designs the suite.

REFERENCES

Association of Operating Room Nurses, Inc.: Recommended practices for operating room environmental sanitation (iii: 9:1-6) and Recommended practices for care of instruments, scopes, and powered surgical instruments (iii: 2:1-8). In AORN standards and recommended practices for perioperative nursing, Denver, 1990, The Association.

Department of Health, Education, and Welfare: Minimum requirements of construction and equipment for hospitals and medical facilities, DHEW Pub. No. (HRA) 79-14500, Washington, D.C., 1978, U.S. Government Printing Office, p. 34.

Hardy, K.: Windows in operating theaters. Br. Med. J. 2:205, 1978.

Keep, P.J.: Stimulus deprivation in windowless rooms. Anesthesia, 35:257-62,1980.

Spooner, R.B.: Hospital electrical safety simplified, Research Triangle Park, N.C., 1983, Instrument Society of America, p. 109.

BIBLIOGRAPHY

Adams, R.H., and Fry, D.E.: Surgical suite reconstruction, AORN J. 39:868, 1984.

Association of Operating Room Nurses, Inc.: Recommended practices for traffic patterns in the surgical suite. In AORN standards and recommended practices for perioperative nursing, Denver, 1990, The Association.

Barton, A.K.: Mainstreaming inpatients and outpatients, AORN J. 41:386, 1985.

Beck, W.C.: Choosing surgical illumination, Am. J. Surg. 140:327, 1980.

Beck, W.C.: Lighting systems. In Laufman, H., editor: Hospital special care facilities, New York, 1981, Academic Press, Inc.

Beck, W.C.: Operating room illumination: the current state of the art, Bull. Am. Coll. Surg. 66:10, 1981.

Doody, L., and Payne, W.P.: Revamping surgical suites to latest standards, Dimens. Health Serv. 57:13, 1980.

Harvey, C.K.: Street clothes don't belong in O.R. peripheral corridor, AORN J. 38:574, 1983.

Joint Commission on Accreditation of Healthcare Organizations: Accreditation manual for hospitals, Chicago, 1990, The Commission.

Kaufman, J., editor: Illuminating Engineering Society handbook, New York, 1981, The Society.

Laufman, H., editor: Hospital special care facilities, New York, 1981, Academic Press, Inc.

National Fire Protection Association: National electric code, NFPA code no. 70, Boston, 1985, The Association.

National Fire Protection Association: Safe use of electricity in patient care areas of hospitals, NFPA code no. 76B, Boston, 1985, The Association.

National Fire Protection Association: Standard for the use of inhalation anesthetics, NFPA code no. 56A, Boston, 1985, The Association.

Porter, D.R.: Hospital architecture: guidelines for design and renovation, Ann Arbor, Mich., 1982, Aupha Press.

Schultz, J.K.: Traffic and commerce in the surgical suite. In Laufman, H., editor: Hospital special care facilities, New York, 1981, Academic Press, Inc.

Stanley, P.E., editor: Handbook of hospital safety, Boca Raton, Fla., 1981, CRC Press, Inc.

Thomas, R.: Unidirectional flow vs. traditional system, AORN J. 31:722, 1980.

4 Procedural and environmental safety

JAYNE HENRY

Hospital liability problems are increasing in the operating room, necessitating a clear understanding of risk management by perioperative nursing personnel. Described as a systematic way of detecting potential problems and ensuring safe patient care, risk management has become important in the health care environment. Numerous intrinsic hazards can be prevented, reduced, or controlled by adherence to sound policies and procedures, thereby managing risk.

Policies and procedures are designed to ensure the safety of patients and personnel and to provide a setting in which all activities of the surgical team and ancillary personnel fit together to result in an efficient course of action for the benefit of each patient. Organizational structure, delegation of responsibilities, and authority of staff members are considered in Chapter 2.

SAFE ENVIRONMENT

People, rather than equipment, are the real obstacles to the creation and maintenance of a safe environment. Incidental to this factor is the architectural design of a hospital and surgical suite. The design of a surgical suite in terms of systems, materials, and human needs is described in Chapter 3. The design incorporates physical and mechanical means of reducing and controlling infection in the suite.

The cause and effect of infectious microorganisms and basic principles of sterilization, disinfection, and aseptic technique are described in Chapter 5.

Administrative control measures

The perioperative nursing staff actively participates with the hospital administrative and medical staffs in creating and maintaining standards, usually through scheduled meetings with the surgical, infection control, and safety or disaster committees.

Each nurse should understand the professional, legal, and ethical responsibilities to each patient as established by the Nurse Practice Act of each state.

Records and forms

The operating room policy and procedure manual should contain current and accurate directions to protect patients and personnel. Protection of patients' personal, moral, and legal rights begins at the time of admission. The course of action involves correctly identifying patients, safeguarding their right to privacy, and keeping confidential all records and reports. Conditions of admission to the hospital and consent forms for treatment or operations are important records that protect both the patients and the persons who render care to them.

The hospital administration provides appropriate forms that are legally acceptable. Personnel who obtain consents or witness them should be aware of the conditions that ensure validity and their personal responsibility to appear in a court of law if necessary. A signed consent must also be an informed consent, which implies adequate communication with the patient regarding the procedure for which the consent is being signed. No surgical procedure should be performed without a signed and witnessed informed consent. The surgeon is responsible for informing the patient about the proposed operation, inherent risks, and complications. The ultimate responsibility for obtaining consent is the surgeon's. In some states consent forms must be signed before the administration of preoperative medications. On the patient's arrival in the operating room, the circulating nurse and the anesthesiologist are responsible for ensuring that the consent is on the chart, correct, and properly signed and witnessed.

Special permits for specific operations, such as sterilization, therapeutic abortion, disposal of severed body parts, and autopsy, provide additional safeguards for patient, staff, and hospital. In case of a death in the operating room or postanesthesia care unit (PACU), the nursing policy manual should state the course of action to be carried out in regard to informing the hospital authorities; notifying physicians, family, and clergy, referring to the medical examiner; and so forth.

Documentation

The Joint Commission on Accreditation of Healthcare Organizations requires that a record be kept of each operation, including the preoperative diagnosis, the surgery performed, a description of findings, the specimens removed, the postoperative diagnosis, and the names of all persons participating in intraoperative care. The AORN

Recommended Practices for Documentation of Perioperative Nursing Care suggests that the intraoperative patient care record should also include, but not be limited to, the following:

1. Evidence of a patient assessment upon arrival to the operating room, as well as an assessment of the patient's skin condition immediately before and after the surgical procedure
2. Any sensory aids or prosthetic devices worn by the patient on admission to the operating room and their subsequent disposition
3. Patient position, including supports or restraints used
4. Location of dispersive electrode pad placement and identification of electrosurgical unit and settings used
5. Location of temperature control device placement with identification of unit used and recording of time and temperature
6. Placement of monitoring electrodes
7. Medications administered or dispensed by the registered nurse
8. Presence of catheters, drains, packing, and dressings
9. Location of tourniquet cuff placement, identification of unit, pressure setting, and inflation and deflation times
10. Fluid output, including blood loss estimates, as appropriate
11. Type, size, and appropriate identifying information (for example, serial number) of implants
12. Sponge, sharp, and instrument counts taken and results obtained
13. Wound classification
14. Time of discharge and disposition of patient from operating room, including mode of transfer and patient status

Using the AORN recommended practices as guidelines, perioperative nurses can achieve objective documentation that accurately reflects assessment and planning, perioperative care given, and evaluation of outcomes. The operative record becomes a permanent part of the patient's chart.

Admission of the patient to the operating room

The operating room policy and procedure manual should contain the procedure and delegation of responsibilities for admitting a patient to the operating room. The admission procedure should include the following:

1. The perioperative nurse should verify the patient's identification verbally with the patient (if feasible) and by reviewing the chart. Information on the patient's identification band, the chart, and the tag on the stretcher or bed should be accurate and identical with the patient's name, hospital number, and room number and the physician's name.
2. The operative consent form, history, and physical and laboratory examination results should be complete. The governing body of the facility determines which examinations are mandatory as part of the patient's preoperative preparation. These may include completed records for physical examination, health history, recent determinations of blood and urine testing, and chest x-ray and ECG examinations. A preoperative checklist is frequently used to prevent oversights and omissions and is designed to protect patients and staff. Any allergies, previous unfavorable reactions to anesthesia or blood transfusions, or religious preferences related to no blood administration must be carefully noted.
3. The patient should be examined for personal effects, including clothing, money, jewelry, wigs, religious symbols, and prostheses such as dentures, lenses, glass eyes, and hearing aids. The nurse is responsible for ensuring their safe handling and proper disposition.
4. The perioperative nurse should review the orders and results concerning nutrition and elimination, such as enema given and amount of urine voided or catheterized. Determining whether preoperative dietary and fluid restrictions have been maintained is important. Aspiration of gastric contents during anesthesia induction is a danger. Every precaution should be taken to prevent such an accident by ensuring that the suctioning apparatus is functional and by having personnel present to assist the anesthesiologist as necessary during induction.
5. The nurse should meticulously chart any medications, fluids, blood, or plasma administered as ordered during the immediate preoperative period.
6. The nursing staff should apply side rails and restraint straps on stretchers and operating room beds to prevent falls and injury to the patient during transportation, transfer, and positioning.
7. Nursing personnel can bestow peace of mind and reassurance in their care of and concern for the patient. By judicious use of *directions* and *self*—assuming a calm, confident manner and a quiet voice; using gentle, precise movements in execution of activities; and providing spiritual assistance as requested—perioperative nursing personnel can help the patient face surgery with equanimity.

Safety measures

All perioperative nursing personnel adhere to the hospital safety program. A representative of the surgical services department should serve on the hopsital safety committee. Each staff member should be prepared to carry out special duties in the care of patients in emergencies and disasters. Periodic review of duties, fire and disaster drills, and safety education programs should be initiated. All personnel should be aware of the hazards peculiar to operating room activities and working conditions.

Minimizing human error helps to eliminate hazardous conditions. In the operating room, where the patient is relatively helpless, nursing personnel must always be alert.

Failure to communicate vital medical information to the surgical team members could be dangerous to the patient. An allergy identification band can prevent the administration of drugs or the use of materials that would evoke a sensitive reaction in the patient.

Preoperative medication errors can occur if both the surgeon and the anesthesiologist write orders; therefore, orders should be written by only one of them and should be time dated. All medications must be checked three times before administration: (1) when removed from the drug cabinet, (2) before being drawn up in the syringe, and (3) before being given to the patient.

The patient's hearing tends to become more acute after the administration of the preoperative medication and in the induction stage of anesthesia. A quiet environment is essential for all patients awaiting surgery. A sudden loud noise can be distorted and frightening. High noise levels interfere with accurate communication among members of the surgical team and may increase the likelihood of error. Noise in the operating room can be controlled and should be kept to a minimum.

Stretchers and operating room beds must be stabilized by locking the wheels and by personnel actions when a patient is moving from one to the other. The patient should be instructed and assisted to prevent injury or a fall. One person should stabilize the stretcher while another stands on the opposite side of the operating room table to receive the patient. All safety devices on stretchers and operating room tables must be in proper working order. These devices—locking mechanisms, side rails, knee straps, intravenous standards, hydraulic controls, and armboards—should be used whenever necessary.

Electrical and fire hazards

Electrical and fire safety regulations pertinent to the operating room should be approved by the operating room committee and hospital administration. Perioperative nursing management should be delegated the responsibility and authority to see that the regulations are put into effect by all operating room staff members. The regulations may include the following:

1. Neither smoking nor the use of any apparatus or device producing an open flame is permitted.
2. Preliminary evaluation and testing of all new equipment should ensure optimum safety and performance.

3. All electrical equipment, regardless of source, should be inspected for safety and proper functioning before use and be labeled with an inspection sticker according to hospital procedure.
4. The biomedical technician or electrical safety officer should determine whether electrical equipment, cameras, lights, and electrosurgical units are safe for use in a given situation.
5. Inventory control, regular inspection, preventive maintenance, and safety approval systems should be established.
6. Personnel must receive instruction in the safe use of all equipment and must demonstrate their proficiency in return. A standard procedure for care and use of electrical equipment should include the following:
   a. The plug, cord, and connections of electrical equipment must be checked before each use.
   b. All electrical cords should be of adequate length and flexibility to reach an outlet without stress and without use of extension cords. Kinks and curls should be removed from electrical cords before they are plugged into wall outlets.
   c. The plug, not the cord, should be handled when electrical cords are plugged into or removed from an outlet. Pulling on the cord may cause it to break at the point where the wire is attached to the plug.
   d. Cords and connections should be handled in accordance with their delicacy. They cannot withstand pulling or rough treatment. Cord breakage is inconvenient and dangerous, and replacing broken cords is extremely expensive.
   e. Cords should not be wrapped tightly around equipment, which causes the protective covering to wear and breaks the wires inside the covering.
   f. Cords should always be removed from pathways before equipment such as a bed or a machine is moved. If the position of electrical equipment necessitates cords lying on the floor where persons will be walking during surgery, the cords should be taped down to prevent tripping.
7. All personnel must be familiar with the procedure for prompt removal from use and expeditious repair of defective equipment.
8. A qualified electrician should inspect electrical outlets and equipment at designated intervals or as requested and should file written reports with the director of surgical services.

Most hazardous situations in surgical suites are caused by the combination of electrical equipment and combustible materials found there. Because flammable anesthetics are rarely used today, environmental safety precautions associated with their use are not presented in this chapter.

For surgery areas in which only nonflammable inhalation anesthetic agents are used, signs indicating this practice must be posted at all entrances to the area. Conductive flooring and footwear are not required in the area. However, if conductive flooring exists, annual testing of conductivity must be performed and test reports kept on file.

Isolated power system

An isolated power system may be provided in anesthetizing locations. These systems may reduce the hazard of shock or burn from electric current flowing through the body to ground. Each isolated power system must be provided with a continually operating line isolation monitor that indicates possible leakage or fault currents to ground. Most monitors are designed with green and red signal lamps. The green lamp remains lighted when the system is isolated from ground. When the monitor detects a ground fault, the red lamp and an audible warning signal are activated. All operating room personnel must know the procedure to follow when this occurs:

1. The last electrical device to be plugged in must be shut off and unplugged.
2. If the red lamp remains lighted, each piece of non-essential equipment must be systematically unplugged until the defective device is found.
3. A replacement must be obtained and the defective device removed from service, properly labeled as to the problem, and sent to the appropriate department for inspection and repair.
4. If a defective device cannot be identified and the red lamp remains lighted, the operating room must be shut down following the completion of that patient's surgery until the situation is corrected.
5. Individuals responsible for ensuring electrical safety must be notified.

Volatile liquids

Flammable solutions must be properly stored. Volatile liquids such as acetone and aerosol sprays are prohibited for cleaning and incidental use in hazardous locations. Skin preparation solutions should be applied with care to prevent pooling, which can lead to a chemical burn. In addition, the solution may be ignited by a spark from an active electrode of the electrosurgical unit or from a charge of static electricity. Ignition of the vapors can occur as the solution evaporates. All solutions used for skin prepping should be nonflammable whenever an electrosurgical unit is used.

Electrosurgery

High-frequency current from an electrosurgical unit (ESU) is frequently used to cut tissue and to coagulate bleeders. Advanced technology has dramatically improved electrosurgical capabilities with the development of solid-state generators and isolated systems (Fig. 4-1). These units significantly decrease the burn potential and the shock hazards that were inherent in the original spark gap units. Personnel must understand the proper use of electrosurgical equipment.

Before each use, the ESU and associated safety features should be inspected for signs of damage and tested to ensure that they are functioning properly. The patient's skin integrity must be assessed before and after ESU use, particularly at positional pressure points and in the area under the dispersive pad (inactive electrode).

After the patient has been positioned, the desired connection between the patient and the ESU is established by placing the dispersive ("ground") pad on a nonhairy area of clean, dry skin. The pad should be placed as close to the operative site as possible, on the same side of the patient's body as the operative site, and over a large muscle mass if possible; bony prominences and scar tissue should be avoided. If a dispersive pad requiring gel is used, the pad must be checked before placement to identify any dry spots on its surface. Placement should ensure that the pad's entire surface area maintains uniform body contact, without tenting or gapping. The ESU power settings should be as low as possible for each procedure, as determined by the surgeon in conjunction with the manufacturer's recommendations, and confirmed orally by the circulating nurse before activation.

The current supplied by the ESU is dispersed by the active electrode (for example, electrosurgical pencil) through the body and is directed back to the generator by the dispersive electrode. In a nonisolated system, failure of this electrical pathway can result in current traveling in alternate pathways and causing burns in the area of contact. A faulty return pathway should be suspected if the surgeon requests higher settings because of inadequate cutting or coagulation. The connection from the patient to the machine should be checked immediately. A faulty return pathway may result from (1) inadequate patient contact with the dispersive pad, (2) poor placement of the pad, (3) inadequate connection of the cable to the pad, or (4) inadequate connection at the unit.

Electrosurgical burns may result from the unit's action on other electrical equipment. When an electrocardiogram monitor is used, the electrodes should be placed on the patient's shoulders and upper chest. Electrode placement should always be as far as possible from the operative site. Distant positioning minimizes the alternate flow of electrosurgical current through the electrodes and monitor to ground.

Some contemporary electrosurgical units possess a patient return electrode monitoring sytem. Current flowing from the active electrode is measured and compared with current returning from the patient return electrode. If the currents are not balanced, the circuit determines that the patient return electrode is not functioning properly, and the unit is deactivated. The most recent innovation in electrosurgical safety is the expanded capability of the return

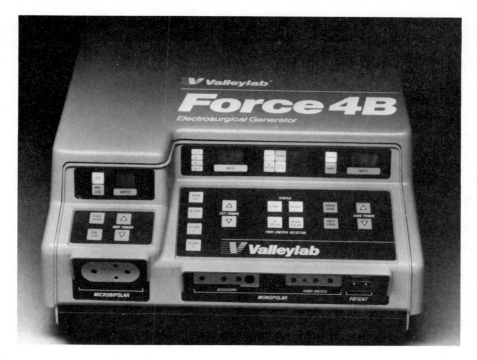

Fig. 4-1. Microprocessor-based electrosurgical unit includes the REM® Contact quality monitoring system, providing safety against electrosurgical burns under the return electrode; dual independent "simultaneous" hand-switching monopolar outputs, allowing two surgeons to coagulate simultaneously yet independently, all from one unit; independent settings for monopolar and micropolar power, allowing for alternative bipolar and monopolar applications without repeated adjustments of power levels; and precise digital wattage controls and displays, offering exact power adjustments. (Courtesy Valleylab, Inc., Boulder, Colo.)

electrode monitoring system to measure the potential for current concentration that may result in a burn at the return electrode site. It identifies inadequate electrode application or reduction of electrode contact area. It also measures the continuity of the entire electrical circuit (patient-pad-cord) for safe current flow. This capability represents a vital patient safety feature.

Radiation safety

Numerous sources of radiation exposure, such as x-ray machines (ionizing) and lasers (nonionizing), are used in the operating room. Members of the surgical team should avoid unnecessary exposure to these sources and be cognizant of practices that reduce the potential for exposure. Personnel present in the operating room must maintain the greatest practical distance from the radiation source when ionizing radiation is used during surgery. Nonessential personnel should leave the room, and members of the scrubbed team should move as far from the radiation source as is aseptically safe.

When feasible, appropriate devices should be used to hold patients or x-ray cassettes during radiography procedures to limit exposure of the surgical team. Otherwise, leaded shields, aprons, and gloves should be used to reduce the intensity of radiation exposure. Careful handling and periodic examination of leaded garments can ensure the

integrity of shielding. Because a fetus is particularly susceptible to injury from radiation exposure, women in the childbearing years should protect their reproductive organs from excessive exposure.

Radiation-monitoring devices should be used in accordance with radiation safety standards and as deemed appropriate in the policies of individual facilities. Periodic staff development programs on radiation safety serve to correct misconceptions or unrealistic practices relating to radiation exposure and monitoring.

Nonionizing radiation (laser) safety is discussed in Chapter 10.

Prevention of accidents and infections

All personnel should be instructed in the use of good body mechanics to avert common falls and strains when reaching, stretching, lifting, or moving heavy patients or articles. Good body mechanics and application of work simplification principles conserve human energy, protect the worker, and thereby promote good performance.

All personnel should be instructed and supervised in the proper use of equipment to prevent injury such as cuts from knife blades, needle sticks, burns from autoclaves and electrical equipment, and abrasions from contact with metal accessory levers and swinging doors.

Steam, electrical, vacuum, hydraulic, ventilation,

plumbing, and emergency generator systems should be inspected by the maintenance or engineering departments according to an established schedule.

The maintenance and cleaning program should be clearly defined and understood by the nursing staff. Prompt attention to spills, prompt drying of wet floors, use of warning signs in danger areas, and keeping the corridors and all traffic areas clear of obstacles are important housekeeping duties.

Cleaning, disinfection, and sterilization of equipment, control of contaminants, and application of aseptic techniques are basic to an effective infection control program. Breaks in asepsis may also result from the intrusion of pests, vermin, insects, noxious substances, chemicals, gases, and infectious body fluids and wastes into the protected areas.

Effective disposal procedures for soiled materials and debris are essential to render the area safe for patients and personnel. All surgical procedures are treated as potentially contaminated; the outmoded "dirty case" rituals have been eliminated and a safe environment ensured.

The professional nursing staff has a responsibility to work with the infection control committee in establishing policies and reporting incidents.

ROUTINE PROCEDURES
Procedure for administering local anesthetics

Local anesthesia refers to the administration of an anesthetic agent to one part of the body by topical application, local infiltration, or subcutaneous injection (see also Chapter 9). It is usually administered by the surgeon. Local anesthesia is preferred if the patient's cooperation is necessary or the patient's physical condition warrants its use. The patient does not lose consciousness and may be aware of the surroundings. Local anesthesia is economic and eliminates the undesirable effects of general anesthesia. However, adverse reactions may occur from large amounts of local agents. If the agent enters the bloodstream directly, convulsion, circulatory and respiratory distress, cardiovascular collapse, or even death can result.

The topical agent may be cocaine hydrochloride, tetracaine, or lidocaine applied to the mucous membranes of the nose, throat, trachea, or urethra, or it may be ethyl chloride sprayed onto a specific area of the skin. Lidocaine, 0.5% to 2%, with or without epinephrine, is the drug most commonly used for infiltration and local injection anesthesia. Epinephrine, a vasoconstrictor, acts to control bleeding and prolong the local anesthetic effects. It should be used with caution in patients with hypertension, diabetes, or heart disease. All local anesthetic containers or syringes should be labeled when on the sterile table.

Patients must be carefully observed for drug reactions; and emergency drugs, suction apparatus, and resuscitation equipment should be readily available. Symptoms of adverse drug reactions include restlessness, unexplained anxiety or fearfulness, diaphoresis, complaints of nausea, palpitation, disturbed respiration, pallor or flushing, syncope, and convulsive movements.

Setup

Anesthetic drugs as ordered
Sterile local anesthesia tray that includes the following items:
  2 Luer-Lok syringes, 10 ml
  1 Luer-Lok syringe, 2 ml
  1 Needle, 25 gauge, ⅝ inch
  1 Needle, 25 gauge, 1½ inches
  1 Needle, 22 gauge, 1½ inches
  1 Medicine cup, graduated, 2 oz
  1 Cup, 6 oz
  1 Basin, 4-inch diameter
  Medication labels

Procedure

The patient should be monitored by a registered nurse or an anesthesiologist when a local anesthetic is used. A general recommendation is that no more than 50 ml of 1% solution or 100 ml of 0.5% solution of an anesthetic drug such as lidocaine be injected per hour for local anesthesia.

In the absence of an anesthesiologist or anesthetist, the circulating nurse or an additional "monitor nurse" is responsible for monitoring the patient's vital signs, cardiac readings, and intravenous infusion. These data as well as the total amount of anesthetic and supplementary drugs administered to the patient should be documented. Psychologic support must be given to the patient throughout the operation.

Procedure for handling blood

Maintenance of circulating blood volume is imperative during surgical procedures in which excessive blood loss may occur. Appropriate precautions must be taken to reduce the hazards of administration of blood and blood components.

When requesting blood or blood components, the appropriate institutional "blood grouping Rh" requisition should be sent to the blood bank. Included on or with this requisition should be the number of units desired. If the patient is sent to the operating room directly from the emergency department without a chart, all patient information must be plainly printed on a piece of paper. The blood bank should be contacted by the nurse in charge to explain the situation. Proper communication facilitates release of the needed units.

Before the administration of blood, the circulating nurse and the anesthesiologist or anesthetist should confirm:

1. That the number on the unit of blood corresponds with the number on the blood requisition
2. That the name and number on the patient's identification band agree with the name and number on the unit of blood

3. That the patient's name on the unit of blood corresponds with the name on the requisition
4. That the blood group indicated on the unit of blood corresponds with that of the patient
5. That the date of expiration has not been reached

When it becomes apparent that more blood will be needed than was originally anticipated, the blood bank should be requested to stay ahead a specific number of units. This procedure allows the blood bank to cross-match the units on a routine basis without jeopardizing the patient. Cross-match requisitions should be sent for the additional units requested. A new, properly labeled sample with a blood grouping requisition may also be needed to have adequate serum for cross-matching.

The need for rapid blood transfusion necessitates the warming of blood to prevent hypothermia, which may induce cardiac arrest. "Warming of blood should be accomplished during its passage through the transfusion set. The warming system must be equipped with a visible thermometer and, ideally, with an audible warning system. Blood must not be warmed above 38.0 C" (American Association of Blood Banks, 1989).

The probability of a transfusion reaction increases in direct proportion to the number of units transfused. The circulating nurse should be alert to any signs of reaction. If any suspicious reactions occur, the circulating nurse should assist the anesthesiologist with the following:

1. Stopping the transfusion
2. Reporting the reaction to the surgeon and the blood bank
3. Returning the unused blood and a sample of the patient's blood to the blood bank
4. Sending a urine sample to the lab as soon as possible
5. Completing an incident report covering the details of the reaction

Unused blood should be returned as soon as the patient leaves the operating room suite. Returned blood can be reissued if it has not been allowed to warm above 10° C.

Autotransfusion, the reinfusion of a patient's own blood, is being used with increasing frequency (see Chapter 12). The blood may be collected days or weeks before surgery. Intraoperative autotransfusion facilitates recovery of blood as it is lost during the surgical procedure and retransfusion to the patient. Special sterile equipment simultaneously suctions, filters, anticoagulates, defoams, and returns blood from the operative site to the patient. This technique can be lifesaving in emergency situations such as major trauma.

Procedure for estimating blood loss

Measurement of blood loss is a vital procedure in the surgical management of infants, critically ill or elderly patients, and patients undergoing complex, extensive surgery. The gravimetric method of weighing sponges provides a reliable means of judging the amount of blood to be replaced. The weight of the unit of dry sponges and the plastic bag for the soiled sponges must be known. Grams are converted to milliliters on a one-to-one basis.

Setup

Blood loss record
Gram scale
Plastic bags and twisters to hold soiled sponges

Procedure

1. Allowing for the weight of the unit of dry sponges and the plastic bag, the scale is adjusted to register at zero.
2. Bagged sponges are placed on the scale.
3. The scale reading is recorded: 1 gram equals 1 ml of blood loss.
4. The blood loss is noted on the record.
5. The new weight is added to the preceding weight each time sponges are weighed so that a current total blood loss from sponges is available.
6. Blood in the suction bottles is measured at regular intervals, and the amount of blood loss is added to the total recorded from sponges. Allowances must be made for any irrigating solutions that may have been used.

Procedure for care and handling of specimens

It is the responsibility of the circulating nurse to identify, document, and properly care for specimens collected in the operating room. Blood, soft tissue, bone, body fluid, and foreign bodies are examples of specimens commonly handled.

Each specimen is cared for according to the specific protocol established by the laboratory that will receive the specimen. Generally all tissue should be kept moist and transported to the laboratory as soon as possible.

When immediate diagnosis is needed, specimens are quick-frozen, sliced, and stained—a method of tissue examination known as frozen-section. The extent or direction of surgery can be determined by frozen-section reports as they are communicated to the surgeon intraoperatively.

All specimens are considered a potential source of infection. The outside of specimen containers must be kept clean to prevent contamination of the individuals transporting or receiving specimens. Gloves should always be worn when handling specimens.

A mislabeled specimen could result in misdiagnosis and subsequent inappropriate treatment of the patient. The circulating nurse must assure each specimen is labeled with the proper patient name and identification number, specimen name, and origin of the specimen. (Example: Jane Doe, 100001, Right breast biopsy.) The surgeon should provide descriptive information about the specimen. All specimens collected are documented on the OR record.

Procedure for sponge, sharp, and instrument counts

Every operating room should establish specific written policies and procedures for sponge, sharp, and instrument counts that define materials to be counted, the times when counts must be done, and the documentation required. Certain general guidelines pertain to counting all three types of items. The scrub nurse and the circulating nurse should count all items in unison and aloud, quietly, as the scrub nurse touches each item. Counting should not be interrupted. If any uncertainty exists about a count, it should be repeated. The circulating nurse should immediately record the count for each type of item on the count record or worksheet. If additional items are dispensed during the procedure, the circulating nurse should record the number and initial it. The names of the circulating nurse and the scrub nurse should be recorded as soon as each total count is completed. Linen or waste containers should neither be emptied nor their contents removed from the operating room until the procedure is completed and the patient has been taken out of the room. Extreme patient emergencies sometimes necessitate omission of counts, the occurrence of which should be documented on the operative record.

Sponge counts

All types of sponges should be counted in all procedures. The scrub nurse and the circulating nurse should count them before the beginning of the operation, before closure begins, and when skin closure is started. Additional counts may be indicated according to individual hospital policy and circumstance. Additional counts should always be taken before a cavity within a cavity is closed, for example, when the uterus is closed during a cesarean section. Types and sizes of sponges used should be kept to a minimum. All soft goods that are used within a wound and that are not intended to be left in the wound after closure must contain an element detectable by x-ray. Radiopacity facilitates finding any item that may be presumed lost or left in the cavity when an incorrect count occurs. Along the same line, x-ray–detectable sponges should never be used for dressings to eliminate the possibility of a seemingly foreign body appearing on postoperative x-ray studies that may be done.

Each type and size of sponge should be kept separate from the other types. Sponges must be kept away from other supplies such as towels and drapes to prevent a sponge from being carried inadvertently into the wound or misplaced. Counted sponges should never be taken from the operating room for any reason during surgery to eliminate the possibility of an incorrect count.

If an incorrectly numbered package of sponges is dispensed to the field, it should be handed off the field, marked as not included in the count, and placed in an isolated spot. This practice reduces the potential for error by using only standard multiples of sponges.

During surgery the scrub nurse should discard soiled sponges into a plastic-lined bucket or receptacle. The circulating nurse transfers the discarded sponges into impermeable plastic bags or other appropriate containers, according to type and prescribed number after counting with the scrub nurse. The bag is then closed, secured, and labeled with the type and number of sponges and the initials of the persons who counted them. The bag can be set aside, and, unless a discrepancy occurs, the sponges need not be taken out and counted again at the time of the closure sponge counts. Bagging of sponges reduces the possibility of airborne contaminants arising from the sponges as they become dry and enables the anesthesiologist to make a visual assessment of the patient's blood loss.

The circulating nurse should tally the numbers of each type of sponge dispensed, as recorded on the count worksheet, before the closure counts are taken. As the first layer of closure is begun, the scrub nurse and the circulating nurse should count all sponges consecutively, proceeding from the sterile field to the back table and off the field. The circulating nurse should inform the surgeon of the results of the count. The procedure should be repeated as skin closure is begun.

Sharp counts

Sharps should be counted in all procedures by the scrub nurse and the circulating nurse at the same times as sponges are counted. In addition to suture needles, sharps may include scalpel and electrosurgical blades, hypodermic needles, and safety pins. When needles are counted before surgery begins, opening every package of suture dispensed onto the field is not necessary. The needles may be counted according to the number indicated on the package. If a package indicates that five needled sutures are contained within, five needles should be documented on the worksheet. The scrub nurse is responsible for verifying the number of needles at the time the package is opened. The scrub nurse should continually count needles during the procedure and hand them to the surgeon on an exchange basis.

Collecting used needles on a needle pad or container helps to ensure their containment on the table. In procedures that may require use of a high volume of needles, the scrub nurse can count any filled needle pads with the circulating nurse and hand them off the field. The circulating nurse should then bag them and label them with the number of needles contained and the initials of the individuals who counted them.

Needles broken during the procedure must be accounted for in their entirety. Like sponges, needles should never be taken from the room for any reason during a procedure. Closure counts are conducted in the same format as that for sponges.

Instrument counts

Instrument counts for all procedures are recommended. However, the policy of some hospitals specifies that instrument counts be taken only when a major body cavity is entered or when the depth and location of the wound are such that an instrument could accidentally be left in the patient. Individual hospital policy must be followed without deviation. Instrument sets should be standardized for ease in counting, with the minimum number and type of instruments in each set. Instruments should be counted in the instrument room as the sets are being assembled, in the operating room by the scrub nurse and the circulating nurse before the beginning of the operation, and before closure begins. Additional counts may be indicated according to hospital policy or individual circumstance. Instruments that are broken or disassembled during the procedure must be accounted for in their entirety. No instruments should be taken from the operating room during a procedure. Printed instrument count sheets with the names of all items to be counted help expedite the count procedure.

Incorrect counts

Any incorrect closure count should be repeated immediately. If it remains incorrect, the circulating nurse should notify the surgeon, and a search should be made for the item. All personnel should direct their immediate attention to locating the missing item. If it is not found, an x-ray film is taken. If the x-ray study is negative, the count is recorded as incorrect, and the x-ray results noted. An incident report should be initiated according to hospital policy.

Accurate counting and recording of sponges, needles, and instruments are essential for the protection of the patient, personnel, and the hospital.

Procedure for emergency signals

Every surgical suite should have an emergency signal system that can be activated from within each operating room proper. A light should appear outside the door of the room involved, and a buzzer or bell should sound in a central nursing or anesthesia area. The signals should remain on until the light is turned off at the source. All personnel should be familiar with the system and should know both how to send a signal and how to respond to it. Such a system, restricted to use in life-threatening emergencies, saves invaluable time in bringing additional assistance.

Procedure for cardiopulmonary resuscitation

Cardiopulmonary resuscitation is the immediate restoration of circulatory and respiratory functions by means of manual and mechanical methods and administration of drugs to provide for ventilation and conversion of the heartbeat to normal sinus rhythm.

Cardiac arrest, standstill, or fibrillation may occur in patients undergoing surgery because of the hazards of surgery, such as blood loss and shock, or because of unfavorable reactions to anesthesia, such as hypoxia and poor ventilation.

For survival of the patient, all body organs and tissues must receive sufficient oxygen through the circulatory system. The circulating blood must carry the oxygen supplied by pulmonary ventilation. Ventilation may be reestablished by mouth-to-mouth breathing or by other means of artificial respiration, such as oxygen apparatus, face mask, and intubation (artificial airway and endotracheal tube). Cardiac compression is directed toward reestablishment of circulation.

A well-defined written protocol should be posted in a designated area in each operating room and should be clearly understood by all personnel. Periodic practice sessions for delegated duties should be scheduled as part of the safety program.

Setup

A movable emergency cardiopulmonary arrest cart containing all items that may be needed should be immediately available. The surgical committee, the perioperative nursing staff, and the anesthesiology staff should determine the equipment needed and the plan of treatment to be initiated, stressing the team approach. The following items should be included on or with the emergency cart:

Emergency thoracotomy kit

1 Knife handle no. 4 with blade no. 20
1 Mallet
1 Lebsche knife
1 Rib retractor
1 Finochietto or Harken self-retaining retractor

Ventilation and resuscitation equipment

Ambu resuscitator, anesthesia machine, or mechanical ventilator
Airways—oral and nasal
Endotracheal tubes
Laryngoscope and endotracheal forceps or guidewires
Suctioning apparatus

Syringes (Luer-Lok) and needles

3 Syringes, 3 ml
4 Syringes, 5 ml
4 Syringes, 10 ml
2 Syringes, 20 ml
2 Syringes, 50 ml
5 Needles, 25 gauge, ⅝ inch
5 Needles, 20 gauge, 1½ inches
5 Needles, 18 gauge, 1½ inches
2 Needles, 20 gauge, 3 inches (intracardiac)

Emergency drugs

Where available, commercially prefilled syringes should be used.
Sodium bicarbonate
Lidocaine
Epinephrine
Calcium chloride
Dopamine
Dobutamine
Isoproterenol hydrochloride (Isuprel)
Methylprednisolone sodium succinate (Solu-Medrol)

Atropine
Propranolol hydrochloride (Inderal)
Levarterenol bitartrate (Levophed)
Procainamide (Pronestyl)
Cedilanid-D (Deslanoside)
Aminophylline
Bretylium
Naloxone hydrochloride (Narcan)
Dextrose 50%
Sodium chloride for injection
Water for injection

Infusion equipment

Fluids for intravenous infusion
Venesection tray
Infusion administration sets
Cutdown tray and intracatheters
Stopcocks
Alcohol sponges
Prep swabs
Tourniquets
Infusion pump
Blood sampling kit
Blood tubes
Heparinized syringes

Cardiac support equipment

Defibrillator
External paddles
Sterile internal paddles
Pediatric paddles, if indicated
Cardiac monitoring equipment

Cardiac arrest board

(for use if patient is in a bed)

A *thoracotomy setup* (Chapter 25) should be available in case open heart massage is attempted. Open heart massage is rarely performed today unless the chest is already open and a thoracic surgeon is present. Closed chest massage is considered equally effective with fewer inherent hazards.

Procedure

1. The emergency alarm should be activated to alert the operating room supervisor and appropriate surgical and anesthesia personnel. The exact time of arrest is recorded, and additional assistance procured as required.
2. In the absence of an anesthesiologist or resuscitative equipment, an airway should be established and ventilation of the patient begun by means of mouth-to-mouth resuscitation or other artificial respiration to restore and maintain oxygenation.
3. Closed chest massage is applied to maintain circulation and provision of oxygen to vital tissues.
4. Nursing personnel responding to the alarm should bring the cardiopulmonary arrest cart to the room.
5. As soon as additional personnel arrive, one person should be designated as the charge person (usually the anesthesiologist) and another as recorder. The recorder should maintain ongoing documentation of all medications given and procedures performed.
6. Medications are prepared and administered as ordered.
7. Infusions or transfusions are procured and prepared as ordered.
8. The surgeon and anesthesiologist are assisted as needed.
9. At the conclusion of the procedure, the event, care given, and disposition of patient are documented.
10. Appropriate administrative services are notified as the situation requires. Included would be a request to the service supplying religious rites and notification to the proper services of the change in the patient's condition and the need to inform the patient's family.

REFERENCE

American Association of Blood Banks: Standards for blood banks and transfusion services, ed. 13, Arlington, Va., 1990, The Association.

BIBLIOGRAPHY

Association of Operating Room Nurses: AORN standards and recommended practices for perioperative nursing. Denver, 1990, The Association.

Board of Commissioners of Joint Commission on Accreditation of Healthcare Organizations: Accreditation manual for hospitals, Chicago, 1990, The Commission.

Creighton, H.: Law every nurse should know, ed. 5, Philadelphia, 1986, W.B. Saunders Co.

Davis, D.: Risk management: another O.R. puzzle to solve? AORN J. 38:767, 1983.

Gendron, F.: Burns occurring during lengthy surgical procedures, J. Clin. Engin. 5:19, 1980.

Groah, L.K.: Operating room nursing, Reston, Va., 1983, Reston Publishing Co., Inc.

Harvey, C.K.: Guidelines for placement of patient return electrode, AORN J. 40:252, 1984.

Ivey, D.F.: Local anesthesia: implications for the perioperative nurse, AORN J. 45:3, 1987.

Kneedler, J.A., and Dodge, G.H.: Perioperative patient care, ed. 2, Boston, 1987, Blackwell Scientific Publications, Inc.

Kuhn, P.A., editor: Massachusetts General Hospital Department of Nursing operating room procedure manual, Reston, Va., 1981, Reston Publishing Co., Inc.

LeMaitre, G., and Finnegan J.: The patient in surgery: a guide for nurses, ed. 4, Philadelphia, 1980, W.B. Saunders Co.

Liechty, R.D., and Soper, R.T.: Synopsis of surgery, ed. 5, St. Louis, 1986, The C.V. Mosby Co.

Long, B.C., and Phipps, W.J.: Essentials of medical-surgical nursing, St. Louis, 1985, The C.V. Mosby Co.

Marriner, A.: Guide to nursing management, ed. 2, St. Louis, 1984, The C.V. Mosby Co.

National Fire Protection Association: National electric code, NFPA code no. 70-1985, Boston, 1985, The Association.

National Fire Protection Association: NFPA Standard for health care facilities, NFPA 99, Quincy, Mass., 1984, The Association.

Yanick, C.B., and Lavery, S.: Intraoperative cardiac arrest, AORN J. 41:404, 1985.

5 Principles and procedures of surgical asepsis

SUSAN V. M. KLEINBECK

Asepsis, which literally means the absence of germs, infection, and septic matter, is directed toward cleanliness and the elimination of infectious agents. Surgical asepsis facilitates healing by preventing infectious organisms from reaching a vulnerable body surface. Practices that restrict microorganisms in the environment and on equipment and supplies and that prevent normal body flora from contaminating the surgical wound are termed *aseptic techniques.* The goal of each aseptic technique is to optimize primary wound healing, prevent surgical infection, and minimize the length of recovery from surgery.

Envisioning contemporary surgery without the complex foundation of science is difficult. However, the principles of asepsis as we know them today began during the middle of the nineteenth century. The rudiments of aseptic techniques and surgical asepsis were described as early as 450 BC. Hippocrates, the father of surgery, used wine or boiled water to irrigate wounds. Galen, a Roman who lived during the second century AD, is reported to have boiled his instruments before use.

Although various forms of surgery were practiced throughout the centuries, the first period of surgical prominence occurred during the 1500s when Ambröise Paré developed the use of ligatures to control bleeding. In that same era, Fracastorius, the world's first epidemiologist, proclaimed that diseases were spread in three ways: by direct contact, by handling articles that infected people had handled previously, and by transmission from a distance.

In the middle of the nineteenth century, a new era began that greatly expanded the horizons of surgery. Anesthesia became a beneficial tool of the surgeon, permitting pain-free operations and decreasing the need for speed during surgery. Interest in surgical techniques and the development of new operations flourished. The preservation of life, however, was still not being fulfilled. Wound infections were so common that they were considered normal. When pus appeared in the incision, it was thought to be a healthy sign, signaling the beginning of clinical improvement. Unfortunately, this septic wound often ruined the surgical procedure, lengthened the patient's hospital stay, and frequently threatened the patient's life.

About the same time, Semmelweis made a simple but momentous contribution to infection control by advocating that hands be washed between examinations of patients.

In the 1850s, Louis Pasteur theorized that fermentation was caused by particles of living matter so small that they could not be seen but could be carried freely in the air. He referred to these microorganisms as *germs* and found that heat killed them. The relationship between the fermentation process and the putrefaction of tissue was not understood at that time. In 1860, Joseph Lister learned about Pasteur's work, recognized the analogous relationship between the two processes, and set out to investigate the relationship of the germ theory to the process of infection. By 1867, Lister was advocating carbolic soaks and sprays for hands, wounds, dressings, sutures, and the operating room itself. Even though Lister's antiseptic methods and principles were crude and undeveloped, their use resulted in a drop in surgical mortality from 45% to 15%. The antiseptic era and the modern age of surgery had begun.

CAUSE AND PREVENTION OF INFECTIONS

How can the patient be protected from a hospital-acquired infection? How is surgical asepsis maintained? The answers to these and similar questions are derived from the principles of microbiology and bacteriology, the foundation for infection control.

Effective hospital and operating room infection control programs must be carried out by everyone who cares for patients. Infection control programs involve methods of housekeeping and maintenance of facilities; cleanliness of the air in the suite and of the skin and apparel of patients, surgeons, and personnel; sterility of surgical equipment; strict aseptic technique; and careful observance of well-defined written procedures, rules, and regulations.

An infection control program is based on a knowledge of the nature and characteristics of microorganisms that are capable of producing infection in the surgical patient and an understanding of their transmission in the environment and wound. An ongoing and up-to-date program requires study and critical analysis of the latest accepted information to provide methods that destroy or inhibit specific microorganisms in particular situations.

Definitions of terms should be agreed on and clarified

by the hospital epidemiologist as necessary. Each member of the surgical team must have some understanding of the nature and characteristics of pathogenic and nonpathogenic microorganisms.

Terms related to infection and infecting agents

Pathogens are microorganisms that are capable of producing disease under favorable conditions. In humans, a satisfactory balance may be reached between the invading pathogens and the host, resulting in no noticeable ill effects. The aggressiveness and virulence of pathogens, the size and composition of the microbial population, the physical environment, and the susceptibility of the host determine the occurrence of an infection.

Most pathogenic bacteria are capable of leading a parasitic or saprophytic existence. Some pathogens reside naturally on or within humans without producing disease until the opportunity arises. For example, the enteric microorganisms are a large group of gram-negative, non–spore-forming bacilli whose natural habitat is within the lumen of the intestine of humans and animals. *Escherichia coli,* one of the enteric bacilli, is capable of producing infection on entrance into the peritoneal cavity.

Parasites are microorganisms that reside on or within the bodies of living organisms called *hosts* in order to find the environment and food they require for life and reproduction. Some microorganisms are obligatory parasites, meaning that they are dependent on their hosts for survival and reproduction. Other microorganisms are facultative parasites, meaning that they normally reside on dead matter but may receive nourishment from living matter. All disease-producing microorganisms are parasites; however, not all parasites are disease producing.

Saprophytes are microorganisms that reside on dead or decaying organic matter. They are found in water, soil, and debris—wherever the process of decay occurs. They reduce decaying matter to simple soluble compounds, which in turn become available to bacteria. For example, *Clostridium tetani,* which causes tetanus (lockjaw), cannot survive in healthy tissue but requires dead (necrotic) material.

Certain bacteria, members of the genera *Bacillus, Clostridium,* and *Sporozoa,* form and develop specialized structures called *spores* (endospores) within the cell under specific conditions. One cell generally produces one spore. The specific environment that starts sporulation is still unknown. When conditions are again favorable for growth, the spore germinates to produce one vegetative cell. The spore appears to possess a large number of active enzymes and is especially resistant to heat, chemicals, and drying.

Transient microorganisms are those having a very short life span, such as the normal flora present on the skin surface of humans.

Resident microorganisms are those that habitually live in the epidermis, deep in the crevices and folds of the skin.

Most bacteria produce one or more poisonous materials known as *toxins. Exotoxins* are specific injurious toxins that diffuse freely from the microorganisms into the environment. *Clostridium tetani, C. botulinum,* the sporulating anaerobes isolated from gas gangrene such as *C. perfringens, Streptococcus pyogenes,* and *Staphylococcus aureus* are microorganisms with this property.

Endotoxins are toxins that are part of the cell wall. Endotoxic substances are not secreted to a significant degree into the parasites' environment but are released after death and dissolution of the microorganisms. Their poisonous effect depends on the species. *Salmonella typhosa* and *Neisseria meningitidis* are endotoxic pathogens.

Bacteria differ from one another in their relationship to molecular oxygen. The strictly *aerobic* (obligatory-type) bacteria are unable to live and produce without access to free atmospheric oxygen. *Mycobacterium tuberculosis, Vibrio cholerae* (agent of Asiatic cholera), *Bacillus subtilis,* and *Corynebacterium diphtheriae* are aerobic bacteria. The strictly *anaerobic* bacteria can live only in the absence of air; atmospheric oxygen is poisonous to them. *Clostridium tetani, C. botulinum,* and *C. perfringens* are anaerobic bacteria. However, many facultative bacteria have enzyme systems that permit them to live and produce with, without, or with only a small amount of free oxygen.

An *infectious agent* is a parasite (bacterium, spirochete, fungus, virus, or any other type of organism) that is capable of producing infection. Infection is the process by which living pathogenic microorganisms enter the host's body under conditions favorable for their growth and, by the production of toxins, may act injuriously on the host's tissues.

A *source* is the object, substance, or individual from which an infectious agent passes to a host. In some cases, transfer is direct from the reservoir, or source, to the host. The source may be at any point in the chain of transmission. For example, the nose of an individual may be the reservoir, or source; hands, clothing, or a mask may become the intermediate mechanism for the transfer of the agent to the host.

Nosocomial infections are infections that are acquired by patients during hospitalization, with confirmation of diagnosis by clinical or laboratory evidence. The infective agents may originate from endogenous sources, as from one tissue to another within the patient (self-infection), or from exogenous sources, as acquired from objects or other patients within the hospital (cross-infection) (Fig. 5-1). Nosocomial infections, which are often referred to as *hospital-acquired infections,* may not become apparent until after the patient has left the hospital. Factors that influence the development of nosocomial infections are the source of infection, the microbial agent, the route of transmission, the susceptibility of the host, and the environment.

A *carrier* is a person who harbors one or more specific pathogens in the absence of discernible clinical disease. Carriers may be classified into three groups: convalescent

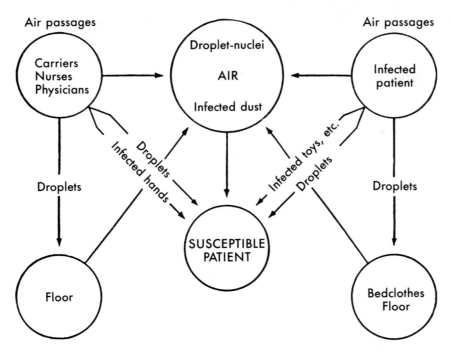

Fig. 5-1. Diagram showing how infections may be accidentally spread in hospitals. (Adapted from Medical Research Council War Memorandum No. 11. Reproduced by permission of the Comptroller of His Britannic Majesty's Stationery Office.)

carriers who continue to harbor or shed microorganisms for variable periods during recovery from the disease; chronic or permanent carriers who harbor microorganisms usually for the duration of life; and transitory or temporary carriers who, without a recognized attack of the disease, harbor microorganisms for short periods.

Contamination is the presence of pathogenic microorganisms on or in an animate or inanimate vector. This term generally is used in reference to a specific object, substance, or tissue that contains microorganisms, especially disease-producing microorganisms. For example, a person's skin or an instrument may be contaminated by contact with pathogenic microorganisms, but it is not infected. Contamination is merely the presence of a microorganism, whereas infection is the implantation and successful reproduction of a microorganism on or in a susceptible human host.

Inflammation is a defense reaction by the body to an injury or abnormal stimulation caused by a physical, chemical, or biologic agent. Frequently the tissue of the host cells, assisted by phagocytes, localizes and destroys the pathogenic invader. This reaction is observed as a local inflammation. Nature provides many barriers for protection against disease-producing microorganisms, such as intact skin and mucous membranes.

Normally the leukocytes (white blood cells) remove debris, including bacteria, from the blood by devouring these foreign particles. This process is called *phagocytosis,* and the devouring cells are called *phagocytes.* In some cases the white cells are killed in the process and accu-

mulate at the site of the infection. This accumulation of decayed cells and serum is called *pus.* The inflammatory battle is an overall reaction of the body to injury. The action of the phagocytes, the bactericidal substances in the blood, and the action of the tissues to localize the infection result in production of the cardinal signs of inflammation: redness, heat, swelling, and pain.

When tissue injury or the body's response to the implantation and successful reproduction of a microorganism results in symptoms of illness, an infection occurs. The stages that lead to overt symptoms of an infection are definable but vary in duration according to the infectious agent. The *latent stage* follows invasion of the cells by a microorganism and lasts until the infection is evident (patent) and the organism can be shed. The *incubation stage,* the phase in which the organism is multiplying, also starts with microorganism invasion and persists until the disease process is present. The *disease stage* may be asymptomatic (subclinical) or have observable presenting symptoms.

A *local* infection is one in which the causative agent is limited to one locality of the body and becomes circumscribed in a boil or abscess. *Primary* infection is the first infection that develops after microbial invasion. In *secondary* infection the microorganisms invade tissues in which there is an existing primary infection. When the infectious agents spread throughout the body tissues, the condition is termed a *systemic* infection. A *bacteremia* is the result of a singular or intermittent dissemination of microorganisms from a primary focus of infection into the bloodstream. In *septicemia* the microorganisms or their toxins are distributed more or less constantly and are continually present in the blood.

Sepsis is a generalized reaction to pathogenic microorganisms, their poisons, or both. The septic condition may be evident clinically by the signs of inflammation and the systemic manifestations of the patient.

An *antigen* is a foreign substance in the body that encourages specific immunity by production of specific substances called *antibodies*. General antibodies, which are proteins, appear to be produced mainly in the spleen, lymph glands, and bone marrow.

Microorganisms that cause infection
Staphylococci

The two recognized species of staphylococci are *Staphylococcus aureus* and *S. epidermidis*.

Numerous disease processes are associated with *S. aureus*. The portals of entry are the skin, the respiratory tract, and the genitourinary tract. Staphylococci survive for long periods in the air, in dust, in debris, in bedding, and in clothing. Pathogenic staphylococci grow in the sweat, urine, tissue, and skin of humans. They are resistant to heat and chemicals, including high concentrations of sodium chloride. They are more difficult to destroy than many other non–spore-forming microorganisms.

Staphylococci are called *coagulase positive* (pathogenic) if they are capable of clotting plasma and *coagulase negative* (usually nonpathogenic) if clumping by the plasma occurs. *S. aureus* is hemolytic, parasitic, pathogenic, and coagulase positive; *S. epidermidis* is parasitic, less pathogenic, and coagulase negative.

Studies of the response of staphylococci to various bacteriophages indicate that certain strains have epidemic potentials and that some are particularly virulent and drug resistant. Two strains classified in this manner that are known to be highly virulent are 80/81 type and 77 type. In the past, there were only one or two epidemic strains, whereas today there are several. Staphylococci vary in their resistance to antibiotics. For example, resistance of staphylococci to penicillin differs from their resistance to other antibiotics. Many formerly nonpathogenic strains are now disease-producing microorganisms.

Pathogenic staphylococci are capable of causing rapid suppuration. In many cases the staphylococci have a tendency to remain localized as an abscess and then break through to the outside. Eventually healing occurs. Wound sepsis is not the only manifestation of staphylococcal infection. Patients may suffer staphylococcal pneumonia, enterocolitis, urinary tract infection, or skin infection. Patients who undergo operations on the heart and great vessels seem to be particularly susceptible to coagulase-negative staphylococci.

Staphylococcal pneumonia may develop in patients who contract influenza in the hospital, especially surgical patients with advanced chronic bronchitis, uremia, or some other type of debilitating disease. If the pneumonia has been classified as caused by an epidemic strain of staphylococci, the patient may become a potent source of infection for other people. A patient with enterocolitis may suffer an acute onset of tachycardia, fever, and profuse diarrhea after surgery. For this reason, terminal disinfection and zoning environmental principles, including adequate air changes, are important factors in an infection control program.

The skin surface is the most common site of staphylococci. Studies indicate that 30% to 70% of people carry staphylococci on their skin, which may lead to contamination of clothing and dispersal of the microorganisms.

For no known reason, people who are skin carriers of staphylococci differ in their ability to shed the microorganisms. No difference is obvious in hygiene and skin condition between light and heavy shedders, and no other contributing factor is apparent. Heavy shedders appear to be in normal good health.

The nasal and throat cavities are the most important reservoirs that continually replenish the external environment. Studies indicate that 40% of adults and 60% of persons under 20 years of age are carriers. Colonization of staphylococci occurs within 8 days after birth in 80% of infants. Among hospital personnel the carrier rate may vary from 10% to 70%. The potential for patient infection increases greatly as the personnel carrier rate increases. Up to 70% of hospital personnel are intermittent carriers; 15% to 20% are permanent or long-term carriers; 15% never become carriers. At least 50% of nasal carriers are also skin carriers. Carriers usually harbor either coagulase-positive (pathogenic) or coagulase-negative (nonpathogenic) staphylococci, seldom both types, and rarely more than one strain. Because an individual may be a carrier of staphylococci one day and a noncarrier the next, frequent swab testing of the nose as a check to the spread of the microorganisms is impractical. Cleanliness of the environment, proper handling and sterilization of linens and equipment, and adherence to adequate washing techniques are important controls to prevent transmission of infection.

The severity of a staphylococcal infection in human beings is determined by many factors: type and size of the invading population, route of transmission, properties of the toxic products, and previous exposure and susceptibility of the host. Other contributing factors are the amount of physical trauma, the general health and nutritional state of the patient, the possibility of allergic states, and the presence of uncontrollable diabetes or toxemia.

Streptococci

Most streptococci are gram-positive, nonmotile, non–spore-forming microorganisms. Streptococci are classified according to their action on red blood cells (alpha, beta, or gamma hemolysis), their resistance to physical and chemical factors (for example, growth at 45° C, growth in 6.5% NaCl), and biochemical tests (for example, group-specific C carbohydrates). Alpha-hemolytic streptococci produce a number of toxic substances resulting in partial hemolysis of red blood cells. When alpha-hemolytic streptococci are present, a greenish discoloration surrounds the colony. Beta-hemolytic streptococci produce toxins that completely hemolyze red blood cells; when they are cultured on blood agar plates (preferably containing sheep blood), a colorless, clear zone surrounds the colony. Gamma-hemolytic streptococci do not hemolyze blood.

According to the immunologic differentiation proposed by Lancefield, group A hemolytic streptococci are primarily pathogens of humans, whereas group C hemolytic microorganisms are occasionally pathogens of humans. Other species are entirely saprophytic for humans. Virulent streptococci are more serious invaders than are staphylococci because the former tend to involve wide areas of tissue and to cause necrosis without localization. However, this tendency is partially counterbalanced by the fact that, whereas these virulent streptococci are usually sensitive to penicillin, staphylococci may not be. Streptococci also occur in mixed infections with other pathogens.

In wounds, a streptococcal infection is introduced through the skin, spreads by way of the lymph vessels and nodes, and results in inflammation, cellulitis, and sometimes suppuration. Alpha-hemolytic, or viridans type, streptococci, which normally reside in the respiratory tract or throat of humans, may produce a localized infection such as an abscess in the gums or teeth or subacute bacterial endocarditis. Alpha-hemolytic streptococci may also produce meningitis, although they are not very virulent, in contrast to pyogenic beta-hemolytic streptococci. Nonhemolytic streptococci or enterococci occasionally produce atypical pneumonia, endocarditis, or urinary tract infection.

Transmission of streptococci from the infected person to the susceptible host is accomplished in part by direct contact and in part by contamination of the environment. Direct contact may occur by inhalation of infectious droplets expelled from the nose and mouth or by hand-to-hand contact. Indirect contact is by means of infected air and dust in the environment. Most upper respiratory tract infections appear to be caused by airborne microorganisms. The most dangerous carrier by far is the nasal carrier, who contributes large numbers of streptococci to the environment (Fig. 5-1).

Prevention of streptococcal infections, via persons and via wounds, can be accomplished by adherence to aseptic techniques, including proper handling of contaminated clothing and masks, adequate ventilation with frequent air changes, exclusion from patient contact of personnel with acute sinusitis, and effective sterilization of supplies and instruments.

Streptococcus (Diplococcus) pneumoniae is a nonmotile, generally gram-positive, non–spore-forming diplococcus that produces no toxins of real significance. Pneumococci are the normal inhabitants of the upper respiratory tract of humans. Between 20% and 70% of people are at some time carriers of pneumococci. The carrier state is not permanent but sporadic and intermittent. Most carriers tend to carry the less virulent types of microorganisms. An individual may carry two or more types simultaneously. A healthy carrier is more important in dissemination of infection than is an infected patient.

Pneumococci are the primary cause of lobar pneumonia in humans. In this disease, pneumococci do not remain in the lung but migrate from the source of infection through the nasal passages or are distributed by means of the vascular system to other parts of the body and then appear as a localized infection. Sinusitis, parotitis, conjunctivitis, peritonitis, and pyogenic infection such as arthritis are frequently caused by pneumococci.

Pneumococci are transmitted primarily by direct contact with and inhalation of droplets expelled into the air from the throat of the infected person or the carrier. Indirect transmission by way of contaminated objects is also possible. Prevention of pneumococcal infection is accomplished through environmental sanitation, exclusion of carriers from the operating room, effective care of patients, strict adherence to surgical and medical asepsis, and use of chemotherapy.

Neisseria

Neisseria species are gram-negative, nonmotile, non–spore-forming diplococci. *N. catarrhalis* is found frequently in the nasopharynx of healthy people and in people with colds and other respiratory infections; *N. sicca* is present on the mucous membrane of the respiratory tract and may be a causative agent of kidney infection.

N. gonorrhoeae usually gains entrance to tissues after being deposited on and by burrowing through the mucous membranes, from which it is spread by the lymphatic or blood vessels. It may invade the bloodstream by means of local lesions. Gonorrheal vulvovaginitis is transmitted by bedding, clothing, and other inanimate vectors, whereas gonorrhea is spread by direct contact. Prophylaxis and control are accomplished by environmental sanitation and chemotherapy.

N. meningitidis, the meningococcus, is a pathogenic organism capable of producing acute meningitis in humans. Meningococci may gain access to the central nervous system via the nasopharynx. The method by which the meningococci leave the nasopharynx, invade the bloodstream, and reach the central nervous system is not known. Meningococcal meningitis is disseminated by direct contact and by droplet infection from secretions of the mouth, nose, and throat. Some persons are temporary carriers, whereas others are chronic meningococcal carriers.

Clostridium

Members of the genus *Clostridium* are anaerobic, spore-forming bacilli, many of which are pathogenic for humans. The species include *C. tetani, C. perfringens, C. novyi,*

C. histolyticum, C. septicum, and *C. botulinum; C. sporogenes* is one of the nonpathogenic species.

C. tetani produces tetanus (lockjaw) in humans. The bacilli normally reside in the soil and in the intestinal contents of some animals and humans. Tetanus toxin is a potent poisonous substance to humans. Tetanus is characterized by spasms of the voluntary muscles, particularly those of the jaw and neck—thus the name *lockjaw.* The bacilli gain entrance to the tissues by way of a deep, dirty wound and set up a localized infection. The toxin is disseminated throughout the body; when it reaches the nervous system, lockjaw occurs. Surgical tetanus may occur postoperatively and usually results from faulty sterilization of equipment or dressings. Puncture wounds provide anaerobic conditions that facilitate multiplication of tetanus bacilli. Injection-related tetanus in narcotic addicts is a contemporary public health problem. Tetanus of the newborn (tetanus neonatorum) may follow infection of the umbilicus. Treatment includes the use of antitoxin and an active immunization program.

Gaseous gangrene is produced by spores of *Clostridium* species present in contaminated wounds, especially those involving fracture or extensive tissue necrosis. Although usually associated with traumatic injuries, it sometimes develops in hospitalized patients in situations in which necrosis, vascular insufficiency, and possible fecal contamination occur. Accidental injuries, puerperal sepsis, and ruptured appendix may be accompanied by gaseous gangrene, which is usually caused by anaerobic, toxin-producing, spore-forming bacilli. The gangrenous process results from the activity of the sporulating obligate anaerobes and the exotoxins they produce. Several species of *Clostridium* may infect wounds and produce gaseous gangrene. The most common are *C. perfringens, C. novyi,* and *C. septicum; C. sporogenes,* although considered nonpathogenic, is found in many cases.

C. perfringens is an anaerobic pathogen capable of producing gaseous gangrene alone or with other anaerobic microorganisms in a closed abscess in uterine, gastrointestinal, genitourinary, or biliary infections. This microorganism is a normal inhabitant of the intestinal tract of humans. Entrance of *C. perfringens* into a wound does not always produce gaseous gangrene. The pathogenicity of a *Clostridium* species depends on the amount of powerful exotoxins it produces either within the body or in circumscribed tissues. In gaseous gangrene, the gas in the tissues causes them to expand. This expansion creates pressure, thereby decreasing the flow of blood to the tissues, and necrosis results. The powerful exotoxins also weaken the general condition of the patient.

Pseudomonas

The best-known pathogenic, aerobic species of *Pseudomonas* for humans is *P. aeruginosa.* It is frequently found in soil, water, sewage, debris, and air and occasionally in the normal flora of the skin and intestines. Its incidence increases in the intestine when the coliform microorganisms are suppressed. Until recently, it was considered a harmless saprophyte or possibly a microorganism of slight pathogenic power. It is now known to be associated with a great many suppurative infections in humans. *P. aeruginosa* appears to be a pathogen only when it is introduced into areas devoid of normal defenses, when it is superimposed on staphylococcal infection, or when it is present in a mixed infection. It may attack a debilitated patient who has extensive burns or traumatic injuries.

P. aeruginosa is resistant to most antimicrobial agents. Environmental sanitation and strict adherence to aseptic techniques are important preventive measures.

Salmonella

Salmonella species are members of a large general classification of microorganisms that are often called *enteric* (or *coliform*) bacilli because they inhabit the intestinal tract of humans. These microorganisms are gram-negative, non–spore-forming, aerobic bacteria. Other well-known members are *Shigella* species (the dysentery bacilli), *Escherichia* species, and *Proteus* species (the paracolon bacilli).

Salmonella species are all pathogenic to a greater or lesser degree and are non–spore-forming, gram-negative, motile bacteria. They do not form exotoxins, but all of them possess endotoxins. *Salmonella* infection in humans is acquired by ingestion of the microorganism, usually in contaminated food or water. These bacteria may produce either clinical or subclinical infection. The three major diseases for which *Salmonella* are causative microorganisms are enteric fever, gastroenteritis, and septicemia.

S. typhosa is the causative agent of typhoid fever. About 3% of patients with typhoid fever become carriers for some time. The bacteria remain in the gallbladder and intestine and occasionally in the urinary tract.

Escherichia

Escherichia coli is one of the most common causes of septicemia, inflammation of the liver, and infections of the gallbladder and urinary tract, especially when the host's defenses are inadequate, as in infants or elderly patients with terminal diseases. These microorganisms may also cause infection after radiation treatment and may escape through the wall of the bowel to cause secondary peritonitis. However, most strains of *E. coli* are nonpathogenic in the normal, healthy host.

Proteus

Proteus vulgaris is often associated with *Pseudomonas aeruginosa. Proteus* microorganisms are gram-negative, motile, aerobic bacilli, usually found free-living in water, soil, dust, and sewage.

P. vulgaris is frequently found in the normal fecal flora

of the intestinal tract. These bacilli also produce infection in humans only when they leave the intestinal tract. This species may become the causative agent of cystitis and is most resistant to heat and antimicrobial agents. Specific antibiotics are active agents against *Proteus*.

Mycobacterium

Mycobacterium tuberculosis is a non–spore-forming aerobic bacillus. Disease is produced by establishment and proliferation of virulent microorganisms and interactions with the host. Tubercle bacilli spread in the host by direct extension through the lymphatic channels and bloodstream and by way of the bronchi and gastrointestinal tract. These bacilli can infect almost any tissue, including skin, bones, kidney, lymph nodes, intestinal tract, and fallopian tubes.

Tubercle bacilli are transmitted directly by means of discharge from the respiratory tract, less frequently through the digestive tract, by inhalation of droplets expelled during coughing, or by kissing. They are transmitted indirectly by means of contaminated articles and dust floating through the air.

Prevention and control programs include rigid environmental hygiene, disinfection and sterilization of contaminated equipment, and isolation of people with active infections.

Viruses

The smallest infectious agents of humans are categorized as viruses. They are classified as small particles, rather than living cells, because viruses have no metabolic activity and must receive all sustenance for survival from a host cell. Viral pathogens are transmitted via the oral and respiratory tract (for example, pox virus and rhinovirus), the intestinal and/or urinary tract (such as poliovirus and hepatitis A virus [HAV]), the genital tract (including herpes simplex 2 and human immunodeficiency virus [HIV]), and through blood and some blood products (for instance, HIV, hepatitis B virus [HBV], and hepatitis C virus, formerly designated non-A, non-B hepatitis virus [NANB]). Some viruses have multiple routes of transmission. For example, HIV may be acquired through contact with blood, semen, or mother's milk or across the placenta.

Once a virus invades a host cell, it commingles with the host cell's nucleic acid (DNA or RNA) and reprograms the host cell metabolism to accommodate virus replication. If the host cell dies, all the viruses are released; if the host cell lives, one virus at a time is released. This process approximates the latent stage of infection. Virus replication stimulates antibody defense in the host. Testing for the presence of the virus, in increasing order of difficulty and expense, may be by detecting virus-specific antibodies that are produced by the infected person's immune system, by detecting the antigens elaborated by the virus and present in the blood, or by culturing the virus itself. Detection of virus-specific antibodies or antigens is termed *seropositivity* or *seroconversion*. Viruses are susceptible to destruction by high-level disinfection, a process that destroys most disease-producing microorganisms.

INFECTION CONTROL PRACTICES FOR OPERATING ROOM PERSONNEL

Statistics prove that the economics of wound infection are awesome. Large quantities of bacteria are present in the nose and mouth, on the skin, and on the attire of personnel who enter the restricted areas of the operating room suite. Proper design of facilities and regulations for use of operating room attire are important ways of preventing transportation of microorganisms into operating rooms, where they may infect patients' open wounds.

Areas should be provided where staff members may remove personal clothing, don operating room attire, and enter the semirestricted area of the surgical suite directly, without passing through a contaminated area.

Daily body cleanliness and clean, dandruff-free hair help prevent superficial wound infections. Hair is a fertile source of bacteria. The hair of the head and of other areas of the body may shed debris and dead cells that may be transported to an open wound. The person who is well rested and healthy is less subject to infectious diseases. Personnel who have nose or throat infections, are known to be carriers, or have open sores should not be permitted in the operating rooms.

Proper operating room attire

Every operating room department should have a written policy and procedure regarding proper attire in the surgical suite. Many points should be considered in establishing regulations for proper operating room apparel.

Street clothes should never be worn within semirestricted or restricted areas of the surgical suite. There should be a point of demarcation between unrestricted and semirestricted areas past which no one may go unless properly attired. All persons who enter semirestricted or restricted surgical areas should be required to wear clean operating room apparel made of materials that meet the National Fire Protection Association standards. This apparel should include hat or hood, one- or two-piece pantsuit, shoe covers, and face mask (Fig. 5-2). Apparel should cover as much skin as possible to protect against shedding and should be flame resistant, lint-free, cool, and comfortable.

When visibly soiled or wet, operating room attire should be changed to reduce the potential of cross-infection. All reusable attire should be laundered after each use in a laundry facility approved and monitored by the hospital, and it should be protected from contamination during transfer and storage.

The first item of apparel donned should be a clean, lint-free surgical hat or hood that completely covers all head

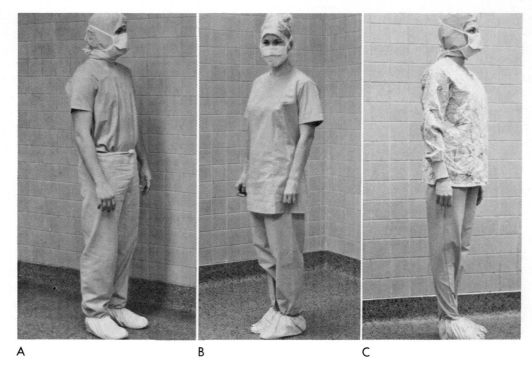

Fig. 5-2. Proper surgical attire consists of a two-piece pant suit or a one-piece coverall suit. Shoe covers may be worn; they should be changed whenever they become wet, torn, or soiled. All head and facial hair should be covered in the semirestricted and restricted areas. In the restricted area, all personnel should wear masks. Jewelry should be removed or totally confined. Nail polish or artificial nails should not be worn. **A,** When a two-piece scrub suit is worn, loose fitting scrub tops should be tucked into pants or, **B,** tunic tops that fit close to the body may be worn outside of pants. **C,** Nonscrubbed personnel should wear long-sleeved jackets that are buttoned or snapped closed.

and facial hair. It eliminates the possibility of hair or dandruff being shed on the scrub suit. The design and composition of the hat or hood should minimize dispersal of bacteria and be comfortable to wear. All hair must be confined as well as covered. Skullcaps that fail to cover the side hair above the ears and hair at the nape of the neck should not be worn in the operating room. Net caps should not be used because they do not provide a barrier to dandruff and hair fallout.

Hair acts as a filter when left uncovered and collects bacteria, which are released into the air during activity. Hair attracts, harbors, and sheds bacteria in proportion to its length, curliness, and oiliness. If reusable hats or hoods are worn, they should be laundered after each use in a laundry facility approved and monitored by the hospital. Disposable headgear should be discarded in a designated receptacle immediately after use. Headgear should not be worn outside the suite. It should always be worn in areas where equipment and supplies are processed and stored.

Scrub suits should be made of a closely woven fabric that minimizes bacterial shedding. They should fit well for comfort and appearance. Care must be taken when donning

scrub pants to avoid dragging the pant legs on the floor. The top of a scrub suit should be secured at the waist, or tucked into the pants, or fit close to the body. Scrub pants may be designed with close fitting cuffs or ankle closures to decrease dispersal of bacteria (Fig. 5-2, *A* and *B*). Loose, flapping folds or shirttails and baggy trousers are sources of possible contamination as personnel move; bacteria are freed by friction. One-piece coverall suits may be worn as alternatives to two-piece suits.

Nonscrubbed personnel should wear warm-up jackets to prevent shedding from bare arms (Fig. 5-2, *C*). Jackets should be snapped at all times in the operating room to eliminate the possibility of the material brushing against a sterile field.

Footwear should provide support and protection for the feet and should be easy to clean. Shoe covers may be worn by personnel entering the semirestricted or restricted areas of the surgical suite. The primary reason for the use of shoe covers is sanitation, because even the most conscientious person has difficulty keeping shoes clean all the time in a busy operating room. Shoe covers should only be worn within the semirestricted or restricted areas; shoe covers should be changed when they are soiled, wet, or torn, which will reduce tracking and facilitate good housekeeping.

Shoe covers should be kept in an area adjacent to the semirestricted area entrance. They should be removed on leaving the semirestricted area, and clean shoe covers should be put on when returning to that area. Cross-contamination from other areas of the hospital must be prevented. Clogs, sandals, and soft shoes present a safety hazard and are unacceptable footwear for use in the operating room.

Masking in the operating room is vital to prevention of infection. Everyone should wear high-filtration masks at all times in the operating room and other designated areas where open sterile supplies or scrubbed people may be located. One mask is worn. Double masking provides a barrier rather than a filter and therefore is unacceptable.

Cloth or gauze masks are not acceptable for use in the

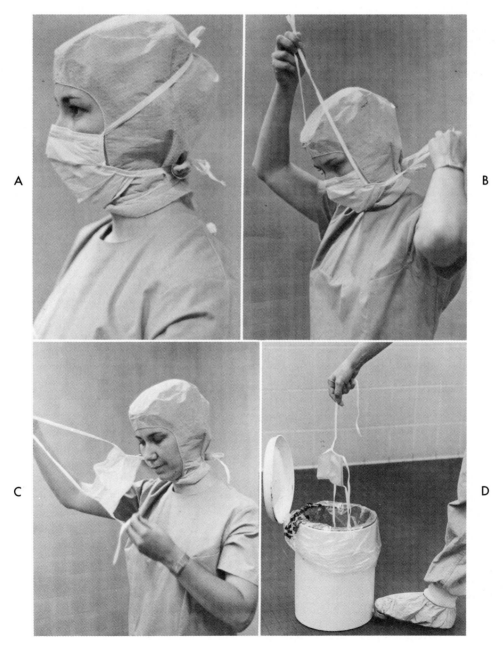

Fig. 5-3. Proper handling of mask. **A,** Edges of properly worn mask conform to facial contours when mask is applied and tied correctly. **B** and **C,** Personnel should avoid touching filter portion of mask when removing it. **D,** Masks should be discarded upon removal.

operating room. They have a very low filtration efficiency and may become ineffective as a bacterial barrier within 30 minutes of wear. The wearer who breathes through a face mask that is thickly inoculated with expired bacteria may expel a higher number of microorganisms into the atmosphere than does the individual who breathes normally and quietly without a mask. Forceful expulsion of the breathing during talking, laughing, or sneezing propels large concentrations of microorganisms into the air.

When choosing a mask, select one with a microbial filtration efficiency of 95% or above. The most effective filter mask is relatively useless if worn incorrectly and can be dangerous if handled improperly. Before handling or donning a mask, the person should wash the hands to prevent contamination of the mask. The mask must cover the mouth and nose entirely, have facial compliance, and be tied securely to prevent venting (Fig. 5-3, *A*). The strings should not be crossed when tied because the sides of the mask will gap and permit nonfiltered air to escape. A pliable metal strip in the top hem of most masks provides a firm, contoured fit over the bridge of the nose. This strip also helps prevent fogging of eyeglasses.

Air should pass only through the filtering system of the mask. Masks should be either on or off. They should not be saved from one operation to the next by being left hanging around the neck or being tucked into a pocket. Bacteria that have been filtered by the mask will become dry and airborne if the mask is worn necklace fashion. Touching only the strings when removing the mask reduces contamination of the hands (Fig. 5-3, *B* and *C*). Masks should be changed between procedures and sometimes during a procedure, depending on the length of the operation and the amount of talking done by the team.

To remove a mask, the wearer should handle only the ties. The facepiece, which is highly contaminated with droplet nuclei, should not come in contact with the hands of personnel. Immediately after removal, masks should be discarded directly into a designated, covered waste receptacle (Fig. 5-3, *D*). After discarding the mask, the wearer must wash and dry the hands thoroughly.

All jewelry should be confined within scrub attire or removed when personnel enter the semirestricted or restricted areas of the surgical suite. Before handwashing, rings, watches, and bracelets should be removed to eliminate harboring organisms. Total confinement of jewelry reduces the potential of it falling into a sterile field or wound.

Because nail polish may crack or chip during performance of intraoperative functions and subsequently harbor organisms, it should be removed before handwashing. Operating room personnel should not wear acrylic or artificial nails because they may also harbor organisms and prevent effective handwashing. Numerous state boards of cosmetology report that fungal growth occurs frequently under artificial nails.

Operating room attire should not be worn outside the operating room department. However, if this practice is not feasible, the scrub suit should be covered by a clean cover gown with a back closure when a person leaves the department. A front opening "lab" coat is less suitable for protecting scrub attire outside the department. The head and shoe coverings should always be removed. When the person returns to the department, the scrub suit should be changed because the cover gown or lab coat is not an effective barrier to bacteria and other potential external contaminants.

Universal precautions

The concept of universal precautions assumes that all recipients of health care are infectious. The Centers for Disease Control recommends that the blood and body fluids of all humans be considered contaminated and that the same safety precautions be followed whether or not the patient has a medically confirmed contagious disease. The difficulty in identifying patients with the blood-borne human immunodeficiency virus (HIV) is the impetus for this recommendation. All patients who receive care might not have been tested for the virus; for those who have been tested, the reliability of the laboratory results may be questionable. The National Institutes of Health reports that false-positive results are possible when individuals do not have HIV, and false-negative results may occur when persons possess all other criteria for AIDS (acquired immunodeficiency syndrome). Further research is necessary before nursing actions can be selected based upon the laboratory denial or confirmation of the presence of HIV.

Another influencing factor may perpetuate universal precautions indefinitely, even when testing is reliable. The latent phase of these HIV infections, shortly after exposure, is likely characterized by a lack of antibodies and low levels of virus proteins that fall below the threshold of detection. This information would dictate that health care professionals in the 1990s, as a safety measure, continue to presume all patients infectious. Although the national focus has been on HIV, the risk of acquiring the hepatitis B virus (HBV) is statistically greater than that for any of the other blood-borne viruses because the incidence of the disease is higher and it is more readily transmitted between hosts. Universal precautions are not exclusively directed at the control of AIDS; rather, they are intended to control cross-infection of any pathogen, virus, or microorganism.

The procedure for universal precautions states that all personnel should wear gloves for direct contact with mucous membranes, blood, body fluids, or nonintact skin. Other protective wear is recommended as necessary to avoid direct contact with any potentially infectious body substance. Intraoperatively, these guidelines suggest the use of goggles or eye coverings for anyone who might be splashed in the eyes by blood, an irrigant, or any other fluid; either sterile or unsterile gloves when handling blood or any other bodily fluid; and protective, fluid-impervious cover gowns when exposed to gross contaminants. The highest risk for transmission of HIV or HBV in the workplace involves parenteral exposure to a needle or other sharp instrument contaminated with an infected patient's blood. Sharp items (needles, knife blades, dermatome blades) should routinely be considered infectious and handled with extreme care. Hypodermic needles should not be recapped or removed from a syringe; rather, all needles should be placed in a puncture-resistant container. To prevent cuts, a clamp should be used to disassemble the knife blade and handle. These intraoperative safety measures are directed toward confining the patient's organisms to the patient or the immediate patient area.

Universal precautions serve to protect the health care provider and to minimize cross-infection of pathogens between patients (Table 5-1). Thus, the circulating nurse should not wear the same pair of gloves during the entire surgical procedure, touching first the patient and then the sterile supply cart. All equipment and supplies, as well as all laundry and trash, that have been in contact with the patient are considered contaminated and should be considered infectious. Local health codes for trash and waste disposal should be consulted; all waste and trash should be confined in readily identifiable plastic bags. The im-

Table 5-1. Universal precautions: intraoperative examples applicable to circulating nurses

Nursing action	Potential contaminant	Precaution
Changing the refuse receptacle for pulsatile irrigation	Irrigation splashes out of container	Goggles, nonsterile gloves
Positioning of a multiple trauma patient with active bleeding	Direct contact with blood or excreta on the skin or scrub attire	Goggles, nonsterile gloves, waterproof apron or nonsterile gown
Removing drapes following a surgery with an estimated blood loss of 50 cc	Direct contact with contaminated drape	Nonsterile gown and gloves, impervious container

plementation of universal precautions in the operating room requires nursing judgment.

Basic aseptic technique

An object or substance is considered sterile when it is completely free of living microorganisms and is incapable of producing any form of life. The basic principles of aseptic technique prevent contamination of the open wound, isolate the operative site from the surrounding unsterile physical environment, and create and maintain a sterile field in which surgery can be performed safely.

The surgical team is composed of scrubbed and circulating persons. Those who scrub their hands and arms and don sterile gowns and gloves are referred to as the *scrubbed* persons; those who supply the needs of the scrubbed team members, coordinate room activities, and attend to patient needs are referred to as the *circulating* persons (nurses).

Proper adherence to aseptic technique eliminates or minimizes modes and sources of contamination. Certain basic principles must be observed during surgery to provide a well-defined margin of safety for the patient.

1. All materials in contact with the wound and used within the sterile field must be sterile. The inadvertent use of unsterile items may introduce contaminants into the wound. When using or dispensing a sterile item, personnel must be assured that the item is sterile and will remain sterile until used. The circulating nurse should check the package integrity, the expiration date, and the chemical process indicator before dispensing a sterile item.

2. Gowns of the surgical team are considered sterile in front from chest to the level of the sterile field. The sleeves are also considered sterile from 2 inches above the elbow to the stockinette cuff. The cuff should be considered unsterile because it tends to collect moisture and is not an effective bacterial barrier. Therefore, the sleeve cuffs should always be covered by sterile gloves. Other areas of the gown that must be considered unsterile are the neckline, shoulders, areas under the arms, and back. These areas may become contaminated by perspiration or by collar and shoulder surfaces rubbing together during head and neck movements. Wraparound gowns that completely cover the back may be sterile when first put on. The back of the gown, however, *must not* be considered sterile because it cannot be observed by the scrubbed person and protected from contamination.

   The sterile area of the front of the gown extends to the level of the sterile field because most scrubbed personnel work adjacent to a sterile table. For this reason the scrubbed person should avoid changing levels, as would occur while moving from footstool to floor. To maintain sterility, scrubbed persons should not allow their hands or any sterile item to fall below the level of the sterile field. Scrubbed persons should neither sit nor lean against unsterile surfaces because the threat of contamination is great. The only time scrubbed persons may be seated is when the entire surgical procedure will be performed at that level.

3. Sterile drapes are used to create a sterile field. Only the top surface of a draped table is considered sterile. Although a bacterial barrier may be draped over the sides of a table, the sides cannot be considered sterile. Any item that extends beyond the sterile boundary is considered contaminated and cannot be brought back onto the sterile field. A contaminated item must be lifted clear of the operative field without contacting the sterile surface and must be dropped with minimum handling to an unsterile person, area, or receptacle. Interpretation of sterile areas versus unsterile areas on a draped patient requires astute observation and use of good judgment.

4. Items should be dispensed to a sterile field by methods that preserve the sterility of the items and the integrity of the sterile field. Good judgment must be used when dispensing items either by presenting them to the scrubbed person or by placing them securely on the sterile field. Items should not be tossed onto a sterile field because they may roll off the edge and become contaminated, displace other items, or penetrate the drape.

   After a sterile package or container is opened, the edges are considered unsterile. Sterile and unsterile boundaries are often intangible. A 1-inch safety margin is usually considered standard on package wrappers, whereas the sterile boundary on a wrapper used to drape a table is at the table edge. On peel-back packages, the inner edge of the heat seal is the line of demarcation. Being hypothetical, these boundaries may not apply to every situation.

   The edge of a bottle cap is considered contaminated once the cap has been removed from the bottle. The sterility of the bottle contents cannot be ensured if the cap is replaced on the bottle. Therefore, when sterile liquids are dispensed, the entire contents of a bottle must be poured or the remainder discarded. Interpreting sterile boundaries requires good judgment based on an understanding of aseptic principles.

5. Motions of the surgical team are from sterile to sterile areas and from unsterile to unsterile areas. Scrubbed persons and sterile items contact only sterile areas; circulating nurses and unsterile items contact only unsterile areas. All members of the surgical team must understand which areas are considered sterile and which are considered unsterile. All must

maintain a continual awareness of these areas. Scrubbed persons must guard their sterile fields to prevent any unsterile item from contaminating the fields or them. Circulating nurses must neither touch or reach over a sterile field nor allow any unsterile item to contaminate the field.

When a circulating nurse opens a package, hand and arm motions are always from unsterile to unsterile objects. The hands are placed under the cuff to provide a protected wide margin of safety between the inside of the pack (sterile) and the hands (unsterile) (Fig. 5-4). When the circulating nurse opens a sterile article that is wrapped sequentially in two wrappers with the corners folded toward the center of the article, the corner farthest from the body is opened first, and the corner nearest the body last (Fig. 5-5).

When a scrub nurse opens a sterile wrapper, the side nearest the body is opened first. This portion of the drape then protects the gown and enables the individual to move closer to the table to open the opposite side (Fig. 5-6).

If a solution must be poured into a sterile receptacle on a sterile table, the scrub nurse holds the receptacle away from the table or sets it near the edge of a waterproof-draped table (Fig. 5-7). This procedure eliminates the need for the circulating nurse to reach over the sterile field. Maintaining a safe margin of space can reduce accidental contamination in passing items between sterile and unsterile fields. An instrument may be used as an extension of a team member's hands to ensure a safe margin between fields. The use of transfer forceps, however, is unacceptable. Maintaining the sterility of these forceps is questionable because of the many variables, such as sterilization method, type of container, and type and amount of soaking solution used. Incorrect handling of soaked forceps is always a problem. Transfer forceps have been replaced by a packaged sterile instrument that is used once and then considered contaminated.

6. Movement around a sterile field must not cause contamination of that sterile field. The patient is the center of the sterile field during an operation; additional sterile areas are grouped around the patient. If contamination is to be prevented, patterns of movement within or around this sterile grouping must be established and rigidly practiced. Scrubbed persons stay close to the sterile field. If they change positions, they turn face to face or back to back while maintaining a safe distance between. Accidental contamination is a threat to any scrubbed person who wanders into a traffic pathway or out of the clean area of the operating room.

Circulating nurses approach sterile areas facing

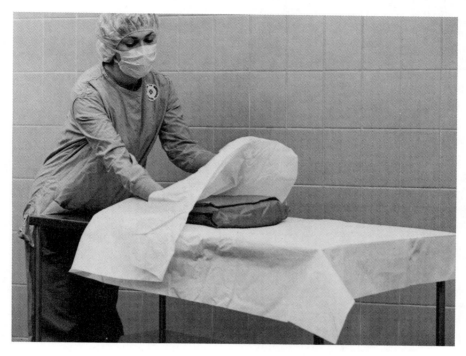

Fig. 5-4. Circulating nurse is shown opening outer cover of pack containing sterile drapes for surgery. Cover is cuffed to provide protection for sterile contents. Circulating nurse avoids contact with sterile area by keeping all fingers under cuff as cover is drawn back over table to expose inner pack.

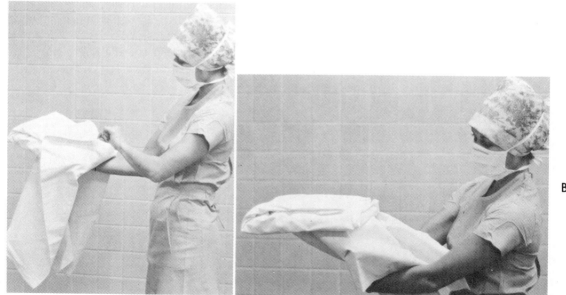

Fig. 5-5. A, When opening sterile package, circulating nurse opens corner nearest body last to avoid potential contamination of inner pack. **B,** To prevent unsterile corners of outer wrapper from touching scrub nurse or sterile field, circulating nurse draws back corners of opened wrapper when presenting inner package.

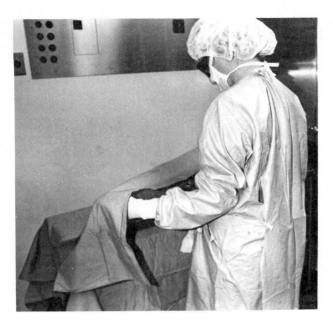

Fig. 5-6. Scrub nurse protects gloves with cuff of drape when opening inner wrapper of pack, which will serve as sterile table cover.

them and never walk between two sterile fields. Keeping sterile areas in view during movement around the area and maintaining at least a 1-foot distance from sterile fields help to prevent accidental contamination. Bacterial fallout from the body or clothing is a source of contamination when a circulating nurse leans over a sterile field. All operating room personnel must maintain a vigilant watch over sterile areas and point out any contamination immediately.

7. Whenever a sterile barrier is permeated, it must be considered contaminated. This principle applies to packaging materials as well as to draping and gown-

ing materials. Obvious contamination occurs from direct contact between sterile and unsterile objects. Other less apparent modes of contamination are the filtration of airborne microorganisms through materials, the passage of liquids through materials, and the undetected perforations in materials. When moisture soaks through a drape, gown, or package, *strike-through* occurs, and the item must be considered contaminated. Potential contaminants can be curtailed by the use of effective barrier materials, the characteristics of which are discussed later in this chapter.

8. Every sterile field should be constantly monitored and maintained. Items of doubtful sterility must be considered unsterile. In practice, the state of sterility is an absolute; items are either sterile or unsterile. Any item that falls on the floor or into any area of questionable cleanliness must be considered unsterile.

Preparation of sterile setups hours before needed and the subsequent covering of these setups with sterile sheets are not acceptable for two reasons: the setups are usually left unguarded and thus become prey to sources of contamination, and removal of the cover sheets without contaminating the sterile setups is almost impossible. Therefore, sterile fields should be prepared as close as possible to the scheduled time of use. If sterile setups are covered or left unguarded, they should be considered contaminated.

Close adherence to principles of asepsis and consistent observance of the boundaries established in the principles provide protection against infection. Application of the basic principles of aseptic technique depends primarily on the individual's understanding and conscience. Every per-

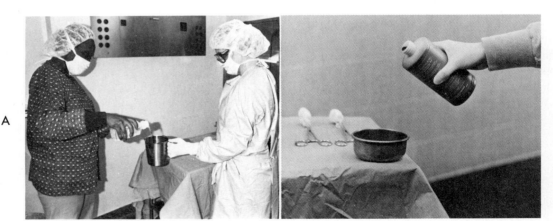

Fig. 5-7. A, When pouring solution into receptacle held by scrub nurse, circulating nurse maintains safe margin of space to avoid contamination of sterile surfaces. **B,** Care must be used when pouring solution into receptacle on sterile field to avoid splashing fluids onto sterile field. Placement of receptacle near edge of table permits circulating nurse to pour solution without reaching over any portion of sterile field.

son on the surgical team must share the responsibility for monitoring aseptic practice and initiating corrective action when a sterile field is compromised.

INSTRUMENT DECONTAMINATION METHODS FOR PREVENTION OF INFECTION

To prevent infection, all items that come in contact with the patient and/or sterile field should be systematically decontaminated after a surgical procedure. Instruments should be immediately submersed in water or a germicidal solution at the close of the procedure to prevent blood and other substances from drying on the surfaces or in the crevices. The cleaning method should be economic and must provide protection from cross-contamination, damage to the instrument, and injury to the worker. Terminally washed and sterilized instruments are then inspected, reassembled into sets, placed in containers or wrapped, and sterilized or stored for future use.

Mechanical washing

During the surgical procedure instruments should be kept as free of body substances (bioburden) as possible by wiping off the gross material with a moistened sponge. Sterile water is selected because saline causes corrosion and deterioration of the instrument surfaces. When the procedure is completed, all instruments that can be immersed are placed in a basin, disassembled or box locks opened, and covered with water or a detergent/germicidal solution. If a detergent/germicide is added to the basin, the decontamination process begins immediately.

One of three methods may be selected for decontamination of instruments and equipment. The optimum method is to cover and transport all items used during the surgery to a centralized location for processing. The cover should be watertight and remain intact during transport to the central decontamination area. Examples of covers include case carts, plastic bags, and impervious surgical drapes.

Soiled instruments should be handled by gloved personnel only. Appropriate apparel for personnel in the central decontamination area includes scrub attire, cap and mask, protective eyewear, a waterproof apron or coverall suit, and long, cuffed, heavy-duty rubber gloves. Upon arrival, the instruments are uncovered, arranged loosely in an open mesh tray with the lightest instruments on the top, and placed directly into a washer-sterilizer (Fig. 5-8). If gross debris is present, a hand prewash in a detergent/germicide solution is recommended. All hand washing and brushing of gross debris should be accomplished while the instrument is immersed to prevent aerosolization of potentially contaminated material.

A pressure instrument washer-sterilizer agitates a water bath containing a detergent and, after the water bath is drained, sterilizes the contents for 3 to 6 minutes at 132° C (270° F) (Fig. 5-9). The efficiency of the process de-

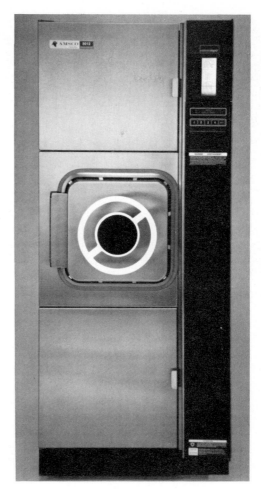

Fig. 5-8. Automatic washer-sterilizer. This type of equipment decontaminates instruments by first cleaning and then subjecting them to a sterilization process using saturated steam. It is usually used immediately after a surgical procedure to protect personnel and prevent cross-contamination. It is specifically designed for this function; however, it may be used in the sterilization mode only to flash sterilize unwrapped instruments for the recommended 3- and 10-minute exposure times for gravity displacement steam sterilizers. (Courtesy of American Sterilizer Company [AMSCO], Erie, Pa.)

pends on the kind of foreign material (bioburden) present and the number of instruments in the load. Complete removal of all soilage from the serrations and crevices depends on the construction of the instrument, the time of exposure, and the pH and efficiency of the detergent. The worker should always follow the manufacturer's operational instructions. When the decontaminated instruments are removed from the washer-sterilizer, they may be transported to the ultrasonic cleaner.

When a centralized area is not available, the instruments must be decontaminated by another method. Two options are available. One requires an autoclave in the substerilizing room; the other involves a thorough hand washing.

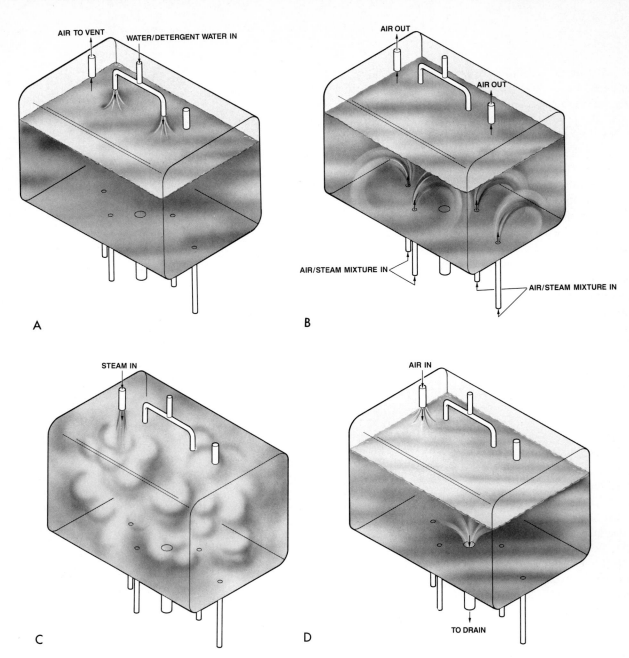

Fig. 5-9. Automatic washer-sterilizer. **A,** The cycle in this machine begins with a cold water rinse, entering through the top of the chamber, to loosen and remove gross soil such as blood and tissue without coagulating proteinaceous material, which would cause it to adhere to instruments. Then, warm water and detergent enter the chamber to a level to cover the instruments. **B,** Next, jets of steam and air are injected into the filled chamber through ports in the floor of the chamber. Violent turbulence in the detergent-water solution removes any debris remaining on the instruments after the initial rinse. **C,** At the conclusion of the wash time, the water drains out of the chamber. Newer model washer-sterilizers may have microprocessor controls that allow the user to set the duration of wash time based on the nature of soil on the instruments. A final water rinse, coming in through the top of the chamber, carries any detergent residues and soil away from the instruments and out the drain. **D,** Finally, saturated steam begins to fill the chamber. Air in the chamber and load is heavier than the steam and, because of gravity, is displaced downward and out the drain. As pressure builds in the chamber from the incoming steam, the temperature rises to 132° C (270° F), the chamber drain closes, and that temperature is held for the duration of the sterilization exposure time preselected by the user. Then steam is exhausted through the automatic condenser exhaust. Some machines have the capability of selecting drying times for the instruments. At the conclusion of the cycle, an audible signal indicates the unit is ready for unloading. Instruments and the inside of the sterilizer are very hot and, if no dry time was used, the instruments and trays are also wet. Use extreme caution in handling. (Courtesy of American Sterilizer Company [AMSCO], Erie, Pa.)

The latter is time-consuming, less efficient, and higher in labor expense.

When using a substerile room, the instruments that were immersed immediately following surgery are carefully rinsed in the operating room by gloved personnel to remove gross soil, placed in a perforated tray, and autoclaved for 3 minutes at 132° C (270° F) or 15 to 20 minutes at 121° C (250° F). Instrument trays that must be transported outside the operating room to the autoclave are contained in impermeable plastic bags to prevent contamination by dripping water or direct contact. The soiled water is discarded directly into the basin of a flushing hopper. The circulating nurse has to flush the hopper before the soiled solution is actually emptied into the hopper by the gloved staff member. Health codes may specify the entry point of contaminated solutions into the sewer system. If the contaminated or soiled solution must be transported to another location before it can be discarded, it must be covered and handled by gloved personnel with protective eye wear. At the completion of the autoclave cycle, the instruments have been decontaminated, can be handled by unprotected personnel, and may be transported to the washer-sterilizer for terminal cleaning.

If neither a washer-sterilizer nor a flash autoclave is readily available in the substerile room or an adjacent room, a centralized decontamination area in the "dirty" utility room or in the "dirty" section of central supply should be established. The procedure would be to transport the instruments to this area, autoclave to decontaminate, and then thoroughly hand wash. Transportation and cleaning of instruments should follow all the precautions recommended for a centralized area, to include eye wear, gloves, mask, and impervious clothing. The practice of hand washing instruments in an operating room delays successive cases and has questionable efficacy.

Ultrasonic cleaning

Once the terminal sterilization is complete, the second phase of instrument processing with an ultrasonic cleaner may begin. The ultrasonic cleaning process removes tenacious soil that remains on instruments after they have been mechanically or manually washed. This process is based on electronic engineering principles. An electric current, usually 230 volts and 60 cycles, is fed into an electronic generator, where the frequency is raised to a rate of 18,000 to 20,000 cycles per second. This electrical energy then flows into a magnetic device known as a *transducer,* which converts the electrical energy into mechanical energy. The ultrasonic waves passing through the fluid in the bath form very small bubbles that expand until they are unstable and then collapse quickly, creating a negative pressure action on all surfaces of the instruments in the bath. By means of this pulling action, called the *cavitation process,* debris and material are removed from all surfaces of the instruments without damage to the instruments. The

purpose of the hot water rinse is to remove suspended debris particles from the instrument surface. Most manufacturers' instructions warn against placing instruments of dissimilar metals (such as stainless steel, copper, and titanium) in the ultrasonic cleaner at the same time. When the ultrasonic cycle is completed, the instruments are removed and dried.

If an ultrasonic cleaner is not available or not recommended for use with particular instruments, they can be washed manually with a noncorrosive detergent to remove any remaining soil. Ultrasonic cleaning is not recommended for some delicate instruments, chrome-plated instruments, or powered surgical equipment. Cleaning instructions prepared by the manufacturer of special surgical equipment or instruments should be followed.

Rearrangement, the final phase of instrument processing, occurs in a designated clean area. Instruments are inspected, and all movable parts are lubricated with an antimicrobial, water-soluble lubricant to protect against rusting, staining, or corrosion. Instruments are then rearranged into sets, placed in containers or wrapped, and sterilized or stored for future use.

STERILIZATION METHODS FOR PREVENTION OF INFECTION

Modern surgery demands increasingly intricate and delicate instruments and more effective supplies and equipment. Methods of sterilization of surgical items must result in complete destruction of microbial life, including spores, and the absence of toxic residue on the objects, as well as little or no deterioration or damage to heat- and moisture-sensitive instruments and other items.

Steam sterilization

Saturated steam under pressure is recognized as the safest, most practical means of sterilizing surgical supplies, fluids, the majority of instruments, and other inanimate objects. Steam under pressure permits permeation of moist heat to porous substances by condensation and results in destruction of all microbial life.

Saturated steam exerts the maximum pressure for water vapor at a given temperature and pressure.

Theory of microbial destruction

Microorganisms are believed to be destroyed by moist heat through a process of denaturation and coagulation of the enzyme-protein system within the bacterial cell. Microorganisms are killed at a lower temperature when moist heat is used than when dry heat is used. This fact is based on the theory that all chemical reactions, including coagulation of proteins, are catalyzed by the presence of water.

Compressed steam results in effective sterilization because moisture and heat are always present. When steam comes in contact with a cold object, condensation takes place immediately. As the steam condenses, it gives off latent heat that heats and wets the object; in other words, both moisture and heat are provided.

Principles and mechanism

Pure steam at sea level atmospheric pressure has a temperature of 100° C (212° F). When water is boiled in a vessel from which the steam cannot escape, a higher temperature is reached. To attain steam under pressure, a vessel that can be closed tightly must be used. A home pressure cooker generates steam from the water inside the tightly closed vessel when it is placed over a gas flame or electric plate. In the hospital autoclave, the steam coming from the boilers is compressed and gives off latent heat.

The higher the steam pressure, the higher the temperature. The steam is the sterilizing agent, not the compressed hot air. If steam is mixed with air at the same pressure, the temperature will be lower than pure steam at atmospheric pressure. For example, if the mixture is two-thirds steam and one-third air, the temperature at 15 pounds pressure per square inch (psi) will be 115° C (240° F) instead of 121° C (250° F). The air acts as a barrier to steam penetration.

Generally the autoclave consists of two metal cylinders (the chamber and the shell), one within the other. Between the cylinders is an enclosed space (the jacket) in which steam and heat can be maintained. This steam jacket facilitates fast, efficient, and effective drying of the load following sterilization.

In the conventional steam sterilizer, the sterilization process may be divided into five distinct phases:

1. Loading phase, in which the objects are packaged and loaded in the sterilizer
2. Heating phase, in which the steam is brought to the proper temperature and allowed to penetrate around and through the objects in the chamber
3. Destroying phase, or the time-temperature cycle, in which all microbial life is exposed to the killing effects of the steam
4. Drying and cooling phase, in which the objects are dried and cooled, filtered air is introduced into the chamber, the door is opened, and the objects are removed and stored
5. Testing phase, in which the efficiency of the sterilization process is checked.

Phase 1

Packaging of surgical supplies and their arrangement in loads in the sterilizer are factors that govern the effectiveness of steam sterilization.

The prime function of a package containing a surgical item is to permit sterilization of the contents and to ensure the sterility of the contents up to the time the package is intentionally opened. Provision must be made for the con-

tents to be removed without contamination. Numerous factors should be considered in selecting an effective packaging material. It must be suitable for the method of sterilization used, that is, permit adequate air removal and steam penetration when steam sterilization is used, and adequate penetration and release of sterilant gas and moisture when gas sterilization is used. It should be durable enough to resist tearing or puncture and be free of pinholes. It also should be moisture resistant. An effective wrapper should be flexible and memory-free to allow easy aseptic presentation with assurance of no particulate contamination when the package is opened. It should establish a barrier to microorganisms or their vehicles.

Sterilization container systems are one way of packaging instruments. As rigid packaging systems that can be sterilized, stacked, and stored, they offer a simple yet effective method of packaging. Because they are rigid, they cannot be punctured, abraded, or easily contaminated by environmental microbes. Studies have indicated that, properly initiated, container systems are a cost effective packaging method. Recommendations for sterilizing containers in various sterilizers should be obtained from the manufacturer. Performance testing should be carried out in the sterile processing department of the health care facility to assure that all conditions essential for both sterilization and drying are effectively achieved. Before opening a container, the perioperative nurse should check for evidence of integrity and sterility. The lid should be removed with care. The scrub nurse should maintain a margin of safety between self and the unsterile outer container when removing the inner basket.

If textile wrappers are used, they must be laundered between sterilization exposures to ensure sufficient moisture content of the fibers, which prevents superheating and absorption of the sterilizing agent. By rehydrating woven materials, laundering also reduces their deterioration rate. All wrappers must be checked for torn areas and holes before they are used.

Many in-hospital packaging materials—woven and nonwoven, reusable and disposable—are marketed today. Available materials should be carefully evaluated before a product is chosen. The present standards for steam sterilization are based on a 140-thread-count woven fabric. Manufacturers of all packaging materials should be able to show that sterilization can be achieved with practical sterilizer operating cycles.

The size and density of woven textile packs must be restricted to ensure uniform steam penetration. The pack should not exceed 12 × 12 × 12 inches and should not weigh more than 12 pounds. When the items in the pack are being assembled, the lighter materials should be placed near the center of the pack. Each succeeding layer of dry goods should be placed crosswise on the layer below to promote free circulation of steam and removal of air. Pack density should not exceed 7.2 pounds per cubic foot. A chemical indicator that accurately reflects one or more of the physical parameters of sterilization should be inserted in the center of each pack. The parameters for steam sterilization include time, temperature, and steam saturation and purity.

The pack should be wrapped sequentially in two barrier-type wrappers, which may be disposable or reusable. A single textile reusable wrapper is defined as one layer of 270- to 280-thread-count woven fabric. Cross-stitching and raw edges are not acceptable. Sequential double wrapping creates a package within a package, providing a better bacterial barrier and ease in presenting the wrapped item to the sterile field. Wrappers are made in suitable dimensions for the various items that must be packaged. The familiar envelope wrap is made by placing the article diagonally in the center of the wrapper. The near corner, which should point toward the worker, is brought over the item, and the triangular tip is folded back to form a cuff. The two side flaps are folded to the center in like manner. The far corner of the wrapper is then folded on top of the other three. The process is repeated with the second wrapper, and the package secured with autoclave indicator tape. When the pack is opened for use, the flaps at the corners are used to form a protective cuff over the nurse's hands during dispensing of the sterile contents. When the items are wrapped, the wrappers should not be folded tightly about the contents, but the package should be firm and sealed securely to prevent contamination in handling and storage.

Before being wrapped and sterilized, instruments should be placed in trays that have mesh or perforated bottoms. Tubes, needles, and drains must have moisture in the lumens that can turn to steam and prevent trapping of air, which creates a barrier against effective sterilization. Their containers must be covered with a material that permits penetration of steam to all inside surfaces of the containers.

Sterilization process (chemical) indicator tape should be used to hold wrappers in place on packages and to indicate that the packages have been exposed to the physical conditions of a sterilization cycle. When packages are opened, these tapes should be removed from reusable wrappers because they create laundry problems, such as stopping up screens and filters. In some cases the tapes leave a dye on the wrappers that may cause deterioration of the material.

Every package intended for sterile use should be imprinted or labeled with a load control number that identifies the date of sterilization, the sterilizer used, the cycle or load number, and the date of expiration. Load control numbers facilitate identification and retrieval of supplies, inventory control, and appropriate rotation to ensure that older packages are used first.

When the chamber of the sterilizer is loaded, the bundles and packages should be arranged to allow little resistance to the passage of steam through the load from the top of the chamber toward the bottom of the sterilizer. All packages should be placed in the sterilizer on edge in a vertical, loose-contact position to allow free circulation and penetration of steam, enhance air elimination, prevent entrapment of air or water, and preclude excessive condensation. A second or upper layer may be placed crosswise on the first or lower layer.

All jars, tubes, canisters, and other nonporous objects should be arranged on their sides with their covers or lids removed to provide a horizontal path for the escape of air and the free flow of steam and heat.

To guard against superheating, surgical packs and supplies should not be subjected to preheating in the sterilizer with steam in the jacket before sterilization.

Phase 2

When the steam enters the autoclave, it is at the same pressure as the atmosphere. With closure of the valves and doors to the outside, the pressure of the steam inside rises, increasing the temperature of the steam.

Gauges on traditional autoclaves register the pressure in both the jacket and the chamber. Most vacuums are designated in terms of inches of mercury. A perfect vacuum is represented by a column of mercury 29.92 inches high. Standard gauges indicate vacuum starting with 0 (at room or normal atmospheric pressure). As the air is removed, the gauge registers down to 30 inches.

Evacuation of air from the conventional sterilizer is necessary to permit proper permeation of steam. A common method for removal of air is the downward or gravity displacement method. This method is based on the principle that air is heavier than steam. The steam that is piped into the sterilizer through a multiport valve is introduced into the chamber. The steam forces the heavier air ahead of it, down and forward, until all the air is discharged from a line at the front of the sterilizer. If a sterilizer is improperly loaded, mixing of air with steam acts as a barrier to steam penetration and prevents attainment of the sterilization temperature.

Phase 3

The destruction period is based on the known time-temperature cycle necessary to accomplish sterilization in saturated steam. Authorities have shown that the order of death in a given bacterial population subjected to a sterilizing process is determined by definite laws. If the temperature is increased, the time may be decreased. The minimum time-temperature relationships in terms of sterilizing efficiency are as follows:

2 minutes at 132° C (270° F)
8 minutes at 125° C (257° F)
18 minutes at 118° C (245° F)

To provide a safety margin, the minimum estimated exposure is extended to cover the lag between the attainment of the selected temperature in the chamber and the temperature of the load. The length of exposure varies with the type of sterilizer, cycle design, altitude, bioburden, packaging, and size and composition of items to be sterilized.

In a gravity-displacement sterilizer, instruments (metal only) in an unwrapped, perforated tray should be exposed for 3 minutes at 132° C (270° F) or 15 minutes at 121° C (250° F). When metal instruments are combined with porous instruments or materials in an unwrapped perforated tray, they must be exposed for 10 minutes at 132° C or 20 minutes at 121° C. Instruments wrapped in four thicknesses of muslin should be exposed for 15 minutes at 132° C or 30 minutes at 121° C. All types of linen packs should be exposed for 30 minutes at 121° C. Bulk loads of supplies, with the exception of rubber gloves and solutions, can be sterilized safely and practically at 121° C for 30 minutes.

In a prevacuum sterilizer, supplies should be exposed for 4 minutes after the temperature reaches at least 132° C at the center of the pack.

The recording thermometer, not the pressure gauge, is the important guide to the sterilizing phase. The recording clock on the sterilizer gives information about the run of the load and to what temperature the goods were exposed. The temperature inside the chamber must be maintained throughout the determined time of exposure.

Phase 4

At completion of the sterilization cycle, the steam inside the chamber is removed immediately so that it will not condense and wet the packs. To assist in the drying process, the jacket pressure should be maintained to keep the walls of the chamber hot as the steam from the chamber is exhausted to 0 gauge pressure. When chamber pressure has been exhausted, the door may be opened slightly to permit vapor to escape. Another method is to introduce clean, filtered air by means of a vacuum dryer (ejector) device in conjunction with the operating valve on the sterilizer. The minimum drying time for all methods is approximately 15 to 20 minutes.

Following removal from the sterilizer, freshly sterilized packs should be left untouched on the loading carriage until adequately cooled. If a loading carriage has not been used, the packs should be placed on edge on wire mesh surfaces that are covered with several layers of woven material to prevent condensation and subsequent contamination. Likewise, freshly sterilized packages should not be placed on cold surfaces such as metal tabletops. Because bacteria are capable of passing through layers of wet material, any packages that are wet must be considered unsterile.

A written record of existing conditions during each sterilization cycle should be maintained. It should include the sterilizer number, the cycle or load number, the time and temperature of the cycle, the date of sterilization, the contents of the load, and the initials of the operator. These records should be retained for the length of time designated by the statute of limitations in each state.

Sterile packages must be handled with care and only as necessary. They should be stored in clean, dry, dustproof, verminproof, limited-access areas that are well ventilated and have controlled temperature and humidity. Closed cabinets are preferred to open shelves for sterile storage. If open shelves must be used, the lowest shelf should be 8 to 10 inches from the floor and the highest should be at least 18 inches from the ceiling. All shelves should be at least 2 inches from outside walls. Shelving should be smooth and well spaced, with no projections or sharp corners that might damage the wrappers. Sterilized packs should never be stacked in close contact with each other. Their arrangement on the shelves should provide for air circulation on all sides of each package. Excessive handling, crowding, dropping, and pummeling of sterile packs tend to force particles through the mesh or matrix of the wrapping material, which might contaminate the contents. For proper rotation, the most recently dated sterile packages should be placed behind those already on the shelves.

Shelf life refers to the length of time a pack may be considered sterile. It is actually event related, not time related. Variables that must be considered in determining shelf life are the type and number of layers of packaging material used, the presence or absence of impervious protective covers, the number of times a package is handled before use, and the conditions of storage. Double-wrapped 140-thread-count woven fabric, nonwoven fabric, and paper-wrapped items may be considered sterile for 21 to 30 days. Plastic or plastic-paper combination wraps that are heat sealed maintain sterility for 6 months to a year. Impervious protective covers may extend shelf life to 6 months or more, depending on the sealing method used. When used to protect sterilized items, impervious covers should be designated as such to prevent their being mistaken for a sterile wrap. They should be applied only to thoroughly cooled, dry packs at the time of removal from the sterilizer cart, following the required cooling period.

Many commercially prepared sterile disposable drapes, packs, and materials are sealed in nonwoven envelopes that are encased in plastic, sealed wrappers. They theoretically maintain sterility for indefinite periods; their sterility, however, is dependent on their exposure during storage, the amount of handling, and the kind and condition of the wrapper.

Supply standards should be planned to maintain adequate stock with prompt turnover. Appropriate volume and proper rotation of supplies reduce the need for concern about shelf life. The longer an item is stored, the greater the chances of contamination.

Phase 5

All mechanical parts of sterilizers, including gauges, steam lines, and drains, should be periodically checked by a competent engineer. Reports of these inspections should be kept by the person responsible for the sterilizers. Temperature, humidity, and vacuum should be measured with control equipment, independent of the fixed gauges. There are several methods of keeping a constant check on the proper functioning of a sterilizer and ensuring the efficiency of the sterilizing process.

Mechanical controls such as thermometers and automatic controls assist in identifying and preventing malfunction of the sterilizing equipment and operational errors made by personnel. Indicating thermometers, located on the discharge line of the sterilizer, show the temperature throughout the sterilizing cycle on a dial on the front of the sterilizer. The device indicates a drop in temperature when and if it occurs and can act as a warning of sterilizer failure. Because lowering of the temperature may be intermittent and is not recorded permanently, it must be seen by those responsible for operating the sterilizer. This device cannot detect air pockets within the load or pack. Air is a poor conductor of heat; therefore, it is one of the most common causes, other than human error, of sterilization failure.

Recording thermometers indicate and record the same temperature as the indicating thermometers. They record the time the sterilizer reaches the desired temperature and the duration of each exposure. The recording thermometer can be helpful if several individuals are using the sterilizer or if the operator should forget to time the load. Its recordings are proof that the exposure time of loads has been correct and proper temperature limits have been maintained. The daily record should show the number of the sterilizer, the number of cycles run, the time, and the date. This evidence can be used to correct discrepancies, should error occur. Like the indicating thermometer, the recording thermometer does not detect cool air pockets; therefore, additional controls are necessary for complete safety.

Automatic controls are devices that, by a predetermined plan, control all phases of the sterilizing process. The controls allow the steam to enter, time the sterilizing cycle, exhaust the steam, and initiate drying. Some lock the door so that it cannot be opened until the cycle is complete. A thermocouple may be placed within the pack or load to indicate whether the required temperature has been reached and maintained within the contents throughout the sterilizing cycle.

Chemical controls or sterilizer indicators, such as sealed glass tubes, sterilizer indicating tape, and color-change cards or strips, can be used to detect cool air pockets inside the sterilizing chamber. They can be useful in checking packaging and loading techniques on a package-by-package or load-by-load basis, as well as the mechanical functioning of the sterilizer. One chemical control is a sealed glass tube that contains a pellet that melts when favorable time and temperature conditions for sterilization are achieved. These tubes are placed in the center of each linen pack. Chemical indicator cards and strips are impregnated with a dye that changes color when steam initiates a chemical reaction in the dye. Indicators that are sensitive to ethylene oxide are also available.

Because chemical indicators vary in their abilities to monitor the parameters of sterilization, their inclusion in all packages to be sterilized is questionable on a cost-effectiveness basis. Every facility must formulate its own policy on the use of internal chemical indicators by considering the cost-benefit ratio, performance limitations, and personnel knowledge of sterilization principles. Tapes, labels, or legends printed on packaging materials may have lines, squares, or words that change color when exposed to the sterilizing agent for a certain time and temperature and identify packages that have been exposed to the physical conditions of a sterilization cycle.

An external chemical indicator should be clearly visible on every package to be sterilized. However, these indicators do not *prove* sterilization because some of them react even when the temperature is inadequate for sterilization. The sensitivity of chemical indicators to temperature can be checked by exposing them to steam in a sterilizer set at 115° C (240° F) for 30 minutes. Because this temperature is inadequate for sterilization, the indicators should not react.

A biologic indicator is the most accurate method of checking sterilization effectiveness. Commercially prepared biologic indicators (manufactured in accordance with minimum performance criteria of the *United States Pharmacopeia*) should be stored and used according to the manufacturer's written instructions. They contain a known population of *Bacillus stearothermophilus*, a highly heat-resistant, spore-forming microorganism that does not produce toxins and is nonpathogenic.

Biologic testing for steam sterilizer loads should be conducted at least weekly on the first run of the day. The biologic indicator should be placed in a test pack that is positioned on edge in the front bottom section of a routinely loaded steam sterilizer, the area of the sterilizer that will most challenge all sterilization parameters. The test pack for gravity displacement and prevacuum steam sterilizers should consist of three muslin gowns, twelve towels, thirty 4 × 4 gauze sponges, five 12 × 4 laparotomy sponges, and one muslin drape sheet. Two biologic indicators and an internal chemical indicator are placed in the center of the pack, separated by towels. Commercially prepared test packs are available.

Following the sterilization cycle, the biologic indicators are removed from the pack and incubated according to the manufacturer's instructions. Negative reports indicate that wrapping techniques, loading procedures, and sterilizing conditions are correct and that the sterilizer is functioning properly. Results of these tests should be filed as a permanent record. A positive report does not necessarily indicate sterilizer failure because false-positives sometimes occur. However, the sterilizer should immediately be retested and taken out of service until it is operationally inspected and the results of retesting are negative. If a sterilizer malfunction is found, all items prepared in the suspect load should be considered unsterile. They should be retrieved if possible and washed, repackaged, and resterilized in another sterilizer. Biologic indicators should also be used after a major sterilizer repair, when evaluating sterilization of a new product, and when sterilizing implantable materials.

Spore control ampules containing *B. stearothermophilus* are used for steam sterilization only and cannot be used in hot air (dry heat) sterilizers, because 121° C (250° F) would also sterilize them without sterilizing the load itself. In general, hot air sterilization is not as good as either steam or ethylene oxide and should be avoided whenever possible. Spore strips containing *B. subtilis* should not be used to check steam sterilizers because they are not sufficiently heat resistant. They may be used, however, to check ethylene oxide and dry heat sterilizers.

High-speed (flash) sterilization

The high-speed steam sterilizer, commonly referred to as a *flash sterilizer,* is adjusted to operate at 132° C (270° F) and 27 psi (Fig. 5-10). Although it can be used for sterilizing packs and solutions, it is most frequently used in the operating room for the sterilization of urgently needed unwrapped instruments. It should be used only when time does not permit sterilization of wrapped sets. Implantable devices should not be flash sterilized because the reliability of sterilization is reduced by the speed of the cycle. If, in an emergent situation, an implantable must be flash sterilized, a biologic indicator should be included in the tray.

The operational process consists of the following steps:

1. Steam is maintained in the jacket of the sterilizer before and during the daily operating schedule.
2. Soiled instruments are cleaned with warm tap water containing a detergent and then rinsed thoroughly in a fat-solvent solution.
3. The opened instruments are placed in a perforated metal tray or flash sterilization container with a chemical indicator, the tray positioned in the sterilizer, and the door of the sterilizer closed and locked. The chemical indicator is not considered porous material.
4. The chamber steam supply valve is opened, and the operating valve is turned to the sterilizing setting. Time exposure begins when the thermometer records 132° C (270° F). If the sterilizer is a gravity displacement type and automatic, the timer is set for a 3- or 10-minute exposure period (based on the composition of the instruments), and the selector switch is turned to the fast exhaust setting. Air-powered drills and other specialty instruments require different exposure times, as directed by the manufacturer.
5. On completion of the exposure period, the chamber steam valve is closed and the operating valve turned to exhaust. The exposure time and temperature of the cycle as recorded on the sterilizer recording device should be checked before opening the sterilizer door.
6. The door is opened when the exhaust valve registers zero.
7. The instruments are removed and delivered to the surgical field by aseptic technique.

Prevacuum, high-temperature sterilization

The automatic prevacuum, high-temperature sterilization method has replaced, in many instances, the downward displacement method of sterilization. Prevacuum,

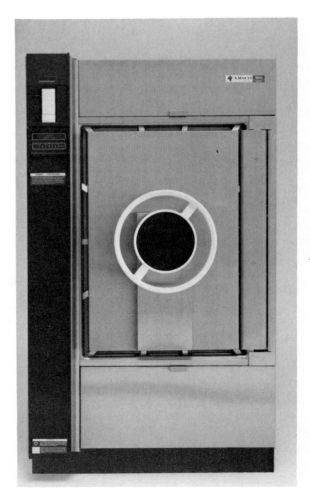

A

Fig. 5-10. For legend see opposite page.

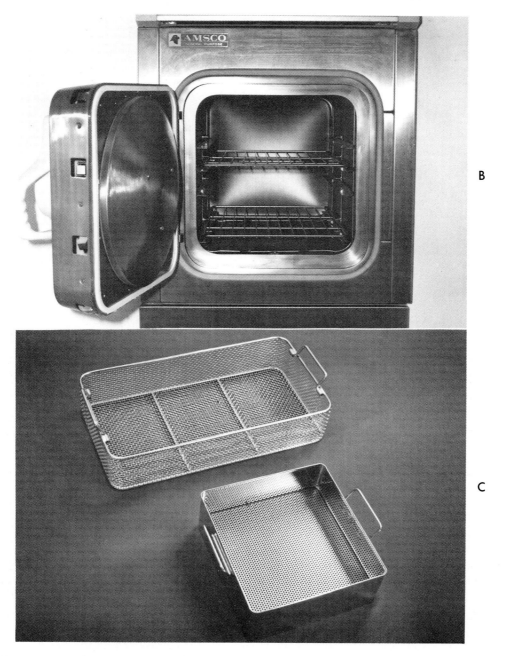

B

C

Fig. 5-10. General-purpose gravity air displacement steam sterilizer. This type of sterilizer can be used to sterilize wrapped or unwrapped instruments and utensils, linen packs, and solutions in specially designed vented flasks. **A,** These units come in several sizes, from the small unit similar in size to the washer-sterilizer in Figure 5-8 to large floor-loading units. A medium-sized unit is pictured here. Newer units have sophisticated microprocessor controls that allow maximum flexibility in selecting sterilization and drying times and help in troubleshooting, should a problem occur during a cycle. Digital readouts and heat-sensitive paper printouts have replaced the round chart and ink pen found on older models. These changes have helped the operator more easily determine and document that the conditions needed for proper sterilization were met. **B,** Adjustable racks and loading cars with adjustable shelves are designed to permit maximum loading efficiency. **C,** Instrument baskets or trays should have either wire mesh bottoms or a sufficient number of perforations in sheet metal to allow for air removal and drainage of condensate during the sterilization cycle. (Courtesy of American Sterilizer Company [AMSCO], Erie, Pa.)

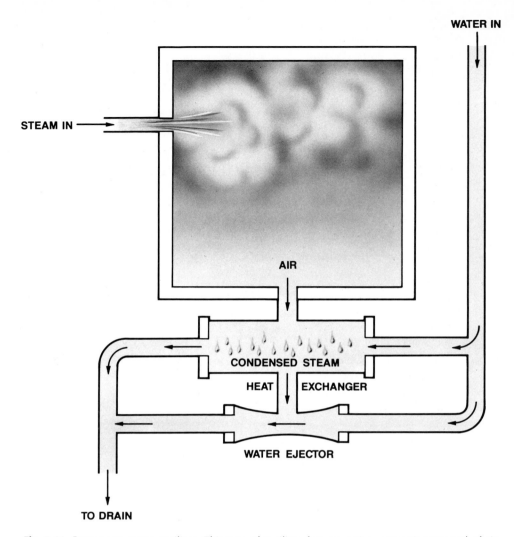

Fig. 5-11. Prevacuum steam sterilizer. This type of sterilizer features active, aggressive removal of air, rather than relying upon the passive action of gravity. The process has undergone several stages of development; therefore several cycle designs are in use. Newer models have the cycle characteristics described here. Steam flows into the chamber for a brief time and then rapidly drains, producing a partial vacuum. This process is repeated several times and deepens the level of vacuum drawn with each pulse. The effect of this pulsing cycle is to displace any air in the load and rapidly increase the chamber and load temperatures. At the conclusion of this conditioning phase, steam flows into the chamber and raises the temperature to sterilization levels, usually 132° C (270° F). The temperature is maintained for at least 3 minutes for unwrapped, nonporous materials or 4 minutes for wrapped or porous items. Steam is then removed from the chamber to draw a partial vacuum once again. Heated, filtered air is introduced into the chamber to dry the load. Drying times are selected and set by the user, depending on the nature of the load. Some newer units have a special cycle designed for rapid sterilization of an instrument tray in a single wrapper. This express cycle has fewer conditioning pulses, a 4-minute exposure time, and 1 or 2 minutes of dry time, for a total cycle time of approximately 12 minutes. Although the wrapper feels warm and dry to the touch, the contents may not be totally dry. Thus this package should be handled by persons wearing sterile gloves and using sterile towels for protection from burns. The instruments sterilized in this express cycle must be used immediately. Because the contents are not dry, the package is not suitable for any length of storage. (Courtesy of American Sterilizer Company [AMSCO], Erie, Pa.)

high-temperature sterilization is usually accomplished by means of an air-blasted, oil-sealed rotary pump, protected by a condenser and coupled with an automatic control mechanism (Fig. 5-11).

Air removal is accomplished by means of a powerful vacuum pump that draws a near-absolute vacuum in the chamber in the first 5 minutes of the cycle, before the steam is introduced. This mechanism reduces the time necessary to accomplish all phases of the sterilizing process.

The prevacuum, high-temperature steam sterilizer provides a system that is automatically controlled and reduces the total cycle time to as little as 20 minutes. The cycle time varies with the size of the sterilizer, the adequacy of the steam, and the supply of water. Faulty packaging and overloading or incorrect placement of objects in the chamber is not likely to interfere with air removal, and full heating of the load takes place more rapidly than with the downward displacement method. The prevacuum, high-temperature steam sterilizer permits more supplies to be sterilized within a given time.

The Bowie-Dick test should be used to evaluate the effectiveness of a prevacuum steam sterilizer in reducing air residuals from the chamber, preventing air reentrainment into the load, and detecting the presence of air pockets, which would result in the absence of sterilizing conditions. It should be used daily before the first sterilization cycle or at a designated time each day if sterilizers are used 24 hours a day. The test pack consists of hydrated surgical towels that are folded no smaller than 9 × 12 inches and are stacked to a height of 10 to 11 inches. A commercially prepared Bowie-Dick–type test sheet is placed in the center of the stack, and a single wrapper is loosely applied. Disposable test packs and devices are also available. The pack is placed horizontally in the bottom front of the sterilizer rack near the door in an otherwise empty chamber. The cycle is then run according to the sterilizer manufacturer's directions. At the completion of the cycle, the test sheet is removed from the pack and examined by a person trained in its interpretation. A uniform color change throughout the test sheet indicates a satisfactory test. The Bowie-Dick test does not measure the efficacy of the sterilization process.

Boiling water (nonpressure)

Boiling does *not* sterilize instruments or other inanimate objects. The boiling point of water varies at different altitudes. For example, at sea level the boiling point of water is 100° C (212° F); at 5000 feet above sea level it is 94.5° C (202° F); and at 10,000 feet above sea level it is 89° C (192° F). Heat-resistant microorganisms, bacterial spores, and certain viruses can withstand boiling water at 100° C (212° F) for many hours.

Dry heat sterilization

Dry heat sterilization is rarely used in hospitals today. However, when the physical characteristics of certain materials, such as powders, grease, and anhydrous oils, do not permit permeation of steam, dry heat sterilization may be used. As the proteins become dry during exposure to dry heat, their resistance to denaturation increases. For this reason, at a given temperature, dry heat sterilization is much less effective than moist heat.

Dry heat sterilization may be accomplished by means of a mechanical convection hot air sterilizer. The time/temperature ratio required to achieve sterilization is based on the items in the load, the method of preparation and packaging, and the loading of the sterilizer. One time/temperature ratio that is considered adequate is 160° C (320° F) for 2 hours. The exposure time does not include heat-up time. The sterilizer should be equipped with a blower for forced air circulation. Overloading delays heat convection and circulation.

An autoclave can be used on a temporary basis as a hot air sterilizer. However, the maximum temperature that can be maintained in the chamber is 121° C (250° F), and the minimum exposure time is 6 hours, preferably longer. Also, the true temperature of the chamber is difficult to determine because the thermometer on the autoclave does not record the temperature when moist heat is not present in the chamber.

Incineration, or actual burning of materials, is the most drastic application of dry heat. It is used for the disposal of contaminated gloves, dry goods, and other inorganic and organic wastes and materials.

Chemical sterilization

New materials that cannot be heat sterilized are continually being introduced for use in hospitals. They require the use of other methods of sterilization. An effective alternative method is based on the use of chemical agents.

Sterilization can be achieved by many agents when only vegetative cells are present. If the microbial population is unknown, however, a sporicidal agent must be employed to ensure sterilization. An antimicrobial agent must exhibit a wide microbiologic spectrum and sporicidal activity to qualify as a chemosterilizer. The use of chemosterilizers is governed by the U.S. Environmental Protection Agency and has been restricted to ethylene oxide (a gaseous chemosterilizer) and aqueous glutaraldehyde (a liquid chemosterilizer).

Chemical sterilization is frequently referred to as *cold sterilization*. This term refers to the maximum temperature of 54° C (130° F) to 60° C (140° F) of gaseous sterilization as compared with the 121° C (250° F) to 132° C (270° F) temperatures of steam sterilization.

Gaseous chemical sterilization

In recent years, gaseous chemical sterilization has had considerable application in sterilization of heat-labile and moisture-sensitive items, such as intricate, delicate surgical instruments, large pieces of equipment used in the hospital, plastic and porous materials, and electrical instruments—all of which are difficult to steam sterilize without deterioration and damage.

Ethylene oxide is the most frequently used gas. It is colorless at ordinary temperatures, has an odor similar to that of ether, and has an inhalation toxicity similar to that of ammonia gas. It is easily kept as a liquid that will boil at 10.73° C (51.3° F) and freeze at −111.3° C (−168.3° F).

Ethylene oxide is highly explosive and very flammable in the presence of air. These hazards are greatly reduced by diluting the ethylene oxide with inert gases such as carbon dioxide or fluorinated hydrocarbons (Freon). Neither of these two inert gases appears to affect the bactericidal activity of the ethylene oxide but serves only as an inert diluent that prevents the flammability hazard.

Several theories on how ethylene oxide kills bacteria have been proposed. The killing rate of bacteria is generally believed to be relative to the rate of diffusion of the gas through their cell walls and the availability or accessibility of one of the chemical groups in the bacterial cell walls to react with the ethylene oxide. The killing rate is also dependent on whether the bacterial cell is in a vegetative or spore state. Destruction takes place by alkylation through chemical interference and probably inactivation of the reproductive process of the cell.

The automatic control cycle of the sterilizing process consists of air evacuation, humidification, sterilization, gas evacuation, and admission of filtered air to relieve the vacuum.

In general, ethylene oxide sterilization should be used only if the materials are heat sensitive and unable to withstand sterilization by saturated steam under pressure. Any item that can be steam sterilized should never be gas sterilized.

As a sterilizing agent, ethylene oxide has the advantages that it is easily available; is effective against all types of microorganisms; easily penetrates through masses of dry material; does not require high temperatures, humidity, or pressure; and is noncorrosive and nondamaging to items.

Sterilization with ethylene oxide also has numerous disadvantages. The long exposure and aeration periods make it a lengthy process. When compared with steam sterilization, ethylene oxide sterilization is expensive. Liquid ethylene oxide may produce serious burns on exposed skin if not immediately removed; insufficiently aerated materials can cause skin irritation, burns of body tissue, and hemolysis of blood; and diluents used with ethylene oxide cause damage to some plastics. Human error and mechanical breakdown are also contributing factors to these disadvantages.

Factors affecting sterilization with ethylene oxide are time of exposure, gas concentration, temperature, humidity, and penetration. The time exposure required depends on temperature, humidity, gas concentration, the ease of penetrating the articles to be sterilized, and the type of microorganisms to be destroyed. Manufacturers of gas sterilizers have developed recommended exposure periods for various ethylene oxide concentrations in relation to the material to be sterilized. In general, an exposure period of 3 to 7 hours is necessary for complete sterilization. Exposure time is set for absolute destruction of the most resistant microorganisms, which is a very slow process.

Gas concentration is affected by the temperature and humidity inside the sterilizing chamber, which also affect the exposure period. Concentration is considered effective within the margin of 450 to 1000 mg/liter of chamber space. If the concentration of gas is doubled, the exposure time may be shortened. The concentration and pressure of the ethylene oxide gas vary with types of sterilizers used; therefore, the manufacturer's instructions should be followed.

Temperature has a marked influence on the destruction of microorganisms. It is important in gaseous sterilization with ethylene oxide because it affects the penetration of the gas through bacterial cell walls, as well as through wrappings and packaging material. The temperature for sterilizing is 21° to 60° C (70° to 140° F), and automatically controlled ethylene oxide sterilizers are usually preheated to 54° C (130° F).

Humidity of 35% to 70% is recommended with ethylene oxide to ensure enough moisture to kill microorganisms. Dry spores are most difficult to kill, but, when moistened, their resistance to gas penetration is lowered. Dehydration makes some microorganisms nearly immune to ethylene oxide sterilization, whereas droplets of moisture can inhibit the action of the gas by protecting the organism. Ethylene oxide sterilizers with automatic controls provide for moisture injection to raise the relative humidity within the chamber.

Items to be sterilized must be thoroughly cleaned and towel or air dried so that no visible droplets remain. Drying inhibits the formation of ethylene glycol during the sterilization cycle. Lumens of tubing, needles, and the like should be dry and open at both ends. Caps, plugs, valves, or stylettes should be removed from instruments or equipment to permit the gas to circulate through the items. The packaging material used should possess the characteristics described previously in this chapter. An ethylene oxide–sensitive chemical indicator should be used with each package to indicate only that the package was exposed to the gas; it does not indicate achievement of sterilization.

Specific instructions from the manufacturer of items to be sterilized should be followed closely. Penetration of gas throughout the load is essential. Care must be taken to avoid overloading the sterilizer. Compression of packages prevents penetration of the gas; if packages are wrapped in plastic, compression hinders evacuation of air and causes packages to open during the decrease in chamber pressure when a vacuum is drawn.

The sterilizer manufacturer's recommendations relating to opening the sterilizer door after completion of the sterilization cycle and subsequent transferring items to the aerator must be closely followed. Excessive exposure to ethylene oxide represents a health hazard to personnel, as it has been linked to cancer, reproductive problems, and other disorders in animals. Therefore, inhalation of ethylene oxide should be avoided or minimized, and direct contact with items sterilized by ethylene oxide should be avoided during transfer to the aerator. Various safety features such as a purge system, an audible alarm at the end of the sterilization cycle, and automatic door locking and sealing mechanisms are used on ethylene oxide sterilizers to protect personnel.

In June 1984, the Occupational Safety and Health Administration (OSHA) issued a new standard relating to ethylene oxide. The standard reduces the permissible exposure from 50 parts per million (ppm) of air over 8 hours to 1 ppm averaged over 8 hours. It requires that routine monitoring and surveillance be performed if the exposure exceeds a 0.5 ppm "action level" over 8 hours. Ethylene oxide monitoring badges are available to facilitate monitoring. Adherence to these guidelines will help protect patients and hospital personnel from problems associated with ethylene oxide sterilization.

Smoking is prohibited in the sterilizer and aerator area. Because ethylene oxide is highly explosive and flammable, the sterilizer and aerator should be installed in a well-ventilated room and should be vented to the outside atmosphere as recommended by the manufacturer and required by the National Institute for Occupational Safety and Health.

The adequacy of every ethylene oxide cycle should be verified by the use of biologic monitors that contain *Bacillus subtilis*. Where feasible, implantable or intravascular items should not be used until the results of the test are known.

When the sterilized items are removed from the sterilizer, they should be transferred immediately to the aerator or aeration area. The length of aeration required depends on the composition and porosity of the items, the sterilization wrap, the concentration of the diluent used with ethylene oxide for the sterilization process, and the airflow rate and temperature during aeration. Materials aerated in a mechanical aerator that provides a minimum of four air changes per hour and elevates the temperature within the cabinet to 50° to 60° C (122° to 140° F) require 8 to 12 hours of aeration based on the composition of the sterilized items and the aerator manufacturer's instructions. If a mechanical aerator is not available, items should be aerated at ambient room temperature for 7 days. Ambient aeration should be carried out in a limited access, well-ventilated room with controlled temperature between 18° and 22° C (65° and 72° F) and vented to the outside. Intravenous or irrigation fluids packaged in plastic bags should not be stored in this area.

Liquid chemical sterilization

When used properly, liquid chemosterilizers can destroy all forms of microbial life, including bacterial and fungal spores, tubercle bacilli, and viruses. Only two liquid chemosterilizers are capable of causing sterilization: aqueous glutaraldehyde and aqueous formaldehyde. Although formaldehyde is one of the oldest chemosterilizers known to destroy spores, it is rarely used because it takes from 12 to 24 hours to be effective and its pungent odor is objectionable. Glutaraldehyde is more rapid and less irritating than formaldehyde solutions.

Activated aqueous glutaraldehyde 2% is recognized as an effective liquid chemosterilizer. It is most useful in the disinfection of lensed instruments such as cystoscopes and bronchoscopes because it has minimal deleterious effects on the lens cement and is noncorrosive. Its low surface tension permits easy penetration and rinsing. Glutaraldehyde is not inactivated by organic matter and will not coagulate blood or protein. This agent does not affect the sharpness of delicate instruments.

Instruments must be free of bioburden and completely immersed in activated aqueous glutaraldehyde solution for 10 hours to achieve sterilization. Any period of immersion less than 10 hours will not kill spores that may be present and must be considered as only a disinfection procedure. During immersion, all surfaces of the instrument must be contacted by the liquid chemosterilizer. Following immersion, instruments must be rinsed *thoroughly* with sterile distilled water before being used.

DISINFECTION

Disinfection is the process of destroying or inhibiting disease-producing microorganisms outside the body. It is most frequently achieved by chemicals in solution. The disinfection process may destroy tubercle bacilli and inactivate hepatitis viruses and enteroviruses but usually does not kill resistant bacterial spores.

Hospital disinfection is divided into two segments. When chemicals are used to disinfect inanimate materials, the chemical is called a *disinfectant;* when used to disinfect body surfaces, the chemical is called an *antiseptic*. Some chemicals can be used for both purposes. A *germicide* is any solution that will destroy germs, or microorganisms. Many germicides can be employed on living tissue as well as on inanimate objects.

Concurrent disinfection refers to the immediate disinfection process following discharge of infectious materials from the body of an infected person or after contamination of articles by an infectious agent. *Terminal disinfection* is the process of rendering all articles, materials, and their immediate physical environment incapable of conveying infectious agents to other persons after the patient has left the room.

In recent years, physicians and hospital personnel have been faced with an array of new germicides, many of which are claimed to be ideal for diverse purposes. Research data, however, do not support these claims.

Process

Disinfection is brought about by various types of reactions or by combinations of them. These include denaturation and coagulation of proteins in the cell, halogenation, poisoning of vital enzymes, hydrolysis, oxidation, and combination with proteins to form salts. The microbial destruction depends on the concentration of the chemical and the effects on the microorganism.

Selection of a disinfectant

Selection of a disinfectant depends on the type and population of microorganisms to be killed and the nature of the application. For disinfection purposes, microorganisms may be grouped into three classes; nonsporulating, vegetative bacteria, which possess the least resistance; tubercle bacilli, which have more resistance than the vegetative microorganisms; and spores, which are extremely resistant to any disinfectant.

Most disinfectants are capable of destroying vegetative bacteria and tubercle bacilli but not spores. The vegetative forms of molds and yeast, as well as animal parasites, are susceptible to disinfectants. Some fungi and antibiotic-resistant staphylococci have been shown to be as resistant as bacterial spores. Viruses vary in their resistance to disinfectants. At present, prolonged time frames are required to deactivate the hepatitis virus. However, several liquid germicides commonly used in hospitals have been shown to kill HIV at concentrations much lower than are used in practice.

Disinfectants are categorized as high, intermediate, and low level. High-level disinfectants can kill bacteria and viruses *if* contact time is sufficient. Intermediate-level agents kill the more resistant bacteria and viruses. Low-level disinfectants kill only the less resistant bacteria and viruses. Neither intermediate- nor low-level disinfectants kill spores.

A strong concentration kills more rapidly than a weak one. A disinfectant is primarily bacteriostatic when the range of concentration over which inhibition of growth occurs is relatively wide; it is primarily bactericidal when the range is narrow. When the microorganisms are killed within a short period of time, the antimicrobial activity is termed *lethal*. When the rate of microbial death is slow, some microorganisms survive for a considerable time without multiplication. For those surviving, the antimicrobial activity is termed *growth inhibiting* or *bacteriostatic*.

Products selected for use as surgical disinfectants are registered with the Environmental Protection Agency and should be used according to the manufacturer's instructions. A disinfectant should be used at the lowest effective bactericidal concentration, because a concentration rapidly lethal for microorganisms may corrode and dull the blades of delicate instruments. However, the disinfecting power of a weak concentration is ineffective.

The larger the number of microorganisms present, the longer the disinfection time required to kill the resistant cells. According to genetic principles, when the population is large, the proportion of highly resistant bacteria is correspondingly greater than when the population is small. However, when the size of the population is *extremely* large, it may contain fewer highly resistant cells.

Temperature and surface tension of disinfectants

Increased temperature accelerates the rate of disinfection. The only practical value of this fact is in disinfection of inanimate objects. With some disinfectants, antimicrobial activity is increased when the chemical agent is added to warm water. The surface tension (wetness) of a disinfectant or antiseptic promotes contact between the agent and the microorganisms. A tension-reducing disinfectant, when combined with other chemicals, enhances the disinfecting power of that solution, thus decreasing the time-exposure rate.

Procedure for disinfection

An object must be thoroughly clean and as dry as possible to provide for effective disinfection and to avoid dilution of the disinfectant. A high-level disinfectant should be used for disinfection of surgical instruments when sterilization is not possible. All surfaces of an item must be in contact with the disinfectant solution for the recommended exposure time. Construction and composition of the object influence the disinfection time. A hard, flat, smooth-surfaced object requires less disinfection time than an uneven-surfaced object or a porous material. The disinfectant coagulates the proteins in blood and other organic debris present on the object. Thus organic material creates a barrier on the object against the disinfecting solution.

High-level disinfection of instruments and equipment should be carried out immediately before use of the items and after terminal cleaning prior to storage. Before use, disinfected items should be aseptically removed from the disinfectant solution, rinsed thoroughly, and dried sufficiently to minimize the risk of significant contamination. Because some disinfectant solutions can be irritating to skin and eyes, personnel should use caution when handling solution containers and disinfected items to avoid potential injury. Disinfectant solutions should be kept covered and used only in a well-ventilated area. The expiration date of an activated disinfectant should be determined according to the manufacturer's recommendations and marked on the container. Disinfectants become ineffective after multiple uses because of dilution, inactivation, or instability.

Types of disinfectants

The various disinfectants on the market may be divided into the following major groups.

Halogens and halogen compounds

Of the halogen compounds, the hypochlorites and iodines are widely used in hospitals. The hypochlorites are available as powders containing calcium hypochlorite and sodium hypochlorite, in combination with hydrated trisodium phosphate, and as liquids containing sodium hypochlorite. Because of their unstable characteristics, preparations containing calcium hypochlorite (chlorinated lime) have been replaced by other detergents for cleaning purposes. Sodium hypochlorite 5% (household bleach) is effective in deactivation of HIV (the AIDS virus) and the hepatitis B virus.

Chlorine acts primarily by oxidation, and its odor may therefore be objectionable. The many organic chlorine compounds that liberate their chlorine more slowly (such as chloride of lime) are effective as mild disinfecting agents. Inorganic chlorine is valuable in the disinfection of water.

Iodine acts directly by iodination and oxidation reactions. It is the most active antimicrobial of the halogens and combines readily with organic material. Because of its insolubility in water, it is prepared in various ways; the tinctures, or alcoholic solutions, are the most common forms.

Several syntheses of many organic iodine compounds in which iodine is held in dissociant complexes are available. The iodophors are iodine-detergent combinations capable of killing vegetative bacteria and tubercle bacilli if used in sufficient concentration (450 ppm of available iodine). Iodophors are not good sporicides.

Heavy metals

All metallic ions inhibit microorganisms if applied in sufficiently high concentrations.

The ions of the heavy metals have such a strong affinity for proteins that the bacterial cells absorb them out of the solution. However, the property that makes these ions appear lethal limits their usefulness because their activity is reduced in the presence of organic matter. The ions are also irritating to tissues and are poisonous.

Attempts have been made to decrease the toxic, corrosive, and irritating qualities of mercuric disinfectants by incorporating mercury in complex organic molecules in preparations such as merbromin (Mercurochrome), thimerosal (Merthiolate), and nitromersol (Metaphen). Data indicate that aqueous solutions of both inorganic and organic mercurials are ineffective in reducing cutaneous flora. Mercurials are poor disinfectants and have no place in modern surgical disinfection.

Phenols and phenol derivatives

Phenol in the pure state (carbolic acid) is not used as a disinfectant because many of its derivatives are more effective. Like phenol, its derivatives act mainly by coagulation and partly by lytic and toxic effects that are not clearly understood. Because phenols appear to have a greater affinity for nonaqueous than for aqueous media, their action is believed to depend on their selective concentration at cell surfaces, resulting in the denaturation of proteins and an increase in permeability.

The aliphatic homologs of phenol have greater antimicrobial power than does phenol itself. Of this group, the methyl phenols—orthocresol, metacresol, and paracresol—and the halogenated phenols have phenol coefficients of three or more, but they are poorly soluble in water. The bisphenols have become the most useful of the phenolic disinfectants. The most important of these compounds are orthohydroxydiphenyl and chlorinated methylene and sulfur compounds. Of the chlorophenes, hexachlorophene is commonly used in soap. The bisphenols are relatively insoluble in water but are soluble in dilute alkali and in many organic solvents.

Synthetic detergent disinfectants

The quaternary ammonium compounds (often called *quats*) are among many surface-active detergents; they are not effective as disinfectants. These compounds are amines that contain pentavalent nitrogen and may be considered derivatives of ammonium chloride in which certain radicals are substituted for the hydrogen. The three types of surface-active detergent substances are: those in which the organic radical is a cation, those in which the organic group is the anion, and those that do not ionize (nonionic).

These compounds possess bacteriostatic power in high dilutions and are not highly irritating or toxic. They are effective surface-tension reductants. Their antimicrobial activity is affected by the kind of water (acid or alkaline, hard or soft) used and the material or substance involved. In the presence of hard, acid, or iron-rich waters, the antimicrobial activity is lowered, especially for the cationic compounds. Quaternary ammonium compounds may be mixed with nonionic detergents that have good solubilizing activity to provide effective cleansing agents.

Alcohols

Ethyl (grain) alcohol and isopropyl (rubbing) alcohol are much more useful as antiseptics than as disinfectants. Alcohol is an active germicide against tubercle bacilli in concentrations of 70% to 90%, but it is not sporicidal.

Frequently alcoholic solutions are prepared by volume instead of by weight. The latter is the more accurate method of preparation. Alcohol is lighter than water and expands in the presence of heat.

Ethyl alcohol is nontoxic, colorless, tasteless, and nearly odorless and acts by denaturation of proteins. It may precipitate a protein covering around bacterial cells present in blood, pus, and mucus. Ethyl alcohol is less effective as a fat solvent than is isopropyl alcohol. A 70% solution of ethyl alcohol by weight is a satisfactory disinfectant for ordinary vegetative bacteria. It is more expensive than isopropyl alcohol.

Formaldehyde

An aqueous solution of formaldehyde (formalin) is highly germicidal and sporicidal in a strong concentration. When a combination of 8% formaldehyde and 70% isopropyl alcohol is used, the action is even greater. Tubercle bacilli and viruses (except the hepatitis virus, whose destruction with certainty is not known) are promptly killed.

Irritating fumes limit formaldehyde's usefulness. It is

also toxic to tissues; therefore, materials treated with formaldehyde must be thoroughly rinsed before use.

Glutaraldehyde

Glutaraldehyde is related to formaldehyde but is more active. An aqueous solution of 2% is equivalent to an 8% solution of formaldehyde and alcohol. It is a high-level disinfectant that is useful in disinfecting lensed instruments. Manufacturers' recommendations should be consulted for length of immersion time in glutaraldehyde.

SKIN CLEANSING AND DISINFECTION

To prevent bacteria on the skin surfaces from entering the surgical wound, the skin area of and around the proposed incision, as well as the hands and forearms of the members of the operating team, must be cleansed and disinfected. Proper skin cleansing and disinfection depend on knowledge of the physiology and bacteriology of the skin and of the action of soaps, detergents, and antiseptic agents.

Objectives and influencing factors

Skin preparation methods vary, but all are based on the same principles and share the same objectives: to remove dirt and transient microbes from the skin, to reduce the resident microbial count as much as possible in the shortest time and with the least amount of tissue irritation, and to prevent rapid rebound growth of microbes.

The same general principles of skin cleansing apply whether the situation is preparation of the patient's skin at the operative site or preparation of the hands and arms of the members of the operating team. In either case, factors to be considered in skin disinfection are (1) the condition of the involved area, (2) the number and kinds of contaminants, (3) the characteristics of the skin to be disinfected, and (4) the general physical condition of the individual.

Structure and physiology of the skin

The skin consists of two distinct layers: the epidermis, which is a stratified squamous epithelium, and the true skin, or dermis. The outer layer, or epidermis, is the tissue to be treated by cleansing and disinfecting procedures (Fig. 5-12).

The *epidermis* constantly sheds the cells that form its horny outer layer, which are replaced by the multiplication and upward movement of cells from the lower levels. It has no blood vessels, although hair shafts, glandular ducts, and fine nerves reach through it. The *dermis* is a connective tissue containing blood and lymph vessels, sweat and sebaceous glands, nerves, and hair follicles.

Bacteria are found in all levels of the skin and comprise

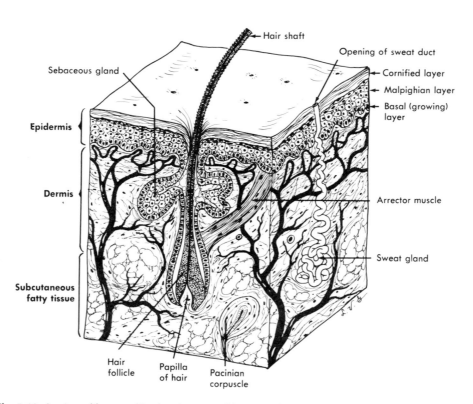

Fig. 5-12. Section of human skin showing several layers and many other structures appearing in skin. (From Schottelius, B.A., and Schottelius, D.D.: Textbook of physiology, ed. 18, St. Louis, 1978, The C.V. Mosby Co.)

two groups, the transient and resident flora. *Transient* bacteria are usually limited to exposed areas of skin. They may be free on the skin or be loosely attached by grease or dirt, especially in the subungual areas. The transient flora are easily removed by mechanical cleansing of the skin.

Bacteria that inhabit the deep structures of the dermis, the glands, and the hair follicles are considered the *resident* flora. They tend to move out and are shed with the old cells and skin secretions. The epidermal layers contain this debris from the dermis as well as soil and bacteria picked up by contact with various objects.

The resident flora of the skin are forced to the surface with perspiration and other secretions. This action is one way in which the skin disinfects and reconditions itself. The bacteria accompanying these secretions from the deep layers may, however, become a source of infection. The activity of sweat glands is increased by external heat, emotional stress, and certain diaphoretic drugs.

Generally, the acidity of perspiration acts as a protective barrier against the growth of certain microorganisms. However, the perspiration in axillary and pubic regions has a higher pH and may permit more bacterial growth. Bacteria are also protected by the folds, ridges, and crevices of the skin from which detritus is not as readily shed as from smoother surfaces.

Agents for skin cleansing and disinfection

Many soaps and detergents are available for skin cleansing. Although most of them produce similar results in the immediate removal of soil and microorganisms, certain factors need further consideration in selecting a product for surgical use. Equally important, an effective antimicrobial agent should be used to achieve appropriate disinfection of skin.

Soaps and detergents

Most soaps and detergents emulsify and peptize other waste products and oils that are absorbed in surface soil and permit the detritus to be rinsed off the skin with running water. The product selected should hydrolyze in the presence of water and yield a pH that corresponds to that of average, normal skin. An odorless agent that produces a good lather for easy, comfortable use is usually preferred. It should not irritate the skin or in any way interfere with normal functioning. Careful rinsing and drying help to minimize skin irritation resulting from frequent scrubbing.

Hexachlorophene added to agents used for cleansing the skin has been found to suppress bacterial growth on the skin. Hexachlorophene retains its antibacterial power in the presence of soap and is combined with it in numerous liquid and solid forms. However, it has known toxic effects that make it less popular today.

Sterilizing the skin is impossible because chemicals that have the power to destroy bacteria are also injurious to the living tissues of the skin. Thus new bacterial populations are constantly being brought to the surface of normal skin.

Antiseptic agents

The antimicrobial agent employed for disinfection of the skin should be selected according to its ability to decrease rapidly the microbial count of the skin and its capability of being applied quickly and remaining effective throughout the operation. It should not cause irritation or sensitization and should not be incompatible with or inactivated by alcohol, organic matter, soap, or detergent.

Povidone-iodine, a complex of polyvinylpyrrolidone and iodine, is a common antimicrobial agent used for skin disinfection. It possesses the potent germicidal effect of iodine without many of its irritating properties. The activity of this agent is prolonged because it is released gradually from the binding polymer as the brownish iodine color fades from the skin. It is effective in the presence of pus, whereas the activity of the iodine complex is of somewhat shorter duration in the presence of blood or serum. It can be safely used on mucous membranes but should not be allowed to pool on the skin or in body cavities.

Tincture of iodine is an effective agent for skin disinfection, although not as commonly used as povidone-iodine. The modern iodine tincture (USP XVIII) contains 2% iodine, 2.4% potassium iodide, and 44% to 50% alcohol by volume. Iodine is a good bactericide but stains fabric and tissue. In combination with alcohol, iodine is tuberculocidal and appears to increase the efficiency of the alcohol as a skin antiseptic. Iodine has the disadvantage of potentially causing tissue irritation and sensitization.

The effectiveness of alcohol as an antiseptic is probably derived from the solution of lipoidal secretions of the skin and consequent mechanical removal of microorganisms. Absolute alcohol has little or no germicidal activity. For skin disinfection, 70% alcohol is the concentration usually used. Because of flammability, it is used in small quantities, applied with sponges or applicators, and not allowed to pool. A 70% alcohol solution is relatively safe to use and is a cost-effective skin-defatting agent and antiseptic.

Hexachlorophene has been popular as a skin antiseptic. It is virtually insoluble in water, but it is soluble in alcohol. Hexachlorophene is a bacteriostatic agent that is active against gram-positive microorganisms but only minimally active against gram-negative microorganisms. If the skin surface is washed frequently each day with hexachlorophene, a relatively low flora population may gradually be achieved and maintained.

Hexachlorophene forms a long-lasting, imperceptible bacteriostatic film on the skin and develops a cumulative suppressive action with routine use. With the increasing problem of *Pseudomonas* and other gram-negative microorganisms as sources of wound infection, and because of studies demonstrating the toxicity of hexachlorophene, its use should be carefully evaluated.

Benzalkonium chloride (Zephiran) in a concentration of 1:1000 is bacteriostatic to vegetative bacteria but has no effect on tubercle bacilli or spores. It should not be considered a satisfactory disinfectant because it has marked incompatibility with anionic soaps, which causes its antibacterial activity to disappear, and it has very limited action against gram-negative microorganisms and fungi.

Preoperative skin preparation
Nursing considerations

The preoperative skin preparation of a surgical patient is the first step in the prevention of wound infection. Because the procedure may be alarming, embarrassing, or uncomfortable for the patient, every effort should be made to minimize these features by proceeding in a considerate, methodical, and professional manner.

If the preoperative skin preparation is done when the patient is awake, the nurse should explain the purpose and method of the procedure. Every effort should be made to allay any fears the patient may express and to answer questions in a reassuring manner. During the procedure, the nurse should observe the patient's general condition, particularly the condition of the skin under treatment. Any contraindication to the procedure because of an abnormal skin condition or an adverse reaction by or injury to the patient should be documented and reported to the physician.

In carrying out the procedure, the nurse should provide for the comfort, safety, and privacy of the patient. Good alignment of the patient's body should be maintained, and special supports for positioning should be used, as indicated.

Initial preparation of operative area

In the immediate preoperative period, the skin of the involved part of the body is prepared by special cleansing. Hair should be removed from the operative site only as necessary. Three alternatives for hair removal are clipping, use of depilatory, and wet shaving. Studies show that the wound infection rate is considerably higher for patients who are shaved preoperatively than for patients who have no preoperative shave preparation or a small amount of hair clipped, or for patients on whom a depilatory is used. If a shave is ordered by the surgeon, the patient should be shaved immediately before surgery, preferably in a holding area within the surgical suite that affords privacy and is equipped with good lighting facilities. The amount of time between the preoperative shave and the operation has a direct effect on the wound infection rate. In shaving the site, great care should be taken to avoid scratching, nicking, or cutting the skin because cutaneous bacteria will proliferate in these areas and increase the chances of

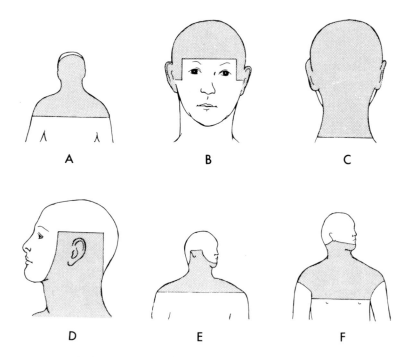

Fig. 5-13. Preparation for head, major neck, and upper thorax surgery. **A,** For posterior craniotomy. **B** and **C,** For craniotomy, frontal tumor excision. **D,** For major otological operations. **E,** For removal of lesions of neck and glands. **F,** For esophageal diverticulectomy, esophagotomy, scalenectomy, cervicothoracic anterior approach, thyroidectomy, and laryngectomy. (Modified from Pate, M.O.: The preparation manual, Long Island City, N.Y., Edward Weck & Co., Inc.)

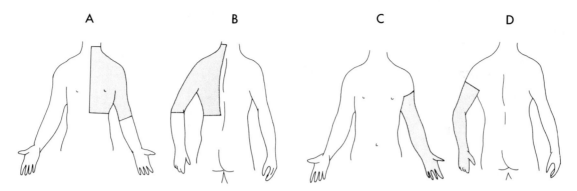

Fig. 5-14. Preparation for surgery of upper extremity. **A** and **B,** For major operations on shoulder and uppermost part of extremity, skin area is prepared from neckline to elbow line and axilla to midline anteriorly and posteriorly. **C** and **D,** For operations on forearm, preparation includes entire arm from fingertips to and including axilla. (Modified from Pate, M.O.: The preparation manual, Long Island City, N.Y., Edward Weck & Co., Inc.)

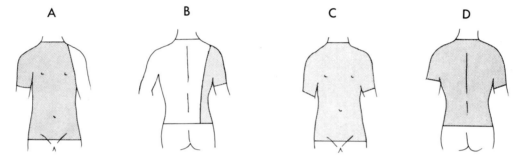

Fig. 5-15. A and **B,** For unilateral chest operations and radical mastectomies, affected chest, shoulder, and upper arm are prepared, from nipple on unaffected side to bedline on affected side. **C** and **D,** For combined thoracoabdominal operations, chest and shoulder are prepared bilaterally, anteriorly, and posteriorly. For cardiac surgery, this preparation may be extended to include legs. (Modified from Pate, M.O.: The preparation manual, Long Island City, N.Y., Edward Weck & Co., Inc.)

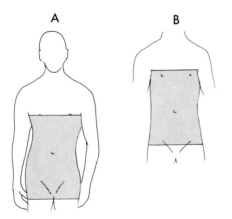

Fig. 5-16. Preparation for abdominal surgery. **A,** Skin area is cleansed and disinfected from nipple line to 3 inches below symphysis pubis, including external genitals, and from bedline to bedline. This preparation is done for gastrointestinal, biliary, and liver operations; splenectomy; herniorrhaphy; appendectomy; and surgery on great vessels of trunk. **B,** Skin prepared from above nipple line to above symphysis pubis. This preparation is done for gastrointestinal, biliary, and liver operations. (Modified from Pate, M.O.: The preparation manual, Long Island City, N.Y., Edward Weck & Co., Inc.)

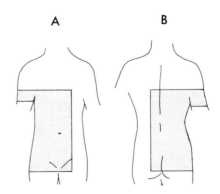

Fig. 5-17. Lateral preparation for operations on kidney and upper ureter. **A,** Anterior view. **B,** Posterior view. (Modified from Pate, M.O.: The preparation manual, Long Island City, N.Y., Edward Weck & Co., Inc.)

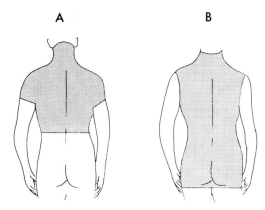

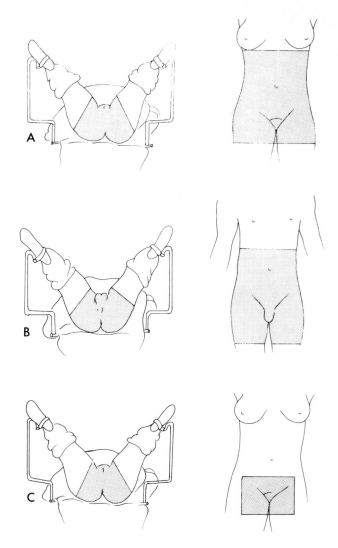

Fig. 5-18. **A,** Preparation for cervical laminectomy. **B,** Preparation for lumbar laminectomy. Preparation includes hairline to fold of buttocks and to bedlines laterally. (Modified from Pate, M.O.: The preparation manual, Long Island City, N.Y., Edward Weck & Co., Inc.)

infection. The decision of where and by whom the procedure is performed depends on when it is to be done, the facilities and personnel available, the patient's reactions, and the philosophy and policies that have been determined and established by the surgical committee.

Although specific orders for the skin preparation are written by the surgeon, a manual with diagrams and instructions concerning the preoperative skin shave is useful for the guidance and information of the personnel to whom the task is delegated (Figs. 5-13 to 5-21). The extent of the area to be shaved is determined by the site of the incision and the nature of the operation.

Shaving the face and neck of children or female patients is rarely necessary. The eyebrows are not shaved unless specifically ordered by the physician. The head and neck are not generally prone to wound infection because of the generous blood supply to this area. For cosmetic and psychologic reasons, preparation for head and neck surgery may be done in the operating room after the induction of anesthesia.

For orthopedic surgery on the extremities, the shave preparation usually extends from one joint above to one joint below the area of incision. If a pneumatic tourniquet will be used during surgery, the entire extremity may be prepared to facilitate proper draping technique. Preparation and draping of the entire extremity also permit manipulation of the limb during surgery. Great care should be exercised in the preparation for surgery on bones because wound infection resulting from improper cleansing may cause a stubborn condition leading to crippling, disfigurement, and permanent dysfunction. The skin may be difficult to clean if it has been affected by casts, splints, or braces that interfere with normal skin care or cause skin damage. Daily soaking may help to clean badly soiled feet in preparation for surgery, just as daily washing is advisable in preparation for general elective surgery.

Fig. 5-19. Pelvic and perineal preparation for gynecological and genitourinary operations. **A,** Preparation for combined vaginal and abdominal operations. **B,** Preparation for suprapubic prostatectomy and bladder operations. **C,** Preparation for minor vaginal and rectal operations. (Modified from Pate, M.O.: The preparation manual, Long Island City, N.Y., Edward Weck & Co., Inc.)

Patients with traumatic injuries that may be excessively painful, such as fractures, burns, and soft tissue lacerations, may require anesthesia for skin preparation. Traumatic wounds usually require copious irrigation to flush out foreign matter. In cleansing the injured area, the surrounding skin is first carefully washed with an antimicrobial detergent. The open wound is irrigated with an isotonic solution, and the area is treated with an antimicrobial solution.

If a patient must be shaved in the operating room, a heavy lather should be used on the skin to control hair clippings and epithelium removed by the razor. Skin preparation in the operating room has the disadvantages that the patient's anesthesia time is prolonged, optimum use

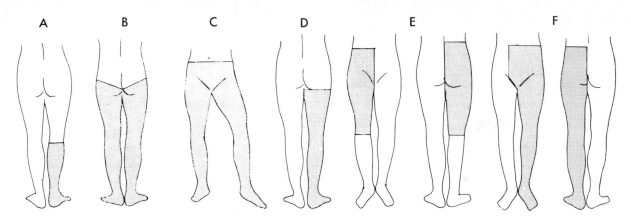

Fig. 5-20. Preparation for surgery of lower extremity. **A,** For operations on ankle, foot, or toes, lower leg is prepared anteriorly and posteriorly. **B** and **C,** For bilateral leg operations such as varicose vein ligation and skin and bone grafts. **D,** For operations on foot and lower leg, entire leg is prepared anteriorly and posteriorly. **E,** For unilateral hip operations. **F,** For unilateral operations involving hip and thigh. (Modified from Pate, M.O.: The preparation manual, Long Island City, N.Y., Edward Weck & Co., Inc.)

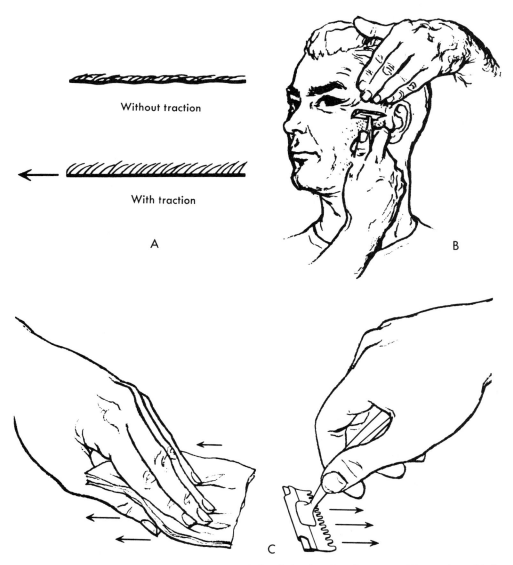

Fig. 5-21. Skin shaving. **A,** Skin traction is provided with free hand in direct opposition to slant of hair to tighten and smooth skin and raise hairs in more upright position. **B,** Hair and horny layer of skin are shaved off. **C,** Traction is applied with sponge, and hoe-type razor head is held against skin, as shown in **B.** (From Pate, M.O.: The preparation manual, Long Island City, N.Y., Edward Weck & Co., Inc.)

of the operating room is infringed on, loose hair remaining on the surrounding linen may get into the wound, and water used to wash the skin can result in sterile drapes becoming wet.

Procedure for preoperative shave

Individual supplies are used for each patient. Commercially prepared kits that contain the basic essentials for shaving the site of incision are available. The use of disposable preparation trays and razors can help ensure a safe, personal technique. The use of disposable gloves is a safeguard for the patient and for the worker. Blankets and supports for the patient's position, as well as the necessary lighting and handwashing facilities, should be provided in the area where shaving is performed. Basic equipment includes gloves, basins for warm water and soap, a disposable razor, sponges for washing, and towels or waterproof pads for draping. Solvent solution may also be required to remove adhesives or nail polish. Volatile liquids such as alcohol and acetone should be strictly regulated because of the danger of fire or burns.

Antimicrobial soap or detergent should be applied to the skin area using sponges moistened with water. A lather is created by using a circular motion and light friction, beginning with the proposed site of incision and working toward the periphery of the area. The principle is progression from cleansed areas to uncleansed ones. Sponges are discarded as they become soiled, and the process is continued with fresh sponges. Application of lather to skin hair for several minutes before shaving enables the keratin of the hair to absorb three to four times its weight in water. The water absorbtion makes the hair softer and easier to shave.

A disposable razor with a sharp blade is used to shave off the lathered hair. Holding the soft areas and loose skin taut with the free hand raises the hair and permits easier access to the area. A clean shave can be obtained without injury to the skin by gently stroking in the direction of the hair growth (Fig. 5-21). Nicks or cuts resulting from the shave should be reported as incidents, and the surgeon should be notified.

The surgeon may order a 5-minute scrub of the prepared area with an antimicrobial soap or detergent after it has been shaved. If so, the shaved area is scrubbed and rinsed carefully, and the skin is blotted dry to prevent chapping and irritation.

At the conclusion of the preparation, the patient should be made comfortable, the unit left in order, and the equipment disposed of or cleaned. Reusable items should be washed and sterilized. Expendable materials should be disposed of according to procedure. The worker should follow the principles of aseptic technique for the removal of gloves and for terminal handwashing before proceeding to the care of other patients.

Final skin disinfection of operative area

After the patient has been positioned on the operating room bed, final skin cleansing and disinfection are performed. If the patient has not showered with an antimicrobial detergent or soap immediately before leaving for the operating room, the operative area may be prepared with an antimicrobial scrub solution. While this is being carried out, the shave can be inspected and touched up or extended, as needed. Skin cleansing is followed by prepping with an antimicrobial solution.

Procedure for final skin prepping

The supplies required for the final skin prepping may be arranged on a separate sterile prepping table. The items should include stainless steel cups for the cleansing agent and the selected antimicrobial agent, sterile sponges, and sponge-holding forceps, if desired. Cotton-tipped applicators are needed to clean the umbilicus thoroughly, and a scrub brush may be required for nails, callused skin, or traumatic injuries of the hands and feet. Final skin disinfection may be done by the circulating nurse or the surgeon.

The skin scrub begins at the line of the proposed incision and proceeds to the periphery of the area. The antimicrobial agent is applied by sponges held in sponge-holding forceps or in the gloved hand. The gloved-hand method requires that the glove be sterile at the beginning of the skin scrub and that the surface of the patient's skin not be permitted to come into contact with the gloved hand. The sponges used in scrubbing are discarded as they become soiled, and fresh ones are taken. A soiled sponge is never brought back over a scrubbed surface. The lather is wiped off with dry, sterile sponges. Depending upon the surgeon's preference, an antimicrobial tincture or "paint" may be carefully applied, avoiding any pooling beneath the patient. All wet drapes should be removed from the patient area after the skin scrub is complete.

Sponges used to cleanse or disinfect a wound, sinus, ulcer, intestinal stoma, the vagina, or the anus are applied once to that area and immediately discarded. After prepping of the area, intestinal fistulas are generally walled off, using one of the plastic transparent adhesive drapes. In contrast to the principle of working from the proposed incision to the periphery, open wounds and body orifices are potentially contaminated areas and as such are prepped after the peripheral intact skin is cleansed. The surgical principle is always to scrub the cleanest area first.

SURGICAL SCRUB
General considerations

The objectives of the surgical scrub are to remove dirt, skin oil, and microbes from hands and lower arms; to reduce the microbial count to as near zero as possible; and to leave an antimicrobial residue on the skin to prevent growth of microbes for several hours. The skin can never be rendered sterile, but it can be made *surgically clean* by reducing the number of microorganisms present. A lengthy mechanical scrub, even with strong antiseptics, will fail to remove all microorganisms. Friction and rinsing significantly decrease the number of bacteria on the epidermis, but their numbers are constantly replenished by the continuous secretory activity of the skin glands.

Only persons who feel well and are free of upper respiratory infections and skin problems should scrub. Cuts, abrasions, and hangnails tend to ooze serum, which is a medium for prolific bacterial growth and can endanger the patient by increasing the hazards of infection.

Hospital procedures govern the selection of materials and the methods used for the surgical scrub. The selection of a reusable or disposable brush for scrubbing should be based on realistic considerations of effectiveness and economy. Studies show no significant difference in scrub effectiveness between reusable brushes and disposable brushes or sponges.

Individually prepackaged disposable brushes and sponges provide a cost-effective, labor-saving alternative to reusable brushes. The use of synthetic sponges in place of brushes has gained wide acceptance, especially where long and repeated scrubbing may be traumatic to the skin. Some disposables are available with one of several antimicrobial soap or detergent solutions impregnated in the sponge. If a reusable brush is desired, it should be easy to clean and maintain and should be durable enough to withstand repeated heat sterilization without the bristles becoming soft or brittle.

The antimicrobial soap or detergent used for the surgical scrub should act rapidly, have a broad spectrum, not depend on cumulative action, have minimal harsh effect on skin, and inhibit rapid growth of microbes.

Two popular antimicrobial agents used for surgical hand scrubs are povidone-iodine and chlorhexidine gluconate. Both are rapid-acting, broad-spectrum antimicrobials that are effective against gram-positive and gram-negative microorganisms. For individuals who have demonstrated skin sensitivity to these agents, another broad-spectrum antimicrobial agent, parachlorometaxylenol (PCMX), is being used as an effective alternative agent for surgical scrubbing. Many persons who previously were unable to use any surgical hand scrub other than hexachlorophene (which is ineffective against gram-negative microorganisms) are now safely using PCMX. It significantly reduces skin flora with an antibacterial effect that persists even after prolonged surgery. Moisturizing agents are now being incorporated into various surgical scrubs to reduce the potential of skin irritation resulting from multiple scrubs.

In scrubbing, light friction is effective in removing the detritus of the epithelium. The friction produces heat, dilation of the blood vessels, and better circulation, which help to recondition the skin. Hard scrubbing and harsh bristles tend to cause desquamation, leaving a bleeding or weeping dermis that is painful and predisposes to infection. It also may massage bacteria into the deeper dermal layers.

An anatomic scrub using a prescribed amount of time or number of strokes plus friction is employed for effective cleansing of the skin.

A properly executed surgical scrub, using the anatomic counted brush stroke method, usually takes approximately 5 minutes. Studies indicate no significant difference in microbial reduction between scrubs of 5 minutes' duration and those of 10 minutes' duration. Individual attention to detail is essential. The same scrub procedure should be used for every scrub, whether it is the first or last scrub of the day.

The prescribed number of strokes with a brush is usually 30 strokes to the nails and 20 strokes to each area of the skin. When scrubbing, the fingers, hands, and arms should be visualized as having four sides; *each* side must be scrubbed effectively.

The number of deep-resident flora is reduced by frequent scrubbing, but the number is increased when the surgical scrub is done only occasionally.

Procedure

Surgical scrub techniques that personnel must observe should be defined in writing.

Before beginning the surgical scrub, members of the surgical team inspect their hands to assure their nails are short and free of polish, their cuticles are in good condition, and no cuts or skin problems exist. All jewelry is removed from the hands and forearms. The cap or hood is adjusted to cover and contain all hair. A fresh mask is carefully placed over the nose and mouth and tied securely to prevent venting. Goggles or protective eye wear is comfortably adjusted to ensure clear vision and to avoid lens fogging. Personnel confirm that the scrub shirt is fitted, tied, or tucked into the trousers to prevent potential contamination of the scrubbed hands and arms from brushing against loose garments.

The basic steps of the procedure follow:

1. The faucet is turned on, and the water brought to a comfortable temperature. Most scrub sinks have automatic or knee controls for the faucets.
2. The hands and forearms are dampened.
3. By a foot control, a few drops of the antimicrobial soap or detergent are dispensed into the palms. Small amounts of water are added to make a lather.
4. The hands and forearms are washed to a level well above the elbows. The amount of time needed varies with the amount of soil and the effectiveness of the cleansing agent.
5. If a prepackaged scrub brush or sponge is used,

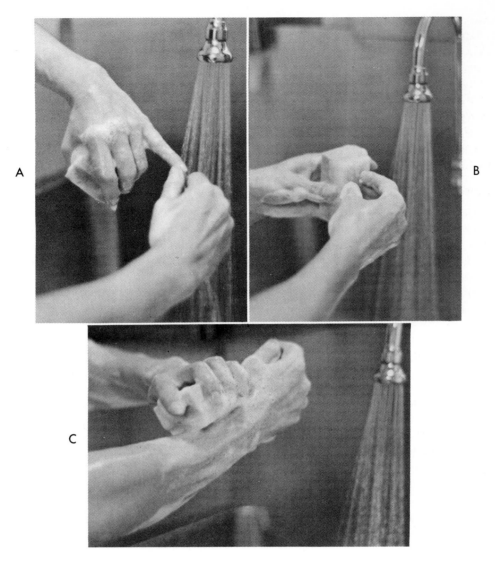

Fig. 5-22. Surgical scrub technique. **A,** Cleaning nails with plastic nail cleaner. **B,** Holding brush perpendicular to nails facilitates thorough scrubbing of undersides of nails. **C,** Holding brush lengthwise along arm covers maximum area with each stroke.

the package is opened, the brush and nail cleaner removed, and the package discarded. The brush is held in one hand while the nails are cleaned with the other hand (Fig. 5-22, *A*). All nails and subungual spaces are cleaned. If a disposable nail cleaner is not available, a metal nail file can be used. Orangewood sticks are prohibited because they cannot be sterilized after use.

6. The hands and arms are rinsed thoroughly; care is taken to hold the hands higher than the elbows. Splashing water onto the scrub suit should be avoided because this moisture causes subsequent contamination of the sterile gown.

7. If the brush or sponge is impregnated with antimicrobial soap, it should be moistened and scrub-

bing begun. If the brush or sponge is not impregnated with soap, antimicrobial soap or detergent solution is applied to hands. Starting at the fingertips, the nails are scrubbed vigorously while the brush is held perpendicular to them (Fig. 5-22, *B*). All sides of each digit are scrubbed, including the web spaces between them. The palm and back of the hand are then scrubbed.

8. Each side of the arm, including the elbow and antecubital space, is scrubbed with a circular motion to 2 inches above the elbow (Fig. 5-22, *C*).

9. The hands are held above the level of the elbows while scrubbing to allow the water and detritus to flow away from the first-scrubbed and cleanest area. The hands and arms are also held away from

the body. Small amounts of water are added during the scrub to develop suds and remove detritus.

10. The hands and arms are rinsed thoroughly. The brush is discarded in a proper receptacle.

11. If the sink is not automatically timed, the faucet is turned off by using the knee control or by using the edge of the brush on a hand control.

12. The hands and arms are held up in front of the body with elbows slightly flexed while entering the operating room.

Drying the cleansed area

Moisture remaining on the cleansed skin after the scrub procedure is dried with a sterile towel before a sterile gown and gloves are donned. The towel must be used with care to avoid contaminating the cleansed skin. The procedure for opening the sterile towel to dry the hands and forearms will vary, depending on the method used in folding the towel before sterilization. One method frequently used is to fold the towel to half its width, then to half its length, and then to half its length again.

The folded towel is grasped firmly near the open corner and lifted straight up and away from the sterile field without dripping contaminated water from the skin onto the sterile field. The person steps away from the sterile field and bends forward slightly from the waist, holding the hands and elbows above the waist and away from the body. The towel is allowed to unfold downward to its full length and width (Fig. 5-23).

The top half of the towel is held securely with one hand, and the opposite fingers and hand are blotted dry,

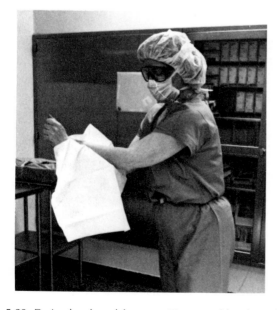

Fig. 5-23. Drying hands and forearms. Fingers and hand are dried thoroughly before forearm is dried. Extending arms reduces possibility of contaminating towel or hands.

making sure they are thoroughly dry before moving to the forearm. To avoid contamination, a rotating motion is used while moving up the arm to the elbow, and an area is not retraced. The lower end of the towel is grasped with the dried hand, and the same procedure is used for drying the second hand and forearm. Care must be taken to prevent contamination of towel and hands. The towel is discarded.

GOWNING AND GLOVING PROCEDURES

Before scrubbed personnel can touch sterile equipment or the sterile field, they must put on sterile gowns and sterile surgical gloves to prevent microorganisms on their hands and clothing from being transferred to the patient's wound during surgery. The sterile gowns and gloves also protect the hands and clothing of personnel from microorganisms present in the patient or in the atmosphere.

Design and packaging of the gown

The gown should be made of a material that establishes an effective barrier, minimizing the passage of microorganisms between unsterile and sterile areas. Reusable fabrics must allow complete penetration of steam during the sterilization process and should withstand multiple inhouse processes and multiple launderings. Tests indicate that 280-count, quarpel-treated materials lose their barrier quality after laundering and sterilizing 75 times. The material should be resistant to tearing and puncture and as lint-free as possible to reduce the dissemination of particles into the wound and the environment. It should facilitate aseptic technique and avoid excessive heat buildup. Regardless of the gown's material, the shape and size should fit the wearer and allow freedom of movement. To provide extra protection, the gown's front from the waist upward and the forearms of the sleeves are made of a water-repellent material. Each sleeve should be finished with a tight-fitting wristlet that prevents the inner side of the sleeve from slipping down onto the outer side of the sterile glove. Cotton tapes or Velcro fasteners are attached to the back of the gown to hold it closed. A wraparound gown should be used to achieve better coverage of the back.

Because the outer side of the front and sleeves of the gown come in contact with the sterile field during surgery, the gown must be folded so that the scrubbed person can put it on without touching the outer side with bare hands. For in-house wrapping and sterilization, the gown is folded with the inner side out and the back edges together. The sleeves are not turned inside out; consequently, they remain within the folded gown. The side folds of the gown are folded lengthwise toward the center back opening, overlapping slightly at the center. With the open edges of the gown remaining on the inside, the bottom third of the gown is folded upward and the top third of the gown is folded over the bottom portion. The gown is then folded in half widthwise so that the inside front neckline of the gown is visible on top.

Gowns with wraparound backs are prepared in the same manner, with care taken to tie the tape securely on the wraparound back flap to the external side tie of the gown before initial folding. A folded hand towel with its free corners facing up is usually placed on top of the folded gown before the gown is wrapped and sterilized.

Procedure for donning the sterile wraparound gown

Scrubbed personnel use the following procedure for donning the sterile wraparound gown:

1. The sterile gown is grasped at the neckline with both hands and lifted from the sterile gown wrapper; the scrub nurse steps into an area where the gown may be opened without risk of contamination.
2. The gown is held away from the body and allowed to unfold with the inside of the gown toward the wearer.
3. The gown is completely unfolded while the hands are kept on the inside of the gown (Fig. 5-24, *A*).
4. Both hands are slipped into the open armholes at the same time, keeping the hands at shoulder level and away from the body.
5. The hands and forearms are pushed into the sleeves of the gown, the hands advanced only to the proximal edge of the cuff if the closed gloving technique is used. If the open gloving technique is employed, the hands are advanced completely through the cuffs of the gown.
6. The circulating nurse pulls the gown over the shoulders and touches only the inner shoulder and side seams (Fig. 5-24, *B*).

7. The circulating nurse ties or clasps the neckline and ties the inner waist ties of the gown by touching only the inner aspect of the gown (Fig. 5-24, *C*).
8. After gloving, the scrub nurse hands the tab attached to the back tie of the gown to the circulating nurse (Fig. 5-25, *A*). The scrub nurse then makes a three-quarter turn to the left while the circulating nurse extends the back tie to its full length. This action effectively wraps the back panel of the gown around the scrub nurse and covers the previously tied inner waist ties. The scrub nurse retrieves the back tie by carefully pulling it out of the tab held by the circulating nurse (Fig. 5-25, *B*) and ties it with the other tie, which had been secured to the front top of the gown.
   a. If another scrubbed person is gowned and gloved, that individual, instead of the circulating nurse, may assist with the "wraparound" procedure. The assisting person must extend the back tie to its fullest length before the scrub nurse turns to avoid any potential contamination.
   b. When a reusable gown is utilized, an alternative method of tying a gown that does not have snaps should be used by the scrub nurse. If the closed gloving technique and commercially prepared, double-wrapped gloves are employed, the inner wrap can be used as a protective extension for the gown tie when the circulating nurse assists with tying a wraparound gown. After gloving, the scrub nurse unties the exterior gown ties (which were tied at the front of the gown before it was folded, wrapped, and sterilized) and holds

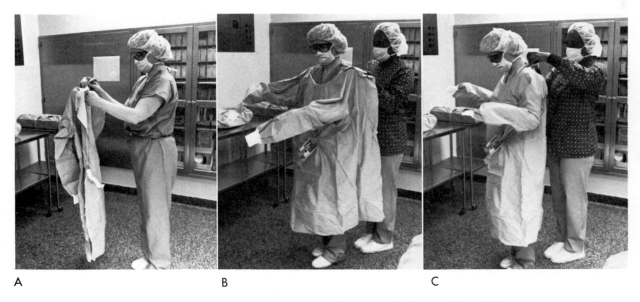

A B C

Fig. 5-24. Gowning procedure. **A,** Scrub nurse keeps hands on inside of gown while unfolding it at arm's length. **B,** Circulating nurse reaches under flap of gown to pull sleeves on scrub nurse. **C,** Circulating nurse snaps neckline of gown, touching only snap section of neckline.

both in the hands. The end of the back tie is placed in the center crease of the empty glove wrapper, approximately two thirds the way up to the edge of the opened wrapper (Fig. 5-25, *C*). The glove wrapper is then closed so that the tie is concealed. The closed wrapper is handed to the circulating nurse, who firmly grasps the folded edge of the wrapper without touching the tie (Fig. 5-25, *D*). The scrub nurse then pivots in the opposite direction from the circulating nurse, who extends the back tie to its full length. The scrub nurse grasps the exposed portion of the back tie, pulls it out of the glove wrapper while taking care to avoid touching the glove

wrapper or the circulating nurse (Fig. 5-25, *E*), and ties both ties. If a sterile glove wrapper is not available, a sterile hemostat may be clamped to the back tie and used in the same manner as a glove wrapper. After the gowning procedure has been completed, the circulating nurse retains the hemostat in the room to avoid problems with the subsequent instrument count.

Use of glove lubricants

The use of powder as a glove lubricant should be abolished because of two primary hazards: the postoperative complication of powder granulomas is an ever-present danger, and powder fallout from hands and gloves provides

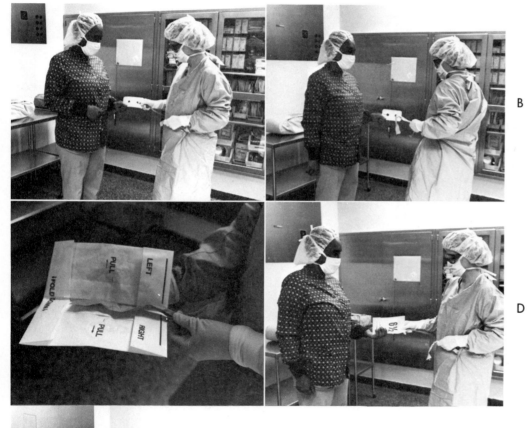

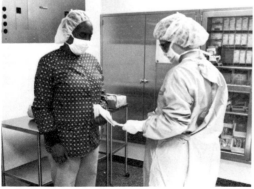

Fig. 5-25. Methods of tying wraparound gown. **A,** After handing tab on back tie of gown to circulating nurse, scrub nurse makes three-quarter turn toward left. **B,** Sterile back panel now covers previously tied unsterile ties; scrub nurse retrieves back tie by carefully pulling it out of tab held by circulating nurse and ties it securely with other tie. **C,** Using sterile inner glove wrapper, scrub nurse places end of back tie in crease of wrapper. **D,** After closing wrapper, scrub nurse hands it to circulating nurse, who grasps it carefully, touching neither tie nor gloved hand. **E,** After making three-quarter turn to left, scrub nurse carefully pulls back tie from wrapper.

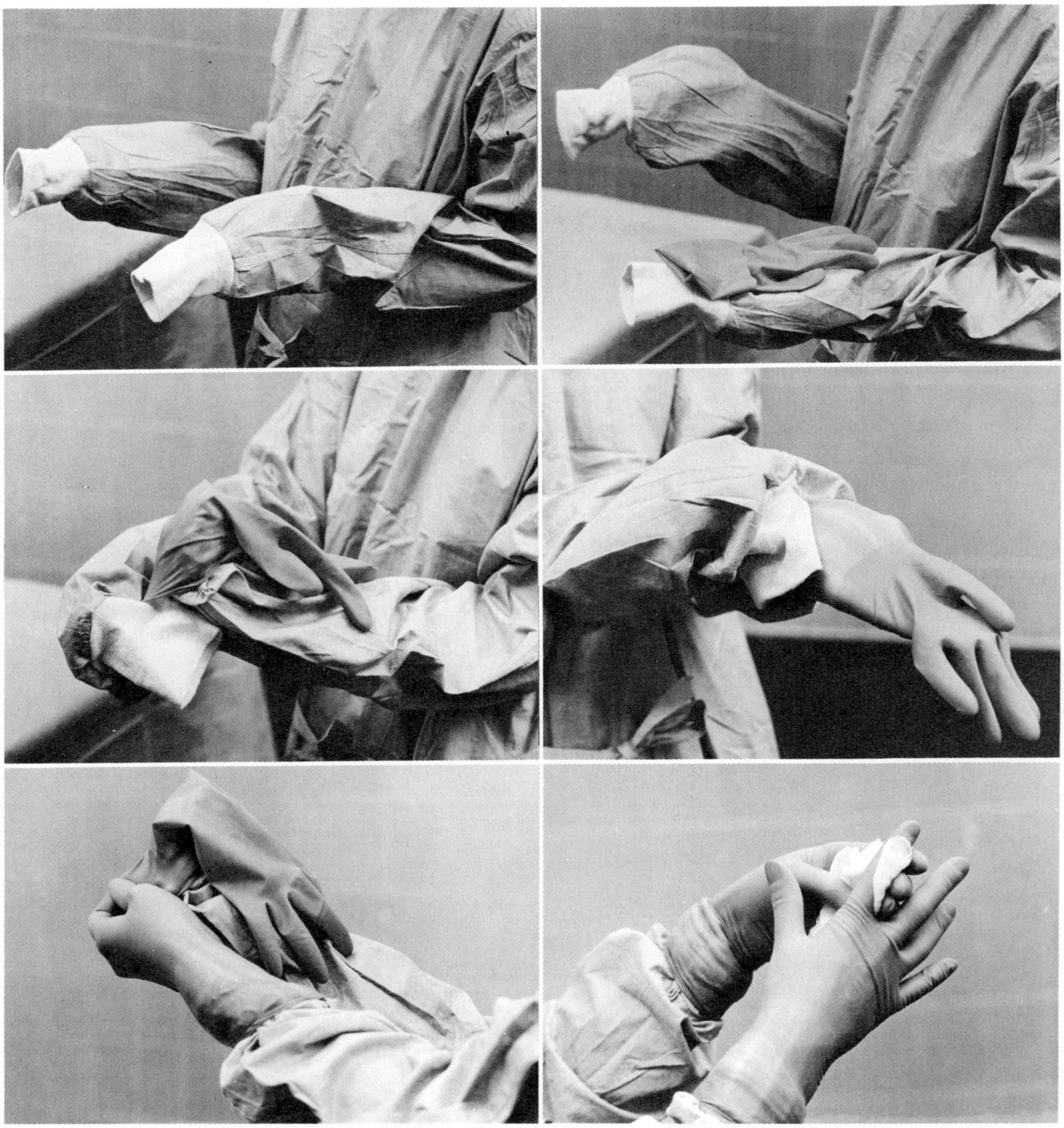

Fig. 5-26. Closed gloving procedure. **A,** When donning gown, scrub nurse does not slip hands through wristlets. Hands are not extended from sleeves. **B,** First glove is lifted by grasping it through fabric or sleeve. Cuff on glove facilitates easier handling of glove. Glove is placed palm down along forearm of matching hand, with thumb and fingers pointing toward elbow. Glove cuff lies over gown wristlet. **C,** Glove cuff is held securely by hand on which it is placed, and, with other hand, cuff is stretched over opening of sleeve to cover gown wristlet entirely. **D,** As cuff is drawn back onto wrist, fingers are directed into their cots in glove, and glove is adjusted to hand. **E,** Gloved hand is then used to position remaining glove on opposite sleeve in same fashion. Glove cuff is placed around gown cuff. Second glove is drawn onto hand, and cuff is pulled into place. **F,** Fingers of gloves are adjusted, and gloves are wiped with wet gauze sponge or commercially prepared sterile disposable glove wipe to remove any powder that may be on gloves.

a convenient vehicle for dissemination of microorganisms throughout the hospital. In order to remove any glove film or powder, the gloves must be wiped thoroughly after they are put on and before the surgical team member approaches the sterile field.

Cream or liquid lubricants of various types have been developed. Some of these contain antiseptic or bacteriostatic agents that assist in keeping the gloved hands relatively free of bacterial growth. Manufacturers of surgical gloves have also used silicone films to eliminate stickiness. Little or no lubrication of the hands is needed to don these gloves easily. Assessing these new products and practices requires determining their effectiveness for the purpose and their harmlessness to the skin and other body tissues of both patients and personnel.

Procedure for donning sterile gloves
Closed method (Fig. 5-26)

The closed method of gloving has the advantage of preventing the bare hands from coming in contact with the outside of the glove, which must remain sterile. The gloves are handled through the fabric of the gown sleeves. The hands are not extended from the sleeves and wristlets when the gown is put on. Instead, the hands are pushed through the cuff openings as the gloves are pulled in place.

Open method (Fig. 5-27)

The everted cuff of each glove permits a gowned person to touch the glove's inner side with ungloved fingers and to touch the glove's outer side with gloved fingers. Keeping the hands in direct view, no lower than waist level, the gowned person flexes the elbows. Exerting a light, even pull on the glove brings it over the hand, and using a rotating movement brings the cuff over the wristlet.

Assisting others with gowning (Fig. 5-28)

A gowned and gloved scrub nurse may assist another person in donning a sterile gown. The gown is opened in the manner previously described. The inner side with the open armholes is turned toward the individual who is to

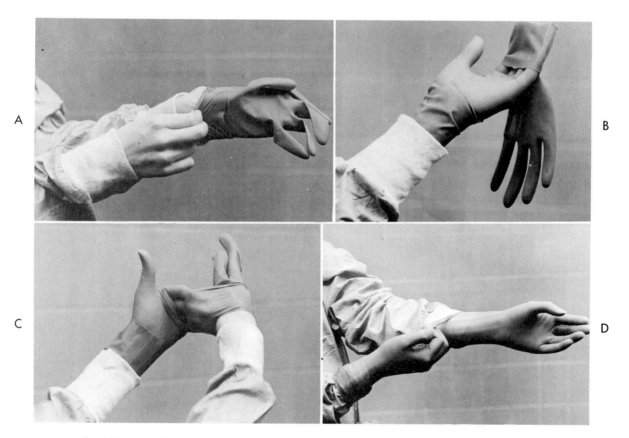

Fig. 5-27. Open gloving procedure. **A,** Scrub nurse takes one glove from inner glove wrapper by placing thumb and index finger of opposite hand on fold of everted cuff at a point in line with glove's palm and pulls glove over hand, leaving cuff turned back. **B,** Scrub nurse takes second glove from inner glove wrapper by placing gloved fingers under everted cuff. **C,** Scrub nurse, with arms extended and elbows slightly flexed, introduces free hand into glove and draws it over cuff of gown and upper part of wristlet by slightly rotating arm externally and internally. **D,** To bring turned-back cuff on other hand over wristlet of gown, scrub nurse repeats **C.**

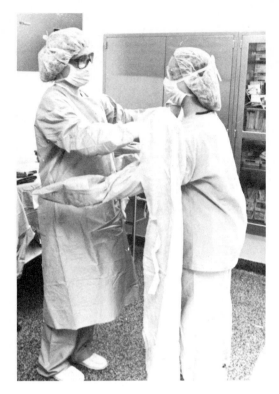

Fig. 5-28. Gowning another person. Gowned and gloved scrub nurse cuffs neck and shoulder area of gown over gloved hands to prevent contamination as scrubbed person puts hands and forearms into sleeves.

be gowned. A cuff is made of the neck and shoulder area of the gown to protect the gloved hands. The gown is held until the person's hand and forearms are in the sleeves of the gown. The circulating nurse assists in pulling the gown onto the shoulders, adjusting the back, and tying the tapes. The wraparound back on the gown is fixed into position by the scrubbed person after gloving is completed.

Assisting others with gloving (Fig. 5-29)

A gowned and gloved scrub nurse may assist another gowned individual with gloving according to the following procedure:

1. The glove is grasped under the everted cuff.
2. The palm of the glove is turned toward the other individual's hand; the thumb of the other glove is opposed to the thumb of the person's hand.
3. The cuff is stretched to open the glove.
4. The gowned person exerts a slight upward pressure on the cuff while inserting the hand into the glove.
5. The gowned person brings the cuff over the wristlet of the gown while slipping the hand well into the glove.
6. The procedure is repeated to don the other glove.

Removing soiled gown, gloves, and mask (Fig. 5-30)

To protect the forearms, hands, and clothing from contacting bacteria on the outer side of the used gown and gloves, members of the scrubbed surgical team should

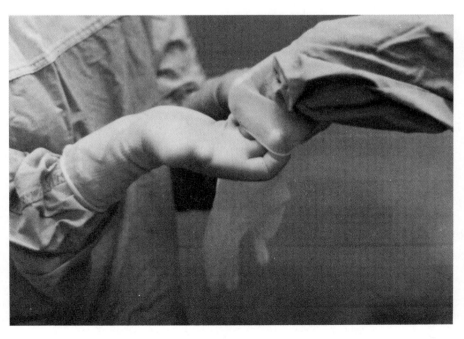

Fig. 5-29. Gloving another person. Gowned and gloved scrub nurse places fingers of each hand beneath everted cuff, keeping thumbs turned outward and stretching cuff as gowned person slips hand into sterile glove, using firm downward thrust.

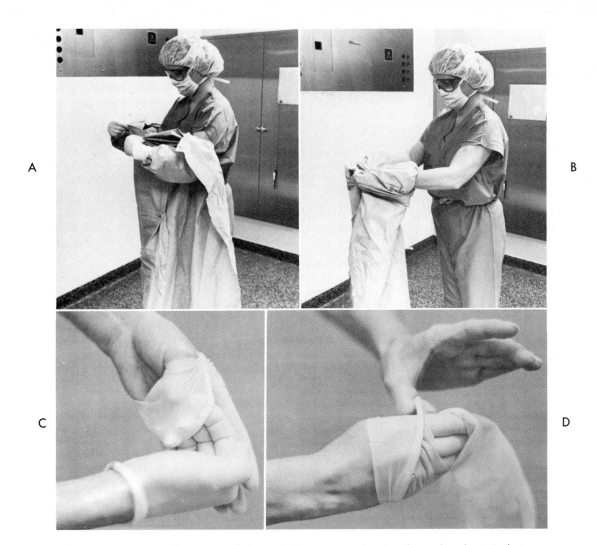

Fig. 5-30. Removing soiled gown and gloves. **A,** To protect scrub suit and arms from bacteria that are present on outer side of soiled gown, the gown is grasped without touching the scrub clothes. **B,** Scrub nurse turns outer side of soiled gown away from body, keeping elbows flexed and arms away from body, so that soiled gown will not touch arms or scrub suit. **C,** To prevent outer side of soiled gloves from touching skin surfaces of hands, scrub nurse places gloved fingers of one hand under everted cuff of other glove and pulls it off hand and fingers. **D,** To prevent ungloved hand from touching outer side of soiled glove, scrub nurse hooks bare thumb on inner side of glove and pulls glove off.

follow these steps to remove soiled gowns, gloves, and masks:

1. The gloves are wiped with a clean, wet sponge.
2. If a wraparound gown is worn, the front or side external waist tie is untied.
3. The circulating nurse unfastens the back closures of the gown.
4. The gown is grasped at one shoulder seam without touching the scrub clothes.
5. The neck of the gown and sleeve are brought forward and over and off the gloved hand, turning the gown inside out and everting the cuff of the glove.

6. Touching only the outside of the gown, step 5 is repeated for the other side, and the gown is pulled off completely.
7. The arms and soiled gown are kept away from the body while the gown is folded inside out and discarded carefully inside the linen hamper.
8. The gloved fingers of one hand are placed under the everted cuff of the other glove, and care is taken not to touch skin with the soiled surface of either glove.
9. The glove is inverted as it is pulled off and then discarded in the appropriate receptacle.
10. The fold of the everted cuff on the remaining glove is grasped with the bare fingers of the ungloved

hand; the glove is pulled off in the same way and discarded.

After leaving the restricted area, the person removes the mask by touching only the strings and discards it in the designated receptacle.

The hands and forearms are washed. If immediately scrubbing for another operation is necessary, the individual dons a fresh mask and repeats the prescribed scrub procedure.

SURGICAL DRAPING

Draping procedures create an area of asepsis called a *sterile field*. All sterile items that come in contact with the wound must be restricted within the defined area of safety to prevent transportation of microorganisms into the open wound.

The sterile field is created by placement of sterile sheets and towels in a specific position to maintain the sterility of surfaces on which sterile instruments and gloved hands may be placed. The patient and operating room bed are covered with sterile drapes in a manner that exposes the prepared site of incision and isolates the area of the surgical wound. Objects draped include instrument tables, basin and Mayo stands, trays, and some surgical equipment.

Draping materials

Draping materials are selected to create and maintain an effective barrier that minimizes the passage of microorganisms between nonsterile and sterile areas. To be effective, a barrier material is resistant to blood, aqueous fluid, and abrasion, as lint-free as possible, and drapable. It should maintain an isothermic environment that is appropriate to body temperature. It should meet or exceed the requirements of the current National Fire Protection Association standards so that no risk from a static charge exists. Fabric draping materials must be penetrable by steam under pressure or by gas to achieve sterilization within hospital facilities.

Several reusable and numerous disposable materials that are currently available exhibit barrier qualities. However, they do not remain equally impermeable to moist contaminants for given periods of time. Barrier properties vary, depending on the stresses applied to the draping materials during actual use.

Reusable drapes

The performance characteristic of primary concern for drapes (or gowns) to be used repeatedly is fluid impermeability under the conditions of use. Bleached and preshrunk muslin with a thread count of 140 to 160 per square inch has been available as a drape for years. Although it conforms easily to body contours and remains in place when draped, muslin does not retard the passage of fluid effectively. Heavy twill, denim, and canvas materials inhibit

steam penetration, are difficult to handle, and retain heat on the patient. These factors prohibit the use of these materials as surgical drapes.

Chemically treated cotton cloth and tightly woven 100% cotton with an approximate thread count of 280 per square inch provide a barrier to liquids and are abrasion resistant. Quantitative data verifying the impervious quality of a textile drape should be furnished by the manufacturer. Care should be taken with reusable drapes to eliminate pinholes caused by towel clamps, needles, or sharp objects. Should breaks in the fabric occur, a heat-sealed patch may be used for repair. Reusable materials with heat-applied vulcanized patches can be effectively sterilized. The limit to the percentage of exposed surface that can be patched depends on the mode of sterilizing, positioning in the sterilizer, and the number of layers of patched fabric.

As in the case of reusable gowns, laundering eventually impairs the barrier quality of the drape. Most manufacturers report a loss of barrier quality after 75 laundry and/ or sterilization cycles. The process of steam sterilizing and laundering swells the fabric, whereas drying and ironing shrinks the fibers. This cycle increases the propensity for loosened fibers that alter the fabric structure. A system to monitor the number of times an item has been laundered is essential for barrier quality control.

Disposable drapes

Numerous synthetic disposable drapes prevent bacterial penetration and fluid breakthrough. These versatile materials can be manufactured to meet different specifications in both absorbent and nonabsorbent forms. The successful disposable drapes currently on the market are soft, lint free, lightweight, compact, moisture resistant, nonirritating, and static free. These products are available prepackaged and presterilized from commercial sources. White and colored drapes are available.

Lightness and compactness of synthetic drapes prevent heat retention by patients, contribute to ease in handling and storage, and conserve storage space and personnel's time.

Disposable drapes reduce the hazards of contamination in the presence of known infectious microorganisms in body fluids and excretions and in situations in which laundering of grossly contaminated textiles is a problem.

The danger inherent in the use of synthetic drapes is that solvents, volatile liquids, and sharp instruments tend to penetrate the barrier. Loss of effectiveness may be caused by cracking at the folds or by pinholes from the use of regular towel clamps. Manufacturers are continually improving disposable flat sheets, fenestrated drapes, and towels to permit easy handling and adaptability to the body.

When considering the purchase of disposable drapes, the buyer must determine whether they will satisfy the needs of surgery, be acceptable to the users, and be cheaper than the cost of laundering reusable drapes. If the cost is not lower, other significant advantages may warrant the purchase of disposable drapes. Availability of items, storage facilities, and disposal method must be analyzed.

Preassembled, sterile, disposable custom packs are now used in many operating rooms. Advantages of these packs include shorter setup and reduced turnover times, less risk of contaminated waste because fewer individually wrapped items are dispensed, improved inventory control, and fewer lost charges. Although custom packs may be more expensive than multiple separate items, indirect savings related to increased efficiency can offset those costs.

Compactors provide a relatively inexpensive method of discarding disposable drapes. They accept any material and reduce the volume by at least a 4:1 ratio. Collection, transportation, and storage of waste materials can be a problem. Hospital engineers must establish methods of controlling odor and maintaining sanitation in the compactor area. Because a portion of the compacted material may be grossly contaminated, city or county codes may prohibit transporting this potentially infectious material through city streets or dumping it at landfills.

Incineration is an alternative method for destroying waste disposables. If incinerators are used, they must be properly managed to prevent environmental contamination. Many hospital incinerators do not meet federal pollution standards; therefore their use is prohibited.

The ecologic impact of disposable items can be only roughly estimated. Each hospital must carefully evaluate its capabilities and restrictions in the handling of disposable drapes before a conversion is implemented.

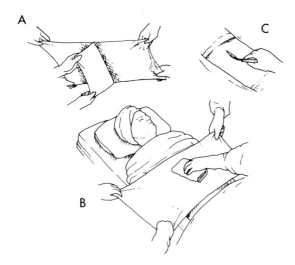

Fig. 5-31. Sterile impermeable adhesive drape. For maximum sealing to prevent wound contamination, prepped skin must be dry and drape applied carefully, preventing wrinkles and air bubbles. **A,** Surgeon and assistant hold plastic drape taut while another assistant peels off back paper. **B,** Surgeon and assistant apply plastic drape to operative site, and, using folded towel, apply slight pressure to eliminate air bubbles and wrinkles. **C,** Surgeon makes incision through plastic drape.

Plastic incisional drapes

Several types of impermeable polyvinyl sheeting are available in the form of sterile, prepacked surgical drapes.

These plastic drapes are useful adjuncts to the conventional draping procedure. They can be applied after the fabric drape, alleviating the need for towel clamps. They obviate the need for skin towels and sponges to separate the surgeon's gloves from contact with the patient's skin. Skin color and anatomic landmarks are readily visible, and the incision is made directly through the adherent plastic drape. These materials facilitate draping of irregular body surfaces, such as neck and ear regions, extremities, and joints. The draping procedure for an impermeable adhesive drape is demonstrated in Fig. 5-31.

Standard drapes

Careful planning by nursing and surgical departments helps to determine the desired types and sizes of sheets and towels required for surgery. The variety of drapes should be kept to a minimum. The most effective sheets and towels are simple and economic in terms of time, body motions, and materials. Standard methods provide management control that ensures the safety of patients, simplifies teaching of staff, and conserves human and material resources.

A *whole,* or *plain, sheet* is used to cover instrument tables, operating tables, and body regions. The sheet should be large enough to provide an adequate margin of safety between the surrounding physical environment and the prepared operative field. Usually two sizes of sheets suffice.

Surgical towels in one or two sizes should be available to drape the operative site. Four surgical towels of woven or nonwoven material are usually sufficient (Fig. 5-32).

Fenestrated, or *slit, sheets* are used for draping patients. They leave the operative site exposed. A typical fenestrated (laparotomy) sheet is large enough to cover the patient and operating bed in any position and to extend over the anesthesia screen at the head of the bed and over the foot of the bed (Figs. 5-33 to 5-35). In some cases it may incorporate the Mayo stand that has been placed over the patient.

The typical fenestrated laparotomy sheet can be used for most procedures on the abdomen, chest, flank, and back. This type of sheet for adults should measure 9 to 10 feet long and 6 feet wide. A rectangular slit 10 inches long by 4 inches wide beginning 4 feet from the uppermost end of the sheet at a point in the center line of the sheet is usually suitable for a routine laparotomy sheet.

Other types of fenestrated sheets similar in length and width but with smaller or split fenestration may be used for the limbs, head, and neck with the patient supine or prone. The size of the fenestration is determined by the use for which the sheet is intended. The fenestrated sheet is fanfolded and handled as a typical laparotomy sheet.

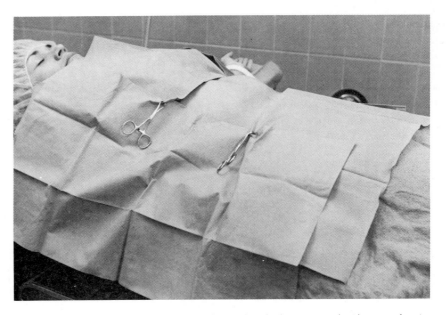

Fig. 5-32. Abdomen may be draped with four sterile towels, which are secured with nonperforating towel clamps. Standard method of placement of disposable towels is used.

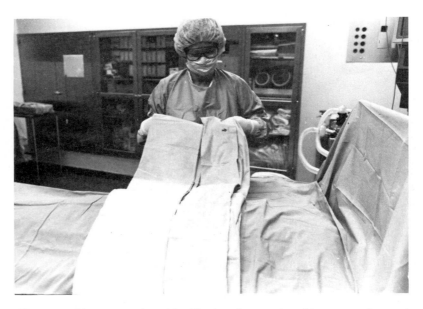

Fig. 5-33. Placement of laparotomy sheet. Identification of top portion of laparotomy sheet assists scrub nurse in readily determining correct placement of drape. After placing folded laparotomy sheet on patient, with fenestration of sheet directly over site of incision outlined by sterile towels, scrub nurse unfolds drape over sides of patient and bed.

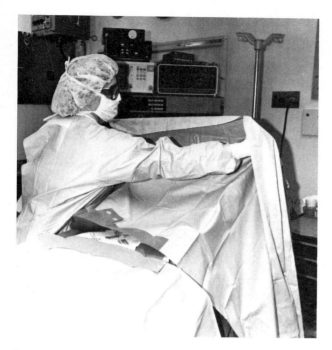

Fig. 5-34. Laparotomy draping continued. Scrub nurse protects gloved hands under cuff of fanfolded laparotomy sheet and draws upper section above fenestration toward head of bed, draping it over anesthesia screen. Bottom portion of fanfolded sheet is then extended over foot of bed in similar manner.

A *perineal drape* is needed for operations on the perineum and genitalia with the patient in lithotomy position. A lithotomy drape consists of a fenestrated sheet and two triangular leggings. The leggings may be attached to the sides of the sheet. The three-piece drape is less costly and is easier to handle and launder. A commercial, disposable lithotomy drape pack, including fenestration sheet, two leggings, absorbent and nonaborbent towels, and a small sheet, is suitable for delivery, cystoscopy, hemorrhoidectomy, and vaginal procedures.

Folding drapes for use

Drapes should be folded so that the gowned and gloved members of the team can handle them with ease and safety. The larger, regular sheet is usually fanfolded from bottom to top. The bottom folds may be 4 inches wider than the upper ones. The small sheet is folded in half and then quartered, and the top corners of the sheet may be turned back or marked for easy identification and handling.

To provide for safe, easy handling and a wide margin of safety between the unsterile item and the scrub nurse's gloved hands, the open end of the Mayo stand cover should be folded back on itself (Fig. 5-36).

Most fenestrated sheets are fanfolded to the opening from the top and the bottom, and then the folds are rolled or fanned toward the center of the opening. The edges of the top and bottom folds of the sheet are fanned to provide a cuff under which the scrub nurse may place gloved hands. The top and lower sections should be identified by a marking to facilitate easy handling.

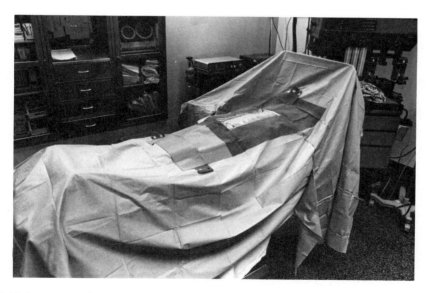

Fig. 5-35. Laparotomy draping completed. Fenestration provides exposure of prepped operative site. Special fabric surrounding fenestration is both absorbent and impermeable. Built-in instrument pad prevents instrument slippage. Perforated tabs provide means of controlling position of cords and suction tubes.

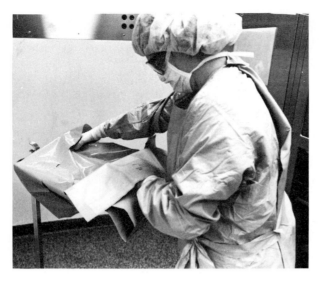

Fig. 5-36. Draping Mayo stand. Folded cover is slipped over frame. Scrub nurse's gloved hands are protected by cuff of drape. Cover is unfolded to extend over upright support of stand.

Draping procedure

If a sterile field is to be created and maintained, numerous important points must be remembered when draping for a surgical procedure:

1. Allow sufficient time and space to permit careful draping of the patient and proper aseptic technique.

2. Handle sterile drapes as little as possible.
3. Carry the folded drape to the operative site, where the drape is carefully unfolded and placed in proper position. After a drape has been placed, it should not be moved.
4. Hold sterile drapes above waist level until properly placed on the patient or object being draped. If the end of a drape falls below waist level, it should not be retrieved because the area below the waist is considered unsterile.
5. Immediately discard a drape that becomes contaminated during the draping procedure without contaminating the gloves or other sterile items.
6. Protect the gown by distance and the gloved hands by cuffing drapes over them (Fig. 5-37). The scrub nurse should have all parts of the drape under positive control at all times during placement and should use precise and direct motions. Draping is always done from a sterile area to an unsterile area and by draping nearest first. The scrub nurse should never reach across an unsterile area to drape. When the opposite side of the operating room bed must be draped, the scrub nurse must go around the bed to drape.
7. Do not flip, fan, or shake drapes. Rapid movement of drapes creates air currents on which dust, lint, and droplet nuclei may migrate. Shaking a drape also causes uncontrolled motion of the drape, which may cause it to come in contact with an unsterile surface or object. A drape should be carefully unfolded and allowed to fall gently into po-

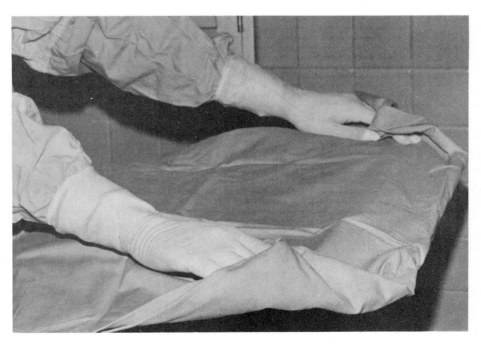

Fig. 5-37. When placing sterile drape on unsterile surface, scrub nurse rolls corners of drape over hands to avoid contamination.

sition by gravity. The low portion of a sheet that falls below the safe working level should never be raised or lifted back onto the sterile area.

8. Drape the incisional area first and then the periphery.
9. Use nonperforating towel clamps or devices to secure tubing and other items on the sterile field.
10. When sterility of a drape is questionable, consider it contaminated.

Arrangement of items on sterile tables

The standard arrangement of instruments, drapes, sutures, and other items on sterile tables for particular operations should be determined by nursing personnel. Factors to be considered include the surgeon's method of working; ease in handling, preparing, and transporting items; and reduction in human energy. Methods of work are based on work simplification and aseptic principles.

The arrangement of the various setups should be clearly defined and understood by operating room personnel. Visual aids are excellent tools for teaching personnel proper procedural methods.

OPERATING ROOM ENVIRONMENTAL SANITATION

Effective sanitation techniques should be established to control and reduce the possibility of cross-infection of patients in the operating room. Blood and tissue fluids from any patient may contain microorganisms that are pathogenic to other persons. Operating room practices should be developed to provide complete isolation for each patient. This isolation is accomplished by considering every surgical wound to be potentially contaminated.

Principle of confine and contain

The principle of confine and contain was originally introduced to perioperative nurses in the early 1970s. This principle recommends that personnel restrict all patient microorganisms to an area of 3 feet around the patient and that, when patient microorganisms leave that limited area, they should be either confined to an impervious container or destroyed. Establishment of procedures to implement this principle prevents the transfer of microorganisms and protects patients and personnel. Adherence to this principle also eliminates the costly practice of special decontamination procedures for "dirty" cases.

Procedure

During the surgical procedure, traffic within and through the room should be kept to a minimum to reduce air turbulence and to minimize human shedding. Efforts should be made to confine contamination to as small an area as possible around the patient. Sponges should be discarded in plastic-lined containers. As they are counted, they should be contained in an impervious receptacle. The circulating nurse must use gloves, instruments, or both when collecting and counting sponges or handling contaminated items. Spillage should be cleaned up immediately with a broad-spectrum detergent-germicide. The exterior surfaces of all specimen containers should be wiped with a disinfectant before removal from the operating room.

Between surgical procedures, personnel must remove their gowns and gloves and place them in the proper receptacles before leaving the operating room. All linens from open packs, whether soiled or not, should be discarded in fluid-impervious bags. The use of fluid-impervious bags eliminates potential contamination from wet linen soaking through to the outside of the bag. Used disposable and expendable items should be discarded in plastic bags and placed in containers for disposal.

The scrub nurse should place all instruments directly in wire mesh–bottom trays for processing in a washer-sterilizer. Basins, cups, and trays should also be washed and terminally sterilized. If a washer-sterilizer is not adjacent to the operating room, all these items should be contained for transportation to a central cleanup area, either in the surgical suite or in central service, for terminal sterilization or high-level disinfection. Wall suction units should be disconnected by the circulating nurse to eliminate contamination of the wall outlet. Suction contents should be disposed of by the scrub nurse during the flushing of a hopper by the circulating nurse. If a flushing type of hopper is not available, the suction contents should be decontaminated with a detergent-germicide and disposed of in a toilet rather than in a conventional sink. Spillage during transport should be prevented. Glass suction containers should be rinsed and terminally sterilized with basins and trays. Disposable suction tubing should be discarded. Use of reusable suction tubing should be avoided because of difficulties in cleaning the lumen properly.

Surgical lights and the horizontal surfaces of furniture and equipment that have been involved in the surgical procedure should be cleaned with a detergent-germicide. The floor should be cleaned with a detergent-germicide using the wet-vacuum method. If a wet vacuum is not available, a clean mophead and clean solution should be used after each patient. The wheels and casters of furniture used during the surgical procedure should be pushed through the solution used for floor cleaning.

At the end of each day's operative schedule, a complete housekeeping program should be initiated to ensure that every operating room, scrub room, and service room is properly cleaned.

BIBLIOGRAPHY

Alexander, J.W., and others: The influence of hair-removal methods on wound infections, Arch. Surg. 118:347, 1983.
American College of Surgeons: Manual on control of infection in surgical patients, ed. 2, Philadelphia, 1984, J. B. Lippincott Co.
Association for the Advancement of Medical Instrumentation: National

standards and recommended practices for sterilization, ed. 2, Arlington, Va., 1988, The Association.

Association of Operating Room Nurses: Standards and recommended practices for perioperative nursing, Denver, 1990, The Association.

Atkinson, L.J., and Kohn, M.L.: Berry and Kohn's introduction to operating room technique, ed. 6, New York, 1986, McGraw-Hill Book Co.

Ayliffe, G.: Surgical scrub and skin disinfection, Infect. Control 5:23, 1984.

Beck, W.C.: Aseptic barriers in surgery, Arch. Surg., 116:240, 1981.

Block, S.S.: Disinfection, sterilization and preservation, Philadelphia, 1983, Lea & Febiger.

Burns, S.: A multiple evaluation study on artificial nails, J. Nurs. Quality Assurance, 2:77, 1988.

Burrows, W.: Textbook of microbiology, ed. 22, Philadelphia, 1985, W.B. Saunders Co.

Centers for Disease Control: Update: Universal precautions for prevention of transmission of human immunodeficiency virus, hepatitus B virus, and other bloodborne pathogens in health-care settings, MMWR, 37:381, 1987.

Centers for Disease Control: Recommendations for prevention of HIV transmission in healthcare settings, MMWR, 34:6S, 1987.

Centers for Disease Control: Guidelines for the prevention and control of nosocomial infections, Atlanta, 1985, CDC.

Christensen, P., and Kropp, D.: Care and processing of surgical instruments, Hosp. Topics, 63:32, 1987.

Copp, G., and others: Covergowns and the control of operating room contamination, Nurs. Res., 35:263, 1986.

Copp, G., and others: Footwear practices and operating room contamination, Nurs. Res., 36:366, 1987.

Crow, S., and others: Disinfection or sterilization? Four views on arthroscopes, AORN J. 37:854, 1983.

Daschner, F.D.: The transmission of infections in hospitals by staff carriers, methods of prevention and control, Infect. Control 6:3, 1985.

Favero, M.S.: Biological hazards in the laboratory, Lab. Med., 18:665, 1987.

Fay, M.F.: Glove powders on trial, Todays OR Nurse 5:9, Nov. 1983.

Fogg, D.M.: Clinical issues: universal precautions and disinfection of endoscopes, AORN J. 49:652, 1989.

Grundler, C.: Clinical issue: "dirty case" is outdated, AORN J. 43:686, 1986.

Jamner, H.: Care and handling of surgical instruments, J. Hosp. Supply, 2:47, 1984.

Joint Commission on Accreditation of Healthcare Organizations: Accreditation manual for hospitals, Chicago, 1990, The Commission.

Kahn, M.A., and others: Suture contamination by surface powders on surgical gloves, Arch. Surg. 118:738, 1983.

Kneedler, J.A. and Dodge, G.H.: Perioperative patient care, ed. 2, 1987, Boston, Blackwell Scientific Publications.

Liechty, R.D., and Soper, R.T.: Synopsis of surgery, ed. 5, St. Louis, 1985, The C.V. Mosby Co.

Moylan, J., and Kennedy, B.: The importance of gown and drape barriers in the prevention of wound infection, Surg. Gynecol. Obstet. 151:465, 1980.

Moylan, J.A., and others: Reducing wound infections, improved gown and drape and barrier performance, Arch. Surg. 122:152, 1987.

National Institutes of Health: The impact of routine HTLV-III antibody testing on public health. In The NIH Consensus Development Conference Statement, 6:5, New Fairfield, Conn., 1989, National Organization for Rare Disorders.

Olderman, G.M.: Liquid repellency and surgical fabric barrier properties, Eng. Med., 13:35, 1984.

O'Neal, M.: Contain and confine technique for OR cleanup, AORN J., 45:979, 1989.

Perkins, J.J.: Principles and methods of sterilization in health sciences, ed. 2, Springfield, Ill., 1983, Charles C Thomas.

Rosenberg, A., Alatary, S.D., and Peterson, A.F.: Safety and efficacy of the skin antiseptic chlorhexidene gluconate, Surg. Gynecol. Obstet. 143:789, 1976.

Spry, C.: Essentials of perioperative nursing, Rockville, Md., 1988, Aspen Publishers, Inc.

Thompson, J.M., and others: Infectious diseases, clinical nursing, ed. 2, St. Louis, 1989, The C.V. Mosby Co.

Tucci, V.J., and others: Studies of the surgical scrub, Surg. Gynecol. Obstet. 145:1977.

Wenzel, R.: Prevention and control of nosocomial infections, Baltimore, 1987, Williams & Wilkins.

Youmans, G.P., Paterson, P.Y., and Sommers, H.M.: The biologic and clinical basis of infectious disease, ed. 3, Philadelphia, 1985, W.B. Saunders Co.

Young, R., and Walsh, P.: Sterilization of powered surgical instruments, AORN J. 37:945, 1983.

6 Positioning the patient for surgery

LESLIE EILEEN RICKER

Surgery is performed on various parts of the human anatomy. The body has to be placed into multiple configurations so that the procedure can be done with accuracy and with the desired outcomes. Positioning the surgical patient is both an art and a science and is as well a key factor in the performance of a safe and efficient surgical procedure. All members of the surgical team have a duty to protect the patient from any deleterious effects of the surgical position.

Although the choice of patient position is usually determined by the surgical approach, the responsibility for overall patient well-being rests with the surgeon, the anesthesiologist, and the nurse, who constantly monitor the patient's physiologic status. The circulating nurse may coordinate the details of restraints, support to the extremities, and safe transfers. The surgeon and the circulating nurse determine the position for patients who receive local anesthetics.

The patient's position should provide optimum exposure and access to the operative site; should sustain body alignments and circulatory and respiratory function; must provide access to the patient for administration of intravenous fluids, drugs, and anesthetic agents; should not compromise neuromuscular structures; and should afford as much comfort to the patient as possible. Good positioning promotes patient well-being and safety while meeting these needs.

SURGICAL ANATOMY

The nurse must be cognizant of the anatomic and physiologic changes associated with anesthesia, positioning of the patient, and the operative procedure. These changes most frequently involve (1) the musculoskeletal system, (2) the nervous system, (3) the circulatory system, and (4) the respiratory system.

The *musculoskeletal system* of the patient may be subjected to unusual and exaggerated stress during operative positioning. Normal range of motion is maintained in the alert patient by pain and pressure receptors that warn against stretching and twisting of ligaments, tendons, and muscles. The tone of opposing muscle groups also acts to prevent strain and stress to the muscle fibers. When phar-

macologic agents such as anesthetics and muscle relaxants depress the pain and pressure receptors and loss of tone causes muscular relaxation, the normal defense mechanisms cannot guard against joint damage and muscle stretch and strain. Obvious resistance to unusual range of motion is often noted only in patients whose arthritic changes prevent even slight exaggeration of the position. Bony prominences of the human anatomy are particularly vulnerable to injury by rubbing and sustained pressure. The position chosen should provide physiologic alignment while protecting the patient from pressure, abrasion, and other injuries.

Nervous system depression accompanies the administration of anesthetic agents and many other drugs. The degree of depression depends on the type of regional anesthesia or the level of general anesthesia. Pain and pressure receptors may be affected either regionally or systemically. The most important factor for the nurse to remember is that when nervous system depression occurs, the body's communication and command system is rendered totally or partially ineffective. Changes in physical status and compensatory actions are no longer possible. Lifesaving, physiologic adaptive mechanisms do not function; the stresses of operative positioning are not automatically compensated. Pressure on superficial nerves must be prevented.

The *circulatory system* is most dramatically affected by anesthesia, causing a lack of nervous system control of vascular dilatation and constriction. It is also affected by direct peripheral pressure on the venous return; blood pools in veins to decrease circulating volume, and blood flow is distributed along variations of the horizontal body plane and follows laws of gravity in other manners than when it is upright. Blood pressure responds to redistribution of blood flow and the horizontal body plane in addition to inherent pathophysiologic processes.

Poor positioning of the patient can adversely affect pulmonary function and therefore the *respiratory system*. Diaphragmatic movement may be impeded, or shifting visceral pressure may occur. The horizontal body plane changes the airflow and functional characteristics of the lungs. Not only airflow but also flow of secretions is affected. The combination of circulatory changes and the compromised respiratory effort affects the oxygen saturation of the blood.

PERIOPERATIVE NURSING CONSIDERATIONS
Assessment/nursing diagnosis

Nursing assessment begins preoperatively with a review of the proposed schedule for the room to which the nurse is assigned. Based on the planned surgical intervention and the operating surgeon's preferences, the basic patient position is anticipated. During the preoperative patient assessment, the nurse reviews the patient's record and determines the patient's height, weight, and general physical condition. Skin integrity and range of motion of all extremities are assessed. Any reddened or ecchymotic areas, lesions, or decubiti must be documented. Limitations in mobility should be noted, as should any preexisting neurovascular problems and complaints of discomfort.

A key issue in patient positioning is prevention of injury. Nursing assessment therefore involves recognition of potential patient problems (vulnerable situations and patients).

Vulnerable situations include

1. Long surgical procedures (time is a critical factor)
2. Vascular surgery (optimal blood perfusion may already be compromised)
3. Demineralizing bone conditions such as malignant metastasis or osteoporosis
4. Excessive sustained pressure to certain body areas because of the surgical procedure or retraction

Vulnerable patients include

1. Geriatric patients whose thin skin layer and circulatory system make them more prone to skin breakdown due to pressure
2. Patients who are malnourished, anemic, obese, hypovolemic, paralyzed, arteriosclerotic, or diabetic are also prone to skin breakdown due to pressure
3. Patients with prosthetic or arthritic joints
4. Patients with edema, infection, cancer, or conditions of lowered cardiac or respiratory reserves

Nursing diagnoses can be derived from the data collected during the preoperative assessment. The primary nursing diagnosis concerned with patient positioning is *potential for injury* related to sustained pressure to certain body areas during surgery.

Planning

Specific nursing care is planned to encompass the surgeon's specifications for the given basic position and to alleviate or prevent an individual patient problem. Planning may involve determining the appropriate mode of patient transport and transfer, determining equipment and positioning aids, or determining the need for ancillary person-

---

Sample Care Plan

NURSING DIAGNOSIS:
Potential for injury related to sustained pressure to certain body areas during surgery.
GOAL:
Patient will be free of injury at the completion of the surgical procedure.
INTERVENTIONS:
Check operating room bed for proper functioning.
Gather positioning aids.
Assist in proper positioning, maintaining proper body alignment.
Pad and protect bony prominences, pressure sites, and vulnerable nerves.
Document in detail patient position, including:
· Type and placement of restraints
· Position of extremities
· Type and placement of positioning aids
· Site of electrosurgical dispersive pad
· Positional changes made during the procedure (for example, supine to lithotomy to supine)

---

nel to accomplish the positioning. The care plan should be individualized for specific patient problems such as diabetic, malnourished, or paralyzed patients.

Implementation

The nurse must be familiar with the normal functions, maintenance, various uses, and potential hazards of the operating room beds, their attachments, and other mechanical adjuncts to both patient position and the operative procedure (such as electrosurgical devices, drills, and radiologic procedures). Mechanical malfunctions must be recognized and corrected for the patient's safety.

Providing patient safety encompasses more than overseeing mechanical functions; it also includes direct patient care. The restraint strap should be snug but should not compromise venous circulation or exert pressure on bony prominences or nerves. It should never be placed directly on the patient's skin but rather over the blanket covering the patient. If possible, patient transfers should be made when the patient is awake. When the patient is anesthetized or unable to assist, a four-person lift or a Davis roller should be used to provide support to the torso, head, and all extremities. Mayo tables should be positioned high enough to prevent pressure on the toes, knees, or legs. The surgical team should be reminded not to lean on the patient's trunk or extremities, because pressure may compromise anatomic and physiologic functions.

Modern operating room beds (operating room tables)

Modern operating room beds are specifically designed to meet the peculiar and highly specialized requirements of surgical therapy. Modern manufacture and design have done much to facilitate safe and effective positioning of the patient while providing the surgeon with anatomic accessibility. Judicious manipulation of the operating room bed obviates untoward manipulation of the patient.

Describing all types of operating room beds available is not feasible. Perioperative nursing personnel have the responsibility of being well versed in the use of all types of operating room beds available in the institution. Nurses should keep abreast of new developments and evaluate their usefulness in actual practice.

In common surgical use are the general operating room bed, the orthopedic (fracture) table, and the urology table. The modern general operating room bed (Fig. 6-1) is so versatile that the need for specialty tables is declining. An operating room bed that is adaptable to a wide range of uses is an economic investment and permits flexibility in the use of operating facilities. The orthopedic table, with its multiple movable and removable parts and suspension frames, remains one of few specialty tables required (Fig. 6-2).

The urology table, designed for cystoscopic procedures, has radiologic equipment attached which facilitates intraoperative x-rays of the genitourinary system.

Modern general operating room beds can be adjusted for height and length and can be tilted laterally to either side and horizontally at the head and foot. They are divided into three or more sections that support the major body parts and permit their placement in flexion or extension. The head section is usually removable, and foot extensions may be added.

Controls and accessories may be employed to maintain the patient in standard or modified dorsal, lateral, or prone positions. Headrests of various designs enable the general operating room bed to be used for cranial and eye surgery. Electrically powered models make bed movements swift and smooth.

Perineal cutouts and drainage trays fitted to the lumbar section adapt the general operating room bed for the perineal approaches used in gynecologic, urologic, and proctologic surgery. Most operating room beds are available with x-ray penetrable tunnel tops that permit insertion of cassette holders at any position along the bed.

Additional accessories for operating room beds include pillows, pads, bolsters, and doughnut cushions of various sizes and shapes. They are made to fit the different anatomic structures of patients and thereby facilitate physiological functions and operative accessibility. All positioning devices should perform three functions: absorb compressive forces, redistribute pressure, and prevent excessive stretching.

Some accessories are soft and made of conductive foam rubber; others are firm, made of conductive rubber, and filled with kapok, "beanbag" material, or fine sand. If not disposable, all of these accessories should be designed to

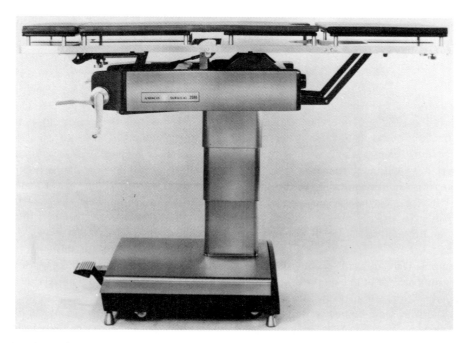

Fig. 6-1. Surgical OR bed with x-ray–penetrable top. (Courtesy AMSCO— American Sterilizer Co., Erie, Pa.)

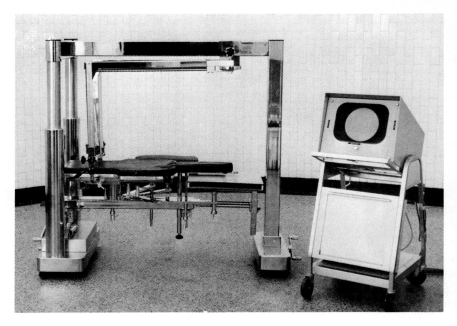

Fig. 6-2. Orthopedic fracture table. (Courtesy Chick Orthopedic, Oakland, Calif.)

permit terminal cleansing between patient usages. If these devices are readily available in the surgical suite, the nurse can save time gathering positioning supplies and thus have more time to individualize patient care.

STANDARD POSITIONS AND PHYSIOLOGIC CONSIDERATIONS

Because operative procedures are performed with the patient resting on the back, abdomen, or side, three basic positions are described: dorsal, prone, and lateral. These basic positions can be modified in many ways. The following discussion of operative positioning is general; there is room for individuality to meet specific needs or preferences.

Dorsal position

In the *dorsal position* the patient's back and spinal column are resting on the surface of the operating room bed mattress. Modifications of the position allow approach to the major body cavities (cranial, thoracic, and peritoneal), the four extremities, and the perineum.

The *dorsal recumbent (supine) position* is the most common position. It is the most natural position of the body at rest. The patient is usually anesthetized in this position (Fig. 6-3), and modifications are made after induction of anesthesia.

The patient lies supine (face upward) with the arms at the sides (either on armboards or at the sides of the body) and the legs extended. The position of the head should place the cervical, thoracic, and lumbar vertebrae in a straight, horizontal line. A small pad placed under the head allows the strap muscles to relax and prevents neck strain. Flexion or twisting may cause contractures in the

neck and may interfere with a clear airway. Small, soft pillows may be placed under the small of the back and under the knees to maintain normal lumbar concavity and to prevent strain on the back muscles and ligaments; such strain may occur if the muscles and ligaments are allowed to assume the configuration of the flat operating room bed surface. The hips are parallel. The legs are parallel and uncrossed to prevent peroneal and tibial nerve injury, rubbing, and compromised circulation. The legs are slightly separated so skin surfaces are not in contact, because moisture from antiseptics, irrigating solutions, and body fluids contributes to irritation and maceration of the skin. The leg restraint (table strap) is placed across the middle to upper thighs, 2 inches above the knees to prevent their flexion, so that the patient is secured but superficial venous return is not impaired. Heel prominences also need protection from prolonged pressure. Doughnut cushions, ankle rolls, or foam heel protectors may be used.

The soles of the feet are usually supported on a firm foam rubber support or padded footboard that extends beyond the toes to prevent plantar flexion (foot-drop) and to guard the toes from the weight and pressure of drapes.

The arms should rest easily at the sides of the body with the palms against the padded body or with the hands pronated (palms down and fingers extended) on the mattress surface. A broad liftsheet can be used to tuck around the arms to support the full length of each arm. The elbows should neither be flexed nor rest on the metal edge of the bed. An elbow resting on the edge may cause pressure to the ulnar nerve as it passes over the epicondyle of the humerus. If the hands are placed under the buttocks, the fingers may be compressed. Wristlets used to restrain the hands endanger the nerves and the blood supply to the

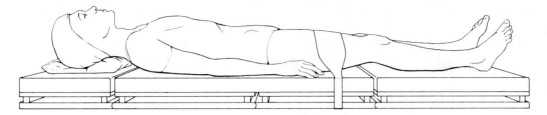

Fig. 6-3. Dorsal recumbent (supine) position.

hands. Leather restraints also may chafe and abrade the skin. When wrist restraints are necessary, the padded cloth clove hitch produces the least trauma.

Frequently, one or both arms rest on armboards. Abduction, extension, and external rotation may stretch the brachial plexus. Hyperabduction of the arm is to be avoided to prevent stretching of the subclavian and axillary vessels under the coracoid process of the scapula, or compression between the clavicle and the first two ribs. To avoid potential injury, the arm should always be placed at less than a 90-degree angle to the body, with palms up to diminish the pressure on the median and ulnar nerves. The mattress and armboard pad should be of the same height. The armboard should be the type that locks into position on the bed to prevent inadvertent angle changes or sudden loss of support to the arm.

When the head is turned to one side or the other, it should be supported to keep the spine in alignment and secured in the desired position with a doughnut cushion, sandbag, or special headrest. Pressure on the ear and other bony prominences where nerves and blood vessels run superficially must be prevented. The eyes must be guarded against pressure; and as drapes are placed, the eyes must be protected to prevent corneal irritation from textiles, solutions, and other foreign objects.

The circulatory system may be compromised in the dorsal recumbent position, not only by a tight restraint but also by the overall effect of the horizontal body posture and the changed effects of gravity. Depending on the degree of medullary and autonomic nervous system depression by general anesthesia, homeostatic compensatory mechanisms may not function to dilate and constrict blood vessels in response to cardiac or blood volume changes. The increased pressure of abdominal viscera or masses on the inferior vena cava may decrease blood return to the heart; blood pressure would then be lowered. Whenever possible, patient position should encourage venous drainage and avoid obstruction to the major veins. An example is tilting the supine cesarean section patient slightly to the left to prevent excessive pressure on the inferior vena cava before the baby is delivered, particularly with spinal anesthesia.

Respiratory function is also compromised in the dorsal recumbent position because the vital capacity is less than that in the erect posture, notwithstanding the effects of anesthesia. Although anterior and upward excursion of the chest during inspiration is not greatly impeded, diaphragmatic excursion may be lessened by the abdominal viscera. The dorsal recumbent position does allow a more even distribution of ventilation from apex to base of the lungs.

Trendelenburg's position is a variation of the dorsal recumbent position (Fig. 6-4). Occasionally in this position the knees are flexed by "breaking" the lower portion of the bed, and the patient must be positioned with knees over the break in the bed to maintain safe anatomic positioning. Another modification is that of keeping the trunk

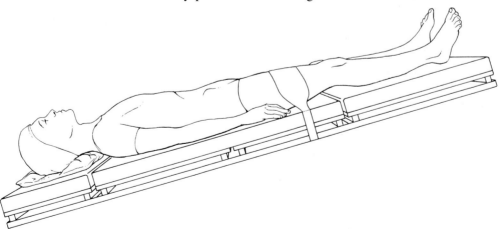

Fig. 6-4. Trendelenburg's position.

level and elevating only the legs by raising the lower part of the bed.

Trendelenburg's position is used either to provide better visualization of the pelvic organs or to improve circulation to the cerebral cortex and basal ganglia when blood pressure is suddenly lowered. In the latter instance, the position enhances arterial blood flow to the cranium, but the venous return pressure is also increased because of necessary venous antigravity flow. Both purposes for this position can be accomplished by occasionally modifying the standard, time-honored, "head down–toes up," tiltboard slant to a position more conducive to physiologic homeostasis.

To reduce pooling of venous blood in the lower extremities, the legs and thighs may be elevated either by pillows or by adjusting the bed. When placing the entire trunk in Trendelenburg's position, the effects of gravitational pull can be improved by flexing the head on the headrest or on a small pillow to promote cranial venous drainage. Although the head-downward position facilitates drainage of secretions from the bases of the lungs and the oropharyngeal passages, the weight of the abdominal viscera further impedes diaphragmatic movement.

The less drastic slant of this modified Trendelenburg's position negates the need for wrist bracelets and shoulder braces that, when improperly placed, would put pressure on the brachial plexus and blood vessels in the neck. This variation of Trendelenburg's position should be maintained only as long as necessary. The patient should be returned slowly to the dorsal recumbent position. Slow, smooth postural transitions allow sufficient time for the body to adjust to the imposed physiologic changes.

Reverse Trendelenburg's position is frequently used to provide access to the head and neck and to facilitate gravitational pull on the viscera away from the diaphragm and toward the feet. When the foot of the bed is tilted toward the floor, the patient's body must be supported by the padded footboard, by nonconstrictive body restraints, and by a liftsheet that supports the arms from above the elbows to the fingers. Lumbar and popliteal pads also tend to prevent the body from slipping. In this position the tilted, head-up bed is usually in a straight line, the opposite of Fig. 6-4.

When a modification of this position is used for thyroid or parathyroid surgery (Fig. 6-5), the neck may be hyperextended by raising the patient's shoulders (using an inflatable pillow, bolster, foam roll, or sandbag), by lowering the headpiece of the bed, or both. There should be no gaps in the support of the neck in this position. When this position is used for biliary surgery, the right side of the patient may be elevated in the horizontal plane by a lengthwise bolster, inflatable gallbladder bag, or tapered foam pad (lemon slice). To prevent twisting of the spine, the full length of the trunk needs support. The hips and shoulders are kept in the same plane.

In the reverse Trendelenburg's position, respiratory function is more like that in the erect position. Venous circulation may be compromised by extended time in the legs-downward position. When this situation is anticipated, the superficial venous return can be aided by the preoperative application of support hose, elastic bandages, or inflatable stockings. If the legs are wrapped, compression of the common peroneal nerve at the head of the fibula must be avoided. Return to the dorsal recumbent position from the reverse Trendelenburg's position should be accomplished slowly and smoothly.

Modified Fowler's (sitting) position causes most of the patient's weight to be on the dorsum of the body. Extra padding should be placed under the buttocks and the small of the back. A potential problem with prolonged pressure on the dorsum is sciatic nerve damage. The position of the body in relation to the breaks in the operating room bed must be carefully adjusted to prevent abnormal pressures. The backrest is elevated, the knees are flexed, and the footboard is set in place. The more erect the patient's posture, the greater the need to support the shoulders and torso. Such support requires adequate padding to protect the axilla and brachial plexus. Frequently, a special headrest is used for cranial ventricular procedures and for posterior fossa craniotomy (Chapter 23). Air embolism is a potential threat in this position due to negative venous pressure in the patient's head and neck area. A Doppler and a central venous pressure line are usually used to monitor the patient during neurosurgical procedures.

The sitting position requires special attention to posi-

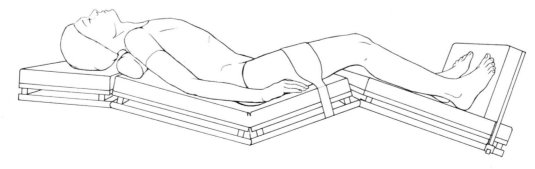

Fig. 6-5. Position for operations on thyroid and neck area.

tioning the arms. Depending on the surgery, the arms may be flexed across the abdomen, resting on a large pillow in the lap, or placed in front of the patient on a padded stand. Hyperextension of the shoulder region must be prevented, and the arms must be secure from falling or pressing against hard surfaces. The vascular system of the arms and legs may require additional supportive measures.

The *lithotomy position* is the most extreme variation of the dorsal recumbent posture (Fig. 6-6). With the patient supine, the legs are raised and abducted to expose the perineal region to gain a surgical approach to the pelvic organs and genitals. This unnatural posture is fraught with danger and discomfort for the patient, and these hazards increase as the position is exaggerated for radical surgery of the groin, vulva, or prostate. Extreme flexion of the thighs impairs respiratory function by increasing intraabdominal pressure against the diaphragm and therefore decreasing the tidal volume. Gravity flow of blood from the elevated legs causes blood to pool in the splanchnic region during the operative procedure. Blood loss during surgery may not be immediately manifested because of this increased splanchnic volume. However, when the legs are lowered and 500 ml or more of blood is diverted to more total leg circulation, the circulating volume is depleted, and the blood pressure may decrease. Normal compensatory mechanisms are depressed by the effect of anesthesia on the nervous system, and homeostasis may not be achieved easily.

Supports for the legs must be carefully chosen and applied. By placing the patient's anterior iliac spine on a line with the leg holder and the buttocks level and on a line with the edge of the break in the operating room bed, a good position can be achieved with a minimum of effort. A small lumbar pad helps to maintain the physiologic concavity of this area.

Modern leg holders provide secure support for the legs without the popliteal pressure of knee crutches and without undue external rotation and abduction, which stretch the abductor muscles and capsule of the hip joint.

The stirrups must be level. The height is adjusted to the length of the patient's legs. This adjustment prevents pressure at the knee and the lumbar spine. The patient's position must be symmetrical. The perineum is in line with the longitudinal axis of the bed; the pelvis is level, and the head and trunk are in a straight line. This position aids the surgeon in identifying anatomic landmarks. Support is provided for the head and neck as previously described.

When a patient is being placed in the lithotomy position, the patient's legs are raised simultaneously. Each leg is raised by grasping the sole of the foot in one hand and supporting the leg near the knee in the other. The leg is raised, and the knee is flexed slowly. The padded foot is secured in the holder by loops of canvas slings. One loop of the canvas sling is placed around the sole at the metatarsals, and the other loop around the ankle. The lower

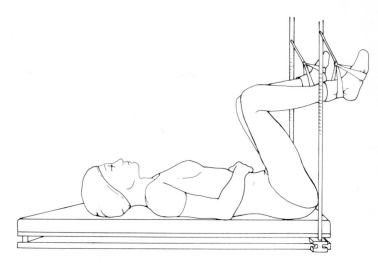

Fig. 6-6. Lithotomy position for vaginal and rectal operations. Stirrups or feet must be padded to prevent patient's skin from touching metal.

part of the leg should be free from pressure against the leg holders to prevent pressure on the common peroneal nerve. Some stirrups may require foam rubber padding between the calves of the legs and the metal posts. Pressure against the soft tissues of the leg may predispose the patient to venous thrombosis. For high lithotomy position during extensive surgery or for patients with ankylosed hip joints, knee and footrest stirrups may be required.

Special care is needed for the patient who has hip prostheses. Severe hip flexion, as well as adduction of the joint, must be avoided in the lithotomy position. The stirrups should be as low as possible and tilted slightly outward, if appropriate. Again, slow and smooth movements are required.

If desired, the patient can be placed in the lithotomy position before anesthesia induction. The patient then has a chance to voice any discomfort or pain, especially of the back, before the procedure begins, and appropriate therapeutic measures can be taken. Because of the exaggeration of this position, any changes in circulatory status or blood pressure can be monitored and treated by the anesthesiologist before induction. With proper explanation regarding this maneuver and adequate covering of the patient's perineal area, the nurse can facilitate the procedure and ease the patient's anxiety.

Arms require special care in the lithotomy position. They should not lie along the sides of the operating room bed because the hands will extend below the break of the foot section of the bed and be in danger of injury when the foot section is raised. They may be folded loosely across the abdomen and supported by the folded gown or a cover sheet, or they may be extended on armboards. Arms must not impede chest movement and respiration. The weight of the limbs on the chest, especially in infants and children, may fatigue the muscles used in respiration and induce respiratory problems.

Adequate assistance must be available for placing the patient in the lithotomy position and for releasing the patient from the position. Any change in body position affects hemodynamics and should be verified beforehand with the anesthesiologist. Movements must be slow and deliberate to allow gradual adjustment to the change. Muscles and joints must be protected from abnormal strain in their relaxed state. The legs should be raised simultaneously to place the feet in the loops of the canvas slings or into padded stirrups. They also must be lowered or taken out of stirrups simultaneously, with support given to the joints above and below to prevent strain on the lumbosacral musculature, which can stretch and tilt, thereby placing the pelvis and limbs in imbalance.

Prone position

In the *prone position* the patient is lying with the abdomen on the surface of the operating room bed mattress. Surgical approaches can then be made to any dorsal surface. Modifications of the position allow approaches to the cervical spine, back, rectal area, and lower extremities. After induction of anesthesia with the patient in the dorsal recumbent posture on a stretcher, the patient is turned onto the abdomen when transferred to the operating room bed. Before the patient is turned, the anesthesiologist secures the endotracheal tube with tape, applies eye ointment into each eye, and then tapes the closed eyelids to prevent corneal abrasions.

"Logroll" turning can be accomplished safely, smoothly, and gently by four persons. The anesthesiologist supports the head and neck during the turn. One assistant stands at the side of the stretcher with hands at the patient's shoulders and buttocks to initiate the roll of the patient. A second assistant stands at the opposite side of the operating room bed, with arms extended to support the chest and lower abdomen as the patient is rolled forward and over. The third assistant stands at the foot of the stretcher to support and turn the legs. At the completion of the turn, the stretcher is removed.

An armboard is provided on each side of the bed, and the patient's arms are brought down and forward to rest on the armboards with elbows flexed and hands pronated. This movement is done to prevent shoulder dislocation and brachial plexus injury. Elbows should be padded and carefully checked for pressure areas. The head is positioned on a foam pillow or towels, with the neck kept in alignment with the spinal column. The eyes are carefully protected.

Body rolls extending lengthwise from the acromioclavicular joint to the iliac crests raise the chest and permit the diaphragm to move freely and the lungs to expand. Supports must not press against the female breasts. Women's breasts and men's genitalia should be checked after final positioning to ensure that they are free from pressure. A bolster or pillow under the pelvis will decrease abdominal pressure on the inferior vena cava. A cushion or pillow is placed under the ankles to prevent pressure on the toes and plantar flexion of the feet. The restraining strap is again placed across the thighs and blanket so that the patient is secured but superficial venous return is not impaired.

The prone posture is initially hazardous as the anesthetized patient is turned from the dorsal recumbent position to the prone position. Normal compensatory mechanisms are depressed, and the patient cannot readily adjust to imposed hemodynamic changes.

Neuromuscularly, the radial nerve may be compressed against the humerus if the forearm is allowed to hang over the side of the bed. The shoulders may be overextended unless the elbows are flexed and the palms pronated. The venous return may be compromised by a tight leg restraint, dependent lower extremities, and visceral compression of the inferior vena cava.

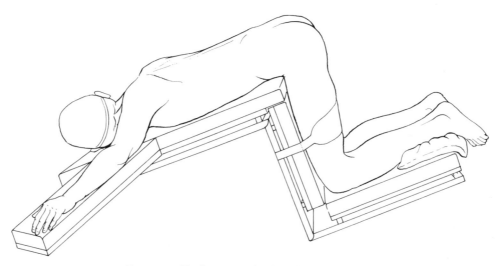

Fig. 6-7. Jackknife position for proctologic operations.

The respiratory system is most vulnerable in the prone position because normal anterolateral respiratory movement is restricted and normal diaphragmatic movement is inhibited by the compressed abdominal wall.

For spinal operations the prone position may be modified to flex the affected part of the spine, for example, the knee-chest position. The hips also may be flexed at one break in the operating room bed and the leg section raised to facilitate a "kneeling" position. The surgeon specifies the modifications preferred.

The *jackknife* or *Kraske's position* is a modification of the prone position that is used for proctological procedures (Fig. 6-7). The patient's hips are placed on a bolster or pillow over the break in the operating room bed, and the bed is flexed at a 90-degree angle, raising the hips and lowering the head and body. The patient's head, chest, and feet need the usual supports in this position. The restraint strap is across the thighs.

The buttocks may be separated with broad straps of adhesive tape secured firmly at the level of the anus a few inches from the midline on either side. These straps are pulled tight simultaneously and are fastened to the underside of the bed surface. The straps are released at the end of the procedure to facilitate the approximation of the wound edges.

If the patient is to be placed on the recovery stretcher in the dorsal recumbent position, the operating room bed is first straightened, and the turning is accomplished by reversing the four-person roll described earlier.

Lateral position

In the *lateral position* the patient is lying on the unaffected side, and the surgical approach may be to the uppermost chest, the kidney, or the upper ureter (Figs. 6-8 and 6-9). Positioning of the extremities and trunk facilitates the desired approach. In lateral positioning, a special

pad or "beanbag" device may be utilized on the operating room bed. The pad is placed prior to the patient's transfer and is to be under the patient's torso. The head and foot portions of the bed are padded to a height equal to the bag to prevent hyperextension of the body when the patient is supine on the bag.

After induction of anesthesia with the patient in the dorsal recumbent position on the operating room bed, the patient is turned to the side. A four-person team is necessary to accomplish a safe, smooth, gentle turn. The anesthesiologist supports the head and neck during the turn. One assistant stands at the shoulder of the operative side facing the patient's head; the assistant's arm and hand nearer the patient cross the chest and grasp the patient's shoulder; the other hand is placed under the nearer shoulder. The second assistant stands at the hips of the operative side, facing the patient's head; the assistant's arm and hand nearer the patient cross the hips and grasp the patient's opposite buttock; the other hand is placed under the nearer buttock. The third assistant stands at the foot of the bed to support and turn the legs. A lifting sheet under the patient can be used by the team to facilitate the turn. At a signal from the anesthesiologist, the first and second assistants lift and bring the patient to his or her side at their edge of the operating room bed; the patient is then placed in the center of the bed. A pillow is placed under the patient's head to maintain good alignment with the cervical spine and the thoracic vertebrae. Another pillow is placed between the patient's legs, the bottom leg flexed at the knee and hip, and the top leg straight or slightly flexed. The lateral aspect of the bottom knee must be padded to prevent pressure on the peroneal nerve, located superficially at the head of the fibula. One assistant should remain at the patient's back to steady and support the torso during positioning of the extremities.

The *lateral chest position* (Fig. 6-8) allows operative

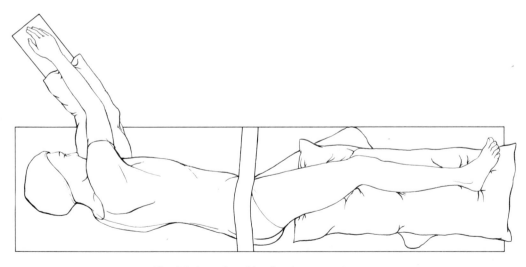

Fig. 6-8. Lateral position for chest operations.

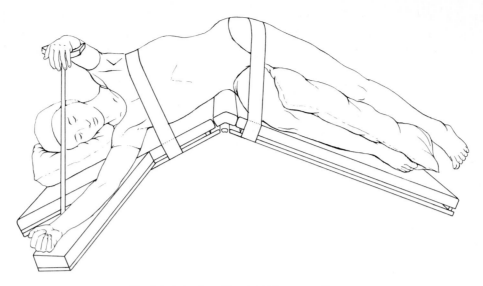

Fig. 6-9. Lateral position for kidney operations.

approach to the uppermost thoracic cavity. The upper arm is flexed slightly at the elbow and raised above the head to elevate the scapula, provide access to the underlying ribs, and widen the intercostal spaces. This arm may be supported on a special raised armboard. The lower shoulder is brought slightly forward to prevent pressure on the brachial plexus and is flexed at the elbow. The lower shoulder may rest on a thin foam pad to prevent tissue pressure from the bony prominence. In chest surgery, infusion and monitoring lines may be placed in the upper or lower arm. Care must be taken to prevent compression of venous return in that arm.

The torso may be stabilized on the bed by well-padded body braces, sandbags, or beanbags. Some surgeons prefer to secure the arms, hips, and legs with wide tape and not use torso supports, which may impede respiratory expansion and decrease the surface area for the surgical approach. A soft roll may be placed at the apex of the scapula in the axillary space to relieve pressure on the arm and allow more chest movement with respirations. True "axillary rolls" are controversial and seldom used. Slanting the upper section of the bed downward places the trachea and mouth at a lower level than the lungs. This slanting of the bed enables bronchial secretions and fluids from the lung bases to drain into the mouth and not pass into the unaffected side of the chest.

For torso stabilization, the legs may be positioned in several ways, according to the surgeon's preference: (1) both legs may be flexed at 90-degree angles at the hips and knees, a pillow placed between the legs, and adhesive tape placed across the hip area to both sides of the top of the bed; (2) the lower leg may be extended straight on the bed, the upper hip and knee flexed at 90-degree angles with two pillows supporting the thigh and calf, the uppermost ankle secured in a padded restraint to the bed top at the patient's back, and adhesive tape placed across the

hip area to both sides of the top of the bed; or (3) the lower hip and knee may be flexed at 90-degree angles, two or more pillows supporting the extended upper leg, the uppermost ankle secured in a padded restraint to the top of the bed at the patient's back, and adhesive tape placed across the upper hip, between the iliac crest and greater trochanter, to both sides of the top of the bed.

The *lateral kidney position* (Fig. 6-9) allows approach to the retroperitoneal area of the flank. After the anesthetized patient is turned from the dorsal position to the lateral position, the patient is moved so that the lower iliac crest is just below the kidney elevator. To render the kidney region readily accessible, the bridge (kidney rest) of the operating room bed is raised and the bed is flexed, so that the area between the twelfth rib and the iliac crest is elevated. A well-padded kidney brace may be placed against the iliac crest. Elevating is dependent on the cardiovascular response of the body to the increased pressure transmitted from this area. The kidney rest is slowly raised; blood pressure is monitored frequently by the anesthesiologist. The bed is then flexed to lower the patient's head and legs. In this position the patient's affected side presents a straight horizontal line from shoulder to hip.

The upper arm is placed on a special raised armboard. The lower shoulder is brought slightly forward, and the arm is flexed to rest on an armboard or near the head on the mattress. A small bolster is placed under the lower axilla to facilitate chest expansion. The lower extremity is flexed and supported by a sandbag or pillow. Two or more pillows support the extended upper leg. The feet should be protected against plantar flexion and the ankles or heels protected from undue pressure. In this position the gravitational force on the head and torso opposes that on the extended limb to facilitate operative exposure. To stabilize the body, a restraining belt or adhesive strap is placed across the shoulder and hip areas and is secured to the bed top. Before wound closure, the adhesive strap is released, the kidney rest lowered, and the bed straightened to facilitate approximation of the wound edges.

Physiologic changes in the lateral position occur in the healthy, alert person but may be more dramatic and stressful in the anesthetized patient. Normally systolic and diastolic pressures decrease when the lateral position is assumed. Because normal compensatory mechanisms are depressed by pharmacologic agents and pathophysiologic processes, the patient may not readily compensate for abrupt postural changes. The acute angulation of the body in the lateral kidney posture and the effect of gravity may also decrease blood return to the right side of the heart.

Respiratory function is compromised by the weight of the body on the lower chest; chest movements are limited, and chest size may be decreased. Diaphragmatic movement is limited by the flexion of the lower limbs toward the abdomen. Another disadvantage of this position is that the weight of the body must rest on the unaffected side, which makes controlling the patient's aspiration of secretions from the lung more difficult on this side. In the lateral kidney position, pressure on the lower thorax and increased tension on the upper intercostal and lumbar musculature interfere with intercostal breathing.

The hazards of neuromuscular damage can largely be prevented through careful manipulation and adequate protective padding. Again, the brachial plexus and common peroneal nerve deserve thoughtful consideration.

EVALUATION

The evaluation of the nursing care plan should be ongoing during the procedure and conclude with a written and verbal report to the postanesthesia care unit nurse. As the outcome of successful implementation of the care plan, the patient is free of injury at the completion of the surgical procedure, as evidenced by

- No redness or change in skin integrity at bony prominences, pressure areas, and the electrosurgical dispersive pad site
- No patient complaints of strained muscles or ligaments, altered range of motion, or compressed or injured nerves postoperatively
- Circulation in extremities matching preoperative status
- No adverse change in hemodynamics related to positioning

Any abnormalities noted should be documented on the postoperative assessment and reported to the surgeon and the postanesthesia care unit nurse.

Positioning is near the top of the list of requirements for safe, successful surgical procedures. Perioperative nurses play a significant role in ensuring uncompromised and physiologically satisfactory patient positioning.

BIBLIOGRAPHY

Anthony, C.P., and Thibodeau, G.A.: Textbook of anatomy and physiology, ed. 12, St. Louis, 1987, The C.V. Mosby Co.

Gendron, F.: "Burns" occurring during lengthy surgical procedures, J. Clin. Eng. 5:19, 1980.

Gruendemann, B.J.: Positioning plus: a clinical handbook on patient positioning for perioperative nurses, Chatsworth, Calif., 1987, Education Department of Devon Industries Inc.

Kneedler, J.A., and Dodge, G.H.: Perioperative patient care, ed. 2, Boston, 1987, Blackwell Scientific Publications, Inc.

Long, B.C., and Phipps, W.J.: Medical-surgical nursing: a nursing process approach, ed. 2, St. Louis, 1989, The C.V. Mosby Co.

Nelson, S.L., Producer: Positioning the surgical patient, Danbury, Conn., 1982, Davis & Geck, American Cyanamid Co. (film).

Phippen, M.: OR nurse's guide to preventing pressure sores, AORN J. 36:205, 1982.

Schmaus, D., Nelson, S., and Davis, D.: Positioning the surgical patient, Denver, 1987, The Association of Operating Room Nurses, Inc.

Sutures, needles, and instruments

JANE C. ROTHROCK

HISTORY AND EVOLUTION OF SURGICAL SUTURES (2000 BC TO PRESENT)

The development of surgical sutures has been closely allied with the development of the art of surgery. Medical writing of ancient Egyptian and Assyrian cultures dating back to 2000 BC mention the various materials used, to a limited extent, for suturing and ligating. *Suture* is a generic term for all materials used to bring severed body tissue together and to hold these tissues in their normal position until healing takes place. A *ligature* is a strand of suture material used to "tie off" (seal) blood vessels to prevent hemorrhage and simple bleeding or to isolate a mass of tissue to be excised (cut out).

The concept of suturing and ligating is also recorded in the writings of the father of medicine, Hippocrates, born in 460 BC. Gut of sheep intestines was first mentioned as suture material in the writings of Galen about AD 200. The Arabian surgeon Rhazes is credited with first employing surgical gut, or catgut, in AD 900 for suturing abdominal wounds. The word *catgut* is a misnomer; it has no relation to a cat but instead originated from the word *kitgut*. The Arabic word *kit* means a dancing master's fiddle, and "kit" strings were originally used for sutures.

Despite these promising early beginnings, the science of surgery, including suturing and ligating, progressed and then regressed, with several cultures never advancing much beyond the rudimentary stages. The principal reasons surgery and its allied practices did not progress in early times were the critical problems of hemorrhage, pain, and infection. Even Ambroïse Paré, the famous French army surgeon of the middle 1500s who developed the technique for ligating to replace cautery in treatment of traumatic war injuries, was confronted with the grim fact that severe pain and subsequent infection markedly curtailed the advancements made possible by surgical repair and correction.

Surgery offered little promise of developing as a truly effective healing science until the nineteenth century, when an American surgeon, Crawford W. Long of Georgia, demonstrated the use of ether as an anesthetic (1842) and Joseph Lister of England first used carbolic acid solution to attempt antiseptic surgery (1865). Lister also experimented with surgical gut as an absorbable suture material and recognized the need for sterile surgical sutures.

Progress in the development of surgical sutures was rapid after the middle 1800s. By 1901, catgut and kangaroo gut were available to the surgeon in sterile glass tubes. Since then, numerous materials have been employed as sutures and ligatures. Gold, silver, metallic wire, silkworm gut, silk, cotton, linen, tendon, and intestinal tissue from virtually every creature that walks, swims, or flies have been used at one time or another throughout the evolution of surgery. During the twentieth century, surgical gut, silk, and cotton emerged as the most commonly used suture materials.

As late as the 1930s, the sterility of sutures commercially prepared and sterilized by manufacturers was subject to question. In addition, sutures varied considerably in their physical properties, such as diameter and strength. From the 1940s to the present, great strides have been made in the uniform preparation and sterilization of suture materials. Today the surgical team is assured of sterility, relatively uniform physical properties, and predictable performance in the sutures received in the operating room.

Since the early 1950s, the trend has been toward individually packaged and presterilized suture materials delivered to the surgical suite in a ready-to-use form. This trend has relieved perioperative nurses of the time-consuming and consequently expensive tasks of preparing sutures and needles for sterilization and then sterilizing them.

SUTURE MATERIALS

A variety of suture materials are available for ligating, suturing, and closing the wound (Table 7-1). The appropriate suture is selected according to a number of characteristics: whether it is absorbable or nonabsorbable, its breaking strength, whether it is monofilament or multifilament, its knot-tying facility, and its tissue reactivity. An understanding of these characteristics of suture materials is essential for the perioperative nurse.

Characteristics of suture material

The three main ways to evaluate the general properties of suture material are: (1) physical characteristics, (2) han-

Table 7-1. General features of absorbable (A) and nonabsorbable (NA) suture materials

Suture	Raw material	Tensile strength (in vivo)	Tissue reaction	Frequent uses
Surgical gut (A) plain	Collagen from sheep or beef intestine	Lost within 7-10 days; faster with severe inflammation; varies with patient characteristics	Moderate	Suture subcutaneous and rapidly healing tissues
Surgical gut (A) chromic	Collagen from sheep or beef intestine; treated to resist digestion	Lost within 21-28 days; varies with patient characteristics	Moderate; less than plain surgical gut	May be used in infected tissues; intended use as an absorbable suture in slowly healing tissues
Polyglactin (A) coated (Vicryl)	Copolymer of lactide and glycolide coated with polyglactin and calcium stearate	Approximately 60% remains at 2 weeks, and 30% at 3 weeks	Mild	Used where an absorbable suture is desired
Polydioxanone (A) (PDS)	Polyester polymer	Approximately 70% remains at 2 weeks, 50% at 4 weeks, and 25% at 6 weeks	Slight	Abdominal and thoracic closure; subcutaneous tissue, colorectal surgery; can be used in infected tissues
Polyglycolic acid (A) (Dexon "S")	Glycolic acid polymer	Approximately 45% remains at 3 weeks	Mild	Peritoneal, fascial, and subcutaneous closures; ligature replaces surgical gut in most applications
Surgical silk (NA)	Protein fiber spun by silkworm	Loses most or all in about 1 year	Moderate	Suturing and ligation; contraindicated in infected tissues; avoid in biliary and urinary tracts
Surgical cotton (NA)	Long staple cotton fibers	Loses 50% in 6 months, and 70% in 2 years	Minimal	Suturing and ligation in most body tissues; contraindicated in infected tissues
Surgical steel (NA)	Alloy of iron-nickel-chromium	Indefinite	Low	Abdominal and sternal closures, retention, tendon repair
Nylon (NA) (Ethilon, Dermalon)	Polyamide polymer	Loses 15-25% per year	Extremely low	Skin closure, retention, microsurgery, tendon repair, pull-out suture
Polypropylene (NA) (Prolene, Surgilene)	Polymer of propylene	Indefinite	Minimal	General closure, vascular anastomoses, pull-out suture
Polyethylene terephthalate (NA) (Dacron, Mersilene Ethibond, Ti·Cron)	Polyester polyethylene terephthalate	Indefinite	Minimal	Ti·Cron and Ethibond are coated, supple in handling, and are especially useful in implanting heart valves and vascular prostheses; general closures; retention

From Davis, C.V., and others: Clinical surgery, St. Louis, 1987, The C.V. Mosby Co.

CHARACTERISTICS OF SUTURE MATERIAL

I. Physical characteristics
Physical configuration
Capillarity
Fluid absorption ability
Diameter (caliber)
Tensile strength
Knot strength
Elasticity
Plasticity
Memory

II. Handling characteristics
Pliability
Tissue drag ⎫
Knot tying ⎬ Related to coefficient of friction
Knot slippage ⎭

III. Tissue reaction characteristics
Inflammatory and fibrous cell reaction
Absorption
Potentiation of infection
Allergic reaction

From Bennett, R.G.: Selection of wound closure materials, J. Am. Acad. Dermatol. 18:619, 1988.

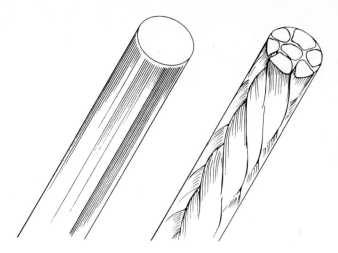

Fig. 7-1. *Left,* Monofilament suture; *right,* multifilament (braided) suture.

dling characteristics, and (3) tissue reaction characteristics (box above). Bennett (1988) describes these as follows:

Physical characteristics

Physical characteristics of suture are officially defined and described by the United States Pharmacopeia (USP). They can be measured or visually determined and include the following properties:

- *Physical configuration:* whether the suture is single-stranded (monofilament) or multistranded (multifilament) (Fig. 7-1)
- *Capillarity:* ability to soak up fluid along the strand
- *Diameter:* determined in millimeters, and expressed in USP sizes with zeroes; the smaller the cross-sectional diameter, the more zeroes
- *Tensile strength:* the amount of weight (breaking load) necessary to break a suture (breaking strength); varies with type of suture material (Table 7-2)
- *Knot strength:* the force necessary to cause a given type of knot to slip, either partially or completely
- *Elasticity:* inherent ability to regain original form and length after having been stretched
- *Memory:* capacity to return to its former shape after being re-formed, such as when tied; high memory yields less knot security

Handling characteristics

Handling characteristics of suture material are related both to pliability, or how easily the material bends, and coefficient of friction, or how easily the suture slips through tissue and ties. A suture with a high friction coefficient tends to "drag" through tissue. It is more difficult to tie because knots do not set easily. Some suture materials are coated to reduce their coefficient of friction. This coating not only improves the way they pull through tissue on insertion, but also affects the force needed to remove the suture after the wound is healed. The coefficient of friction cannot be too low, however, because knots may more easily slip undone.

Tissue reaction characteristics

Because it is a foreign substance, all suture material causes some tissue reaction. Tissue reaction begins when the suture inflicts injury to the tissue during insertion. In addition, tissue reaction to the suture material itself occurs (Table 7-3). This reaction begins with an infiltration of white blood cells; macrophages and fibroblasts then appear; by about the seventh day, fibrous tissue with chronic inflammation is present. The reaction persists until the suture is encapsulated (nonabsorbable material) or absorbed (absorbable material).

Types of suture materials

Suture materials are usually classified into two broad groups: absorbable and nonabsorbable.

Absorbable suture materials

Absorbable suture can be digested or hydrolyzed and assimilated by the tissues during the healing process. The United States Pharmacopeia (USP) defines an absorbable surgical suture as a

Table 7-2. Relative straight pull tensile strength of suture materials

	Nonabsorbable	Absorbable
G ↑	Steel	
R	Polyester	Polyglycolic acid
E	Nylon (monofilamentous)	Polyglactin 910
A	Nylon (braided)	
T	Polypropylene	Polydioxanone
E	Silk	
R		Catgut

From Bennett, R.G.: Selection of wound closure materials, J. Am. Acad. Dermatol. 18:619, 1988.

Table 7-3. Relative tissue reactivity to sutures

	Nonabsorbable	Absorbable
M ↑		Catgut
O	Silk, cotton	
S	Polyester coated	Polyglactin 910
T	Polyester uncoated	Polyglycolic acid
	Nylon	
	Polypropylene	

From Bennett, R.G.: Selection of wound closure materials, J. Am. Acad. Dermatol. 18:622, 1988.

. . . sterile, flexible strand prepared from collagen derived from healthy mammals, or from a synthetic polymer. . . . It is capable of being absorbed by living mammalian tissue, but may be treated to modify its resistance to absorption. . . . It may be modified with respect to body or texture. It may be impregnated with a suitable coating, softening, or antimicrobial agent. It may be colored by a color additive approved by the federal Food and Drug Administration.

Absorbable sutures vary in treatment, color, size, packaging, and resistance to absorption, according to their purpose. Types of absorbable suture include plain or chromatized catgut, collagen, and glycolic acid polymers (Table 7-4).

Surgical gut

Surgical gut, or catgut, is obtained from the collagen of the submucosal layer of the small intestine of sheep or the intestinal serosa of cattle (Hardy, 1988). Catgut sutures may be either type A suture (plain catgut) or type C suture. Both types consist of processed strands of collagen, but type C suture is processed by physical or chemical means (chromatization) to provide greater resistance to absorption in living mammalian tissue, hence its name, *chromic catgut.*

Proper chromatizing of gut ensures the integrity of the suture and maintenance of its strength during the early stages of wound healing. It enables the wound with slow healing power to gather sufficient strength of its own before the suture is entirely absorbed. To chromatize the gut strands, the tanning process is applied either to the submucosal ribbons before they have been twisted into the strand or to the finished strand after it has been formed from the ribbons. The strength of the chromium salt content and the duration of the chromatizing process are accurately controlled and tested.

The absorption rate of surgical gut is also influenced by the type of body tissue it contacts and, to some extent, by the patient's general physical condition. Studies also show that surgical gut is absorbed faster in serous or mu-

cous membranes than in muscular tissues. When fine chromic gut is properly buried in successive layers of the gastrointestinal tract, for example, it retains its strength long enough for primary union to take place.

The elaborate processes of mechanical and chemical cleaning of the raw gut are followed by sterilization, usually with cobalt 60 irradiation, and storage in hermetically sealed packages. Modern manufacturing processes also ensure tensile strength, more controlled absorption, and predictable results.

Restoring pliability. To provide maximum pliability of surgical gut sutures, the gut should be used immediately after removal from the packet. When a gut suture is removed from its packet and is not used at once, the alcohol evaporates, which causes the strand to lose its pliability. The strand's pliability may be restored just before use by immersing it in sterile water or normal saline solution, preferably at 37° C (98.6° F). If the latter method is used, the gut strand should be immersed for only a few seconds.

Collagen sutures

Collagen sutures are extruded from the tendon of cattle. They are chemically treated to remove noncollagenous material, purified, and processed into strands that have physical properties superior to surgical gut (*Wound Closure Manual,* 1988). Collagen suture is most often used as a fine suture material for the eye.

Synthetic absorbable sutures

To produce synthetic absorbable sutures, specific polymers are extruded into suture strands that range in size from no. 10-0 to no. 2. These sutures are packaged dry and are not to be dipped or soaked in water or saline. Moisture reduces the tensile strength. Polyglactin 910 (Vicryl) suture is a copolymer of lactide and glycolide. The precisely controlled combination of these two substances results in a molecular structure that maintains sufficient tensile strength for efficient approximation of tissues dur-

Table 7-4. Comparison of absorbable sutures

Trade name	Company	Material	Configuration	Tensile strength	Tissue reactivity
Collagen (plain)	Davis & Geck	Beef flexor tendon	Twisted	Poor (0% at 2-3 weeks)	Moderate
Collagen (chromic)	Davis & Geck	Beef flexor tendon	Twisted	Poor (0% at 2-3 weeks)	Moderate
Surgical gut (plain)	Ethicon; Davis & Geck	Animal collagen	Twisted	Poor (0% at 2-3 weeks)	High
Surgical gut (chromic)	Ethicon; Davis & Geck	Animal collagen	Twisted	Poor (0% at 2-3 weeks)	Moderately high
Coated Vicryl	Ethicon	Polyglactin 910 (coated with calcium stearate and polyglactin 370)	Braided	Good (50% at 2-3 weeks)	Low
Dexon "S"	Davis & Geck	Polyglycolic acid	Braided	Good (50% at 2-3 weeks)	Low
Dexon Plus	Davis & Geck	Polyglycolic acid (coated with poloxamer 188)	Braided	Good (50% at 2-3 weeks)	Low
PDS	Ethicon	Polydioxanone	Monofila-mentous	Good (50% at 2-3 weeks)	Low

Reproduced and modified from Bennett, R.G.: Fundamentals of cutaneous surgery, St. Louis, 1988, The C.V. Mosby Co.

ing wound healing and then absorbs rapidly. Polyglycolic acid (Dexon) suture, a homopolymer of glycolic acid, is a popular suture material and was the first synthetic absorbable suture on the market. It absorbs slightly faster than the Polyglactin 910 suture.

The newest synthetic absorbable sutures are PDS, prepared from the polyester poly(*P*-dioxanone), and Maxon, prepared from polyglycomate. These soft, pliable monofilament materials provide wound support twice as long as other synthetic absorbable sutures. Absorption is minimal until about 3 months postoperatively. Maxon and PDS are useful when prolonged patient wound healing is expected, as with fascial closures or surgery performed on elderly or oncological patients. The PDS suture combines two desirable qualities: absorbability and extended wound support.

Synthetic absorbable sutures are absorbed by slow hydrolysis in the presence of tissue fluids. Hydrolysis is the chemical process whereby the polymer reacts with water to cause an alteration of breakdown of the molecular structure. These sutures are degraded in tissue by this process at a more predictable rate than surgical gut (or collagen) and with less tissue reaction.

Nonabsorbable sutures

Nonabsorbable sutures are strands of material that effectively resist enzymatic digestion in living animal tissue.

A single strand may be composed of metal or of organic material. Each strand is of substantially uniform diameter throughout its length. It may be composed of a single filament or of filaments of fibers rendered into a thread by spinning, twisting, braiding, or any combination thereof. It may be coated or uncoated. It may be untreated for reduction of capillarity and designated type A, untreated and capillary; or it may be treated to reduce capillarity and designated type B, treated and noncapillary. It may be uncolored, naturally colored, or dyed with a suitable dyestuff (Table 7-5).

The USP classifies nonabsorbable surgical suture as:

Class I suture is composed of silk or synthetic fibers of monofilament, twisted, or braided construction. . . .

Class II suture is composed of cotton or linen fibers or coated natural or synthetic fibers where the coating significantly affects thickness but does not contribute significantly to strength.

Class III suture is composed of monofilament or multifilament metal wire.

Nonabsorbable suture materials are not absorbed in tissues during the process of wound healing. Generally, the material remains encapsulated or walled off by the tissues around it. In suturing skin, for which nonabsorbable materials are often the choice, the sutures are removed before healing is complete.

Handling	Knot security	Memory	Absorption	Degradation	Comments
Fair	Poor	Low	Unpredictable (12 weeks)	Proteolytic	Less impure than surgical gut
Fair	Poor	Low	Unpredictable (12 weeks)	Proteolytic	Less impure than surgical gut
Fair	Poor	Low	Unpredictable (12 weeks)	Proteolytic	May be ordered as "fast-absorbing gut" (Ethicon) for percutaneous sutures
Fair	Fair	Low	Unpredictable (14-80 days)	Proteolytic	Darker, more visible (Davis & Geck): mild or extra chromatization (Davis & Geck)
Good	Fair	Low	Predictable (80 days)	Hydrolytic	Clear, violet, coated
Fair	Good	Low	Predictable (90 days)	Hydrolytic	Uncoated
Good	Fair	Low	Predictable (90 days)	Hydrolytic	Clear, green, coated
Poor	Poor	High	Predictable (180 days)	Hydrolytic	Violet, clear

Types of nonabsorbable suture materials

The most common nonabsorbable suture materials are silk, cotton, nylon, polyester fiber, polypropylene, and stainless steel wire.

Silk

Silk is prepared from thread spun by the silkworm larva in making its cocoon. Top-grade raw silk is processed to remove the natural waxes and gum, manufactured into threads, and dyed with a vegetable dye. The strands of silk are either twisted or braided to form the suture. Modern silk is braided, which gives it high tensile strength and better handling qualities. Silk handles well, is soft, and forms secure knots. Untreated silk has a capillary action through which body fluids may transmit infection along the length of the suture strand. For this reason surgical silk is treated to render it noncapillary (able to withstand the action of body fluids and moisture). It is available in sizes 9-0 to 5, in sterile packets or precut lengths and with or without swaged needles. The sterile precut type relieves the nurse from having to expend time preparing strands. Silk should be kept dry by the scrub nurse. Wet silk loses up to 20% in strength.

In the strict sense, silk is not a true nonabsorbable material. In a wound it loses its tensile strength after about a year and may disappear after several years. Silk sutures occasionally migrate gradually to a wound's exterior, pro-

ducing "spitting." Spitting is annoying and sometimes frightening to the patient but has no deleterious effect on wound healing.

Cotton

Surgical cotton sutures are made from individual cotton fibers that are combed, aligned, and twisted to form a finished strand. They differ from other sutures in that twisted cotton gains 10% in tensile strength when wet. Therefore, cotton sutures should be moistened before use. Fine cotton sutures, when buried in tissue, produce minimum tissue reaction but should not be used in the presence of infection. Cotton handles much like silk but is not as strong.

Surgical nylon

Surgical nylon (Dermalon, Ethilon, Surgilon, Nurolon) is a synthetic polyamide material. It is available in two forms: multifilament (braided) and monofilament strands. Multifilament nylon is relatively inert in tissues and has a high tensile strength. It is used in conditions similar to those in which silk and cotton are used. Because of its elasticity, the surgeon usually ties three knots in small sutures and a double square knot in large sutures. It has excellent knot security. Monofilament nylon is a smooth, noncapillary material particularly well suited for closing skin edges and also for tension sutures. It is strong, rel-

Table 7-5. Comparison of nonabsorbable sutures

Generic or trade name	Company	Material	Configuration	Tensile strength
Cotton	—	Cotton	Twisted	Good
Silk	Ethicon; Davis & Geck	Silk	Braided	Good
Ethilon	Ethicon	Polyamide (nylon)	Monofilamentous	High
Dermalon	Davis & Geck	Polyamide (nylon)	Monofilamentous	High
Surgamid	Look	Polyamide (nylon)	Monofilamentous or braided	High
Nurolon	Ethicon	Polyamide (nylon)	Braided	High
Surgilon	Davis & Geck	Polyamide (nylon) (coated with silicone)	Braided	High
Prolene	Ethicon	Polyolefin (polypropylene)	Monofilamentous	Fair
Surgilene	Davis & Geck	Polyolefin (polypropylene)	Monofilamentous	Fair
Dermalene	Davis & Geck	Polyolefin (polypropylene)	Monofilamentous	Good
Novafil	Davis & Geck	Polybutester	Monofilamentous	High
Mersilene	Ethicon	Polyester	Braided	High
Dacron	Deknatel; Davis & Geck	Polyester	Braided	High
Polyviolene	Look	Polyester	Braided	High
Ethibond	Ethicon	Polyester (coated with polybutilate)	Braided	High
Ti·Cron	Davis & Geck	Polyester (coated with silicone)	Braided	High
Polydek	Deknatel	Polyester (coated with Teflon-light)	Braided	High
Tevdek	Deknatel	Polyester (coated with Teflon-heavy)	Braided	High
Stainless steel	Ethicon	Stainless steel	Monofilamentous, twisted, or braided	High

From Bennett, R.G.: Selection of wound closure materials, J. Am. Acad. Dermatol. 18:4, 1988.

atively inert, and nonirritating in tissues. It is frequently used in ophthalmology and microsurgery because it can be manufactured in fine sizes. Size no. 11-0 nylon is one of the smallest suture materials available.

Surgical polyester fiber

Surgical polyester fiber (Ti·Cron, Dacron, Mersilene, Tevdek, Polydek, Ethibond) is available in two forms: a nontreated polyester fiber suture and a polyester fiber suture that has been specifically coated or impregnated with a lubricant. Polyester fiber is available in fine filaments that can be braided into various suture sizes. They are closely braided to provide good handling properties.

This material has many advantages over other braided, nonabsorbable sutures. It has greater tensile strength, minimum tissue reaction, maximum visibility, and nonabsorbency of tissue fluids. The treated polyester fiber suture offers additional advantages of smooth passage through tissue and smooth tie-down on each throw of the knot. Polybutilate, a polyester surgical lubricant, adheres tightly to the polyester suture (Ethibond). Other commercial lubricants are used, but they are not specifically designed for suture use. Coated polyester sutures are used in cardiovascular surgery for valve replacements, graft-to-tissue anastomoses, and revascularization procedures.

Polybutester (Novafil), a special type of polyester su-

Tissue reactivity	Handling	Knot security	Memory	Comments
High	Good	Good	Poor	Obsolete
High	Good	Good	Poor	Predisposes to infection; does not tear tissue; D & G suture is silicone treated; Ethicon is waxed
Low	Poor	Poor	High	Cuts tissue; nylon 6,6; black, clear, or green
Low	Poor	Poor	High	Nylon 6,6
Low	Poor	Poor	High	Nylon 6,6
Moderate	Good	Fair	Fair	May predispose to infection; black or white; waxed; nylon 6,6
Moderate	Fair	Fair	Fair	Nylon 6,6
Low	Poor	Poor	High	Very low coefficient of friction; cuts tissue; blue or clear
Low	Poor	Poor	High	—
Low	Poor	Poor	High	—
Low	Fair	Poor	Low	Blue or clear
Moderate	Good	Good	Fair	Green or white
Moderate	Good	Good	Fair	—
Moderate	Good	Good	Fair	Green or white
Moderate	Good	Good	Fair	Green or white
Moderate	Poor	Poor	Fair	—
Moderate	Good	Good	Fair	—
Moderate	Poor	Poor	Fair	—
Low	Poor	Good	Poor	May kink

ture, was introduced in the 1980s. This suture possesses many of the advantages of both polyester and polypropylene. Because it is a monofilament, it induces little tissue reaction.

Polypropylene

Polypropylene is a clear or pigmented polymer. This monofilament suture material (Prolene, Surgilene) is used for cardiovascular, general, and plastic surgery. Because polypropylene is a monofilament and is extremely inert in tissue, it may be used in the presence of infection. It has high tensile strength, causes minimal tissue reaction, and holds knots well. Surgeons have indicated that polypropylene sutures can be tied into more secure knots than most other synthetic suture materials. Sizes range from no. 10-0 to no. 2, swaged to needles.

Surgical stainless steel

Surgical stainless steel is formulated to be compatible with stainless steel implants and prostheses. This formula, 316L (L for low carbon), ensures absence of toxic elements, optimal strength, flexibility, and uniform size.

Monofilament and multifilament surgical stainless steel has an enviable reputation among nonabsorbable sutures for strength, inertness, and low tissue reaction. However, the stainless steel suturing technique is very exacting. Steel

Table 7-6. Steel suture comparison

Size (USP)	B&S gauge	Size (USP)	B&S gauge
6-0	40	0	26
6-0	38	1	25
5-0	35	2	24
4-0	34	3	23
4-0	32	4	22
000	30	5	20
00	28	7	18

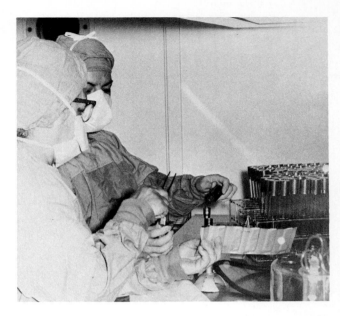

Fig. 7-2. Preparation of individual packages of suture. (Courtesy Ethicon, Inc., Somerville, N.J.)

can pull or tear out of tissue, and necrosis can result from too tight a suture. Barbs on the end of steel can tear gloves, thus breaking sterile technique, or they can traumatize surrounding tissue. Kinks in the wire can render it practically useless. For this reason, packaging has played a unique part in the development of surgical stainless steel sutures.

Surgical stainless steel is available on spools or in packages of straight, precut, sterile lengths, with or without swaged needles. This packaging affords protection to the strands and delivery in straight, unkinked lengths.

Before surgical stainless steel's availability from suture manufacturers, it was purchased by weight with the Brown and Sharp (B&S) scale for diameter variations. Today the B&S gauge, along with USP size classifications, is used to distinguish diameter size ranges. Table 7-6 gives comparisons of steel sutures.

Packaging and storage methods

Manufacturers now supply almost all suture materials in some form of sterile package ready for immediate use (Fig. 7-2). The USP specifies, "Preserve . . . dry or in fluid, in containers so designed that sterility is maintained until the container is opened." The obsolete so-called wet pack method consisted of sealing the sutures in glass tubes, foil, or plastic packets, immersing them in a chemical solution, and storing them in glass jars or metal cans.

In the current dry packaging method, the suture material is sealed in a primary inner packet, which may or may not contain fluid, inside a dry, outer, peel-back packet. This unit is sterilized. This method permits easy dispensing onto the sterile field. Various forms of foil, plastic, and special paper are used for both the inner and outer packets. Packages are stored in moistureproof and dustproof containers.

Each primary suture packet is self-contained, and its sterility for each patient is ensured as long as the integrity of the packet is maintained. Some suture packets have expiration dates that relate to stability and sterility.

Suture packets may contain single or multiple strands, with or without a needle swaged to the strand. The smaller

sutures are in greater demand because the finer diameter provides better handling qualities and small knots. Improved suturing techniques are possible with sutures of finer diameter. Studies indicate that wounds heal more quickly and with less tissue reaction when sutures of a finer gauge are used.

Skin staples

Skin staples are one of the most frequently chosen methods of skin closure. They can be used on many types of surgical incisions. These staples are disposable and easy to use. They reduce both operating time and tissue trauma, allowing uniform tension along the suture line and less distortion from the stress of individual suture points. However, they leave unsatisfactory skin marks if they are placed too tightly or allowed to remain in the skin longer than 1 week (Miller, 1988). They are prepackaged in various assortments of numbers of and types of staples, depending on the length of the incision and the type of tissue encountered. An extractor is required for their removal.

Skin tapes

The selection of surgical tape for skin closure is based on the tape's adhesive ability, tensile strength, and porosity. The tape must provide a firm tape-to-skin bond in order to keep the wound edges closely adherent. The tensile strength must be sufficient to maintain wound approximation. A tape that is too occlusive limits moisture vapor transmission; fluid may accumulate under the tape and lead to maceration and bacterial growth. Microporous tapes prevent this. Wounds that are subjected to minimal static and dynamic tension are easily approximated with skin tape. The tape must be applied to dry skin; an adhesive adjunct (for example, tincture of benzoin) may be applied in a thin film to the skin at the wound edges prior to tape application. Tapes are applied perpendicular to the wound edge, on one side and then the other, so that the edges can be pulled together.

SELECTION OF SUTURES

Suture use is dependent on the procedure, the tissue being sutured, the general condition of the patient, and the surgeon's preferences.

An operating room committee or surgical group may be responsible for establishing standard suture uses for various operations. Current guides published by suture manufacturers should be consulted. These guides list the specific suture materials recommended for various wounds and are based on current clinical practices and research.

To develop standards related to suture usage, nurses may use a collecting data sheet that is divided into columns with the desired headings, such as sutures for subcutaneous use. A code or symbols may be used to identify the types and sizes of sutures. Suture cards may be obtained from some manufacturers.

SURGICAL NEEDLES

Surgical needles vary considerably in shape, size, point design, and wire diameter (Fig. 7-3). The appropriate needle is selected depending on the surgical procedure being performed and the type of tissue being sutured. In general, cutting-edge needles are used on tough tissue (skin or eye tissues) and taper needles are used on soft tissue (bowel or subcutaneous tissues).

Surgical needles are made from either stainless steel or carbon steel. They must be strong, ductile, and able to withstand the stress imposed by tough tissue. Stainless steel is the most popular, not only because it provides these physical characteristics but also because it is non-corrosive.

Surgical needles fall into three general categories: (1) eyed needles, in which the needle must be threaded with the suture strand and two strands of suture must be pulled through the tissue; (2) spring or French eyed needles, in which the suture is secured through the spring; and (3) eyeless needles, a needle-suture combination in which a needle is swaged onto one or both ends of the suture material.

The most universally used needle type is the swaged, or atraumatic, needle (Fig. 7-4). The surgeon draws a single strand of suture material through the tissue, and tissue damage is thereby minimized. Swaged needles also eliminate threading eyed needles before and during surgery. Studies indicate that swaged needles provide greater safety to patients and economic use of materials and time. The swaged needle, permanently attached to the suture strand, must be cut off with scissors. A needle swaged for

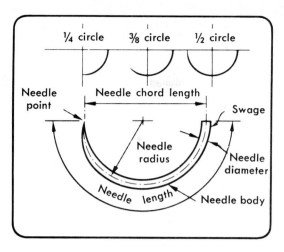

Fig. 7-3. Surgical needle differentiation by type, shape, and point. (Courtesy Ethicon, Inc., Somerville, N.J.)

controlled release of the suture (semiswaged) facilitates interrupted suturing techniques. The needle remains attached until the surgeon releases it with a straight tug of the needle holder.

The body of the needle may be round, triangular, or flattened. The body of a round needle gradually tapers to a point. It tends to tear tissue less than cutting needles and leaves a small hole in the tissue. Triangular needles have cutting edges along three sides. The cutting action may be conventional or reverse cutting (Fig. 7-5). The reverse cutting needle is preferred for cutaneous suturing. When it transects the skin lateral to the wound, the outside edge is pointed away from the wound edge, and the inside flat edge is parallel to the edge of the wound. This cutting action creates less of a tendency for suture to tear through tissue (Bennett, 1988). The conventional cutting needle has its cutting edge directed along the inner curve of the needle, facing the wound edge when suturing.

Surgical needles may also be straight or curved; the curve is described as part of an imaginary circle (Fig. 7-

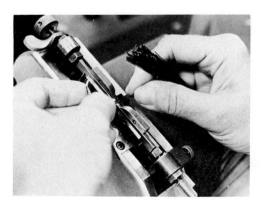

Fig. 7-4. Process of swaging needle to suture during manufacture. (Courtesy Ethicon, Inc., Somerville, N.J.)

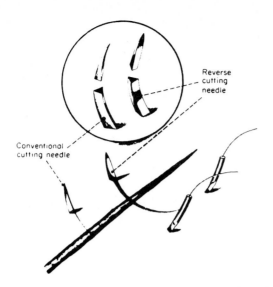

Fig. 7-5. Comparison between conventional cutting needle and reverse cutting needle. Conventional cutting needle has cutting edge directed toward wound and flat surface away from wound; reverse cutting needle has flat surface toward wound and cutting edge away from wound. (From Bennett, R.G.: Selection of wound closure materials, J. Am. Acad. Dermatol. 18:632, 1988.)

3). As the radius of the imaginary circle increases, the size of the needle also increases.

For certain types of delicate surgery, needles with exceptionally sharp points and cutting edges are used. Microsurgery, ophthalmology, and plastic surgery require needles of this type; special honing wheels provide needles of precision-point quality for surgeons in these specialties.

In addition, developments in the 1980s included the application of a microthin layer of plastic to the needle surface, providing for easier penetration and a reduction in drag of the needle through the tissue.

Most operating rooms have instituted standardization programs to reduce the variety of needle-suture combinations available for different types of surgical procedures.

TYPES OF SUTURE LINES AND SUTURING METHODS
Closure of wounds

The *primary suture line* refers to sutures that hold the edges of the wound in approximation until healing takes place. The *secondary suture line* refers to sutures that supplement the primary suture line, obliterate dead space, and prevent serum from accumulating in the wound.

Buried sutures, usually referred to as *subcuticular*, are those placed completely under the epidermal layer of the skin.

A *ligature* is a strand of suture material used to encircle or close off the lumen of a vessel, effect hemostasis, close off a structure, or prevent leakage of materials.

A *suture ligature, stick tie,* or *transfixion ligature* is a strand of suture material threaded or swaged on a needle. The needle is used to prevent the ligature from slipping off the end of the vessel or structure, especially when the vessel is fairly large.

When two ligatures are used to ligate a large vessel, usually a free ligature is placed on the vessel and then a suture ligature is placed distal to the first ligature. To ligate a blood vessel situated in deep tissues, the strand must be of sufficient strength and length to allow the surgeon to tighten the first knot.

Any one of several techniques can be used to secure a ligature in deep tissues:

1. A hemostat is placed on the end of the structure; the ligature secured in a forceps is then placed over the vessel. The knot is tied and tightened by means of the surgeon's fingers or with the aid of forceps.
2. A slipknot is made, and its loop is placed over the involved structure by means of a forceps or clamp.
3. A forceps or clamp is applied to the structure; then transfixion sutures are applied and tied.

The preparation of ligatures and suture ligatures is discussed in a later section of this chapter.

An interrupted suture is inserted in tissues or vessels in such a way that each stitch is self-contained and tied. This type of suture is widely used and generally considered the most efficient (Fig. 7-6). The various techniques used for the insertion of interrupted sutures in the tissue result in a mattress suture, vertical, horizontal, or crossed in a figure-of-eight stitch (Fig. 7-7, A). These techniques are designed to alter the angle of pull and the relationship of the wound's edges to each other. Such maneuvers cause the edges of the wound either to invert or to evert and aid in wound healing because fewer sutures are used.

A continuous suture consists of a series of stitches, of which only the first and last are tied (Fig. 7-8). This type of suture is not widely used because a break at any point may mean a disruption of the entire suture line. It is used, however, to close a tissue layer such as the peritoneum, which does not have great strength but requires a tight closure to prevent the intestinal loops from protruding.

A purse-string suture is a continuous circular suture placed to surround an opening in a structure and cause it to close. This type of suture may be placed around the appendix before its removal or in an organ such as the cecum, gallbladder, or urinary bladder before opening it so that a drainage tube can be inserted, followed by tightening of the purse-string suture.

A retention or stay suture provides a secondary suture line (Fig. 7-9). These sutures, which are placed at a distance from the primary suture line, relieve undue strain and help obliterate dead space. They are placed in the wound in such a way that they include most if not all layers of the wound. A simple interrupted or figure-of-

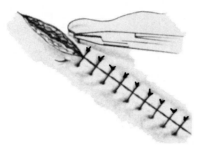

Fig. 7-6. Interrupted suture technique. (Courtesy Ethicon, Inc., Somerville, N.J.)

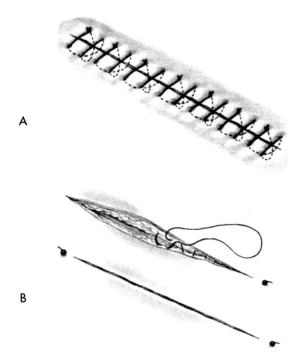

Fig. 7-7. Two types of skin closure. **A,** Interrupted figure-of-eight sutures. **B,** Continuous subcuticular closure anchored with lead shot. (Courtesy Ethicon, Inc., Somerville, N.J.)

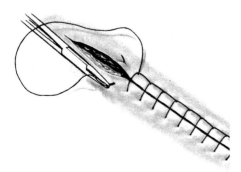

Fig. 7-8. Continuous suture technique. (Courtesy Ethicon, Inc., Somerville, N.J.)

eight stitch is used. Usually heavy, nonabsorbable suture materials such as silk, nylon, polyester fiber, or wire are used to close long, vertical abdominal wounds and lacerated or infected wounds. To prevent the suture from cutting into the skin surface, a small piece of rubber tubing or other type of "bumper" is passed over or through the exposed portion of the suture (Fig. 7-9, *C*), or the suture is tied over a plastic bridge. The bridge device allows the surgeon to adjust tension over the wound postoperatively.

Holding a drain in place

If a drainage tube is inserted in the wound, the tube may be anchored to the skin with a nonabsorbable suture so that it will not slip in or out. A tube left in a hollow viscus, such as the gallbladder or common duct, may be secured to the wall of that organ with an absorbable suture.

Knot-tying technique

The successful use of the many varieties of suture materials depends, in the final analysis, on the skill with

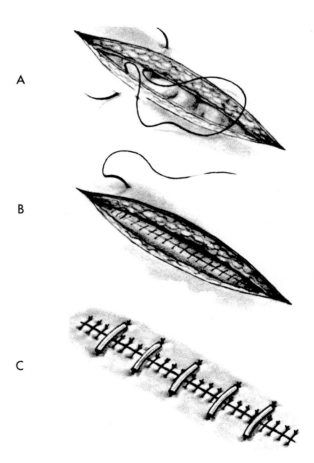

Fig. 7-9. Retention suture technique. **A,** Surgeons may place retention sutures from inside peritoneal cavity through to skin. **B,** Other surgeons prefer to close peritoneum first, then place retention sutures to penetrate only layers from fascia to skin. **C,** To prevent heavy materials from cutting into skin, "bolsters" or "bumpers" are used with retention sutures. (Courtesy Ethicon, Inc., Somerville, N.J.)

which the surgeon or RN first assistant (RNFA) ties the knot. The completed knot should be firm to prevent slipping and small with ends cut short to minimize the bulk of suture material in the wound. The suture may be weakened by excessive tension, sawing, friction between the strands, and inadvertent crushing with clamps or hemostats.

Ligating clips

Ligating clips may be made of several metals, such as stainless steel, tantalum, and titanium. Stainless steel clips are the most economic to use. Although more expensive, titanium clips are used frequently in specific surgical procedures because the "starburst" effect on postoperative radiographic scans is less with titanium than with other metals.

Ligating clips are available in several sizes; each size requires its own size of applier (Fig. 7-10). Ligating clips afford the surgeon or RN first assistant a rapid and secure method of accomplishing hemostasis or of ligating arteries, veins, nerves, and other small structures. These clips are available in disposable, prepackaged units. Absorbable clips made of PDS (synthetic absorbable suture material) are also available.

Metal Cushing or Frazier clips are made of small-diameter pieces of stainless steel or silver wire and are heat sterilized. In neurosurgery and other orthopedic procedures, Frazier clips are applied to the ends of severed nerves and blood vessels by means of a forceps designed for the purpose.

Perioperative nursing considerations

In the preparation and use of sutures in surgery, every precaution must be taken to keep the sutures sterile, to prevent prolonged exposure and unnecessary handling, and to avoid waste. Before the nurses prepare the sutures, they should review the sutures listed in the card file for a particular procedure and surgeon. The scrub nurse should prepare only one or two sutures during the preliminary preparation, but the circulating nurse should have an adequate supply of sutures available for immediate dispensing to the sterile instrument table. Use of suture materials in dry packages provides sterile sutures ready for use, reduces the time previously needed to prepare them, and decreases wasted motion (Fig. 7-11).

Customized suture kits that contain a designated number and variety of sutures for particular procedures, surgeons, or both are available for use when suture preferences are consistently the same. These kits may be more economic because of reduced packaging costs, decreased "pulling" and dispensing times, less waste, and less capital outlay for inventory.

Opening primary packets

The scrub nurse tears the foil packet across the notch near the hermetically sealed edge and removes the suture (Fig. 7-12). Plastic packets may be torn along designated lines or opened with suture scissors.

Handling suture materials

To remove a suture that does not have a needle, the loose end is pulled out with one hand while the folder is grasped with the other hand. To straighten a long suture, the free end is grasped (using the thumb and forefinger of the free hand) and the kinks are removed by pulling gently. The free ends are secured in one hand and the center loop in the other, and then slowly the arms are abducted slightly to straighten the strands.

Kinks should never be removed by running gloved fingers over the strand because this action causes fraying. The tensile strength of a gut suture should not be tested before it is handed to the surgeon. Sudden pulls or jerks used to test the tensile strength of a suture may damage it so that it will break when in use.

To prepare individual ligatures and sutures, the strand is folded in equal parts and held between the fingers; then the strand is divided (Fig. 7-13). Sutures are also provided in 12- to 30-inch precut lengths by the manufacturer.

In many institutions, spiral wound sutures are used. Long sutures are wound on cylindrical or circular reels supplied by suture manufacturers (Fig. 7-14). The surgeon holds the reel while ligating the bleeding vessels. This

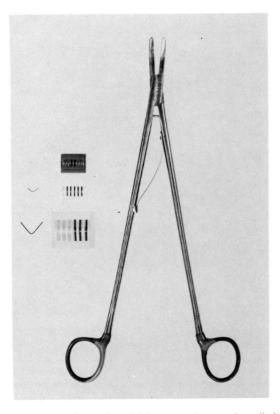

Fig. 7-10. Ligating clip applier with large, medium, and small clips.

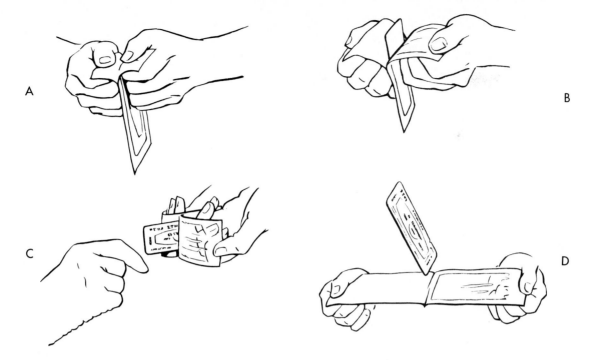

Fig. 7-11. Opening suture packet. **A,** Circulating nurse grasps two flaps between extended thumbs; **B,** rolls thumbs outward, peeling overwrap halfway down sealed edges; **C,** offers sterile inner pact to scrub nurse; **D,** or flips it onto sterile surface. (Courtesy Ethicon, Inc., Somerville, N.J.)

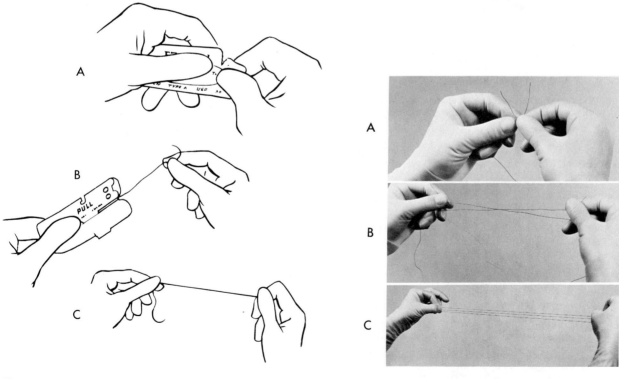

Fig. 7-12. Preparation of prepackaged individual suture. **A,** Opening sterile package. **B,** Swaged-on needle and suture strand are removed from package as a unit. **C,** Suture strand is grasped at both ends. (Courtesy Ethicon, Inc., Somerville, N.J.)

Fig. 7-13. Preparation of individual "freehand" ligatures. **A,** Free ends of ligature are grasped in each hand and gently pulled to remove kinks. **B,** Ligature is folded in equal parts of desired length. **C,** Ligatures are divided into individual strands. (Courtesy Ethicon, Inc., Somerville, N.J.)

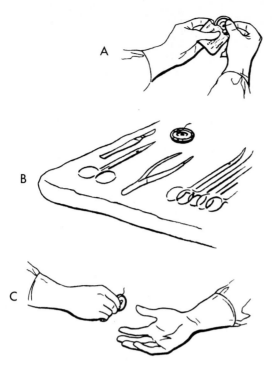

Fig. 7-14. Preparation of continuous ties on plastic disk type of reel. **A,** Foil packet containing appropriate material on reel is torn open. **B,** End of strand is extended slightly for easy grasping. Reel is placed conveniently on Mayo tray. **C,** Scrub nurse passes reel to surgeon as needed, being certain end of ligating material is free to be grasped. (Courtesy Ethicon, Inc., Somerville, N.J.)

technique eliminates the need to rewind sutures on reels, saves nurses' time, and eliminates wasted motions.

To remove a suture-needle combination, the scrub nurse grasps the needle of the suture with a needle holder and gently pulls the strand to remove it. To straighten the suture in a suture-needle combination, the scrub nurse grasps the suture 1 to 2 inches distal to the needle and pulls gently on the end of the strand. The jaws of the needle holder are placed on the flattened surface of the needle to prevent breakage and bending. To facilitate suturing, the needle is secured near the tip of the needle holder (Fig. 7-15). The opening of a multiple suture packet is shown in Fig. 7-16.

Cutting suture lengths

A suture or free ligature should not be too long or too short. A long suture is difficult to handle and increases the possibility of contamination because it may be dragged across the sterile field or fall below it. A short suture makes tying difficult, and if threaded on a needle it may slip out of the eye.

The depth and distance to the site of tying or suturing, along with good judgment, guide the scrub nurse in preparing ties or sutures of the correct length. In deep cavities, ties are often "mounted" on the tips of clamps to facilitate

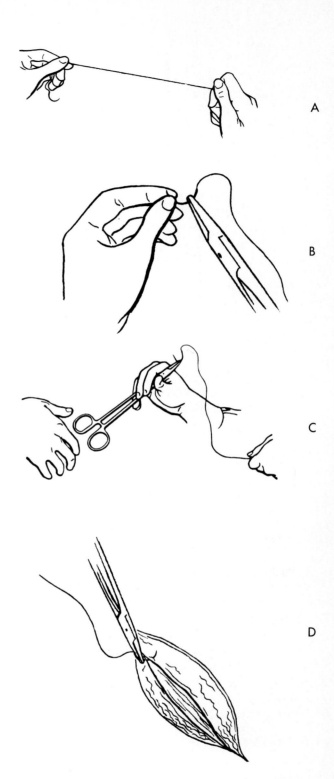

Fig. 7-15. Preparation of swaged suture. **A,** If necessary to straighten, strand is grasped 1 to 2 inches away from needle-suture junction and pulled gently. **B,** Needle holder is clamped about three fourths of distance from needle point. It should be clamped at swaged area. Needle is placed near tip of holder to facilitate suturing. **C,** Surgeon or assistant receives needle holder with needle point toward thumb to prevent unnecessary wrist motion. Scrub nurse controls free end of suture. **D,** Surgeon or assistant begins closing with swaged needle and suture. (Courtesy Ethicon, Inc., Somerville, N.J.)

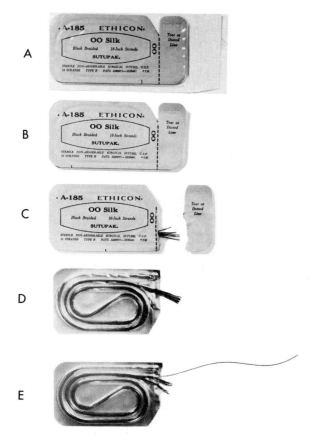

Fig. 7-16. Steps in opening multiple suture packet. **A,** Plastic packet enclosed in overwrap. **B,** Plastic packet as presented to scrub nurse. **C,** Packet torn open along dotted line. **D,** Reverse of packet showing strand packaging. **E,** Individual strand removed from packet. (Courtesy Ethicon, Inc., Somerville, N.J.)

reaching the site where the use of only the hands would be cumbersome.

For general surgery a continuous suture threaded on a needle is usually about 24 inches long and its short end is 3 to 4 inches long. An interrupted suture is 12 to 14 inches long with 2 or 3 inches threaded through the needle. To ligate a vessel in the epidermal and subcutaneous layers, the ligature may be 12 to 15 inches long. However, vessels or structures deep in the wound are ligated with a suture or ligature that is 24 to 30 inches long.

Threading surgical needles

The scrub nurse pulls the suture about 4 inches through the eye of the needle to prevent the suture from being pulled out of the eye during suturing. A curved needle is threaded from within its curvature so the short end falls away from the outside curvature. This practice helps to prevent easy pullout. To keep the needle secure in the jaws of the needle holder and to prevent damage to the eye of the needle, the needle holder is placed on the flattened surface of the needle at least ⅛ inch from its eye.

Counting needles

Different institutions vary in their policies regarding needle and sharp counts during operative procedures. Initial counts, prior to the start of the procedure, provide the basis for subsequent counts. The count should be performed audibly and with each sharp visualized by the scrub and circulating nurses. During the procedure, needles should be accounted for by the scrub nurse as they are handed to the surgeon on an exchange basis. Subsequent counts should be performed by the scrub and circulating nurses when sharps are added to the field, prior to closure of a body cavity or deep, large incision, after closure of a body cavity, when either of the nurses is relieved by other personnel, and immediately before completion of the surgical intervention. Used needles should be kept on a needle pad or in a container on the scrub nurse's table. Broken or missing needles must be reported to the surgeon and accounted for in their entirety. All sharps should be accounted for and properly disposed of prior to preparing the room for the next patient.

INSTRUMENTS
Historical perspective

The history of surgical instruments dates back to 2500 BC. The first instruments were sharpened flints and fine animal teeth. Ancient Greek, Egyptian, and Hindu instruments are amazing in their resemblance to present-day instruments.

In the late 1700s, to be equipped for the practice of surgery, the surgeon had to employ various skilled artisans such as coppersmiths, steelworkers, needle grinders, turners of wood, bone, and ivory, and silk and hemp spinners. The surgeon had to explain the mechanisms of the instruments and supervise their manufacture. The resulting instruments were crude, expensive, and time-consuming to make. Each artisan used hand labor exclusively, devoted time to making only one type of instrument, and thereby gained proficiency. For example, a cutter would keep a small supply of surgical knives. Thus began physician's supply houses and surgical instrument making in America.

In the mid-1800s, physicians' principal tools were their eyes and ears. Official records show that amputation, the trademark of the Civil War, was the result in three of four operations. Surgeons were scarce and medical instruments almost nonexistent. Kitchen knives and penknives, carpenter saws, and table forks did the job. After the Civil War the advent of the administration of ether and chloroform brought a demand for new ideas and methods in surgery and instruments. The division of general surgery into specialties took place in the late 1800s and early 1900s. Delicate instruments were seen as more useful than the force of crude and heavy instruments. So that instruments could withstand repeated sterilization, handles of wood, ivory, and rubber were discontinued.

During World War II the development of stainless steel

in Germany ensured a better material for surgical instruments and other equipment. Today, surgeons and perioperative nurses assist manufacturers in research for new and better instrumentation.

Composition of surgical instruments

Perioperative nurses are responsible for the use, handling, and care of hundreds of surgical instruments a day. A basic knowledge of how these instruments are manufactured can help in their selection and maintenance. Surgical instruments are expensive and represent a major investment for every hospital.

Instruments are manufactured from stainless steel. Stainless steel is a compound of iron, carbon, and chromium, which means that stainless steel can be of varying qualities. These qualities are designated by grading the steel into series by the American Iron and Steel Institute (AISI). For example, the 400 series stainless steel has some noncorrosive characteristics and good tensile strength. It resists rust, produces a fine point, and retains a keen edge. Handheld ringed instruments, such as scissors and clamps, should be 420 series stainless steel.

The raw steel is converted into instrument blanks by a machinist. These blanks, male and female halves, are then die forged into specific pieces. This process makes an impression of the piece in the stainless steel blank. The excess metal is trimmed away, and the instrument parts are ready for the final steps.

The two halves are then milled to prepare the box lock fittings, jaw serrations, and ratchets. After this step is done, the halves are assembled by hand. The pin is inserted through the box lock, and the jaws and shanks are properly aligned. Final grinding and hardening accomplished by heat treating bring the object to proper size, weight, spring temper, and balance. The final inspection testing is for hardness, proper jaw closure, and smooth lock and ratchet action.

There are three types of instrument finishes. The first is the bright, highly polished mirror finish, which tends to reflect light and may restrict the vision of the surgeon. The second is the satin or dull finish, which tends to eliminate glare and lessen eyestrain for the surgeon. The third finish is ebonizing, which produces a black finish.

The last part of the process is called *passivation*. The instruments are put in nitric acid to remove any residue of carbon steel. The nitric acid also produces a surface coating of chromium oxide. Chromium oxide is important because it produces a resistance to corrosion in the stainless steel instrument. The instrument is then polished and ready for sale.

Instruments used today are made in the United States and in other countries such as Germany, France, and Pakistan. The United States does not have an agency that reviews or sets standards for surgical instruments. The quality is set by the individual manufacturer. If the instruments are inferior, they will not withstand normal usage, and the customer will not receive full return for investment. A properly cared for instrument should last 10 years or more. A reputable company stands behind its product.

Instrument companies have brought highly skilled instrument makers to the United States and have bought instruments from plants in other countries. A limited number of 5-year apprentice programs now exist to train instrument makers. Most instrument manufacturers will design any instrument to a physician's specifications. The high cost of instruments is easily explained by the small number of skilled artisans available and the amount of time necessary to make an instrument, as well as by the cost of raw materials.

Perioperative nursing considerations

Nursing personnel have a responsibility to know surgical instruments and their proper uses and care.

Instrument categories

Although there is no standard nomenclature for specific instruments, there are four main categories: sharps, clamps, holding instruments, and retractors.

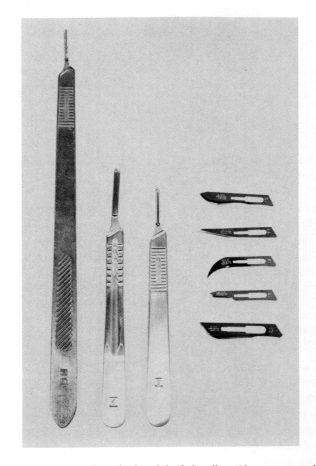

Fig. 7-17. Long and regular-length knife handles with assortment of blades. Blades, *top to bottom*, nos. 10, 11, 12, 15 and 20.

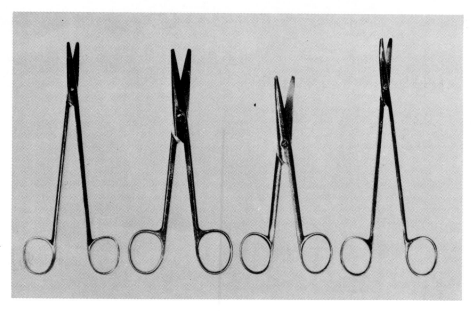

Fig. 7-18. Commonly used scissors. *Left to right,* Straight, blunt dissecting scissors; heavy or suture scissors; Mayo scissors; Metzenbaum scissors.

Sharps include scissors and scalpels. Scalpels are probably the oldest of all surgical instruments (Fig. 7-17). Most scalpels are handles with one end suited to the attachment of disposable blades. During an operation the blades may be conveniently changed by the scrub nurse as often as necessary. The blades come prepackaged and sterile and are passed onto the sterile field as needed by the circulating nurse. Careful disposal of blades at the end of a procedure is important in the implementation of universal precautions (see Chapter 5).

Scissors are designed in short, long, small, and large sizes and in various shapes for different purposes in cutting body tissues and surgical materials (Fig. 7-18). The basic design consists of two blades, each having a chisel-shaped edge with the bevel consistent with the structure it has to cut. Scissors tips may be blunt or sharp and the blades straight or curved. Conventional scissors require two movements in use: one to open and another to close the jaws. Other scissors may have a spring action in the body design that holds the jaws in an open position. A single movement pressing the spring together closes the jaws to cut. Scissors designed for delicate plastic and eye surgery are often of the latter type. A basic instrument set usually includes a curved Mayo scissors for dissection of heavy tissues, a Metzenbaum scissors for dissection of delicate tissues, and straight scissors for cutting the suture. For surgery in deep areas of the body, a scissors with long handles and short blades is used for better control and easier use.

Clamps are generally used for achieving hemostasis (Fig. 7-19). These instruments make surgery possible by preventing excessive blood loss in the course of dissection.

The well-designed modern instrument is styled for the lightness, balance, and security that yield maximum efficiency in closing the severed ends of each vessel with a minimum of tissue damage. The grasping ends have deep transverse cuts so that bleeding vessels may be compressed with sufficient force to stop the bleeding from smaller vessels if left for a couple of minutes. The serrations must be cleanly cut and perfectly meshed to prevent the clamps from slipping from the tissue to be held. Special jaws that have finely meshed, multiple rows of longitudinally arranged teeth are made for vascular clamps to prevent leakage and to minimize trauma to the vessel walls when the severed vessels are anastomosed. The surgical service usually selects a hemostat or clamp design according to the surgeons' preferences.

The apposition of the clamp tips is necessary for its functioning and must be periodically checked. When the instrument is held up to the light and the handles are fully closed, no light should be visible between the jaws. These instruments, if used for purposes other than that for which they are intended, will be useless and need to be repaired.

The instrument's joint must also be checked. Instruments made up of two halves may have three types of joints. The screw joint is the most popular. The two halves are connected only by a screw or pin. The joint must be checked and tightened periodically because the screw may work itself loose. Screw joint instruments are easy to make and comparatively inexpensive.

The second kind is the box lock joint instrument. One arm passes through a slot in the other arm. This kind is needed where accurate approximation of the tips is necessary, as in vascular forceps.

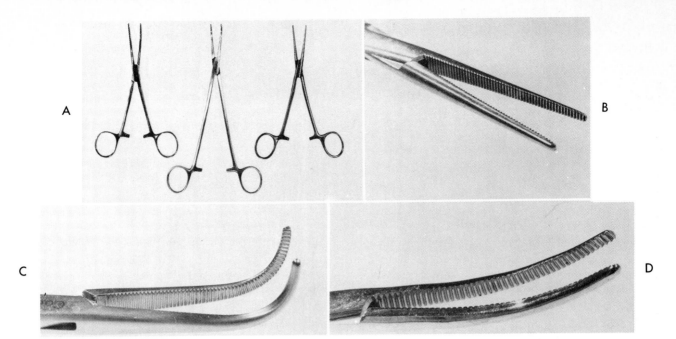

Fig. 7-19. A, Commonly used hemostatic clamps. **B,** Straight Kelly. **C,** Right-angle. **D,** Curved Kelly.

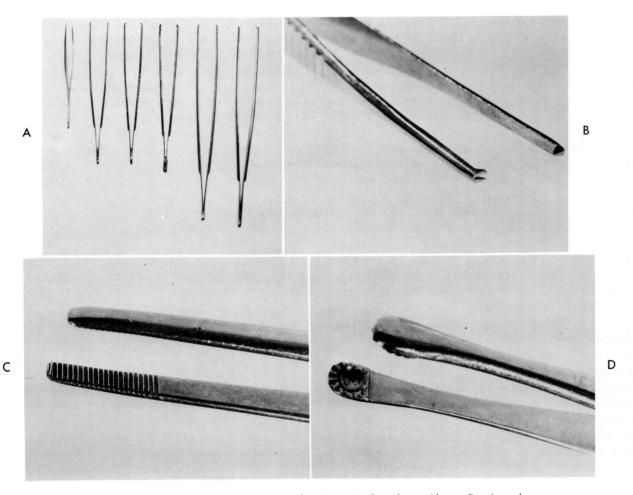

Fig. 7-20. A, Various types of tissue forceps or "pickups," ranging from those with very fine tips to heavy tips. **B,** Tips with teeth. **C,** Smooth tip. **D,** Tips of Russian forceps.

The final and least popular type is the semibox or aseptic joint. It has the advantage that the two halves can be separated for easy cleaning.

These joints must be cleaned regularly, and any protein deposits or rust collecting at the site must be removed to ensure proper functioning.

The grasping or holding instruments are used for tissue retraction or suturing. They must have a firm grip while inflicting a minimum of trauma to the tissues they hold. The most common kinds are the various simple two-armed spring forceps (Fig. 7-20). They vary in length and thickness and are available with and without teeth. Nontoothed forceps create minimal damage and hold delicate, thin tissues. Toothed forceps hold thick or slippery tissues that need extra grip.

Other holding forceps have handles like clamps with specialized tips or jaws (Fig. 7-21). These jaws may be triangular, straight, angular, or T-shaped. The Allis forceps has multiple teeth that do not crush or damage tissue in its grasp. The Babcock forceps has curved, fenestrated blades with no teeth, and it grips or encloses delicate structures such as a ureter or fallopian tube. Sponge-holding forceps with ring-shaped jaws are available in 7- and 9-inch lengths. They can be used to grasp or handle tissue but are usually used as sponge holders. A gauze sponge is folded and placed in the jaws and is then used to retract tissue or to absorb blood in the field.

Needle holders (Fig. 7-22) are frequently used and are put through many different motions, even in a routine surgical operation. Because they must grasp metal rather than soft tissues, they are subject to greater damage. As a result, needle holders must be repaired and replaced regularly.

For maximum usage, needle holders must retain a firm grip on the needle. Many types of jaws have been designed to meet this need but all eventually become worn down and damaged beyond repair. The so-called diamond jaw needle holder has a tungsten carbide insert designed to prevent rotation of the needle. A longitudinal groove or pit in the jaw of the needle holder releases tension, prevents flattening of the needle, and holds the needle firmly in needle holders of standard design. Needle holders may have a ratchet similar to that of a hemostat, or they may be of a spring action and lock type.

Towel clamps are also considered holding instruments. Of two basic types, the first is a nonpenetrating towel clamp used for holding in place barrier draping materials. The other type has sharp tips used to penetrate drapes and tissues but is damaging to both. The use of sharp towel clamps to penetrate drapes is highly discouraged.

Retractors determine the exposure of the operative field. A surgeon needs the best exposure possible while inflicting a minimum of trauma to the surrounding tissue. Retractors are either self-retaining (Fig. 7-23) or held in place by a member of the surgical team. The two types of self-retaining retractors are those with frames to which various blades may be attached and those with two blades held apart with a ratchet. An example of the latter is a Weitlaner

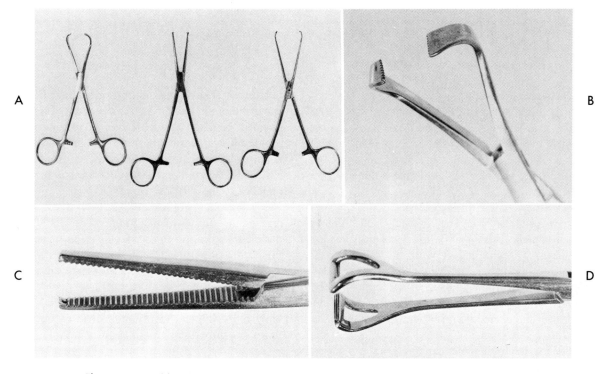

Fig. 7-21. A, Holding forceps with special jaws. **B,** Allis. **C,** Kocher or Ochsner. **D,** Babcock.

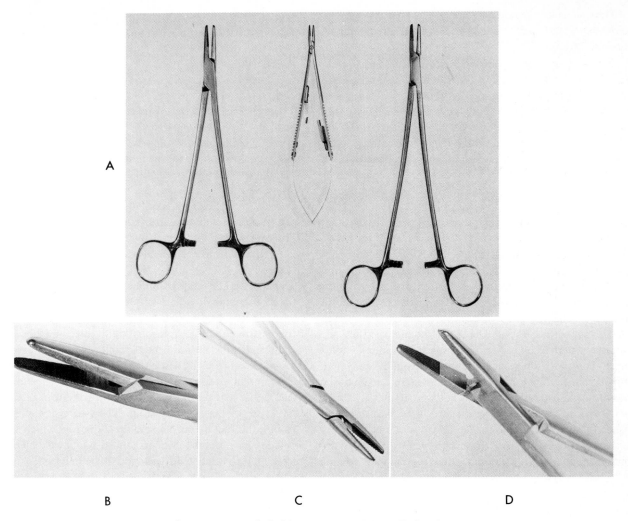

Fig. 7-22. A, Needle holders. **B,** Heavy. **C,** Fine. **D,** Regular.

retractor. With handheld retractors (Fig. 7-24), the handles may be notched, hook shaped, or ring shaped to give the holder a firm grip without tiring. The blade is usually at a right angle to the shaft and may be a smooth blade, rake, or hook. A malleable (ribbon) retractor is one that may be shaped by the surgeon at the field, with the original shape being a flat ribbon.

Many miscellaneous instruments or specialty items are particular to a certain service, such as mallets and screwdrivers in orthopedic surgery. Microsurgical instruments are extra fine for vascular and nerve repair; they are extremely delicate and should be handled separately from other instruments. Instruments used in specialty surgery and the instruments that compose various instrument sets are discussed in the chapters on surgical interventions in Part Two.

When nursing team members can analyze the planned surgical procedure and approach, they are able to identify each instrument and its specific function. They can select instrument sets without omitting necessary items and without including items that will not be used. This intelligent, planned approach ensures economy of time and motion, protects instruments from abuse, and prevents unnecessary handling. During the operation the informed nurse who anticipates instrument needs becomes a more valuable member of the surgical team.

Designated operating room or central supply personnel arrange the various instrument trays or sets. The trays are named according to their functions. For example, a local (or plastic surgery) set includes instruments needed for a simple superficial incision, excision, and suturing. A basic laparotomy set includes instruments to open and close the abdominal cavity and repair any gross defects in the major body musculature. An example of three basic operating room instrument sets would be major, minor, and plastic.

According to each patient's needs, more individualized instruments, such as an intestinal set or a vascular set, may be added. In the same way, basic instrument sets may

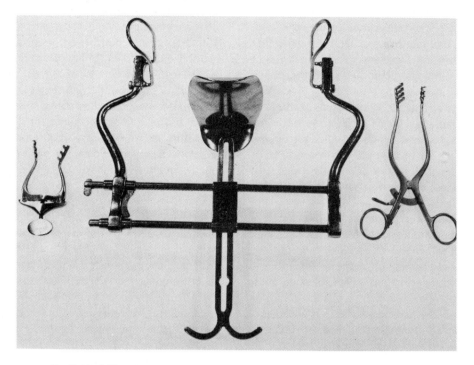

Fig. 7-23. Self-retaining retractors. *Left to right,* Mastoid, Balfour, and Weitlaner.

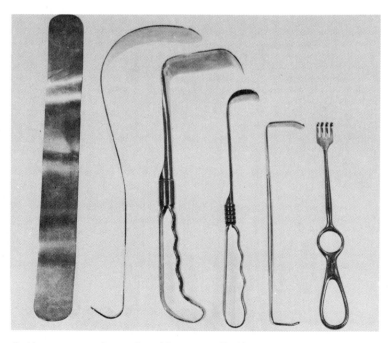

Fig. 7-24. Handheld retractors. *Left to right,* Ribbon, or malleable; Deaver; two sizes of Richardsons; Army-Navy, or USA; and rake.

be selected for opening other body cavities, such as the skull, chest, and pelvis.

Selecting and preparing instruments for patient use

Instruments are selected according to the size of the patient's body structures and the nature of the organs involved. Proper selection requires a general understanding of surgical procedures and approaches and knowledge of anatomy, possible pathologic conditions, and the design and purpose of instruments.

For example, the nurse needs to know that instruments for incising and penetrating bones differ from those designed to cut soft tissues. Instruments designed for surgery on infants and for surgery of the eye, ear, blood vessels, nerves, brain, and facial structures are smaller, finer, and more delicate than those designed to handle thick, fibrous tissues such as cartilage and bone.

This knowledge is reinforced during the orientation of new personnel to the operating room. New personnel learn basic technique first in general surgery and then proceed to the specialty services, where different instruments and devices are added but the same basic principles are used.

In most operating rooms the instruments are set up on Mayo stands (Fig. 7-25) and back tables in a planned, standardized, organized, functional manner to maintain continuity when the original scrub nurse is replaced by another. The teaching manual should have illustrations or diagrams to which all personnel may refer. Each item used by the scrub nurse should have its own placement on the table to prevent the mass clutter that would occur if instruments and supplies were placed randomly.

A proficient and experienced scrub nurse must know the instrument inventory of the department, the routine instruments needed for each type of operation, the individual surgeon's preferences, correct use and handling, method of preparation, and aftercare of the instruments. A file of preference cards may list the procedures each physician performs, the physician's glove size, the preferred skin preparation solution, specific draping instructions, and instruments required for the procedure.

Before an operative procedure, the scrub nurse may assist the circulating nurse in gathering the needed supplies, equipment, and sutures. The scrub nurse scrubs, dons gown and gloves (Chapter 5), and begins to set up the sterile tables with drapes, instruments, supplies, and sutures. A Mayo stand is set up for use at the immediate operative site. Once the patient is on the operating room bed and is draped, the Mayo stand is brought across the patient. One or two back tables, according to the number of instruments and supplies, are also set up.

Instruments are arranged with those most frequently used on the Mayo stand (Fig. 7-25). The scrub nurse prepares the sutures and ligatures and places the knife blades on the handles. Other supplies needed are suction tubing and tips, electrosurgical cord and tip, drains, basins,

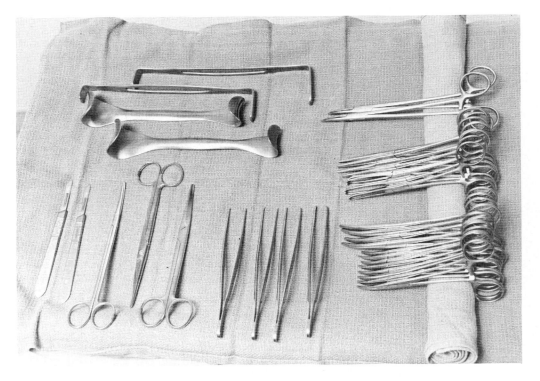

Fig. 7-25. Mayo stand setup.

gowns, gloves, drapes, sponges, and needles, all of which are sterile and set up on a back table according to standardized hospital policy (Fig. 7-26).

The scrub nurse must be attentive to the sterile field in order to anticipate the surgeon's needs. Instruments should be passed in a positive and decisive manner. Each instrument is placed or slapped firmly into the surgeon's or RNFA's palm in such a manner that it is ready for immediate use with no wasted motion. For example, when a needle holder with a needle is passed to the surgeon or RNFA, the needle should be pointing in the direction of the surgeon's or RNFA's thumb; there should be no need for readjustment. Knowing if a surgeon or the assistant is left- or right-handed is necessary in order to pass a needle holder correctly.

Often the surgeon or assistant signals with hand motions for the type of instrument desired to eliminate unnecessary talking and help the scrub nurse pass the instruments quickly.

Care and handling of instruments

An instrument should be used only for the purpose for which it is designed. Proper use and reasonable care prolong its life and protect its quality. Scissors and clamps, which are most frequently abused, can be forced out of alignment, cracked, or broken when used improperly. Tissue scissors should not be used to cut suture or gauze dressings. Hemostatic clamps should not be used as towel clamps or to clamp suction tubing.

Instruments must be handled gently. Bouncing, dropping, and setting heavy equipment on top of them should be avoided. At the end of a procedure, the instruments should not be thrown together in a tangled heap. They should be handled individually or in small groups. Sharps and delicate instruments should be set aside for individual handling and cleaning.

Each instrument should be inspected before and after each use to detect imperfections. An instrument should function perfectly to prevent needlessly endangering a patient's life and increasing operative time because of instrument failure. Before surgical use, instruments must be completely clean to ensure effective sterilization.

Forceps, clamps, and other hinged instruments must be inspected for alignment of jaws and teeth and for stiffness. Ratchets should hold firmly yet release easily when necessary. The tips of jaws and teeth should meet perfectly, and instrument joints should work smoothly. The serrations on the ends of forceps must mesh perfectly so that blood flow may be occluded but a vein or artery will not be injured or cut.

The edges of scissors should be tested for sharpness. To cut, they must be beveled smoothly. All instruments should be checked for worn spots, chipping, dents, cracks, or sharp edges.

While instruments are on the sterile field, the scrub nurse wipes them with a damp sponge to prevent blood and other substances from drying in the crevices or on the surfaces. At the conclusion of the surgical procedure, uni-

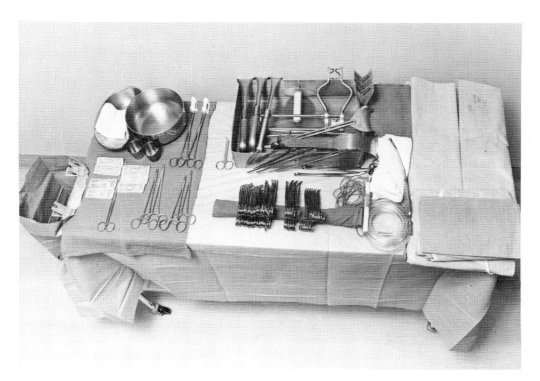

Fig. 7-26. Back table setup.

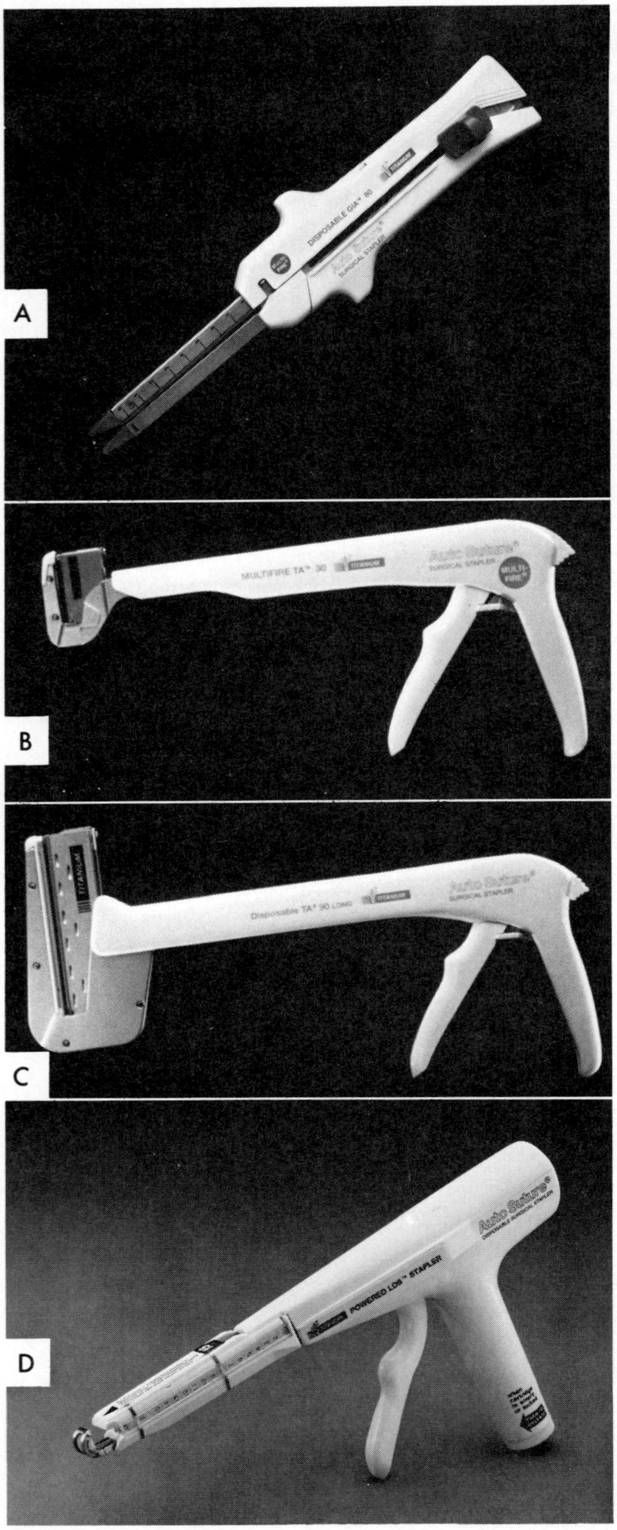

Fig. 7-27. Set of Auto Suture instruments. **A,** GIA instrument. **B,** TA-30 instrument. (TA-55 size instrument is also available.) **C,** TA-90 instrument. **D,** LDS instrument. (Courtesy United States Surgical Corp., Norwalk, Conn.)

versal precautions are implemented. Instruments are taken to the appropriate location for washing and terminal sterilization and then are reassembled and sterilized for future use (Chapter 5).

Instrument counts

Most institutions perform sponge, sharp, and instrument counts as standard practice. Establishing standardized instrument sets with the minimum numbers and types of instruments in them facilitates instrument counts. Initial counts should be carried out concurrently by the circulating and scrub nurses before the procedure. Subsequent counts should be taken when instruments are added to the sterile field, before closure of a cavity or large, deep incision, when the nurses are relieved by other personnel, and at the completion of the procedure. Instruments that are disassembled during surgery, such as certain retractors, must be accounted for in their entirety.

Storing instruments

Instruments should be stored safely. The use of locked cabinets or cupboards located in designated areas prevents theft and indiscriminate use. Cabinet shelving should be adjustable and properly spaced for storage of various sizes and types of instruments. Attached labels and diagrams in cabinets assist personnel. An inventory should be taken at periodic intervals. Damaged instruments should be set aside and sent for repair or replacement. An instrument repair service should be selected carefully and used for regular maintenance, such as sharpening and realignment of instruments.

Stapling instruments

Within the past decade, internal stapling devices have been refined and are now widely used (Fig. 7-27). Sets are composed of various instruments used to suture tissue mechanically. These instruments are used for ligation and division, resection, anastomoses, and skin and fascia closure (Figs. 7-28 to 7-30). They are employed in thoracic, abdominal, and gynecologic surgery. Because of the mechanical application of these instruments, tissue manipulation and handling are reduced. The edema and inflammation that usually accompany anastomoses are also reduced.

Mechanical staplers (nondisposable and disposable) utilize cartridges of tiny stainless steel or absorbable, nonmetallic staples that are commercially preloaded, presterilized, and prepackaged. The staples are essentially nonreactive, and their use thereby minimizes the probability of tissue reaction or infection. Because of the noncrushing B shape of the staples, nutrients can pass through the staple line to the cut edge of the tissue. This characteristic reduces the possibility of necrosis and promotes healing. The use of staplers significantly decreases operating time and may shorten postoperative stays.

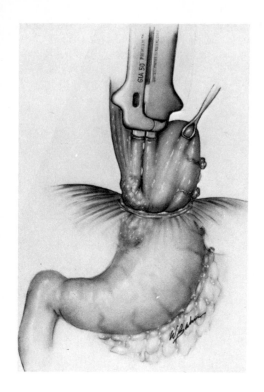

Fig. 7-28. GIA instrument used to perform esophagogastrostomy. Forks of the instrument are inserted into stab wounds made in the lateral wall of the esophagus and the medial wall of the gastric fundus. The instrument is closed and staples are fired. (Courtesy United States Surgical Corp., Norwalk, Conn.)

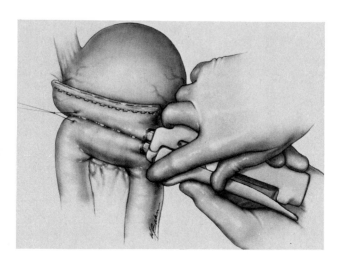

Fig. 7-29. Using GIA to staple and join stomach and jejunum. At same time, blade in GIA cuts between double staple lines, creating stoma for gastrojejunostomy. (Courtesy United States Surgical Corp., Norwalk, Conn.)

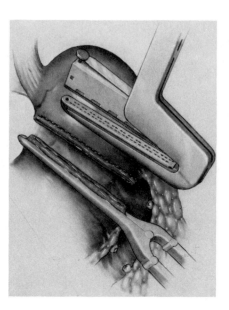

Fig. 7-30. Using TA-90 to close gastric pouch. Jaws of TA-90 are slipped around stomach at level of transection, the instrument is closed, and staples are fired. (Courtesy United States Surgical Corp., Norwalk, Conn.)

REFERENCES

Bennett, R.G.: Selection of wound closure materials, J. Am. Acad. Dermatol. 18:4, 1988.

Hardy, J.D., Kukora, J.S., and Pass, H.I.: Hardy's textbook of surgery, Philadelphia, 1988, J.B. Lippincott Co.

Miller, T.A.: Physiologic basis of modern surgical care, St. Louis, 1988, The C.V. Mosby Co.

Wound closure manual: use and handling of sutures, needles and mechanical wound closure devices, Somerville, N.J., 1988, Ethicon, Inc.

BIBLIOGRAPHY

Anderson, R.M., and Romfh, R.F.: Techniques in the use of surgical tools, New York, 1980, Appleton-Century-Crofts.

Association of Operating Room Nurses: Recommended practices for sponge, sharp, and instrument counts. In AORN standards and recommended practices for perioperative nursing, Denver, 1990, The Association.

Brooks Tighe, S.M.: Instrumentation for the operating room, ed. 3, St. Louis, 1989, The C.V. Mosby Co.

The care and handling of surgical instruments, Randolph, Mass., 1981, Codman & Shurtleff, Inc.

Davis, C.V., and others: Clinical surgery, St. Louis, 1987, The C.V. Mosby Co.

Day, T.G.: A guide to surgical instruments and suture materials, Contemp. Obstet. Gynecol. 16:87, 1980.

Sabiston, D.C.: Textbook of surgery: the biological basis of modern surgical practice, Philadelphia, 1986, W.B. Saunders Co.

Stapling techniques: general surgery, ed. 3, Norwalk, Conn., 1988, United States Surgical Corporation.

8 Wound healing, dressings, and drains

JAYNE HENRY

WOUND HEALING

One of the most fundamental and marvelous defensive properties of living organisms is the power to heal wounds. This process is infallible in the absence of endogenous and exogenous infections, mechanical interferences, or certain disease processes. Apposition and maintenance of the edges of a cleanly incised wound almost always result in prompt healing.

Etiology of wounds can be described in three categories:

Surgical: caused by an incision or excision
Traumatic: caused by an injury (mechanical, thermal, or chemical)
Chronic: caused by an underlying pathophysiology, such as pressure sores or venous leg ulcers, over time.

Clean wound healing is an intricate, exact biologic process that takes place in an orderly sequence. First, an exudate containing blood, lymph, and fibrin begins clotting and loosely binds the cut edges together. Blood supply to the area is increased, and the basic process of inflammation is set in motion. Leukocytes increase in number to fight bacteria in the wound area and by phagocytosis help to remove damaged tissues. The severed tissue is quickly glued together by strands of fibrin and a thin layer of clotted blood, forming a scab. Plasma seeps to the surface to form a dry protective crust. This seal helps to prevent fluid loss and bacterial invasion. During the first few days of wound healing, however, the seal has little tensile strength.

After 3 to 4 days, connective tissue cells (fibroblasts) rapidly proliferate and give strength to the wound by producing collagen, a tough fibrous protein responsible for the structural integrity of skin. At the same time small blood vessels regenerate and build new blood channels. Granulation tissue (fibrous connective tissue) includes blood vessels and lymphatics that proliferate from the base of the wound. Rapidly growing and multiple epithelial cells begin to restore the epithelial continuity of the skin. At this stage the wound appears healed; however, healing is not complete until the granulation tissue organizes into scar tissue. By the ninth or tenth day, the wound is moderately well healed and then becomes progressively stronger. The whole process of repair takes 2 weeks or more, depending on factors such as physical condition of the patient, size and location of the wound, and stresses put on the incisional area. During this time the scar (cicatrix) strengthens as the connective tissue shrinks.

The amount of tissue loss, the existence of contamination or infection, and damage to tissue are all factors that determine the type of wound healing that will occur. This process of healing takes place in one of three ways.

Healing by primary (first) intention

When wounds are created aseptically, with a minimum of tissue destruction and postoperative tissue reaction, healing occurs through primary intention (Fig. 8-1). Postoperative complications, such as dehiscence, infection, excessive discharge or swelling, or abnormal scar formation, do not occur during the healing process.

Healing by first intention takes place under the following conditions:

1. Edges of an incised wound in a healthy person are promptly and accurately approximated.
2. Contamination is held to a minimum by impeccable aseptic technique.
3. Trauma to the wound is minimal.
4. After suturing, no dead space is left to become a potential site of infection.
5. Drainage is minimal.

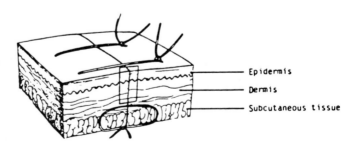

Fig. 8-1. Healing by primary intention (surgically closed wound). (Courtesy of Johnson & Johnson Patient Care, Inc., New Brunswick, N.J.)

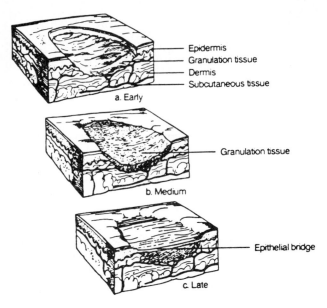

Epidermis
Granulation tissue
Dermis
Subcutaneous tissue
a. Early

Granulation tissue
b. Medium

Epithelial bridge
c. Late

Fig. 8-2. Three stages in secondary intention healing. (Courtesy of Johnson & Johnson Patient Care, Inc., New Brunswick, N.J.)

Healing by secondary intention (granulation)

When surgical wounds are characterized by tissue loss with inability to approximate wound edges, healing occurs through secondary intention (Fig. 8-2).

This type of wound is usually left open and allowed to heal from the inside toward the outer surface. In infected wounds, this process allows the proper cleansing and dressing of the wound as healthy tissue builds up from the inside. The area of tissue loss gradually fills with granulation tissue (fibroblasts and capillaries).

Scar tissue is extensive because of the size of the tissue gap that must be closed. Contraction of surrounding tissue also takes place. Consequently, this healing process takes longer than primary intention healing.

Healing by delayed primary closure (third intention)

As the name implies, this healing process takes place when approximation of wound edges is delayed by 3 to 5 days or more after injury or surgery. The conditions that contribute to a decision for a delayed closure are:

1. Removal of an inflamed organ
2. Heavy contamination of wound

Factors influencing wound healing

The patient's nutritional status and overall recuperative power are of utmost importance in tissue repair and healing. Especially significant is an adequate supply of protein, which is necessary for the growth of new tissues, the regulation of the osmotic pressure of blood and other body fluids, and the formation of prothrombin, enzymes, hormones, and antibodies. Also important is vitamin C, which

aids connective tissue production and strong scar formation.

Healthy tissues are able to tolerate and counteract a certain amount of contamination, but devitalized tissues have little resistive power. Large numbers of or very virulent microorganisms can, however, overpower the body defenses of even a healthy person and interfere with wound healing. Therefore, scrupulous aseptic technique must be used to prevent any wound infection—the most common cause of delayed wound healing.

Theories abound as to the genesis of wound infection. Cross-contamination from operating room, postanesthesia care unit (PACU), and unit personnel is believed to be a primary source. Adherence to aseptic principles and maintenance of operating room environmental conditions are significant factors. Length of time that the wound is open in the operating room has also been mentioned. Authorities are now suspecting, however, that the most common source of infection may be the patient, because many infections can be traced to the patient's own endogenous flora. This source points out the importance of meticulous preoperative antimicrobial preparation of the patient, thorough preparation of the surgical site, and careful observation of sterile technique, not only in the operating room but also during postoperative dressing changes.

Wound healing can be impaired by poor surgical technique. Rough handling of tissue causes trauma that can lead to bleeding and other conditions conducive to infection. Examples of meticulous surgical technique that promote wound healing are adequate hemostasis, precise cutting and suturing techniques, elimination of dead spaces, and minimal pressure from retractors and other instruments.

Other factors affecting wound healing are the patient's age, stress level, and preexisting conditions such as diabetes, anemia, malnutrition, cancer, obesity, advanced age, or cardiovascular or respiratory impairments—in other words, overall physical and psychologic condition.

Following are terms used in connection with wound healing:

keloid Dense, unsightly connective tissue or excessive scar formation that is often removed surgically

"proud flesh" Overgrowth of granulation tissue

gangrene Anaerobic infection process that may occur instead of healing; implies necrosis (death of tissue) and putrefaction (decomposition); usually caused by failure of nutriment or blood to reach a part

adhesions Adherence of serous membranes to one another, causing fibrous tissue to form; sometimes occurring in healing and inflammatory processes; commonly occurring in or about gastrointestinal tract, where adhesions may form bands and cause obstructions and subsequent surgical emergencies

dehiscence Separation of layers of surgical wound (Fig. 8-3)

evisceration Extrusion of internal organs, or viscera, through gaping wound (Fig. 8-3)

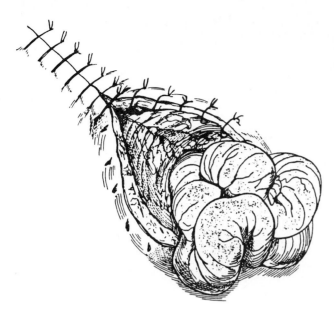

Fig. 8-3. Wound dehiscence and evisceration. (Courtesy of Johnson & Johnson Patient Care, Inc., New Brunswick, N.J.)

WOUND CLASSIFICATION

The Centers for Disease Control (CDC) recommends four surgical wound classifications: clean wounds, clean contaminated wounds, contaminated wounds, and dirty or infected wounds. This classification scheme reflects the probability of infection and thus enables appropriate preventive measures to be taken. "AORN Recommended Practices for Documentation of Perioperative Nursing Care" states that the patient record should reflect the surgical wound classification (AORN, 1990). Following are descriptions of each classification. The associated infection risk rate has been determined by numerous studies (Garner, 1985).

Clean wounds

In these wounds the respiratory, alimentary, and genitourinary tracts are not entered. They are primarily closed and can be drained with a closed wound drainage system. They show no sign of infection. Examples are breast biopsy, total hip replacement, or open heart surgery. The risk of infection is 1% to 5%.

Clean contaminated wounds

In these wounds the respiratory, alimentary, or genitourinary tract is entered under controlled conditions. There is no sign of infection and no break in surgical aseptic technique. Examples of clean contaminated wounds are nonperforated appendectomy, hysterectomy, or thoracotomy. The risk of infection is 3% to 11%.

Contaminated wounds

These wounds are open, fresh, accidental wounds or operations with major breaks in aseptic technique. Incisions with signs of infection or gross spillage from the gastrointestinal tract are also included. Some examples are an appendectomy for ruptured appendix, a penetrating abdominal trauma involving bowel, or a gunshot wound to the abdomen. The risk of infection is 10% to 17%.

Dirty or infected wounds

These wounds include old traumatic wounds with retained devitalized tissue and wounds that involve an existing clinical infection or perforated viscera. Examples of dirty or infected wounds are excision and drainage of abscess or delayed primary closure of ruptured appendix. The risk of infection is greater than 27%.

DRESSINGS

After surgery a dressing may be applied to the wound. Following are the purposes of a dressing:

1. To cushion and protect the wound from trauma and gross contamination
2. To absorb drainage
3. To support, splint, or immobilize the body part and incisional area
4. To aid in hemostasis and minimize edema, as in a pressure dressing
5. To enhance the patient's physical comfort and esthetic appearance
6. To maintain a moist environment and prevent cell dehydration
7. To apply medications

Dressings are as varied as operations but can be grouped into two main categories: *primary* and *secondary* dressings.

Primary dressings are placed directly over the wound. A variety of dressing materials are available on the market today. The function of these dressings is to absorb drainage and allow it to wick away from the wound edge. Cotton gauze or synthetic dressings are often used for this purpose. These dressings are usually nonocclusive and allow exposure of the wound to air. The layer of the dressing directly contacting the wound should be nonadherent unless debridement is desired.

Secondary dressings are placed directly over the primary dressing. These function to absorb excessive drainage, provide hemostasis by compression, and protect the wound from further trauma. These functions are usually accomplished with a bulky dressing such as an abdominal pad. These pads have a cotton filling that provides extra absorbency.

Dressings are most commonly secured with tape. Tape is available with a variety of backing materials (cloth, paper, taffeta, plastic) and with regular or nonallergenic

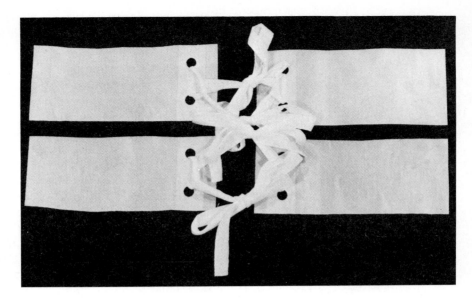

Fig. 8-4. Montgomery straps.

adhesive. The amount of strength, elasticity required, patient allergies, and anticipated frequency of dressing change influence which type is selected. When frequent dressing changes are anticipated, Montgomery straps can be selected to secure the dressing (Fig. 8-4). When compression of the wound for hemostasis or reduction of edema is desired, an elastic tape or elastic bandage is used to secure the secondary dressing. Immobilization is accomplished with the addition of soft padding, splints, elastic bandages, and casting materials. These immobilizing dressings are discussed in more detail in Chapter 22.

Several varieties of transparent "biologic" synthetic dressings are now available and are quite popular. Most are vapor and oxygen permeable, conform to irregular body surfaces, prevent gross outside contamination, and allow visibility of the wound itself. These transparent semiocclusive films keep the wound moist and thereby enable epidermal cells to move more quickly across the wound and bridge the incision. The "scab" stage of wound healing is avoided. Although these film types of dressings cannot be used on heavily draining wounds, their skinlike

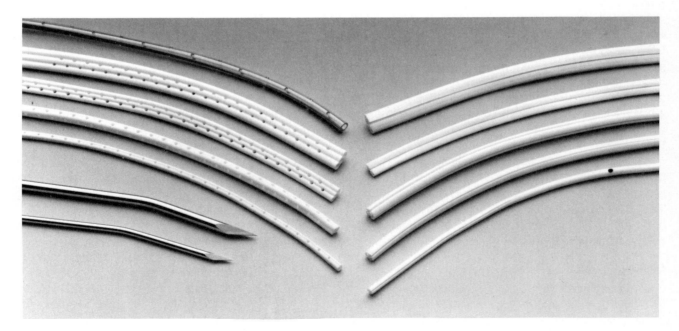

Fig. 8-5. Drains are available in a variety of styles. Pictured are round PVC, flat and round silicone, trocars, and a variety of fluted silicone drains. (Courtesy of Johnson & Johnson Patient Care, Inc., New Brunswick, N.J.)

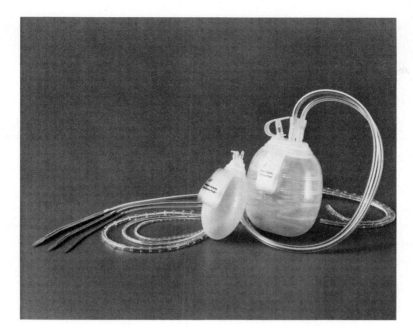

Fig. 8-6. Portable, self-contained closed wound drainage system. (Courtesy Zimmer, Inc., Warsaw, Ind.)

qualities seem to aid wound healing and protect delicate healing skin edges.

In some situations the wound is not dressed at all. The air-exposed wound will heal, and having no dressing: (1) allows for optimum observation of the incisional area, (2) aids bathing, (3) prevents possible adhesive tape reactions, (4) increases comfort and maneuverability for many patients, and (5) seems to minimize adverse responses by the patient to the operation.

DRAINS

Drains provide exits through which air and fluids such as serum, blood, lymph, intestinal secretions, bile, and pus can be evacuated from the operative site. Drains may also be used to prevent the development of deep wound infections. They are usually inserted at the time of surgery, directly from the incision or through a separate small incision, known as a *stab wound,* close to the operative site.

In some instances (chest, common bile duct, bladder), drainage is directly through the tube. In other instances (peritoneal cavity), drainage of pus or blood is primarily along the outside surface of the drain by capillary action and gravity (as with the Penrose drain). One specialized type of drain inserted into the bladder during many types of surgery is the Foley retention catheter, commonly used to monitor urinary output and aid the healing process, especially in pelvic and genitourinary surgery.

Many types of drains are available. The most common are made of latex, PVC (polyvinyl chloride), or silicone (Fig. 8-5). For many wounds, a portable, self-contained, closed wound suction unit is selected. These units create a negative pressure in a reservoir attached to the drain. Fluid is then gently drawn out of the wound and collected in the reservoir (Fig. 8-6).

The perioperative nurse must clearly document the location and type of drains on the operative record. This information is important to nurses caring for the patient in the postanesthesia and postoperative nursing units.

REFERENCES

Association of Operating Room Nurses: Recommended practices for documentation of perioperative nursing care (iii: 4:1–4). In AORN standards and recommended practices for perioperative nursing, Denver, 1990, The Association.

Garner, Julia S.: Guidelines for prevention of surgical wound infections, Atlanta, 1985, U.S. Department of Health and Human Services.

BIBLIOGRAPHY

Association of Operating Room Nurses, AORN standards and recommended practices for perioperative nursing, Denver, 1990, The Association.

Carey, K., editor: Nursing photobook: caring for surgical patients, Springhouse, Pa., 1982, Intermed Communications.

DiNoble, C.: Wound drainage, past, present, future, Todays OR Nurse 6, 1984.

Flynn, M., and Rovee, D.: Promoting wound healing, Am. J. Nurs. 82:1544, 1982.

Johnson and Johnson Products Inc.: A practical guide to wound care, New Brunswick, N.J., 1985.

Johnson and Johnson Products, Inc.: Dynamics of wound healing and treatment: workbook, New Brunswick, N.J., 1985.

Peacock, E.: Wound repair, ed. 3, Philadelphia, 1984, W.B. Saunders Co.

Westaby, S.: Wound care, St. Louis, 1985, The C.V. Mosby Co.

Wysocki, A.: Surgical wound healing: a review for perioperative nurses, AORN J. 49:502, 1989.

9 Anesthesia

JOHN LEE HOFFER

Without anesthesia, most modern surgical procedures would not be feasible. Therefore, the perioperative nurse must be familiar with the principles and practices of anesthesia and the perioperative functions of the anesthesiologist. This chapter presents an overview of the modern practice of anesthesia, the factors involved, and the interrelationship with the perioperative nurse. Included are the major types of anesthesia, an introduction to the more commonly used drugs, descriptions of the anesthesia machines and monitoring equipment so that the perioperative nurse is familiar with their basic functions when minor cases are done without anesthesia services, a review of the standards of anesthesia care, and an overview of some of the problems that can occur during the perioperative period. Forms of anesthesia that are rarely used, including hypnoanesthesia (usually hypnosis) and acupuncture (commonly used in Asian countries) are not discussed.

HISTORY OF ANESTHESIA

The early history of modern anesthesia was fraught with controversy. Surgeons in the early nineteenth century frequently used alcohol or opium to intoxicate the patient for procedures involving intense pain or when muscle relaxation was needed. In some cases, hypnotism was also employed. Therefore, the success of surgery was commonly correlated with the speed of the surgeon.

In March 1842, Crawford W. Long, a physician in Danielsville, Georgia, using ether as an anesthetic, removed a cystic tumor from the neck of James Venable. As confirmed by other physicians in the area, Dr. Long subsequently used ether for other procedures but did not publish reports of his experiences.

In 1844, Horace Wells, a dentist in Hartford, Connecticut, began to use nitrous oxide for anesthesia and communicated his results to his former partner, William T.G. Morton. However, following a fatality with nitrous oxide, Wells quit the practice of dentistry and later committed suicide. Morton subsequently studied medicine and learned of the anesthetic effects of chloric ether from his preceptor, Charles T. Jackson, a chemist. In July 1844, while employing this new drug, Morton was able to fill a tooth without the patient experiencing pain. He later learned from Jackson that sulfuric ether had similar properties and utilized it while extracting a deeply rooted bicuspid tooth from another patient.

Morton then contacted John C. Warren, a surgeon at Massachusetts General Hospital, and persuaded him to give the new anesthetic a trial during a surgical procedure. With Morton as the anesthetist, this historic operation took place in the amphitheater (subsequently renamed The Ether Dome) of Massachusetts General Hospital on October 16, 1846. In 5 minutes, Warren operated on an unconscious, still patient and dissected "a congenital but superficial vascular tumor just below the jaw on the left side of the neck." As the patient regained consciousness, Warren exclaimed "Gentlemen, this is no humbug." The next day, a large fatty tumor on the shoulder of another patient was removed by Haywood with Morton as the anesthetist.

Based on these events, the first medical report of anesthesia was announced to the world on November 18, 1846, by Henry J. Bigelow in the *Boston Medical and Surgical Journal*. An era had ended in which successful surgery was largely predicated on the lightning speed of the surgeon while working on a struggling, distressed patient. Anesthetic techniques gave the surgeon more time to operate and permitted new procedures that would have been impossible before. Thus, many modern surgical techniques have been feasible because of advancements in the art and science of anesthesia.

The word *anesthesia* is derived from the Greek word *anaisthesis*, which literally means "not sensation." Anesthesia was listed in *Bailey's English Dictionary* in 1721. When the effects of ether were discovered, Oliver Wendell Holmes suggested "anesthesia" be used as a name for the new phenomenon. Some believed that he coined this term; others think he knew of the Greek word Plato had employed. In any case, in the new era of surgery for which it became a cornerstone, anesthesia was, in the memorable phrase of Werr Mitchell, the "death of pain."

From these early beginnings, anesthesia has expanded to a more precise and sophisticated science that interrelates with many other medical specialties.

ANESTHESIA PROVIDERS

In the United States, anesthesia care is usually provided by an anesthesiologist (a physician with 4 or more years of specialty training in anesthesiology after medical school) or by a certified registered nurse anesthetist (CRNA) working under the direction and supervision of an anesthesiologist or a physician. The CRNA must have 2 years of training in anesthesia. The anesthesiologist is frequently said to be the patient's advocate in the perioperative period; as such, the anesthesiologist must be concerned with many divergent factors when the patient's own sensory and cerebral functions have been obtunded by anesthesia. The field of anesthesia has become so complex that in many large hospitals an anesthesiologist may further specialize in such areas as obstetric, neurosurgical, pediatric, cardiovascular, or ambulatory anesthesia.

PATIENT SAFETY

Patient risk and safety are always concerns during surgery and anesthesia. About 25 million anesthetics are administered each year in the United States. Of these, an anesthetic misadventure is a primary cause of death in only about 2000 cases. For healthy individuals, the risk factor is only about 0.01%. Data from a number of studies of deaths caused principally by anesthesia indicate a death rate ranging from 1 per 20,000 to 1 per 35,000, although one study reported a rate of 1 per 85,000. These rates represent approximately a fourfold decline over the last 30 years, even though surgical procedures are undertaken on increasingly sicker and much higher risk patients than in the past. However, for several reasons the general public still seems to consider anesthesia a major risk. Sensationalized reports have appeared in the news media and magazine articles. Also, anesthesia-related deaths often occur acutely, whereas surgical problems may not result in mortality or morbidity until hours or even days after the surgery. In addition, anesthesiologists have been willing to report, analyze, and study anesthetic misadventures in an effort to improve the overall quality of patient care. Awareness of potential problems and constant vigilance are crucial to good patient care.

PREOPERATIVE PREPARATION
Patient evaluation

Before surgery the anesthesiologist reviews the patient's chart, evaluates the laboratory data and diagnostic studies such as the electrocardiogram and chest x-ray, verifies the surgical procedure, examines the patient, discusses the options for anesthesia and the attendant risks, and orders premedications if appropriate. The analysis and significance of abnormal laboratory data and diagnostic studies are beyond the scope of this chapter; however, many standard anesthesia texts provide extensive discussions. The patient's physical status is assessed, and the most appropriate anesthetic technique is selected. Before elective surgery the patient should be in optimal medical condition. Occasionally, the anesthesiologist may feel that a patient's physical status could be improved to reduce the risk in-

volved. In such cases this opinion is discussed with the patient's primary physician, and if necessary elective surgery is deferred until the patient's condition can be improved. If the intended surgery is emergent, any benefits to be gained from delay must be weighed against the attendant hazards of waiting.

The assignment of a physical status classification by the anesthesiologist is based upon the patient's physiologic condition independent of the proposed surgical procedure. The physical status classification was developed by the American Society of Anesthesiologists (ASA) to provide uniform guidelines for anesthesiologists. It is an evaluation of anesthetic morbidity and mortality related to the extent of systemic diseases, physiologic dysfunction, and anatomic abnormalities. Intraoperative difficulties occur more frequently with patients who have a poor physical status classification. The ASA classification is given in Table 9-1.

Choice of anesthesia

The choice of anesthesia for a given surgical procedure is primarily made by the anesthesiologist. Numerous factors influence this decision, including the patient's understanding and wishes regarding the type of anesthesia that could be used, the type and duration of the surgical procedure, the patient's position during surgery, the patient's physiologic status and stability, the presence and severity of coexisting diseases, the patient's mental and psychologic status, the postoperative recovery from various kinds of anesthesia, options for management of postoperative pain, and any particular requirements of the surgeon. It is often said that there is major and minor surgery but only major anesthesia.

Types of anesthesia care

A frequently used classification of anesthesia care is the following:

1. *General anesthesia.* This reversible, unconscious state is characterized by amnesia (sleep, hypnosis, or basal narcosis), analgesia (freedom from pain), depression of reflexes, muscle relaxation, and manipulation of physiologic systems and functions. This "trip toward the edge of life" is carefully controlled and orchestrated by the anesthesiologist. Most patients think of general anesthesia when they are scheduled to have a surgical procedure; that is, they expect to be "put to sleep."

2. *Regional anesthesia.* In the broad sense it includes any instance in which a local anesthetic is injected to block or anesthetize a nerve or nerve fibers. Typically, regional anesthesia implies a major nerve block administered by an anesthesiologist (such as spinal, epidural, caudal, or major peripheral block).

3. *Monitored anesthesia care.* Infiltration of the sur-

Table 9-1. Physical (P) status classification of the American Society of Anesthesiologists

Status*†	Definition	Description and examples
P1	A normal healthy patient.	No physiologic, psychologic, biochemical, or organic disturbance.
P2	A patient with a mild systemic disease.	Cardiovascular disease with minimal restriction on activity. Hypertension, asthma, chronic bronchitis, obesity, or diabetes mellitus.
P3	A patient with a severe systemic disease that limits activity, but is not incapacitating.	Cardiovascular or pulmonary disease that limits activity. Severe diabetes with systemic complications. History of myocardial infarction, angina pectoris, or poorly controlled hypertension.
P4	A patient with severe systemic disease that is a constant threat to life.	Severe cardiac, pulmonary, renal, hepatic, or endocrine dysfunction.
P5	A moribund patient who is not expected to survive 24 hours with or without the operation.	Surgery is done as last recourse or resuscitative effort. Major multisystem or cerebral trauma, ruptured aneurysm, or large pulmonary embolus.
P6	A patient declared brain dead whose organs are being removed for donor purpose.	

Reprinted with permission from the American Society of Anesthesiologists, ASA, 515 Busse Highway, Park Ridge, Ill., 60068.
*In status 2, 3, and 4, the systemic disease may or may not be related to the cause for surgery.
†For any patient (P1 through P5) requiring emergency surgery, an E is added to the physical status, for example, P1E, P2E.

gical site with a local anesthetic is frequently performed by the surgeon. The anesthesiologist may supplement the local anesthesia with intravenous drugs that provide systemic analgesia and sedation and depress the response of the patient's autonomic nervous system. The anesthesiologist also monitors the patient's vital functions and may titrate additional intravenous drugs to optimize the patient's physiologic status. This technique can be used for critically ill patients who may not tolerate a general anesthetic as well as for healthy patients undergoing relatively minor surgical procedures. *Local standby* or *anesthesia standby* are formerly used equivalent terms.

4. *Local anesthesia.* This type is usually employed for minor procedures in which the surgical site is infiltrated with a local anesthetic such as lidocaine or bupivacaine. For such procedures the anesthesiologist is not involved in the patient's care. A perioperative nurse usually monitors the patient's vital signs and in addition may inject intravenous sedative or analgesic drugs as the surgeon directs.

Premedications

The purpose of premedication before anesthesia is to sedate the patient and reduce anxiety. Premedications may be classified as sedatives and hypnotics, tranquilizers, analgesics or narcotics, and anticholinergics. A single drug may possess the properties of several classes. An analgesic or narcotic may be ordered if preoperative discomfort is anticipated during invasive procedures or administration of a regional anesthetic. An anticholinergic such as atropine or glycopyrrolate may be included for pediatric patients, for surgery involving the oropharynx, or when a cardiac reflex may cause bradycardia.

Depending on the anesthesiologist's preference and the drugs ordered, either an intramuscular (IM), intravenous (IV), or oral (with 15 to 30 ml of water) premedication may be used. However, for many cases no premedication is ordered. An oral premedication is less painful for the patient; the absorption and uptake are more predictable than with an IM injection; and the small amount of water is readily absorbed directly across the gastric mucosa. With an oral premedication, an antacid or an H_2 receptor-blocking drug such as cimetidine (Tagamet) or ranitidine (Zantac) may be included to decrease gastric acid production and thus make the gastric contents less acidic. Should aspiration occur, this premedication decreases the resultant pulmonary damage.

Premedications are usually given 60 to 90 minutes before surgery but may be given intravenously after the patient arrives in the surgical suite. Except for the small amount of water needed to swallow any medications, adult patients are usually kept NPO (nothing by mouth) for a minimum of 6 hours before elective surgery.

Although pharmacologic premedications are commonly used, studies have shown that visits before surgery by the anesthesiologist and the perioperative nurse are far more important in decreasing the patient's anxiety. Patients' major fears include the unknown, relinquishing control of their lives to someone else, and never awakening from anesthesia (that is, dying). Often premedication is not given to older patients because their anxiety levels seem to be lower, their responses to medications may be unpredictable, and additional sedation can be given intravenously in the operating room suite if required. Preoperative sedation is usually not given to ambulatory patients because residual effects of the drugs are present long after the patients have been discharged and gone home.

Perioperative monitoring

The last few years have brought more advancements in perioperative monitoring than the previous two decades. Among the medical specialties, anesthesiology has been a pioneer in the review and analysis of perioperative mishaps and implementation of improved monitoring techniques and guidelines. These improvements have resulted in significant decreases in mortality and morbidity. In several states the malpractice insurance carriers have recognized the significance of these improvements and decreased their premiums if certain monitors such as pulse oximeters and end tidal carbon dioxide ($ETCO_2$) monitors are routinely employed.

The American Society of Anesthesiologists has adopted the Standards for Basic Intra-Operative Monitoring (in the box on pp. 150-151) as guidelines for good patient care. The perioperative nurse must be familiar with these standards and understand their significance in patient safety. If routine or frequent deviation from such standards occur, then a Q.A. alert (notification through the hospital's quality assurance program) should be considered.

For patients under general anesthesia, monitors that are considered appropriate by most anesthesiologists include: (1) inspired oxygen analyzer (F_1O_2), which is calibrated to room air and 100% oxygen on a daily basis; (2) low-pressure disconnect alarm, which senses pressure in the expiratory limb of the patient circuit; (3) inspiratory pressure; (4) respirometer (these four devices are an integral part of most modern anesthesia machines); (5) electrocardiograph; (6) blood pressure (frequently measured with an automated unit); (7) heart rate; (8) precordial or esophageal stethoscope; (9) temperature; (10) peripheral nerve stimulator if muscle relaxants are used; (11) pulse oximeter; and (12) end tidal carbon dioxide monitor. Many hospitals also analyze respiratory and anesthetic gases with a mass spectrometer.

In addition, a Foley catheter may be used. For selected cases with a potential risk of venous air embolism, a doppler probe may also be placed over the right atrium. Based on the cardiovascular and pulmonary status of the patient, the surgical procedure, and the chance of significant physiologic changes, additional invasive monitors may be used. They include direct arterial pressure measurements, central venous pressure measurements, pulmonary artery catheter, and continuous mixed venous oxygen saturation measured

with a special pulmonary artery catheter. For special conditions other monitors, such as transcutaneous O_2 and CO_2, transesophageal echocardiography, evoked potentials, electroencephalogram, and cerebral or neurologic function monitors may be used.

Despite some controversy, most anesthesiologists believe that the extent of noninvasive and invasive monitoring employed depends upon the physiologic status and stability of the patient; the surgical procedure planned and its potential for sudden changes in cardiorespiratory functions, acute blood loss, or major fluid shifts; and the anticipated monitoring needs for postoperative management as opposed to whether a general or regional anesthetic technique will be used. However, monitoring of some parameters is negated by the anesthetic technique selected. For example, a low-pressure disconnect alarm is unnecessary with regional anesthesia when a patient is breathing spontaneously. A peripheral nerve stimulator is not needed if muscle relaxants are not used.

The perioperative utilization of pulse oximetry and end tidal capnography has grown exponentially. Therefore, a brief overview of the principles involved will aid in understanding their use.

Pulse oximetry

Pulse oximetry is based on the principles of spectrometric oximetry, plethysmography, and the Lambert-Beer law, which relates the concentration of solute in suspension to the intensity of light transmitted through the solution. It provides a continuous noninvasive indication of the arterial oxygen saturation of functional hemoglobin and the pulse rate and thus provides an early warning of hypoxemia. Maintenance of an arterial O_2 saturation above 90% corresponds to a PaO_2 of 60 torr or greater.

The sensor combines two low-intensity light-emitting diodes (LED) as light sources and a photodiode as a receiver or light detector. One LED emits red light (approximately 660 nanometers [nm]), and the other LED emits infrared light (approximately 940 nm). These light sources alternate approximately 480 times a second. When transmitted through blood and tissue, the two frequencies are absorbed differently by the tissue components and by the reduced hemoglobin and the oxyhemoglobin. Because absorption by the other tissue components is essentially constant, the major variable is the saturation of the hemoglobin with oxygen. The internal microprocessor analyzes the variations in the absorption of light emitted from both LEDs and provides a readout of the percent saturation of hemoglobin with oxygen. The pulse rate is incidentally derived. Several units also provide a waveform that correlates with the arterial pulsations.

The response of the pulse oximeter can be adversely affected by any event that significantly reduces vascular pulsations, such as hypoperfusion, hypotension, hypovolemia, vasoconstriction, or hypothermia. Electrosurgery,

STANDARDS FOR BASIC INTRA-OPERATIVE MONITORING

These standards apply to all anesthesia care although, in emergency circumstances, appropriate life support measures take precedence. These standards may be exceeded at any time based on the judgement of the responsible anesthesiologist. They are intended to encourage high quality patient care, but observing them cannot guarantee any specific patient outcome. They are subject to revision from time to time, as warranted by the evolution of technology and practice. This set of standards addresses only the issue of basic intraoperative monitoring, which is one component of anesthesia care. In certain rare or unusual circumstances, 1) some of these methods of monitoring may be clinically impractical, and 2) appropriate use of the described monitoring methods may fail to detect untoward clinical developments. Brief interruptions of continual† monitoring may be unavoidable. *Under extenuating circumstances, the responsible anesthesiologist may waive the requirements marked with an asterisk (*); it is recommended that when this is done, it should be so stated (including the reasons) in a note in the patient's medical record.* These standards are not intended for application to the care of the obstetrical patient in labor or in the conduct of pain management.

Standard I

Qualified anesthesia personnel shall be present in the room throughout the conduct of all general anesthetics, regional anesthetics and monitored anesthesia care.

Objective

Because of the rapid changes in patient status during anesthesia, qualified anesthesia personnel shall be continuously present to monitor the patient and provide anesthesia care. In the event there is a direct known hazard, e.g., radiation, to the anesthesia personnel which might require intermittent remote observation of the patient, some provision for monitoring the patient must be made. In the event that an emergency requires the temporary absence of the person primarily responsible for the anesthetic, the best judgement

of the anesthesiologist will be exercised in comparing the emergency with the anesthetized patient's condition and in the selection of the person left responsible for the anesthetic during the temporary absence.

Standard II

During all anesthetics, the patient's oxygenation, ventilation, circulation and temperature shall be continually evaluated.

Oxygenation

Objective

To ensure adequate oxygen concentration in the inspired gas and the blood during all anesthetics.

Methods

1) Inspired gas: During every administration of general anesthesia using an anesthesia machine, the concentration of oxygen in the patient breathing system shall be measured by an oxygen analyzer with a low oxygen concentration limit alarm in use.*

2) Blood oxygenation: During all anesthetics, a quantitative method of assessing oxygenation such as pulse oximetry shall be employed.* Adequate illumination and exposure of the patient is necessary to assess color.*

Ventilation

Objective

To ensure adequate ventilation of the patient during all anesthetics.

Methods

1) Every patient receiving general anesthesia shall have the adequacy of ventilation continually evaluated. While qualitative clinical signs such as chest excursion, observation of the reservoir breathing bag and auscultation of breath sounds may be adequate, quantitative monitoring of the CO_2 content and/or volume of expired gas is encouraged.

2) When an endotracheal tube is inserted, its correct positioning in the trachea must be verified. Clinical assessment is essential and end-tidal CO_2

Reprinted with permission from the American Society of Anesthesiologists, ASA, 515 Busse Highway, Park Ridge, Ill., 60068.
†Note that "continual" is defined as "repeated regularly and frequently in steady rapid succession" whereas "continuous" means "prolonged without any interruption at any time."

STANDARDS FOR BASIC INTRA-OPERATIVE MONITORING—cont'd

analysis, in use from the time of endotracheal tube placement, is encouraged.

3) When ventilation is controlled by a mechanical ventilator, there shall be in continuous use a device that is capable of detecting disconnection of components of the breathing system. The device must give an audible signal when its alarm threshold is exceeded.

4) During regional anesthesia and monitored anesthesia care, the adequacy of ventilation shall be evaluated, at least, by continual observation of qualitative clinical signs.

Circulation
Objective
To ensure the adequacy of the patient's circulatory function during all anesthetics.

Methods
1) Every patient receiving anesthesia shall have the electrocardiogram continuously displayed from the beginning of anesthesia until preparing to leave the anesthetizing location.*

2) Every patient receiving anesthesia shall have arterial blood pressure and heart rate determined and evaluated at least every five minutes.*

3) Every patient receiving general anesthesia shall have, in addition to the above, circulatory function continually evaluated by at least one of the following: palpation of a pulse, auscultation of heart sounds, monitoring of a tracing of intra-arterial pressure, ultrasound peripheral pulse monitoring, or pulse plethysmography or oximetry.

Body Temperature
Objective
To aid in the maintenance of appropriate body temperature during all anesthetics.

Methods
There shall be readily available a means to continuously measure the patient's temperature. When changes in body temperature are intended, anticipated or suspected, the temperature shall be measured.

---

motion, or ambient light may also artifactually decrease the readout. Carboxyhemoglobin (carbon monoxide bound to hemoglobin) falsely elevates the saturation, and methemoglobin (hemoglobin that has an oxidized iron molecule and cannot reversibly combine with oxygen) falsely lowers the saturation. Intravenous dyes affect the pulse oximeter. Methylene blue may cause a drop to 65% for 1 to 2 minutes, indigo carmine a very slight decrease, and indocyanine green a slightly greater decrease.

The sensor is usually placed on the third or fourth finger, although various manufacturers have other sensors for the ear lobe and the bridge of the nose, as well as smaller ones for infants and children. The pulse oximeter does not require user calibration. Care must be taken to prevent localized neurovascular or ischemic damage. For example, a hard-cased sensor placed on a finger when the arms are tightly secured at the patient's side during a long procedure may cause ischemia.

Capnography

A capnometer measures carbon dioxide, and a capnograph has a waveform display. In patients with normal circulation and pulmonary function, it provides an excellent method to evaluate alveolar ventilation. There is only a small gradient from the arterial to the alveolar CO_2, and

with forced expiration the $ETCO_2$ provides a close approximation of the arterial CO_2 ($PaCO_2$). However, because an anesthetized patient only passively expires and the point of measurement is near the connection between the patient circuit and the endotracheal tube, there is approximately a 5 to 8 torr gradient between the $ETCO_2$ and the $PaCO_2$ measured with an arterial blood gas.

The $ETCO_2$ can be measured by a mass spectrometer or an infrared analyzer. Recent advances in the technology and application of infrared analyzers and microprocessors have resulted in compact units that provide a continuous indication of the $ETCO_2$ and have made these the most widely used units for perioperative monitoring. They measure the amount of infrared light (426 microns) absorbed by CO_2 in the sample of gas. Two general types of monitors are in use. In the *mainstream* unit, all respired gas passes through the detector, whereas with the *sidestream* unit a portion of the gas is aspirated at a constant rate (50 to 250 ml/min) through a small-bore tubing into the unit. Each design has advantages. Most units display a waveform of the expiratory CO_2 partial pressure versus time after a short sampling and processing delay. The waveform is important for correctly interpreting the output data. Digital readouts usually give the $ETCO_2$ and respiratory rate. Daily user calibration is rarely required with the newer units. Nitrous oxide also absorbs infrared near the same frequency, but most units have empirically compensated for nitrous oxide usage. Clinically, the units are useful to verify endotracheal intubation, circuit disconnection, alveolar ventilation, early return of muscle function after muscle relaxants are used, and acute alterations in metabolic functions such as malignant hyperthermia or thyrotoxicosis.

GENERAL ANESTHESIA
Mechanism of action

Numerous theories have been proposed to explain the action of general anesthetics. Many of the recent investigations have involved the inhalation anesthetics. (The terms *volatile anesthetic* and *potent agent* are synonymous with *inhaled anesthetic*.) Most evidence indicates that the synaptic transmission of nerve impulses is reversibly inhibited in several areas of the central nervous system. The extent of inhibition and consequently the progressive depression of function are correlated with the partial pressure of the inhaled anesthetic at various sites. The inhibition is believed to occur at a lipophilic site on the biologic membrane of synapses and possibly on small, unmyelinated nerve fibers. Suppression of spinal reflex activity is thought to produce some relaxation of skeletal muscles. Although no single concept explains all the phenomena, a few theories explain many of the actions that have been observed. The following are some of the more widely accepted theories:

1. The *protein receptor theory* proposes that hydrophobic areas of specific proteins in the central nervous system act as receptor sites. The steep dose-response curve of inhaled anesthetics seems to support this theory by indicating that a critical number of receptor sites must be occupied before patient movement in response to a noxious stimuli is obtunded.
2. The *Meyer-Overton theory* is also called the *critical volume hypothesis* to explain the correlation between the lipid solubility (oil/gas partition coefficient) and the anesthetic potency. This theory proposes that when enough anesthetic molecules dissolve (that is, a critical volume is reached) at a crucial hydrophobic site such as the lipid cellular membrane, anesthesia is achieved. As the cell membrane expands in response to the dissolved anesthetic molecules, changes in the ionic channels occur and alter the sodium flux involved in cellular depolarization. However, because some lipid-soluble compounds are not anesthetics, this theory does not give a complete explanation of anesthetic action.
3. *Endogenous endorphins* or opiate-like substances suppress various pain pathways. Several classes of endorphins have been identified. The action of beta-endorphins is antagonized by naloxone (a specific

narcotic antagonist), but the relative potency of inhaled anesthetics is not altered. Although some degree of analgesia may be explained by this mechanism, it does not correlate well with the anesthesia caused by inhaled anesthetics.

Intravenous anesthetics may function by some of the mechanisms proposed for the inhaled anesthetics. Factors involved in the pharmacokinetics of intravenous drugs include the volume of distribution, biotransformation, and clearance of the drug by metabolism, excretion, or elimination of the drug and its metabolites. The concept of half-life (distribution and elimination) of a drug is used to correlate the decline of a drug's action with the concentration of the drug in the blood.

In summary, no single theory for the mechanism of action can explain all the effects observed with anesthetic agents. The spectrum of anesthetic activity varies with the different anesthetics; the effects on the central nervous system and skeletal muscles are similar but not identical; structural and spatial differences exist among agents; changes at both the membrane and cellular levels occur; and optical isomers produce different responses. Although similar in many respects, anesthetic agents are individually unique and probably work through numerous mechanisms and at multiple sites to produce their effects.

Levels of general anesthesia

Guedel integrated the signs and stages of ether anesthesia into a system (Fig. 9-1) that was used clinically for more than 60 years. This system applied only to unpremedicated patients breathing spontaneously during ether anesthesia, a technique that is rarely used in modern medicine. By evaluating the physiologic changes and reflex responses listed in Fig. 9-1, one can estimate the depth of anesthesia. Stage 1 is from the initial administration of anesthetic agents to loss of consciousness. Stage 2 is from the loss of consciousness to onset of regular breathing and loss of the eyelid reflex. Stage 2 is also called the *delirium* or *excitement* stage, and thrashing movements may occur. No auditory or physical stimulation should take place during this stage. Stage 3, which begins with onset of a regular breathing pattern and lasts until cessation of respiration, is divided into four planes and is the stage of surgical anesthesia. Stage 4 is from cessation of respiration to circulatory failure that leads to death.

Although Guedel's system gives us an appreciation for the interrelationships of numerous signs during anesthesia, the variety of drugs and anesthetic techniques used today do not provide such uniform responses suitable for estimating the exact depth of anesthesia. Opioids and anticholinergic drugs given as premedicants alter the pupillary responses. Evaluation of respiratory responses and muscle tone is not valid when controlled ventilation and muscle relaxants are used. Today, general anesthesia is usually begun with the intravenous injection of a rapid-acting drug

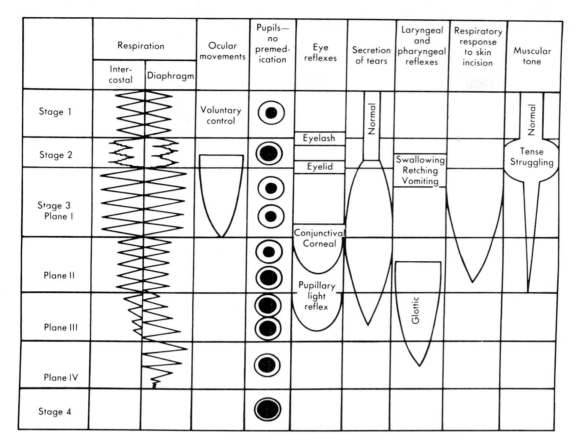

Fig. 9-1. Changes occurring during anesthesia as seen with ether anesthesia. The actions of different anesthetics vary slightly from this. (After Guedel; from Atkinson, R.S., Rushman, G.B., and Lee, J.A.: A synopsis of anaesthesia, London, 1982, John Wright & Sons, Ltd., Medical Publishers.)

such as thiopental that takes the patient to stage 3 and eliminates the untoward responses often seen during stage 2.

For optimal anesthesia and good surgical conditions, several different but interrelated factors are involved: hypnosis (sleep), analgesia (freedom from pain), amnesia (lack of recall), appropriate surgical conditions such as muscle relaxation and positioning of the patient, and continued homeostasis of the patient's vital functions such as the respiratory, cardiovascular, and renal systems. Different drugs and anesthetic agents possess various properties that facilitate the above conditions. Thus, combinations of drugs are used to obtain the desired effect. For example, diazepam is a hypnotic and amnestic, thiopental and etomidate are hypnotics, morphine and fentanyl are analgesics, and pancuronium and succinylcholine are muscle relaxants. Muscle relaxants primarily affect only skeletal muscles and not cardiac or smooth muscles; however, some relaxants may cause side effects such as tachycardia via the autonomic nervous system or hypotension secondary to release of histamine. The potent inhalational anesthetics (halothane, enflurane, and isoflurane) provide sleep, am-

nesia, analgesia, and muscle relaxation in varying degrees. Hypotensive or hypertensive drugs and cardioactive agents may also be included to achieve the optimum depth of anesthesia while affecting physiologic homeostasis as little as possible. Some of the drugs commonly used in anesthesia are briefly described in Table 9-2.

Phases of general anesthesia

General anesthesia may be divided into three phases: induction, maintenance, and emergence. Induction begins with administration of anesthetic agents and continues until the patient is ready for surgical manipulation, skin preparation, or incision. This exact point may vary with the surgical procedure. The maintenance phase continues from this point until near completion of the procedure and may be accomplished with inhalation agents and/or with titrated doses of intravenous drugs. Emergence varies in length and depends on the depth and duration of anesthesia and on the patient's position and condition. Emergence starts as the patient begins to "emerge" from anesthesia and usually ends when the patient is ready to leave the operating room. Intubation occurs during the induction

Table 9-2. Commonly used anesthetic drugs

	Common usage	Advantages	Disadvantages	Comments
INHALATIONAL AGENTS				
Oxygen (O₂)	Essential for life	Can slightly increase amount available to tissues in low cardiac output states	Can cause retinopathy in premature infants	High concentrations hazardous with lasers in surgery of head and neck and pulmonary areas Hypoxia if overdose given
Nitrous oxide (N₂O)	Maintenance; occasionally for induction	Rapid induction and recovery; additive effects to other anesthetics	No relaxation; can depress myocardium	
Enflurane (Ethrane)	Maintenance; occasionally for induction	Good relaxation; allows larger amounts of epinephrine to be used than with halothane; 2.4% metabolized	Can cause increased heart rate and hypotension; lowers seizure threshold; slightly irritating odor	Abnormal EEG at high concentrations
Halothane (Fluothane)	Maintenance; occasionally for induction	Rapid induction and recovery; pleasant, nonirritating odor, fair relaxation	Narrow margin of safety—sensitizes myocardium to epinephrine; rare cause of liver damage; 15-20% metabolized.	May cause bradycardia and hypotension; PVCs and ventricular fibrillation may occur if epinephrine is used
Isoflurane (Forane)	Maintenance; occasionally for induction	Good relaxation; allows larger amounts of epinephrine to be used than with halothane; maintains cardiac output; 0.2% metabolized	Increases heart rate; slightly irritating odor	Isomer of enflurane
DEPOLARIZING MUSCLE RELAXANTS				
Succinylcholine (Anectine)	Intubation; short cases	Rapid onset; short duration	Requires refrigeration; may cause muscle fasciculations, postoperative myalgias and arrhythmias; increase in serum K⁺ with burns, tissue trauma, paralysis and diseases affecting muscles; slight histamine release	Prolonged muscle relaxation with pseudocholinesterase deficiency and certain antibiotics

NONDEPOLARIZING MUSCLE RELAXANTS—Intermediate onset and duration				
Atracurium (Tracrium)	Intubation; maintenance of relaxation	No significant cardiovascular effects; no cumulative effects; good with renal failure	Requires refrigeration; slight histamine release	Breakdown by Hofmann elimination and ester hydrolysis
Vecuronium (Norcuron)	Intubation; maintenance of relaxation	No significant cardiovascular effects; no cumulative effects and no histamine release	Requires mixing	Mostly eliminated in bile, some in urine
NONDEPOLARIZING MUSCLE RELAXANTS—Longer onset and duration				
d-Tubocurare (Curare, tubocurarine)	Maintenance of relaxation		May cause histamine release and transient ganglionic blockade	
Metocurine (Metubine)	Maintenance of relaxation	Good cardiovascular stability	Slight histamine release	Large bolus may cause hypotension
Pancuronium (Pavulon)	Maintenance of relaxation		May cause tachycardia and hypertension	Mostly dependent on renal elimination
INTRAVENOUS ANESTHETICS				
Etomidate (Amidate)	Induction	Good cardiovascular stability; fast, smooth induction and recovery	May cause pain with injection and myotonic movements	
Diazepam (Valium)	Amnesia; hypnotic; preoperative medication	Good sedation	Prolonged duration	
Ketamine (Ketalar)	Induction, occasional maintenance (IV or IM)	Short acting; patient maintains airway; good in small children and burn patients	Large doses may cause hallucinations and respiratory depression	Need darkened quiet room for recovery; often used in trauma cases
Midazolam (Versed)	Hypnotic; anxiolytic sedation often used as adjunct to induction	Excellent amnesia; water soluble (no pain with IV injection); short acting	Slower induction than thiopental	
Propofol (Diprivan)	Induction and maintenance	Rapid onset; awakening in 4 to 8 min.	May cause pain if injected in small vein	Short elimination half-life (34 to 64 min)
Sodium methohexital (Brevital)	Induction	Ultrashort-acting barbiturate	May cause hiccups	Can be given rectally
Thiopental sodium (Pentothal)	Induction	Fast, smooth induction and recovery	Large doses may cause apnea and cardiovascular depression	May cause laryngospasm; can be given rectally

Continued.

Table 9-2. Commonly used anesthetic drugs—cont'd

	Common usage	Advantages	Disadvantages	Comments
LOCAL ANESTHETICS				
Bupivacaine (Marcaine, Sensorcaine)	Epidural, spinal, or local infiltration	Good relaxation; long acting	Overdose can cause cardiac collapse	Maximum dose: 200 and 150 mg/70 kg with and without epinepherine, respectively
Chloroprocaine (Nesacaine)	Epidural anesthesia	Ultrashort acting; good relaxation	May cause neurotoxicity if injected into CSF	Maximum dose: 1000 and 800 mg/70 kg with and without epinepherine, respectively
Lidocaine (Xylocaine)	Epidural, spinal, peripheral, IV blocks and local infiltration	Short acting; good relaxation; low toxicity	Overdose can cause convulsions	Also used for ventricular dysrhythmias; maximum dose: 7 and 5 mg/kg with and without epinepherine, respectively
Tetracaine (Pontacaine)	Spinal anesthesia	Long acting; good relaxation		Maximum dose: 1-1.5 mg/kg (epinepherine rarely used)
ANTICHOLINERGICS				
Atropine	Blocks effects of acetylcholine; decreases vagal tone; reverses muscle relaxants; treats sinus bradycardia	Increases heart rate; suppresses salivation, bronchial and gastric secretions	Depresses sweating; may cause dry mouth, flushing, dizziness, CNS symptoms	Quite selective at muscarinic receptor in smooth and cardiac muscle and exocrine glands
Glycopyrrolate (Robinul)	Similar to atropine	Small increase in heart rate; does not cross blood-brain barrier; can raise gastric pH more than atropine	Prolonged duration of effects	Lower incidence of dysrhythmias than atropine

phase, and extubation is usually performed during emergence. Recovery from anesthesia can be considered as a fourth phase of general anesthesia.

Types of general anesthesia

The type of general anesthesia employed for maintenance is often described as intravenous, inhalation (with a volatile anesthetic agent), or a combination of both intravenous and inhalation anesthetics (also referred to as *balanced*). For example, an intravenous technique includes an induction agent such as thiopental, followed by 30% to 40% oxygen with nitrous oxide, an amnestic drug such as midazolam or diazepam, an analgesic such as fentanyl or morphine sulfate, and a muscle relaxant. In contrast, an inhalation technique may utilize thiopental to faciliate a rapid induction, or the patient may "breathe himself down" with increasing concentrations of a potent agent such as halothane, enflurane or isoflurane plus oxygen. An inhalation induction is often used with children to avoid inserting an intravenous catheter before induction, which can be traumatic. Depending upon the kind of surgical procedure, maintenance of anesthesia may be accomplished with only an inhalation agent and spontaneous, assisted, or controlled ventilation. Effects of the volatile agents are dose related and provide differing levels of sleep, amnesia, analgesia, muscle relaxation, and cardiovascular system responses. If supplemental muscle relaxation is needed, the dose required is significantly less than the dose necessary during intravenous anesthesia. In the past, the term *balanced anesthesia* was used when various combinations of intravenous drugs were "balanced" to provide complete anesthesia. Today, the term is most often used to describe a combination of both intravenous drugs and inhalation agents employed to obtain specific effects in each patient and procedure.

Typical sequence of general anesthesia

After arriving in the operating room suite, the patient is identified, the chart is checked for a signed consent or operative permit, and the latest results of laboratory tests and diagnostic studies are reviewed. Depending on the policy of the anesthesia department, an intravenous infusion may be started in a preoperative area or after the patient is transferred to the operating room bed. In the perioperative period, nearly all anesthesia-related drugs are given intravenously, except, of course, the inhalation agents. The appropriate intraoperative monitoring devices are usually connected to the patient before induction of anesthesia.

At induction, the patient is usually preoxygenated (actually denitrogenated) through a mask with 100% oxygen for 3 to 5 minutes. This practice permits washout of most of the gaseous nitrogen from the body and provides a large reserve supply of oxygen in the lungs, should any difficulties be encountered during induction or intubation. A test dose of the induction agent (for example, 50 mg of thiopental) is given to check for any unusual or exaggerated response. If succinylcholine will be used for intubation, then a small pretreatment dose of a nondepolarizing muscle relaxant (such as 3 mg of *d*-tubocurarine or 0.5 to 1 mg of pancuronium) is usually given. When given approximately 5 minutes before the succinylcholine, this small dose is usually sufficient to block most of the muscle fasciculations seen with succinylcholine and thereby decrease the resultant postoperative myalgias.

To induce anesthesia and to move the patient rapidly to stage 3, a short-acting barbiturate such as thiopental (2 to 6 mg/kg) is given. When the patient becomes apneic and the eyelid reflex is gone, the airway is checked for patency by ventilating the patient with a mask. Depending on several factors such as an adequate airway and the type and duration of surgery, oxygen and anesthetic gases may be delivered to a spontaneously breathing patient via a mask that is held in place with a head strap. Positioning of the head and an oral or nasal airway may be used to maintain a patent airway. If mask anesthesia is not suitable, then an endotracheal tube may be used to facilitate ventilation or to protect the airway from aspiration. Typical equipment used for intubation and airway control is shown in Fig. 9-2. An intubating dose of a muscle relaxant such as succinylcholine (1 to 1.5 mg/kg) is then given. The muscle relaxant causes temporary paralysis of the jaw and diaphragmatic muscles as well as other skeletal muscles.

To facilitate intubation, a laryngoscope held in the left hand is inserted into the right side of the mouth and then moved to the midline, "sweeping" the tongue to the left. The endotracheal tube is introduced on the right side of the mouth and gently inserted into the trachea so that the cuff is approximately 1 cm below the vocal cords. The cuff is inflated just enough to occlude any air passage with the peak pressures used for ventilation. Correct location of the endotracheal tube is verified by listening for bilaterally equal breath sounds with a stethoscope, by absence of sounds over the stomach, by symmetrical movement of the thorax with positive pressure ventilation, by condensation of moisture from expired air in the endotracheal tube and breathing circuit, and by an appropriate level and waveform of $ETCO_2$. Proper placement of the endotracheal tube is shown in Fig. 9-3. The vocal cords are the narrowest portion of an adult trachea; however, the smallest portion of a child's airway is below the vocal cords. Therefore uncuffed endotracheal tubes are usually used for children because the internal diameter of cuffed tubes in these small sizes would have too much resistance to ventilation and could easily become obstructed. After the paralysis from the succinylcholine has worn off, the patient may be allowed to breathe spontaneously with intermittent assistance, or additional muscle relaxant may be given and the ventilation controlled either manually or mechanically.

If the procedure is an emergency or the patient is at

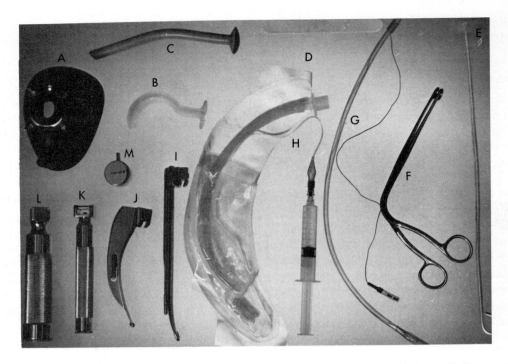

Fig. 9-2. Commonly used anesthesia equipment. **A,** Mask. **B,** Oral airway. **C,** Nasal airway. **D,** Tongue blade. **E,** Stylet for endotracheal tube. **F,** McGill forceps. **G,** Esophageal stethoscope with temperature monitor. **H,** Endotracheal tube. **I,** Miller blade. **J,** MacIntosh blade. **K,** Pediatric laryngoscope handle. **L,** Laryngoscope handle. **M,** Precordial stethoscope.

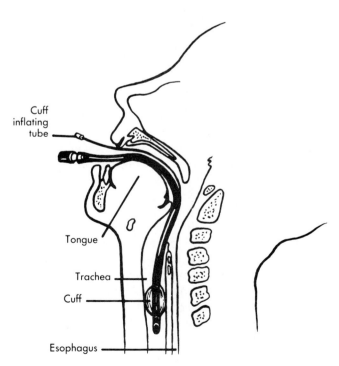

Fig. 9-3. Endotracheal tube in position.

risk for aspiration (for example, in cases of intestinal obstruction, full stomach, hiatal hernia), the anesthesiologist may undertake a rapid sequence induction. Standing on the patient's right side, the perioperative nurse must be ready to assist as necessary by applying downward pressure on the cricoid cartilage with the thumb and index finger of the right hand while the left hand is placed under the patient's neck for stability. The cricoid cartilage is the only complete ring in the trachea, and downward pressure occludes the esophagus, which lies immediately posterior to the trachea. If, after assessment of the patient's airway, the anesthesiologist feels that rapid intubation of the trachea may be difficult, an awake intubation, using a fiberoptic bronchoscope or other techniques, may be chosen.

Maintenance of anesthesia can be accomplished with either intravenous or inhalational anesthetic techniques or a combination of both, with or without additional muscle relaxant. A variety of factors are considered by the anesthesiologist in selecting the anesthesia technique for each situation.

Many factors also influence emergence, but typically the objective is to have the patient ready to be moved from the operating room bed to the postanesthesia care unit (PACU) bed as soon as the dressing is completed. During emergence, the anesthesiologist suctions the oropharynx to decrease the risk of aspiration or laryngospasm following extubation, reverses any residual paralysis from the

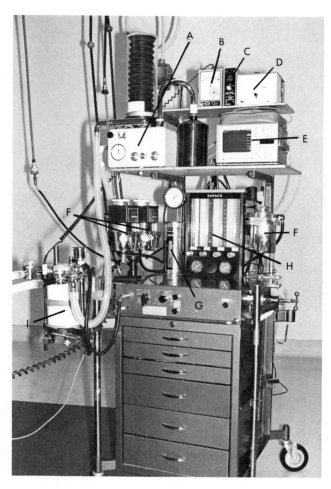

Fig. 9-4. Older anesthesia machine. **A,** Ventilator. **B,** Oxygen analyzer. **C,** Disconnect alarm. **D,** Temperature monitor. **E,** ECG monitor. **F,** Flow-through vaporizers. **G,** Copper Kettle vaporizer. **H,** Flowmeters. **I,** CO_2 absorber and circle system.

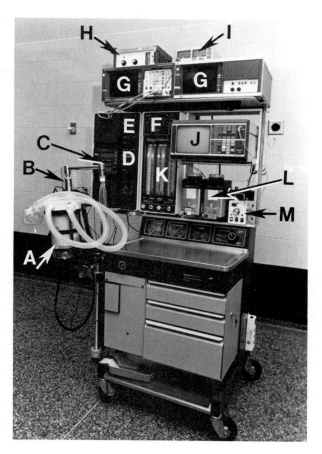

Fig. 9-5. Modern anesthesia machine. **A,** CO_2 absorber and circle system. **B,** Ventilator. **C,** Pulse oximeter. **D,** Oxygen analyzer. **E,** Expired flow monitor. **F,** Ventilator controls. **G,** ECG and direct pressure monitor. **H,** Doppler. **I,** Temperature monitor. **J,** $ETCO_2$ and respiratory gases monitor. **K,** Flowmeters. **L,** Flow-through vaporizers. **M,** Peripheral nerve stimulator.

nondepolarizing muscle relaxant with an anticholinesterase such as neostigmine and an anticholinergic such as atropine, and allows the washout of nitrous oxide and volatile anesthetic agents by giving 100% oxygen for several minutes before extubation. The patient is then transported to the PACU to awaken from the anesthetic experience.

Untoward events that can occur with general anesthesia include hypoxia; respiratory, cardiovascular, or renal dysfunction; hypotension; hypertension; imbalance of fluids or electrolytes; residual muscle paralysis; neurologic problems; and malignant hyperthermia. The anesthesiologist usually directs the treatment and management of such events.

Anesthesia machines

The first apparatus resembling an anesthesia machine was used in 1905. Since then, innumerable changes and improvements have been incorporated. The anesthesia machine used for general anesthesia looks more complicated

than it is, but the basic functions of all anesthesia machines are similar and simple to understand. Perioperative nurses should comprehend the basic function of anesthesia machines because they may need to administer oxygen during local procedures. Many anesthesia machines are still in service after 10 to 25 years. An older model is shown in Fig. 9-4 and a newer one in Fig. 9-5. A typical schematic is shown in Fig. 9-6. Anesthesia machines sold in the United States after January 1, 1984, are required to meet the criteria set forth in the Amerian National Standards Institute (ANSI) Standard Z79.8. This standard incorporates many safety features that were not required on earlier machines. Because diagrams of anesthesia machines are difficult to find in reference books, the pneumatic circuit for the Ohmeda Modulus II Plus is shown in Fig. 9-7 and the piping diagram for the North American Drager Narkomed models 2B and 3 in Fig. 9-8. These references will enable perioperative nurses to become familiar with the anesthesia machines used at their hospital.

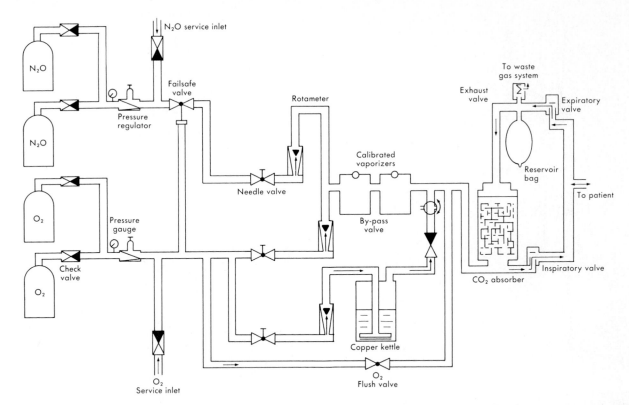

Fig. 9-6. Anesthesia machine circuit. Oxygen and nitrous oxide enter the machine from cylinders or from the hospital service supply. Pressure regulators reduce cylinder pressure to about 50 psi. Check valves prevent transfilling of cylinders or gas flow from cylinders to service line. The fail-safe valve prevents flow of nitrous oxide if the oxygen supply fails. Needle valves control flows to rotameters. Calibrated vaporizers provide a preselected concentration of volatile anesthetics. An interlock allows only one vaporizer to be on at a time. The Copper Kettle delivers the saturated vapor of any agent; thus the effluent must be diluted. The bypass valve vents vapor from the Kettle when it is not in service. Gases are delivered to the circle absorber, where unidirectional valves assure flow from patient through carbon dioxide absorber. Excess gas is vented through the exhaust valve into a waste gas scavenger system. The reservoir bag compensates for variations in respiratory demand. (From Dripps, R.D., Eckenhoff, J.E., and Vandam, L.D.: Introduction to anesthesia: the principles of safe practice, ed. 6, Philadelphia, 1982, W.B. Saunders Co.)

Oxygen and nitrous oxide are usually supplied from the hospital pipelines to the anesthesia machine at pressures of 50 to 55 psi. The gas hoses going to the machine are color-coded, and the connectors are specific for each gas so that nitrous oxide cannot be inadvertently connected to the oxygen hose or vice versa. If a central gas supply is not available or the hospital piping system fails, the machines are equipped with E-size cylinders of both gases. One or two cylinders of each gas are connected to yokes on the machine. These yokes are pin indexed so that only the correct gas (oxygen or nitrous oxide) can be connected in that position. In the pin-indexing safety system, two steel pins are in a unique location on the yoke assembly. The mating gas cylinder (for example, the oxygen tank) has two matching holes in the same locations so that the cylinders cannot be mounted in the wrong place.

In cylinders, oxygen is stored as a compressed gas. A full E-size cylinder contains about 660 L of oxygen at 2000 psi. As the oxygen is used, the pressure falls in direct

proportion to the remaining volume. Because the E-size cylinder is used to provide oxygen while transporting patients, knowing how much oxygen is left in a partially used tank is important. Thus 1000 psi would indicate 330 L remaining, and 500 psi would indicate 165 L remaining or sufficient oxygen for 5 L/min flow for more than 25 minutes. When the pressure has dropped to about 250 psi, the cylinder should not be used because it no longer has an adequate reserve.

Nitrous oxide is stored as a liquid in cylinders, and the pressure above the liquid is 750 psi. A full, E-size cylinder contains about 1600 L of nitrous oxide. As the nitrous oxide is used, the pressure above the liquid remains constant. Only when the liquid has been completely vaporized does the pressure begin to fall. Therefore the nitrous oxide can be almost gone but still show the same pressure. In contrast to oxygen, the amount remaining in the tank cannot be readily determined.

The gases in the cylinders flow through regulators that

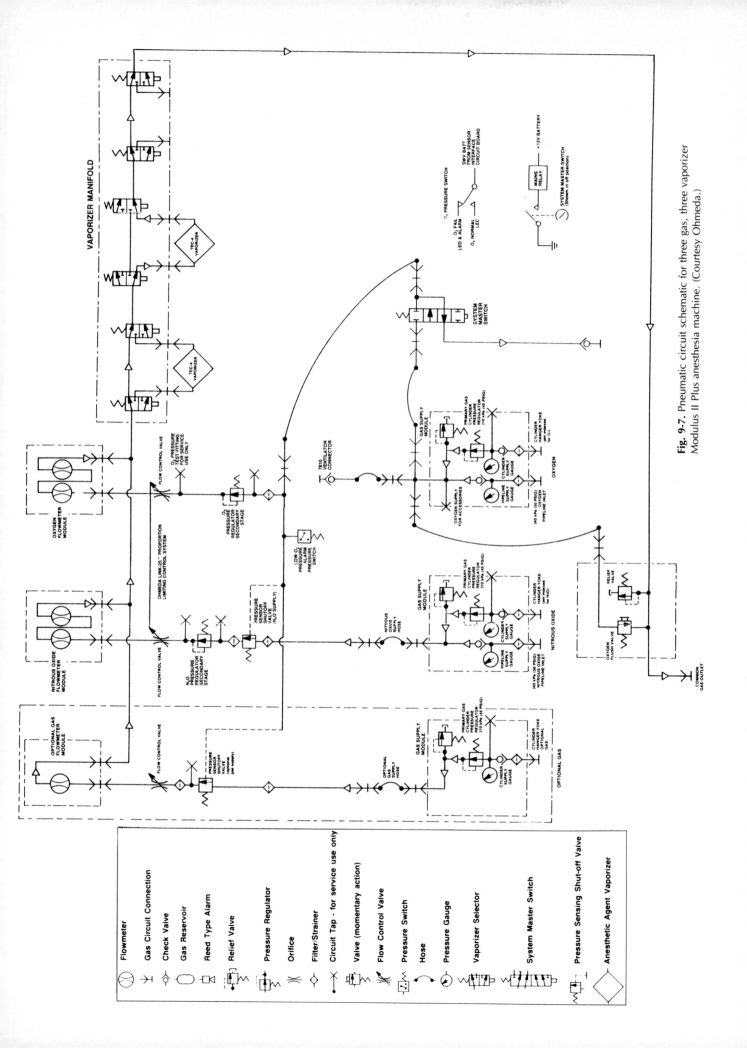

Fig. 9-7. Pneumatic circuit schematic for three gas, three vaporizer Modulus II Plus anesthesia machine. (Courtesy Ohmeda.)

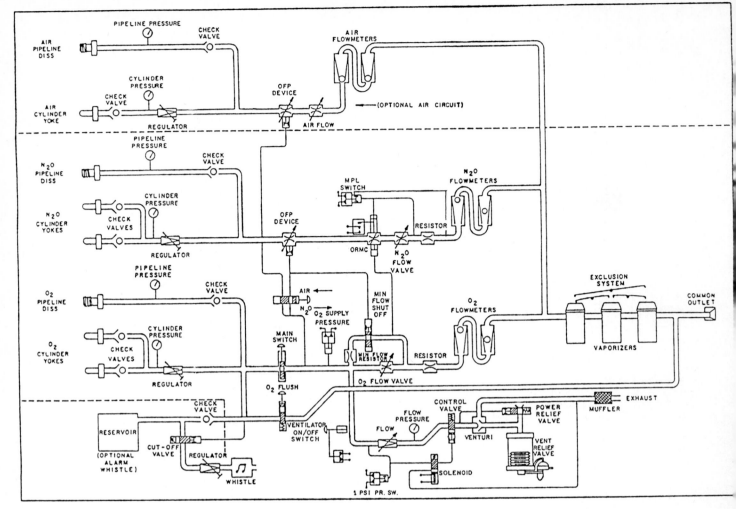

Fig. 9-8. Piping diagram for Narkomed models 2B and 3 anesthesia machines. (Courtesy North American Drager.)

reduce the pressure to about 50 psi. The hoses from the hospital gas sources are connected to the machine at the outlet of these regulators. In most machines of recent vintage, a pressure interlock device shuts off the nitrous oxide flow if oxygen pressure is not present. The gases then flow through individual *flowmeters* (or rotameters) on the front of the machine so that the gas flows and the ratio of oxygen to nitrous oxide can be selected by the anesthesiologist. From the top of the flowmeters, the gases are mixed and then flow through a vaporizer in which the inhalational anesthetic of choice is vaporized and added to the oxygen–nitrous oxide mixture. The total gas flow is then delivered from the machine to the patient. With a *flow-through vaporizer*, by definition, all of the fresh gas going to the patient from the anesthesia machine flows through the vaporizer. The control dials are usually located on top of these vaporizers and are calibrated in percentages. Most recently manufactured vaporizers are flow and temperature compensated, meaning that they are reasonably accurate

at all flows and temperatures used clinically. The filling ports on the vaporizers are usually key indexed so that only the appropriate volatile agent can be used.

Although no longer approved (by the ANSI Z79.8 standard) for sale in the United States, another type of vaporizer, the *bypass vaporizer,* functions in a different manner. The Copper Kettle is one type of bypass vaporizer that may still be found on many older machines. A low flow of oxygen (usually less than 1 L/min) goes through a separate flowmeter and then through the bypass vaporizer, where this oxygen is totally saturated with the anesthetic vapor. The saturated oxygen is then combined with the oxygen–nitrous oxide mixture from the other flowmeters, and the total mixture flows from the machine to the patient. To calculate the concentration of anesthetic going to the patient, the anesthesiologist must know the barometric pressure, the vapor pressure of the anesthetic agent being used, the oxygen flow through the bypass vaporizer, the temperature of the anesthetic liquid in the

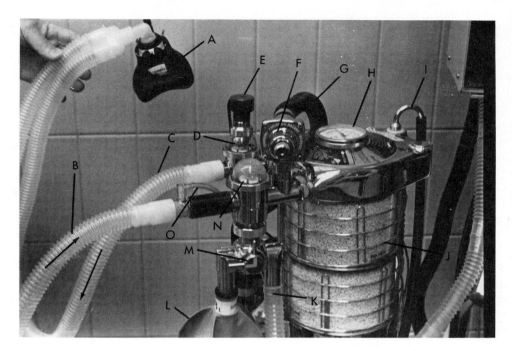

Fig. 9-9. A typical circle system. **A,** Anesthetic mask. **B,** Expiratory limb of patient circuit. **C,** Inspiratory limb of patient circuit. **D,** One-way inspiratory valve. **E,** Inspired oxygen sensor. **F,** Adjustable pop-off valve. **G,** Waste gas tubing to scavenging system. **H,** Inspiratory pressure gauge. **I,** Fresh gas supply. **J,** Carbon dioxide absorber. **K,** Connection to ventilator. **L,** Reservoir bag. **M,** Reservoir bag/ventilator selector. **N,** One-way expiratory valve. **O,** Sensing line for low-pressure alarm.

vaporizer, and the combined flow of the oxygen–nitrous oxide mixture. The major advantage of bypass vaporizers is that any volatile anesthetic agent can be used in them. However, serious accidents have occurred when the "wrong" anesthetic was in the vaporizer and the concentration of anesthetic was thus incorrectly calculated.

Another important feature of the anesthesia machine is the *oxygen flush button.* With all new machines and on most earlier models, pushing the oxygen flush button allows 100% oxygen from the 50 psi line to flow directly to the *fresh gas outlet* on the machine and thus to the patient. This oxygen flow completely bypasses the flowmeters and vaporizers. Caution must be exercised, because the pressure is 50 psi.

In most hospitals in the United States, a semiclosed circle system is used to deliver the fresh gas flow (including anesthetic gases) to patients. The circle system is composed of a container filled with a CO_2-absorbing material (such as soda lime or baralime), *two unidirectional valves,* an *adjustable pressure limiting valve (APL),* a *reservoir bag,* an inlet connection for fresh gas flow, and two connections to the patient through corrugated breathing (or anesthesia) hoses. As the patient inspires, gases are drawn through the CO_2 absorber and from the fresh gas supply through the inspiratory limb of the corrugated hoses. As the patient exhales, the one-way valve on the inspiratory limb prevents backflow, and the exhaled gases flow through the expiratory limb and through the expiratory one-way valve. The expiratory limb and valve are easily identified by the condensation of water vapor along this portion of the circuit. The 3-L reservoir bag absorbs the peak flow of expired gases and allows the anesthesiologist to force gas through the CO_2 absorber along the inspiratory limb of the circuit and thereby ventilate the patient. The expired gases flow through the CO_2 absorber, where the carbon dioxide is removed from them. Any excess gas is vented through the APL valve, which is usually mounted just ahead of the CO_2 absorber. A typical circle system is shown in Fig. 9-9.

The F_IO_2 sensor is usually mounted in the inspiratory limb just after the one-way valve. It measures the fraction of inspired O_2 and can be set to alarm if a low concentration is detected. A low pressure sensor is usually mounted in the expiratory limb near the other one-way valve to detect a ventilator malfunction or a disconnection in the circuit.

The advantage of the circle system is that much lower flows of oxygen, nitrous oxide, and anesthetic gases can be used, thereby reducing the cost. The compounds used in the CO_2 absorber include an indicator that changes color as the substance becomes exhausted. For example, the soda lime may turn from white to blue, indicating that the absorbent material must be changed to prevent a buildup of CO_2 in the patient.

A semiclosed circuit (or circle system) is typically used

where the fresh gas flow into the system may range from 1 to 6 L/min. During exhalation, some of the expired gases recycle through the CO_2 absorber, and the excess gas is scavenged or eliminated (hence *semiclosed*). With a *closed-circuit system,* all CO_2 is absorbed, no gas is vented from the system, and only enough oxygen to meet the basal requirements of the patient (3.5 ml/kg/min) is added to the system. Measured quantities of volatile anesthetics may be injected into a closed-circle system. In an *open circuit* (such as the Ayres T-piece, Magill, or Bain circuits), a relatively high flow of fresh gas is used, and most of the exhaled gas is vented from the circuit. The fresh gas flow rates vary from approximately two thirds of the patient's minute volume with the Magill circuit to at least 100 ml/kg for the Bain or T-piece circuits. The open-circuit system is commonly used for neonates, infants, and small children.

With all these circuits, the final connection to the patient is via a mask or endotracheal tube. A mask may be used for a patient with a good airway and at minimal risk of aspiration, for relatively short procedures, and when the surgical site is not around the head or neck. An endotracheal tube is inserted into the trachea (intubation) to ensure a patent airway during surgery on the head or neck or when the patient is paralyzed. In such cases the ventilation is usually controlled during the procedure.

REGIONAL ANESTHESIA

Preoperative preparation is essentially the same for both general and regional anesthesia except that an analgesic such as morphine sulfate may be added to the preoperative medications before regional anesthesia to blunt any discomfort during placement of the regional block. The criteria for monitoring during general and regional anesthesia are also similar. Whenever regional anesthesia is performed, resuscitative equipment and drugs must be immediately available. Regional anesthesia can be accomplished by injecting a local anesthetic anywhere along the peripheral nerve pathways from the spinal cord (spinal anesthesia), epidurally, peripherally, or topically. Comparative locations for the needle and catheter relative to the dura for spinal and epidural anesthesia are shown in Fig. 9-10.

Spinal anesthesia

A local anesthetic (usually lidocaine, tetracaine, or bupivacaine) is injected into the cerebral spinal fluid (CSF) in the subarachnoid space. The anesthetic is generally mixed with a dextrose solution for total of 1 to 4 ml to make a hyperbaric solution. For short procedures, lidocaine with 7.5% dextrose may be used. A 25- or 22-gauge × 3½-inch spinal needle is usually inserted in the L2-3, L3-4, or L4-5 interspace with the patient either lying on one side curled into a fetal position or in a sitting position. These mixtures are hyperbaric (heavier than the

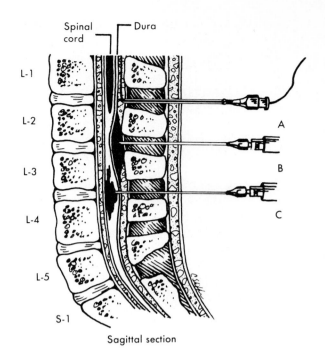

Fig. 9-10. Location of needle point and injected anesthetic relative to dura. **A,** Epidural catheter. **B,** Single injection epidural. **C,** Spinal anesthesia. (Interspaces most commonly used are L4-5, L3-4, and L2-3.)

CSF) and settle in a gravity-dependent manner. Thus, by changing the patient's position, the block can be directed up, down, or to one side of the spinal cord. For example, with prostate surgery the patient may remain in the sitting position for a minute or so after the local anesthetic is injected. A bilateral block of the S1-5 dermatomes results.

For surgery in the upper abdomen, the patient may be placed in a slightly (5-degree) head-down position to allow the anesthetic to move cephalad while the anesthesiologist carefully checks the level of sensory block. When an adequate level is obtained, the bed is leveled to minimize further spread. After 10 minutes, the block is usually "set" and will not extend farther. The sympathetic nervous system is usually blocked two dermatomes higher and the motor block two dermatomes lower than the sensory block. The patient may then be positioned as necessary for surgery.

Spinal anesthesia may evoke several physiologic responses that can result in major problems if not properly managed by the anesthesiologist.

1. Rapid decline in blood pressure may occur after the local anesthetic is injected. It is caused by vasodilation as the sympathetic nerves that control vasomotor tone are blocked, with peripheral pooling of blood causing reduced venous return to the heart and a decrease in cardiac output. This hypotensive response can usually be avoided by infusing 750 to 1500 ml of balanced salt solution immediately be-

fore the block and placing the patient in a 5-degree head-down position to improve venous return to the heart. A vasopressor such as ephedrine may also be administered.

2. An inadvertently high (or "total") spinal may cause paralysis of the respiratory muscles and necessitate immediate intubation and ventilation. An amnestic agent should also be given. The anesthesiologist and the circulating nurse should be vigilant for any symptoms of respiratory distress after administration of a spinal anesthetic.

3. Because pain and sensory input to a portion of the patient's body are blocked, care must be taken in positioning the patient intraoperatively to avoid neurologic damage, burns, or other trauma.

4. Although the problem is not related to the regional anesthetic technique as such, the patient may become disoriented or incoherent during cases such as transurethral resection of the prostate (TURP) and be incorrectly treated with additional sedation. This alteration in mental status is caused by extensive resection across venous sinuses and use of copious irrigation fluid, which is absorbed into the vascular system. Dilutional hyponatremia occurs as the sodium-free irrigation solution is mixed with blood. Treatment may include diuretics, sodium infusion, or both.

One of the most frequent postoperative complaints following spinal anesthesia is a "postspinal headache." The incidence is greatest in young parturients or other individuals less than 40 years of age, but even in these patients it is only about 1% when a 25- or 26-gauge needle is used and is unrelated to how soon the patient is ambulated. The headache is thought to result from leakage of cerebrospinal fluid through the hole in the dura and typically occurs when the patient assumes an upright position. The headache is usually in the occiput and generally resolves over 1 to 3 days. Various treatment modalities are used, including strict bedrest for 24 to 48 hours, vigorous hydration, abdominal binders, epidural infusion of saline, and injection of 5 to 20 ml of autologous blood into the epidural space at the puncture site (that is, a "blood patch").

Epidural and caudal anesthesia

The epidural space is between the ligamentum flavum and the dura and extends from the foramen magnum to the sacrococcygeal membrane. This potential space is filled with epidural veins, fat, and loose areolar tissue. For epidural anesthesia the local anesthetic is usually injected through the intervertebral spaces in the lumbar region, although it can also be injected in the cervical or thoracic regions. The anesthetic spreads both cephalad and caudad from the site of injection. A comparative location of the needle points and injected anesthetic is shown in Fig. 9-10.

For caudal anesthesia the local anesthetic is also injected into the epidural space, but the approach is through the caudal canal in the sacrum. This approach requires a significantly greater volume of anesthetic to fill the epidural space to the same level as an anesthetic injected epidurally in the lumbar area. Caudal anesthesia also has a 5% to 10% technical failure rate; however, it may be employed for pediatric surgery on the lower extremities or for perineal surgery in adults.

Several techniques may be used, including a malleable needle, a "single-shot epidural" injected through the needle before its removal, intermittent injections through a catheter threaded into the epidural space (followed by withdrawal of the needle), and continuous infusion through the catheter with a calibrated pump. Technical skill is required to identify the epidural space with the needle point. Such techniques include "hanging drop" and "loss of resistance" to injection of either air or saline as the needle point is slowly advanced through the ligamentum flavum.

For the hanging drop technique, the epidural needle is filled with sterile saline or local anesthetic with a meniscus at the needle hub. As the needle is slowly advanced into the epidural space, a negative (less than atmospheric) pressure draws the fluid inward toward the epidural space. Location of the needle tip within the epidural space is verified by injection of 1 to 2 ml of air or saline.

When the local anesthetic is injected into the epidural space, the major sites of action are probably the dorsal root ganglia and the nerve roots as they leave the spinal cord and proceed out the intervertebral foramina beyond the meningeal sheath. However, some of the anesthetic diffuses into the subarachnoid space itself. Because the local anesthetic diffuses superiorly and inferiorly from the site of epidural injection, segmental anesthesia may be possible in specific areas. In contrast to spinal anesthesia, much larger volumes of local anesthetic are needed with epidural anesthesia; the head-up, head-down, or lateral position of the patient does not have as much effect on the level of the epidural anesthetic; and onset of the block is much slower with epidural anesthesia. As with spinal anesthesia, hypotension can occur with epidural anesthesia, but the onset is much slower, and the hypotension can usually be managed with rapid intravenous infusion of a balanced salt solution and repositioning of the patient.

The most frequently used local anesthetics are lidocaine (with or without epinephrine), bupivacaine, and chloroprocaine. Depending on the concentration of the anesthetic agent, the effect can range from loss of sensory input to complete motor blockade. To help verify that the anesthetic is not being injected into the subarachnoid space or into an epidural vein, a test dose of 3 to 5 ml of lidocaine with a 1:200,000 concentration of epinephrine is frequently used. Injected intravascularly, this test dose causes a transient tachycardia; if injected into the subarachnoid space, it produces onset of spinal anesthesia. Neurologic sequelae have been reported when chloroprocaine was inadvertently injected into the subarachnoid space, and cardiac arrest has occurred when bupivacaine was injected intravascularly.

With epidural anesthesia several problems can occur.

1. Inadvertent puncture of the dura with the large (17- or 18-gauge) epidural needle, called a *wet tap,* can cause a postdural puncture headache. This headache is significant in about 50% of patients, and the intensity can be incapacitating. Treatment is essentially the same as discussed previously for postspinal headache.

2. If the needle or catheter is unintentionally inserted into the subarachnoid space and the large volume of local anesthetic typically used for epidural anesthesia is injected as a bolus, it causes a "total spinal" anesthesia. The anesthetic effect moves all the way to the brain and results in rapid hypotension caused by vasodilation, profound bradycardia as the vagus nerves to the heart are blocked, and a totally paralyzed and anesthetized, but awake, patient. Treatment includes intubation, control of ventilation, support of blood pressure and the cardiovascular system, and amnestic drugs until the block has resolved. If properly managed, this problem is not life threatening, but use of the test dose described previously usually averts it. With patient movement over time, the epidural catheter can migrate through the dura. Therefore, a small test dose should be given each time additional anesthetic solution is injected through the catheter.

3. The local anesthetic may be inadvertently injected into an epidural vein. This problem can occur with the initial injection or any subsequent dose. As stated previously, bupivacaine can cause cardiac arrest and cardiovascular collapse. Toxicity from other local anesthetic agents can cause sudden and profound hypotension, convulsions from the effects on the central nervous system, and tachycardia if the solution contains epinephrine. The convulsions usually dissipate rapidly as the local anesthetic is redistributed throughout the body, and thiopental or diazepam can be given intravenously to reduce the effects. A vasopressor (such as phenylephrine or ephedrine) can be used to restore blood pressure, and the patient may be paralyzed, intubated, and ventilated until the toxic effects are gone. Use of the test dose with each injection usually prevents these problems.

Peripheral nerve block

A wide variety of peripheral nerves can be effectively blocked by injecting local anesthetic around them to provide adequate surgical anesthesia. Anesthesia of the upper extremities can be easily provided in this manner. Onset and duration of the block are related to the drug used, its concentration and volume, and the addition of epinephrine. Complications are usually caused by an inadvertent intravascular injection or an overdose of the local anesthetic. Rarely, nerve damage may also occur from trauma by the needle or compression from the volume of local anesthetic.

Intravenous regional anesthesia

Intravenous regional anesthesia was first described by August Bier in 1908 and is frequently referred to as a *Bier block.* Although it can be used on a lower extremity, it is more often used on the upper extremities. It is highly reliable.

A small intravenous catheter is inserted as distally as feasible, and a single- or double-cuffed pneumatic tourniquet is placed around the limb proximal to the surgical site. The limb is raised upward, and the blood is then exsanguinated from the limb by wrapping with an Esmarch bandage. The tourniquet is then inflated to approximately 100 mm Hg above the patient's systolic blood pressure, and the Esmarch bandage is removed. Approximately 50 ml of 0.5% lidocaine is injected into the catheter. Onset of anesthesia is rapid and lasts until the tourniquet is deflated.

When a double-cuffed pneumatic tourniquet is used, the proximal cuff is initially inflated. When the patient experiences discomfort from the cuff pressure (usually about 35 to 40 minutes after inflation of the cuff), the distal cuff, which is located over an anesthetized area, is inflated. Then the proximal cuff is deflated. The proximal cuff must remain inflated until the distal cuff has been inflated to prevent loss of the intravenous anesthetic from the limb.

The patient may feel pain from the tourniquet, and an intravenously administered analgesic or sedative can be used to supplement the Bier block. Although problems can occur from an overdose or toxic reaction to the lidocaine, such problems are rare if the tourniquet has been inflated more than 20 minutes and is intermittently deflated for only a few seconds at a time for several cycles when the surgical procedure is over. This deflation procedure reduces the transient blood level of the local anesthetic in the central nervous system and the heart. Obviously, loss of pneumatic pressure in the tourniquet can cause both toxic reactions and loss of anesthesia.

MONITORED ANESTHESIA CARE

A gentle and patient surgeon can safely accomplish minor and even some major procedures when the surgical site is infiltrated with a local anesthetic. This technique can be employed both for normal, healthy individuals and for sicker, unstable patients who may not easily tolerate general anesthesia.

During monitored anesthesia care, the anesthesiologist

may supplement the local anesthetic with an intravenous analgesic such as fentanyl and with sedative and amnestic agents as needed. In addition, the anesthesiologist carefully monitors the patient's vital signs, respiratory and cardiovascular status, and positioning, and may give supplemental low-flow oxygen. Depending on the clinical situation, the anesthesiologist may have to induce general anesthesia or utilize one of the regional techniques described previously if a greater degree of anesthesia is necessary.

LOCAL ANESTHESIA

For selected patients a regional nerve block, "field" block, or infiltration with a local anesthetic is done by the surgeon. Other physicians such as cardiologists, pulmonologists, proctologists, or gastroenterologists may also schedule local cases in the operating room suite.

For these patients the physician may order a premedication. The physician is responsible for monitoring the patient and for all perioperative drugs used. The terms *local anesthesia, local,* and *straight local* are used interchangeably to describe these procedures. The anesthesiologist is not involved in such procedures. Hospitals and ambulatory facilities have established guidelines for monitoring, perioperative drugs, and the types of procedures that can be done with the patient under local anesthesia. A perioperative nurse is usually responsible for monitoring the patient and administering drugs as directed by the physician.

Patients receiving local anesthesia may have an intravenous infusion started before the procedure. Whenever feasible, intraoperative drugs are given intravenously and carefully titrated as their effects are monitored. Adequate venous access can be critical in life-threatening situations when resuscitative drugs must be given immediately.

The nurse should have a basic knowledge of the monitoring equipment that will be used, including the function, patient connections, and interpretation of the outputs and displays. As a minimum, this monitoring should include an ECG, heart rate, blood pressure, and pulse oximetry.

The nurse should be familiar with the drugs to be administered during the procedure. This knowledge should include the usual dosages, limits on both the rate of injection and maximum dosage (usually stated on a per kilogram basis), the duration of action, the physiologic and psychologic changes to be expected, normal and abnormal reactions to the drugs used, and the appropriate action to take should an untoward reaction occur. In addition to continuous or very frequent assessment of the patient's status, the vital signs should be recorded at least every 15 minutes. The drug dosage, route and time of administration, and patient monitoring performed should also be properly documented.

Should any significant change occur in the patient's physiologic or psychologic status, the nurse must immediately notify the physician. Good communication is essential for optimal patient care. Because the patient is awake during the procedure, extraneous or irrelevant conversation and noise pollution should be kept to a minimum.

Following completion of the procedure, the patient's postoperative status must be carefully assessed. The patient may be transferred to the PACU for recovery and observation or may be returned directly to the hospital room. This evaluation and decision should be properly documented on the chart, and a report called to the receiving unit prior to the patient's transfer. The report should include the type and amount of drugs given and any adverse reaction noted, the site and condition of the intravenous infusion (if applicable) as well as the type and amount of solution infused in the operation room, the range of intraoperative vital signs, the surgical procedure performed and the condition of the dressing, any special postoperative orders, and a general statement on the patient's tolerance of the procedure.

MALIGNANT HYPERTHERMIA

First identified in the late 1960s, malignant hyperthermia is a rare, life-threatening complication that may be triggered by drugs commonly used in anesthesia. Halothane and succinylcholine are the most frequently implicated triggering agents. Malignant hyperthemia may also be induced by trauma, strenuous exercise, or emotional stress. It is genetically transmitted as an autosomal dominant trait with variable expression in affected individuals. The syndrome begins with a hypermetabolic condition in skeletal muscle cells that involves altered mechanisms of calcium function at the cellular level. Characteristics of the syndrome include cellular hypermetabolism resulting in hypercarbia, tachycardia, hypoxia, metabolic and respiratory acidosis, cardiac dysrhythmias, and elevation of body temperature at a rate of 1 to 2° C every 5 minutes. It must be emphasized that the rise in body temperature is one of the late manifestations of malignant hyperthermia. These signs may occur during induction or maintenance of anesthesia, although the syndrome can occur postoperatively or even after repeated exposures to anesthesia. It is most frequently seen in children and adolescents.

Although malignant hyperthermia is rare, time is crucial when it does occur, and all operating room and anesthesia personnel should be familiar with the protocol for its management. In the past, mortality ranged from 50% to 80%, but the immediate infusion of dantrolene and proper treatment have significantly reduced the incidence of fatalities and complications. In addition to dantrolene, the major modalities of treatment include cooling the patient with ice packs and cold intravenous solutions, administering diuretics, treating cardiac arrhythmias, correcting the acid-base and electrolyte imbalances, and monitoring fluid intake and output and the body temperature.

Patients known or suspected to have this syndrome can

be anesthetized with minimal risk if appropriate precautions are taken. If the syndrome is suspected, a muscle biopsy should be done to make a definitive diagnosis. For their own safety, relatives of persons with malignant hyperthermia should be evaluated and tested for presence of the disease.

OPERATING ROOM POLLUTION

Contamination and pollution of the operating room environment can come from many sources. Every chemical should be considered potentially harmful until proven otherwise. Reaction to chemicals and irritants may vary with age, sex, race, season of the year, and concurrent exposure to other substances. Disinfectants, antiseptics, soaps, aerosol or pressurized sprays, and other compounds contribute to the potential for pollution. Recent attention is also being placed on noise pollution. Of particular interest in the present context is the pollution of the operating room with anesthetic gases such as nitrous oxide and the halogenated agents halothane, enflurane, and isoflurane. Various surveys taken among personnel exposed to these anesthetic gases (anesthesiologists, other anesthesia personnel, perioperative nurses, dentists, and dental assistants who work with anesthetic gases) and their spouses have implicated such pollution as a possible contributing factor to an increased abortion rate and incidence of lymphoma and other conditions. However, the interpretation of these surveys is controversial.

To minimize the hazards of bacteria and other airborne pollutants, as well as waste anesthetic gases, many operating room suites receive 100% fresh "conditioned" air with up to 25 air exchanges each hour. To reduce pollution from trace anesthetic gases and contain costs, many anesthesiologists use "low-flow" anesthetic techniques that greatly reduce the volume of waste gases. However, air pollution with waste anesthetic gases is still a major concern, and all anesthesia machines should have a waste gas scavenging system. In older systems the waste anesthetic gases may be vented through the air exhaust vent in each room. In modern operating room suites, a dedicated vacuum line is used to scavenge such gases. One such scavenging system is shown in Fig. 9-11. It has a reservoir bag so that less instantaneous suction or vacuum is needed, a positive pressure-relief valve that prevents excessive back pressure in the patient's lungs and that vents excess gas into the room air should the vacuum be occluded or inadequate, a negative pressure-relief valve that prevents excessive vacuum from damaging the patient's lungs, and a needle valve to adjust the vacuum. Evacuation hoses are connected to the ventilator and the APL valve. When the patient is not intubated, however, air pollution may occur from a loose mask fit on the patient's face. According to the National Institute for Occupational Safety and Health (NIOSH), pollution levels should be less than 25 ppm for nitrous oxide and 0.5 ppm for halogenated agents. Often

levels cannot be continuously kept this low during induction and emergence.

Chronic occupational exposure to trace concentrations of anesthetic gases is of particular concern to pregnant women. A safe exposure level below which one can be assured that no adverse effects will occur has not been established. Individuals with questions about exposure levels should consult a knowledgeable member of the anesthesia department for the latest information.

PERIOPERATIVE NURSING CONSIDERATIONS RELATED TO ANESTHESIA

Care of the surgical patient is a cooperative effort, and personnel involved in the perioperative period should function as a smooth, well-coordinated team. The nurse who checks the chart must verify the patient's identity and the scheduled procedure, confirm that the operative permit is properly signed, determine any allergies the patient may have, and ensure that current reports of laboratory tests and diagnostic studies are complete and on the chart.

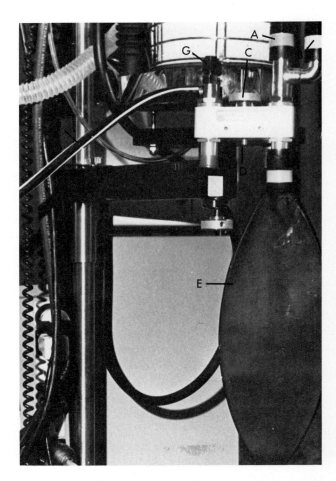

Fig. 9-11. A typical scavenging system for waste anesthetic gases. **A,** Scavenging hose from ventilator. **B,** Scavenging hose from pop-off valve. **C,** Positive pressure relief valve. **D,** Negative pressure relief valve. **E,** Reservoir bag. **F,** Vacuum line. **G,** Vacuum adjustment valve.

A patient must never be left alone in an operating room. For example, when an anesthesiologist has an anesthetized patient in the operating room, a perioperative nurse should always be immediately available to provide assistance if needed.

During insertion of intravenous, central venous pressure, arterial, or pulmonary artery catheters, the nurse should assist as appropriate.

During induction of anesthesia, particularly with a traumatized patient or for an emergency procedure, the nurse should stand at the right side of the patient and be ready to apply cricoid pressure to prevent regurgitation of stomach contents and to assist the anesthesiologist in visualizing the vocal cords. When cricoid pressure is used to prevent aspiration, it should not be released until the intubation is accomplished, the cuff on the endotracheal tube has been inflated, and proper placement of the endotracheal tube has been verified.

Operating room personnel should never move an unconscious patient without first obtaining permission from the anesthesiologist.

When the patient is appropriately positioned for surgery, the nurse should always check the arms and legs to ensure that no pressure points exist and that the extremities are appropriately positioned and padded.

As a team member, the nurse may be asked by the anesthesiologist to perform specific duties during the anesthetic induction or emergence. Throughout the surgical procedure, the circulating nurse is keenly aware of all aspects of the patient's care and assists the anesthesiologist as necessary.

Prior to the patient being transported to the PACU following completion of the procedure, the circulating nurse calls the PACU to give a preliminary status report of the patient's condition. That report includes the surgical procedure performed, type of anesthesia care provided, information specific to the patient's preoperative diagnosis and subsequent outcome related to intraoperative intervention, and any special equipment, such as a ventilator, that will be needed in the PACU.

POSTANESTHESIA RECOVERY

Recovery from anesthesia usually takes place in the PACU. In the past it was called the recovery room. Critically ill patients are usually transferred directly to the surgical intensive care unit for recovery and postoperative management. The PACU should be immediately adjacent to the operating room suite for rapid access by the anesthesiologist, should any untoward event occur. The PACU is staffed (ideally one nurse per patient) by nurses specially trained in prompt recognition and management of postoperative complications. Equipment and drugs must be available for routine postoperative care such as supplemental oxygen, suctioning, monitoring of vital signs, and

fluids management, as well as for full resuscitation if necessary.

When the patient arrives in the PACU, the anesthesiologist provides the PACU nurse with pertinent information, including name, age, surgical procedure and complications, type of anesthesia, preoperative medications and anesthesia drugs, preoperative and intraoperative vital signs, estimated blood loss and intraoperative fluid intake and output, allergies, orders for analgesia during recovery, and any special instructions. Any analgesics, sedatives, or other drugs given in the PACU are usually ordered by the anesthesiologist.

The initial vital signs and patient status are usually recorded on the anesthesia record. Supplemental oxygen (2 to 5 L/min) is usually given via nasal cannulae. Vital signs are recorded every 15 minutes or less and charted with other pertinent information on a separate PACU record. To facilitate recovery, the PACU nurse encourages the patient to wake up, cough, breathe deeply, and change positions. For a graphic summary of the patient's recovery, many institutions use some variation of the post anesthetic recovery score (PARS) originally proposed by Aldrete. The PARS is recorded every 15 to 30 minutes until discharge. A score of 9 or 10 usually indicates that the patient is ready for transfer to the postoperative nursing unit. The parameters typically evaluated are shown in Fig. 9-12. Before transfer back to the room, the patient is evaluated and discharged from the PACU by the anesthesiologist.

Common problems

A number of problems can occur during recovery from anesthesia. The PACU nurse must be aware of the potential problems and frequently assess the patient's status so that early intervention therapy can be initiated.

Nausea and vomiting

Nausea is believed to be caused by stimulation of the vomiting center in the medulla by impulses from the gastrointestinal tract, other cerebral centers, or drugs. It occurs more frequently in females than males. Contributing factors include a history of motion sickness, pain, perioperative medications, anesthetic technique, gastric distention, duration of surgery, surgical site (upper abdomen or thorax more than lower abdomen or extremities), perioperative hypotension, respiratory insufficiency, obesity, patient positioning, and rapid patient movement.

Prophylactic measures that decrease the instance of nausea and the risk of aspiration include nonparticulate antacids (0.3 M sodium citrate), H_2 antagonists (cimetidine or ranitidine) to reduce gastric acid secretion, gastrokinetic agents (metoclopramide) to improve gastric emptying, and the choice of anesthetic agents and drugs.

Postoperative management for nausea is directed toward minimizing rapid patient movements, prompt and satisfactory relief of pain, ensuring adequate respiratory

CRITERIA	At arrival			

ACTIVITY
 	
    Able to move 4 extremities voluntarily or on command = 2
    Able to move 2 extremities voluntarily or on command = 1
    Able to move 0 extremities voluntarily or on command = 0				

RESPIRATION
 	
    Able to deep breathe and cough freely = 2
    Dyspnea or limited breathing   = 1
    Apneic = 0				

CIRCULATION
 	
    BP ± 20% of preanesthetic level   = 2
    BP ± 20% to 50% of preanesthetic level = 1
    BP ± 50% of preanesthetic level = 0				

CONSCIOUSNESS
 	
    Fully awake   = 2
    Arousable on calling = 1
    Not responding = 0				

COLOR
 	
    Pink   = 2
    Pale, dusky, blotchy, jaundiced, other = 1
    Cyanotic = 0				

TOTALS				

Fig. 9-12. Postanesthetic recovery score form. (Modified from Aldrete, J.A., and Kroulik, D.: Anesth. Analg. 49:924, 1970.)

function and stable vital signs, use of antiemetics, and prevention of aspiration.

Pain

Unsatisfactory pain relief is a common complaint from patients. An adequate amount of promptly administered analgesics that are appropriate for the kind of pain experienced is necessary for satisfactory pain control. Generally, all medications in the PACU should be given intravenously because the absorption and onset of intramuscular drugs are delayed and highly variable. However, newer methods of pain relief, including intrathecally or epidurally administered narcotics and patient-controlled analgesia (PCA) given intravenously, are commonly used. Studies have shown that, with proper education and usage, these newer modalities result in shorter intensive care unit and hospital stays and a decrease in the total amount of drug required.

Alteration in mental status

Abnormal neurologic function is common in the first hour. Agitation, shivering, hyperreflexia, hypertonicity, and clonus are commonly observed. Common causes include pain, respiratory dysfunction, gastric or urinary distention, perioperative medications, anesthetic technique, electrolyte imbalance (for example, dilutional hyponatremia after prostatic resection), drug abuse, and preexisting psychologic factors. These changes usually resolve with

treatment of the contributing factors and additional recovery time. However, sedation and restraint of the patient may be necessary on an interim basis.

Hypoxemia

Hypoxemia is defined as inadequate oxygenation of the blood or a decrease in the arterial oxygen content. Hyperoxia is rarely a problem in the PACU except with premature infants or adults with prolonged (greater than 24 hours) exposure to F_IO_2 above 0.5. Increasing age, obesity, preexisting pulmonary disease, and smoking increase the risk for hypoxemia. Recognition of hypoxemia in the PACU can first be made by pulse oximetry, then cyanosis, and confirmed by arterial blood gases.

The causes of hypoxemia can be organized as problems with oxygen delivery to the lungs, the pulmonary system, or delivery of oxygen from the lungs to the tissues. Inadequate F_IO_2 can reduce the amount of oxygen delivered to the lungs. Hypercarbia can displace oxygen in the alveoli.

Obstruction of the airway is a common cause of hypoxemia. Pharyngeal obstruction is usually caused by the tongue, surgery on the head or neck, or abnormal anatomy. Management includes supplemental oxygen, anterior displacement of the mandible, positioning the patient on the side, or use of an oral or nasal airway. Laryngeal obstruction can be caused by spasm, edema, secretions triggering glottic response, or surgery on the airway. Management includes supplemental oxygen or a mixture of helium and oxygen, suctioning of secretions, positive airway pressure with a mask or assisted ventilation, racemic epinephrine, or reintubation.

Pulmonary causes of hypoxemia are numerous. Hypoventilation secondary to drugs, splinting from surgical pain (particularly on the upper abdomen or thorax), obesity, or positioning can reduce oxygenation. Intrapulmonary shunting of blood past obstructed or poorly oxygenated alveoli reduces the oxygen content of arterial blood. Difficulties in the diffusion of oxygen from the alveoli to arterial blood can be caused by atelectasis, aspiration, adult respiratory distress syndrome, bronchospasm caused by allergies or asthma, pulmonary edema, pneumonia, pneumothorax, or pulmonary embolism.

Changes in the delivery of oxygen from the lungs to the tissues can be caused by inadequate cardiac output, bleeding, hypovolemia, anemia, or increased oxygen consumption from fever or disease processes such as malignant hyperthermia, thyrotoxicosis, or sepsis.

If the simple maneuvers discussed previously do not improve the oxygenation, the anesthesiologist should be called immediately.

Carbon dioxide elimination

Tachypnea resulting in a decrease in $PaCO_2$ is rarely a problem in the PACU but can be caused by splinting with pain, anxiety, or elevated CO_2 production. More commonly, hypoventilation occurs resulting in elevated $PaCO_2$. Changes in $PaCO_2$ can be recognized by $ETCO_2$ monitoring and confirmed with arterial blood gases.

Causes of hypoventilation include the operative procedure and surgical site as discussed previously, preexisting pulmonary disease, depression of the respiratory center (by drugs, narcotics, sedatives, or residual anesthetics), obesity, disease states, muscle weakness secondary to residual muscle relaxants, and increased carbon dioxide production from shivering, hyperthermia, or excitement on emergence.

Treatment should begin with determination of the cause and then appropriate management should be initiated.

Hypotension

Verification of the blood pressure (for example, properly sized BP cuff, transducer calibration) and an assessment of the rapidity of the change are essential factors in the initial diagnosis and management of hypotension. Hemodynamic stabilization of the patient may be necessary before the precipitating factor can be determined. Possible causes can be organized as problems with preload to the heart, intracardiac difficulties, cardiac afterload, and miscellaneous factors.

A decreased preload secondary to hypovolemia is probably the most common cause. Hemorrhage or inadequate fluid replacement should be considered first, but decreased venous return (position, compression of major vessels, pulmonary embolism, or pneumothorax) and response to venodilators or diuretics must also be considered.

Intracardiac causes of hypotension include ischemia, myocardial infarction, arrhythmias, congestive heart failure, tamponade, cardiomyopathy, valvular dysfunction, and the effects of myocardial depressants.

Decreased afterload can be caused by vasodilation from epidural or spinal anesthesia, drugs or other anesthetics, allergic reactions, or transfusion reactions. Miscellaneous factors include septic shock and Addison's disease.

Treatment depends upon the diagnosis, but the ECG, peripheral pulses, jugular venous engorgement, changes or alterations in the cardiac or pulmonary auscultatory findings, and urinary output should be quickly evaluated.

Hypertension

As with hypotension, verification of the blood pressure and the rapidity of the change must be done first. Pain, hypoxia, hypercarbia, and preexisting hypertension are common causes. Other causes include hypervolemia, bladder distention, drug effects, hypoglycemia (reflex sympathetic response), reflex vasoconstriction from hypothermia, autonomic hyperreflexia, and elevated intracranial pressure. Diseases such as malignant hyperthermia, thyrotoxicosis, or pheochromocytoma can also cause acute hypertension.

Treatment of hypertension depends upon the etiology and the rapidity of onset. Unless the cause can be readily identified (for example, pain, hypoxia, hypercarbia or bladder distention), the anesthesiologist should be immediately notified.

Cardiac dysrhythmias

Multiple cardiac dysrhythmias can occur postoperatively, and their diagnosis and management is beyond the scope of this overview. Common predisposing factors include preexisting cardiac disease, pain, hypothermia, respiratory dysfunction resulting in hypoxia, hypercarbia or acidosis, and imbalance of fluids, electrolytes, or acid-base status.

ANESTHESIA FOR AMBULATORY SURGERY

In recent years increasing numbers of surgical procedures have been done on an ambulatory basis, and many health professionals believe that ambulatory surgery will comprise 40% to 60% of all elective surgery in the near future. Reasons for this change include evolving concepts for delivery of health care, a significant reduction in the overall cost for such surgical procedures, an increased emphasis on personal attention to patients' needs, and the overwhelming satisfaction of patients who have ambulatory surgery. Depending on many factors, ambulatory surgery may be performed in a regular operating room, elsewhere in the same facility, in a separate building adjacent to the hospital, or at a freestanding facility not directly associated with a hospital.

In an effort to reduce health care costs, many hospitals are admitting patients the day of surgery for major elective procedures. Because the postoperative hospitalization is scheduled in advance, these patients are not true ambulatory patients. To distinguish them from inpatients, however, these patients and procedures are frequently called *ambulatory-admit, ambulatory-inpatient, a.m. admit,* or *admission day surgery.*

Although the anesthetic technique may be similar for the inpatient and ambulatory surgery, the concepts of anesthesia care are very different. Because ambulatory surgery is usually reserved for relatively healthy individuals, the preoperative evaluation may be done several days before the surgery, on the day of surgery, or by telephone. Many laboratory tests and diagnostic studies, such as electrocardiograms and chest x-ray studies, are no longer done routinely before ambulatory surgery because they have not been cost-effective for healthy asymptomatic individuals. In most instances, the commonly used preoperative medications are omitted because they tend to prolong the postoperative recovery period and may have residual effects for 1 to 3 days after surgery. The goal is to provide high-quality health care in a pleasant, personal, safe, and expeditious manner with minimal disruption of the patient's usual level of activity.

One typical scenario illustrates the general concepts of ambulatory surgery. After an examination in the physician's office, the patient and physician agree that the surgery is needed. A specialized history and physical examination form is completed by the surgeon and the consent for operation is signed and witnessed. The patient is given a brochure about ambulatory surgery and then scheduled for the elective procedure. Two to five days before the date for the surgery, the patient visits the ambulatory surgery center for a preoperative interview, appropriate laboratory tests, and diagnostic studies. An evaluation by the anesthesiologist may take place on that day or on the day of surgery. The patient is instructed to be NPO after midnight the evening preceding surgery. On the day of surgery, the patient arrives 1 hour before the procedure and changes into an operating room gown plus a robe. In the preoperative area a nursing assessment is done, an intravenous infusion is started and the patient reads magazines, listens to music, or visits with family or friends until going to the operating room. The surgeon usually speaks with the patient in the preoperative area. The patient walks to the operating room and lies down on the operating room bed. Induction of anesthesia commences. Generally, only short-acting anesthetic drugs are used, and all medications are given intravenously. After surgery, the patient is transferred to a stretcher and taken to the phase I PACU. When recovered significantly, the patient is assisted to the phase II recovery area and sits in a reclining chair. In phase II, a family member or responsible adult joins the patient, and the patient is offered water, ginger ale, cola, tea, or coffee. When ready to go home, the patient is evaluated by the anesthesiologist and receives discharge instructions from the PACU nurse. A mail-in questionnaire is also given to the patient for comments about the ambulatory surgery experience. The patient may not drive and must be taken home by a responsible adult. Typical times from completion of surgery to discharge are 1½ to 2½ hours. Two to five days after surgery, a follow-up telephone call is made to the patient by one of the nursing staff.

BIBLIOGRAPHY
Anesthesia

Anderton, J.M., Keen, R.I., and Neave, R.: Positioning the surgical patient. Boston, 1988, Butterworths.

Atkinson, R.S., Rushman, G.B., and Lee, J.A.: A synopsis of anaesthesia, ed. 10, Bristol, England, 1987, Wright.

Atlee, J.L.: Perioperative cardiac dysrhythmias: mechanisms, recognition, management, ed. 2, Chicago, 1989, Year Book Medical Publishers.

Barash, P.G., Cullen, B.F., and Stoelting, R.K.: Clinical anesthesia, Philadelphia, 1989, J.B. Lippincott Co.

Benumof, J.L.: Anesthesia for thoracic surgery, Philadelphia, 1987, W.B. Saunders Co.

Berry, F.A.: Anesthetic management of difficult and routine pediatric patients, New York, 1986, Churchill Livingstone.

Bevan, D.R., Bevan, J.C., and Donati, F.: Muscle relaxants in clinical anesthesia, Chicago, 1988, Year Book Medical Publishers.

Birch, A., and Tolmie, J.B.: Anesthesia for the uninterested, ed. 2, Baltimore, 1986, University Park Press.

Bishop, M.J., editor: Problems in anesthesia (2:2): physiology and consequences of tracheal intubation, Philadelphia, 1988, J.B. Lippincott Co.

Blitt, C.B.: Monitoring in anesthesia and critical care medicine, ed. 2, New York, 1990, Churchill Livingstone.

Brown, D.L., editor, Risk and outcome in anesthesia, Philadelphia, 1988. J.B. Lippincott Co.

Brown, D.L., editor. Problems in anesthesia (2:3): perioperative analgesia, Philadelphia, 1988. J.B. Lippincott Co.

Bruner, J.M.R., and Leonard, P.S.: Electricity, safety, and the patient, Chicago, 1989, Year Book Medical Publishers.

Churchill-Davidson, H.C., editor: Wylie and Churchill-Davidson's a practice of anaesthesia, ed. 5, Chicago, 1984, Year Book Medical Publishers.

Corssen, G., Reves, J.G., and Stanley, T.H.: Intravenous anesthesia and analgesia, Philadelphia, 1988, Lea & Febiger.

Cottrell, J.E., and Turndorf, H.: Anesthesia and neurosurgery, ed. 2, St. Louis, 1986, The C.V. Mosby Co.

Cousins, M.J., and Bridenbaugh, P.O.: Neural blockade in clinical anesthesia and management of pain, ed. 2, Philadelphia, 1988, J.B. Lippincott Co.

Datta, S., and Ostheimer, G.W.: Common problems in obstetric anesthesia, Chicago, 1987, Year Book Medical Publishers.

Davenport, H.T.: Anesthesia and the aged patient, Boston, 1988, Blackwell Scientific Publications.

Dorsch, J.A., and Dorsch, S.E.: Understanding anesthesia equipment: construction, care and complications, ed. 2, Baltimore, 1984, Williams & Wilkins.

Dripps, R.D,, Eckenhoff, J.E., and Vandam, L.D.: Introduction to anesthesia: the principles of safe practice, ed. 7, Philadelphia, 1988, W.B. Saunders Co.

Eger, E.I., II: Nitrous oxide/N_2O, New York, 1985, Elsevier.

Eriksson, E.: Illustrated handbook in local anaesthesia, ed. 2, Philadelphia, 1980. W.B. Saunders Co.

Firestone, L.L., Lebowitz, P.W., and Cook, C.E.: Clinical anesthesia procedures of the Massachusetts General Hospital, ed. 3, Boston, 1988, Little Brown & Co.

Gilman, A.G., and others: Goodman and Gilman's the pharmacological basis of therapeutics, ed. 7, New York, 1985, Macmillan Publishing Co.

Gravenstein, N., editor: Problems in anesthesia (1:1): monitoring, Philadelphia, 1987, J.B. Lippincott.

Gravenstein, J.S., and Paulus, D.A.: Clinical monitoring practice, ed. 2, Philadelphia, 1987, J.B. Lippincott Co.

Gravenstein, J.S., Paulus, D.A., and Hayes, T.J.: Capnography in clinical practice, Boston, 1989, Butterworths.

Gregory, G.A.: Pediatric anesthesia, ed. 2, New York, 1989, Churchill Livingstone.

Kaplan, J.A.: Cardiac anesthesia, ed. 2, New York, 1987, Grune & Stratton.

Katz, J., Benumof, J.L., and Kadis, L.B.: Anesthesia and uncommon diseases, ed. 3, Philadelphia, 1989, W.B. Saunders Co.

Katz, J., and Steward, D.J.: Anesthesia and uncommon pediatric diseases, Philadelphia, 1987, W.B. Saunders Co.

Keys, T.E.: The history of surgical anesthesia, Huntington, N.Y., 1978, Robert E. Krieger Publishing Co.

Lake, C.L.: Cardiovascular anesthesia, New York, 1985, Springer-Verlag.

Martin, J.T.: Positioning in anesthesia and surgery, ed. 2, Philadelphia, 1987, W.B. Saunders Co.

Miller, R.D., editor: Anesthesia, ed. 3, New York, 1990, Churchill Livingstone.

Moller, A.R.: Evoked potentials in intraoperative monitoring, Baltimore, 1988, Williams & Wilkins.

Mueller, R.A., and Lundberg, D.B.A.: Manual of drug interactions for anesthesiology, New York, 1988, Churchill Livingstone.

Nimmo, W.S., editor: Anaesthesia, London, 1989, Blackwell Scientific Publications.

Nunn, J.F., Utting, J.E., and Brown, B.R., Jr.: General anaesthesia, ed. 5, Boston, 1989, Butterworths.

Nuwer, M.R.: Evoked potential monitoring in the operating room, New York, 1986, Raven Press.

Orkin, F.K., and Cooperman, L.H.: Complications in anesthesiology, Philadelphia, 1983, J.B. Lippincott Co.

Petty, C.: The anesthesia machine, New York, 1987, Churchill Livingstone.

Raj, P.P.: Practical management of pain, Chicago, 1986, Year Book Medical Publishers.

Reves, J.G., and Hall, K.D.: Common problems in cardiac anesthesia, Chicago, 1987, Year Book Medical Publishers.

Ryan, J.F., and others: A practice of anesthesia for infants and children, New York, 1986, Grune & Stratton.

Saidman, L.J., and Smith, N.T.: Monitoring in anesthesia, ed. 2, Boston, 1984, Butterworths.

Shapiro, B.A., and others: Clinical application of blood gases, ed. 4, Chicago, 1989, Year Book Medical Publishers.

Shnider, S.N., and Levinson, G.: Anesthesia for obstetrics, ed. 2, Baltimore, 1987, Williams & Wilkins.

Smith, N.T., and Corbasico, A.N.: Drug interactions in anesthesia, ed. 2, Philadelphia, 1986, Lea & Febiger.

Stephen, C.R., and Assaf, R.A.E.: Geriatric anesthesia: principles and practice, Boston, 1986, Butterworths.

Stoelting, R.K.: Pharmacology and physiology in anesthetic practice, Philadelphia, 1987, J.B. Lippincott Co.

Stoelting, R.K., Dierdorf, S.F., and McCammon, R.L.: Anesthesia and co-existing disease, ed. 2, New York, 1988, Churchill Livingstone.

Stoelting, R.K., and Miller, R.D.: Basics of anesthesia, ed. 2, New York, 1989, Churchill Livingstone.

Vandam, L.D.: To make the patient ready for anesthesia: medical care of the surgical patient, Menlo Park, Calif., 1980, Addison-Wesley Publishing Co.

Wetchler, B.V., editor: Anesthesia for ambulatory surgery, Philadelphia, 1985, J.B. Lippincott Co.

Wetchler, B.V., editor: Problems in anesthesia (2:1): outpatient anesthesia, Philadelphia, 1988, J.B. Lippincott Co.

Winnie, A.P.: Plexus anesthesia: perivascular techniques of brachial plexus block, Philadelphia, 1983, W.B. Saunders Co.

General

Addleman, A.: What do you look for in the pediatric postanesthesia patient? J. Post Anes. Nur. 3(1):3, 1988.

Aldrete, J.A., and Kroulik, D.: A postanesthetic recovery score, Anes. Analg. 49:924, 1970.

Association of Operating Room Nurses: Recommended practices for cleaning and processing anesthesia equipment. In AORN standards and recommended practices of perioperative nursing, Denver, 1990, the Association.

Association of Operating Room Nurses: Recommended practices for monitoring the patient receiving local anesthesia. In AORN standards and recommended practices of perioperative nursing, Denver, 1990, the Association.

Atsberger, D.B., and Shrewsbury, P.: Postoperative pain management: the PACU nurse's challenge, J. Post Anes. Nurs. 3(6)399, 1988.

Bland, D.: Pulse oximetry: monitoring arterial hemoglobin oxygen saturation, AORN J. 45:964, 1987.

Brown, S.L.: Postanesthetic management of regional anesthesia, J. Post Anes. Nurs. 1:87, 1986.

Brown, S.L.: Obesity: implications for postanesthesia care, J. Post Anes. Nurs. 1(4):248, 1986.

Burden, N., and Amiyer, J.: Local anesthesia: not always benign, J. Post Anes. Nurs. 2(1):45, 1987.

Cottrell, J.E., editor: Occupational hazards to operating room and recovery room personnel, Int. Anes. Clin. 19:1, 1981.

Cramer, C.: Postanesthetic management of regional anesthesia, J. Post Anes. Nurs. 1:236, 1986.

DiNobile, C.: Patient-controlled analgesia: a new trend in pain control, J. Post Anes. Nurs. 3(3):154, 1988.

Ehrenwerth, J., and Donielson, D.: Pulse oximetry in the postanesthesia care unit, J. Post Anes. Nurs. 2(1):9, 1987.

Feldman, M.E.: Inadvertent hypothermia: a threat to homeostasis in the postanesthetic patient, J. Post Anes. Nurs. 3(2):82, 1988.

Fernsebner, B.: Monitoring nitrous oxide in the OR, AORN J. 45:1166, 1897.

Fezer, S.J.: Cricoid pressure: how, when and why, AORN J. 45:1374, 1987.

Gatch, G.: Caring for children needing anesthesia, AORN J. 35:218, 1982.

Hildebrand, R.: Muscle relaxants: a review, J. Post Anes. Nurs. 3(3):165, 1988.

Ivey, D.F.: Local anesthesia: implications for the perioperative nurse, AORN J. 45:682, 1987.

Jacobs, M.: Patient-controlled analgesia: who really benefits? J. Post Anes. Nurs. 3(6)404, 1988.

Kolb, M.E., Horne, M.L., and Martz, R.: Dantrolene in human malignant hyperthermia, Anesthesiology 56:254, 1982.

Kulb, T.K., and DeFalque, R.J.: Axillary block: an anesthetic alternative for upper extremity injuries, AORN J. 46:672, 1987.

Lewis, J.M., and Beaulieu, J.B.: Application of nursing diagnosis to the PAR scoring system, J. Post Anes. Nurs. 2(4):237, 1987.

Litwack, K.: Practical points in the use of midazolam, J. Post Anes. Nurs. 3(6):408, 1988.

Litwack, K., and Parnass, S.: Practical points in the management of postoperative nausea and vomiting, J. Post Anes. Nurs. 3(4):275, 1988.

Litwack, K., and Zeplin, K.: Practical points in the management of laryngospasm, J. Post Anes. Nurs. 4(1):36, 1989.

Luczun, M.E.: Postanesthesia nursing: a comprehensive guide, Rockville, Md., 1984, Aspen Publications.

Pesci, B.R.: Neuromuscular blockade and reversal agents: a primer for postanesthesia nurses, J. Post Anes. Nurs. 1(1):42, 1986.

Rosenberg, H.: Malignant hyperpyrexia, Am. J. Nurs. 81:1484, 1981.

Saufel, N.F., and Garmon, J.D.: Assessment and management of the multiple-trauma patient in the PACU, J. Post Anes. Nurs. 3(5):305, 1988.

Schoeppel, S.L., and others: Effects of myocardial infarction on perioperative cardiac complications, Anesth. Analg. 62:493, 1983.

Seaman, D.J.: Shortcuts to a more complete postanesthesia room transfer: summary, Nursing 83:47, 1983.

Summers, S., Dudgeon, J., and Dubin, J.S.: Postanesthesia care unit hypertension in normotensive young adult males: a pilot study, J. Post Anes. Nurs. 3(5):324, 1988.

Tobias, R.: Circulator, you can help your anesthetist, Point of View 17:14, 1980.

Toledo, L.W.: Pulse oximetry: clinical implications in the PACU, J. Post Anes. Nurs. 2(1)12, 1987.

Trounson, L.: Hypertensive crisis, J. Post Anes. Nurs. 3(2):102, 1988.

Weis, O.F., and others: Reduction of anxiety in postoperative analgesic requirements by audiovisual instruction, Lancet 1:43, 1983.

Wetchler, B.V.: Managing pain in the postanesthesia care unit, J. Post Anes. Nurs. 1(1):52, 1986.

10 Lasers

KAY A. BALL

Perioperative nursing, perhaps more than any other nursing specialty, has been tremendously affected by the technologic explosion of the past several decades. Nurses practicing in the operating room during the past 25 to 30 years have witnessed and participated in a vast number of changes in the procedures performed and the instrumentation and equipment used in state-of-the-art surgery. Throughout this transition, the primary concern of perioperative nurses has been the care, comfort, and safety of patients encountering surgical intervention. Continual advances in technology have, however, forced nurses to improve their organizational skills and mechanical aptitudes to cope competently with the myriad sophisticated and often complex devices used, while still ensuring high-quality perioperative patient care.

One of the health care revolutions that has occurred in the last three decades is the birth and evolution of an amazing tool called the *laser*. The perioperative nurse of the 1990s must be keenly aware of the responsibilities associated with laser applications. The laser is radically changing surgery by developing less invasive procedures, decreasing inpatient hospitalization, diminishing postoperative complications, and saving health care dollars.

LASER BIOPHYSICS
Historical perspective

During the early 1900s, Albert Einstein first described the theory that involved the stimulation of matter to cause the release of energy. In 1958, Schawlow and Townes used this concept of stimulated emission to develop the principle of laser, meaning *Light Amplification by the Stimulated Emission of Radiation.*

In 1962, Theodore Maiman developed the first laser for medicine and surgery using a ruby crystal. The ruby laser was used for dermatologic applications and for retinal photocoagulation in patients with diabetic retinopathy. It was not very efficient, however. Other lasing media, such as the argon, carbon dioxide, and neodymium: yttrium aluminum garnet (Nd: YAG) lasers, were developed and are now used in many surgical disciplines. New lasers, such as the excimer and free electron lasers, continue to be investigated and refined for clinical use. Advancements in laser technology have provided the physician with a precision tool for cutting, coagulating, vaporizing, and welding tissue during surgical intervention.

Principles of light

Laser is an acronym that describes a process in which light energy is produced. This term also refers to the device that generates the laser energy.

Light is a form of electromagnetic energy that can be graphically illustrated on a continuum known as the *electromagnetic spectrum* (Fig. 10-1). The unit of measurement that delineates the continuum is called a *wavelength,* which is the distance between two successive peaks of a wave. Wavelength determines color and is usually measured in nanometers (10^{-9} meter) or microns (1000 nanometers). The various wavelengths of laser energy extend from the shorter waves in the ultraviolet area to the longer waves in the infrared region along this perpetual line. The visible laser wavelengths occupy only a small portion of this continuum.

Briefly, the laser functions in the following way. A negatively charged electron orbits a positively charged nucleus while the atom is in its ground or resting state. An outside source of energy can excite the atom and cause an electron to jump to a higher, less stable orbit. The electron almost immediately returns to the resting state. As it does so, it spontaneously emits a tiny bundle of surplus energy called a *photon*. If an atom that is already excited is struck or stimulated by a photon of equal energy, two identical photons are emitted. This process is "stimulated emission" (Fig. 10-2).

This activity occurs in the resonating chamber of the laser, where the lasing medium is contained. The name of the laser is derived from the actual medium that causes the lasing action. The stimulation of radiation continues as the number of excited atoms surpasses the number of resting atoms. The photons are reflected back and forth between two mirrors at each end as the process is amplified, until the state of "population inversion" has been reached. One mirror is partially reflective and when activated allows a stream of laser photons to escape the unit. These photons are then introduced to the target area via a special delivery system.

175

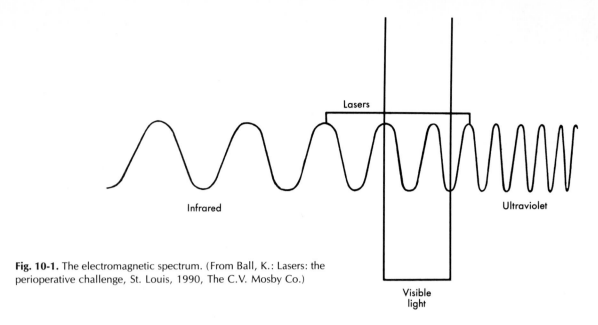

Fig. 10-1. The electromagnetic spectrum. (From Ball, K.: Lasers: the perioperative challenge, St. Louis, 1990, The C.V. Mosby Co.)

Characteristics of laser light

Three distinct characteristics distinguish laser light from ordinary light. Laser light is monochromatic, collimated, and coherent.

Monochromatic light is composed of photons of the same wavelength or color. In contrast, ordinary light consists of many different colors or wavelengths.

A *collimated* laser beam consists of waves parallel to each other that do not diverge significantly and thus minimize any loss of power. When a collimated beam is passed through a lens, the light is focused into a tiny spot that tremendously concentrates the energy. In comparison, the light waves from a flashlight are not parallel and lose intensity as they travel away from the source. A lens cannot readily focus all the waves to concentrate the light into a small area.

Laser light is *coherent,* as all the waves are in phase with each other as they travel in the same direction. All peaks and troughs of the waves are opposite each other in both time and space. This property has an additive effect and gives the laser beam power. Ordinary light is inco-herent, as the waves radiate in many different directions from the source.

Laser power

The power, or energy, of a laser beam is measured in watts. One of the most critical factors in laser application is the concept of *power density* or irradiance of the beam. Power density is the amount of power that is concentrated within an area and is described by the following formula:

$$\text{Power density} = \frac{\text{Watts}}{\text{Spot size (cm}^2)}$$

The spot size of the laser beam can be controlled by passing the beam through a special lens that causes the beam to converge. The configuration of the lens determines where the beam is most intense; this is the focal point. If the beam extends over a large spot, the laser energy is spread over a larger area, decreasing the intensity of the beam. In contrast, a small spot size concentrates the power into a smaller area, increasing the intensity of the beam.

A *joule* is the unit of measurement used to describe the

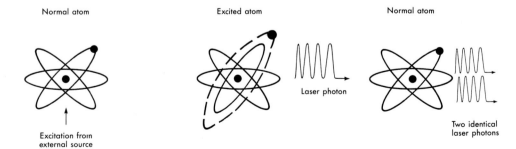

Fig. 10-2. Laser energy is produced when an external source excites the atom to emit a photon spontaneously. This photon can then "stimulate" the emission of two identical photons. (From Ball, K.: Lasers: the perioperative challenge, St. Louis, 1990, The C.V. Mosby Co.)

total energy used. A joule is expressed by the power multiplied by the time duration of beam exposure. *Fluence* is a term that involves the power and duration of exposure of the beam and measures the specific amount of energy that is delivered to the tissue. The following equation calculates the fluence:

$$\text{Fluence} = \frac{\text{Watts} \times \text{Duration time}}{\text{Spot size (cm}^2)}$$

The *transverse electromagnetic mode* (TEM) determines the precision of the beam by the distribution of the power over the spot area. The most precise or fundamental mode, TEM 00, evenly distributes the power over the spot with the most concentrated energy in the center and the intensity of the beam decreasing toward the periphery.

Tissue interaction

When laser energy is delivered to the target area, four different interactions can occur: reflection, scattering, transmission, or absorption (Fig. 10-3). The extent of the reaction of the beam on the target depends upon the laser wavelength, power settings, length of time the beam is in contact with the tissue, and the characteristics of the tissue.

Reflection of the laser beam occurs when the direction of the beam is changed after it impacts an area. Specular reflection occurs when the angle of the incoming light is equal to the angle of the reflected light. Laser light can be intentionally reflected in this manner off a reflective mirror to impact hard-to-reach areas. This type of reflection can also pose safety problems if not controlled at all times.

Scattering of the laser light occurs when the beam spreads over a large area as the tissue causes the beam to disperse. The intensity of the beam is decreased as the waves travel in different directions. The Nd: YAG laser beam can backscatter up an endoscope and possibly cause damage to the end of the scope, the optics, or the operator's eye.

Transmission of the laser beam occurs when the beam passes through fluids or tissue without thermally affecting the area. For example, the argon beam can be transmitted through the clear fluids and structures of the eye to impact the retina and cause a thermal photocoagulation. The lens and vitreous are unaffected by the transmission of the beam.

Absorption of the laser light results when the tissue is altered from the impact of the beam. This reaction is usually thermal but can sometimes be acoustic in effect. The consistency, color, and water content of the target tissue often determine the rate of absorption of the laser energy. Specific laser light, such as that from the argon laser, is highly absorbed by pigmented tissues. The CO_2 laser, however, is independent of color-selective absorption. The CO_2 laser light is absorbed superficially by tissue to a shallow depth of 0.5 mm. Argon laser light is absorbed by pigmented tissue to a depth of 0.5 to 2 mm, while that of the Nd: YAG is more readily absorbed by darkened tissue to a depth of 2 to 6 mm.

Tissue reaction becomes more pronounced as the temperature of the impact area increases (Table 10-1). During this thermal reaction, the laser energy is absorbed, causing the cellular water to be heated. Intracellular protein is

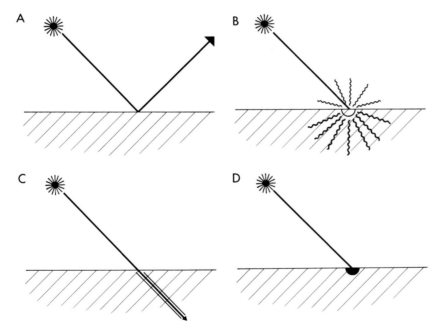

Fig. 10-3. Laser tissue interaction: reflection, scattering, transmission, absorption. (From Ball, K.: Lasers: the perioperative challenge, St. Louis, 1990, The C.V. Mosby Co.)

Table 10-1. Tissue changes with temperature increases

Temperature	Visual change	Biological change
37-60° C	No visual change	Warming, welding
60-65° C	Blanching	Coagulation
65-90° C	White/grey	Protein denaturization
90-100° C	Puckering	Drying
100° C	Smoke plume	Vaporization, carbonization

From Ball, K.: Lasers: the perioperative challenge, St. Louis, 1990, The C.V. Mosby Co.

destroyed; as the temperature rises, the water inside the cell turns to steam. Eventually, the membrane ruptures from increased pressure, spewing cellular debris and plume (laser smoke) from the tissue. The surrounding tissue is also heated because it borders the impact site. The degree of adjacent tissue damage depends on the duration of the laser beam exposure that causes the thermal injury.

LASER SYSTEMS

New laser systems are being introduced into the health care arena regularly. Constant efforts by researchers and physicians to explore the use of different wavelengths are changing surgical approaches in a variety of specialties. Table 10-2 describes some of the more popular lasers used in medicine and surgery today.

The five major components to a laser system are the excitation source, laser head, ancillary components, control panel, and delivery system. When a laser malfunctions, an organized investigation of each of these components (Fig. 10-4) can usually determine the source of the problem.

The *excitation source* supplies the energy to the laser. Different sources include flash lamps, electricity, battery, chemicals, or another laser system. For example, the CO_2 laser is excited by electrical current, and the Nd: YAG laser is excited by flash lamps.

The *laser head* or optical resonator is the chamber where the laser energy is generated. The laser head contains the active medium or substance that actually produces the photons that generate the laser light. The active medium can be a gas (CO_2 or argon), a solid (Nd: YAG), a liquid (tunable dye), or a semiconductor crystal (diode laser).

The *ancillary components* are the other laser parts that are needed to help produce the laser energy. The cooling system maintains the appropriate temperature of the laser head to keep the unit from overheating. Usually lasers are

Table 10-2. Description of laser color and wavelength

Laser	Color	Wavelength, nm
Excimer	Ultraviolet	
ArF		193
KrCl		222
KrF		248
XeCl		308
XeF		351
Helium-cadmium		325
Argon	Blue	488
	Green	515
Frequency doubled YAG (KTP)	Green	532
Krypton	Green	531
	Yellow	568
	Red	647
Dye laser	Variable with dyes	
	Red	632
	Yellow/green	577
Gold vapor	Red	628
Helium neon	Red	632
Ruby	Deep red	694
Nd:YAG	Infrared	1064
		1318
Holmium-YAG	Infrared	2100
Erbium YAG	Infrared	2900
Carbon dioxide	Infrared	10,600

From Ball, K.: Lasers: the perioperative challenge, St. Louis, 1990, The C.V. Mosby Co.

either air-cooled or water-cooled. A vacuum pump may be required in a CO_2 laser to pull the gas mixture from an external cylinder into the laser head for laser light production.

The *control panel* is the board that regulates the delivery of laser energy. Various power settings, modes, time durations, and other parameters can be selected as desired. Many laser panels are now computerized, allowing the laser to be quickly and accurately controlled. The laser team should be extremely familiar with the operation of the laser control panel.

The *delivery system* of the laser is the device or accessory that actually conducts the laser energy from the laser head to the target area. Carbon dioxide laser energy is delivered to the tissue through an articulated arm with a series of special mirrors at each joint. Argon and Nd: YAG lasers deliver energy through a fiber system. Advancements in laser technology are refining delivery systems to make them more adaptable, convenient, and comfortable for the physician.

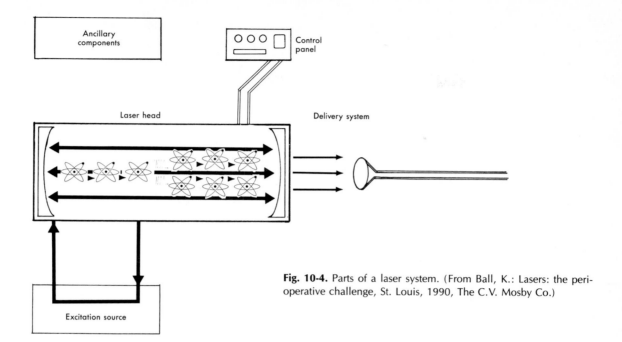

Fig. 10-4. Parts of a laser system. (From Ball, K.: Lasers: the perioperative challenge, St. Louis, 1990, The C.V. Mosby Co.)

COMMON SURGICAL LASERS

The *carbon dioxide laser* is versatile and widely used. Its wavelength of 10,600 nm (nanometers) is located in the infrared region of the electromagnetic spectrum. Because this light is invisible, a visible helium neon laser beam is usually transmitted coaxially with the CO_2 energy to serve as an aiming beam.

The CO_2 laser is characterized by its superficial tissue interaction, as the beam is highly absorbed by water. The degree of tissue response is related to the amount of heat buildup from the absorption. Therefore, the longer the CO_2 beam impacts the tissue, the more destruction is noted. The depth of penetration by the CO_2 energy is very superficial and might be described as "what you see is what you get." The CO_2 beam is also absorbed by any color of tissue; therefore, lighter tissue can absorb the beam as readily as darker tissue.

Currently, two types of CO_2 lasers are available. The free-flowing system requires an external cylinder of a special gas mixture of carbon dioxide, helium, and nitrogen. The concentrations must be precise so that the laser operates properly. The gas is pulled into the laser head by a vacuum pump, generates laser energy, and is then discharged as dissociated by-products. The cylinder is replaced when empty.

The other type of CO_2 laser is the sealed-tube system, which contains the special mixture of carbon dioxide, helium, and nitrogen within a tube that is sealed. A catalyst is added to the tube and causes regeneration of the mixture so that lasing action is produced again. The shelf life (functional period) of this type of tube is usually from 1 to 4 years. At the end of this time, the tube can be reprocessed by the manufacturer to replace the special gas and catalyst mixture.

The CO_2 laser light is delivered to the target area through a hollow tube called an *articulated arm*. Mirrors are positioned within the arm to reflect the laser energy forward. Because the helium-neon aiming beam runs coaxially with the CO_2 beam, care must be taken when moving the laser so that the mirrors are not jarred out of alignment.

The articulated arm can be attached to a microscope or a special handpiece. A lens system within these attachments causes the beam to converge at a certain point called the *focal point*. At the focal point, the beam is most intense, because all the energy is concentrated into a very small spot. The size of the spot can be changed by focusing or defocusing the lens to allow the spot to become larger or smaller. Sometimes tubing is connected to the handpiece or microscope adapter to conduct a purge gas, or compressed air, that blows the laser smoke away and keeps the lens cool and free from debris.

The CO_2 laser energy can be delivered to tissue in a variety of modes. The continuous mode allows the laser energy to be delivered continuously as long as the foot-pedal is depressed. A pulsed mode delivers the energy in an interrupted manner that allows the adjacent tissue to cool so that tissue destruction is controlled. Some lasers pulse the delivery so quickly that it may appear to be a continuous mode.

The *neodymium: yttrium aluminum garnet* (Nd: YAG) laser wavelength is in the infrared region of the electromagnetic spectrum at approximately 1064 nm. This invisible wave is usually accompanied by a visible helium neon beam or white light to provide an aiming source. The Nd: YAG laser has a solid crystal of yttrium aluminum that is laced with neodymium, which produces the lasing energy when exposed to bright flash lamps.

The Nd: YAG energy is delivered to the tissue through a fiber system. The core fiber may be surrounded by a catheter sheath that can be used to conduct a purge gas, air, or fluid to cool the end of the fiber and keep debris from accumulating.

The Nd: YAG wavelength is transmitted through clear fluids and structures and is more highly absorbed by darker tissue. This laser light tends to scatter within the tissue and cause thermal damage to approximately 6 mm. Tissue absorption produces a homogeneous coagulative effect as tissue is heated to the point of coagulation without vaporization occurring. Like other lasers, the Nd: YAG beam can easily backscatter, posing an eye safety concern when used through an endoscope.

A synthetic sapphire contact probe or scalpel can be attached to the end of a fiber to deliver the Nd: YAG energy directly to the tissue in a more concentrated manner. These contact tips are available in a variety of geometric configurations. Depending upon the desired tissue effects, the appropriate contact tip is chosen. A scalpel is used to cut, and a rounded probe is used to vaporize. A flat probe may be used to coagulate tissue. Contact tip technology provides precision, as the power output of the beam is confined to a very small area. It causes less thermal buildup so that adjacent tissue is relatively unaffected. The beam does not scatter as readily as the free Nd: YAG energy, and less plume is generated.

Another Nd: YAG wavelength being investigated is in the 1318-nm range. This laser causes minimal heat dissipation and allows greater cutting precision.

Besides the continuous mode Nd: YAG laser, a special pulsed mode Nd: YAG laser for ophthalmologic applications delivers the energy to the tissue in extremely short pulsations of nanoseconds in duration. This laser works by an acoustic effect instead of a thermal effect. For example, a clouded membrane behind an artificial lens implant can be ruptured quickly and painlessly with the use of this system.

The *argon laser* is another popular laser system. This laser produces an intense, visible blue/green light of approximately 488 and 515 nm, respectively. In clinical applications, this combination of light wavelengths allows more complete tissue absorption. The aiming system is low-power argon laser energy because the beam is visible.

The argon energy is highly absorbed by hemoglobin, melanin, or other similar pigmentation and is less absorbed by lighter tissue. The absorbed laser energy is then converted to heat to cause coagulation or vaporization. Because of the high color selectivity of the beam, adjacent tissue injury is reduced significantly.

The argon wavelength, like the Nd: YAG laser, is transmitted through clear fluids and structures. The argon laser energy is delivered to the target area through a fiber sys-

tem. The fiber can be attached to a slit lamp, microscope, or handpiece, depending upon the surgical approach. Because the argon light diverges 10 to 14 degrees when exiting the fiber, the size of the spot can be altered by changing the distance of the fiber tip to the tissue. Special handpieces that contain an internal lens can be adjusted to change the spot size of the beam.

SAFETY

Because laser systems are capable of concentrating high amounts of energy within very small areas, they present potential hazards. Safe and appropriate use of the laser during surgical intervention is the responsibility of the entire health care team. Each member must be acutely aware of the many controls needed to prevent accidental injury.

The laser is a class III medical device that is subdivided into four subclasses. The lasers designated as subclass III and IV have the potential to cause injury. Some of the ophthalmologic Nd: YAG lasers that cause an acoustic instead of a thermal reaction are classified in the subclass III category and can cause injury with sustained interaction. Most of the lasers used in surgical applications today are known as subclass IV lasers and can cause thermal reactions that can lead to fire, skin burns, and optical damage by either direct or scattered radiation. Specific safety precautions must be followed to prevent injury from these laser systems.

Many agencies are beginning to address the regulation of laser safety. Health care facilities must develop safety protocols in anticipation of mandates by these regulatory agencies as the technology advances and grows.

The American National Standards Institute (ANSI), a nongovernmental organization of experts, published the ANSI Z136.1 standards in 1973 as safety guidelines for laser use in warfare, industry, and health care. In 1988, ANSI Z136.3 standards were established to provide specific recommendations for laser use in health care environments. The appendix of ANSI Z136.3 discusses a consensus on laser safety in each of the specialty areas of medicine and surgery.

Other guidelines have been suggested by the Center for Devices and Radiological Health (CDRH), Association of Operating Room Nurses (AORN), American Society for Laser Medicine and Surgery (ASLMS), Laser Institute of America (LIA), Food and Drug Administration (FDA), and individual state and local regulatory bodies.

Hospitals and other health care delivery facilities need to formulate laser safety policies and procedures using these groups of experts as resources. When developing safety guidelines for a facility, protocols should individually address situations without being too general or too specific. Facilities must realize that they can be held liable for following their own safety policies and procedures. Therefore, basic in-services for all personnel in the operating room environment (including orderlies and house-keeping personnel) should be mandatory. National standards and guidelines are currently being developed as the technology continues to grow and mature.

Eye protection

Because the eye is extremely sensitive to laser radiation, great care must be taken to protect the eyes during laser intervention. Even low levels of laser radiation can lead to permanent optical damage. The area of possible ophthalmologic injury is dependent upon the type of wavelength. The CO_2 laser can damage the cornea of the eye, as this beam is readily absorbed by the surface cells. Immediate pain is associated with this injury. The argon and Nd: YAG laser beams, in contrast, are transmitted through the clear optical structures and fluids and can be refocused by the lens of the eye. The intensity of the beam after refocusing can permanently damage the retina. Sometimes pain is not even felt during this destruction (Fig. 10-5).

Adequate eye protection requires understanding the two concepts of maximum permissible exposure (MPE) and nominal hazard zone (NHZ). According to the ANSI Z136.3 standards, the MPE is the level of laser radiation to which a person may be exposed without hazardous effects to the eye or skin. The MPE levels are determined by considering the laser wavelength, exposure time, and pulse repetition. The NHZ is the space where the level of the direct, reflected, or scattered radiation during normal laser operation exceeds the MPE; therefore, eye, skin, and fire safety precautions must be followed while within this hazard zone.

Recommendations suggest that protective goggles, glasses, and endoscope lens covers should be inscribed with the appropriate filtering capabilities and adequate optical densities for the specific wavelength being used. For example, a pair of Nd: YAG goggles may be inscribed, "1064 nm, optical density 4." The optical density of the lens is the ability of the lens material to absorb a specific wavelength. The darker lens shades do not necessarily have higher optical density or give more protection. Technology has introduced lighter lens shades with high optical densities that provide adequate safety. Therefore, the perioperative nurse must ensure that the eye wear is properly labeled and handled so that scratching or damage is avoided.

During a microscopic procedure, an automatic lens shutter can be connected to the microscope head. During the laser activation the shutter allows a lens filter to drop in place to provide a shield from any laser backscatter. When this device is attached to the microscope head, an observer tube must also be placed above the filter so that all portal optics have protection provided.

A lens filter can be placed over the eyepiece of a rigid or flexible endoscope. The lens must offer the appropriate protection for the specific laser being used. Guidelines

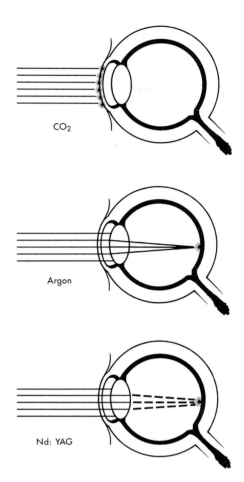

Fig. 10-5. The CO_2 laser beam can damage the cornea; the argon and Nd: YAG beams can injure the retina. (From Ball, K.: Lasers: the perioperative challenge, St. Louis, 1990, The C.V. Mosby Co.)

suggest that the other surgical team members also wear eye protection, even though the laser energy appears to be confined within an enclosed cavity. Optical injury is always possible if a fiber or articulated arm becomes separated from the endoscope while the laser is activated.

The ANSI standards recommend that a baseline eye examination, noting visual acuity and retinal health, be performed on those health care professionals who routinely work with laser systems. Another eye examination can be performed after an ophthalmologic accident or upon termination of employment. The baseline exam then provides a foundation for comparison with any abnormal findings from subsequent examinations. This preventive procedure protects the facility from a potential worker's compensation claim for retinal damage from incidental beam reflection, should the problem occur.

The patient's eyes must also be protected during laser intervention. Patients under general anesthesia should have their eyes covered with wet gauze, eye pads, or a towel; the eyes should be taped closed. If awake or under local

---

GUIDE TO EYE SAFETY DURING LASER SURGERY

- Make sure that everyone in the operating room is wearing the appropriate eye protection before activating the laser. The eye wear should have the laser wavelength protection and optical density of the lens material inscribed on the side.
- A special lens cover can be placed over the eyepiece of an endoscope to protect the physician's eye from laser backscatter.
- An automatic lens shutter can be connected to a microscope head to provide eye protection for persons viewing the procedure through the microscope.
- When general anesthesia is used, cover the patient's closed eyes with moistened gauze sponges. When the patient is awake, place the appropriate glasses or goggles on the patient. Explain the need for eye protection to the patient.
- During laser surgery near the eye, a lead eye shield may be placed directly on the anesthetized eye surface.
- Make sure that the appropriate protective eye wear is available at all entrances to the laser room for anyone entering the area.
- When storing protective eye wear, guard against scratches and mishandling.

GUIDE TO CONTROLLED ACCESS DURING LASER SURGERY

- Hang laser warning signs at all entrances to the laser room to prevent unauthorized persons from entering.
- The warning sign should include "Danger" and "Laser in Use."
- Cover windows or ports with the appropriate protection for the specific laser wavelength being used.
- Do not store the laser key in the laser. The laser key must be available only to authorized persons.

---

anesthesia, the patient should wear appropriate eye protection. Explanations should be provided to the patient regarding this safety action. If the laser is to be used in the immediate vicinity of the eye, such as to lighten a portwine stain on the eyelid, a lead eye shield can be placed on the surface of the eye after instilling a drop of an ophthalmologic local anesthetic. The box above summarizes actions to promote eye safety during laser surgery.

Controlled access

Inadvertent access into rooms where laser treatments are being performed should be prevented. Laser warning signs must be placed at all entrances to the treatment area so that access is granted only to those individuals who have been appropriately educated in laser safety. The word *danger* should be listed on any laser warning sign to indicate the possibility of hazards. Laser signs should be removed when the procedure has been completed.

Windows or ports into rooms where lasers are utilized must be covered with the appropriate protection for the specific laser being used. The CO_2 laser beam is stopped by clear glass or Plexiglas panels, but the argon and Nd:YAG laser wavelengths can be transmitted through this glass. Therefore, the windows or ports must be covered with a blocking barrier that stops the transmission of specific beams.

The laser key must not be left in the laser during storage. The key should be available only to authorized personnel who have the appropriate education and training to operate the laser. Laser keys can be stored in the narcotics cabinet or in a special key lockbox to control access. The box above summarizes actions that should be initiated to control access to laser rooms.

Fire safety

An awareness of laser biophysics and tissue interaction is necessary to understand the actions needed to prevent laser fires. A fire can be started by a reflected beam as easily as from a direct impact. The laser team must be able to respond quickly if a fire occurs. Immediate action is the key to minimize injury to the patient and the surgical team.

The box on p. 183 summarizes important measures to support fire safety during laser surgery.

Sterile water or saline is usually readily available to douse a small fire. A halon fire extinguisher should be available to control a fire within the laser system. This fire extinguisher contains halogenated hydrocarbons that do not produce a residue that could harm the internal delicate components of the laser. In contrast, a CO_2 fire extinguisher can cause thermal damage to the components from the extremely cold temperature of the residue that is emitted. A dry chemical fire extinguisher is not appropriate, as it discharges a fine dust that damages the optics and circuitry of the laser system.

During the surgical intervention, dry combustibles,

such as sponges or towels, near the laser tissue impact site should be kept wet to prevent ignition. The scrub nurse or RN first assistant should constantly monitor the moisture level of the sponges or other materials to prevent drying that could eventually support a fire.

Flammable draping material can be easily ignited by a laser beam. Some water-repellent drapes are able to withstand a laser impact, and thus the flammability of the material is decreased. If the restrictions of draping material or any other supplies are questionable, an article can be tested for flammability in the manufacturer's or researcher's laboratory. The laser beam can be directed to the material with different power settings to determine any limitations before clinical use. Water should be immediately available during these experiments.

Instrumentation used in the immediate vicinity of the laser tissue impact site should be nonreflective to decrease the chance of the laser beam bouncing off the surface and accidentally impacting another area. The laser beam can easily be reflected off shiny instrument surfaces and can cause skin or eye injury or ignite flammable materials. An instrument may be ebonized by coating the instrument with a special substance (usually black) to decrease reflectivity. Many companies offer this service at a low cost. The instrument should be inspected regularly to ensure the integrity of the coating. Any scratched surface or area where the ebonization has worn off should be recoated as necessary.

An instrument may also be anodized or given a matte finish to decrease reflectivity. Other coatings and surfaces are being introduced that cause the laser light to scatter and diffuse upon impact. Larger retractors can be covered with wet sponges or towels so that the laser beam cannot accidentally reflect from a shiny surface.

Other instrumentation will provide a backstop for the laser energy to decrease adjacent tissue damage and the chance of fire. Titanium rods are effective backstops and can be reprocessed easily. Quartz rods are often used as backstops for the CO_2 laser beam, but the argon and Nd:YAG beams are transmitted through them. Glass rods must never be used with a CO_2 laser because the glass material heats and shatters when continuously impacted by the beam. Teflon backstops should not be used as they melt and produce toxic fumes. Wet sponges can also be used as backstop material.

Special laser mirrors have been introduced that directly reflect the beam onto a hard-to-reach area. Mirrors may be made of rhodium or stainless steel. Glass-surface mirrors do not withstand laser impact and instead shatter. Using a laser mirror requires skill, as the beam must be focused on the target area and not on the mirror in order to deliver the full impact of the laser energy. A laser beam that is misdirected off a mirror can easily cause a fire.

Flammable skin preparations should not be used for laser procedures. During the skin cleansing, an alcohol-based preparation can pool underneath a patient, and ethanol vapors become trapped beneath the drapes. The volatility of these vapors increases the risk of a surgical drape fire.

When a laser is used in the rectal area, a wet pack may be used to tamponade the methane gas that could enter the surgical area and cause an explosion. The wet sponges used for the pack must be counted so that the packing is not inadvertently left in place after the surgery is completed.

Airway explosion caused by the laser beam igniting the endotracheal tube can be a potentially lethal accident for

---

GUIDE TO FIRE SAFETY DURING LASER SURGERY

- Sterile water or saline should be immediately available to douse a small fire.
- A halon fire extinguisher should be available in the department in case the laser catches on fire.
- Do not place dry combustibles in the vicinity of the laser impact site. Use wet towels or nonflammable drapes near the laser target area. Moisten these items with sterile saline or water to prevent ignition. Constantly monitor the moisture level throughout the procedure.
- Utilize nonreflective instrumentation in or near the laser tissue impact site to decrease accidental direct reflection of the laser beam. Cover larger instruments, such as retractors, with wet sponges or towels to protect against reflection.
- Do not prep with flammable skin preparations, such as alcohol.
- A wet pack may be inserted into the rectum to provide a tamponade to prevent methane gas from escaping into the surgical area.
- Use a specially prepared or a commercially manufactured laser endotracheal tube during laser procedures of the oropharynx. An unprotected PVC endotracheal tube can readily be ignited from an inadvertent laser beam impact. Protect the endotracheal tube cuff with wet gauze sponges.
- Place the laser in the standby mode when not in use.
- Identify the laser footpedal to avoid accidental activation.
- Do not place fluids or solutions on the laser unit. Protect the laser system from spillage or splatter that could cause short-circuiting and fire.

the patient. A polyvinylchloride endotracheal tube is highly flammable, especially as a high concentration of oxygen flows through it during anesthesia administration. Special red rubber, foil-wrapped endotracheal tubes or specific laser-retardant endotracheal tubes should be used during oral, tracheal, or esophageal laser procedures that require general anesthesia. The laser power limitations of a commercially prepared endotracheal tube must be followed closely to ensure proper performance of the tube. New materials are being developed that can be applied to a regular endotracheal tube so that penetration by the laser beam is not a problem. The cuff of the endotracheal tube should be inflated with sterile saline to provide a heat sink and retard a fire if perforated by the laser beam. A protocol should be developed that describes the emergency procedure needed to control an endotracheal fire. Immediate considerations include the following:

1. Remove the flaming endotracheal tube and instruments. Stop the flow of oxygen by pinching the oxygen tube or shutting off the supply valve.
2. Reintubate immediately to prevent laryngospasm.
3. Inspect the mouth, oral cavity, and bronchial tree.

Endoscope safety

Special precautions should be followed when using the laser during an endoscopic procedure. When a laser fiber is introduced through the biopsy port of a flexible or rigid endoscope, the operator must view the tip of the fiber before activating the laser. If the end of the fiber is still within the sheath of the endoscope and the laser is fired, the heat from the laser energy will quickly damage the optics and channel of the endoscope.

When a "bare" fiber is placed down the biopsy channel of a flexible endoscope, the sharp tip can possibly tear the inside lumen of the channel. A length of medical grade tubing can be placed over the fiber with the tip recessed within the sheath. The entire unit is then passed through the endoscope. Once the end of the tubing is observed, the medical grade tubing is withdrawn to expose the end of the fiber. This procedure effectively protects the inside lumen of the endoscope channel.

Smoke evacuation

Smoke evacuation and odor control must be adequate when laser plume is generated. Research has conclusively determined that the size of the particulate matter in laser plume is extremely small and could coat lung alveoli if inhaled over a period of time. Controversy exists today as to the viability of the laser plume. Laser plume contains carbonized particles, water, and odor; therefore, adequate smoke evacuation is necessary to remove the potentially viable contaminants from the air. Small amounts of laser plume can be evacuated with a special in-line suction filter positioned between the wall outlet and the suction canister.

GUIDE TO SMOKE EVACUATION DURING LASER SURGERY

- Use the appropriate smoke evacuation system for the amount of plume generated. Never use a nonfiltered in-line suction system to remove the laser plume.
- Change the smoke evacuation filter(s) as often as recommended.
- Maintain the smoke tube or evacuation device as close as possible to the laser tissue impact site.
- Wear surgical masks that provide adequate filtration when a laser plume is generated.

If the amount of plume is significant, an individual smoke evacuation unit that can filter particulate matter as small as 0.3 microns in size and larger should be used. The smoke evacuation filters should be changed regularly as specified by the manufacturer.

Contamination by the laser plume and tissue splatter is also decreased when the surgical team wears gloves, gowns, and masks. Laser masks that provide a higher percentage of air filtration than standard surgical masks are available.

The key to adequate smoke evacuation and elimination of inhalation hazards is to evacuate the plume at the laser-tissue impact site. Constant vigilance is mandatory to ensure that the smoke evacuation wand or suction device is very close to the laser target area. Research continues in this area to develop devices to control the plume so that the surgical team and the patient are not subjected to inhalation contaminants and offensive odors. The box above summarizes important measures for smoke evaluation during laser surgery.

Other safety measures

Footpedals can also present safety problems if mistakenly activated. Technology has given the physician more pedals to control devices and instrumentation. The number of footpedals placed on the floor for the physician can often be confusing and may lead to accidents. The laser pedal should be clearly identified for the physician and should be used by only the physician who is actually delivering the laser energy to the target area.

Laser team members should appreciate the potential for electrical hazards because the laser is a high-voltage piece of equipment. Water and other solutions should not be placed on the laser unit, and the components of the laser should be protected against spillage or splatter that could cause short circuit. The outside housing of the laser should never be removed by unauthorized personnel as the potential for electrical shock or electrocution is high.

Transportation hazards are always a potential threat as most of the laser systems are heavy. When these units need to be moved from one area to another, proper body mechanics must be employed to prevent injury to the transporter. The laser should never be bumped against a wall because the internal components can be damaged or thrown out of alignment.

Documentation

Complete and accurate documentation that notes the safety parameters followed during a laser procedure is critical. Documenting laser safety is important for the med-

---

SAMPLE LASER LOG

Date _____ O.R. Room No. _____

Patient Information:

Name _____ Hospital No. _____

Zip Code _____ Sex: M F Age _____

Status: IP OP

Insurance _____ Total Charges _____

Surgery Information:

Physician _____ Anesthesia: General Local

Procedure _____

Laser Information:

Laser _____

Power _____ Duration _____

Total Spots _____ Total Energy _____

Laser Time On _____ Laser Time Off _____

    Total Laser Time _____

Laser Fiber _____

Contact Tip _____

Smoke Evacuation _____

Comments: _____

_____

_____

_____

LASER SAFETY OFFICER _____

---

icolegal reasons when a potentially hazardous piece of equipment is used. Documentation can be on a laser log form or as part of the existing intraoperative nursing notes. Either record should be placed on the patient's chart so that safety activities that were performed can be recorded. A sample laser log is shown in the box at left.

DEVELOPING A LASER PROGRAM

As the popularity of the laser continues to grow, laser programs are also growing and developing. Initiating or expanding a laser program requires careful and intense planning. Dedication and enthusiasm by physicians, administration, and laser team members are essential for the success of a laser program. Forming a laser committee, providing appropriate staffing, procuring laser systems, monitoring reimbursement, and fostering utilization through marketing are all vital elements in laser program development.

Laser committee

The first action in developing a laser program is to form a laser committee. The laser committee can initially be part of the surgical committee but eventually, as the program expands, the laser committee will become an independent committee of the health care facility. The membership on this committee includes but is not limited to a representative from administration, physicians from different specialty areas, laser safety officers, operating room director, facility risk manager, librarian, and a public relations or marketing representative. Others can be invited to attend as mandated by the agenda of each meeting. Meetings should be held on a regular basis (at least monthly) and may be open to anyone interested in the laser program to encourage participation by more people.

The purpose of the laser committee is to provide guidance to the laser program so that laser technology is expanded and enhanced to benefit patients. The success of the laser program is usually in direct response to the activities of the laser committee.

One of the responsibilities of the laser committee is to plan for the expansion of the laser program. Feasibility studies should be conducted regularly to note physicians' needs and interests. For example, if another laser system is to be purchased, a survey should be sent to physicians to note preferences and forecast usage. Potential volume and revenue can then be projected to justify the procurement of a specific system. The utilization trends of the laser program can note the need to expand into a local anesthesia laser center or determine the support from different specialty areas.

Another responsibility of the laser committee is to formulate a physician credentialing policy. The specific laser credentialing protocol is determined by each facility because no national regulations mandate a standard. Recommendations of ANSI suggest that a physician receive didactical laser information including laser physics, safety, tissue interaction, and clinical application. Laser technology is beginning to be introduced in medical schools as part of the students' initial education process. Currently, many specialty laser courses are available for practicing physicians to attend. Usually a facility requires the physician to attend one of these courses and then have a preceptor (one who is already credentialed to use the laser) oversee one or more laser procedures to document the physician's safe and appropriate use of the laser. The physician's credentialing is sometimes reviewed by the specialty department and then is approved by the governing board of the hospital. Written credentialing approval should be kept on record in the physician's file in the medical staff office.

The laser committee should also address a credentialing protocol for residents who want to become involved with laser technology. Written guidelines should be established to allow a resident to participate in clinical laser applications.

Because laser technology is continually changing, an annual credentialing review process may be developed by the laser committee. This procedure involves determining the number of laser procedures that each credentialed physician has performed within the year. Because laser use requires skill, a physician who uses the laser infrequently may need a refresher course to decrease the chance of any problems. Sometimes an annual credentialing review determines why a physician is using the laser at another facility more often. This information can be used to help market the laser program to encourage more physician participation.

Formulating safety policies and procedures is another responsibility of the laser committee. Guidelines must be set to provide consistency within the laser program. These rules must be openly communicated to the laser team so that compliance can be enforced. Often the laser committee gives the laser safety officer the responsibility and authority to shut down a laser system if safety procedures are not being followed. Safety policies and procedures should be reviewed annually for appropriateness and should reflect the standard of care followed during laser procedures.

Staffing

The laser team provides the backbone of a successful laser program. Some of the many responsibilities include:

- Set up and test fire the laser system.
- Operate the laser control panel.
- Monitor and enforce laser safety.
- Perform preventive maintenance and minor troubleshooting on the laser.
- Document the laser procedure, laser charges, and laser service.

- Inventory and maintain laser supplies and accessories.
- Attend laser committee meetings.
- Assist with patient education.
- Help monitor physician credentialing.
- Stay abreast of laser technology by attending continuing education conferences or reading laser publications.
- Actively assist with laser system evaluation.
- Act as the laser resource person for the surgical team.
- Act as the liaison to the operating room, radiology, outpatient clinic, and other areas that are involved in the laser program.
- Make suggestions to enhance the laser program.
- Assist with a laser marketing program to increase visibility and utilization.

The clinical laser nurse is involved with perioperative patient education. The nurse reinforces to the patient what the physician has described before the laser procedure. When the patient is told that surgery is needed, the patient is often anxious because of the unknown. When a patient is told that "laser surgery" is needed, the anxiety may be compounded, as the patient is confronted with two alarming unknowns. Many patients develop anxiety about laser procedures based on information through science fiction movies, talk shows, and other such sources. The patient should always have the opportunity to discuss the laser procedure to allay any worries. After the physician has explained the procedure to the patient and has had the surgical consent form signed, the clinical laser nurse may provide additional information if the patient has any further questions. The consent form should reflect that the laser will be used during the surgical experience.

An adequate amount of time should be allotted for patient questions before the procedure. If local anesthesia is used, the patient should understand what to anticipate during the surgery, what sounds or odors will be present, why eye protection is needed, and what the patient's role is during the procedure. If the patient understands the application, the role of the laser, and his or her responsibility during and after the procedure, the nurse can expect better compliance. Discharge instructions are required for any ambulatory procedure; therefore, laser discharge instructions may be preprinted for each surgical application. These written instructions should be reviewed and given to the patient upon discharge. A follow-up phone call helps the nurse evaluate the care delivered during the laser intervention and the patient's compliance with the postoperative instructions.

Sometimes the laser nurse is placed in a compromising position by being expected to circulate during the surgical procedure and also operate the laser. The laser nurse then has the tremendous responsibility of being accountable for two critical roles in the operating room, and the risk of a laser incident is increased. In the traditional setting, one nurse circulates while another operates the laser. The health care facility must determine what procedures will require more staffing to handle each role.

According to ANSI Z136.3 standards, the laser safety officer (LSO) is the individual who has the responsibility to monitor and enforce laser safety. This person is usually a nurse but can be a technician or even a physician. The LSO reports safety infractions to the laser committee for evaluation and resolution.

The LSO training involves attendance at an educational offering that focuses on laser physics, tissue interaction, safety, and clinical application. The LSO is the generalist who must understand laser applications in all specialty areas. Unlike physicians who focus on their own specialty, the LSO must be able to provide support during all types of laser procedures. This expertise level is achieved by constant review of the literature to understand new techniques and developments.

Documentation is a critical responsibility of the LSO. Laser utilization must be documented on the patient's chart according to the hospital protocol. A laser log can be designed to be a permanent part of the patient's record and could include such information as the laser used, power, pulse duration, and other laser parameters. The use of smoke evacuation, fibers, and contact tips should also be documented, especially if charges for these items are made. Sometimes a third-party carrier does not reimburse for an item if its use is not documented.

A biomedical laser technician may be needed as part of the laser team as the number of laser systems increases. Initially a service contract may be purchased after the warranty period has expired on the laser, if only a few lasers are in the program. As the number of systems grows, however, the economic rationale to add the position of biomedical laser technician may be justified. This person usually has attended a training school or program for laser and optics technology. The addition of this position allows preventive maintenance to be performed on a regular basis and laser malfunctions to be addressed immediately.

Laser procurement

Planning and budget manipulation is required to procure a laser system. Because these highly technologic pieces of equipment can be very expensive, creative financing is often needed. Procuring a laser system is a two-phase process involving justification and acquisition.

The justification phase is conducted by the laser committee. This process determines the need for the laser system and which system will fulfill this need. A justification survey is sent to physicians who might use the system. The written responses are tallied to decide the need and interest. After the determination has been made that a system is needed, then several lasers are usually evaluated. A comparison sheet can be developed to note the features of the different laser systems. The advantages and dis-

advantages are thoroughly examined for each unit. Often lasers are brought into the hospital for a clinical trial period. This evaluation should be stringently controlled and organized, as the cost to the manufacturer or distributor to provide this evaluation is usually high. The opinions of physicians and laser team members are considered in open discussions. Some factors for deciding which system to buy can involve the laser warranty package, cost of service contracts, service response time, availability of the laser system and accessories, cost of laser supplies, FDA-approved procedures, future laser applications, ongoing research and development, and the cost of the system. Usually a laser is purchased that will address the needs of more than one specialty area to ensure utilization after the laser is procured. Sometimes a laser is purchased because of one physician's wishes. Later, the utilization does not produce the expected return on investment for the hospital. Intense planning by the laser committee to justify the laser procurement is vital to guarantee utilization.

The acquisition phase is usually the responsibility of the financial department after the laser procurement has been justified and the specific laser system has been determined. Several methods, including outright purchase, leasing, developing a foundation, and promoting donations, can be used to procure a laser system.

The outright purchase method of laser procurement offers immediate possession of the laser unit. The laser can be purchased from capital equipment funds and then a tangible asset is immediately realized. Monthly budgeting for cash expenditures is not necessary because one lump sum is used to buy the system. Two disadvantages of this method are loss of potential investment monies and early outdating of an owned, highly technologic piece of equipment.

Because laser technology continues to change at a rapid pace, ownership of the laser system may not be desirable. Leasing the laser is an option that can be designed to spread the payment over a period of time. Usually a laser is leased for 3 to 5 years. At the end of the lease, a buy-out option can be arranged. Laser leases are offered by the manufacturer, the distributor, or a third-party financier who is in the business of leasing medical equipment. Some manufacturers even lease the laser system per each use, but this method is associated with difficulty in tracking the utilization. Whichever leasing agreement is used, the facility should scrutinize the leasing contract carefully.

A limited partnership may be formed by physicians to purchase the laser if the hospital is unable or unwilling to purchase or lease the system. The physician group can then set up a fee schedule for the hospital to repay the group as the laser is used. This method of procurement ensures that the physicians use the laser because the investors have a vested interest in its use. As tax laws and regulations are introduced, physicians must be aware of changes concerning physician limited partnerships that own equipment that will generate revenue and also be used in their practices.

Donations can also be used to help procure a laser system. If a hospital is a nonprofit organization, the donations may be tax deductible. Benevolent gifts and fund-raising events can make funds available to defray the cost of expensive laser systems. Because laser technology is considered futuristic and has been shown to benefit patients, community organizations and individuals are usually eager to donate funds to help medical advancement in their community.

Whenever an order is placed for a laser, plans must be made to accommodate the system when it arrives. Special water or electrical hookups that may be required should be installed before the system is delivered so that it can be used immediately. If a hospital is not prepared for the laser when it arrives, the warranty period begins to lapse, and the period of return on investment for the laser is prolonged.

Reimbursement

The amount of reimbursement for the laser procedure determines how quickly return on investment can be expected. Because laser technology can be expensive, the amount that is reimbursed often decides the growth of the laser program. The cost to perform the laser procedure should be less than the reimbursed amount.

The first consideration when exploring the economics of a laser program is to determine the cost of performing the procedure. Direct and indirect expenses, including the cost of the laser system, fibers, smoke evacuation, sterile supplies, unsterile supplies, ancillary equipment, drugs, staffing, physical plant, and other related expenses must be calculated. After the cost has been determined, a charge for the laser and the procedure can be developed. Charges for the laser unit can be based on a per use basis or on time increments. The charge should be comparable to other laser charges in the geographic area.

Laser technology has decreased hospitalization for some procedures and has even converted inpatient surgeries to outpatient status. The trends in laser usage have helped to decrease the health care dollars spent as less invasive procedures are introduced, fewer complications are realized, and fewer ancillary supplies are needed.

Reimbursement is divided into inpatient and outpatient status. Inpatient reimbursement is often determined by the discharge diagnosis and the diagnosis related group (DRG). This prospective payment system provides a specified amount of reimbursement no matter how long the patient is hospitalized. If the laser is used and hospitalization is decreased, then the expenses are less but the reimbursement remains the same. Therefore, the laser helps to control costs and makes the DRG system more profitable for the hospital.

Outpatient reimbursement controls are gradually enter-

ing into the prospective payment system in the 1990s. Ambulatory surgery procedures have been grouped into different classifications depending upon the severity of the procedure. Reimbursement is determined for each grouping independent of any charges or costs. This system continues to be refined as more third-party carriers are investigating the possibility of implementing this type of reimbursement method.

When the amount of reimbursement is compared to the costs of performing a procedure, profitability can be determined. Cost-containment measures can be encouraged to decrease the expense related to each procedure. Cost containment requires the continuing efforts of everyone involved in the laser program, including laser safety officers, perioperative nursing staff members, department directors, and physicians. Awareness of the actual expense related to the laser system or special supplies, coupled with an understanding of the amount of reimbursement, can help the laser team manage costs through creative implementation and administration.

Marketing

Marketing can be critical to a laser program. Many times a carefully planned laser program is implemented and does not begin to grow because a marketing plan to encourage utilization has not been initiated or followed. Therefore, the "dusty laser syndrome" occurs as large amounts of money are expended to meet the needs of the laser program, but due to the lack of marketing the laser is not used. Physicians become distressed because they have no patients on whom to use the laser, the administration becomes disappointed because the return on investment is not happening, and the laser team members are discouraged because their special laser training is not being employed. The missing link is a marketing program to promote the laser to the community and to referring physicians.

A marketing program begins with an external assessment to analyze the laser market. This assessment should document historical trends of laser technology, potential clinical applications of the laser, community needs, and competition in the area. An internal assessment determines physician interest in the laser and the knowledge and willingness of referring physicians to send patients to specialists who use the laser. After a comprehensive review, the determination of where the laser program can fit into the overall marketplace and into local competition can be made. Opportunities for the laser program can be highlighted, and threats to the program can also be disclosed.

Developing a marketing plan based on a strategic survey starts with defining the objectives of the laser program. These objectives must be measurable so that the degree of achievement can be evaluated. The objectives should be formed through the coordinated efforts of everyone involved with the laser program. The finalized written objectives should be communicated so that everyone is working toward the same goals. When more people are involved with this phase of marketing, "ownership" in the program is widely felt and commitment is fostered.

The target audience for laser marketing must be determined so that the marketing plan is designed specifically to reach this group. Usually marketing programs designate the patient as the primary target audience, with referring physicians as the secondary group.

In formulating the plan of action for the marketing program, characteristics of the laser program should be designed to reflect the uniqueness of the services that are offered. Also, budgetary commitments to marketing efforts should be resolved so that financial limitations can be realized and the best marketing can be achieved for the money to be spent.

Implementing a marketing plan for a laser program can be accomplished through advertising, personal selling, sales promotion, and publicity. A combination of these methods is usually the most cost-effective manner to promote a laser program.

An advertising campaign usually is most successful if the primary emphasis is on the benefits of laser surgery and the secondary emphasis is on the laser program itself. The consumer needs to hear or read of the advantages and benefits of laser technology before getting involved with the services of a specific laser program. The consumer must believe in the product before the service will be used. The various media available to advertise a laser program include newsprint, radio, television, billboards, and direct mail. Personal selling of laser services can be achieved through speaking engagements and personal contacts with physicians. Publicity is another method to promote the laser program as news releases to the media, a booth display at a health fair, and informational brochures carry the message about the laser program.

A marketing program should be evaluated on a regular basis to determine the results and the continuity of the activities. The success of each endeavor should be documented so that strengths and weaknesses are noted. Alterations to a marketing plan should be expected as the laser program grows and changes. Successful marketing depends upon the financial commitment from administration and the energies of the laser team and physicians.

BENEFITS OF LASER TECHNOLOGY

Laser technology continues to evolve as more surgical applications are developed. Once controversial, the laser has now become a respected and valued medical device that is revolutionizing surgery. As physicians become more adept in laser applications, utilization continues to grow. As techniques are introduced, less invasive procedures are preferred over the former more invasive methods. The true potential of the laser has yet to be realized as health care practitioners explore different applications of laser technology. The following list describes some of the advantages that have been associated with laser technology, depending upon the procedure performed.

- Seals small blood vessels (less intraoperative and postoperative blood loss)
- Seals lymphatics (decreases postoperative edema and the chance of spread of malignant cells in the lymphatic system)
- Seals nerve endings (on selective procedures, to decrease postoperative pain)
- Sterilizes tissue (from the heat generated at the laser tissue impact site)
- Decreases postoperative stenosis (from decreasing the amount of scarring)
- Minimal tissue damage (from precision of the laser beam)
- Reduced operative and anesthesia time
- Shift to more outpatient procedures
- More use of local anesthesia instead of general anesthesia
- Quicker recovery and return to daily activities

As new laser technology is introduced and refined, perioperative nurses will have the responsibility of expanding their knowledge base by keeping current with the safety requirements and operation of these systems. Laser technology is a challenge to the perioperative nurse's professional growth. It offers the opportunity to develop creative methods of nursing practice to deliver high-quality patient care during laser procedures. The full potential of laser use is still being realized, and the perioperative nurse will continue to have an instrumental role in the development of this technology in the 1990s.

BIBLIOGRAPHY

Absten, G.T., and Joffe, S.N.: Lasers in medicine: an introductory guide, London, 1985, Chapman and Hall.

American National Standards Institute, Inc.: American national standard for the safe use of lasers in health care facilities, ANSI Z136.3, New York, 1988, The Institute.

Apfelberg, D.B., editor: Evaluation and installation of surgical laser systems, New York, 1987, Springer-Verlag.

Baggish, M., Laser plume danger? Questions remain, caution advised, Clinical Laser Monthly, October: 111, 1988.

Ball, K.A.: The evolution of surgical lasers, Today's OR Nurse, 8:6, 1986.

Ball, K.: Developing a laser program, Today's OR Nurse, 8:16, 1986.

Ball, K.: Laser marketing, Today's OR nurse, 9:26, 1987.

Ball, K.: Lasers: the perioperative challenge, St. Louis, 1990, The C.V. Mosby Co.

Dubuque, S.: Advertising a laser program, Clinical Laser Management Postconference, August 27, 1988, New York City.

Fuller, T.A., editor: Surgical lasers, a clinical guide, New York, 1987, Macmillan Publishing Co.

Garden, J.M., and others: Papillomavirus in the vapor of carbon dioxide laser-treated verrucae, JAMA 8:1199, 1988.

Goldman, L., editor: The biomedical laser, technology and clinical applications, New York, 1981, Springer-Verlag.

Joffe, S.N., and Oguro, Y., editors: Advances in Nd: YAG laser surgery, New York, 1988, Springer-Verlag.

Joint Commission on Accreditation of Healthcare Organizations: Accreditation manual for hospitals, Chicago, 1990, The Commission.

Lobraico, R.V., Schifano, M.J., and Brader, K.R.: A retrospective study on the hazards of the carbon dioxide laser plume, J Laser Applications, Fall: 6, 1988.

Mackety, C.: Laser nursing, Thorofare, N.J., 1984, Slack, Inc.

Mihashi, S., and others: Some problems about condensates induced by CO_2 laser irradiation, Karume, Japan, 1975, Department of Otolaryngology and Public Health, Karume University.

Pfister, J.I., Kneedler, J.A., and Purcell, S.K.: The nursing spectrum of lasers, Denver, 1988, Education Design, Inc.

Ratz, J.L.: Lasers in cutaneous medicine and surgery, Chicago, 1986, Year Book Medical Publishers.

Reeves, W.G., Forrest, D., and Nezhat, C.: Smoke from laser surgery: Is there a health hazard? 185 (reprint).

Swergold, Chevitz, and Sinsabaugh, Inc.: Experts predict strong laser market over next five years, Clinical Laser Monthly 5:1, 1987.

Part Two

SURGICAL INTERVENTIONS

11 Abdominal incisions and closures, laparotomy, and gastrointestinal surgery

KAREN S. McNEELY

The most frequently performed procedure is the laparotomy, by which various disease processes can be diagnosed or treated. Many different procedures involving the GI tract are performed using a laparotomy approach; examples include resection of a portion of the bowel due to disease or obstruction, procedures performed on the stomach such as gastrectomy, or procedures performed to diagnose a problem that has resulted in physiologic symptoms.

Surgical procedures involving the GI tract are usually performed through an abdominal incision. The surgeon chooses an incision that affords maximum exposure of the involved structures, ensures minimal trauma and postoperative discomfort, and provides for primary wound healing with maximal wound strength. Although surgical interventions have changed drastically over the years, the types of incisions used to expose the affected organs of the GI tract have remained relatively constant. In few other types of surgery can attention to detail and technique so profoundly affect the ultimate result as in the opening and closing of abdominal incisions. This chapter examines these incisions and the indications for each.

Anatomy of the abdominal wall. The abdominal wall consists of various tissue layers through which dissection is necessary to enter the abdominal cavity. (Figs. 11-1 and 11-2). Beneath the skin and subcutaneous fat, the layers include fascia, muscles (external and internal oblique, rectus abdominis, and transversus abdominis), preperitoneal fat, and peritoneum. Fascia, which consists of bands of tough, fibrous connective tissue, surrounds the muscles anteriorly and posteriorly (Fig. 11-3). The peritoneum is a serous membrane lining the abdominal cavity. Incision of this tissue layer exposes abdominal cavity contents.

Types of abdominal incisions
Vertical midline incision

The vertical midline incision is the simplest abdominal incision to perform. It is an excellent primary incision and generally preferred because it offers good exposure to any part of the abdominal cavity. With this incision, hemostasis is easily achieved, and fewer layers are traversed. The incision can be extended from just below the sternal notch, distally around the umbilicus (which is avascular, tough connective tissue), back to the midline, and down to the symphysis pubis (Fig. 11-4). The peritoneum is incised, and the round ligament of the liver may be divided.

To close the wound, the peritoneum and posterior fascia are usually sutured as a single layer. Sometimes the suture line is supported by using retention sutures, which extend through most or all layers of the wound. Anterior fascia, subcutaneous tissue, and skin are closed as layers. An alternative closure uses figure-of-eight sutures of a monofilament, nonabsorbable suture.

Oblique incisions
McBurney muscle-splitting incision

The McBurney muscle-splitting incision is used for removal of the appendix. It is an 8-cm oblique incision that begins well below the umbilicus, goes through McBurney's point, and extends upward toward the right flank (Fig. 11-4). The external oblique muscle and fascia are split in the direction of their fibers and are retracted. The internal oblique muscle, transversalis muscle, and fascia are split and retracted. The peritoneum is incised transversely, and closure is as described, later in the chapter, for laparotomy. This incision is quick and easy to close and allows a firm wound closure. However, it does not permit good exposure and is difficult to extend. To extend the incision medially, the inferior epigastric vessels are ligated, and the rectus sheath is incised transversely.

Subcostal incision

The subcostal incision is usually made on the right side and may be used for operations on the gallbladder, common duct, or pancreas. When made on the left side, it is used for splenectomy. This incision usually gives only limited exposure unless the patient is short with a wide abdomen and wide costal margins. The advantages of this type of incision are that it provides good cosmetic results because it follows the skin lines and the nerve damage is limited because only one or two nerves are cut, most commonly the eighth intercostal nerve. Also, tension on the incisional edges is less than in a vertical incision, it can readily be extended for wide exposure, and it causes less respiratory impairment.

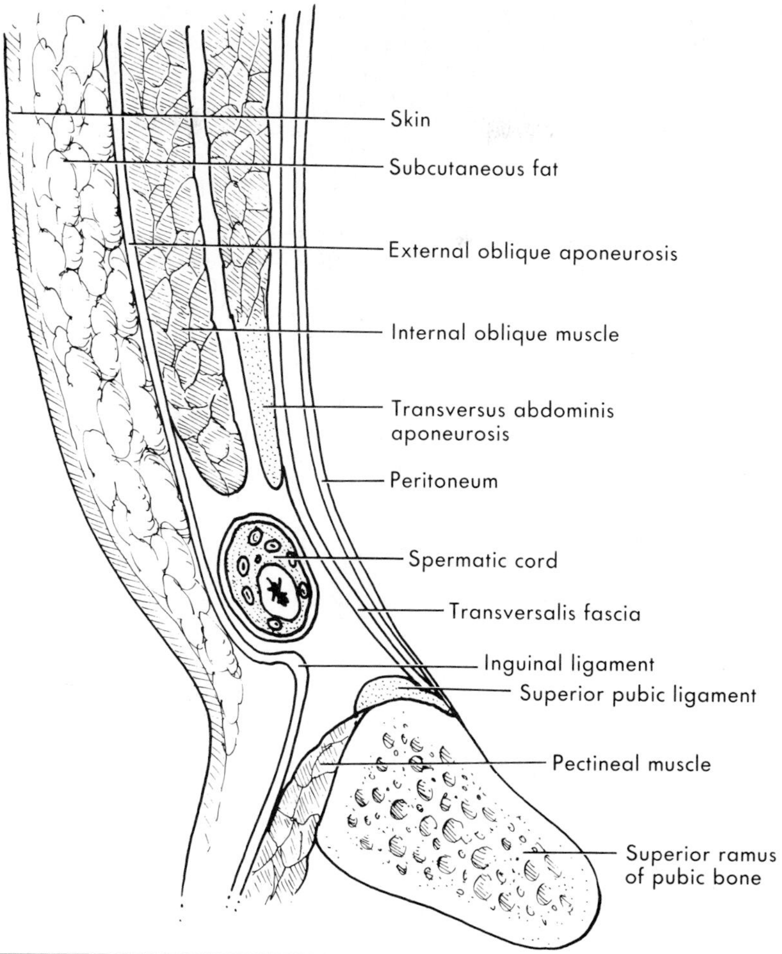

Fig. 11-1. Vertical section of abdominal wall. (Redrawn from Lichtenstein, I.L.: Hernia repair without disability, St. Louis, 1970, The C.V. Mosby Co.)

Skin

Subcutaneous fat

External oblique aponeurosis

Internal oblique muscle

Transversus abdominis aponeurosis

Peritoneum

Spermatic cord

Transversalis fascia

Inguinal ligament

Superior pubic ligament

Pectineal muscle

Superior ramus of pubic bone

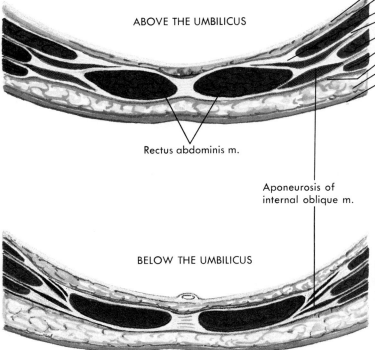

Nine layers:

9-Peritoneum
8-Preperitoneal fat
7-Transversalis fascia
6-Transversus m.
5-Int. oblique m.
4-Ext. oblique m.
3-Scarpa's fascia
2-Camper's fascia
1-Skin

ABOVE THE UMBILICUS

Rectus abdominis m.

Aponeurosis of internal oblique m.

BELOW THE UMBILICUS

Fig. 11-2. Horizontal section of abdominal wall. Aponeurosis of internal oblique muscle splits into two sections, one lying anterior and the other posterior to rectus abdominis muscle, thereby forming encasing sheath around muscle above umbilicus. Below umbilicus, aponeuroses of all muscles pass anterior to rectus. (From Thibodeau, G.A.: Anthony's textbook of anatomy and physiology, ed. 13, St. Louis, 1990, The C.V. Mosby Co.)

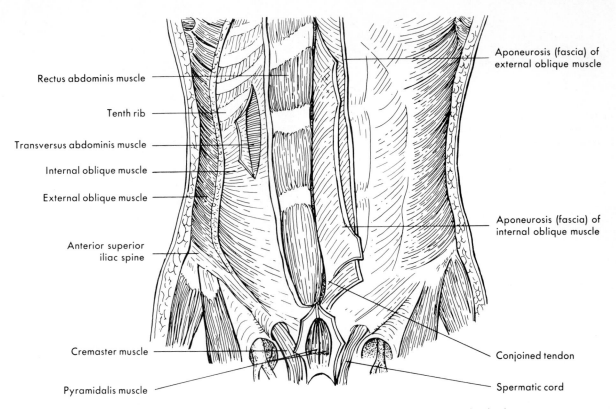

Rectus abdominis muscle

Tenth rib

Transversus abdominis muscle

Internal oblique muscle

External oblique muscle

Anterior superior
iliac spine

Cremaster muscle

Pyramidalis muscle

Aponeurosis (fascia) of
external oblique muscle

Aponeurosis (fascia) of
internal oblique muscle

Conjoined tendon

Spermatic cord

Fig. 11-3. Superior muscles of abdominal wall. (Redrawn from Thibodeau, G.A.: Textbook of anatomy and physiology, ed. 10, St. Louis, 1979, The C.V. Mosby Co.)

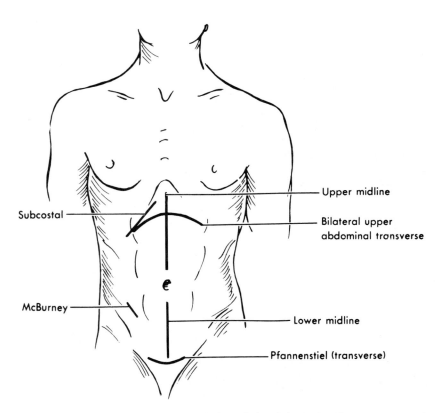

Subcostal

McBurney

Upper midline

Bilateral upper
abdominal transverse

Lower midline

Pfannenstiel (transverse)

Fig. 11-4. Incisions made through the abdominal wall.

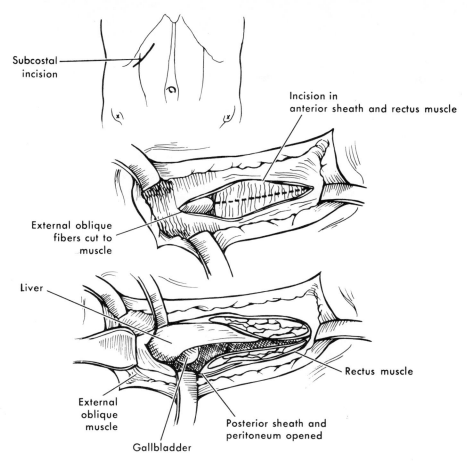

Fig. 11-5. Subcostal incision in upper right quadrant. Anterior sheath has been divided transversely, and muscle is exposed. Posterior sheath and peritoneum have been opened transversely.

This oblique incision begins in the epigastrium, extending laterally and obliquely downward to just below the lower costal margin (Fig. 11-5). Each muscle contains veins and arteries requiring ligation. If more exposure is needed, the incision is extended across the rectus muscle of the other side. The rectus muscle is either retracted or transversely divided. Vessels in the muscle must be ligated.

The closure of this incision includes approximation and closure of the falciform ligament, peritoneum, posterior rectus sheath, and anterior rectus sheath with interrupted, nonabsorbable sutures. The subcutaneous tissue and skin are closed as described for laparotomy. Absorbable sutures may be used in conjunction with staples.

Transverse incisions
Pfannenstiel incision

The Pfannenstiel incision is used frequently for pelvic surgery. It is a curved transverse incision across the lower abdomen through the skin, subcutaneous tissue, and rectus sheaths (Fig. 11-6). This incision is made approximately 1½ inches above the symphysis pubis. The rectus muscles are separated in midline, and the peritoneum is entered through a midline vertical incision. This incision provides for a strong closure; when the rectus muscles contract, there is less strain on the fascial sutures.

Midabdominal transverse incision

The midabdominal transverse incision is used on the left or right side or for a retroperitoneal approach. The incision begins slightly above or below the umbilicus on either side and is carried laterally to the lumbar region at an angle between the ribs and crest of the ilium. The skin and subcutaneous tissue are incised, the anterior rectus sheath is split, the rectus muscle is divided, and the vessels within the rectus are clamped and ligated. The posterior rectus sheath and peritoneum are cut in the direction of the fibers, preserving the intercostal nerves. The peritoneum is incised near the midline, and the incision is extended laterally to the oblique muscle. The lateral muscles are incised to provide wide exposure. The closure is in layers with interrupted sutures; the subcutaneous tissue and skin are closed as for laparotomy (see p. 207). The rectus muscle usually cannot be closed because its fibers run vertically. Approximation of the rectus sheath brings the

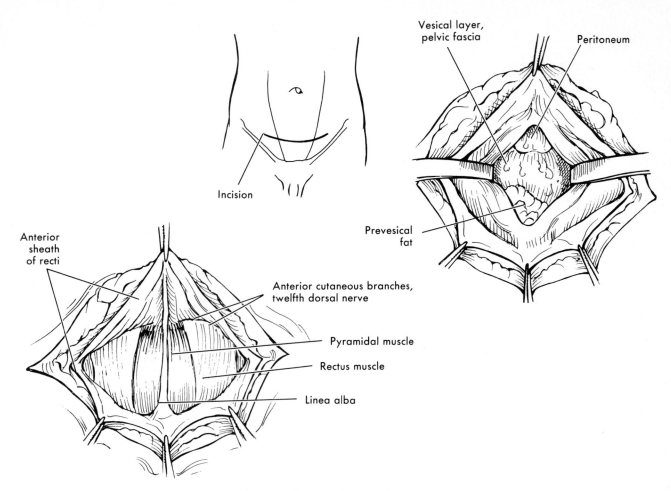

Incision

Vesical layer, pelvic fascia

Peritoneum

Prevesical fat

Anterior sheath of recti

Anterior cutaneous branches, twelfth dorsal nerve

Pyramidal muscle

Rectus muscle

Linea alba

Fig. 11-6. Pfannenstiel incision (transverse).

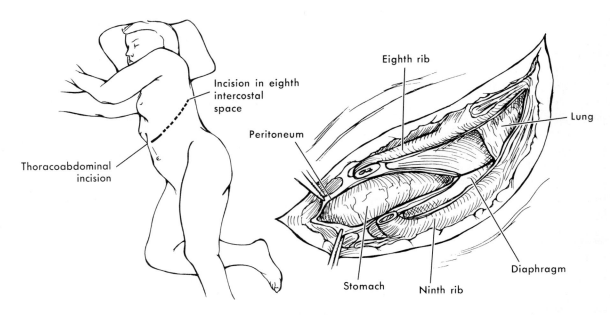

Incision in eighth intercostal space

Thoracoabdominal incision

Peritoneum

Eighth rib

Lung

Stomach

Ninth rib

Diaphragm

Fig. 11-7. Thoracoabdominal incision. Patient is placed on unaffected side. Incision is usually made from point midway between xiphoid process and umbilicus to costal margin at site of eighth costal cartilage. Dissection is carried down to peritoneum and pleura. Costal cartilage and diaphragm are divided, and stomach is exposed.

edges of the rectus muscle into excellent apposition, thus eliminating the need to suture the muscle itself.

Thoracoabdominal incision

The thoracoabdominal incision is used for operations on the proximal portion of the stomach and the distal section of the esophagus. Often the abdominal part of the incision is made first for exploration and then if necessary is extended across the costal margin into the chest.

The incision begins at a point midway between the xiphoid process and the umbilicus and extends across to the seventh or eighth interspace and to the midscapular line. The rectus and oblique abdominal muscles are divided in the line of incision down to the peritoneum and pleura. The costal cartilage and the diaphragm are then divided (Fig. 11-7).

The wound is closed in layers with interrupted sutures. Absorbable sutures may be used for the peritoneum and intercostal muscles. Nonabsorbable suture may be used for the muscle and fascial layers. Skin edges are approximated with staples or a nonabsorbable suture.

Upper inverted-U abdominal incision

An upper inverted-U abdominal incision is seldom used today; however, it can be used for gastrectomy, transverse colon resection, transverse colostomy, and biliary and pancreatic procedures. The incision extends from a point below the costal margin on one side in the anterior axillary line to the same point on the opposite side. It is curved, with the midpoint lying midway between the xiphoid process and the umbilicus. The intercostal nerves are preserved.

An upper abdominal transverse incision is closed by placing interrupted sutures in the peritoneum and anterior and posterior rectus sheaths. The muscle and fat need not be sutured. The skin edges are approximated and closed as described for laparotomy (see p. 207).

SURGICAL ANATOMY

The alimentary canal comprises a series of organs joined to form a tubelike structure that extends the entire length of the trunk (Fig. 11-8). The alimentary tract includes the mouth, pharynx, esophagus, stomach, small intestine consisting of the duodenum, jejunum, and ileum, and large intestine, which is comprised of the cecum, ascending colon, transverse colon, descending colon, sigmoid colon, rectum, and anus. These organs are responsible for the supply of nourishment to the body and the elimination of solid wastes.

The *esophagus* extends from the pharynx, at the level of the sixth cervical vertebra, and passes through the neck, posterior to the trachea and heart and anterior to the vertebral column. The lower portion of the esophagus passes in front of the aorta and through the diaphragm, slightly to the left of the midline, to join the cardia of the stomach.

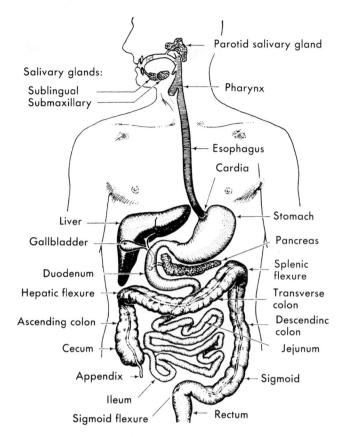

Fig. 11-8. Alimentary canal and its appendages. (Modified from Schottelius, B.A., and Schottelius, D.D.: Textbook of physiology, ed. 18, St. Louis, 1979, The C.V. Mosby Co.)

Blood is supplied to the esophagus from branches of the inferior thyroid, thoracic aorta, and celiac arteries. The nerve supply comes from branches of the vagi and sympathetic chain. The esophagus of an adult is about 10 inches in length and is a collapsible musculomembranous tube.

The *stomach* is situated between the esophagus and the duodenum and lies in the upper left abdominal cavity, slightly to the left of the midline and beneath the diaphragm. The stomach is divided into three parts; the fundus, the body, and the antrum (Fig. 11-9). The *fundus* lies beneath the left dome of the diaphragm, behind the apex of the heart, and the *body* and *antrum* lie in an oblique direction within the abdominal cavity. The stomach is stabilized indirectly by the lower portion of the esophagus and directly by its attachment to the duodenum, which is anchored to the posterior parietal peritoneum. The omentum, the peritoneal ligaments, and branches of the celiac vessel provide additional support to the stomach.

The convex or lower margin of the stomach is known as the *greater curvature,* and the concave margin, the *lesser curvature.* Attached to the greater curvature is the *greater omentum,* which is a double fold of peritoneum

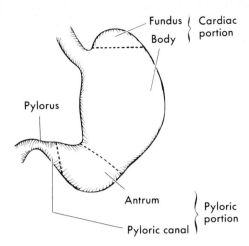

Fig. 11-9. Regional anatomy of stomach.

containing fat. It covers the intestines loosely and is not to be confused with the mesentery, which connects the intestines with the posterior abdominal wall. The left gastroepiploic branch of the splenic artery and the right gastroepiploic branch of the hepatic artery run through the greater omentum. The *lesser omentum,* which is attached to the lesser curvature of the stomach, contains the left gastric artery, a branch of the celiac axis, and the right gastric branch of the hepatic artery (Fig. 11-10). During a gastrectomy, these vessels are clamped and ligated.

The *small intestine* begins at the pylorus and ends at the ileocecal valve (Fig. 11-8). It is also divided into three

Fig. 11-10. Arterial supply of stomach. (After Cutler and Zollinger; from Francis, C.C., and Martin, A.H.: Introduction to human anatomy, ed. 7, St. Louis, 1975, The C.V. Mosby Co.)

parts; the duodenum, which is about 11 inches long; the jejunum, which is about 7½ feet long; and the ileum, which is about 11½ feet long in an adult. The small intestine varies in size with the degree of contraction but is usually about 20 feet in length and 1 inch in diameter (Fig. 11-8). The *duodenum,* the proximal portion of the small intestine, begins at the pylorus, is continuous with the jejunum and is stabilized by a fusion between the pancreas and the posterior parietal peritoneum. The duodenum also communicates with the common bile duct, and the duodenojejunal angle is stabilized by the ligament of Treitz that suspends the duodenum. The ligament of Treitz serves as an important landmark during any abdominal operation.

The middle portion of the duodenum forms an acute angle in its descent. It passes along the right side, and then its inferior portion traverses to the left, so that it lies in front of the right ureter, the inferior vena cava, and the aorta. It then turns upward and forward to become a part of the duodenojejunal flexure that in turn joins the jejunum. The bile and pancreatic ducts enter the descending portion of the duodenum; the blood supply of the duodenum comes from the arterial branches of the celiac axis.

The *jejunum,* which is situated in the upper portion of the abdomen, joins the *ileum,* which is situated in the lower portion of the cavity. The ileum empties into the large

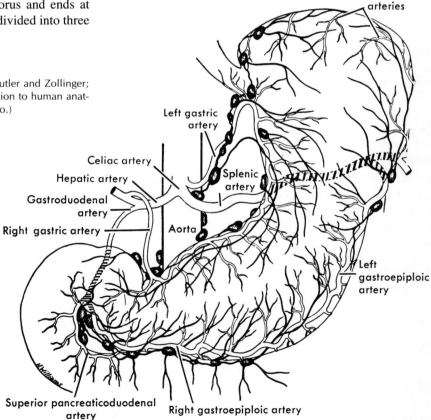

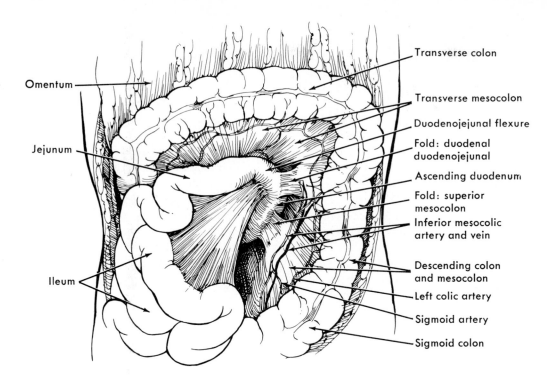

Fig. 11-11. Mesentery, as seen when intestine is pulled aside.

intestine through the ileocecal valve. The jejunum and ileum are suspended by the mesentery, which is attached to the posterior abdominal wall (Fig. 11-11). The free border of the mesentery, which is about 18 feet long, contains branches of the superior mesenteric artery, many veins, lymph nodes, and nerve fibers.

The *large intestine* begins at the ileocecal valve and terminates at the anus. It is divided into the cecum and the colon.

The *cecum* is attached to the ileum and extends about 2½ inches below it (Fig. 11-8). The cecum in an adult is usually adherent to the posterior wall of the peritoneal cavity and has a serosal covering on its anterior wall only. The cecum forms a blind pouch from which the appendix projects.

The *colon* is divided into five parts; the ascending colon; the transverse colon, the descending colon, the sigmoid colon, and the rectum (Fig. 11-12).

The ascending colon is about 6 inches long and extends upward from the ileocecal valve to the hepatic flexure. The upper portion of the ascending colon lies behind the right lobe of the liver and in front of the anterior surface of the right kidney.

The transverse colon, which is about 20 inches long, begins at the hepatic flexure and ends at the splenic flexure. It lies below the stomach and is attached to the transverse mesocolon.

The descending colon extends downward from the splenic flexure to the area just below the iliac crest and is about

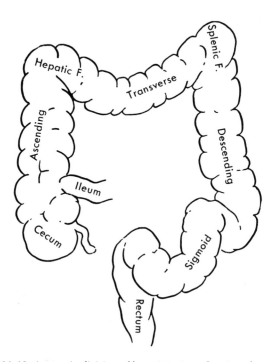

Fig. 11-12. Anatomic division of large intestine, showing placement of ileocecal valve, hepatic flexure, and splenic flexure.

7 inches long. The iliac portion of the sigmoid colon, which is about 6 inches long, lies on the inner surface of the left iliac muscle. The remaining portion of the colon passes over the pelvic brim into the pelvic cavity and lies partly in the abdomen and partly in the pelvis. It then forms an S curve in the pelvis and terminates in the rectum at the level of the third segment of the sacral vertebrae.

The blood supply to the ascending colon, hepatic flexure, and transverse colon comes from the superior mesenteric artery, whereas the blood supply to the descending colon and rectum comes from the inferior mesenteric artery.

The wall of the colon is made up of teniae coli, epiploic appendices, and haustra. The teniae coli are three longitudinal, or axial, strips of muscles distributed around the circumference of the colon. They represent the longitudinal muscle layer, which is not complete in the colon. The small intestine and rectum have both circular and complete longitudinal muscle layers. The epiploic appendices are fatty appendages along the bowel that have no particular function; the haustra are sacculations that are the outpouchings of bowel wall between the teniae coli.

The diameter of the colon varies in size from about 3½ inches in the cecum to an average of about 1½ inches in the sigmoid colon (Fig. 11-12).

The rectum, which is a continuation of the sigmoid colon, terminates in the anus. The rectum, a slightly curved passage about 6 inches long, is surrounded by the pelvic fascia as it lies on the anterior surface of the sacrum and coccyx. In the male the rectum lies behind the prostate gland and the bladder. In the female the rectum lies behind the uterus and the vagina. The rectum dilates just before it becomes the anal canal, and this dilation or ampulla presents folds called Houston's valves. The wall of the rectum consists of four layers, similar to those of the small intestine.

The anal canal is a narrow passage about 1 inch long, which passes downward and backward. It is surrounded and controlled by two circular muscle groups, which form the external and internal anal sphincters. The internal sphincter is a continuation of the longitudinal muscle layer.

The esophagus serves as the route from which food enters the stomach from the mouth. When food enters the stomach, it undergoes chemical and mechanical changes and then enters the duodenum, where it is mixed with bile and pancreatic juices. The stomach is never entirely empty because it always contains some gastric juice, which is acid in nature and produced by numerous tubular glands in the wall of the stomach.

Food enters the stomach by passing through the cardiac sphincter and leaves by passing through the pyloric sphincter. When food is in the stomach, the stomach becomes distended and the rugae, or folds, flatten out. Little absorption takes place in the stomach, and liquid enters the duodenum within half an hour after its ingestion. Food is moved through the stomach and intestines by peristalsis, which consists of waves of motion caused by successive contractions of the muscles in the walls of the stomach and intestines.

Absorption of nutrients is a function of the small intestine. The large intestine absorbs water from the contents and expels the indigestible residue from the body. The residue is composed primarily of cellulose from carbohydrates, connective tissue, and undigested fats. The act of defecation is accomplished by contraction of the rectal and abdominal muscles, the descent of the diaphragm, and the relaxation of the anal sphincter muscles.

The gastrointestinal tract is probably affected by psychological factors at least as much as are other body systems. In our high-pressured society, people tend to overeat or undereat, and the pressures of everyday living frequently show their effects on the gastrointestinal tract. Although there is no conclusive evidence, some disease entities—for example, pylorospasm, peptic and duodenal ulcers, colitis, and obesity—seem to be exacerbated by psychologic factors. Some of these diseases can be treated medically; others require adjunctive psychotherapy. All of them necessitate diagnostic studies, and many require surgery.

PERIOPERATIVE NURSING CONSIDERATIONS
Assessment/nursing diagnosis

Nursing care for patients undergoing gastrointestinal surgery begins with assessment. Individualized care, integrating physiologic with psychologic preparation, is afforded each patient.

Patients undergoing gastrointestinal surgery should understand why they need preoperative preparation, what the intended surgical intervention will be, and how it will affect them postoperatively. A preoperative nursing assessment of the patient is essential for appropriate planning and implementation of intraoperative nursing care and evaluation of patient outcomes. The nurse should ensure that the patient understands the nature of the surgery and the site of the incision. Turning, coughing, and deep breathing are taught preoperatively and reinforced after surgery.

The value of nursing care plans has been well documented in the literature. Perioperative nurses are challenged to diagnose, plan, implement, and evaluate care in a very short time. They must have the ability to prioritize patient needs and act accordingly. The first step in this process, patient assessment, leads to the formulation of nursing diagnoses and is essential to all other steps. Nursing diagnoses appropriate to patients undergoing gastrointestinal surgery are as follows:

· Potential for anxiety related to fear of the unknown.
· Body image disturbance related to potential postoperative ostomy.

- Potential for fluid volume deficit related to loss of blood and electrolyte-rich gastric and intestinal juices.
- Potential for injury related to positioning.
- Hypothermia related to room temperature, skin exposure, and an open wound.

Planning

Preoperative assessment enables the perioperative nurse to plan for the specific needs of the individual patient. For example, the size of the patient influences positioning during surgery and may necessitate additional instruments, such as deeper retractors and longer forceps and scissors. The perioperative nurse has to provide the patient with reassurance and emotional support for effective management of anxiety. The nurse must also understand the potential for altered body image with some gastrointestinal procedures.

Once the nursing diagnosis is made, the care plan is developed. This care plan is an essential component in assuring high-quality perioperative nursing care. The Sample Care Plan on p. 202 is an example of a generic care plan addressing the needs of patients undergoing gastrointestinal surgery through a laparotomy incision.

Implementation

Preoperative mechanical preparation of the gastrointestinal tract is often employed for elective surgery, and often bactericidal and bacteriostatic agents are used in an attempt to eliminate pathogenic microorganisms, especially in the lower gastrointestinal tract. Many patients require nasogastric tubes. Fluid and electrolyte balance must be maintained before, during, and after surgery. Often a Foley catheter is inserted preoperatively or immediately after induction to monitor output and renal function during surgery and to keep the bladder empty, thereby allowing more space in the lower abdomen for the surgeon to perform the operation.

If required, hair removal from the proposed incisional site should be done before the patient enters the operating room. Hair should be removed according to the protocol for the type of surgery the patient is to have, as well as the surgeon's preference (Chapter 5).

If the surgeon anticipates the need to replace blood, the patient's blood is typed and cross-matched before the operation. Preadmission arrangements may have been made for the availability of autotransfused blood (Chapter 12).

The circulating nurse should be well informed of what the procedure will entail and should ensure that all necessary supplies and equipment are on hand and that the integrity of the equipment is uncompromised. An electrosurgical unit and accessories may be used for the cutting and coagulation of tissue (Chapter 4).

As in all surgery, careful consideration should be given to positioning the patient so that the surgeon can gain optimum exposure without compromising the respiratory, circulatory, and nervous systems and without producing undue pressure on any body part (Chapter 6).

Suture materials used on gastrointestinal tissue have traditionally been chromic and silk. With the increased number of synthetic absorbable and nonabsorbable suture materials available, surgeons have a variety of materials from which to choose (Chapter 7). Polyester fiber sutures and polyglycolic acid sutures are frequently employed on gastrointestinal tissue. For ease of reference, chromic and silk are listed as sutures of choice, but synthetic absorbable and nonabsorbable sutures are recognized equivalents. Checking the surgeon's preference card for appropriate suture materials not only ensures the availability of necessary supplies but also is a cost-effective measure.

Irrigating solution is frequently used during gastrointestinal procedures. The surgeon specifies the solution of choice, which frequently contains a broad-spectrum antibiotic. Normal saline, an isotonic solution, may be used to moisten laparotomy sponges and for irrigation. Moist packs are used to isolate open and diseased portions of the stomach and bowel from the abdominal cavity and to protect other viscera. Solutions should be warm when used for these purposes.

As in all operations, the excised specimen is handled carefully and prepared for examination by the pathologist. The surgeon usually determines how the specimen will be handled before examination. It may be sent to the pathology department fresh, in saline, or in a preservative solution. Tissue also may be sent for frozen section examination to verify the pathologic condition and determine whether tissue margins are free of malignant cells.

To reduce tissue trauma, the jaws of heavy intestinal forceps may be protected by pieces of soft rubber tubing or other smooth material. These guards (shods) should fit the jaws firmly but not tightly and should extend slightly beyond the tips of forceps. Before sterilization the rubber shods must be separated from the forceps to facilitate and ensure steam penetration.

Surgical stapling instruments have had a great impact on the technical aspects of gastrointestinal surgery. For some surgeons the use of these devices has to an extent replaced conventional suturing techniques. The stapling instruments can be employed to divide and ligate, resect and anastomose. The B design of the implanted staple does not compromise the vascularity of the resected tissue edges. These devices are available in reusable and disposable models. Personnel must be familiar with the types of available stapling equipment, applications, assembly if indicated, and proper loading (Chapter 7).

Whenever a portion of the gastrointestinal tract is entered, bowel technique must be performed. *Bowel technique* means that any instrument coming in contact with the gastrointestinal mucosa is not used after the lumen of

Sample Care Plan

NURSING DIAGNOSIS:
Potential for anxiety related to fear of the unknown
GOAL:
Patient will verbalize knowledge of the perioperative experience.
INTERVENTIONS:
Explain preoperative procedures that will facilitate the surgery; e.g., intravenous lines, skin preparation, bowel preparation. Explain all procedures done in the OR prior to induction.
Explain postoperative drains, catheters, dressings.
Minimize stimuli in the OR.
Remain with the patient during induction.
Allow time for the patient to verbalize feelings/fears.

NURSING DIAGNOSIS:
Body image disturbance related to potential postoperative ostomy
GOAL:
Patient demonstrates knowledge of the ostomy and a desire to perform self-care.
INTERVENTIONS:
Participate in therapeutic communication during the preoperative visit; include family members if appropriate.
Be aware of nonverbal cues.
Refer patient to ostomy nurse.
Encourage patient participation in all aspects of care.

NURSING DIAGNOSIS:
Potential for fluid volume deficit related to loss of blood and electrolyte-rich gastric and intestinal juices
GOAL:
The patient's fluid and electrolyte balance is maintained.

INTERVENTIONS:
Obtain baseline data from the chart relating to fluid and electrolyte balance.
Assess nutritional status, skin turgor, or medications affecting fluid and electrolyte balance.
Periodically inform the surgical team of estimated blood loss.
Record all solutions being administered from the surgical field.

NURSING DIAGNOSIS:
Potential for injury related to positioning
GOAL:
Patient will be free from injury related to supine position.
INTERVENTIONS:
Align patient's torso in straight line with the head and feet.
Extend arms on padded arm boards at 90 degrees or less.
Place palms up if arms tucked at sides.
Place safety strap 2 inches above the knees with the buckle at the patient's side.
Assure that patient's legs remain uncrossed.
Pad bony prominences to avoid pressure points.

NURSING DIAGNOSIS:
Hypothermia related to room temperature, skin exposure, and an open wound
GOAL:
The patient is free from injury related to heat loss.
INTERVENTIONS:
Provide the patient with a warm blanket prior to induction.
Assure that irrigating solutions are warm.
Keep room temperature at a level that provides for maintenance of body temperature.
Cover the patient with a warm blanket prior to transport to PACU.

the gastrointestinal tract has been restored. These instruments are discarded in a separate basin and do not come in contact with other instruments. For closure, some surgeons may desire a new set of instruments, additional draping materials, and a change of gown and gloves.

Instruments used during GI surgery should include a basic laparotomy set combined with instruments specifically designed for use with gastrointestinal tissue. The basic laparotomy set should include:

Cutting instruments (Fig. 11-13)

2 Knife handles, no. 3 with blade no. 10, and no. 7 with blade no. 15
1 Mayo scissors, straight, 6¼ inches
1 Mayo scissors, curved, 6¼ inches
1 Metzenbaum scissors, 7 inches
1 Suture scissors

Holding instruments (Fig. 11-14)

2 Tissue forceps without teeth, 5½ inches
2 Tissue forceps with teeth, 5½ inches
2 Tissue forceps without teeth, 7 and 10 inches
2 Tissue forceps with teeth, 7 and 10 inches
2 Russian tissue forceps, 7 and 10 inches
2 Adson forceps with teeth
4 Sponge-holding forceps, 10 inches
6 Towel clamps, 3½ or 5½ inches
4 Allis forceps, 6 and 9 inches
4 Babcock intestinal forceps, 6 inches

Clamping instruments (Fig. 11-15)

12 Crile forceps, straight or curved, 5½ inches
12 Rochester-Pean forceps, curved, 6¼ inches
8 Rochester-Pean forceps, curved, 10 inches
4 Ochsner or Kocher forceps, straight, 6¼ inches
4 Ochsner or Kocher forceps, straight, 9 inches

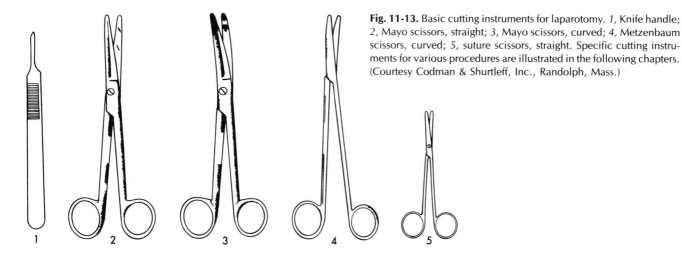

Fig. 11-13. Basic cutting instruments for laparotomy. *1,* Knife handle; *2,* Mayo scissors, straight; *3,* Mayo scissors, curved; *4,* Metzenbaum scissors, curved; *5,* suture scissors, straight. Specific cutting instruments for various procedures are illustrated in the following chapters. (Courtesy Codman & Shurtleff, Inc., Randolph, Mass.)

Fig. 11-14. Basic holding instruments for laparotomy. *1,* Tissue forceps, smooth; *2,* tissue forceps with teeth; *3,* Adson tissue forceps; *4,* sponge-holding forceps; *5,* towel clamps; *6,* Allis forceps; *7,* Babcock intestinal forceps. Specific holding instruments for various procedures are illustrated in the following chapters. (Courtesy Codman & Shurtleff, Inc., Randolph, Mass.)

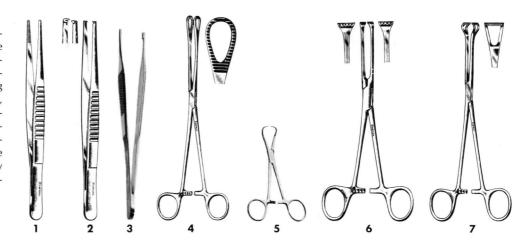

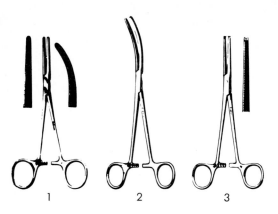

Fig. 11-15. Basic clamping instruments for laparotomy. *1*, Crile hemostatic forceps; *2*, Rochester-Pean hemostatic forceps; *3*, Ochsner or Kocher hemostatic forceps. Specific holding instruments for various procedures are illustrated in the following chapters. (Courtesy Codman & Shurtleff, Inc., Randolph, Mass.)

Exposing instruments (Fig. 11-16)

2 Malleable retractors, 1- to 1½-inch width
2 Vein retractors, small
2 Parker, Roux, Greene, or Army-Navy retractors
6 Richardson or Kelly retractors, small, medium, and large
4 Rake retractors, four- and six-pronged pairs, dull
3 Deaver retractors, small, medium, and large
1 Weitlaner retractor
1 Balfour self-retaining retractor with blades

Suturing instruments (Fig. 11-17)

6 Needle holders, 6 and 8 inches
2 Skin hooks (optional)

Accessory items (Fig. 11-18)

1 Frazier suction tip
1 Poole (sump) suction tube and tubing
2 Yankauer suction tubes and tubing
1 Silver probe
1 Grooved director

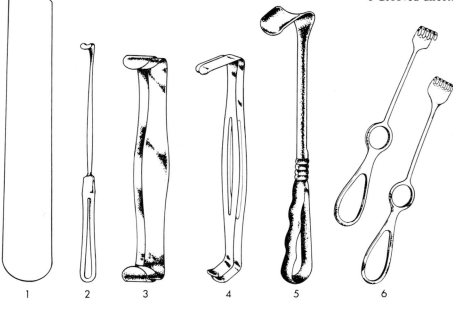

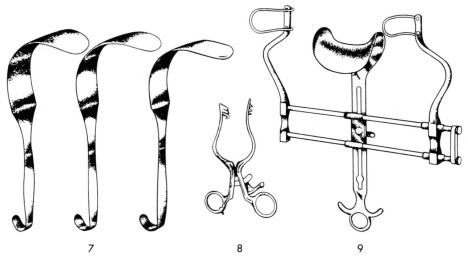

Fig. 11-16. Basic exposing instruments for laparotomy. *1*, Malleable copper retractor; *2*, vein retractor; *3*, Parker retractors; *4*, Army-Navy retractors; *5*, Richardson retractor; *6*, Volkmann rake retractors; *7*, Deaver retractors; *8*, Weitlaner retractor; *9*, Balfour self-retaining retractor with blades. Specific retractors for various procedures are illustrated in the following chapters. (Courtesy Codman & Shurtleff, Inc., Randolph, Mass.)

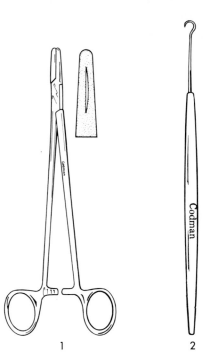

Fig. 11-17. Basic suturing instruments. *1*, Needle holder; *2*, skin hook. Specific needle holders for various procedures are illustrated in the following chapters. (Courtesy Codman & Shurtleff, Inc., Randolph, Mass.)

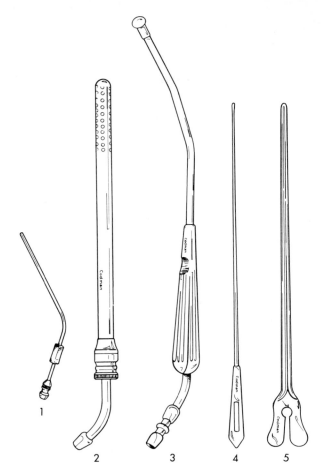

Fig. 11-18. Accessory items. *1*, Frazier suction tip; *2*, Poole suction tube; *3*, Yankauer suction tube; *4*, silver probe; *5*, grooved director. Special accessory items for various procedures are illustrated in the following chapters. (Courtesy Codman & Shurtleff, Inc., Randolph, Mass.)

The GI set should include:

Cutting instruments

1 Metzenbaum scissors, 9 inches
2 Metzenbaum scissors, 5¾ inches, 1 straight and 1 curved
2 Mayo scissors, 9 inches, 1 straight and 1 curved

Clamping instructions (Fig. 11-19)

1 Best colon clamp
4 Allen intestinal anastomosis clamps
4 Rochester-Carmalt forceps, straight, 8 inches
4 Doyen intestinal forceps, longitudinal serrations, 9 inches, 2 straight and 2 curved
2 Mayo vessel clamps, angled, 9 inches
2 Mayo-Robson intestinal forceps, straight
2 Dennis intestinal clamps
6 Ochsner forceps, 6¼ inches
6 Ochsner forceps, 9 inches
1 Pace-potts clamp
4 Gallbladder forceps, right-angled, assorted sizes
4 Rochester-Pean forceps, curved, 8 inches
12 Rochester-Pean forceps, curved, 6¼ inches
12 Crile hemostats, curved, 5½ inches
36 Halsted mosquito hemostats, 5 inches, 24 curved and 12 straight

Holding instruments

2 Tissue forceps without teeth, 5½ inches

2 Fixation or Adson forceps, 5 inches
2 Potts-Smith dressing forceps, 8 inches
6 Babcock intestinal forceps, 6¼ inches
6 Allis forceps, 6¼ inches

Exposing instruments

1 Doyen retractor, large blade, 2¼ inches wide × 3½ inches deep
2 Kelly retractors, large blade, 2½ inches wide × 3 inches deep
Self-retaining retractor and blades

Suturing items

2 Fine needle holders, 6 inches
2 Medium ligating clip appliers with clips
2 Long ligating clip appliers with clips
Suture materials for gastrointestinal operations:
Ligatures for small blood vessels: chromic no. 4-0 and silk no. 5-0, 4-0, or 3-0

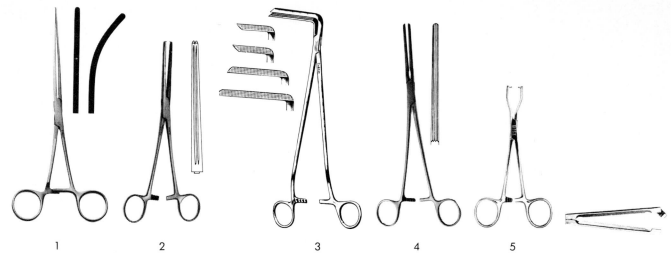

Fig. 11-19. Instruments for stomach and intestinal operations. *1,* Doyen intestinal forceps, straight and curved; *2,* Allen intestinal anastomosis clamp; *3,* Best colon clamps; *4,* Dennis intestinal forceps, *5,* Pace-Potts clamp. (*1, 2,* and *4,* courtesy Codman & Shurtleff, Inc., Randolph, Mass.; *3,* courtesy American V. Mueller, Deerfield, Ill.; *5,* courtesy Edward Weck & Co., Research Triangle Park, NC.)

Ligatures for larger blood vessels: chromic no. 0 or silk no. 2-0 or 0

Closure of gastrointestinal layers:

Mucosal—chromic no. 4-0 or 3-0 with curved atraumatic intestinal needle; usually continuous

Seromuscular—chromic no. 3-0 or 2-0 and silk no. 4-0 or 3-0 with curved or straight atraumatic intestinal needles: interrupted silk sutures on intestinal needles may be used

Abdominal closure and retention sutures, as previously described (Chapter 7)

Accessory items

2 Malecot, Pezzer, or Foley catheters, desired size
1 Robinson catheter, desired size
1 Baker jejunostomy tube
1 Closed wound drainage system
  Sump drain
  Suction drain
2 Poole suction tubes with tubing
1 Yankauer suction tubes with tubing
  Electrosurgical unit with accessories, if desired

Evaluation

As with any surgical procedure, evaluation of nursing care must be done throughout the surgery and before the patient is transported to PACU. The dressing and drains are securely placed to avoid damage during transfer to the PACU stretcher. Skin is assessed for reddened or bruised areas; if such areas are present, treatment is begun immediately. The circulating nurse assures that the patient is covered with a clean, warm blanket before being transported to PACU. Any variances postoperatively are reported to the surgeon, documented in the nursing notes, and included in the report given to the nurse in PACU. Patient outcomes based on the perioperative nursing diagnoses and identified goals should be reviewed. Based on the nursing diagnoses selected for the patient undergoing gastrointestinal surgery, documenting and reporting perioperative patient care might include the following statements:

· The patient's anxiety was reduced.
· The patient verbalized feelings about body image disturbance.
· The patient's fluid volume status was maintained.
· No injury occurred related to positioning.
· Normothermia was maintained.

SURGICAL INTERVENTIONS
Endoscopic procedures

Endoscopic procedures that permit direct visual inspection of the contents and walls of the esophagus, stomach, and colon may be pertinent to establishing a diagnosis or determining preferred treatment of a disease process. A neodymium-YAG laser may also be used in conjunction with endoscopic procedures as a treatment modality for ulcers, esophageal varices, malignancies, and gastrointestinal bleeding (Chapter 10).

Care must be taken in handling fiberoptic equipment. Flexible scopes can be easily damaged if handled improperly. The endoscopic equipment is terminally cleaned according to the manufacturer's instructions (Chapter 25).

Endoscopic procedures may be performed with local anesthesia, with sedation only, or during the course of a procedure being performed with general anesthesia. Although medications may be used for sedation, the nurse must be immediately available to provide emotional support and appropriately monitor the patient's physiologic and psychologic status.

Gastroscopy

Gastroscopy is visual inspection of the stomach, with aspiration of contents and biopsy, if necessary, by an instrument known as a *gastroscope*. When gastroscopy is performed with local anesthesia or sedation, the patient is usually not allowed to eat solid food 4 to 6 hours before the procedure but may take liquids up to 2 hours before it.

Procedural considerations. The patient's position for gastroscopy depends on the areas of the stomach to be visualized. For inspection of lesions in the gastric fundus and cardia, an upright sitting position may be used.

Instrumentation is as follows:

Local anesthesia set	Suction set
Gastroscope	Lubricating jelly
Light source	Aspiration tubes
Biopsy forceps	

Operative procedure

1. The gastroscope is thinly but completely covered with water-soluble lubricating jelly.
2. During introduction of the gastroscope, the patient's head and neck must remain in the sagittal plane of the spine so the axis of the mouth is in line with the esophagus.
3. The gastroscope is slowly passed into the stomach.
4. The stomach is inspected, and stomach contents may be aspirated for cytologic analysis. A biopsy can be performed.

Colonoscopy / sigmoidoscopy

Colonoscopy/sigmoidoscopy is visual inspection of the entire large intestine by means of a colonoscope. The colonoscope is an important diagnostic tool and may be used for biopsy and removal of polyps. The patient must receive a liquid diet for 2 days before the colonoscopy and may receive laxatives. Enemas are given until clear before the procedure.

Procedural considerations. The following instruments are required:

Colonoscope
Light source
Carbon dioxide tank
Biopsy forceps
Snares
Electrosurgical unit and accessories
Lubricating jelly
Suction

Operative procedure

1. Analgesia is induced intramuscularly or intravenously.

2. The well-lubricated colonoscope is passed slowly into the anal canal and advanced continuously until it reaches the cecum.
3. Following the endoscopic examination, the patient should be observed carefully to ensure that neither postprocedural bleeding nor signs of perforation occur.

Laparotomy

An opening made through the abdominal wall into the peritoneal cavity is called a *laparotomy*. Surgical intervention may be necessary to repair or remove traumatized tissue, to cure disease processes by organ removal, and to examine by biopsy or otherwise visualize internal organs for diagnosis. Surgery may be indicated for diagnostic, therapeutic, palliative, or prophylactic reasons. Most procedures requiring a laparotomy involve the organs of the alimentary canal.

Operative procedure
Laparotomy opening

1. The suction tube and tubing are connected, tested, and secured to the field.
2. The skin incision is made and carried to fascia.
3. Hemostats or ligating clips are used to control bleeding vessels. Clamped vessels are ligated with fine absorbable ligatures or silk, or they are electrocoagulated.
4. The wound edges are retracted with small retractors.
5. With tissue forceps and scalpel, the external fascia is incised.
6. With Metzenbaum scissors, the external oblique muscle is split the length of the incision. Bleeding vessels are controlled with hemostats, ligating clips, or medium or fine ligatures.
7. The external oblique muscle is retracted.
8. The internal oblique and transverse muscles are split, parallel to the fibers, up to the rectus sheath with a scalpel or scissors. These muscles are then retracted.
9. The peritoneum is exposed, grasped with smooth tissue forceps, and nicked with scalpel no. 3 and blade no. 10.
10. Sponges, laparotomy pads, and suction are used as needed. Cultures may be taken at this time.
11. The peritoneal incision is extended the length of the wound with Metzenbaum scissors.
12. The peritoneum is retracted with large Richardson retractors for exploration.
13. Once the affected organs are identified, a self-retaining retractor may be used to ensure adequate exposure.

Laparotomy closure

1. Two tissue forceps or clamps are used to approximate the peritoneal edges, and the peritoneum is closed with a continuous absorbable suture or interrupted nonab-

sorbable sutures. The internal oblique fascia is usually closed with the peritoneum. Muscle tissue is approximated and may or may not be sutured.

2. The external oblique fascia is closed with interrupted sutures, staples, or both. Retraction is necessary as the various layers are closed.

3. Fine interrupted absorbable sutures are usually employed to close the subcutaneous tissue. Retraction is provided with laparotomy pads or small retractors.

4. Skin edges are held with Adson forceps, and approximated with interrupted fine silk, nylon or other non-absorbable sutures on a cutting needle. Skin staples or clips are often used to approximate skin edges.

Esophagectomy and intrathoracic esophagogastrostomy

Esophagectomy and intrathoracic esophagogastrostomy involve the removal of diseased portions of the stomach and esophagus through a left thoracoabdominal incision in the left chest—including a resection of the seventh, eighth, or ninth rib or separation of the two appropriate ribs—and establishment of an anastomosis between the esophagus and the stomach (Fig. 11-20). These procedures are performed to remove strictures in the lower esophagus that may develop after trauma, infection, or corrosion or to remove tumors in the cardia of the stomach or in the distal esophagus.

Procedural considerations. The basic thoracotomy set (Chapter 25) and gastrointestinal set are required.

Operative procedure

1. The skin incision is carried downward midway between the vertebral border of the scapula and the spinous processes to the eighth rib and then forward along this rib to the costochondral junction. The extent of the vertical portion of the incision depends on the location of the tumor. The wound is retracted, and bleeding vessels are ligated or coagulated.

2. The chest cavity is opened, and the rib spreader is placed. Moist packs are placed, and the lung is retracted with a Deaver or Harrington retractor.

3. The mediastinal pleura is incised with long Metzenbaum scissors and long plain forceps in line with the esophagus and the lesion. The esophagus is dissected free from the aorta with dry dissectors. Suture ligatures of silk nos. 2-0 and 3-0 are used for controlling bleeding vessels.

4. The diaphragm is opened, and a series of traction sutures is attached. The stomach is mobilized by dissection of its ligamental attachment with long scissors and curved thoracic clamps.

5. The left gastric artery is clamped, cut, and doubly ligated with silk no. 2-0 and a suture ligature of silk no. 3-0.

6. The sterile field is prepared for the open method of

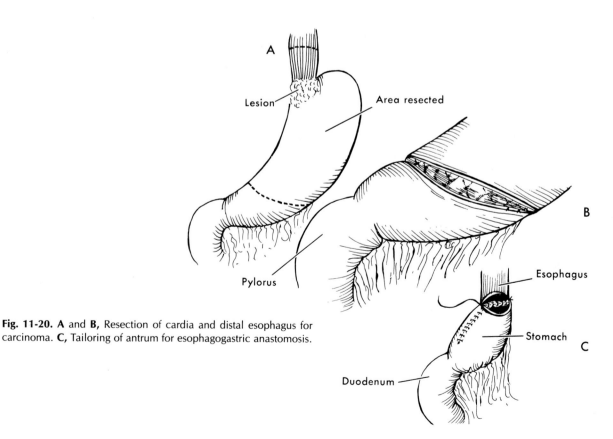

Fig. 11-20. A and **B,** Resection of cardia and distal esophagus for carcinoma. **C,** Tailoring of antrum for esophagogastric anastomosis.

anastomosis. The stomach is transected well below the lesion with the selected resection instruments. Closure of the stomach is completed with two rows of intestinal sutures of chromic no. 2-0 and sometimes with an additional row of silk no. 3-0 sutures for reinforcement. A separate circular opening is usually made in the upper portion of the stomach for anastomosis to the esophagus.

7. Two Allen clamps or a stapler type of clamp is applied above the stricture, and the freed esophagus is divided.
8. The circular opening in the stomach and the transected end of the esophagus are anastomosed. The mucosal layers are approximated. The muscular layers of the esophagus and stomach are closed by two rows of interrupted sutures.
9. A mechanical end-to-end anastomosing surgical stapling device may also be used to accomplish the gastroesophageal anastomosis.
10. The stomach is anchored to the pleura, and the edges of the diaphragm are sutured to the wall of the stomach with interrupted sutures of silk no. 3-0 or 2-0.

11. The pleura is cleansed with warm normal saline irrigation that is suctioned off. A thoracic catheter is inserted for closed drainage. The chest wall is closed as described for thoracotomy (Chapter 25).

Excision of esophageal diverticulum

Excision of an esophageal diverticulum, sometimes referred to as Zenker's diverticulum, is removal of a weakening in the wall of the esophagus that collects small amounts of food and causes a sensation of fullness in the neck. Because diverticula usually occur in the cervical portion of the esophagus, excision gives complete relief of symptoms.

Procedural considerations. A thyroid set (Chapter 16), two Pennington clamps, six Halsted curved mosquito hemostats, two 5-inch Adson forceps, and two lateral retractors are required.

Operative procedure (Fig. 11-21). An incision is made over the inner border of the sternocleidomastoid muscle and is extended from the level of the hyoid bone to a point 2 cm above the clavicle. The sac of the diverticulum is freed and ligated, and the pharyngeal muscle

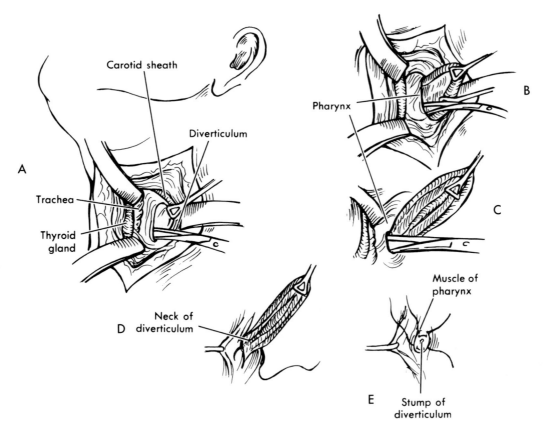

Fig. 11-21. Harrington technique for one-stage esophageal diverticulectomy. **A,** Wound is opened, thyroid is retracted medially, and carotid sheath with sternocleidomastoid muscle is retracted laterally, exposing diverticulum. **B,** Diverticulum is dissected free from surrounding structures down to neck. **C,** True neck of sac is dissected from surrounding muscles of posterior wall of pharynx. **D,** Neck of sac is ligated with chromic sutures. **E,** Stump of sac is invaginated into wall of pharynx, and opening in pharyngeal muscles is closed.

and surrounding tissues are closed. In conjunction with this procedure, an esophageal myotomy is often performed distal to the diverticulum. A myotomy seems to lessen the likelihood of recurrence.

Esophageal hiatal hernia repair/antireflux procedure

Hiatal herniorrhaphy is performed to restore the cardioesophageal junction to its correct anatomic position in the abdomen, to secure it firmly in place, and to correct gastroesophageal reflux.

A hiatal hernia is a special type of hernia in which a defect, either congenital or accidental, in the diaphragm permits a portion of the stomach to enter the thoracic cavity (Fig. 11-22).

Hiatal hernias are usually of two distinct types, paraesophageal hiatal hernias and sliding hiatal hernias. Symptoms vary from none to severe heartburn, reflux (backward flow), regurgitation, and dysphagia. When symptoms are severe enough, a repair of the hernia is done, usually through a transabdominal approach.

An antireflux procedure, which prevents reflux of gastric juices into the esophagus, is also done when the hernia is repaired. The three most frequently performed antireflux procedures are the Nissen, Hill, and Belsey Mark IV procedures.

Procedural considerations. A transthoracic approach is used in patients who previously had left upper quadrant surgery or are extremely obese, or if a Belsey Mark IV procedure is selected.

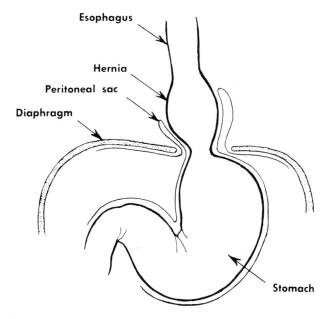

Fig. 11-22. Schematic drawing showing displacement of portion of cardia of stomach through normal hiatus into thoracic cavity in sliding hiatus hernia. (From Anderson, H.C.: Newton's geriatric nursing, ed. 5, St. Louis, 1971, The C.V. Mosby Co.)

Instrumentation is as follows:

Laparotomy set
Thoracotomy set (Chapter 25), if requested
2 Forceps, smooth, extra long
1 Semb ligature carrier
2 Crile nerve hooks
2 Schnidt thoracic forceps, long
2 Vessel clip appliers, long, with clips

Operative procedure
1. Through a transabdominal incision, the hernia is located, and a crural repair is done.
2. The fundus of the stomach is wrapped around the lower 4 to 6 cm of the esophagus and is sutured in place (Nissen fundoplication); the upper part of the lesser curvature of the stomach and the cardioesophageal junction are sutured to the median arcuate ligament (Hill procedure); or the stomach is plicated around approximately 270 degrees of esophageal circumference (Belsey Mark IV procedure).
3. Vagotomy, pyloroplasty, or both may be performed at the same time.
4. The wound is closed.

An alternative to traditional surgical repair of gastroesophageal reflux and sliding hiatal hernia is the use of a silicone prosthesis (Fig. 11-23). Through an upper abdominal vertical incision, the prosthesis is placed around the esophagus under the diaphragm and above the stomach. A radiopaque marker on the device facilitates x-ray location after surgery. Proper placement of the prosthesis allows passage of food into the stomach yet prevents the stomach from sliding into the chest cavity.

Esophagomyotomy (Heller cardiomyotomy)

Esophagomyotomy (Heller cardiomyotomy) is myotomy of the esophagogastric junction and is done to correct esophageal obstruction resulting from cardiospasm.

Procedural considerations. Selection of a transthoracic or transabdominal incision depends on the patient's general condition and other existing pathological factors. The surgeon may elect to perform a pyloroplasty to prevent reflux.

Operative procedure
1. The surgeon uses a transthoracic or a transabdominal incision.
2. After exposure of the esophagogastric junction, a Maloney dilator is inserted to distend the esophagus.
3. A scalpel with a no. 15 blade is used to make a longitudinal incision through the muscular wall of the distal esophagus and proximal stomach, leaving the mucosa intact.
4. A small portion of the fundus of the stomach may be plicated to the lateral wall of the esophagus.
5. The wound is closed.

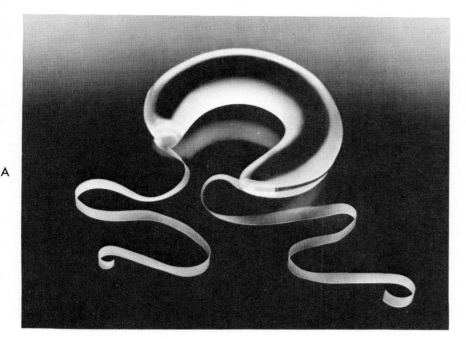

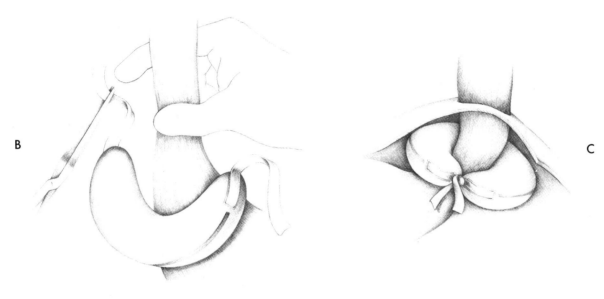

Vagotomy

Truncal vagotomy

Truncal vagotomy is the identification of the two vagal trunks on the distal esophagus and resection of a segment of each, including any additional nerve fibers running separately from the trunks. By interrupting the parasympathetic innervation, this procedure reduces the gastric acid secretion in patients with duodenal ulcers. When truncal vagotomy was initially performed alone, a high incidence of gastric stasis resulted from the loss of cholinergic innervation to the smooth muscle of the stomach; thus pyloroplasty or another gastric drainage procedure almost always accompanies truncal vagotomy. Truncal vagotomy deprives not only the stomach but also the liver, gallblad-der, bile duct, pancreas, small intestine, and half of the large intestine of the parasympathetic nerve supply. Truncal vagotomy with antrectomy or drainage procedure is the most common operation for duodenal ulcers.

Selective vagotomy

Selective vagotomy is the transection of each abdominal vagus at a point just beyond its bifurcation into the gastric and extragastric divisions. Thus the hepatic branch of the anterior vagus and the celiac branch of the posterior vagus are preserved. Selective vagotomy possesses theoretical advantages over truncal vagotomy because vagal innervation of the viscera other than the stomach is preserved. However, selective vagotomy also denervates the entire stomach, so the addition of a drainage procedure is still necessary. Selective vagotomy may cause less postvagotomy diarrhea than truncal vagotomy, but the incidence of dumping syndrome is probably the same or even higher. Both procedures are about equally effective in controlling duodenal ulcers.

Parietal cell vagotomy

Parietal cell vagotomy is the vagal denervation of only the parietal cell area of the stomach. The technique spares the main nerves of Latarjet but divides all vagal branches that terminate on the proximal two thirds of the stomach. The operation has also been called *proximal gastric vagotomy* or *highly selective vagotomy*. Because antral innervation is preserved, gastric emptying is unimpaired and a drainage procedure is unnecessary. The incidence of dumping and diarrhea following parietal cell vagotomy is much lower than after truncal or selective vagotomy.

Procedural considerations. Instrumentation is as follows:

> Basic thoracotomy set (if a thoracoabdominal incision is to be used)
> Gastrointestinal set
> 2 Blunt nerve hooks
> 2 Vessel clip appliers, 10 inches, with clips

Operative procedure

1. A midline incision is made, and the esophagus is identified and retracted with Penrose drains.
2. The vagus nerves or their branches, depending on which type of vagotomy is being done, are identified, clamped with either a ligature or a hemostatic clip, and resected.
3. The wound is closed in layers.

Pyloroplasty

Pyloroplasty is the formation of a larger passageway between the prepyloric region of the stomach and the first or second portion of the duodenum with excision of peptic ulcer, if present. A pyloroplasty may be performed for the treatment of a peptic ulcer under selected conditions but is more frequently employed to remove cicatricial bands in the pyloric ring, thus relieving spasm and permitting rapid emptying of the stomach. In adults a vagotomy is usually performed in conjunction with a pyloroplasty.

Procedural considerations. A gastrointestinal instrument set is required.

Operative procedure

1. The abdominal cavity is opened through a midline incision.
2. An incision is made through the stomach and the duodenum (Fig. 11-24).
3. The pyloroplasty is closed with silk or chromic intestinal sutures.
4. The abdominal wound is closed in layers, and a dressing is applied.

Gastrostomy

In a gastrostomy, through a high left rectus abdominal or midline incision, a temporary or permanent channel is established from the gastric lumen to the skin. This lumen

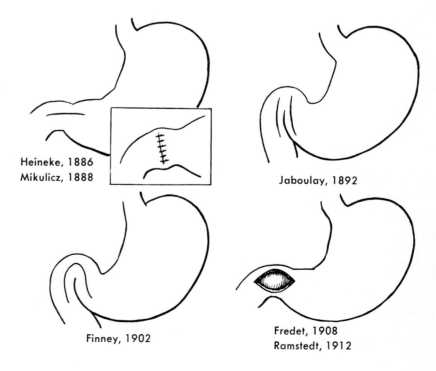

Fig. 11-24. Different types of pyloroplastic procedures: Heineke-Mikulicz longitudinal incision with transverse closure to enlarge lumen; Jaboulay anastomosis of two longitudinal incisions; Finney closure of inverted U incision; Ramstedt longitudinal incision down to muscle layer, with mucosa pouching out to level even with adjoining serosa. (After Waugh and Hood; from Moyer, C.A., and others: Surgery: principles and practices, ed. 3, Philadelphia, 1965, J.B. Lippincott Co.)

Heineke, 1886
Mikulicz, 1888

Jaboulay, 1892

Finney, 1902

Fredet, 1908
Ramstedt, 1912

permits liquid feeding or retrograde dilation of an esophageal stricture. Gastrostomy is a palliative procedure performed to prevent malnutrition and starvation, which may be caused by a lesion or stricture situated in the esophagus or in the cardia of the stomach. A temporary procedure is done when the obstruction is capable of being corrected.

Procedural considerations. For an extensive lesion of the esophagus, some surgeons advise a permanent gastrostomy in which a stomach flap is formed around the catheter. The catheter is brought out of the abdomen through a separate stab wound. When the incisional area is avoided, tissue healing is improved, and the incidence of postoperative wound-healing problems decreases.

Operative procedure (Fig. 11-25)

1. The abdominal cavity is opened through an upper midline or transverse incision.
2. The stomach is held with Allis or Babcock forceps, and a purse-string suture is placed at the proposed site for the catheter.
3. A scalpel with a no. 15 blade is used to make an incision within the purse-string suture, and the contents of the stomach are suctioned.
4. Bleeding points are controlled. The catheter is inserted, and the purse-string suture is tied around it.
5. The catheter is brought through a stab wound in the area of the left rectus muscle.

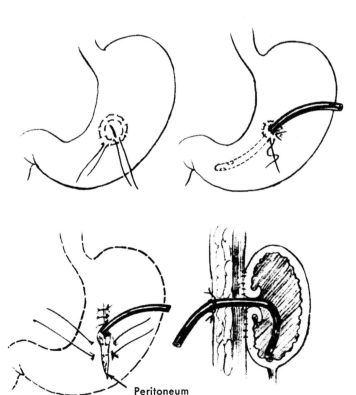

Fig. 11-25. Stamm technique of simple gastrostomy. (From Wilder, J.R.: Atlas of general surgery, ed. 2, St. Louis, 1964, The C.V. Mosby Co.)

6. The stomach may be sutured to the peritoneal layer, and the abdominal wound is closed in layers.

Gastrotomy

Gastrotomy is the opening of the anterior stomach wall through a left paramedian abdominal incision and exploration of the interior. This procedure is usually done to explore for upper gastrointestinal tract bleeding, perform a tissue biopsy, or remove a gastric lesion or foreign body.

Procedural considerations. A gastrointestinal instrument set is required.

Operative procedure

1. A longitudinal incision is made through the anterior wall of the stomach, halfway between the curvatures.
2. The stomach wall is grasped and elevated by Allis or Babcock forceps.
3. An incision is made, and a suction tube is inserted into the stomach to remove gastric contents.
4. The lesion or foreign body is removed, and the stomach wall and abdominal wall are closed.

Closure of perforated gastric or duodenal ulcer

Closure of a perforation in the stomach or duodenum is performed through a high right rectus or midline abdominal incision.

Procedural considerations. A perforated gastric or duodenal ulcer is treated as a surgical emergency, and the operation is performed as soon as the diagnosis is made. The patient's blood should be typed and cross-matched so an adequate supply will be available for emergency replacement. A gastric lavage is not performed, but continuous suction is used. A gastrointestinal set is required.

Operative procedure

1. Through a right rectus or midline abdominal incision, the perforation is located.
2. Suction is used to remove exudate in the peritoneal cavity.
3. The perforation is closed with a purse-string suture by inverting the raw edges and suturing a piece of omentum over the closure.
4. The abdomen is irrigated with warm saline, which may contain a broad-spectrum antibiotic.
5. The abdominal wound is closed in layers, and a dressing is applied.

Gastrojejunostomy

Gastrojejunostomy is the establishment of a permanent communication, either between the proximal jejunum and the anterior wall of the stomach or between the proximal jejunum and the posterior wall of the stomach, without removing a segment of the gastrointestinal tract. It is accomplished through a midline or a paramedian abdominal incision. Gastrojejunostomy may be performed to treat a benign obstruction at the pyloric end of the stomach or an inoperable lesion of the pylorus when a partial gastrectomy would not be feasible. It also provides a large opening without sphincter obstruction.

Procedural considerations. A gastrointestinal instrument set is required.

Operative procedure
1. Through an upper midline or paramedian abdominal incision, exploration of the peritoneal cavity is completed, as described for routine laparotomy. The pathological condition is confirmed.
2. Warm, moist packs are placed, and a loop of proximal jejunum is grasped with Babcock forceps and freed from the mesentery. It is approximated to either the anterior or posterior stomach wall several centimeters from the greater curvature. Silk no. 2-0 traction sutures are placed through the serosal layers at each end of the selected portion of the jejunum and stomach. Gastroenterostomy clamps may be placed before insertion of the posterior interrupted silk no. 3-0 or 2-0 serosal sutures.
3. The field is draped for open anastomosis. The jejunum and stomach are opened. Bleeding points are clamped with mosquito hemostats and ligated with chromic no. 3-0 sutures. The inner posterior row of sutures is placed, using continuous chromic no. 2-0 or 3-0 with atraumatic intestinal needles, and continued for the first anterior row. The anastomosis is completed with anterior serosal sutures of silk no. 3-0 or 2-0. Traction sutures are removed. Interrupted silk no. 4-0 sutures may be used for reinforcement.
4. The contaminated instruments are discarded. The ab-

dominal wound is closed in layers and a dressing applied.

Partial gastrectomy
Billroth I

A Billroth I gastrectomy is the resection of the diseased portion of the stomach through a right paramedian or midline abdominal incision and the establishment of an anastomosis between the stomach and duodenum. It is performed to remove a benign or malignant lesion located in the pyloric, or upper, half of the stomach. One of several techniques may be followed to establish gastrointestinal continuity, including the Schoemaker, the von Haberer-Finney, and other modifications of the Billroth I procedure (Fig. 11-26).

Procedural considerations. A gastrointestinal instrument set is required.

Operative procedure
1. The abdominal wall is incised, and the peritoneal cavity opened and explored. Bleeding vessels are clamped and ligated or coagulated.
2. The abdominal wound is retracted, and the surrounding organs are protected with warm, moist packs.
3. The gastrocolic omentum is freed from the colon mesentery to prevent injury to the middle colic artery. With hemostats and Metzenbaum scissors, the right and left gastroepiploic arteries and veins are clamped, divided, and ligated with silk no. 2-0 and suture ligatures of silk nos. 2-0 and 3-0, thereby freeing the greater curvature of the stomach. The gastrohepatic vessels are

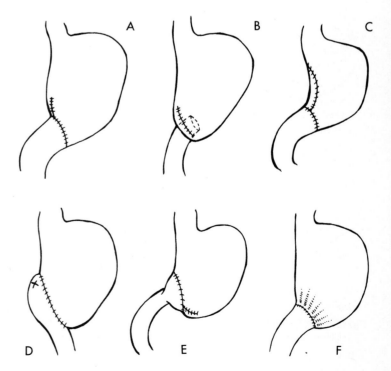

Fig. 11-26. Diagrams illustrating resections of stomach with anastomosis of stomach and duodenum (gastroduodenal anastomosis). All are modifications of Billroth I technique, in which stomach is brought to duodenum. **A,** Billroth I: after pylorus is removed, lesser curvature is partially closed, and duodenum is sutured to open end of stomach at its lower margin. **B,** Kocher: distal end of stomach is closed, and duodenum is brought up to posterior margin of closed stomach. **C,** Schoemaker: lesser curvature of stomach is sutured and brought down to same size as duodenum, and end-to-end anastomosis is done. **D,** von Haberer-Finney: side of duodenum is brought up to end of stomach so that entire end of stomach is open for direct anastomosis. **E,** Horsley: lesser curvature end of stomach is used to suture to duodenum and closes greater curvature end. **F,** von Haberer: modification of operation shown in **D.** Stomach is, so to speak, narrowed or puckered so that it fits end of duodenum. Modification of this is done by some as follows: duodenum is split longitudinally, and its ends are flared open so that opening is large enough to fit open end of stomach.

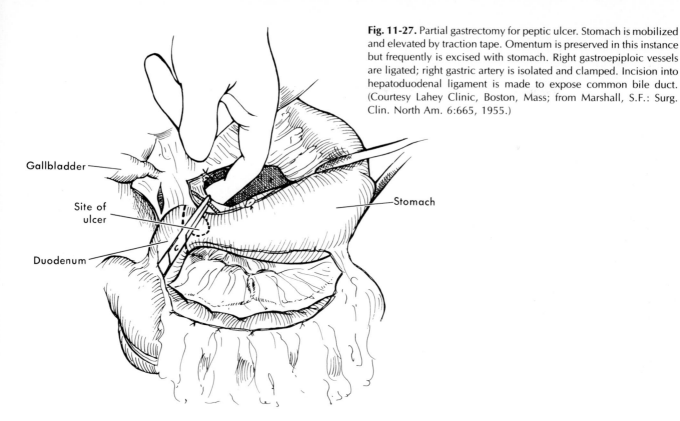

Fig. 11-27. Partial gastrectomy for peptic ulcer. Stomach is mobilized and elevated by traction tape. Omentum is preserved in this instance but frequently is excised with stomach. Right gastroepiploic vessels are ligated; right gastric artery is isolated and clamped. Incision into hepatoduodenal ligament is made to expose common bile duct. (Courtesy Lahey Clinic, Boston, Mass; from Marshall, S.F.: Surg. Clin. North Am. 6:665, 1955.)

Gallbladder

Site of ulcer

Duodenum

Stomach

also clamped, divided, and ligated to free completely the diseased portion of the stomach (Fig. 11-27).

4. The operative field is prepared for open anastomosis. Two Allen intestinal anastomosis clamps or other suitable clamps are placed on the upper portion of the duodenum just distal to the pylorus. Division is accomplished by scalpel or electrosurgery, as preferred. Additional moist packs are placed for protection, and two sets of anastomosis clamps are placed across the stomach. Division is completed by the surgeon's preferred method.

5. At the lower margin the opened stomach is approximated to the duodenum by a series of interrupted sutures placed in the serosa layers. No. 3-0 silk on atraumatic intestinal needles is used. Suture ends are held with hemostats, and the intestinal clamps are removed. Stumps of the stomach and duodenum are cleansed with moist sponges, and bleeding vessels are ligated with fine suture or coagulated. During the anastomosis the involved segments may be held with rubbershod clamps.

6. The excess of the lesser curvature in the stomach is closed on completion of the anastomosis (Fig. 11-27). Soiled instruments are discarded.

7. Routine laparotomy closure is completed.

Billroth II

A Billroth II gastrectomy is a resection of the distal portion of the stomach through an abdominal incision and the establishment of an anastomosis between the stomach and jejunum. It is performed to remove a benign or malignant lesion in the stomach or duodenum. This technique and modifications may be selected because the volume of acidic gastric juice will be reduced, and the anastomosis can be made along the greater curvature or at any point along the stump of the stomach. Modifications of the Billroth II procedure include the Pólya and Hofmeister operations, which also establish gastrointestinal continuity through bypassing the duodenum.

After surgery, duodenal and jejunal secretions empty into the remaining gastric pouch. The stomach empties more rapidly because of the larger opening, and a limited amount of gastric juice remains.

Procedural considerations. A gastrointestinal instrument set is required.

Operative procedure

1. Through an abdominal incision, the distal portion of the stomach is resected, and an anastomosis is established between the stomach and jejunum (Fig. 11-28).

2. The abdomen is closed.

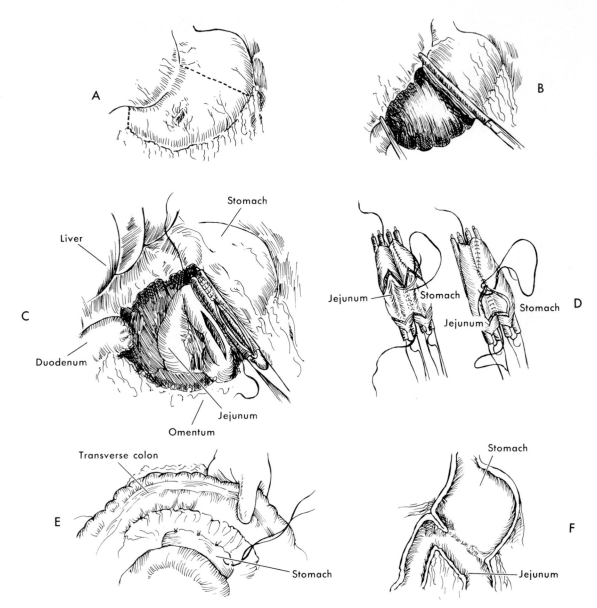

Fig. 11-28. Subtotal gastric resection. **A,** Diagram of stomach showing lesion. *Dotted lines,* Section of stomach to be removed. **B,** Portion of stomach has been clamped and resected. Duodenal stump is now prepared for inversion. **C,** Duodenal invagination is completed. Upper third of stomach is closed. Jejunum is brought through mesocolon. **D,** Anastomosis is established between jejunal loop and lower two thirds of incomplete stomach opening. **E,** Gastrojejunal anastomosis is completed. Stomach is now fixed to edges of slit in mesocolon. **F,** Cross-section demonstrating completed operation, showing anastomosis between stomach and jejunum. (From Manual of operative procedures, Somerville, N.J., 1977, Ethicon, Inc.)

Total gastrectomy

Total gastrectomy is the complete removal of the stomach and establishment of an anastomosis between the jejunum and the esophagus. It may include an enteroenterostomy, if indicated. Total gastrectomy is done as a potentially curative or palliative procedure to remove a malignant lesion of the stomach and metastases in the adjacent lymph nodes.

Procedural considerations. The incision may be bilateral subcostal, long transrectus, long midline, or thoracoabdominal. A basic thoracotomy set (if a thoracoabdominal incision is to be used; Chapter 25) and a gastrointestinal set are necessary. Also, two long blunt nerve hooks and two 10-inch needle holders are used.

Operative procedure

1. The abdomen is opened, and the wound edges are

protected and retracted, as previously described.

2. Careful and complete exploration for the extent of metastasis is carried out.

3. The omentum is freed from the colon, using sharp dissection; vessels are ligated with silk no. 2-0.

4. The splenic vessels are ligated and transfixed with silk nos. 2-0 and 3-0 at the tail of the pancreas; the spleen is left attached to the omentum.

5. The duodenum is mobilized, intestinal clamps are applied, and the operative field is protected for transection and closure of the distal duodenum.

6. The right gastric artery is ligated and transfixed with silk nos. 2-0 and 3-0, and the gastrohepatic omentum is separated from the liver. Following ligation of the left gastric artery, the mobilized stomach, spleen, omentum, and lesser and greater curvature ligamentous attachments are delivered into the wound.

7. Division of the coronary ligament of the left lobe of the liver permits exposure of the diaphragmatic peritoneum over the esophagogastric junction. The liver is protected by moist packs, and gentle retraction is maintained with a Harrington, Deaver, or malleable retractor.

8. A flap of peritoneum is freed from the diaphragm, and branches of the vagus nerves are divided, as in Fig. 11-29.

9. A loop of jejunum is selected and delivered antecolic to the esophagogastric junction for anastomosis. With the specimen for traction, the posterior layer of interrupted silk no. 3-0 sutures is inserted.

10. As the jejunum and the esophagus are incised, bleeding is controlled by mosquito hemostats and ligatures of chromic no. 3-0. The posterior layer is reinforced with chromic no. 3-0, intestinal, interrupted sutures.

11. Division of the esophagus is completed, and the entire specimen is removed. Interrupted, chromic no. 4-0 sutures also are used to approximate the mucosal anterior wall of the anastomosis. A second layer of sutures, silk or chromic no. 3-0, is placed anteriorly in the seromuscular and muscular coat of the intestine. A flap of the peritoneum is attached to the jejunum

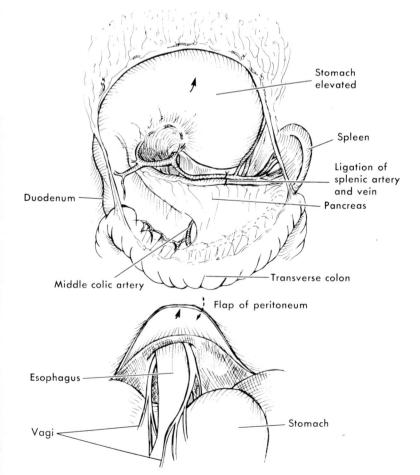

Fig. 11-29. Total gastrectomy. *Top,* Method of detaching greater omentum from transverse colon so that entire lesser peritoneal cavity is exposed. Spleen left attached to omentum and stomach and gastrohepatic omentum are removed in one block. *Bottom,* Flap of peritoneum cut from front surface of esophagus and reflected over diaphragm is diagrammatically shown. This flap will be used to suture to jejunum, reinforce anterior suture line, and take up weight of jejunum anastomosed to esophagus. Vagi also are shown diagrammatically. It is necessary to sever nerves before free delivery of esophagus can be obtained.

Stomach elevated

Spleen

Ligation of splenic artery and vein

Pancreas

Duodenum

Middle colic artery

Transverse colon

Flap of peritoneum

Esophagus

Vagi

Stomach

with interrupted no. 3-0 silk sutures to relieve traction on the anastomosis. A lateral jejunojejunal anastomosis is completed to permit irritating bile and pancreatic fluids to bypass the anastomosis line, thereby preventing esophageal regurgitation (Fig. 11-30). An alternative method of establishing continuity is a combination of a Roux-en-Y jejunojejunostomy and a jejunoesophagostomy (Fig. 11-31).

12. The abdominal wound is closed in layers. If retention sutures are used, they must be placed extraperitoneally because of the absence of omentum to protect the small bowel.

Operation for Meckel's diverticulum

A Meckel's diverticulum is removed to prevent inflammation and obstruction from intussusception of the diverticulum. Meckel's diverticulum consists of an unobliterated congenital duct that is attached to the distal ileum (Fig. 11-32). The diverticulum may contain gastric mucosa, which may ulcerate, perforate, or bleed.

Procedural considerations. A gastrointestinal instrument set is required.

Operative procedure

1. The abdomen is opened, and the diverticulum is identified.

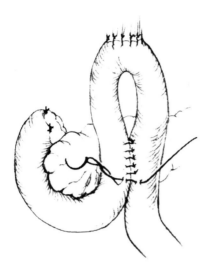

Fig. 11-30. Jejunojejunostomy performed to prevent regurgitation esophagitis. (From Wilder, J.R.: Atlas of general surgery, ed. 2, St. Louis, 1964, The C.V. Mosby Co.)

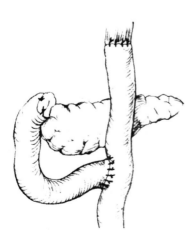

Fig. 11-31. Completed jejunoesophageal anastomosis with Roux-en-Y jejunojejunostomy. (From Wilder, J.R.: Atlas of general surgery, ed. 2, St. Louis, 1964, The C.V. Mosby Co.)

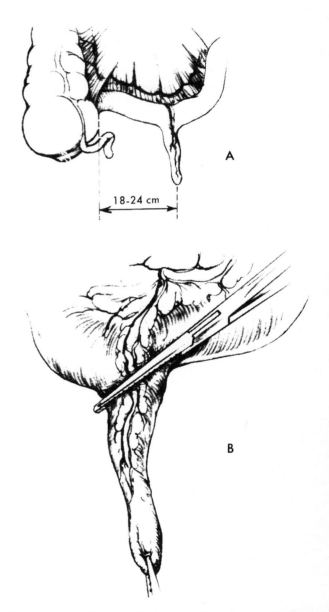

Fig. 11-32. A, Diagrammatic representation of usual location of Meckel's diverticulum. **B,** Ochsner forceps placed across base of diverticulum at its juncture with ileum. (From Wilder, J.R.: Atlas of general surgery, ed. 2, St. Louis, 1964, The C.V. Mosby Co.)

2. If the diverticulum is long and narrow with a narrow base, the procedure is similar to that of an appendectomy.
3. If the base is broad, the loop of bowel containing the diverticulum is isolated from the mesentery, and a limited small bowel resection is performed.
4. An anastomosis of the divided ends is completed with an inner continuous layer of chromic no. 3-0 and an interrupted outer layer of silk no. 4-0 sutures.
5. The wound is closed as in a laparotomy.

Appendectomy

Appendectomy is the severance and removal of the appendix from its attachment to the cecum through a right lower quadrant muscle-splitting (McBurney) incision (Fig. 11-33). This procedure is performed to remove an acutely inflamed appendix, thereby controlling the spread of infection and reducing the danger of peritonitis. A normal appendix is sometimes removed when the abdomen is opened for another procedure.

Procedural considerations. Instrumentation is the same as for a laparotomy.

Operative procedure
1. A right lower quadrant muscle-splitting incision usually is made.
2. Muscles are retracted with Richardson or Parker retractors to expose the peritoneum.
3. The peritoneum is grasped with tissue forceps or

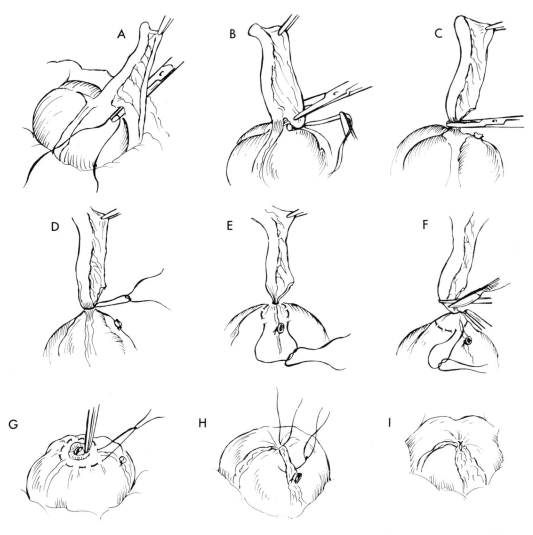

Fig. 11-33. Appendectomy. **A,** Cecum is walled off, and ligature is passed through mesoappendix. **B,** Mesoappendix is ligated and cut. Multiple clamps may be used. **C,** Mesoappendix is separated, and clamp is placed at base of appendix. **D,** Crushing clamp is removed, and groove left in base is now ligated. **E,** Purse-string suture at base. Appendix is ready for amputation. **F,** Clamp is placed distal to ligature. Appendix is amputated with knife. **G,** Appendiceal stump is inverted as purse-string suture is tied. **H,** Suturing of ileocecal fat pad or mesentery protects stump. **I,** Operation is completed. Alternative method omits purse-string suture. (From Manual of operative procedures, Somerville, N.J., 1977, Ethicon, Inc.)

Allis forceps, and a small incision is made with a scalpel and a no. 15 blade. A culture may be taken. The incision is completed with Metzenbaum scissors.

4. The mesoappendix is grasped near the tip with a Babcock forceps or a hemostat for gentle traction. The mesoappendix is dissected from the appendiceal wall by hemostats and ligated with silk no. 3-0. If a suture ligature is required, chromic no. 2-0 on an atraumatic gastrointestinal needle is preferred.

5A. The appendix is elevated as a purse-string suture of chromic no. 2-0 is placed in the cecal wall at the appendiceal base.

   a. The base of the appendix is crushed with a straight hemostat, a chromic no. 3-0 tie is placed over the crushed area, and a hemostat is placed above the ligature.

   b. A basin is provided for the specimen and discarded instruments, which have come in contact with gastrointestinal mucosa.

   c. Protective gauze sponges are placed over the cecum around the base of the appendix. The appendix is amputated between the clamp and chromic suture with a scalpel.

   d. The appendiceal stump may be inverted into the lumen of the cecum as the purse-string suture is tightened and tied by means of a fine straight hemostat and a small sponge on a holder. Soiled instruments are discarded in the basin.

   e. The abdomen is closed in the usual manner.

5B. If the appendix has ruptured, the peritoneum is drained. The drain may be inserted down to the appendiceal bed to allow continuous drainage. Deeper layers are closed, leaving the subcutaneous tissue and skin open. The wound may then be packed open with moist, fine-mesh gauze, and healing by secondary intention is permitted. This packing method may be used in any case in which bowel contamination or abscess formation is present. It allows clean healing and prevents pocketing of pus.

Resection of the small intestine

Resection of the small intestine involves excision of the diseased intestine through an abdominal incision and frequently includes some type of bowel reanastomosis. It is performed to remove certain tumors, a gangrenous portion of the intestine caused by strangulation from bands of adhesions, a herniation of the intestine, or a volvulus.

Procedural considerations. A gastrointestinal instrument set is required.

Operative procedure

1. The abdominal wall is incised and retracted; the peritoneal cavity is explored and protected with moist, warm packs.

2. The clamps are placed above and below the diseased segment of the bowel and mesentery. The involved area is removed with an electrosurgical blade or a scalpel.

3. The continuity of the gastrointestinal tract is established by an end-to-end, an end-to-side, or a side-to-side anastomosis.

4. The wound is closed and dressed.

An alternative approach to a traditional suture anastomosis is the use of a mechanical stapling device (Fig. 11-34). The device allows the surgeon to perform an end-to-end, end-to-side, or side-to-side anastomosis. An enterotomy is made close to the anastomosis site. The stapler is inserted, and the distal bowel is secured between the anvil and the head of the stapler (Fig. 11-35). The anvil is then inserted into the proximal loop of bowel and secured to the center rod. The gap is closed, and the stapler fired. The stapler is extracted through the enterotomy. The integrity of the anastomosis is verified, and the enterotomy is closed with sutures.

Ileostomy

Ileostomy is the formation of a temporary or permanent opening into the ileum. This procedure is generally done when an extensive lesion is present either to reduce activity in the colon by means of diversions or when all the large bowel has been resected.

Procedural considerations. A gastrointestinal instrument set and an ostomy appliance for the stoma are required.

Operative procedure

1. Through a midline incision, the peritoneal cavity is explored and the pathologic condition determined.

2. The ileum is mobilized with Metzenbaum scissors and hemostatic clamps. The mesentery is clamped, divided, and ligated with silk no. 3-0 sutures at the proposed site, usually about 15 cm from the ileocecal junction.

3. Two intestinal clamps are placed on the bowel, and the ileum is divided with a scalpel between the two clamps.

4. The distal end of the ileum is closed with chromic no. 2-0 on a general closure needle.

5. The proximal end is brought out to the skin through an opening on the right side and is held in place by clamps, making sure that the ileum is not overstretched or its blood supply compromised. The mesentery of the ileum is sutured to the parietal wall to eliminate a potential internal hernia. The abdomen is then closed.

6. The stoma is sutured to the skin after the ileum is everted to form a protective cover over the exposed ileal serosa.

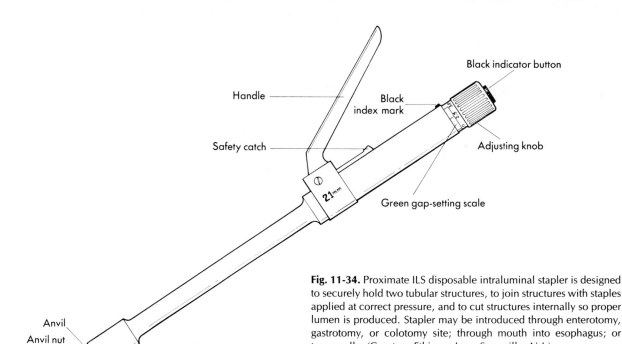

Handle

Safety catch

Black index mark

Black indicator button

Adjusting knob

Green gap-setting scale

21mm

Anvil
Anvil nut

Head

Fig. 11-34. Proximate ILS disposable intraluminal stapler is designed to securely hold two tubular structures, to join structures with staples applied at correct pressure, and to cut structures internally so proper lumen is produced. Stapler may be introduced through enterotomy, gastrotomy, or colotomy site; through mouth into esophagus; or transanally. (Courtesy Ethicon, Inc., Somerille, N.J.)

7. A disposable ostomy appliance is placed over the stoma to collect small bowel contents.

An alternative to a conventional ileostomy for selected patients is the Kock pouch, or continent ileostomy. The internal pouch is constructed of small intestine with an outlet to the skin. When it is functioning properly, no stool spontaneously exits from the stoma. A catheter is inserted into the stoma three or four times daily to evacuate the contents. This procedure eliminates the need for an external appliance.

Colostomy

Colostomy is mobilization of a loop of colon through a right rectus incision to expose the transverse colon. A left rectus incision can also be made to expose the descending sigmoid colon. The layers of the wound beneath or around the colostomy are subsequently closed. A colostomy is performed to treat an obstruction in the sigmoid colon resulting from a malignant lesion. Another possible indication for this procedure is advanced inflammation or trauma that has caused distention or obstruction of the proximal portion of the colon. A temporary colostomy is often done to decompress the bowel or to give the bowel a rest.

Procedural considerations. A gastrointestinal set and stoma appliances as determined by the surgeon are required. These items may include a glass rod, rubber tubing, or a loop ostomy bridge.

Operative procedure
First-stage loop colostomy
1. The abdomen is opened, and the wound edges are protected and retracted. The peritoneal cavity is opened and walled off with moist laparotomy packs, and appropriate retractors are inserted.
2. A small opening is made in the mesentery near the bowel with curved hemostats and Metzenbaum scissors. A piece of tubing is passed around the colon, and the two ends are held with a hemostat to maintain gentle traction.
3. The loop of colon is brought out through an incision made on the left side of the midline.
4. The abdomen is closed.
5. A loop ostomy bridge is used to keep the loop of colon in proper position.
6. The loop of intestine is dressed with petrolatum gauze.

Second-stage loop colostomy. After 48 hours, the loop of colon is completely severed by an electrosurgical blade. By this time, if there is no tension, healing has advanced sufficiently to allow feces onto the wound. This procedure is simple and painless and is usually performed in the patient's room or in a treatment room.

Transverse colostomy
1. A short incision, vertical or preferably transverse, is made to reach the transverse colon.
2. A loop of transverse colon, freed of omentum, is withdrawn (Fig. 11-36). A loop ostomy bridge is

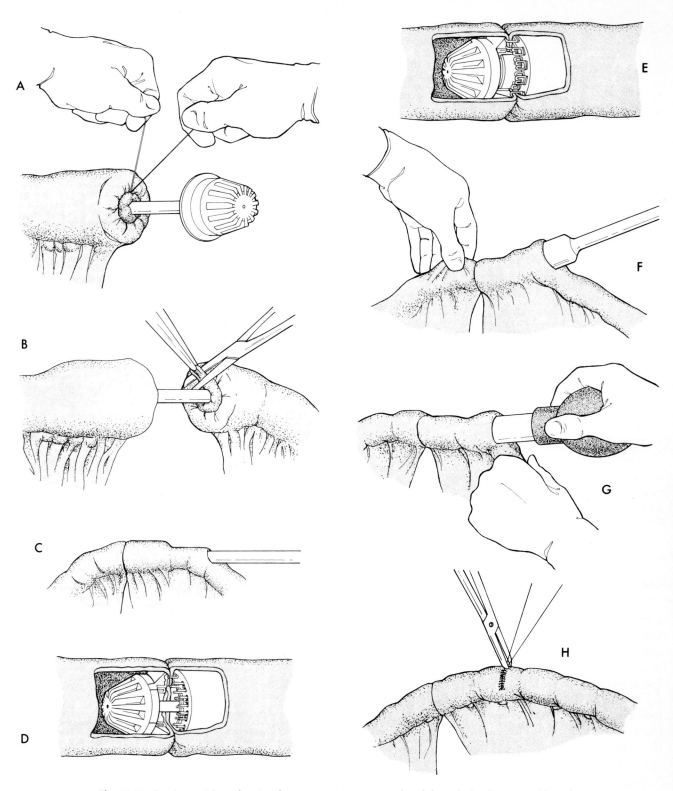

Fig. 11-35. Proximate ILS stapler. **A,** After purse-string suture is placed through distal portion of bowel, stapler is introduced through enterotomy. Distal bowel is secured between anvil and head of stapler. **B,** Anvil is then inserted into proximal loop of bowel and secured to center rod. **C,** Gap is closed, and stapler is fired. **D** and **E,** Staples are driven into tissue and formed against anvil, while knife blade advances to cut uniform stoma through tissue pulled around center rod. **F,** Stapler is extracted through enterotomy. **G,** Integrity of anastomosis is verified. **H,** Enterotomy is closed with sutures. (Courtesy Ethicon, Inc., Somerville, N.J.)

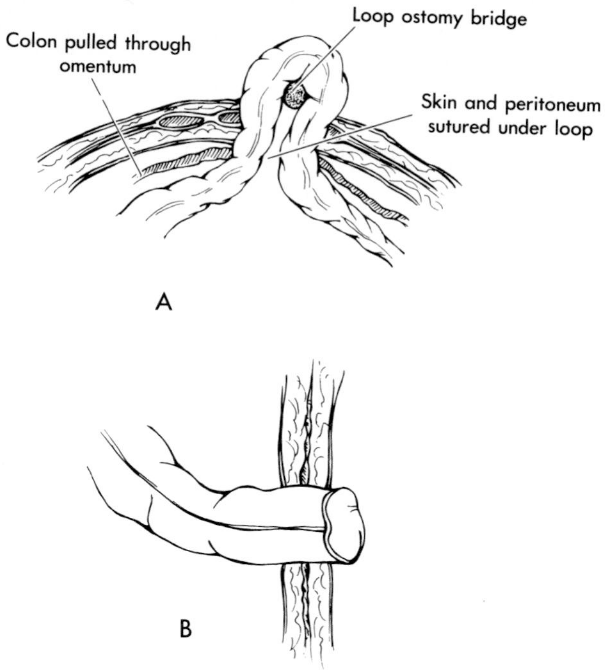

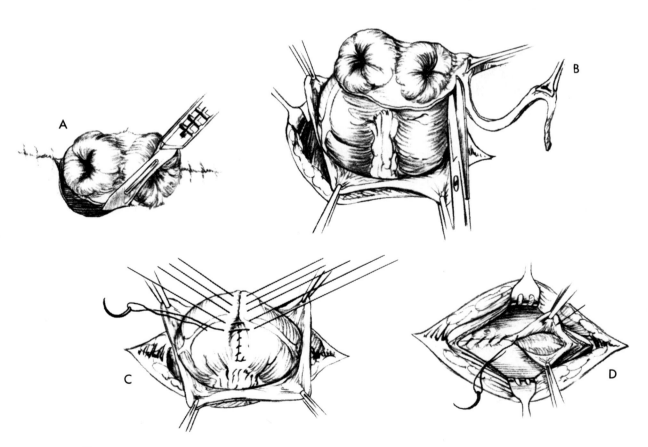

Colon pulled through omentum

Loop ostomy bridge

Skin and peritoneum sutured under loop

A

B

Fig. 11-36. A, Loop colostomy. **B,** Terminal colostomy.

passed through an avascular area of the mesocolon, preventing the loop from returning to the peritoneal cavity. A mushroom catheter, which is held in place with a purse-string suture, brings about immediate decompression.

3. The bowel is opened 24 to 36 hours later.
4. The bridge may be removed in about 10 days.

Closure of a colostomy

Closure of a colostomy involves the reestablishment of internal intestinal continuity and repair of the abdominal wall (Fig. 11-37).

Procedural considerations. When the loop has been completely divided, a closed or open anastomosis may be performed.

A gastrointestinal instrument set is required.

Operative procedure

1. A circumferential incision is made around the colostomy to free the skin margin. Moist packs, a scalpel with a no. 10 blade, Metzenbaum scissors, and Crile hemostats are used as the layers of the abdominal wall are identified and dissected free.

A

B

C

D

Fig. 11-37. Closure of colostomy. **A,** Skin incised close to colostomy bud. **B,** Scar tissue excised. **C,** Bowel closed transversely with interrupted sutures of fine silk and replaced in abdomen. **D,** Wound closed completely with gut or wire sutures. (From Wilder, J.R.: Atlas of general surgery, ed. 2, St. Louis, 1964, The C.V. Mosby Co.)

2. An end-to-end anastomosis is completed in two layers, the inner with chromic no. 3-0 and the outer with silk no. 3-0 on an intestinal needle, using interrupted sutures. This anastomosis may be completed with a surgical stapling device.

3. The abdominal wound is closed in layers. A drain may be inserted, if indicated. A dressing is applied. The surgeon may elect to leave the subcutaneous tissue and skin open. The wound would be packed and permitted to heal by secondary intention.

Right hemicolectomy and ileocolostomy

Right hemicolectomy and ileocolostomy involve the resection of the right half of the colon—including a portion of the transverse colon, the ascending colon, and the cecum—and a segment of the terminal ileum and mesentery. An end-to-end (Fig. 11-38), side-to-side, or end-to-side anastomosis is done between the transverse colon and the ileum. A right hemicolectomy and ileocolostomy are performed to remove a malignant lesion of the right colon and in some cases to remove inflammatory lesions involving the ileum, cecum, or ascending colon.

Procedural considerations. When a side-to-side anastomosis is carried out, the transected stumps of the ileum and the transverse colon are closed before the anastomosis is done. It is completed between the side portions of the ileum and the transverse colon. When an end-to-end anastomosis is performed, the layers of the transected stumps of the ileum and the transverse colon are sutured together.

A gastrointestinal instrument set is required.

Operative procedure

1. The abdomen is opened, and the peritoneal cavity is retracted and packed with warm, moist sponges.

2. The mesentery of the transverse colon and the terminal ileum are incised at the points where the resection is to be done. Moist packs, Metzenbaum scissors, hemostats, and silk no. 3-0 ligatures are used.

3. The lateral peritoneal fold along the lateral side of the right colon is incised, and the right colon is mobilized medially. Metzenbaum scissors, hemostats, and sponges on holders are used. The ureter and duodenum are carefully identified.

4. The same procedure is carried out on the terminal ileum.

5. The mesenteric vessels are clamped and ligated with silk no. 2-0 ligatures.

6. The operative field is prepared for anastomosis. Resection clamps are placed on the transverse colon and ileum. Division is completed with a scalpel, and the specimen is removed.

7. An end-to-end anastomosis is completed between the severed ends of the terminal ileum and the transverse colon.

8. Instruments and supplies that have come in contact with bowel mucosa are discarded.

9. The mesentery and posterior peritoneum are closed with interrupted sutures of silk no. 3-0.

10. The abdominal wound is closed. Retention sutures and a drain may be used. A dressing is applied.

Transverse colectomy

Transverse colectomy is excision of the transverse colon through an upper midline or transverse incision. Bowel integrity is reestablished by an end-to-end anastomosis. A transverse colectomy is performed for malignant lesions of the transverse colon. A more radical procedure may be required when the lesion has perforated the greater curvature of the stomach. If the entire lesion is resectable, a partial gastrectomy may also have to be performed.

Procedural considerations. A gastrointestinal instrument set is required.

Operative procedure

1. The abdomen is opened, and the peritoneal cavity is explored to determine the extent of the pathological area.

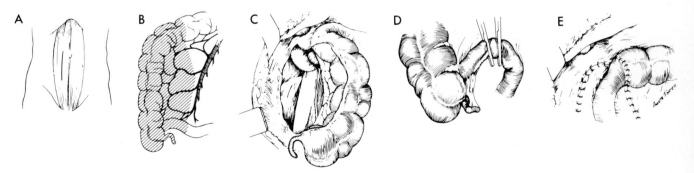

Fig. 11-38. Right hemicolectomy and ileocolostomy. **A,** Right paramedian incision. **B,** Specimen to be resected. **C,** Mobilization of right colon medially. **D,** Clamps on distal portion of ileum. **E,** End-to-end anastomosis of ileum and transverse colon. (Redrawn from Manual of operative procedures, Somerville, N.J., 1977, Ethicon, Inc.)

2. Moist packs are used to wall off surrounding structures to expose the hepatic and splenic flexures.
3. The colon is mobilized by incising the lateral peritoneum on either side and transecting the transverse mesocolon. Hemostats, Metzenbaum scissors, and silk no. 3-0 ligatures are used.
4. The operative field is prepared for resection. Two Allen intestinal resection clamps are applied. Transection is completed with a scalpel, and an end-to-end anastomosis is completed, as previously described.
5. Contaminated articles are discarded. Approximation of mesentery and lateral peritoneum is completed with silk no. 3-0 sutures.
6. The abdominal wound is closed. Retention sutures may be used. The wound is dressed.

Anterior resection of the sigmoid colon and rectosigmoidostomy

Anterior resection of the sigmoid colon and rectosigmoidostomy involve the removal of the lower sigmoid and rectosigmoid portions of the rectum. This is usually done through a laparotomy incision, and an end-to-end anastomosis is completed. This operation is selected to treat lesions in the lower portion of the sigmoid and rectum that permit excision with a wide margin of safety and still retain sufficient tissues with adequate blood supply for a viable rectosigmoid end-to-end anastomosis.

Procedural considerations. A gastrointestinal instrument set is required.

Operative procedure

1. The abdomen is entered through a laparotomy incision. The peritoneal cavity is explored for metastasis and resectability of the lesion.
2. Before the colon is mobilized, the tumor-bearing segment is isolated by ligatures to the lymphovenous drainage (that is, provided these structures are accessible).
3. A loop of sigmoid colon is elevated as the small intestines are walled off with moist packs; retractors are placed.
4. The peritoneum on the left side of the colon is incised with a long scalpel, scissors, hemostats, and sponge forceps. Traction sutures of silk no. 2-0 may be used as the peritoneum is reflected. Bleeding vessels are ligated with silk no. 2-0 or 3-0 ligatures.
5. The pelvic peritoneum is exposed and dissected free to form the left side of the reconstructed pelvic floor. Long dissecting instruments are used. Vessels are ligated with 24-inch silk ligatures. Extreme care must be exercised throughout to protect the ureters from injury.
6. The sigmoid colon is turned toward the left, and the procedure that was described in step 4 is carried out on the right side of the pelvis. The two incisions are then curved and joined in front of the rectum.
7. The rectum is freed anteriorly and posteriorly from the adjacent structures.
8. The sigmoid colon is clamped with resection clamps after mobilization of the proximal portion. As the sigmoid colon is divided distally to the clamp, the transected rectal edges are grasped with Allis or Ochsner forceps, and the rectal opening is exposed. The diseased portion is removed, and the soiled instruments discarded.
9. Continuity is established by an end-to-end anastomosis of the proximal colon and the rectum.
10. The pelvic floor is reperitonealized, and drains may be placed.
11. The abdominal wound is closed in the routine manner, and a dressing is applied.

An alternative to traditional surgical anastomosis is the use of a stapling device. The device can be used intraabdominally through a colotomy approach or transanally (Fig. 11-39). Use of a stapling device may obviate the need for an abdominoperineal resection because a very low anastomosis can be performed.

Abdominoperineal resection

Adbominoperineal resection is the mobilization and division of a diseased segment of the lower bowel through a midline incision, extending from several centimeters above the umbilicus to the pubis. The proximal end of bowel is exteriorized through a separate stab wound as a colostomy. The distal end is pushed into the hollow of the sacrum and removed through the perineal route.

An abdominoperineal resection is performed for malignant lesions and inflammatory diseases of the lower sigmoid colon, rectum, and anus.

Procedural considerations. The choice of patient position depends on the surgeon. Some surgeons prefer to start with the patient in the supine position and move the patient to the lithotomy position for the perineal portion of the operation. Others initially place the patient in a modified lithotomy position; thus surgery may be performed simultaneously by two teams, which may require two scrub nurses with two different setups. A Foley catheter is inserted after induction.

A gastrointestinal set and an ostomy appliance are required for the abdominal portion of the procedure. A perineal set is used for the perineal portion of the procedure; it consists of basic laparotomy instruments plus the following:

2 Volkmann rake retractors, four-pronged, sharp
2 Hill retractors
1 Anal retractor
1 Rectal speculum
4 Pennington forceps, 6 inches

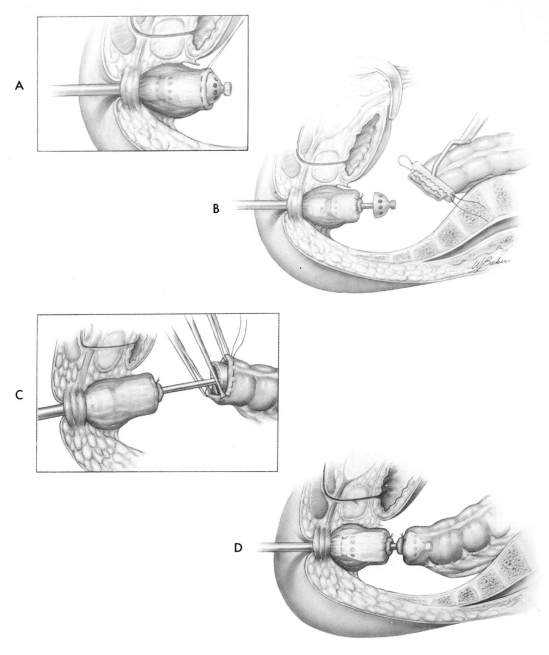

Fig. 11-39. EEA stapling device, used to perform low anterior anastomosis. **A,** Stapler is introduced into anus. **B,** EEA is advanced to level of purse-string instrument. **C,** Anvil portion of EEA is inserted into proximal colon. **D,** Purse-string suture secures bowel to instrument. (Reprinted with the permission of U.S. Surgical Corporation © USSC 1974, 1975, 1980. All rights reserved.)

Operative procedure

1. A midline incision is made.
2. After thorough exploration of the abdominal cavity, the surgeon determines the extent and operability of the lesion.
3. If a resection is to be done, the surgeon retracts the sigmoid colon to the right side. The peritoneum on the left of the mesocolon is divided.

4. The incision into the peritoneum is made opposite the main branches of the inferior mesenteric vessels and extended into the pelvis and around anterior to the rectum.
5. The pelvic peritoneum is mobilized by blunt dissection to form the left side of the new pelvic floor and permit early visualization of the left ureter.
6. The peritoneum is incised on the right side until the

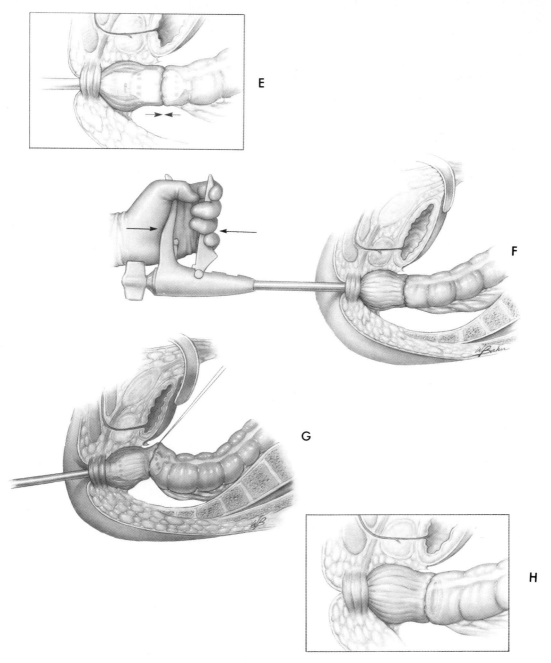

Fig. 11-39, cont'd. E and **F,** EEA is closed and fired. Circular double-staggered row of staples joins bowel; simultaneously, circular blade in instrument cuts stoma. **G,** Instrument is gently removed. **H,** Resulting anastomosis is illustrated with bowel wall transparent to depict reconstruction.

incision connects with that made on the left. The right ureter is identified and protected.

7. The blood supply of the portion of intestine to be removed is isolated and ligated.

8. Care must be taken not to damage the left colic artery, which will supply the blood to the colostomy.

9. The mesentery is tied to permit greater exposure in the operative field.

10. The surgeon frees the rectum, usually as low as the sacrococcygeal junction. Care is taken to avoid injury to the presacral nerves, which may result in sexual and bladder dysfunction.

11. After the bowel is freed, the surgeon prepares the permanent colostomy.

12. The omentum is brought down into the pelvis, and the abdominal wound is closed. Many surgeons repair the pelvic peritoneum.

13. The patient is placed in the lithotomy position.

14. The surgical team changes gowns and gloves. New instrumentation is used for this portion of the procedure.
15. The perineal area is prepped and the patient redraped.
16. To prevent contamination, the anus is often closed with a purse-string suture. An incision is made around the anus.
17. The anus is grasped with Allis or Ochsner forceps and tipped upward to enable its attachment to the coccyx to be severed more readily.
18. The levator ani muscle is exposed; while the finger of the surgeon is held beneath it, it is divided as far from the rectum as possible.
19. All bleeding points are clamped and tied.
20. The Foley catheter allows the surgeon to get as close to the bladder as possible without damaging it.
21. After the anococcygeal raphe is divided, the surgeon's hand is thrust up into the hollow sacrum to free the rectum by blunt dissection, grasp the upper end of the distal fragment, and bring the sigmoid colon into the wound.
22. Finally, the distal fragment with its tumor, the attached mesentery of the lower sigmoid colon, and all structures of the hollow of the sacrum are removed, along with the rectum and anus.
23. When all bleeding is controlled, the incision is closed.

Ileoanal endorectal pull-through

Ileoanal endorectal pull-through is the removal of the entire colon and the proximal two thirds of the rectum. It includes a mucosectomy of the remaining distal rectum, creation of a pouch from the distal small bowel, and anastomosis of the pouch to the anus.

An ileoanal endorectal pull-through is performed to relieve the symptoms of ulcerative colitis and familial polyposis (diarrhea, pain, cramping, bleeding, and others) and to prevent colon malignancies. This procedure is an anal sphincter–saving operation that is done to avoid the need for a traditional ileostomy.

Procedural considerations. The patient is usually placed in a modified lithotomy position. Some surgeons prefer to perform the mucosectomy with the patient in a jackknife position and then place the patient in a modified lithotomy position for the remainder of the procedure.

A gastrointestinal set and a perineal set plus rectal instrumentation are required. Separate instrument sets are used for the rectal and abdominal approaches. Additional draping and gowning supplies should be available because redraping and regowning occur after the mucosectomy and after the ileoanal anastomosis. An epinephrine solution should be available for injection into the submucosal tissue, proximal to the anus, to separate the mucosa from the muscularis layer. An ileostomy appliance is applied immediately postoperatively.

Operative procedure

1. The anal canal is dilated and inspected through an anoscope. Starting at the dentate line, the anal-rectal junction, the epinephrine solution is injected circumferentially, separating the mucosa from the muscularis layer. The mucosectomy is then performed by making a circular incision at the dentate line, cutting only through mucosa. The mucosa is peeled off the muscularis tissue for a distance of 2 to 8 cm and resected. When all bleeding is controlled, the patient is repositioned, if necessary, for the abdominal approach.
2. A midline incision is made, and the abdomen explored. The entire large intestine from the ileocecal junction through the upper two thirds of the rectum is freed and immobilized. All vessels are ligated. The terminal ileum is separated from the cecum using a mechanical cutting and stapling device (GIA). The mesocolon is ligated using suture ligatures or a ligating, dividing, and stapling instrument. The rectum is resected down to the level of the mucosectomy. The colon and resected portion of the rectum are removed en bloc.
3. The pouch is created. Most surgeons use either the J pouch or the S pouch. The J pouch is created at the terminal ileum by folding two adjacent loops of small bowel, approximately 12 to 15 cm each, parallel with each other and anastomosing them using a GIA. An opening is made at the bottom of the pouch, and the pouch is pulled through the rectal stump. The bottom of the pouch is anastomosed to the anus with interrupted absorbable sutures (Fig. 11-40). An S pouch is created by aligning the distal ileum in an S configuration with each of the three limbs approximately 12 cm in length. The most distal 2 cm of the ileum is not incorporated into the pouch but is preserved for the anastomosis to the anus. The three limbs are manually incised and anastomosed to create a pouch. Mucosal tissue is approximated with absorbable suture, and nonabsorbable suture is used for the serosal layer. The preserved distal end of the ileum and the pouch are pulled through the rectal stump and anastomosed to the anus (Fig. 11-41). This completes the anal portion of the procedure.
4. The scrubbed team changes gowns and gloves and completes the abdominal procedure by creating a loop ileostomy on a previously designated site through the abdominal wall (Fig. 11-42). The abdominal incision is closed in the usual manner.
5. Approximately 2 to 6 months are required after the initial operation for adequate healing of the ileoanal anastomosis to occur and to ensure the absence of post-

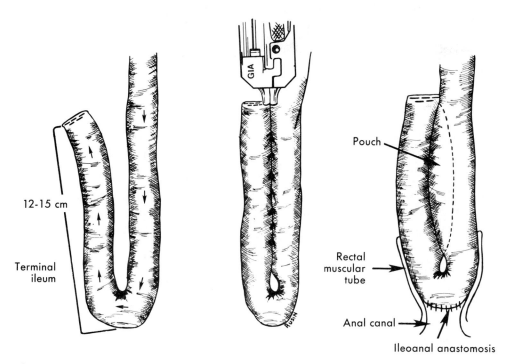

Fig. 11-40. J pouch for ileoanal endorectal pull-through. **A,** The J pouch is created at terminal ileum by folding two adjacent loops of small bowel, approximately 12 to 15 cm each, parallel with each other. **B,** Two loops are anastomosed using mechanical cutting and stapling device (GIA). **C,** Opening is made at bottom of pouch, and pouch is pulled through rectal stump. Bottom of pouch is anastomosed to anus. (Courtesy J.R. Rusin, Lutheran Medical Center, Wheat Ridge, Colo.)

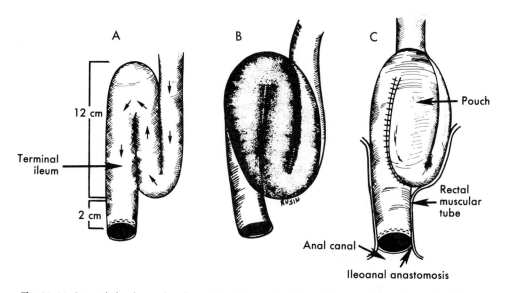

Fig. 11-41. S pouch for ileoanal endorectal pull-through. **A,** Pouch is created by aligning distal ileum in S configuration with each limb (three in total) approximately 12 cm in length. **B,** Three limbs are incised and anastomosed to create pouch. **C,** Distal end of ileum and pouch are pulled through rectal stump and anastomosed to anus. (Courtesy J.R. Rusin, Lutheran Medical Center, Wheat Ridge, Colo.)

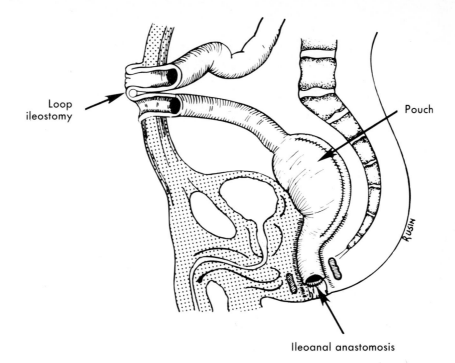

Fig. 11-42. Sagittal view demonstrating anatomical relationship of loop ileostomy, S pouch, and ileoanal anastomosis. (Courtesy J.R. Rusin, Lutheran Medical Center, Wheat Ridge, Colo.)

surgical complications. When the patient's status is determined to be satisfactory, a second procedure is performed to restore bowel continuity and close the loop ileostomy.

Hemorrhoidectomy

Hemorrhoidectomy is the excision and ligation of dilated veins in the anal region to relieve discomfort and control bleeding. The frequency of hemorrhoidectomies performed in the operating room has decreased due to "banding" procedures now being done on an outpatient basis.

Procedural considerations. Preoperative anal dilation aids in exposing the vessels and contributes to the patient's comfort in the immediate postoperative period. Many surgeons prefer to precede the operation with a sigmoidoscopy. Spinal, caudal, or local anesthesia may be used.

A minor set (see Chapter 13) plus two 8-inch tissue forceps without teeth and the following rectal instruments are required:

2 Hill retractors	1 Set of rectal dilators
1 Anoscope	Buie pile forceps
1 Rectal speculum	1 Crypt hook

The CO_2 laser may also be used for vaporization and coagulation of hemorrhoidal tissue.

Operative procedure

1. The patient is usually placed in the lithotomy or jack-knife position.

2. The anal canal is dilated and inspected through an anoscope.
3. Four Allis forceps are applied several centimeters from the anal margin to expose the anus.
4. The base of the hemorrhoid and tissue are grasped with Allis forceps and held.
5. An intestinal suture of chromic no. 2-0 is placed and tied at the proximal end of the hemorrhoid, and a Buie pile forceps is applied across the base and above the proposed incision line. Excision is completed with a scalpel. Suturing is completed by loosely placed continuous sutures over the Buie forceps. The suture is tightened as the forceps is removed, and the suture ends are tied.
6. Traction may be maintained as hemostatic forceps are applied and dissection is completed segmentally. Suture ligatures of chromic no. 2-0 are used as each hemostat is removed.
7. Remaining hemorrhoids are excised in a similar manner.
8. Petrolatum gauze packing is placed in the anal canal. A dressing and a T binder are applied.

Excision of anal fissure

Excision of an anal fissure involves the dilation of the anal sphincter and removal of the lesion. Anal fissures are benign lesions of the anal wall.

Procedural considerations. A minor set and rectal instruments, as listed previously, are required.

Operative procedure

1. The patient is placed in the lithotomy or jackknife position.
2. Dilation of the anal sphincter is completed.
3. The fissure is excised, and bleeders are ligated or electrocoagulated.
4. A lateral incision is made, and the internal sphincter is incised. The mucosa is approximated over the incision.
5. A drain or packing is inserted.
6. A dressing is applied.

Excision of pilonidal cyst and sinus

Excision of a pilonidal cyst and sinus is removal of the cyst with sinus tracts from the intergluteal fold on the posterior surface of the lower sacrum. A pilonidal cyst and sinus, which may have a congenital origin, rarely becomes symptomatic until the individual reaches adulthood. Inflammatory reaction varies from a mild, irritating, draining sinus tract to an acute abscess with secondary recurrences. Treatment consists of drainage in the acute stage and total surgical excision during remission.

The excision of the cyst and sinus tracts must be complete to prevent recurrence. The defect resulting from recurrences may become too large for primary closure. In this case the wound is left open to heal by granulation.

Procedural considerations. A minor set and rectal instruments, as listed previously, are required.

Operative procedure

1. The patient is placed in a jackknife
2. The sinus tracts are identified with probes.
3. An elliptical incision is made down to the fascia. A curette is used to remove gelatinous tissue. Excision of cyst and sinus tracts is completed.
4. Bleeding is controlled.
5A. If the wound is to be left open, it is packed, and a pressure dressing is applied.
5B. If the wound is closed, 2-0 silk sutures are used for stay sutures on the deeper tissue, and fine silk is used on the skin.

BIBLIOGRAPHY

Aimino, P.A.: Perioperative nursing documentation: developing the record and using care plans, AORN J. 46:1, 1987.

Barrett, N.: Ileal loop and body image, AORN J. *36*:712, 1982.

Benjamin, S.B., and others: Complications of the Angelchik antireflux prosthesis, Ann. Intern. Med. 199(4):570, 1984.

Beyers, M., and Dudas, S.: The clinical practice of medical-surgical nursing, ed. 2, Boston, 1984, Little, Brown & Co.

Brunner, L.S., and Suddarth, D.S.: Textbook of medical-surgical nursing, ed. 6, Philadelphia, 1988, J.B. Lippincott Co.

Cello, J.P., and others: Endoscopic neodymium-YAG laser palliation of nonresectable esophageal malignancy, Ann. Intern. Med. 102:610, 1985.

Cohen, D.J., and Starling, J.R.: Surgery for reflux esophagitis: experience with the antireflux prosthesis, AORN J. 43:858, 1986.

Cooperman, M.: Complications of appendectomy, Surg. Clin. North Am. 63:1233, 1983.

Duranceau, A.C.: Symposium on esophageal surgery, Surg. Clin. North Am. 63:4, 1984.

Fleischer, D.: Endoscopic laser therapy for gastrointestinal diseases, Arch. Intern. Med. 144:1225, 1984.

Fleischer, D.: Endoscopic laser therapy for gastrointestinal neoplasms, Surg. Clin. North Am. 64:947, 1984.

Fromm, D.: Gastrointestinal surgery, New York, 1985, Churchill Livingstone.

Gear, M.W., Gillison, E.W., and Dowling, B.L.: Randomized prospective trial of the Angelchik anti-reflux prosthesis, Br. J. Surg 71(9):681, 1984.

Gerber, A., Apt, M.K., and Craig, P.H.: The Kock continent ileostomy, Surg. Gynecol. Obstet. 156:345, 1983.

Given, B.A., and Simmons, S.J.: Gastroenterology in clinical nursing, ed. 4, St. Louis, 1984, The C.V. Mosby Co.

Hrabovsky, E.E., Walne, A.L., and Carrier, J.M.: Changing management in familial polyposis: role of ileoanal endorectal pull-through, Am. J. Surg 147:130, 1984.

Johnson, L.: Vertical banded gastroplasty, Nurs. Times 80(37):24, 1984.

Kleinbeck, S.V.M.: Developing nursing diagnoses for a perioperative care plan: a classroom research project, AORN J. 49:6, 1989.

Leonardi, H.K., and Ellis, F.H., Jr.: Complications of the Nissen fundoplication, Surg. Clin. North Am. 63:1155, 1983.

Myer, S.A.: Overview of inflammatory bowel disease, Nurs. Clin. North Am. 19:3, 1984.

Nyhus, L.M., and Wastell, C.: Surgery of the stomach and duodenum, ed. 4, Boston, 1986, Little, Brown & Co.

Patras, A.Z., and Brozenec, S.: Gastrointestinal assessment, AORN J. 40:276, 1984.

Patras, A.Z., Paice, J.A., and Lanigan, K.: Managing GI bleeding: it takes a two-tract mind, Nursing 84 14(7):26, 1984.

Proximate ILS Disposable Stapler System: reference manual, Somerville, N.J., 1981, Ethicon, Inc.

Ravitch, M.M., and Steichen, F.M.: Symposium on surgical stapling techniques, Surg. Clin. North Am., vol. 64, no. 3, 1984.

Sabiston, D.C., Jr., editor: Davis-Christopher textbook of surgery: the biological basis of modern surgical practice, ed. 13, Philadelphia, 1986, W.B. Saunders Co.

Schoetz, D.D., Jr.: Complications of anorectal operations, Surg. Clin. North Am. 63:1249, 1983.

Schwartz, S., and others: Principles of surgery, ed. 4, New York, 1983, McGraw-Hill Book Co.

Shaw, L.M.: Treating GI reflux with a prosthesis, AORN J. 35:1303, 1982.

Simmons, C.: Using the nursing process in treating inflammatory bowel disease, Nurs. Clin. North Am. 19:11, 1984.

Skellenger, M.E., and Jordan, P.H., Jr.: Complications of vagotomy and pyloroplasty, Surg. Clin. North Am. 63:1167, 1983.

Stapling techniques in general surgery, ed. 3, Norwalk, Conn., 1988, United States Surgical Corp.

Sweet, K.: Hiatal hernia: what to guard against most in postop patients, Nursing 83 13(12):28, 1983.

Thibodeau, G.A.: Anthony's textbook of anatomy and physiology, ed. 13, St. Louis, 1990, The C.V. Mosby Co.

Wilpizeski, M.D.: Helping the osteomate return to normal life, Nursing 81 11(3):62, 1981.

Wilson, C.: The diagnostic work-up for the patient with inflammatory bowel disease, Nurs. Clin. North Am. 19:51, 1984.

Wong, W.D., Rothenberger, D.A., and Goldberg, S.M.: Ileoanal pouch procedures, Curr. Probl. Surg. 22(3):3, 1985.

Wound closure manual: reference manual, Somerville, N.J., 1985, Ethicon, Inc.

Zollinger, R.M., and Zollinger, R.M., Jr.: Atlas of surgical operations, ed. 5, New York, 1983, MacMillan, Inc.

12 Surgery of the liver, biliary tract, pancreas, and spleen

LYNDA R. PETTY

Diseases of the liver, biliary tract, pancreas, and spleen have a great influence on the wellness of the patient. Because they are highly vascular and control many of the metabolic and immune functions of the body, pathology in one or more of these organs requires urgent intervention. Surgical interventions relating to the liver, biliary tract, pancreas, or spleen may be indicated for tumor, infection, cystic anomalies, congenital anomalies, metabolic diseases, or trauma.

Approximately 30% of all abdominal injuries involve the liver. Next to the spleen, the liver is the most commonly injured viscus in blunt trauma, and it is the organ most frequently injured by penetrating wounds of the abdomen (McDermott, 1989).

In the past decade, surgeries of the liver and biliary tract have become more advanced as research and new technology have permitted more complete diagnosis of pathology involving this complex organ and portal system. Resection of the liver for carcinomas has achieved a recognized role for cure or substantial palliation with safety and low morbidity. As of 1987, the operative mortality rate for patients undergoing right hepatic resection was estimated to be less than 5% in the United States (McDermott, 1989).

Cholecystectomy is an operation commonly performed in most hospital operating rooms. Approximately 20 million people in the United States have gallstones, and nearly 300,000 operations are performed each year for this disease and its complications (Way and Pellegrini, 1987).

Laparoscopic laser cholecystectomy is a sophisticated technical procedure performed with increasing frequency. It offers the advantages of reduced trauma to tissues as well as a significant reduction in the length of postoperative recovery.

New diagnostic technology and the intraoperative use of ultrasound, biliary endoscopy, and radiography have enabled surgeons to better treat diseases of the biliary tract.

End-stage liver disease and insulin-deficient diabetes are now surgically treatable. Recent advances in liver transplantation, pancreas transplantation, and the treatment of liver and spleen injuries have resulted in improved survival of patients with diseases of these organs.

SURGICAL ANATOMY

The *liver* is in the right upper quadrant of the abdominal cavity, beneath the dome of the diaphragm and directly above the stomach, duodenum, and hepatic flexure of the colon. The external covering, known as *Glisson's capsule,* is composed of dense connective tissue. The peritoneum extends over the entire surface of the liver, except at the point of posterior attachment to the diaphragm. The arterial blood supply is maintained by the hepatic artery, and venous blood from the stomach, intestines, spleen, and pancreas is carried to the liver by the *portal vein* and its branches (Fig. 12-1). The hepatic venous system returns blood to the heart by way of the inferior vena cava.

Bile, manufactured by the liver cells, is secreted into the fine biliary radicles and in turn flows into the large ducts. It ultimately leaves the liver through the right and left hepatic ducts. These ducts join immediately after leaving the liver to form one common hepatic duct that merges with the cystic duct from the gallbladder to form the common bile duct (Fig. 12-2). The common bile duct opens into the duodenum in an area called the *ampulla* or *papilla of Vater,* located about 7.5 cm below the pyloric opening from the stomach.

Bile contains bile salts, which facilitate digestion and absorption, and various waste products. The liver is essential in the metabolism of carbohydrates, proteins, and fats. It metabolizes nutrients into glycogen stores for regulation of blood glucose levels and energy sources for the brain and body functions.

The liver plays several important roles in the blood-clotting mechanism. It is the organ that synthesizes plasma proteins, excluding gamma globulins but including prothrombin and fibrinogen. Vitamin K, a cofactor to the synthesis of prothrombin, is absorbed by the metabolism of fats in the intestinal tract as a result of bile formation by the liver. Patients with liver disease may have alterations in their blood coagulation abilities.

The liver also synthesizes lipoproteins and cholesterol. Cholesterol is an essential component of the blood plasma. It serves as a precursor for bile salts, steroid hormones, plasma membranes, and other specialized molecules. A

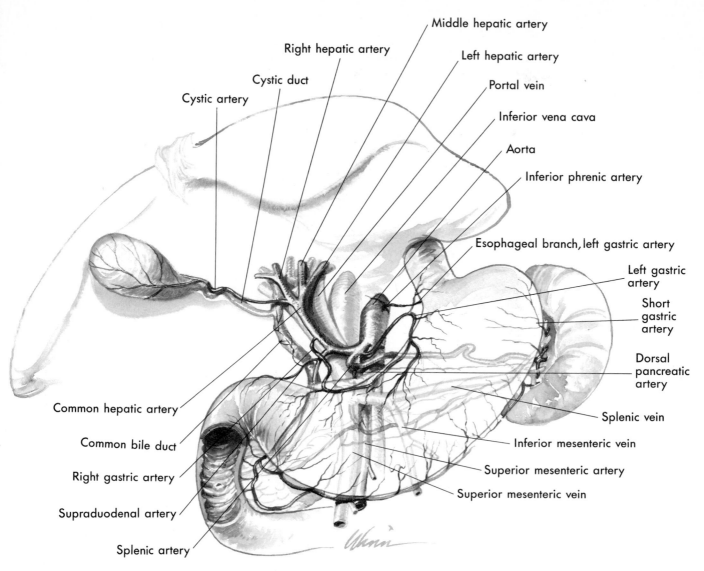

Cystic artery

Cystic duct

Right hepatic artery

Middle hepatic artery

Left hepatic artery

Portal vein

Inferior vena cava

Aorta

Inferior phrenic artery

Esophageal branch, left gastric artery

Left gastric artery

Short gastric artery

Dorsal pancreatic artery

Splenic vein

Inferior mesenteric vein

Superior mesenteric artery

Superior mesenteric vein

Common hepatic artery

Common bile duct

Right gastric artery

Supraduodenal artery

Splenic artery

Fig. 12-1. Illustration of the intricate relationships of the arterial and venous blood supply of the liver, gall bladder, pancreas, spleen, and the biliary ductal system. (From Davis, J.H., and others: Clinical surgery, vol. 2, St. Louis, 1987, The C.V. Mosby Co.)

diet high in cholesterol reduces the amount that must be synthesized by the liver. When diet is deficient in cholesterol, the liver increases synthesis to maintain the levels necessary for the production of the vital chemical molecules.

The liver also serves in the metabolic alteration of foreign molecules or biotransformation of chemicals. The microsomal enzyme system (MES) plays a major role in the body's response to foreign chemicals such as pollutants, drugs, and alcohol. Patients with liver disease may have alterations in their response to chemical substances. This consideration is most important in the induction and management of general anesthesia for patients with liver disorders.

The *gallbladder*, which lies in a sulcus on the under-

surface of the right lobe of the liver, terminates in the cystic duct (Fig. 12-3). This ductal system provides a channel for the flow of bile to the gallbladder, where it becomes highly concentrated during the storage period. As food, especially fats, is ingested, cholecystokinin is released by the duodenal cells when food enters the small intestine. The musculature of the gallbladder contracts, forcing bile into the cystic duct and through the common duct. As the *sphincter of Oddi* in the ampulla of Vater relaxes, bile pours forth, flowing into the duodenum to aid in digestion by emulsification of fats. The gallbladder receives its blood supply from the cystic artery, a branch of the hepatic artery.

The *pancreas* (Fig. 12-3) is a fixed structure lying transversely behind the stomach in the upper abdomen. The

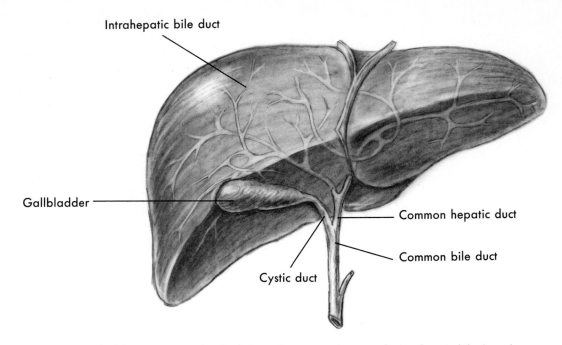

Fig. 12-2. The biliary system can be divided into three anatomic areas: the intrahepatic bile duct, the extrahepatic bile duct (common hepatic and common bile ducts), and the gallbladder and cystic duct. (From Davis, J.H., and others: Clinical surgery, vol. 2, St. Louis, 1987, The C.V. Mosby Co.)

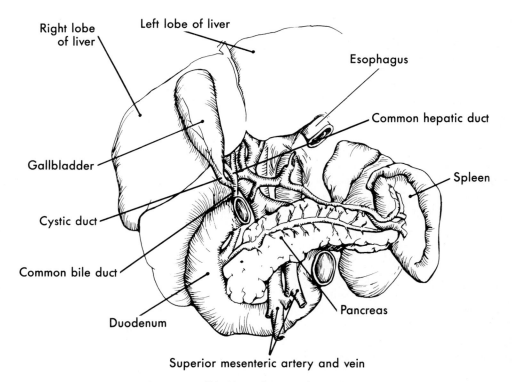

Fig. 12-3. Gallbladder and surrounding anatomy.

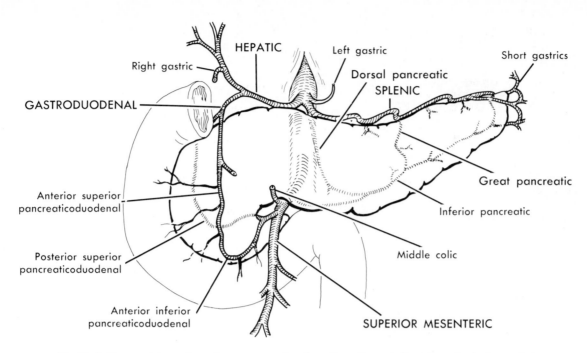

Fig. 12-4. The arterial supply to the pancreas arises from the celiac axis (hepatic and splenic arteries) and the superior mesenteric artery. The blood supply to the head of the gland is via the pancreatico-duodenal (anterior and posterior) arcades, which arise from the gastroduodenal artery (superior) and superior mesenteric arteries (inferior). (From Cooperman, A.M., and Hoerr, S.O., editors: Surgery of the pancreas: a text and atlas, St. Louis, 1978, The C.V. Mosby Co.)

head of the pancreas is fixed to the curve of the duodenum. Blood is supplied to the pancreas and the duodenum via the celiac axis and the superior mesenteric artery (Figs. 12-4 and 12-5). The body of the pancreas lies across the vertebrae and over the superior mesenteric artery and vein. The tail of the pancreas extends to the hilum of the spleen. The pancreatic secretions, containing digestive enzymes, are collected in the pancreatic duct, or duct of Wirsung, which unites with the common bile duct to enter the duodenum about 7.5 cm below the pylorus. The ampulla of Vater is formed by the dilated junction of the two ducts at the point of entry.

The pancreas also contains groups of cells, called *islets* or *islands of Langerhans*, that secrete hormones into the blood capillaries instead of into the duct. These hormones are insulin and glucagon, and both are involved in carbohydrate metabolism.

The *spleen* (Fig. 12-6) is in the upper left abdominal cavity, with full protection provided by the tenth, eleventh, and twelfth ribs; the lateral surface is directly beneath the dome of the diaphragm. The anterior medial surface is in proximity to the cardiac end of the stomach and the splenic flexure of the colon. The spleen is covered with peritoneum that forms supporting ligaments. The arterial blood supply is furnished by the splenic artery, a branch of the celiac axis. The splenic vein drains into the *portal system.*

The spleen has many functions. Among them are the

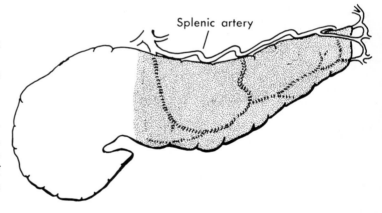

Fig. 12-5. The major arterial supply to the body and tail of the pancreas is derived from branches of the splenic artery. (From Cooperman, A.M., and Hoerr, S.O., editors: Surgery of the pancreas: a text and atlas, St. Louis, 1978, The C.V. Mosby Co.)

defense of the body by phagocytosis of microorganisms, formation of nongranular leukocytes and plasma cells, and phagocytosis of damaged red blood cells. It also acts as a blood reservoir.

PERIOPERATIVE NURSING CONSIDERATIONS
Assessment/nursing diagnosis

The patient with hepatobiliary disease may have extreme jaundice, urticaria, petechiae, lethargy, and irrita-

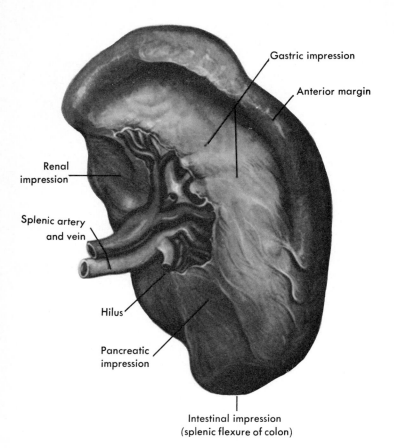

Gastric impression

Anterior margin

Renal impression

Splenic artery and vein

Hilus

Pancreatic impression

Intestinal impression
(splenic flexure of colon)

Fig. 12-6. Spleen, medial aspect. Arrangement of vessels at hilum is highly variable. (From Anthony, C.P., and Thibodeau, G.A.: Textbook of anatomy and physiology, ed. 11, St. Louis, 1983, The C.V. Mosby Co.)

Table 12-1. Laboratory tests for evaluating liver function

Function and test	Normal value
Fat metabolism	
Serum total cholesterol and cholesterol esters	140-220 mg/100 ml blood
Serum phospholipids	150-250 mg/100 ml blood
Protein metabolism	
Total serum protein	6-8 g/100 ml
Albumin	3.4-5 g/100 ml
Protein electrophoresis	
Immunoglobulins	
Blood urea nitrogen (BUN)	10-20 mg/100 ml
Serum prothrombin time (PT)	12-15 sec
Serum partial prothrombin time (PTT)	68-82 sec
Blood ammonia level	7 g/100 ml
Bilirubin metabolism	
Total bilirubin	0.1-1 mg/100 ml
Urine bilirubin	Normally not found
Urine bilinogen	0.2-1.2 units
Fecal urobilinogen	90-280 mg/day
Serum enzymes	
SGOT/AST	Up to 60 units/liter
SGPT/ALT	Up to 40 units/liter
LDH	Up to 220 units/liter
GGT	5-85 units/liter
Alkaline phosphotase	Varies
Antigens and antibodies of hepatitis	Normally not present

Table 12-2. Laboratory tests for evaluating pancreatic disease

Test	Normal value
Amylase	80-150 Somogyi units
Urine amylase	2-50 Wohlgemuth units/ml
24-hr urine amylase	6-30 Wohlgemuth units/ml
Lipase	0-1.5 units
Calcium	4.5-5.75 mEq/L (9.0-11.5 mg/100 ml)
Total serum, proteins	6-8 g/100 ml
Serum glucose	90-120 mg/100 ml

bility. Depending upon the extent of the disease, the patient may have increased bleeding and coagulation times and a decreased platelet count, thus predisposing the patient to bruising easily.

A thorough nursing history is necessary to properly assess the health status of patients with dysfunctions of the hepatobiliary system, the pancreas, or the spleen. Assessment should include data pertaining to the patient's perception of his or her disease, comfort status, nutritional status, fluid and electrolyte balance, bowel and elimination patterns, energy level and independence, and exposure to toxins.

Establishing the objective data base for a person with hepatobiliary or pancreatic dysfunction requires comprehensive assessment. Particular attention should be directed toward observing for characteristic signs of dysfunction. Increased abdominal girth and distention, palmar erythema, distended periumbilical veins, hemorrhagic areas, spider nevi, muscle wasting, and dry mucous membranes are a few of the characteristic signs and symptoms of dysfunction. Vascular volume can be assessed by monitoring vital signs, including orthostatic changes, assessment of skin turgor, temperature, appearance, and weight gain or loss.

Physical examination of the patient's abdomen should include palpation and percussion to evaluate tenderness, ascites, and organ enlargement.

The common laboratory tests to assess liver function are those that evaluate fat metabolism, protein metabolism, blood coagulation properties, bilirubin metabolism, and antigens and antibodies of hepatitis (Phipps, Long, and Woods, 1987) (Tables 12-1 and 12-2).

Radiographic studies commonly used to evaluate function of the liver, pancreas, and spleen include ultrasound studies, computed tomography (CT scan), radioisotope scanning, nuclear magnetic resonance imaging, angiography, cholecystography, and cholangiography. An abdominal flatplate radiograph and upper GI series may also aid in diagnosing gross anomalies of the liver, pancreas, and spleen.

Endoscopy and biopsy are more invasive diagnostic procedures that may be used in evaluation of the liver, pancreas, and spleen. Endoscopic retrograde cholangiopancreatography (ERCP) is a procedure that allows for direct visualization of the biliary tract, the injection of radiographic dye into the ductal system, and biopsy when indicated (Fig. 12-7).

Following a thorough nursing assessment of all subjective and objective data related to the patient with dysfunction of the liver, biliary tract, pancreas, or spleen, nursing diagnoses are formulated. Nursing diagnoses applicable to patients having surgery of the liver, biliary tract, pancreas, or spleen include:

- Anxiety related to impending surgical procedure
- Potential for alteration in body temperature
- Potential for fluid volume deficit related to hemorrhage or large-volume blood loss
- Potential for injury related to immobility and anesthetized state during operative procedure
- Potential for infection

Planning

Planning for the care of the patient having surgery of the liver, biliary tract, pancreas, or spleen requires assimilation of knowledge of the anatomy and subsequent physiologic complications that may occur with surgical interruption of tissues. Principles of proper positioning of the patient, maintenance of asepsis, prevention of biologic and electrical hazards, and providing proper instrumentation and equipment are a few constituents of the plan of care.

An example of a perioperative care plan for the patient having surgery of the liver, biliary tract, pancreas, or spleen is shown in the Sample Care Plan on p. 238.

Implementation

The patient having surgery of the liver, biliary tract, pancreas, or spleen usually undergoes general anesthesia. General procedures of skin preparation and draping are discussed in Chapter 5. The following pertinent factors are to be considered in caring for the patient undergoing biliary surgery.

Positioning the patient

The patient is placed in a supine position with the right upper quadrant elevated with an inflatable "gallbladder bag," folded sheet, or other positioning aid. Some surgeons do not use an elevation device because they do not believe that it aids in exposure, and it may cause backaches postoperatively for the patient.

When an operative cholangiogram is anticipated, the operating room bed is prepared with an x-ray cassette holder before the patient is positioned. A preliminary x-ray film may be taken to ensure correct placement of the cassette. The holder must be directly beneath the patient's right upper quadrant because correct positioning is imperative to ensure accurate visualization of the biliary tract.

Attention is given to proper alignment of the patient's body and extremities. Areas of pressure and bony prominences are padded well to prevent interruption of circulation and pressure injury to tissues. This precaution is especially important with diabetic, circulatory impaired, and elderly patients.

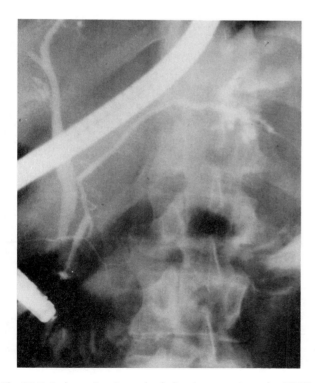

Fig. 12-7. Endoscopic retrograde cholangiopancreatography (ERCP) showing extravasation from the duct of the pancreatic body into a pseudocyst. (From Davis, J.H., and others: Clinical surgery, vol. 2, St. Louis, 1987, The C.V. Mosby Co.)

Sample Care Plan

NURSING DIAGNOSIS:
Anxiety related to impending surgical procedure
GOAL:
Patient will maintain a manageable level of anxiety as evidenced by the patient's ability to follow simple directions and respond appropriately to routine preoperative orientation questions.
INTERVENTIONS:
Complete as much of the setup as possible before the patient's arrival to the OR suite, especially those activities that create noise.
Greet the patient positively and professionally.
Introduce the patient to the OR team
Avoid hasty movements or gestures of indecision.
Speak slowly and clearly when addressing the patient, and use terminology the patient can understand.
Offer emotional reassurance through touch, facial expression, and allowing the patient to talk about feelings.

NURSING DIAGNOSIS:
Potential for alteration in body temperature
GOAL:
Patient will maintain therapeutic body temperature as evidenced by a postoperative temperature reading of not less than 96° F.
INTERVENTIONS:
Adjust room temperature and humidity to accommodate preservation of body temperature.
Cover all possible body surfaces to maintain body heat.
Use only warm irrigation solutions.
Warm IV fluids and blood products prior to infusion.

NURSING DIAGNOSIS:
Potential for fluid volume deficit related to hemorrhage or large-volume blood loss
GOAL:
Patient will maintain fluid volume equilibrium throughout operative procedure.
INTERVENTIONS:
Have available blood products in close, refrigerated storage for timely access.
Measure and record accurate fluid volume loss throughout operative procedure.
Anticipate and communicate potential for fluid volume deficit to blood bank personnel.
Check lab values intraoperatively.

NURSING DIAGNOSIS:
Potential for injury related to immobility and anesthetized state during operative procedure
GOAL:
Patient will maintain neuromuscular function and tissue integrity normal to the individual as a result of proper positioning and body alignment.
INTERVENTIONS:
Assure patient is in optimal anatomic alignment following induction of anesthesia.
Adequately pad all bony prominences.
Secure limbs with nonflexible safety strap to assure position is maintained and to prevent limb from falling from positioning device.
Assure safe and proper placement of electrosurgical dispersive pad.
Assure that no fluid pooling occurs beneath patient during operative procedure.
Assure that no weight or stress is placed upon body parts and structures.
Assure padding beneath all self-retaining retractors.

Instrumentation

Instrumentation includes a basic laparotomy set (Chapter 11) with instruments available for dilating and exploring the ducts adjacent to the pancreas and biliary tract. Vascular clamps, gastrointestinal clamps, ligating clips of all sizes with appliers, and linear stapling instruments should be available. A self-retaining retractor system such as the Bookwalter or the Omni-tract allows optimal safe retraction of tissues and excellent exposure of the abdominal viscera.

Specific biliary tract instruments should be included as follows:

Cutting instruments

1 Metzenbaum or Nelson scissors, 9¼ inches
1 Potts-Smith scissors

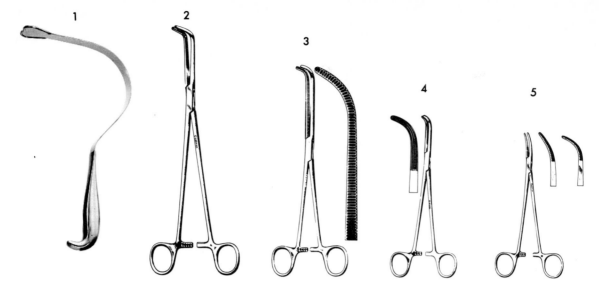

Fig. 12-8. Clamping and exposing instruments for gallbladder surgery. *1,* Harrington retractor; *2,* Mixter (right-angle) gallbladder forceps; *3,* Johns Hopkins gallbladder forceps; *4,* Lahey gall duct forceps; *5,* Schnidt gall duct forceps. (Courtesy Codman & Shurtleff, Inc., Randolph, Mass.)

Clamping and exposing instruments (Fig. 12-8)

2 Harrington retractors
2 Mixter gallbladder forceps, 7¼ inches
2 Johns Hopkins gallbladder forceps, 8 inches, or
2 Lahey gall duct forceps, 7¼ inches
6 Schnidt gall duct forceps

Duct instruments (Fig. 12-9)

1 Mayo common duct scoop, malleable shaft, 10½ inches
1 Set gall duct spoons, malleable, sizes 1 to 5
1 Ochsner gallbladder aspirating trocar
2 Potts-Smith tissue forceps

Stone instruments (Fig. 12-10)

1 Set Randall kidney stone forceps (may be used instead of Blake and Desjardin gallstone forceps)

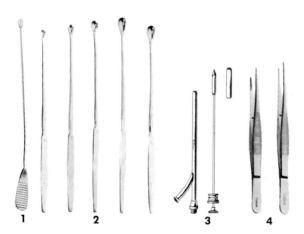

Fig. 12-9. Duct instruments, *1,* Mayo common duct scoop; *2,* gall duct spoons; *3,* Ochsner gallbladder trocar; *4,* Potts-Smith tissue forceps. (Courtesy Codman & Shurtleff, Inc., Randolph, Mass.)

2 Blake gallstone forceps, 1 straight and 1 curved, 8¼ inches
1 Desjardin gallstone forceps, 9¼ inches
1 Set Bakes common duct dilators
1 Moynihan bile duct probe and scoop

Accessory items

Drainage catheters, as desired (Fig. 12-11)
Sutures, surgeon's preferences
Fogarty biliary catheters (Fig. 12-11)
Contrast media (Hypaque, Conray, or Reno-M)
Culture tubes

Equipment and supplies

An electrosurgical unit, laser, argon beam coagulator, surgeon's headlight, intraoperative ultrasound handpiece and unit, CUSA (Cavitron Ultrasonic aspirator) unit, and cell saver system may be required for the operative procedure, according to the surgeon's preference.

Thrombin, Gelfoam, Surgicel, Avitene, and other hemostatic agents should be available in the operating room suite. Radiographic dye and supplies for intraoperative radiography or angiography may also be required.

Drainage materials

Tubes and catheters must be in optimal condition and suitable for the areas to be drained (Fig. 12-11). If a defective drain is used, a free fragment may remain in the wound on removal of the tube.

The scrub nurse should note the condition of all drainage materials and should test them for patency before they are placed in the patient.

Soft rubber or latex tissue drains may be used after a cholecystectomy or a choledochotomy. A latex rubber T tube drain (Fig. 12-11) of suitable size is prepared by the

Fig. 12-10. Stone instruments. *1* to *4,* Randall kidney stone forceps (four shapes); *5,* Blake gallstone forceps; *6,* Desjardin gallstone forceps. *7,* Bakes common duct dilators; *8,* Moynihan gall duct probe and scoop. (Courtesy Codman & Shurtleff, Inc., Randolph, Mass.)

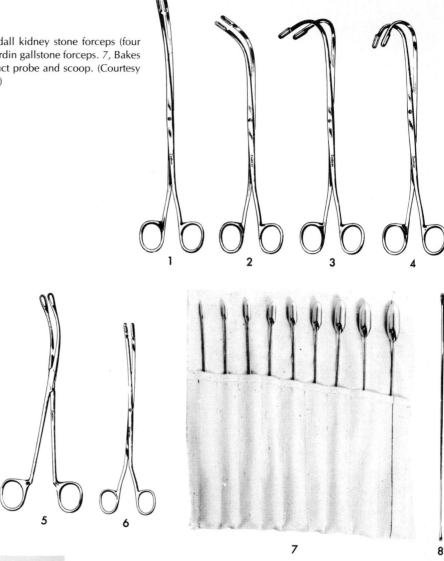

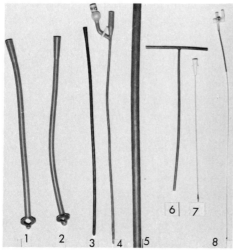

Fig. 12-11. Drainage tubes and catheters for biliary surgery. *1,* Malecot or bat-wing catheter; *2,* mushroom or Pezzer catheter; *3,* red Robinson catheter; *4,* Foley catheter; *5,* Penrose soft latex drain; *6,* T tube (latex); *7,* biliary balloon probe; *8,* cholangiography catheter.

surgeon after the duct has been explored. The center of the crossbar is notched opposite the junction of the vertical limb so that its ends will bend more readily during removal. The ends are beveled and tailored to fit the duct.

Two types of T tube drains are available on the market, and the surgeon may have a preference. The Deaver T tube has the same size crossbar as the drain stem. The Whalen-Moss T tube is designed to have an optional size of crossbar with a larger stem (Fig. 12-12).

Drains are usually exteriorized through separate stab wounds and anchored to skin edges to prevent retraction of the drain.

Aseptic considerations

When the common duct is opened or an anastomosis is established between a duct and other parts of the tract, care should be exercised to isolate contaminated instruments and materials from the remainder of the op-

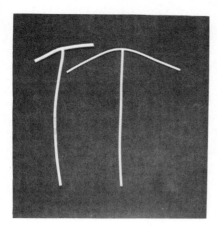

Fig. 12-12. Deaver and Whalen-Moss T tubes.

erative field, as described for gastrointestinal surgery (Chapter 11).

Instruments and materials used for the exteriorization of a drain should be treated as contaminated.

Blood products

The perioperative nurse should be aware of the type and amount of blood products available for the patient having surgery of the liver, biliary tract, pancreas, or spleen. Constant evaluation of blood loss is communicated to the anesthesia and surgical team as well as to the blood bank personnel so that blood products are readily available.

Evaluation

Evaluation of the patient following surgery includes examination of all skin surfaces and comparison to the preoperative assessment data. Abdominal drains, chest drainage systems, urinary drainage systems, and peripheral infusion lines are assessed for patency and labeled appropriately. Fluid volume use and loss are documented and communicated appropriately. A thorough report of the patient's history, preoperative assessment, intraoperative events, and postoperative evaluation is communicated to the PACU nurse.

The evaluation of patient status can be phrased as outcome statements such as:

- The patient expressed a positive recollection of the surgical event upon postoperative visit.
- The patient's body temperature was no lower than 96° F upon arrival at PACU.
- The patient's hematocrit was in the 30% to 35% range; vital signs were stable.
- All skin surfaces were clear, intact, and free of stress markings; capillary filling was noted following blanching of tissues. The patient demonstrated normal range of motion in extremities.
- The patient will be free of nosocomial infection related to the surgical wound.

SURGICAL INTERVENTIONS
Operations on the biliary tract
Cholecystectomy

Cholecystectomy is removal of the gallbladder. It is performed for the treatment of diseases involving the gallbladder, such as acute or chronic inflammation (cholecystitis), stones (cholelithiasis), or the presence of polyps or carcinoma.

Procedural considerations. A basic laparotomy set and biliary instruments are utilized.

Operative procedure (Fig. 12-13)

1. Through a right subcostal, right paramedian, or midline incision, the abdominal cavity is opened, as described for laparotomy (Chapter 11). Retractors and laparotomy packs are employed as the abdominal cavity is carefully examined.

2. The common duct is palpated for evidence of stones, and the pathologic condition determined. Harrington or Deaver retractors, moist laparotomy packs, long tissue forceps, and suction are used.

3. The surrounding organs are walled off from the gallbladder region by laparotomy packs and deep retractors.

4. To facilitate gentle traction, Pean forceps are usually placed on the body of the gallbladder (Fig. 12-13, *A*).

5. The peritoneal fold overlying the junction of the cystic and common duct is incised with a no. 7 knife handle and a no. 15 blade, long Metzenbaum scissors, and forceps. Suction is available, and bleeding points are clamped and ligated or electrocoagulated.

6. Adhesions are separated by blunt dissection with small, round, dry dissector sponges, sponges on holders, and blunt right-angled clamps. Dissection is continued to expose the neck of the gallbladder, the cystic artery, and the cystic duct (Fig. 12-13, *B* and *C*).

7. Dissection is continued to expose the cystic artery as it enters the wall of the gallbladder. On complete exposure and visualization of the branches, the cystic artery is doubly ligated with silk or clamped with ligating clips and divided (Fig. 12-13, *B*). Occasionally a third ligature or clip may be used. If the cystic artery has more than one branch, each is ligated and divided separately. Abnormalities of the arterial and ductal anatomy are common (Fig. 12-14), and the surgeon works with meticulous care to identify these structures.

8. The true junction of the cystic duct with the common bile duct is visualized. The cystic duct is identified and carefully dissected down to its junction with the hepatic duct. Any stones in the cystic duct are milked back into the gallbladder, and a tie is placed around the proximal cystic duct. If necessary, a cholangiogram is performed at this time (see procedure for intraoperative cholangiogram).

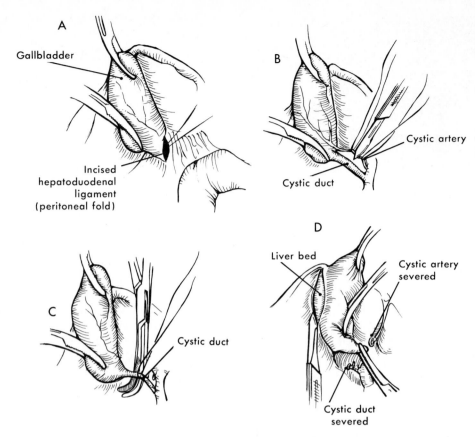

Fig. 12-13. Cholecystectomy. **A,** With Pean forceps in place, gentle traction is maintained as peritoneum over Calot's triangle is incised. **B,** Cystic artery is clearly visualized, doubly ligated, and divided. **C,** Cystic duct is carefully dissected and identified before forceps and ligatures are applied. **D,** Dissection of gallbladder from liver bed is completed.

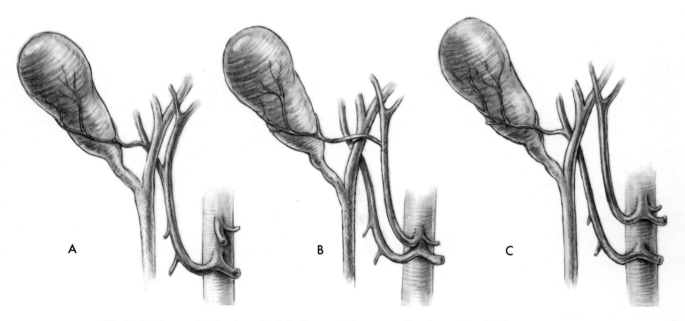

Fig. 12-14. The arterial blood supply of the liver and biliary system is quite variable. **A,** The most common anatomic arrangement is a cystic artery arising from the right hepatic artery. **B,** A dual-hepatic blood supply is found in 15% to 20% of patients, with the right hepatic artery arising from the superior mesenteric artery in a significant number of patients as in **C.** (From Davis, J.H., and others: Clinical surgery, vol. 2, St. Louis, 1987, The C.V. Mosby Co.)

9. If a cholangiogram is not done, the cystic duct is doubly ligated and divided (Fig. 12-13, *C*). A transfixion suture of fine absorbable suture may be used on the stump of the cystic duct near the common bile duct. The gallbladder is freed from the liver, working upward to the fundus, and it is removed (Fig. 12-13, *D*). In some cases working from the fundus downward to the neck of the gallbladder may be necessary.

10. All bleeding is controlled; reperitonealization of the liver bed, if indicated, is accomplished with interrupted or continuous fine absorbable intestinal sutures.

11. A drain may be inserted near the cystic duct stump. The free end of the drain is exteriorized through a stab wound in the lateral abdominal wall.

12. The wound is closed in layers, as described for laparotomy (Chapter 11) and a dressing applied.

Intraoperative cholangiogram

An intraoperative cholangiogram is usually performed in conjunction with cholecystectomy to visualize the common bile duct and the hepatic ductal branches and to assess patency of the common bile duct.

Procedural considerations. An intraoperative cholangiogram requires the use of x-ray. The OR bed should be prepared with radiographic attachments that permit easy insertion of the x-ray film cassette beneath the patient. If the surgeon prefers fluoroscopy to visualize the filling of the ducts, the OR bed is prepared, prior to the patient's arrival to the OR suite, with an image-intensification attachment.

Protective shielding such as x-ray aprons or leaded shields should be readily available for all members of the surgical team.

Because the patient's abdomen remains open while the x-ray equipment is positioned directly over the operative site, appropriate draping to maintain asepsis is necessary. Radiopaque sponges and any unnecessary instrumentation are removed from the abdominal site to avoid obscuring the view of the contrast medium filling the ducts.

A cholangiocath is prepared by the scrub nurse by attaching a stopcock with a 20-cc syringe of saline and a 20-cc syringe of contrast medium to the Luer-Lok ports. All air bubbles are removed, as they may be misinterpreted as gall duct stones on the x-ray.

Operative procedure

1. The cholangiocath is irrigated with saline prior to and during the insertion of the catheter into the cystic and common bile ducts (Fig. 12-15). Irrigation during insertion facilitates dilation and reduces trauma to the ductal lumen.

2. The cholangiocath is anchored in the lumen of the common bile duct by the surgeon's preferred method. The more common methods are applying a ligaclip proximal to the insertion site, tying or suturing the catheter in place, or using a ring-jawed holding clamp,

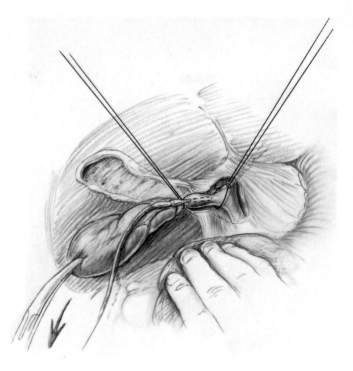

Fig. 12-15. Illustration of a cholangiocath inserted into the cystic duct through a small opening proximal to a silk tie placed at the cystic duct–gallbladder junction. The gallbladder has been dissected from the liver bed, and the cystic duct is dissected down to its junction with the hepatic duct. (From Davis, J.H., and others: Clinical surgery, vol 2, St. Louis, 1987, The C.V. Mosby Co.)

such as a Swenson clamp, that has been designed specifically for this purpose.

3. With placement of the cholangiocath confirmed and anchored, the surgeon informs the surgical team that x-ray is now required.

4. All radiopaque sponges, instruments, and obstructing equipment are removed from the field.

5. The surgical field is draped with a sterile drape sheet to maintain asepsis of the wound and field.

6. The x-ray equipment is positioned, as the surgeon redirects the stopcock to allow for injection of the contrast medium.

7. The surgeon directs the radiology technician as to the precise time to take the radiograph.

8. The x-ray equipment is removed from the operative site and the drapes covering the incisional site are carefully removed and discarded.

9. The x-ray is developed immediately to assure that appropriate visualization of the ductal structures has been achieved. Figs. 12-16 and 12-17 illustrate stones in various locations in the ducts.

10. Once the surgeon studies the radiograph hung on the x-ray view box in the OR, the decision is made to repeat the intraoperative cholangiogram, to explore

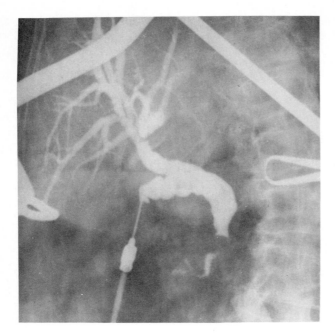

Fig. 12-16. Operative cholangiogram shows multiple stones in the common bile duct and a dilated cystic duct. One stone is partially obstructing the distal bile duct. (From Davis, J.H., and others: Clinical surgery, vol. 2, St. Louis, 1987, The C.V. Mosby Co.)

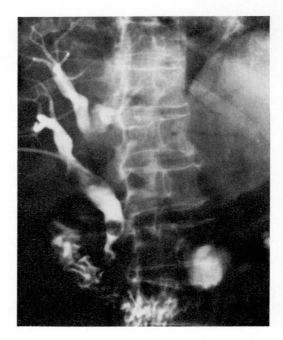

Fig. 12-17. Cholangiogram shows a retained stone in the distal bile duct. (From Davis, J.H., and others: Clinical surgery, vol. 2, St. Louis, 1987, The C.V. Mosby Co.)

the common bile duct, or to proceed with the conclusion of the patient's surgery.

Cholecystostomy

Cholecystostomy is establishment of an opening into the gallbladder to permit drainage of the organ and removal of stones. This procedure is usually selected for patients with acute gallbladder disease and a general physical condition that does not permit more extensive surgery.

Procedural considerations. A large syringe (50 ml) or an Asepto syringe may be needed for irrigation purposes. If a local anesthetic is used, the anesthetic drug and syringes and needles are necessary. Specified drainage tubes or catheters should be available.

Operative procedure

1. Although many surgeons prefer the right subcostal incision, cholecystostomy procedures are often performed as emergencies, and so a quicker midline or transverse incision may be used.
2. The fundus of the gallbladder is grasped with an Allis or Babcock forceps, and the proposed opening is encircled by means of an absorbable purse-string suture, leaving the ends long (Fig. 12-18, *A*).
3. To protect the abdominal cavity from contamination, the gallbladder is isolated with laparotomy packs, and suction is available.
4. Within the purse-string suture, the gallbladder is aspirated by means of a suction tubing attached to a trocar sheath (Fig. 12-18, *A*).
5. As the contents are aspirated, cultures should be

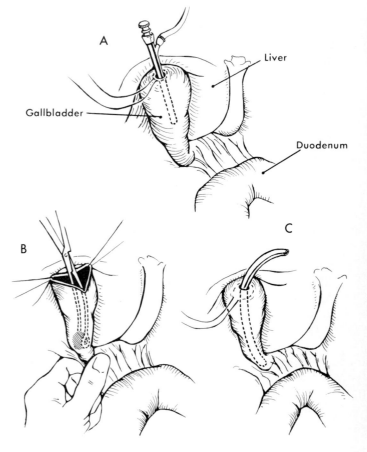

Fig. 12-18. Cholecystostomy. **A,** Purse-string suture and trocar are in place. **B,** Calculus is removed through opening in fundus. **C,** Drainage catheter is in place.

taken. The contaminated trocar and sheath are removed and discarded.

6. The opening can be enlarged with Metzenbaum scissors; gallstones are removed with malleable scoops and stone forceps (Fig. 12-18, *B*). Irrigating the gallbladder with isotonic saline solution is necessary to remove small stones, grit, or pastelike material. A syringe with a catheter or an Asepto syringe may be used for irrigation. Contaminated instruments are placed in a basin on the operative field.

7. A drainage tube is inserted in the gallbladder opening (Fig. 12-18, *C*). The purse-string suture is tightened around the catheter, care being taken not to occlude it. A second purse-string suture or separate mattress sutures may be used to secure the gallbladder to the peritoneum and the posterior rectus fascia.

8. The free end of the catheter or tube is exteriorized through a stab wound and then anchored to the skin edges, as described for cholecystectomy.

9. Drainage of the abdominal cavity is established. The exterior end of each drain is secured.

10. The wound is closed in layers, as described for laparotomy, and dressings are applied without disturbing the drains.

Choledochotomy and choledochostomy (exploration of the common bile duct)

Choledochotomy is an incision made into the common bile duct (Fig. 12-19). Choledochostomy is the establishment of an opening into the common bile duct with placement of a drainage T tube. Choledochotomy with subsequent choledochostomy is performed to treat choledocholithiasis or to relieve an obstruction in the common bile duct.

Procedural considerations. Before exploration is begun, operative cholangiography may be performed to locate all stones within the ductal system. X-ray films are repeated after the T tube drain is in place to confirm the successful evacuation and patency of the ducts.

A subcostal or upper right rectus incision is made. Instrumentation is as described for biliary surgery, with the addition of the following instruments and supplies:

1 Set Bakes common duct dilators, malleable shafts, sizes 3 to 11 mm (Fig. 12-10)
1 Ochsner flexible spiral gallstone probe, 14 inches
1 Malleable silver probe, 8 inches
1 Asepto syringe, 60 ml
4 Syringes, 2, 20, 30, and 50 ml
3 Aspirating needles: 24 gauge, ¾ inch; 19 gauge, 3½ inches; and 16 gauge, 2 inches
1 Catheter adapter for saline solution irrigation
2 Ampules contrast media
3 Robinson catheters, 8, 12, and 16 Fr
3 T tubes, 8 to 26 Fr, as desired (Fig. 12-12)
   Fogarty biliary catheters (Fig. 12-11)

Operative procedure

1. The abdomen is opened as for cholecystectomy. If the gallbladder has not been previously removed, it is exposed and removed, or retracted by means of laparotomy packs and retractors.

2. The common duct may be identified by means of an aspirating syringe and fine-gauge needle to make certain that the suspected duct is not a blood vessel. Cultures may be obtained.

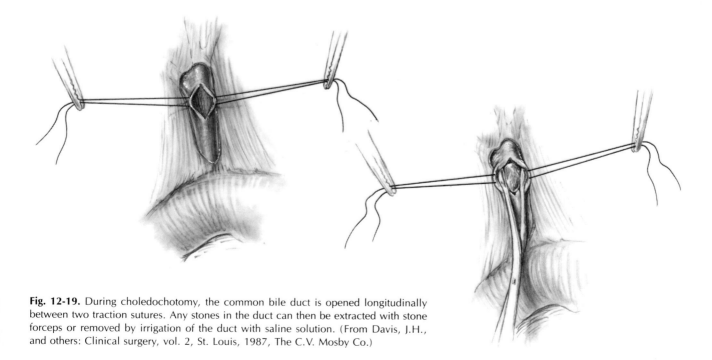

Fig. 12-19. During choledochotomy, the common bile duct is opened longitudinally between two traction sutures. Any stones in the duct can then be extracted with stone forceps or removed by irrigation of the duct with saline solution. (From Davis, J.H., and others: Clinical surgery, vol. 2, St. Louis, 1987, The C.V. Mosby Co.)

3. Two fine traction sutures are placed in the wall of the duct, below the entrance of the cystic duct.
4. The common duct region is walled off with laparotomy packs and narrow blade retractors. A discard basin for contaminated instruments is placed at the lower end of the operative field; a suction apparatus is made ready for immediate use.
5. A longitudinal incision is made in the common duct (Fig. 12-20, *A*), between the traction sutures, with a long no. 3 knife handle and a no. 15 or no. 11 blade. Constant suction is maintained with a Yankauer suction tube to keep the field free of oozing bile as the incision is enlarged with a Potts angled or Metzenbaum scissors. Additional stay sutures may be applied to the ductal opening.

6. Visible stones are removed with gallstone forceps, after which exploration of the duct is begun with small malleable scoops proximal and then distal to the opening. Probing is continued as stones are removed from both the common and hepatic ducts. Isotonic saline solution in an Asepto syringe and a small-lumen catheter or a Fogarty-type, balloon-tipped catheter are used to facilitate the removal of small stones and debris, as well as to demonstrate patency of the common bile duct through to the duodenum (see Fig. 12-20, *B* to *D*).
7. A duodenotomy may be performed if patency of the sphincter of Oddi and ampulla of Vater cannot be demonstrated.
   a. An area of the duodenum is walled off with laparotomy packs. The incision is made longitudinally, using a scalpel with a no. 15 blade and Metzenbaum scissors.
   b. Bleeding vessels are clamped with mosquito hemostats and ligated with fine silk or absorbable sutures or electrocoagulated.
   c. Fine silk traction sutures are inserted, and exploration is carried out.
   d. The duodenal opening is usually closed transversely in two layers with fine absorbable and silk intestinal sutures.
8. The T tube is prepared by the surgeon (Fig. 12-20, *E*), irrigated for patency, and introduced into the common duct with fine vascular forceps.
9. The common duct incision is closed with fine absorbable intestinal sutures. Contaminated instruments are placed in the discard basin.
10. The T tube is irrigated to demonstrate patency (Fig. 12-20, *E*), and a cholangiogram is done.
11. The gallbladder may be removed as described for cholecystectomy.
12. A drain is introduced into the foramen of Winslow. Both drain and T tube are exteriorized through a stab wound.
13. The wound is closed in layers; the T tube and drain are carefully anchored to the skin, and each wound is dressed individually to prevent undue tension that could result in displacement of the tube and drain.
14. Sterile tubing is used to connect the T tube to a small drainage container or bag.

Choledochoscopy

Choledochoscopy is direct visualization of the common bile duct by means of an instrument (choledochoscope, Fig. 12-21) introduced into the common bile duct.

Choledochoscopy may take the place of operative cholangiography. It provides a means for extraction of stones that are difficult to remove from the common bile duct.

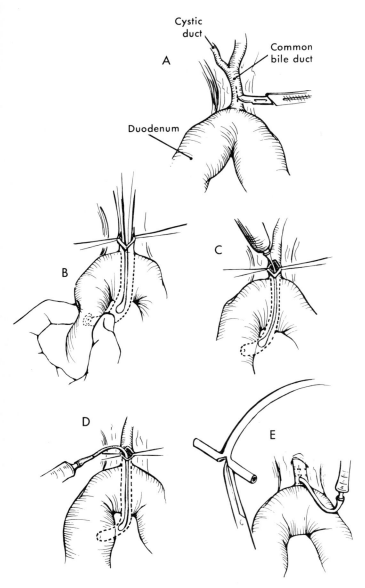

Fig. 12-20. Choledochotomy with choledochostomy. **A,** Opening common duct. **B,** Introducing stone forceps. **C,** Probing common duct. **D,** Irrigating duct. **E,** Preparing and irrigating T tube.

Procedural considerations. Distending the common duct is necessary to better visualize it. This is done by irrigating the duct with copious amounts of sterile saline. To accomplish this, a pressure bag must be used on the saline and pressure applied to 300 mm Hg. Sterile tubing is then attached to the saline and directly to the irrigating stopcock on the scope.

Instrumentation is as described for biliary surgery, with the addition of the following instruments:

Choledochoscope with accessories: biopsy forceps, stone grasping forceps, and a sheath that can be used to direct other instruments into various portions of the biliary tract

Eyepiece protector disk
Light cord
Normal saline, 1000 ml bag
Sterile IV tubing
IV pole
Pressure bag
Light source

Operative procedure
1 to 5. As described for choledochotomy.
6. The choledochoscope is inserted into the duct, and the common duct is flushed with saline. Stones are grasped with the stone forceps and removed. The choledocho-

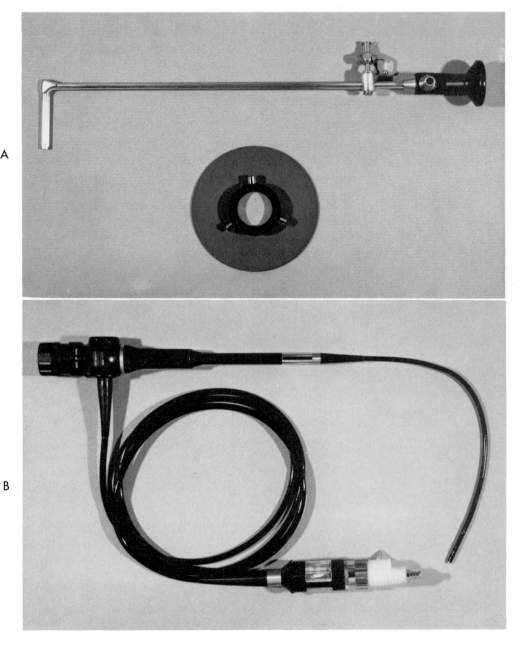

Fig. 12-21. A, Rigid choledochoscope with eyepiece protector disk. **B,** Flexible choledochoscope.

scope allows visualization of the entire duct so no stones will remain. After all stones are removed, the common duct is again thoroughly flushed with saline. Closure of the duct and wound is completed.

Cholelithotripsy

Cholelithotripsy is currently an investigational procedure performed for patients with stones in the biliary system. The procedure presently is not performed in the OR as it is noninvasive and does not require incision into the abdomen.

Cholecystoduodenostomy or cholecystojejunostomy

Cholecystoduodenostomy or cholecystojejunostomy is the establishment of continuity by creating an anastomosis between the gallbladder and duodenum or jejunum to relieve an obstruction in the distal end of the common duct.

An obstruction in the biliary system may be caused by a tumor of the ducts involving the head of the pancreas or the ampulla of Vater, the presence of an inflammatory lesion, a stricture of the common duct, or the presence of stones.

Procedural considerations. Instrumentation is as described for cholecystostomy, plus two Doyen intestinal forceps, curved with guards, or similar nontraumatic holding forceps.

Operative procedure
1. The abdomen is opened, the gallbladder is exposed and aspirated, and the pathological condition is confirmed, as described for cholecystostomy.
2. The anastomosis site is prepared, posterior serosal silk sutures are placed, and open anastomosis is performed. The surgical technique as described for gastrointestinal anastomosis is followed (Chapter 11).
3. Contaminated instruments are placed in the discard basin, and the operative field is prepared for closure.
4. A drain may be introduced; the wound is closed in layers, and dressings are applied.

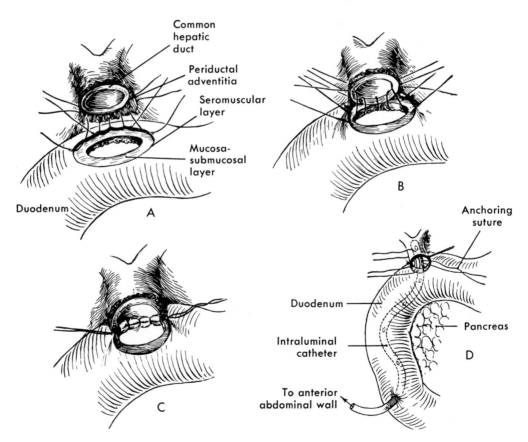

Fig. 12-22. Technique for choledochoduodenostomy. **A,** First posterior row of interrupted, silk sutures approximates adventitia around proximal biliary segment and seromuscular layer of anterior aspect of duodenum. **B,** Second posterior row approximates full thickness of duct and mucosa-submucosal layer of bowel. Knots are on outside of lumen. **C,** Two posterior rows are completed. **D,** Intraluminal catheter is in place, secured by absorbable suture at line of anastomosis. Extra holes in catheter provide egress of bile to bowel. (From Longmire, W.P., Jr., and Lippman, H.N. In Allen, A.W., and Barrow, D.W., editors: Abdominal surgery, New York, 1961, Harper & Row, Publishers.)

Choledochoduodenostomy or choledochojejunostomy

Choledochoduodenostomy or choledochojejunostomy is anastomosis between the common duct and duodenum or jejunum.

These procedures are usually necessary in postcholecystectomy patients to circumvent an obstructive lesion and reestablish the flow of bile into the intestinal tract.

Procedural considerations. Surgical approaches are similar to choledochostomy and cholecystojejunostomy.

Operative procedures

Choledochoduodenostomy

1. The abdomen is opened, and the common duct and duodenum are exposed.
2. The common duct is identified and dissected free.
3. The common duct and duodenum are approximated, either side-to-side or end of common duct to side of duodenum, and an anastomosis is established (Fig. 12-22).
4. An intraluminal catheter is inserted, the wound is closed in layers, and dressings are applied.

Choledochojejunostomy

1. The abdomen is opened, the jejunum is mobilized, and the common duct is identified and opened (Fig. 12-23, A).
2. Anastomosis is established between the common duct and the transected jejunum. A catheter is introduced, as described for cholecystoduodenostomy.
3. Jejunal continuity is reestablished by jejunojejunostomy (Fig. 12-23, B).
4. As an alternative, anastomosis may be fashioned from the end of the severed duct to the side of a loop of jejunum, with a side-to-side jejunal anastomosis.
5. Contaminated instruments are removed from the operative field.
6. A drain is exteriorized, the wound is closed in layers, and dressings are applied.

Repair of strictures of the common and hepatic ducts

Repair of strictures of the common and hepatic ducts relieves biliary obstruction either by resection of a stricture of the duct and an end-to-end anastomosis over a T tube splint (Fig. 12-24) or by means of an anastomosis between the duct or ducts and the intestinal tract. These operations are usually difficult because they follow previous unsuccessful operations on the biliary tract with resultant scarring, stricture, and fistulas.

Operative procedure
1. The abdomen is opened, and the anastomosis to be

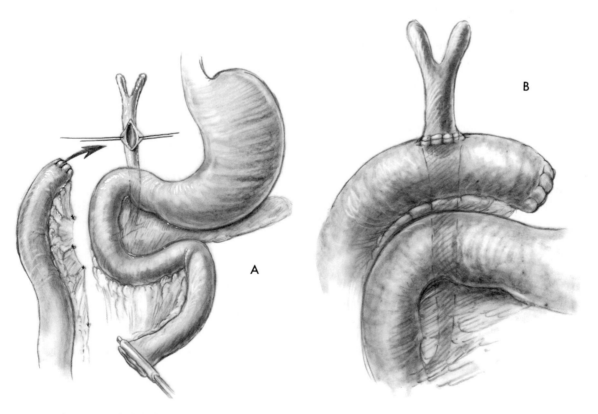

Fig. 12-23. Choledochojejunostomy. **A,** The divided end of the jejunum is closed, and an end-to-side choledochojejunostomy is made in two layers to the jejunum. **B,** A jejunal-jejunostomy completes the operative procedure. (From Davis, J.H., and others: Clinical surgery, vol. 2, St. Louis, 1987, The C.V. Mosby Co.)

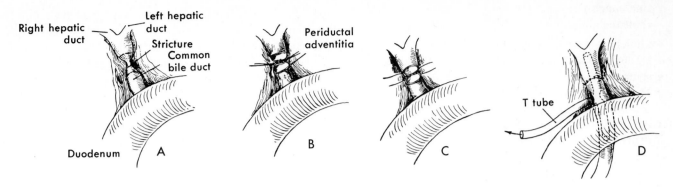

Fig. 12-24. Technique for duct-to-duct anastomosis with T tube in place. **A,** Strictured area is defined; *dotted lines* indicate area to be excised. **B,** First posterior row of sutures has been placed in adventitia around duct. **C,** Posterior inner row of interrupted, absorbable sutures has been completed. **D,** Completed anastomosis with T tube in place, brought out below line of anastomosis. (From Longmire, W.P., Jr., and Lippman, H.N. In Allen, A.W., and Barrow, D.W., editors: Abdominal surgery, New York, 1961, Harper & Row, Publishers.)

performed is selected after careful exploration and evaluation of the existing pathologic condition.

2. After anastomosis, the selected T tube is inserted (Fig. 12-24). Extreme caution is exercised to prevent displacement of the vital drainage tubes.
3. The wound is closed.

Transduodenal sphincteroplasty

Transduodenal sphincteroplasty is a method of producing a choledochoduodenostomy between the distal end of the common duct and the side of the duodenum. The sphincters normally affecting the distal common and pancreatic ducts are rendered functionless because the stoma is noncontractile and remains permanently open.

Indications for transduodenal sphincteroplasty include a history of recurrent bile stones, impacted distal common duct stones, papillary stenosis, distal common bile duct strictures, recurrent idiopathic pancreatitis, and postcholecystectomy pain.

Procedural considerations. Instrumentation is as described for choledochotomy, with the addition of a gastrointestinal set, as the duodenum is entered through a longitudinal incision. The patient is positioned supine on the operating room bed.

Operative procedure

1. The abdomen is prepped from nipple line to pubis.
2. A right subcostal or midline incision is made, and exposure of the biliary tract is achieved.
3. All structures are inspected, and the normal configuration is established before any structure is tied, clamped, or divided during biliary tract dissection (Way and Pellegrini, 1987).
4. Operative cholangiography is then performed by placing a cholangiocath through a small incision made with a no. 11 blade into the cystic duct.
5. The surgeon examines the films and makes the final decision to proceed with the sphincteroplasty.

6. If the gallbladder is present, cholecystectomy is performed.
7. The duodenum is mobilized by dividing the peritoneal reflection that covers the lateral portion of the second part of the duodenum and holds it in place (Way and Pellegrini, 1987).
8. The common duct is incised longitudinally between two stay sutures and explored. Any residual stones are removed.
9. Duodenotomy is performed with a longitudinal incision and the location of the papilla of Vater is identified (Fig. 12-25, *A*).
10. The sphincter of Oddi is divided at 11 o'clock with an angled Potts scissors, and the ductal mucosa is sutured to the duodenal mucosa with a fine absorbable suture on a small urologic needle (Fig. 12-25, *B*).
11. The duodenum is then closed in two layers.
12. The common bile duct is joined to the apex of the mobilized duodenum in a two-layer anastomosis.
13. A T tube is inserted to splint the anastomosis (Fig. 12-25, *C*).
14. The abdominal cavity is drained, and the wound is closed.

Operations on the pancreas
Drainage or excision of pancreatic cysts

Pancreatic cysts may be drained internally into the small intestine or stomach or may require excision or external drainage (marsupialization).

Cysts of the pancreas have been classified according to the following etiological factors: developmental or congenital, inflammatory, traumatic, neoplastic, and parasitic. Their etiology, size, location, and anatomical relationships are important factors in selection of the surgical procedure. Pancreatic pseudocysts result from pancreatic fluid exudate in the lesser sac region.

Procedural considerations. Internal or external drain-

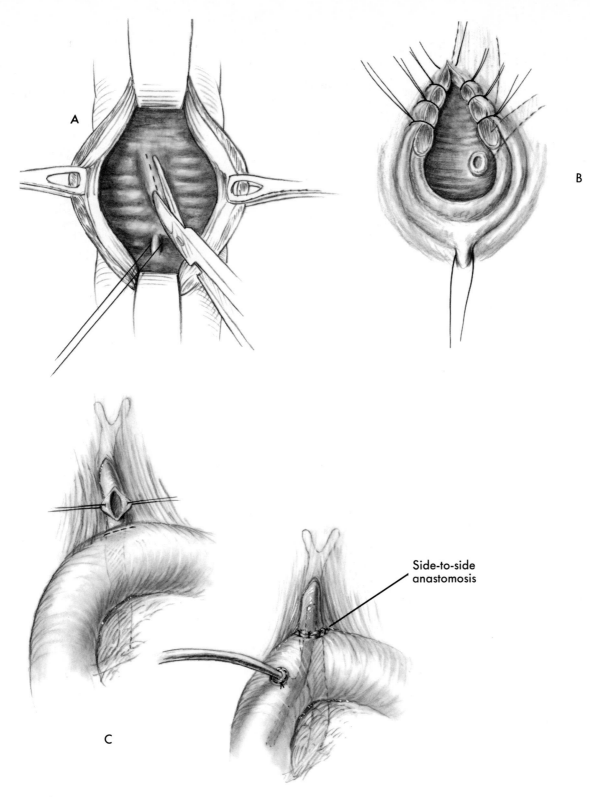

Fig. 12-25. Transduodenal sphincteroplasty. **A,** The duodenum is opened longitudinally. **B,** The sphincter of Oddi is divided at 11 o'clock with an angled Potts scissors, and the ductal mucosa is then sutured to the duodenal mucosa with 4-0 absorbable suture. The duodenum is then closed longitudinally in two layers. **C,** Choledochoduodenostomy. The common bile duct is joined to the apex of the mobilized duodenum in a two-layer anastomosis. A T tube is placed to stent the anastomosis with the external stem of the tube brought out through the bile duct or through the wall of the duodenum. (From Davis, J.H., and others: Clinical surgery, vol. 2, St. Louis, 1987, The C.V. Mosby Co.)

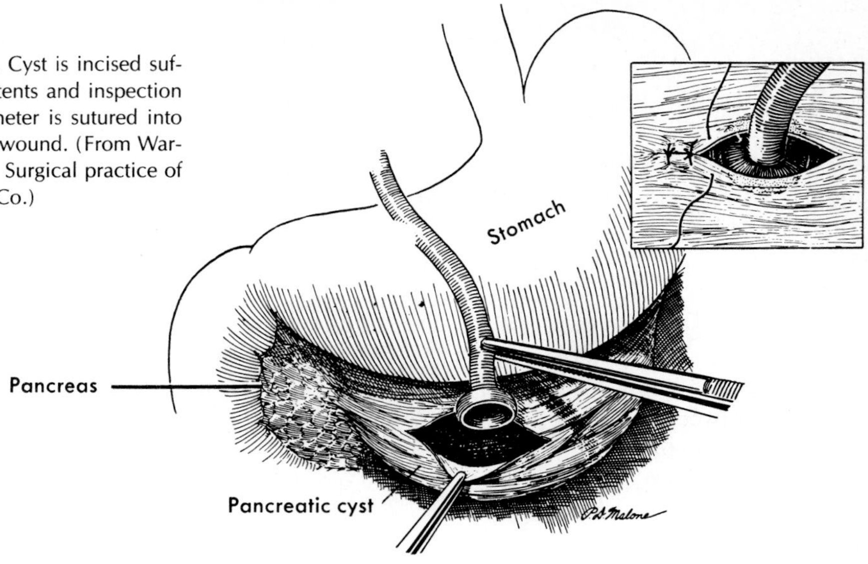

Fig. 12-26. Simple drainage of pancreatic cyst. Cyst is incised sufficiently to permit complete evacuation of contents and inspection of lining of cavity. Flanged end of Pezzer catheter is sutured into cyst, and other end is brought out through stab wound. (From Warren, K.W., and Baker, A.L., Jr. In Lahey Clinic: Surgical practice of the clinic, Philadelphia, 1962, W.B. Saunders Co.)

Fig. 12-27. Treatment of pancreatic pseudocyst by internal drainage by means of anastomosis of cyst to stomach. **A,** Sagittal section showing relationship of cyst of body of pancreas to posterior wall of stomach. **B,** Cystogastrostomy, sagittal view. **C,** Cystogastrostomy, anterior view. Stomach has been lifted cephalad to demonstrate anastomosis between pseudocyst and posterior wall of stomach. (From Dreiling, D.A., Janowitz, H.D., and Perrier, C.V.: Pancreatic inflammatory disease, New York, 1964, Harper & Row, Publishers.)

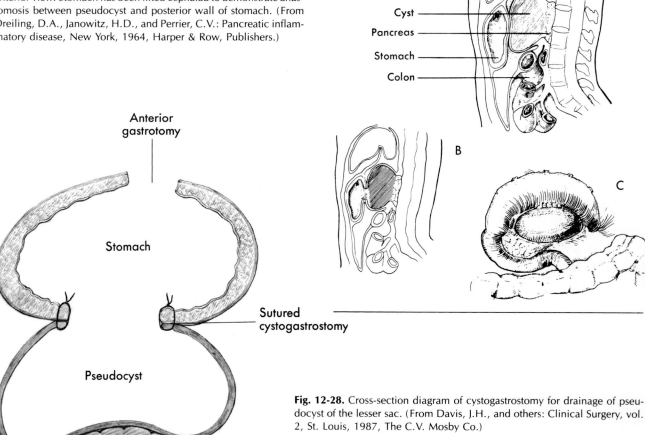

Fig. 12-28. Cross-section diagram of cystogastrostomy for drainage of pseudocyst of the lesser sac. (From Davis, J.H., and others: Clinical Surgery, vol. 2, St. Louis, 1987, The C.V. Mosby Co.)

age of the cyst is the preferred procedure. Appropriate drains must be available.

Operative procedure

1. Simple external drainage is established by direct introduction of a retention catheter into the cyst (Fig. 12-26), following decompression and inspection.
2. Internal drainage may be accomplished by an incision into the anterior wall of the stomach, directly opposite the cyst as it adheres to the posterior wall (Fig. 12-27). A fistula is established between the anterior wall of the cyst and the posterior wall of the stomach, thereby providing drainage through the gastrointestinal tract (Fig. 12-28). Many surgeons prefer an anastomosis between the cyst and a Roux-en-Y loop of jejunum or into the duodenum directly, depending on the location of the cyst.
3. The anterior gastrotomy is closed, and the wound closure is completed.

Pancreatoduodenectomy (Whipple's operation)

Pancreatoduodenectomy is the removal of the head of the pancreas, the entire duodenum, a portion of the jejunum, the distal third of the stomach, and the lower half of the common bile duct, with the reestablishment of continuity of the biliary, pancreatic, and gastrointestinal tract systems.

Radical excision of the head of the pancreas for carcinoma is a technically hazardous procedure because it involves many vital structures and organs. Resectability of the tumor in the presence or absence of metastasis and the general overall condition of the patient are evaluated carefully before resection.

Procedural considerations. General laparotomy and gastrointestinal instruments, plus appropriate drains and catheters, are used for this procedure.

After the surgeon opens and explores the abdomen, including the liver, pancreas, and biliary tree, the blood bank should be advised if the patient will require extensive surgery. Pancreatoduodenectomy may require 5 to 6 hours and the transfusion of many units of blood or blood products. This procedure is one of the most extensive of all abdominal procedures.

After surgery the surgeon must reevaluate the patient's insulin requirements and supplementary pancreatin.

Operative procedure

1. The abdomen is entered through an upper transverse, bilateral subcostal, or long paramedian incision. Laparotomy packs and retractors are used to expose the operative site and protect vital structures.
2. Mobilization of the duodenum is achieved with an adequate Kocher maneuver, which consists of incision of peritoneal reflection, lateral to the second portion of the duodenum, with Metzenbaum scissors and subsequent blunt dissection of loose areolar tissue.

3. Mobilization of the duodenum continues, and bleeding vessels are ligated with silk.
4. The gastrocolic ligament and the gastrohepatic omentum are divided between curved forceps and are ligated or transfixed.
5. The gastroduodenal and right gastric arteries are clamped, divided, and ligated.
6. The prepyloric area of the stomach is mobilized. The operative field is prepared for open anastomosis. By placing two long Allen or Payr clamps near the midportion of the stomach, the transection is completed.
7. The duodenum is reflected, the common duct is divided, and the hepatic end is marked or tagged for later anastomosis.
8. The jejunum is clamped with two Allen forceps, and the duodenojejunal flexure is divided.
9. The pancreas is divided, and the duct is carefully identified.
10. Further mobilization of the duodenum and division of the inferior pancreatoduodenal artery are done to permit complete removal of the specimen.
11. Reconstruction of the gastrointestinal tract is completed by the following anastomoses: retrocolic end-to-end pancreatojejunostomy, retrocolic end-to-side choledochojejunostomy, and an antecolic long-loop isoperistaltic gastrojejunostomy (Fig. 12-29).
12. Drains are introduced, as for cholecystostomy. Some surgeons prefer to place a sump drain near the pancreatic anastomosis.
13. The wound is closed in layers, usually including wire sutures.

Pancreatic transplantation

Pancreatic transplantation is the implantation of a pancreas from a donor into a recipient. This procedure is considered a possible means of treatment for Type I diabetes. Pancreatic transplantation differs from other organ transplants in that it does not have immediate life-saving results. Insulin therapy is a more common alternate medical treatment. Pancreatic transplantation is indicated for long-established, totally insulin-deficient diabetics with end-stage renal disease. As nephropathy, retinopathy, and neuropathy are secondary complications to long-established, insulin-deficient diabetes, pancreatic transplantation may interrupt the progression of those related complications.

Pancreatic transplant can be combined with the renal transplant procedure (Fig. 12-30). Serial transplantation is an alternative for patients who have already received a transplanted kidney.

The surgical technique for pancreatic transplantation varies between segmental pancreatic grafting and whole-organ transplantation. With either procedure, vascular anastomosis and management of the pancreatic duct are performed. Managing pancreatic ductal exocrine secre-

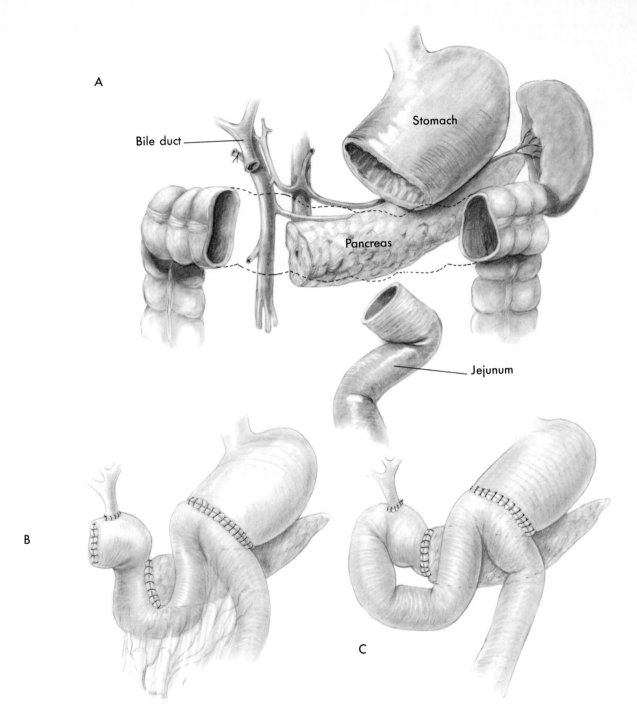

Fig. 12-29. A, Resection margins of bile duct, pancreas, stomach, and jejunum following a Whipple's procedure. **B,** Reconstruction following a Whipple's procedure showing biliary anastomosis preceding pancreas and stomach. **C,** Reconstruction showing pancreatic anastomosis preceding bile duct and stomach. (From Davis, J.H., and others: Clinical Surgery, vol. 2, St. Louis, 1987, The C.V. Mosby Co.)

tions remains one of the major technical problems with the transplantation procedure.

The segmental pancreatic graft can be placed in a paratopic position just superior to the native pancreas of the recipient or in a heterotopic position in the retroperitoneum or intraperitoneum. The pancreatic duct is then routed into the stomach, intestine (Fig. 12-31, *A*), or urinary bladder (Fig. 12-31, *B*). A pancreaticocutaneous fistula, with external drainage via a catheter (Fig. 12-31, *C*), may also be an alternative for managing the exocrine secretions from

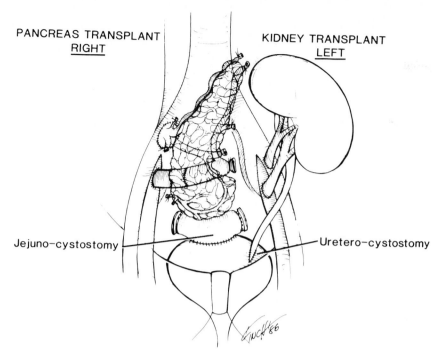

PANCREAS TRANSPLANT
RIGHT

KIDNEY TRANSPLANT
LEFT

Jejuno-cystostomy

UreTERO-cystostomy

Fig. 12-30. Whole pancreas transplantation with simultaneous or serial kidney transplantation illustrating the position of the two donor grafts in the recipient. (From Cerilli, G.J.: Organ transplantation and replacement, Philadelphia, 1988, J.B. Lippincott Co.)

the pancreatic duct. Occlusion of the pancreatic duct with polymer injection (Fig. 12-31, *D*) prior to transplantation or 3 to 6 weeks following the transplant is another means of managing the exocrine secretions.

Whole-organ pancreatic transplantation has achieved popularity over segmental pancreatic transplantation. Better blood supply of the whole-organ graft and an increased number of islet cells for insulin production are the advantages that have changed the trend to whole-organ pancreatic transplantation in recent years.

Procedural considerations. Instrumentation for pancreatic transplantation includes a transplant set as described for kidney transplantation in Chapter 15. In addition to the transplant set, consideration must be given to the resection of the duodenal segment and the management of the pancreatic duct. A gastrointestinal instrument set and linear stapling devices with two loads are required for grafting the duodenal segment that contains the pancreatic duct into an enteric route of drainage.

Operative procedure

1. The whole-organ pancreatic transplantation procedure is performed through an oblique incision opposite the side of the renal transplant in the lower abdominal quadrant. A midline incision may also be used for pancreatic transplant.
2. The external iliac artery and vein are skeletalized, and lymphatics are tied off with 4-0 silk strands.

3. The external iliac vein is clamped with noncrushing vascular clamps, and venotomy is achieved with a no. 11 blade. The venotomy incision is extended with Potts scissors.
4. An end-to-side anastomosis of the donor portal vein to the recipient's external iliac vein is achieved with four double-armed 5-0 polypropylene sutures.
5. The external iliac artery is then clamped, and arteriotomy is achieved with an aortic punch.
6. An end-to-side anastomosis of the recipient's external iliac artery with the donor aortic patch containing the origin of the superior mesenteric artery and the celiac axis is performed with four double-armed 6-0 polypropylene sutures.
7. Management of the pancreatic duct is then performed. The whole-organ pancreatic transplantation may also be performed as a pancreaticoduodenal transplantation or a pancreaticoduodenal-splenic transplantation.

Management of the pancreatic duct is dependent upon the type of "en bloc" procedure performed. Various enteric procedures for drainage of pancreatic duct secretions have been performed with whole-organ transplants en bloc with a segment of duodenum and the spleen. They include cutaneous jejunostomy, drainage into an ileal loop, and duodenojejunostomy with an end-to-end or side-to-side anastomosis.

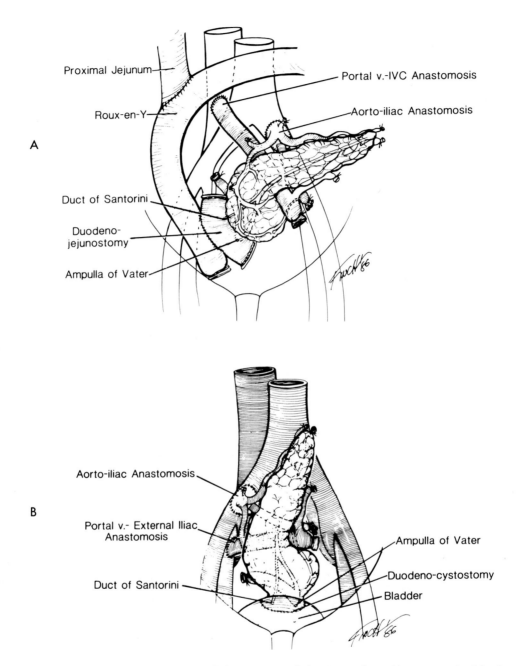

Fig. 12-31. A, Enteric drainage of a whole-pancreas graft showing a side-to-side anastomosis of the donor duodenal patch and the recipient's jejunal segment of a Roux-en-Y. **B,** Whole-pancreas transplantation showing donor duodenal patch anastomosed to dome of urinary bladder. **C,** Enteric drainage of a segmental pancreas graft to a Roux-en-Y limb of the recipient jejunum, showing an external drain exteriorized through the abdominal wall. **D,** Segmental pancreas transplantation showing polymer injection into pancreatic duct of graft. (From Cerilli, G.J.: Organ transplantation and replacement, Philadelphia, 1988, J.B. Lippincott Co.)

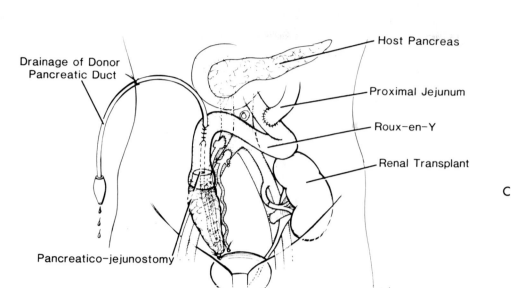

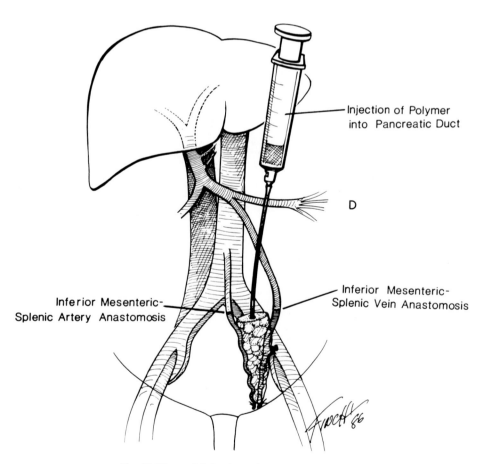

Fig. 12-31, cont'd. For legend see opposite page.

Direct grafting of the pancreatic duct into the enteric or urinary system is also performed for management of exocrine secretions. Surgical procedures would include pancreaticojejunostomy with an established Roux-en-Y loop of jejunum, pancreaticoductoureterostomy, and pancreaticocystostomy.

Operations on the liver

Drainage of intrahepatic, subhepatic, or subphrenic abscess

Abscesses of the liver may require incision and drainage. Hepatic abscesses may be pyogenic or parasitic and single or multiple.

Extreme care is used in removal of an *Echinococcus* (hydatid) cyst because the fluid is under high tension, and any spillage into the peritoneal cavity may result in anaphylactic reaction. Even more important is the possible escape of "daughter" cysts that can spread through the abdomen and produce multiple cysts, an extremely difficult condition to treat. Hydatid cysts of the liver are rare in the United States.

Procedural considerations. Biliary instrumentation, drainage materials, and aerobic and anaerobic culture tubes should be available.

Operative procedure

1. The incision and type of procedure selected depend on the cause and location of the abscess. For the anterior approach, a right transperitoneal incision is made. For the posterior approach, the patient is prepped and the incision selected as described for a posterior thoracotomy.
2. Drainage of an abscess may be treated in one or two stages. In the one-stage procedure, the approach is through the outer third of the right twelfth rib to reach the liver abscess retroperitoneally and extrapleurally.

A two-stage operation, which is rarely done, obliterates the right pleural cavity. The objective of the first stage is to seal off the pleural cavity by stimulating adhesions with the insertion of iodoform packing. When the second stage is performed at a higher level, the chest cavity does not become contaminated.

Hepatic resection

The liver is divided into the left lobe and the right lobe, with the caudate lobe lying in the dorsal segment. Resection of the liver is according to the lobe and segment involved (Figs. 12-32 and 12-33); a small wedge biopsy, excision of simple tumors, or a major lobectomy may be performed. Increased knowledge of liver function and circulatory physiology as well as improved methods of hemostasis now permit the surgeon to offer safe, definitive treatment to the patient with liver disease or trauma.

Procedural considerations. Supplies and equipment should be available for hypothermia, electrosurgery, measurement of portal pressure, thoracotomy drainage, and replacement of blood loss. Special blunt needles for suturing liver tissue are also necessary.

The patient is placed in the supine position. Some surgeons elevate the hepatic area with an inflatable "gallbladder bag," folded sheet, or other positioning aid. A midline abdominal incision, occasionally with division of the lower sternum, provides access to the left lobe, whereas a combined right thoracoabdominal incision is needed to expose the right hepatic region for major resection. Vertical abdominal incisions are also advantageous because they

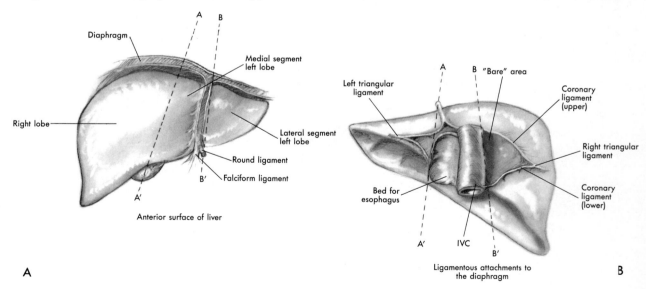

A

B

Fig. 12-32. A, Anterior surface of the liver. Plane A-A divides the liver into the right and left lobes. Plane B-B divides the left lobe into the medial and lateral segments. **B,** The ligamentous attachments to the diaphragm. (From Davis, J.H., and others: Clinical surgery, vol. 2, St. Louis, 1987, The C.V. Mosby Co.)

can be made and closed more rapidly and permit better exposure of all abdominal organs.

Instrumentation is as for portacaval shunt and common duct procedures, plus additional items as follows:

Manometer
2 Chest drainage catheters
12-18 Liver sutures, silk or chromic, according to surgeon's preference
Hemostatic material, such as Gelfoam, Surgicel, Avitene, absorbable collagen sheets

Operative procedure

1. Through an upper midline incision, the abdominal cavity is opened and examined by using items as described for biliary surgery. Pathologic condition is determined, and resectability evaluated (Fig. 12-34, *A*).
2. Moist laparotomy packs are inserted, and a self-retaining retractor is placed.
3. Exposure of the hilar structures is obtained by upward displacement of the right lobe toward the right chest cavity, application of a clamp to the falciform ligament to facilitate traction, and inferior displacement of intestines with moist packs and retractors.

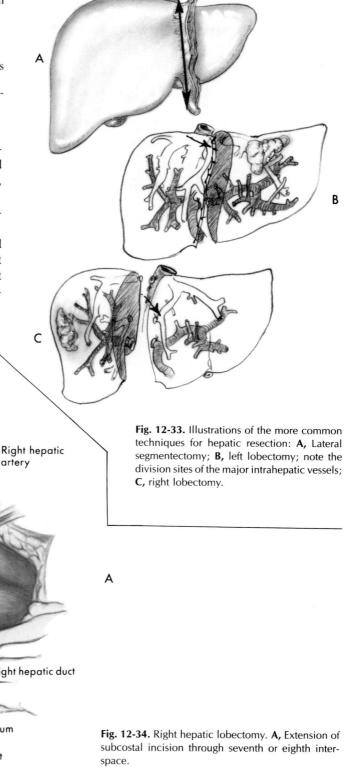

Fig. 12-33. Illustrations of the more common techniques for hepatic resection: **A,** Lateral segmentectomy; **B,** left lobectomy; note the division sites of the major intrahepatic vessels; **C,** right lobectomy.

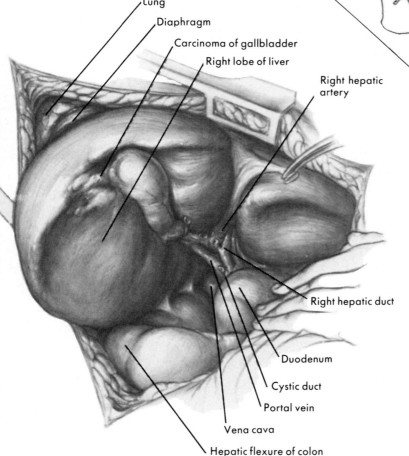

Lung
Diaphragm
Carcinoma of gallbladder
Right lobe of liver
Right hepatic artery
Right hepatic duct
Duodenum
Cystic duct
Portal vein
Vena cava
Hepatic flexure of colon

A

Fig. 12-34. Right hepatic lobectomy. **A,** Extension of subcostal incision through seventh or eighth interspace.

Continued.

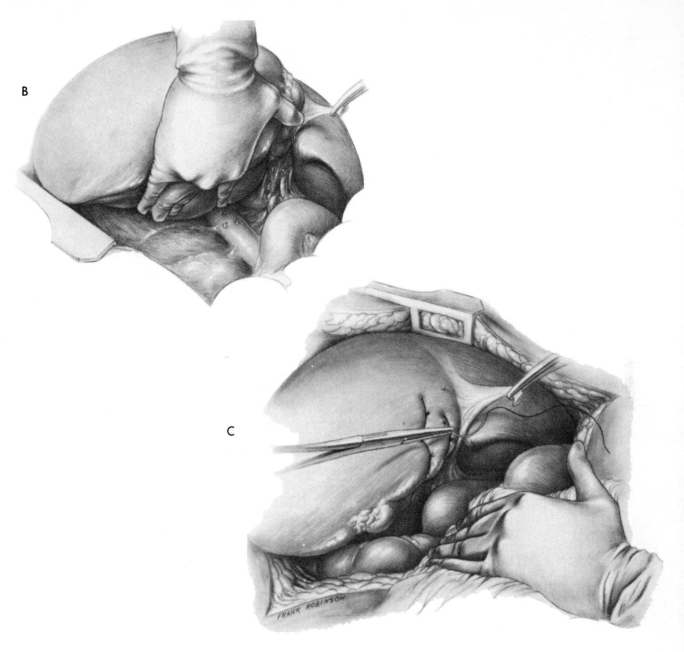

Fig. 12-34, cont'd. B, Hilar structures ligated preparatory to transection of right lobe. **C,** Preparation of devascularized channel for transection by placement of interlocking sutures.

4. The cystic duct is carefully exposed, using Metzenbaum scissors, vascular forceps, small dry dissectors on curved clamps, and fine right-angled forceps. It is clamped, transected, and doubly ligated with chromic or silk ligatures and transfixion sutures (Fig. 12-34, *B*).

5. The involved hepatic duct, branch of hepatic artery, and branch of the portal vein are also transected and doubly ligated with silk ligatures and transfixion sutures.

6. The liver is rotated forward, and the multiple hepatic veins entering the inferior vena cava are carefully identified, clamped, divided, and ligated.

7. A double row of interlocking liver sutures is placed (Fig. 12-34, *C*). Blunt needles are used to prevent undue trauma or tearing of the liver. A scalpel is used to excise the lobe through the devascularized section. Fine suture ligatures may be needed to ligate bile ducts and small blood vessels (Fig. 12-34, *D*). As additional sutures are placed, care should be exercised to avoid injury to other hepatic veins.

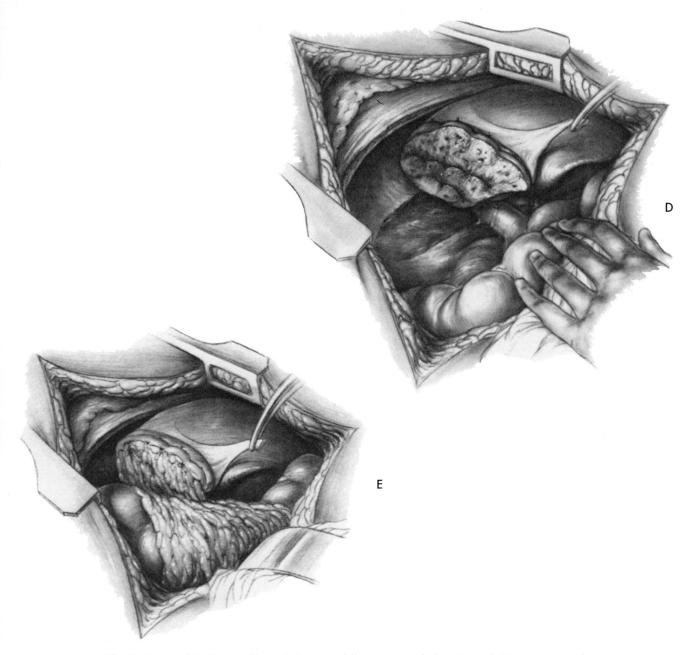

Fig. 12-34, cont'd. D, Pattern of hemostatic sutures following removal of specimen. **E,** Omentum sutured over raw liver surface to decrease bile and serum loss. (From Indications and technique of right hepatic lobectomy, Somerville, N.J., 1964, Ethicon, Inc.)

8. The omentum may be sutured to the raw liver surface to decrease bile and serum loss (Fig. 12-34, *E*).
9. Chest and abdominal drainage tubes are inserted, and wound closure is completed.

Excision of multiple metastatic hepatic tumors

Patients with primary colon or rectal cancer can have metastasis to the liver occur within 5 years of primary resection of the colon or rectal lesion. These patients are followed closely by monitoring carcinoembryonic antigen

(CEA) levels in their blood at scheduled intervals that are dependent upon the findings. When a rise in CEA levels is noted, x-rays, liver scan, and CT scan are often used for diagnosis.

Resection of multiple metastatic hepatic lesions is a relatively new procedure. The criteria for candidacy exempt those who have metastases outside the abdominal cavity, in lungs, or in bones.

Procedural considerations. Intraoperatively, the surgeon can confirm suspicions of liver metastasis by bimanual examination of each lobe, intraoperative ultrasonography, biopsy, and/or Neoprobe scanning of the liver. This procedure is sometimes scheduled as a *CEA-directed second-look procedure*, and equipment and supplies for bowel resection and/or liver resection should always be available.

Operative procedure. An elongated electrosurgical blade with the unit set on a high blend 2 setting is used to initiate the resection of the metastatic tumor. The CO_2 laser with smoke evacuator (Chapter 10), the CUSA aspirator (Fig. 12-35), and the argon beam coagulator (Fig. 12-36), provide current technology found to be of value for resecting multiple metastatic lesions of the liver.

The surgeon's intent is to achieve a 1-cm margin of normal liver tissue dissection around each lesion.

Multiple metastatic lesions may range from 0.5 cm to 20 cm in diameter. When four or more lesions may be from the liver, localized chemotherapy lines may be indicated for postoperative, self-administered chemotherapy.

Following resection and/or excision of the four or more lesions, a Broviac catheter is inserted into the hepatic artery, and a Hickman catheter is inserted into the portal vein via the gastroepiploic artery and vein. The catheters exit the skin in the right upper quadrant of the abdomen and are labeled accordingly.

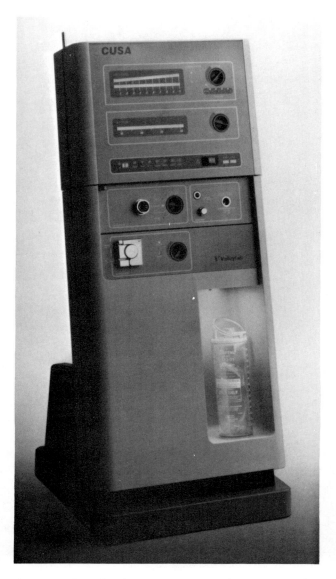

Fig. 12-35. The Valleylab CUSA System 200 ultrasonic surgical aspirator manufactured by Valleylab, Inc., Boulder, Colo. 80301.

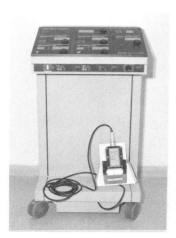

Fig. 12-36. Argon beam coagulator.

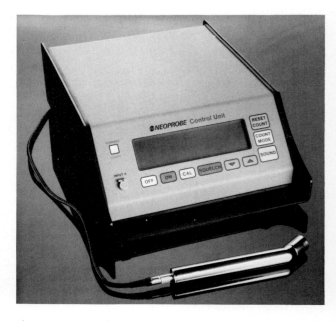

Fig. 12-37. Neoprobe instrument. (Courtesy Neoprobe Corp., Columbus, Ohio.)

Radioimmunoguided surgery (RIGS)™

Radioimmunoguided surgery is a new technique used intraoperatively to detect cancer that may not be readily visible. This technique has been found to be very useful in detecting safe margins in hepatic resections for metastatic colon cancer lesions. Patients receive an intravenous injection of radiolabeled monoclonal antibody, which binds reactive antigen on or near the surface of tumor cells. Consequent concentrations of radioactivity, or gamma emissions, localized in tumor tissue are detected by an intraoperatively used, handheld, gamma-detecting probe that emits an audible signal (Martin and others, 1988).

In the RIGS method of surgery, the patient is injected with the radiolabeled monoclonal antibody 3 weeks before the scheduled surgery date. The uptake and clearing of the radiolabeled antibody take 14 to 21 days to localize in tumor tissue. Ex vivo scanning of the patient's heart and liver is done periodically to determine uptake and clearing; scanning is done with the same type of unit that is used intraoperatively. The Neoprobe instrument (Fig. 12-37) gives a digital reading as well as an audible pitch that rises or lowers in tone when placed on the gamma-emitting tissue.

Procedural considerations. A gastrointestinal instrument set is required.

Operative procedure

1. The operative procedure is identical to the second-look laparotomy procedure as described previously.
2. A midline abdominal incision is made from the xiphoid process to the pubis.
3. Intraoperative scanning of the liver and abdominal viscera is performed using the probe. The digital readings as well as the anatomic structures being scanned are recorded. Great care is taken to scan mesenteric, pelvic, and periaortic lymph nodes individually.
4. The liver is scanned, and areas emitting strong-pitched tones are marked with a sterile marking pen. A very distinct change in pitch may be noted on liver tissue within a 2- to 3-cm radius of the tumor site.
5. Intraoperative ultrasound and a review of the CT scan of the patient's liver are used to further confirm the liver lesions.
6. Margins for resection are drawn using an electrosurgical knife on a blend 2 setting set at 40. Resection of the lesion may be segmental, circumferential, or lobar.
7. Following each resection, the margins of healthy liver tissue adjacent to the resection site are scanned, and readings are recorded.
8. This procedure continues until all tissue emitting high gamma waves has been resected.
9. Specimens are sent to pathology for further pathologic and histologic analysis.

Liver transplantation

Liver transplantation is the implantation of a liver from a donor into a recipient. The total procedure involves re-trieving, or procuring, the liver from a donor, transporting the donor liver to the recipient's hospital, performing a hepatectomy on the recipient, and implanting the donor liver, including reanastomosis of suprahepatic vena cava, infrahepatic vena cava, portal vein and hepatic artery, biliary reconstruction with end-to-end anastomosis of donor and recipient common bile ducts, or Roux-en-Y anastomosis if recipient bile duct is absent as a result of biliary atresia.

Procedural considerations. Successful transplantation requires the cooperative efforts of the organ procurement agency and the staffs of the donor and recipient hospitals. Usually, two members of the surgical team from the recipient's hospital travel to the donor's hospital to procure the donated liver.

The *donor operating room* is set up for a major laparotomy procedure. Basic instrumentation and equipment include the following:

Major abdominal instrument set
Cardiovascular instruments
Nephrectomy instruments
Power sternal saw
Intravenous volumetric pumps on stands
Extra suction bottles

The procurement team provides special Collins' solution for flushing the organs, sterile plastic containers and ice chest for organs, and in situ flush tubing. The liver is generally placed in two Lahey bags immediately after procurement. Common practice is to procure the kidneys as well as the liver; other organs, tissues, and bone may also be procured.

Each transplant surgeon has preferred instruments, supplies, and sutures. In general, the following are needed in the *recipient operating room:*

Major abdominal instrument set
Cardiovascular instrument set
Set of T tubes
Slush unit or means of providing iced lactated Ringer's solution
2 Electrosurgical units
Thermia unit
Temperature probe
Intravenous volumetric pumps on stands
2 Blood warmers or water baths
Foley catheter and urinometer
1 Sterile gown and glove table
Large Mayo stand and tray
Ring stand with basin
Large sterile draped instrument table for scrub nurse
Medium sterile draped instrument table for preparation of liver
Prep table and set
Gram scale for measuring blood loss in sponges and laparotomy pads
4 Calibrated suction reservoirs for measuring blood loss through suction unit

Large-bore cannulae for intravenous monitoring and fluid or blood replacement lines

2 Headlights and light sources

Venovenous bypass system

Extra drape sheets, table covers, gowns, towels, gloves, sponges, and laparotomy pads

50 Tuberculin syringes or 1-cc blood tubes (for blood specimens)

Syringes, 50, 10, and 20 ml, 6 each

Cold intravenous Ringer's solution

1 Sterile intravenous administration set for flushing new liver

Umbilical tape, booties, and vessel loops

Sutures, as designated by surgeon

Loupes, as desired by surgeon

A cart containing sutures and the numerous other small items should be set up and placed in the room for each procedure. This practice eliminates the circulating nurse running for extra supplies.

The procedure requires a bilateral subcostal incision with possible midline extension and removal of the xiphoid. The right side of the chest may be entered to provide more exposure when needed.

In addition to previously noted nursing diagnoses, patient goals, and nursing interventions, the following aspects of implementing the perioperative care plan deserve special attention:

1. *Patient positioning*. The patient is placed in the supine position with knees slightly flexed and padded. Accurate body alignment is essential. Foam eggcrate padding should be used under all potential pressure areas. Heel protectors are applied and an eggcrate pad is placed over both legs and secured with the safety strap. As much body surface as possible should be in contact with the heating blanket to assist in maintaining the patient's temperature. A stocking cap may be helpful in preventing heat loss from the patient's head.

2. *Blood loss and replacement*. Blood loss may be extensive, and replacement must be timely. Blood products normally available at the beginning of the procedure include 10 units each of packed cells, fresh-frozen plasma, and platelets. Sufficient clot should be available in the blood bank to process additional blood products if needed. As in all surgical procedures, care must be exercised by all members of the surgical team in handling bloody sponges and instruments. Nursing and medical team members should have previously been tested for immunity to hepatitis B and should have received Heptavax or another appropriate vaccine if indicated. Needle sticks must be reported and treated according to hospital policy.

3. *Intraoperative laboratory testing*. Thirty to 50 blood specimens can be drawn for analysis during the procedure. This blood must be recorded on the "blood loss" record and calculated into replacement needs. The specimens are delivered to the laboratory immediately. A telephone in the operating room is most useful for receiving reports directly from the laboratory.

4. *Length of procedure*. Procedures may last from 12 to 24 hours but normally last 10 to 16 hours. Special attention must be directed toward maintaining the integrity of the sterile environment from the standpoint of time and the numbers of people moving in and out of the room. Surgical team members can become exhausted, especially when procedures begin after members have completed a regular workday. Adequate staffing enables team members to take rest and nourishment breaks.

5. *Communication with family*. Frequent reports to the family are important. Family members usually are knowledgeable about liver function tests and laboratory values and want this information, in addition to reports on the condition of their loved one. One person should be assigned in advance to make the contacts with family and support persons on a regular basis.

Operative procedure

1. Bilateral subcostal incisions are made with a midline incision extended toward the umbilicus.

2. Initial dissection of the underlying tissues is achieved with electrosurgery and suture ligatures.

3. Isolation of all hilar structures and dissection to mobilize the lobes of the native liver are performed.

4. The retrohepatic vena cava is skeletalized, as are the hepatic artery, portal vein, common bile duct, and inferior vena cava.

5. Nothing irreparable is done to the native liver prior to the arrival and examination of the donor liver.

6. Following the arrival of the donor organ, the patient is prepared for veno-veno bypass, if indicated, by incision into the left external iliac vein and the left axillary vein. Cannulation into both the femoral and axillary sites allows for bypass of the portal system and inferior vena cava.

7. The infrahepatic vena cava and the suprahepatic vena cava are clamped, as are the portal vein, the hepatic artery, and the common bile duct. Native hepatectomy is then performed.

8. Revascularization of the donor organ begins with an end-to-end anastomosis of the suprahepatic vena cava with double-armed 3-0 vascular suture. The infrahepatic vena cava anastomosis is performed, followed by the end-to-end anastomosis of the portal vein. At this point, all venous clamps are removed, and blood flow through the vena cava and portal vein is restored. Hemostasis of the anastomosis sites is then achieved. Veno-veno bypass is discontinued, and the cannulation sites are closed.

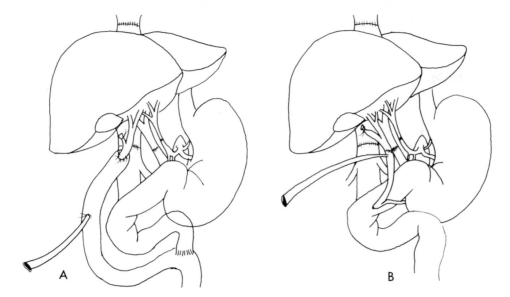

Fig. 12-38. Completed orthotopic liver transplant with **A,** Roux-en-Y biliary reconstruction and **B,** end-to-end anastomosis of the donor-to-recipient common bile ducts. (From Ascher, N.L., and others: In Simmons, R.L., and others, editors: Manual of vascular access, organ donation, and transplantation, New York, 1984, Springer-Verlag.)

9. In situations in which the portal vein anastomosis may obstruct the ability to anastomose the hepatic artery, the hepatic artery anastomosis may be performed before that of the portal vein. Clamps are removed from the vena cava sites, the portal vein, and the hepatic artery simultaneously.

10. Modifications in the method of arterial reconstruction may be necessary, depending on the anatomic structure of the donor organ and the recipient's remaining hepatic arterial stump.

11. The post-revascularization phase focuses on achieving hemostasis. Complete hemostasis may require extensive time at this point. Bleeding may be exacerbated by a fibrinolytic episode associated with the reperfusion of the donor organ.

12. Biliary reconstruction varies with the status of the recipient's biliary tract. If biliary atresia is the cause of the patient's end-stage liver disease, choledochoenterostomy into a Roux-en-Y loop of jejunum is performed (Fig. 12-38, *A*). Sclerosing cholangitis also necessitates this biliary reconstruction procedure. An end-to-end reconstruction of the common bile duct may be possible if the recipient's biliary tract is free of disease and a T tube can be placed in the native duct (Fig. 12-38, *B*).

13. Drains are inserted and exit through the right abdominal wall.

14. The abdomen is then closed.

Donor hepatectomy

Donor hepatectomy is performed for procurement of a healthy liver for transplant into a patient suffering from end-stage liver failure. This procedure occurs only after the donor patient has been determined to be brain-dead and family consent for organ donation has been obtained.

Donor hepatectomy can be performed at any hospital. Organ procurement agencies arrange contact with transplant centers when a viable organ donor has been identified. Candidates for liver transplants are placed on a national network waiting list and are matched according to urgency of need, blood type, and body size.

Procedural considerations. Once the liver transplant candidate has been identified, the procurement team from that transplant center travels to the institution where the organ donor is hospitalized. If multiple organs are being donated, surgeons from several transplant centers may arrive to procure the organs they will be transplanting at their respective centers.

The procedure for procurement of multiple organs may differ according to the transplant centers represented. Most commonly the systemic cooling of the donor's body temperature is started prior to the procurement of the heart. Cannulation sites may also vary according to which organs are procured.

The perioperative nurses at the donor hospital are responsible for supplying a basic laparotomy setup with instrumentation to open the sternum. Basic vascular clamps are also required for clamping the major vascular structures. Cold lactated Ringer's solution for parenteral infusion and cold Ringer's solution for irrigation are usually used in large amounts.

Perioperative nurses involved in organ procurement procedures must first consider their ethical and moral beliefs. Often, the organ donor is a young and otherwise healthy individual who does not exhibit outward signs of death. The donor is brought to the surgical suite on life-support systems. The donor may appear as any patient would under general anesthesia. Strong feelings of uncertainty, denial, and internalization of fear for one's own loved ones must be dealt with appropriately. Perioperative nurses involved with organ procurement procedures must support and respect each person's feelings as that individual may be grieving for the donor and his or her family during and long after the procedure is completed.

Operative procedure

1. The donor is positioned supine on the OR bed. The skin area from neck to mid-thigh is prepped and draped.
2. A midline incision is made from the suprasternal notch to the pubis. A subcostal incision is performed bilaterally on the abdomen for better exposure of the abdominal viscera.
3. Retractors are placed to provide optimal exposure of the organs that will be procured. The aorta and vena cava, superior and inferior to the liver and kidneys, are skeletalized by dissection and ligation of the lymphatics and smaller vasculatures. The porta hepatis is dissected; the superior mesenteric artery and celiac trunk are dissected and delicately exposed as close to the aorta as is convenient.
4. The superior mesenteric vein is dissected and prepared for cannulation. The donor is heparinized and systemically cooled.
5. If the heart is to be procured, at this point in the procedure the patient is pronounced dead, and the procurement of the heart is achieved.
6. Further cooling and flushing of the pancreas, liver, and kidneys are achieved by cannulation and infusion of cold Ringer's lactate via the inferior vena cava just superior to the bifurcation. One to 2 L of lactated Ringer's solution are infused before the organs have been properly cooled.
7. The liver, pancreas, spleen, and a segment of the duodenum harboring the pancreatic duct are procured en bloc by placing clamps on the suprahepatic and infrahepatic venae cavae. The suprahepatic vena cava is transected with a surrounding cuff of diaphragm intact. The infrahepatic vena cava is transected above the level of the renal veins. The celiac axis is detached from the aorta with an aortic patch or taken with a full aortic circumference. The duodenal segment is procured, using a linear stapling device at opposite ends of the segment.
8. The en bloc organs are taken to a back table for further dissection and ligation to separate the liver from the en bloc pancreas, spleen, and duodenal segment graft. Meanwhile, other members of the procurement team continue working to free the kidneys and ureters if they are to be taken.

9. The liver is placed in a basin of very cold Ringer's solution, double-bagged in sterile Lahey bags, and placed in an ice chest for transport to the recipient's hospital.
10. The kidneys are placed in sterile cassettes and mechanically perfused.
11. The pancreatic en bloc graft is also placed in a basin of cold Ringer's solution, bagged, and transported in a thermal chest of ice.
12. The abdomen is closed with a single layer of nonabsorbable no. 1 or 0 suture.
13. Drapes are removed, and the body is cleaned and washed. Tubes and infusion lines are tied off or clamped.
14. Sometimes the family of the donor requests to view the body following organ donation. This factor may be important in helping them face the loss of their loved one. The perioperative nurse can assist them in their grieving process by providing them with a quiet and private environment in which to say good-bye to their family member. Removing the donor's body from the OR where the surgical procedure took place is best. The nurse should make sure that the donor is clothed and covered with a warm blanket and then stay with the family to support them through this most painful realization.
15. Morgue care is performed, and the donor is transported via stretcher to the morgue.

Operation on the spleen
Splenectomy

Splenectomy is removal of the spleen. It is usually performed for trauma to the spleen, for specific conditions of the blood such as hemolytic jaundice or splenic anemia, or for tumors, cysts, or splenomegaly. Another common indication for splenectomy is accidental injury to the spleen during vagotomy or other gastric procedures or operations involving mobilization of the splenic flexure of the colon. If accessory spleens are present, they are also removed, as they are capable of perpetuating hypersplenic function.

Procedural considerations. Massive splenomegaly may occasionally require a thoracoabdominal approach. Abdominal suction apparatus should be available throughout all splenectomies.

Instrumentation is as described for a basic laparotomy, plus two large, right-angled pedicle clamps, long instruments, and hemostatic materials or devices.

Operative procedure

1. The abdomen is opened through an upper midline or left subcostal incision. Retractors are placed over laparotomy packs, and gentle retraction is employed as exploration is carried out. The costal margin is retracted upward.
2. The splenorenal, splenocolic, and gastrosplenic ligaments are clamped and divided with long dressing for-

ceps, long hemostats, sponges on holders, and long Metzenbaum or Nelson scissors. Adhesions posterior to the spleen are freed.

3. The spleen is delivered into the wound after these attachments are freed. The short gastric vessels are now easily identified, clamped, divided, and ligated.

4. The cavity formerly occupied by the spleen is packed with moist laparotomy pads, if necessary.

5. The splenic artery and vein are dissected free with fine dissecting scissors and forceps.

6. The artery is clamped and doubly ligated with silk. The artery is ligated first, and then the vein, thus permitting disengorgement of blood from the spleen and facilitating the return of venous blood to the circulatory system.

7. The splenic vein is clamped, divided, and ligated.

8. The specimen is removed; all bleeding vessels are controlled.

9. The wound is closed in layers, as described for laparotomy, and dressings are applied. Drainage is usually required only if many adhesions to the diaphragm were divided or if significant clotting abnormalities exist.

Trauma

Few patients require as much of a perioperative nurse's expertise as does a trauma patient. Often the demand occurs during the night when the nurse is on call.

Trauma is the third leading cause of death in the United States, following coronary artery disease and cancer. For people under 40 years of age, it is the number one cause of death. Traumatic emergencies include serious injury to the head, chest, or abdomen and loss of a limb. A trauma patient may also require immediate surgery to stop internal bleeding. Gunshots, knife stabbings, and automobile accidents cause many of these life-threatening injuries. Trauma centers have been established, and hospital operating rooms, with specialized equipment and trained staff, are increasingly called on to handle the severely injured patient.

Trauma is a specialty that involves a combination of emergency department, perioperative, and intensive care nursing expertise. Many times the perioperative nurse encounters a situation requiring skills that previously were expected only of intensive care nurses, for example, setting up central venous pressure (CVP) and arterial lines, administering emergency drugs, and performing a nursing assessment of the traumatized patient.

Procedural considerations in care of trauma patients. After receiving notification of the trauma patient's arrival, the perioperative nurse should check with the emergency department personnel or the surgeon to determine exactly what procedure(s) is to be done. If possible, the patient is examined and a nursing assessment that focuses on immediate priorities is performed. A report should be obtained from the emergency department nurse

regarding the patient's allergies, oral intake status, fluid replacement, traumatized parts of the body, and any other pertinent information. An exploratory laparotomy may be scheduled first. The patient may come to the operating room intubated and attached to a respirator, with peripheral intravenous lines or a CVP line, a Foley catheter (which should be attached to a urinometer), a nasogastric tube, and sometimes an arterial line in place.

On the patient's arrival in the operating room, the nurse must remember that this patient is a person and not a "trauma case." Getting caught up in the excitement and forgetting about the human, interpersonal aspects can be easy. The nurse should talk to the patient, even if he or she is unconscious, and explain what is being done.

If the hospital has a helicopter base station, the patient may be received in the helicopter basket, which presents a problem of transferring the patient to the operating room bed. In this case, sterile technique often becomes secondary in importance to the emergency of the situation. Emergency department personnel who help transport the patient may have to enter the operating room suite wearing their uniforms or street clothes.

The patient sometimes arrives wearing a military antishock trouser (MAST) suit. The suit is usually applied at the scene of the accident or in the emergency department. It is used in cases of hemorrhagic injury and is said to increase central venous pressure and improve cardiac filling. The suit is in one piece, similar to a pair of wraparound trousers. The trousers enclose the body from the ankles up to the rib cage. The suit is inflated by a foot pump until the exterior of the suit is smooth. The MAST suit should not be removed by anyone but the surgeon except by the surgeon's specific order. When the suit is deflated, the patient's blood pressure usually drops, sometimes drastically. The abdominal compartment is deflated first, then each leg section. If the blood pressure drops too low after the abdominal compartment is deflated, the leg trousers may be kept inflated during the surgery. If the patient's blood pressure is too low, either a skin prep may not be done or some prepping solution can be quickly applied to the operative site.

The packs, instruments, and needed supplies should be opened before the patient arrives. If possible, the patient's x-ray studies should be in the room. A thermia blanket on the operating room bed is a good idea, as is having the autotransfuser or Cell Saver available and assembled, ready for use.

The perioperative nurse quickly assesses and prioritizes the immediate needs of the surgical trauma patient upon entering the OR suite. Priorities follow the ABCs (airway, breathing, circulation) established by the Committee on Trauma of the American College of Surgeons (Moylan, 1987).

Tracheostomy may be required if intubation is not possible, as in the case of extensive facial injuries. Once a stable airway is established, breathing is most likely accomplished by attachment of a ventilating system.

Hypovolemic shock and the management and/or resuscitation of the circulatory system are the next priority. Large-bore peripheral access cannulae, cutdown trays, and IV solutions of 0.9% saline or lactated Ringer's should be readily available with blood infusion tubing attached. Blood-warming units should also be available.

Blood specimens for typing and cross-matching blood products are sent as quickly as possible. A supply of O-negative blood should be available if the need to reestablish blood volume is crucial. Commercially available ansanguineous solutions such as colloids, crystalloids, and electrolytes may be required to assist in the initial treatment of the hypovolemic patient.

Colloids are suspensions of varying molecular weight particles such as plasma, albumin, dextran, and hydroxyethyl starch. They are sometimes referred to as *plasma expanders* and can assist in initial hypovolemic shock therapy.

Crystalloids are solutions that contain nonionizing particles such as glucose. A most common example is dextrose 5% in water.

Electrolyte solutions, such as 0.9% saline and lactated Ringer's solution, are most often used to treat hypovolemic shock until typed and cross-matched blood products are available.

When patients receive large volumes of blood transfusions (more than 10 units), they may begin to exhibit signs of coagulopathies. Generally, one unit of fresh-frozen plasma (FFP) is given for every 4 to 5 units of packed red blood cells. Ten units of platelets are usually given for every 8 to 10 units of packed red blood cells transfused. A hematocrit of 30% to 35% is the goal for red blood cell replacement. The blood bank should be alerted early as to the potential need for FFP and platelets

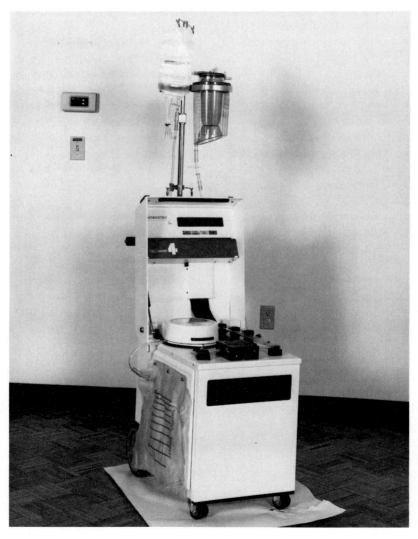

Fig. 12-39. Cell Saver autologous blood recovery system, with Bentley cardiotomy reservoir. (Courtesy Haemonetics Corp., Braintree, Mass.)

so that thawing bath time does not compromise the patient's condition.

Attention is next given to initiation of the operative procedure. Autotransfusion can be used to preserve the patient's own blood loss for reinfusion.

Autotransfusion. The purpose of the autotransfuser is to retrieve blood from and return it to a traumatically injured patient. Autotransfusion is contraindicated if the wounds are more than 4 hours old, if the patient has cancer, or if gross contamination from bowel or stomach contents has occurred. The blood is immediately available, fresh, and type specific for the patient. Hemothorax is the most frequent indication for autotransfusion; others include injury to the liver, spleen, chest wall, heart, pulmonary vessels, kidney, iliac vein, portal vein, and inferior vena cava. Using a patient as a self-donor was first reported in 1818. Since that time, autotransfusers that are safe and relatively simple to use have been manufactured.

Autotransfusion is indicated whenever enough uncontaminated blood is recovered to make transfusion worthwhile, that is, 2 or 3 units. Autotransfusion is especially useful if there is a blood shortage or the patient has a rare blood type. Because the blood is the patient's own, transfusion reactions are decreased.

Growing use and acceptability of autotransfusion have decreased the potential of transferring diseases such as hepatitis and acquired immune deficiency syndrome (AIDS) through donor blood transfusions. Patients can donate their own blood before elective procedures such as total joint replacement or spinal fusion, or surgeons can elect to have a sophisticated system such as the Cell Saver (Fig. 12-39) available during surgical procedures that have potential for large-volume blood loss, such as those associated with trauma. A Cell Saver returns washed red blood cells to the patient; an autotransfusion system returns filtered, anticoagulated blood. Autotransfusion methods

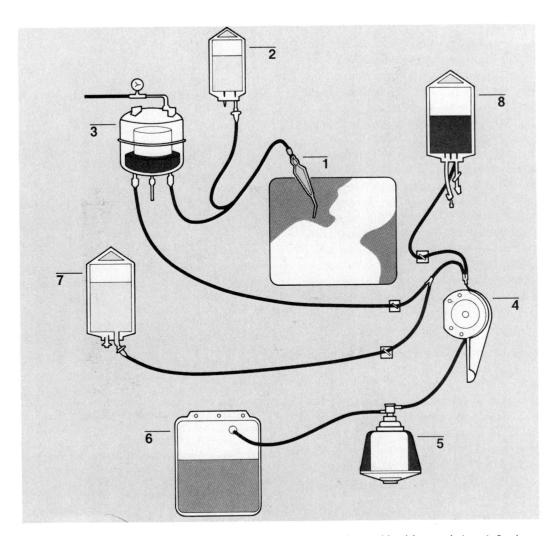

Fig. 12-40. Cell Saver method of recovering and collecting autologous blood for transfusion. *1,* Suction from patient. *2,* Anticoagulant. *3,* Collection reservoir. *4,* Pump. *5,* Centrifuge bowl. *6,* Waste bag. *7,* Sterile saline solution. *8,* Reinfusion bag. (Courtesy Haemonetics Corp., Braintree, Mass.)

provide intraoperative salvage without disease transmission, transfusion reaction, or compatibility testing.

The Cell Saver method of preparing autologous blood for transfusion is shown in Fig. 12-40. During surgery, shed blood is *(1)* suctioned from the surgical field and *(2)* anticoagulated. The sterile collection reservoir *(3)* filters out tissue, clots, orthopedic cement, and other macrodebris and stores the blood, ready for processing or other disposal. Blood from the reservoir is pumped *(4)* into the spinning centrifuge bowl *(5)*. The centrifugal force within the bowl captures the red blood cells (RBCs). Plasma overflows from the bowl into the waste bag *(6)*, taking with it free hemoglobin, irrigation fluids, and activated clotting factors. When the hematocrit within the bowl reaches approximately 50%, sterile normal saline *(7)* is pumped through the centrifuge bowl, washing the packed red cells. At the completion of the wash cycle, packed RBCs suspended in saline are pumped from the centrifuge bowl to the reinfusion bag *(8)* for return to the patient. The procedure is fast and requires minimal supervision by the operator.

Systems such as the autotransfuser and the Cell Saver eliminate the risk of transfusion-related diseases and associated costs, including length of hospital stay, an important factor in the era of diagnosis-related groups (DRGs) and other cost-containment measures. The use of both systems has created positive outcomes for the trauma patient.

Operative procedure for abdominal trauma. Exploratory laparotomy is performed for abdominal trauma following assessment and evaluation of objective data related to the injury. The decision regarding laparotomy is based on physical examination, the condition of the patient, laboratory studies, plain x-ray films, peritoneal lavage, and other special studies such as CT scan, ultrasound, or arteriography (Moylan, 1987).

In cases in which the patient's condition warrants rapid intervention, such as in hypovolemic shock, exploratory laparotomy is performed for visible signs of blunt or penetrating trauma wounds to the abdomen.

1. The patient is positioned supine and prepped and draped as described for laparotomy (Chapter 11).
2. A midline incision is made with a knife blade, and then underlying tissues are dissected and coagulated with an electrosurgical blade.
3. The peritoneal cavity is opened, and a large Richardson retractor is inserted. Visual and manual examination of the large organs and vessels may be facilitated by the use of two suction lines and copious amounts of warm irrigating solution.
4. In the case of profuse abdominal injury, layers of large, thick clots need to be manually removed from the abdominal cavity. These large clots may contain bullet fragments, in the case of a gunshot wound, or other

foreign objects. The volume of clotted blood should be calculated into the blood volume loss for planning fluid replacement therapy.
5. Injuries are surgically repaired by oversewing or resection of the involved anatomy.
6. Drains are inserted, the abdomen is closed, and a protective dressing is applied.
7. The patient's condition is evaluated, and a report is given to the PACU or SICU (surgical intensive care unit) nurse, depending upon which unit the patient is transferred to for postoperative observation.

REFERENCES

McDermott, W.V.: Surgery of the liver, Boston, 1989, Blackwell Scientific Publications.

Martin, E.W., and others: Radioimmunoguided surgery using monoclonal antibody, Am. J. Surg. 156, 1988.

Moylan, J.A.: Trauma surgery, Philadelphia, 1987, J.B. Lippincott Co.

Phipps, W.J., Long, B.C., and Woods, N.F.: Medical-surgical nursing concepts and clinical practice, ed. 3, St. Louis, 1987, The C.V. Mosby Company.

Way, L.W., and Pellegrini, C.A.: Surgery of the gallbladder and bile ducts, Philadelphia, 1987, W.B. Saunders Co.

BIBLIOGRAPHY

Budassi, S.S.: Giving an autotransfusion with MAST, Nursing 81 11(10):50, 1981.

Budassi, S.S., and Barber, J.M.: Emergency nursing: principles and practice, ed. 2, St. Louis, 1985, The C.V. Mosby Co.

Calne, R.Y., and Della Rovere, G.Q.: Liver surgery, Philadelphia, 1982, W.B. Saunders Co.

Cooperman, A.M., and Hoerr, S.O., editors: Surgery of the pancreas: a text and atlas, St. Louis, 1978, The C.V. Mosby Co.

Davis, J.H., and others: Clinical surgery, vol. 2, St. Louis, 1987, The C.V. Mosby Co.

Davis, J.W., McKone, T.K., and Cram, A.: Hemodynamic effects of military antishock trousers (MAST) in experimental cardiac tamponade, Ann. Emerg. Med. 10:185, 1981.

Ellis, H., and Watsell, C.: General surgery for nurses, ed. 2, London, 1980, Blackwell Scientific Publications.

Freeman, M.C., Flanagan, M.E., and Champion, H.R.: Perioperative nursing care of the multiple trauma patient: when seconds count, AORN J. 50:1, 1989.

Gips, C.H., and Krom, R.A.: Progress in liver transplantation, Boston, 1985, Martinus Nijhoff Publishers.

Herlihy, B.: Hepatic and biliary systems, Crit. Care Nurse 4:104, 1984.

Liechty, R.D., and Soper, R.T.: Synopsis of surgery, ed. 5, St. Louis, 1985, The C.V. Mosby Co.

Maddrey, W.C.: Transplantation of the liver, New York, 1988, Elsevier Science Publishing Co.

Minton, J.P., and others: Results of surgical excision of one to 13 hepatic metastases in 98 consecutive patients, Arch. Surg. 124, 1989.

Najarian, J.S., and Delaney, J.P.: Advances in hepatic, biliary and pancreatic surgery, Chicago, 1984, Year Book Medical Publishers.

Ricker, L.E., and others: Colorectal carcinoma: using a gamma counter to find recurrent tumors, AORN J. 50:5, 1989.

Sabiston, D.C., Jr., editor: Davis-Christopher textbook of surgery: the biological basis of modern surgical practice, ed. 12, Philadelphia, 1981, W.B. Saunders Co.

Toledo-Pereyra, L.H.: Pancreas transplantation, Boston, 1988, Kluwer Academic Publishers.

13 Repair of hernias

LYNDA R. PETTY

A hernia is a protrusion or the displacement of intraabdominal tissue or viscus through a congenital or acquired opening or fascial defect in the abdominal wall. In general, hernias of the abdominal wall occur far less frequently in women than in men, with the greatest disparity in the incidence of indirect and direct inguinal hernias.

In the United States, the incidence of hernias has been estimated to be 50 per 1000 population; men are affected (8%) more than women (1%) (Lichtenstein, 1986). Femoral hernias are more evenly distributed between men and women and account for more than 5% of all hernias in both sexes. About 75% of hernias occur in the groin, with the remaining 25% distributed among ventral, umbilical, femoral, and other types. As the frequency and magnitude of abdominal surgery have increased in recent years, so has the incidence of incisional hernia.

Herniorrhaphy is one of the most common operative procedures performed and is the preferred treatment for all population groups when a defect is detected. In the mid-1980s, hernia repair was second only to hysterectomy as the most common major surgical intervention in this country (Lichtenstein, 1986).

Hernias have a tremendous economic significance in the United States. In 1983, 500,000 hernias were repaired, accounting for approximately 10 million lost work days at a staggering cost to the nation's economy (Lichtenstein, 1986). A hernia can occur in several places in the abdominal wall, with protrusion of a portion of the parietal peritoneum and often a part of the intestine. The weak places or intervals in the abdominal aponeurosis are (1) the inguinal canals, (2) the femoral rings, and (3) the umbilicus. Any number of conditions causing increased pressure within the abdomen can contribute to the formation of a hernia. Contributing factors to hernia formation include age, sex, previous surgery, obesity, nutritional state, and pulmonary and cardiac disease. Loss of tissue turgor occurs with aging and in chronic debilitating diseases.

SURGICAL ANATOMY

A *hernia* is a sac lined by peritoneum that protrudes through a defect in the layers of the abdominal wall. Generally, a hernial mass is composed of covering tissues, a peritoneal sac, and any contained viscera. Hernias may be acquired or congenital.

Depending on their location, hernias are classified as direct inguinal, indirect inguinal, femoral, umbilical, or epigastric. Hernias in any of these groups are either *reducible* or *irreducible;* that is, the contents of the hernia sac either can be returned to the normal intraabdominal position or are trapped in the extraabdominal sac *(incarcerated)*. The conditions preventing the return of the hernial contents to the abdomen can result from (1) adhesions between the contents of the sac and the inner lining of the sac, (2) adhesions among the contents of the sac, or (3) narrowing of the neck of the sac. Patients with incarcerated hernias may have signs of intestinal obstruction, such as vomiting and distention. The great danger of an incarcerated hernia is that it may become *strangulated.* In a strangulated hernia the blood supply of the trapped sac contents becomes compromised, and eventually the sac contents necrose. When bowel is trapped in such a hernia, resection of necrosed bowel, in addition to the repair of the hernia defect, becomes mandatory.

Inguinal hernias

The anterolateral abdominal wall consists of an arrangement of muscles, fascial layers, and muscular aponeuroses lined interiorly by peritoneum and exteriorly by skin (Figs. 13-1 and 13-2). The abdominal wall in the groin area is composed of two groups of these structures: a superficial group—Scarpa's fascia, external and internal oblique muscles, and their aponeuroses—and a deep group—the internal oblique transverse fascia and peritoneum.

Essential to an understanding of inguinal hernia repair is an appreciation of the central role of the transversalis fascia as the major supporting structure of the posterior inguinal floor. The inguinal canal, which contains the spermatic cord and associated structures in males and the round ligament in females, is approximately 4 cm long and takes an oblique course parallel to the groin crease. The inguinal canal is covered by the aponeurosis of the external abdominal oblique muscle, which forms a roof (Fig. 13-3). A thickened lower border of the external oblique aponeurosis forms the inguinal (Poupart's) ligament. This ligament stretches from the anterior superior iliac spine to the pubic tubercle. Structures that traverse the inguinal canal enter it from the abdomen by the internal ring, a natural opening in the transversalis fascia, and exit by the external

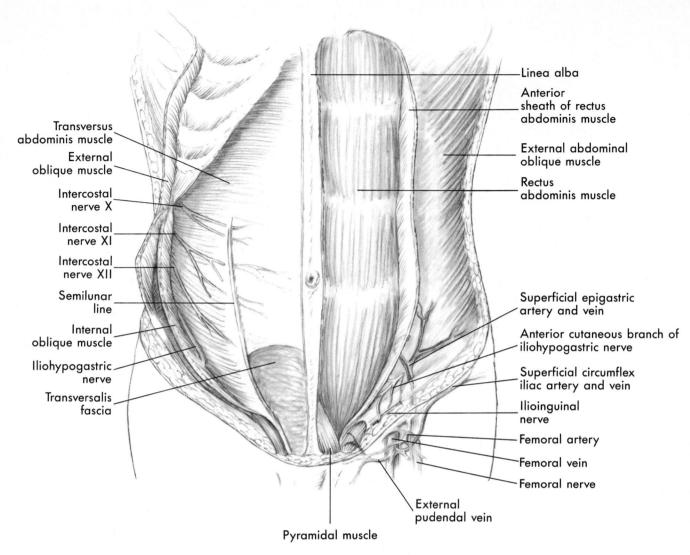

Labels (clockwise from upper left):

Transversus abdominis muscle

External oblique muscle

Intercostal nerve X

Intercostal nerve XI

Intercostal nerve XII

Semilunar line

Internal oblique muscle

Iliohypogastric nerve

Transversalis fascia

Pyramidal muscle

External pudendal vein

Femoral nerve

Femoral vein

Femoral artery

Ilioinguinal nerve

Superficial circumflex iliac artery and vein

Anterior cutaneous branch of iliohypogastric nerve

Superficial epigastric artery and vein

Rectus abdominis muscle

External abdominal oblique muscle

Anterior sheath of rectus abdominis muscle

Linea alba

Fig. 13-1. Perspective of the anterior abdominal wall illustrating the layers of musculature, aponeurotic extensions, vasculature, and innervation. (From Davis, J.H., and others: Clinical surgery, vol. 2, St. Louis, 1987, The C.V. Mosby Co.)

ring, an opening in the external oblique aponeurosis to go to either the testis or the labium. If the external oblique aponeurosis is opened and the cord or round ligament mobilized, the floor of the inguinal canal is exposed. The posterior inguinal floor is the structure that becomes defective and is susceptible to indirect, direct, or femoral hernias.

The key component of the important posterior inguinal floor is the transversalis muscle of the abdomen and its associated aponeurosis and fascia. The posterior inguinal floor can be divided into two areas. The superior lateral area represents the internal ring, whereas the inferior medial area represents the attachment of the transversalis aponeurosis and fascia to Cooper's ligament (iliopectineal line). Cooper's ligament is the site of the insertion of the transversalis aponeurosis along the superior ramus from the symphysis pubis laterally to the femoral sheath. Note

that the inguinal portion of the transversalis fascia arises from the iliopsoas fascia and not from the inguinal ligament.

Medially and superiorly, the transversalis muscle becomes aponeurotic and fuses with the aponeurosis of the internal oblique muscle to form anterior and posterior rectus sheaths. As the symphysis pubis is approached, the contributions from the internal oblique muscle become less and less. At the pubic tubercle and behind the spermatic cord or round ligament, the internal oblique muscle makes no contribution, and the posterior inguinal wall (floor of the inguinal canal) is composed solely of aponeurosis and fascia of the transversalis muscle.

None of the three groin hernias develops in the presence of a strong transversus abdominis layer and in the absence of persistent stress on the connective tissue layers (Nyhus and Condon, 1989).

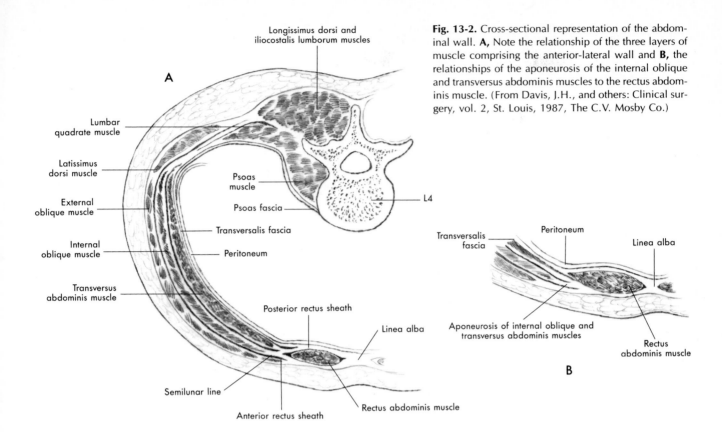

Fig. 13-2. Cross-sectional representation of the abdominal wall. **A,** Note the relationship of the three layers of muscle comprising the anterior-lateral wall and **B,** the relationships of the aponeurosis of the internal oblique and transversus abdominis muscles to the rectus abdominis muscle. (From Davis, J.H., and others: Clinical surgery, vol. 2, St. Louis, 1987, The C.V. Mosby Co.)

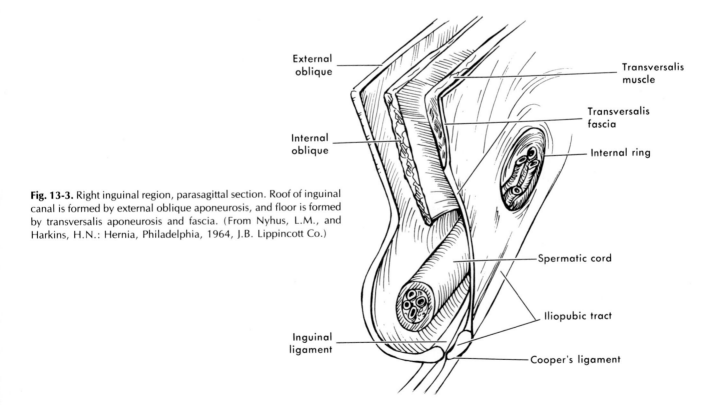

Fig. 13-3. Right inguinal region, parasagittal section. Roof of inguinal canal is formed by external oblique aponeurosis, and floor is formed by transversalis aponeurosis and fascia. (From Nyhus, L.M., and Harkins, H.N.: Hernia, Philadelphia, 1964, J.B. Lippincott Co.)

When a weakening or a tear in the aponeurosis of the transversus abdominis and the transversalis fascia occurs, the potential for development of a direct inguinal hernia is established.

Femoral hernias

When the transversus abdominis aponeurosis and its fascia are only narrowly attached to the Cooper's ligament, a femoral hernia may develop. Dilation of the femoral ring and canal, which allows for the prominence of the ilio-femoral vessels, can also result in femoral herniation.

The walls of the femoral sheath are formed anteriorly and medially from the transversalis fascia, posteriorly from pectineus and psoas fascia, and laterally from iliacus fascia. The pelvic ostium consists of a relatively fixed rim of bone and connective tissue: anteriorly and medially, the iliopubic tract; posteriorly, the superior ramus; and laterally, the iliopectineal arch.

The femoral sheath is subdivided into three compartments. The lateral compartment contains the femoral artery, and the intermediate compartment, the femoral vein. The medial compartment is the smallest and constitutes the femoral canal.

The femoral canal is formed anteriorly and medially by the iliopubic tract. Laterally, this opening is bound by the iliofemoral vessels, and posteriorly, by the superior pubic ramus and pectineus fascia. Superiorly, laterally, and inferiorly, the fossa is formed by the falciform margin of the fascia lata.

Abdominal hernias

The anterior abdominal wall is composed of external abdominal oblique muscles attached to a thick sheath of connective tissue called the *rectus sheath*. The linea alba extends superiorly and inferiorly from above the xiphoid process to the pubis. Beneath the rectus sheath lies the rectus abdominis muscles, lateral to the right and left of the linea alba. Lateral to the rectus abdominis is the linea semilunaris. The transversus abdominis muscles originate from the seventh to the twelfth costal cartilages, lumbar fascia, iliac crest, and the inguinal ligament and insert on the xiphoid process, the linea alba, and the pubic tubercle. The third layer of abdominal wall includes the internal abdominal oblique muscles originating from the iliac crest, inguinal ligament, and lumbar fascia and inserting on the tenth to twelfth ribs and rectus sheath.

Direct and indirect hernias

The deep epigastric vessels (inferior epigastric) arise from the external iliac vessels and enter the inguinal canal just proximal to the internal ring. The triangle formed by the deep epigastric vessels laterally, the inguinal ligament inferiorly, and the rectus abdominis muscle medially is referred to as Hesselbach's triangle (Fig. 13-4).

Hernias that occur within Hesselbach's triangle are called *direct inguinal hernias*. *Indirect inguinal hernias* occur lateral to the deep epigastric vessels. Therefore, both direct and indirect hernias represent attenuations or tears in the transversalis fascia (Fig. 13-5).

Direct hernias protrude into the inguinal canal but not into the cord and therefore rarely into the scrotum. Direct inguinal hernias usually result from heavy lifting or other strenuous activities.

Indirect hernias leave the abdominal cavity at the internal inguinal ring and pass with the cord structures down the inguinal canal. Consequently the indirect hernia sac may be found in the scrotum. Indirect hernias may be either congenital, representing a persistence of the pro-

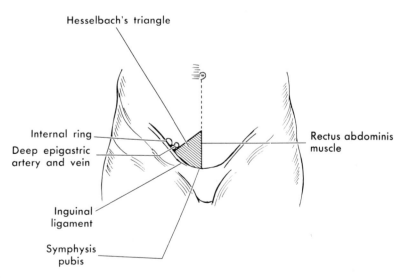

Fig. 13-4. Schematic representation of Hesselbach's triangle. Boundaries of Hesselbach's triangle are deep epigastric vessels laterally, inguinal ligament inferiorly, and rectus abdominis muscle medially.

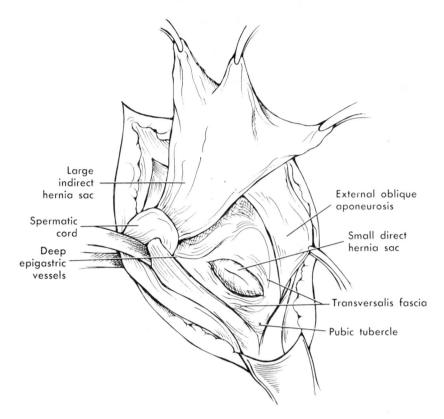

Fig. 13-5. Defect in transversalis fascia, medial to deep epigastric vessels, gives rise to direct hernia. Defect lateral to deep epigastric vessels results in indirect hernia. (From Maingot, R.: Abdominal operations, ed. 6, New York, 1974, Appleton-Century-Crofts.)

cessus vaginalis, or acquired. In a congenital hernia, the hernia sac has a small neck, is thin walled, and is closely bound to the cord structures. In an acquired indirect hernia, the neck is wide, and the sac is both short and thick walled. When both direct and indirect hernias are present, the defect is called a *pantaloon hernia* after the French word for pants, which this situation suggests.

PERIOPERATIVE NURSING CONSIDERATIONS
Assessment/nursing diagnosis

Assessment of the patient with a hernia begins with a nursing history of past surgeries related to the herniated area. The patient's occupation and physical activities may be contributing factors to the development of the hernia. A thorough nursing history includes information relating to a familial history of hernias, the patient's nutritional status, when the symptoms occurred, a history of obesity, and, in the case of females, pregnancy.

Pain is usually the first notable symptom for the patient. An accurate description of the type and degree of pain is included in the assessment.

Physical examination is the most common means for diagnosis. Palpation of the herniated area reveals the contents of the hernia sac. Fingertip palpation allows the nurse to feel the edges of the ring or abdominal wall. Having the patient stand and cough during the examination also assists in the evaluation of the herniated area.

Diagnosis for abdominal hernia is possible with ultrasonic scanning and computerized tomography (CT) when indicated.

A hernia may cause no symptoms; its only sign may be a swelling or protrusion in a restricted area of the abdominal wall. If the hernia is unilateral, the patient notes the lack of a protrusion on the other side in comparison. The area may be visible when the patient stands or coughs and may disappear on reclining.

Nursing diagnoses applicable to the patient anticipating surgery for hernia repair are:

- Anxiety/fear related to the surgical intervention
- Potential for chemical, physical, and electrical injury
- Potential for neuromuscular injury and circulatory impairment related to positioning
- Potential for infection

Planning

The perioperative nurse formulates a plan of care for the patient having surgery for hernia repair by assimilating knowledge pertaining to the anatomy involved and principles of asepsis. Instrumentation, draping, and positioning for the patient's surgery depend on the type of hernia.

Sample Care Plan

NURSING DIAGNOSIS:
Anxiety/fear related to the surgical intervention
GOAL:
Patient will demonstrate a manageable level of anxiety and responds appropriately to events associated with the surgical procedure.
INTERVENTIONS:
Note the patient's preoperative emotional status.
Maintain an atmosphere conducive to relaxation and stress reduction for the patient.
Provide emotional support.
Encourage/assist the patient with anxiety reduction (music, relaxation techniques).
If patient remains awake throughout surgical intervention, explain sequence of events and expectations.
Monitor vital signs, patient's response to stimuli, ECG, and oxygen saturation; report deviations from baseline data.

NURSING DIAGNOSIS:
Potential for chemical, physical, and electrical injury
GOAL:
The patient will be free from injury related to chemical, physical, and electrical hazards.
INTERVENTIONS:
Place electrosurgical dispersive pad on an appropriate skin surface that is dry and free of scars, lesions, hair, and skin folds.
Prevent skin preparation fluids from pooling beneath the patient or at the site of the dispersive pad.
Note the condition of skin surfaces preoperatively and postoperatively.
Keep OR bed dry and wrinkle-free.
Expose only that part of the patient necessary for skin preparation.
Assure patient safety during transport to and from OR bed.

NURSING DIAGNOSIS:
Potential for neuromuscular injury and circulatory impairment related to positioning
GOAL:
The patient will be free from injury related to positioning hazards.
INTERVENTIONS:
Determine baseline neuromuscular and tissue integrity preoperatively, and compare for postoperative variances.
Protect all bony prominences and pressure points with padding.
Place restraining straps snugly but not tightly.
Modify position of OR bed (for example, to slight lawn-chair position) as appropriate.
Provide positioning accessories such as small pillows at the lumbar curve and beneath the head as indicated for patient comfort.
Protect vulnerable neurovascular bundles from compression against hard surfaces.
Assure that all OR bed attachments (for example, arm boards and leg stirrups) are securely engaged and capable of bearing the patient's weight.
Maintain proper anatomic alignment when positioning the patient.

NURSING DIAGNOSIS:
Potential for infection related to surgical disruption of tissues
GOAL:
The patient will be free from postoperative wound infection.
INTERVENTIONS:
Maintain and monitor aseptic technique.
Assure proper ventilation and air exchange of the OR suite.
Classify surgical wound for wound surveillance.
If prescribed, obtain antibiotics for wound irrigation or systemic administration. Label all medications on the sterile field. Check patient allergies prior to the administration of antibiotics.
Document medications administered from the sterile field.

A typical care plan for a patient having surgery for repair of a hernia is shown in the Sample Care Plan.

Implementation

The patient may undergo general anesthesia, spinal or epidural block, regional anesthesia with sedation, or local anesthesia. During inguinal herniorrhaphy the surgeon may want the patient to cough or "bear down."

The patient is usually positioned supine with basic prepping and draping procedures followed (Chapter 5).

Instruments used for herniorrhaphies are those found in standard laparotomy sets (Chapter 11) or minor sets. A typical minor instrument set contains:

    8 Towel clamps, nonperforating
    6 Halsted mosquito forceps, straight
    6 Halsted mosquito forceps, curved
   10 Crile artery forceps, 5½ inches, curved
    4 Allis forceps
    2 Ochsner forceps, straight
    2 Babcock forceps
    2 Mayo-Hegar needle holders, 6 inches
    2 Webster needle holders, 4½ inches
      Metzenbaum dissecting scissors, 5½ inches, curved
      Mayo dissecting scissors, 6¾ inches, straight
      Metzenbaum dissecting scissors, 7 inches, straight
      Forester sponge forceps, 7 inches, straight
    2 Adson tissue forceps, 4¾ inches
    2 Tissue forceps, 5½ inches
      Dressing forceps, 5 inches
    2 Brophy tissue forceps, 8 inches
    2 USA retractors
    2 Volkmann rake retractors, 4 prong, blunt
    2 Volkmann rake retractors, 4 prong, sharp
    2 Richardson retractors, ¾ inch × 1 inch
    2 Richardson retractors, 1⅛ × 1⅛ inches
    2 Senn retractors
    2 Weitlaner retractors, 6½ inches
    2 Cushing vein retractors
    2 Single skin hooks
    2 Double skin hooks
    2 Knife handles, no. 3
      Knife handle, no. 7
      Knife handle, no. 4
    2 Frazier suction tips, 8 Fr and 12 Fr

A self-retaining retractor, such as a Weitlaner, facilitates the separation of tissue layers. A Penrose drain is used to retract the spermatic cord structures for better exposure. Because the peritoneal cavity may be entered in this procedure, accurate sponge, sharp, and instrument counts must be done.

With a sliding hernia or an incarcerated hernia, the possibility of having to enter the peritoneal cavity must be considered. If the hernia is strangulated, necrotic bowel must be resected, and instruments for doing a bowel anastomosis must be ready.

Repair of the inguinal hernia includes approximation of the transversalis fascia with a heavy, nonabsorbable type of suture. With some indirect hernias, only two or three sutures may be necessary. In other cases, however, up to 10 sutures in succession may be needed. Numerous types of needles are used for hernia repair. Mayo and Ferguson needles are frequently requested. Scarpa's fascia is approximated with absorbable sutures, and the skin is closed by one of several methods.

Evaluation

Evaluation of the patient having repair of a hernia should include examination of all skin surfaces to assess variances in comparison to the preoperative assessment data. The patient should awaken from general anesthesia in a reasonable amount of time without exhibiting signs of anxiety or extreme disorientation. Extubation should be timely to avoid stress on the repaired hernia site.

The evaluation of patient status can be phrased as outcome statements such as:
- The patient expressed a positive recollection of the surgical event.
- Patient's skin surfaces were free from burns or reddened areas postoperatively.
- Patient demonstrated neuromuscular function and tissue integrity normal to the individual as recorded in the preoperative baseline assessment data.
- The patient experienced normal wound healing.

The perioperative nurse gives a detailed report to the PACU nurse pertaining to the relative events and patient status during the operative procedure.

Urinary retention may occur after a herniorrhaphy, and measures must be taken to prevent overdistention of the bladder. Early ambulation is permitted to encourage the resumption of bladder and bowel functions. If the bowel has been resected because of strangulation, a nasogastric tube and suction may be required to reduce the incidence of postoperative vomiting and distention with subsequent strain on the suture line.

Postoperative inflammation or swelling of the scrotum from manipulation is reduced with the application of either a scrotal support (suspensory), ice packs, or both. The patient is reassured that ecchymosis and discomfort will diminish within a few days and that sexual functioning should not be affected.

Hospital stays for hernia patients are usually only a day or two. An uncomplicated herniorrhaphy may also be done as an outpatient procedure with the patient going home a few hours following the surgery. A patient who has had elective surgery for a hernia should be restricted from strenuous activity for at least a week and should be informed that good body alignment is necessary. If the patient's occupation involves heavy lifting or straining, some modifications may be necessary.

SURGICAL INTERVENTIONS
Operations for repair of groin hernias
Repair of inguinal hernias

Several operative procedures for repair of inguinal hernias are currently used. Approaches that reestablish the integrity of the transversalis fascia and simultaneously reestablish and strengthen the posterior inguinal floor are favored. A surgical repair in which transversalis fascia is sewn to transversalis fascia accomplishes this goal.

Procedural considerations. The patient is in the supine position for abdominal wall and inguinal and/or femoral hernia repairs. The patient's skin surface area from above the umbilicus to mid-thigh is exposed, prepped with antimicrobial solutions, and draped with sterile drapes.

Operative procedures

McVay or Cooper's ligament repair

A McVay or Cooper's ligament repair approximates transversalis fascia superiorly to the inferior insertion of the transversalis fascia along Cooper's ligament.

1. A 6-cm oblique incision is made parallel to the inguinal ligament, ending two fingerbreadths lateral to the pubic tubercle. Frequently the skin is lightly cross-hatched to facilitate later closure (Fig. 13-6).
2. The incision is carried through the superficial and deep (Scarpa's) fascia to the external oblique aponeurosis. Hemostasis is maintained with fine ties or electrocoagulation.
3. The external oblique aponeurosis is opened in the direction of its fibers to the external ring, and the aponeurotic flaps are reflected back along the iliohypogastric and ilioinguinal nerves, which are usually encountered at this point (Fig. 13-6).
4. The cremaster muscles that form an envelope around the spermatic cord and represent the continuation of the internal oblique muscles are opened and the cord exposed.
5. By gentle dissection the spermatic vessels and the vas deferens are separated. While this is being done, the cord is examined for an indirect hernia, which arises

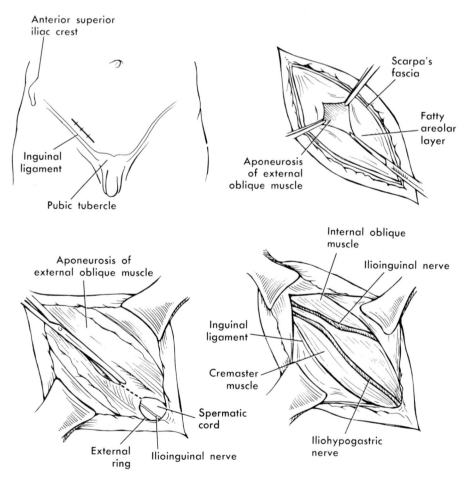

Fig. 13-6. Skin incision with division of superficial muscle and fascial layers. (From Madden, J.L.: Atlas of techniques in surgery, ed. 2, New York, 1964, Appleton-Century-Crofts.)

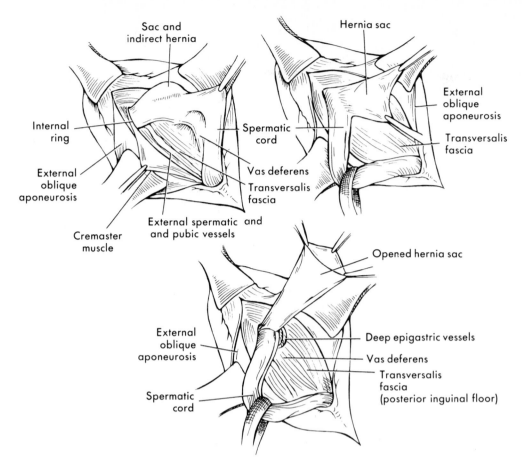

Fig. 13-7. Indirect hernia sac is identified along with cord structures and dissected away from cord. Neck of hernia sac is clearly delineated, and sac opened to check for abdominal contents. (From Madden, J.L.: Atlas of techniques in surgery, ed. 2, New York, 1964, Appleton-Century-Crofts.)

from the internal ring and is initially adherent to the cord.

6. If an indirect sac is identified, it is carefully dissected away from the cord until the neck of the hernia is clearly delineated (Fig. 13-7).

7. The sac is opened, and any abdominal contents are returned to the abdominal cavity.

8. A suture ligature is placed high in the neck of the sac, and the excess peritoneum of the hernia is excised. The ligated stump quickly retracts into the peritoneal cavity. If only a direct sac is present, usually no resection of the hernia is done because the sac easily returns to the abdominal cavity.

9. If transversalis fascia is present on both sides of the hernia defect, it is sutured together (Fig. 13-8). Suturing begins at the symphysis pubis and continues laterally to the internal ring. If the transversalis fascia inferiorly is weak or not present, the superior portion of the transversalis fascia is sutured to Cooper's ligament, the site of insertion of the transversalis fascia. In this case, suturing again begins at the pubic tubercle

and is continued laterally along Cooper's ligament to the medial border of the femoral sheath, where a transition stitch is placed. The repair is then carried laterally, approximating transversalis fascia to inguinal ligament (Fig. 13-9).

10. When the transversalis fascia is pulled down to Cooper's ligament, a relaxing incision in the rectus sheath is sometimes necessary to relieve excess tension. Essentially this incision is 5 to 7 cm long in the anterior rectus sheath. The incision begins immediately above the pubic crest, approximately 1 cm from the midline, and extends cephalad, following the line of fusion of the external oblique aponeurosis with the rectus sheath. The posterior rectus sheath and the rectus muscle itself guard against later herniation at the point where the relaxing incision is made. In some situations a prosthetic material, such as Marlex mesh, may be used to cover the hernia defect to allow repair and healing without undue stress.

11. After the integrity of the posterior inguinal floor has been reestablished, the cremaster muscles are reap-

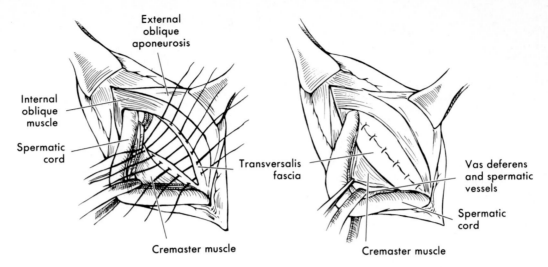

Fig. 13-8. Transversalis fascia on either side of large hernia defect is approximated. (From Madden, J.L.: Atlas of techniques in surgery, ed. 2, New York, 1964, Appleton-Century-Crofts.)

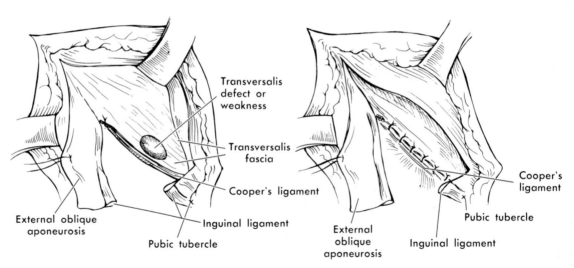

Fig. 13-9. Defect in transversalis fascia repaired by approximation of transversalis fascia to Cooper's ligament. (From Nyhus, L.M., and Harkins, H.N.: Hernia, Philadelphia, 1964, J.B. Lippincott Co.)

proximated around the cord. Repair is completed with the approximation of the external oblique aponeurosis, Scarpa's fascia, and the skin.

Bassini repair

The Bassini repair approach to the hernia and the treatment of the sac is identical to that previously described. The major difference with this repair is that the superior transversalis fascia is sutured to the inguinal ligament with no attempt made to approximate it to the inferior portion of the transversalis fascia or Cooper's ligament. Critics of this procedure claim that it is not anatomical because layers that originally are not one (transversalis fascia and inguinal ligament) now are approximated. Nonetheless, this repair

is extremely popular and is used successfully by many surgeons.

Shouldice repair

Again the approach to the hernia is the same as previously described, but in the Shouldice repair a double layer of transversalis fascia is sutured to the inguinal ligament. It is reinforced by a layer of internal oblique muscle and conjoined tendon approximated to the undersurface of the fascia of the external oblique. At the Shouldice Clinic in Toronto, where this procedure was developed and now is used exclusively, the hernia recurrence rate is about 0.6% (Nyhus and Condon, 1989).

Although the Shouldice repair is controversial as to the

popularity of the procedure, it remains a practiced alternative for those surgeons who have studied the technique.

Repair of inguinal hernias in females

Regardless of the specific technique used, the initial approach to the repair of a hernia in the female is the same as that used in the male. After the cremaster muscles are opened to expose the round ligament, variations that may be encountered include the following: (1) with the sac exposed and cleared from the round ligament, the round ligament and accompanying vessels are dissected free from the inguinal floor to the labium; (2) at the labium the round ligament is clamped, ligated, and divided; (3) the sac at the internal ring is opened, checked to be sure that no abdominal contents are present, and ligated at its neck, together with the round ligament and associated vessels; or (4) the sac distal to the ligature is removed with the distal round ligament, while the ligated stump retracts promptly into the abdomen. The remainder of the repair is the same as that previously described.

Repair of femoral hernias

A femoral hernia protrudes from the groin below the inguinal ligament into the thigh (Fig. 13-10). In its most obvious form, a femoral hernia is an inflamed, tender mass with bowel sounds below the inguinal ligament. Unfortunately, the presentation is frequently more subtle, and the diagnosis is completely missed or confused with enlarged inguinal lymph nodes, a psoas muscle abscess, a saphenous varix, or a lipoma. The defect is usually small and frequently irreducible. Femoral hernias are highly likely to incarcerate and strangulate; elective repair is clearly indicated unless serious contraindications to surgery exist (Davis and others, 1987).

Operative procedure. The general approach is surgical treatment to free the tightly bound hernia, closely examine the contents of the hernia for ischemic change, and repair the hernia defect. The principles for repair of this type of hernia are the same as those described for inguinal herniorrhaphies. Ultimately, repair of the transversalis fascia must be accomplished. Repair of femoral hernia requires approximating the aponeurotic margins of the femoral canal. The sutures are placed through the iliopubic tract superiorly and through the Cooper's ligament and pectineus fascia inferiorly.

Preperitoneal (properitoneal) repair

Preperitoneal (properitoneal) repair also is based on the essential role of the transversalis fascia in the cause and subsequent correction of a hernia. This repair is suitable for direct, indirect, and femoral hernias. It is particularly applicable in dealing with recurrent hernias because exposure is obtained by operating through virgin surgical fields rather than through previous scars.

Operative procedure

1. A transverse incision is made 2 cm above the symphysis pubis, through the rectus abdominis muscle on the affected side (Fig. 13-11, A).
2. The wound is deepened by cutting the external oblique, internal oblique, and transversalis muscles.
3. The transversalis fascia is then cut, and the preperitoneal space is entered. This is the proper plane of dissection for the remainder of the operation.
4. Retraction on the lower side of the incision reveals the posterior inguinal wall and the hernia defect.

Variations in the procedure are performed for different types of hernias.

1. If the hernia is direct, it can be reduced easily, and the superior edge of the hernia defect (the transversalis fascia) is sutured to the iliopubic tract (origin of the transversalis fascia) (Fig. 13-11, B).
2. In an indirect hernia, the sac is gently retracted from the inguinal canal. A purse-string suture is placed around the peritoneal defect as the sac is excised (Fig. 13-11, C). The lateral aspect of the internal abdominal ring is closed, and the posterior wall is reinforced as with the direct hernia.
3. In repair of a femoral hernia, the sac is again reduced by traction. After the sac is inspected for contents, a high ligation is performed. As it approaches Cooper's ligament, the defect in the posterior inguinal floor, the transversalis fascia, is clearly identified and is repaired by direct approximation (Fig. 13-11, D).

After repair of any of the foregoing hernias, the preperitoneal space is irrigated with saline solution, and the appropriate layers are approximated.

Repair of sliding hernias

Direct or indirect hernias may occur as sliding hernias. A sliding inguinal hernia occurs when the wall of a viscus forms a portion of the wall of the hernia. The most common

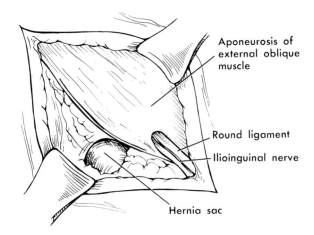

Aponeurosis of
external oblique
muscle

Round ligament

Ilioinguinal nerve

Hernia sac

Fig. 13-10. Bulge from femoral hernia occurring below inguinal ligament. (From Madden, J.L.: Atlas of techniques in surgery, ed. 2, New York, 1964, Appleton-Century-Crofts.)

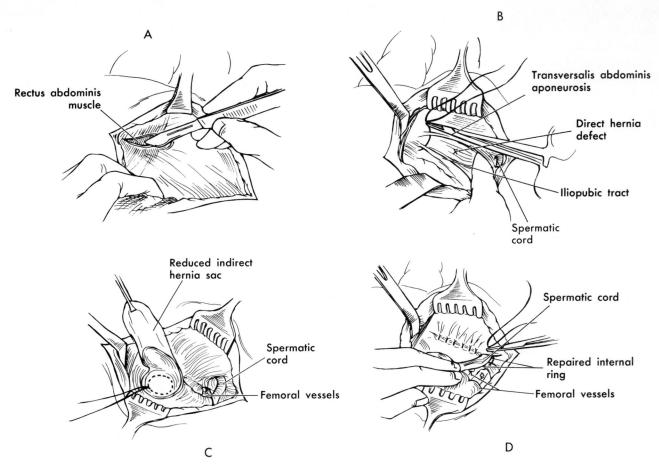

Fig. 13-11. Preperitoneal repair. **A,** Skin incision starts 2 cm above symphysis pubis and is extended through external oblique, internal oblique, and transversalis muscles. **B,** With finger in direct hernia defect, surgeon sutures transversalis abdominis aponeurosis to iliopubic tract. **C,** In case of indirect defect, sac is reduced and then excised, with high ligation being achieved by use of a purse-string suture. **D,** Internal ring is tightened after transversus abdominis aponeurosis has been approximated to iliopubic tract. (From Nyhus, L.M., and Harkins, H.N.: Hernia, Philadelphia, 1964, J.B. Lippincott Co.)

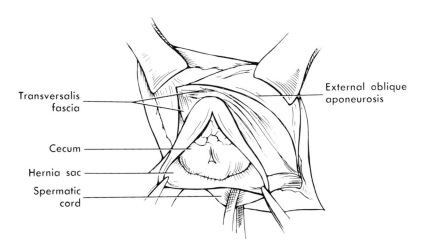

Fig. 13-12. Sliding hernia with cecum forming portion of posterior hernia sac wall. (From Madden, J.L.: Atlas of techniques in surgery, ed. 2, New York, 1964, Appleton-Century-Crofts.)

sliding hernias involve the bladder in direct hernias, the sigmoid colon in left indirect hernias, and the cecum in right indirect inguinal hernias (Fig. 13-12). This hernia must be recognized early in the repair because attempts at surgical removal of the entire sac will injure the sliding viscus.

Operative procedure. All operations designed to repair sliding hernias adhere to the basic principle of repairing the defect in the transversalis fascia. To free the bowel from the sac, the following steps must be taken:

1. The sac is opened in an area where no bowel is present and is excised medially and laterally to a point at which the bowel can be mobilized (Fig. 13-13).
2. The lateral and medial peritoneal margins are approximated.
3. The bowel is reduced to the peritoneal cavity, and high ligation of the sac is performed.
4. Repair of the transversalis fascia is done by one of the methods previously described.

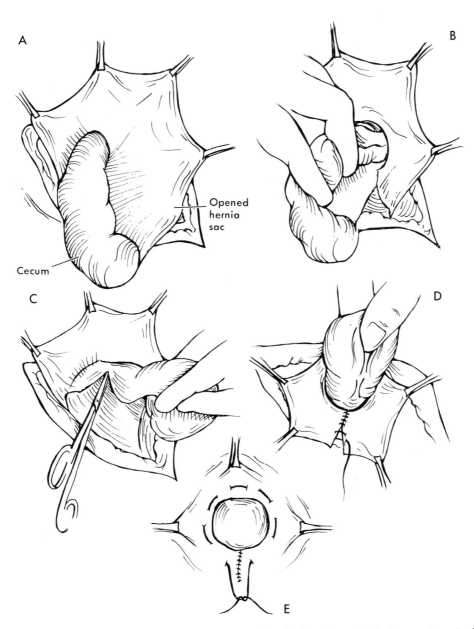

Fig. 13-13. Right sliding hernia. **A,** Cecum forms posterior wall of hernia sac. **B,** Peritoneum is excised medially, **C,** and laterally, **D,** allowing mobilization of cecum for subsequent reduction to peritoneal cavity. Lateral and medial margins are approximated. **E,** After reduction, high ligation is accomplished by using purse-string suture. (Redrawn from Ponka, J.L.: Am. J. Surg. *112*(7):52, 1966.)

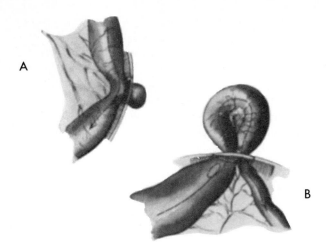

A

B

Fig. 13-14. A, Richter's hernia. Only a portion of bowel passes through hernial ring; *arrow* indicates that bowel need not be obstructed mechanically even with strangulation. **B,** Incarcerated hernia. Distended bowel in hernia cannot return to abdomen through narrow fascial defect. (From Liechty, R.D., and Soper, R.T.: Synopsis of surgery, ed. 5, St. Louis, 1985, The C.V. Mosby Co.)

Littre's hernia, Maydl's hernia, Richter's hernia

An inguinal hernia containing a Meckel's diverticulum is called Littre's hernia, and one containing two loops of bowel is called Maydl's hernia. A special type of strangulated hernia is Richter's hernia (Fig. 13-14). In this case only a part of the circumference of the bowel is incarcerated or strangulated in the hernia. Frequently it is described as a knuckle of bowel that becomes trapped and ischemic. Because initially a very small area is necrotic, diagnosis may be delayed and the probability of mortality becomes significant. Richter's hernia most frequently occurs in femoral hernias because of the small size and sharp, relatively inflexible nature of the fascial ring in this area. A strangulated Richter's hernia may be reduced spontaneously, and the gangrenous piece of intestine may be overlooked at the time of operation. Most commonly, the distal ileum is involved in Richter's hernia; however, omentum is infrequently encountered in the sac. The favored approach for repair is through the preperitoneal space.

Operations for repair of hernias of the anterior abdominal wall
Repair of ventral or incisional hernias

Ventral hernias can appear either spontaneously or after previous operations. Spontaneously occurring ventral hernias include epigastric and umbilical hernias. Postoperative ventral hernias are called *incisional hernias*. Incisional hernias appear more frequently when the original incision was a T-shaped incision or a vertical midline incision. Operations that involve a potential for contamination, such as for acute perforated ulcer or other perforated abdominal viscera, are more prone to developing subsequent ventral

hernias. A poor nutritional state with resulting hypoproteinemia predisposes some individuals to ventral hernia formation. Finally, faulty surgical technique, such as the choice of inappropriate suture materials, may result in the ultimate appearance of a ventral hernia.

Several methods have been developed for repairing ventral hernias. If all layers of the abdominal wall are easily identified, anatomic layer-by-layer repair may be done. Frequently a type of overlap method for repair is employed. Vertical and transverse overlap procedures are referred to as *vest-over-pants repairs*. For large defects, in which approximation of tissue would result in closure with excessive tension or would cause either circulatory or respiratory compromise, synthetic materials such as Marlex mesh or Gore-tex patch are employed.

When a very large fascial defect is present, a recent technique that extrapolates on the principles of tissue expansion may be used. A Tenckhoff catheter is placed percutaneously into the peritoneal cavity. Gradual expansion of the abdominal fascia is accomplished by insufflation of the abdomen with 1 to 2 L nitrous oxide gas, similar to the procedure for laparoscopy. The patient's vital signs are monitored during and after the insufflation procedure, which may be performed on a nursing unit or possibly in an outpatient clinical setting. The graduated expansion of the tissues sometimes allows for primary closure of the defect without the use of synthetic mesh or Gore-tex patch.

Repair of umbilical hernias

Umbilical hernias are extraperitoneal hernias that occur as small fascial defects under the umbilicus. They are common in children and frequently disappear spontaneously by the time a child is 2 years old. If the defect is persistent, a simple approximation of the overlying fascia is all that is necessary for repair. In adults, umbilical hernias represent a defect in the linea alba just above the umbilicus. These hernias tend to occur more frequently in obese people, making diagnosis more difficult. Umbilical hernias are potentially dangerous because they have small necks and frequently incarcerate. Surgical repair is indicated for all adults with asymptomatic umbilical hernias.

Repair of epigastric hernias

Epigastric hernias are protrusions of fat through defects in the abdominal wall between the xiphoid process and the umbilicus. Patients with epigastric hernias can have nausea, vague abdominal pain, or epigastric pain similar to that observed with cholecystitis or duodenal ulcers. Surgical repair of epigastric hernias is simple and very successful.

Repairs of spigelian hernias

The linea semilunaris, often referred to as Spigelius' line, marks the transition from muscle to aponeurosis in the transversus abdominis muscle. The area of aponeurosis that lies between the linea semilunaris and the lateral edge of the rectus muscle is referred to as the *spigelian zone*. Protrusion of a peritoneal sac, preperitoneal fat, or other abdominal viscera through a congenital or acquired defect in this area is called a *spigelian hernia*.

A spigelian hernia is usually located between the different muscle layers of the abdominal wall. For this reason, the spigelian hernia may be referred to as an *interparietal*, *interstitial*, or *intramuscular hernia*.

Spigelian hernias are uncommon and are generally difficult to diagnose. Ultrasonic scanning has improved the diagnosis of such intramural hernias. When ultrasonic scanning is not conclusive, CT can better visualize the hernia orifice.

Repair of interparietal hernias

An interparietal hernia lies between the layers of the abdominal wall. These hernias may be classified by dividing them into those that present with ventral swelling and those without ventral swelling (Nyhus and Condon, 1989).

Diagnosis is often made during an exploratory laparotomy for symptoms of intestinal obstruction.

Repair follows the same procedure as that done for a strangulated hernia. The sac contents are closely examined for ischemia, the sac is resected, and the defect repaired.

Synthetic mesh and patch repairs

Synthetic meshes, such as Mersilene or Marlex, have been particularly helpful in repairing recurrent hernias or large ventral hernias. These synthetic materials are strong and durable. Mersilene and Marlex promote fibrovascular growth within their pores, which lends extra strength to the repair. A major criticism of synthetic meshes is that, as with any foreign body implant, the risk of infection is increased.

Another synthetic material, Gore-tex patch, has become popular for the reconstruction of abdominal wall defects

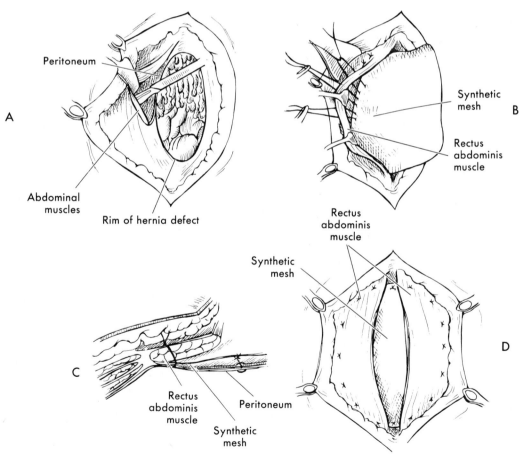

Fig. 13-15. Use of mesh in hernia repair. **A,** After layers of abdominal wall surrounding ventral hernia are identified, **B,** mesh is inserted between rectus and peritoneum. **C,** Mesh is sutured into place on one side. **D,** With moderate tension on mesh, it is inserted between appropriate layers on opposite side and is sutured into place. (From Maingot, R.: Abdominal operations, ed. 6, New York, 1974, Appleton-Century-Crofts.)

and repair of soft tissue. Gore-tex soft-tissue patch comes in both 1-cm and 2-cm thicknesses. It has been found to have reduced incidence of infection.

Essential to the use of mesh or patch in a hernia repair are the identification and cleaning of tissue planes to which the mesh or patch will be attached (Fig. 13-15, *A*). In a ventral hernia the peritoneum is dissected from the undersurface of the rectus abdominis muscle, and the mesh or patch is placed between the peritoneum and the rectus (Fig. 13-15, *B*). After the mesh or patch is positioned, it is sutured in place on one side, using the synthetic suture material compatible with the type of mesh or patch employed (Fig. 13-15, *C*).

At this point the peritoneum can be closed, if possible. If the peritoneum cannot be closed, mesh or patch can be placed directly over the omentum. The mesh or patch is then placed and sutured to the other side of the defect, with moderate tension maintained (Fig. 13-15, *D*). If possible, the mesh or patch is then covered with a fascial or muscular layer before the subcutaneous fat and skin are closed. Closed wound drainage catheters are usually placed in the wound, and antibiotics are frequently used prophylactically. Using mesh or patch to repair inguinal hernias is based on the same principles used for closing ventral hernias. With inguinal hernias the mesh or patch is sutured to transversalis fascia on both sides of the defect.

REFERENCES

Davis, J.H., and others: Clinical surgery, vol. 2, St. Louis, 1987, The C.V. Mosby Co.

Lichtenstein, I.L.: Hernia repair without disability, ed. 2, St. Louis, 1986, Ishiyaku Euroamerica, Inc.

Nyhus, L.M., and Condon, R.E.: Hernia, ed. 3, Philadelphia, 1989, J.B. Lippincott Company.

BIBLIOGRAPHY

Berlinger, S.D.: Surgery annual: 1983, 15:307, 1983.

Dunphy, J.E., and Way, L.: Current surgical diagnosis and treatment, ed. 4, Los Altos, Calif., 1979, Lange Medical Publications.

Grew, H.E., and Kremer, K.: Atlas of surgical operations, vol. 2, Philadelphia, 1980, W.B. Saunders Co.

Kleinbeck, S.V., Developing nursing diagnoses for a perioperative care plan, AORN J. 49:6, 1989.

Liechty, R.D., and Soper, R.T.: Synopsis of surgery, ed. 5, St. Louis, 1985, The C.V. Mosby Co.

Nyhus, L.M.: Symposium on hernias (guest editorial), Surg. Clin. North Am. 64:183, 1984.

Pollak, R., and Nyhus, L.M.: Complications of groin hernia repair, Surg. Clin. North Am. 63:1363, 1983.

Ponka, J.L.: Hernias of the abdominal wall, Philadelphia, 1980, W.B. Saunders Co.

Schumann, D.: How to help wound healing in your abdominal surgery patient, Nursing 80 10(4):34, 1980.

Way, L.W.: Current surgical diagnosis and treatment, ed. 8, Norwalk, Conn., 1988, Appleton & Lange.

14 Gynecologic surgery and cesarean birth

GWEN LYNN NELSON

Historically, advancements in gynecology have been based on increasing the quality of health care provided for women. Descriptions of gynecologic examinations have been traced back to the time of Hippocrates. For years the midwife performed the roles of gynecologist and obstetrician in society. As knowledge increased regarding female anatomy and its abnormalities, surgeons began to develop techniques in abdominal and pelvic surgery. In 1794, Jesse Bennett is recorded as having performed one of the earliest pelvic surgeries. Effective surgical corrections of gynecologic disorders continued in the nineteenth century. With the efficiency of laparoscopy, improvements in diagnostic and surgical interventions were marked.

Today's gynecologic surgery has built on this foundation. Some of the gynecologic specialties that have evolved include oncology, endocrinology, and infertility. The numerous developments and techniques within each of these specialty areas represent challenges for today's perioperative nurse.

Operations on the structures of the reproductive system in the female are performed for diagnostic or therapeutic purposes, for conditions such as abnormal bleeding from any of the female reproductive organs, for suspected malignant or benign neoplasms, or for infertility. Procedures are also done to remove or repair weakened anatomic structures.

SURGICAL ANATOMY

The female reproductive organs and their relationships are shown in Fig. 14-1. The adult female structures, as associated with the process of reproduction, are the bony pelvis, the associated ligaments and muscles, the soft tissues and contents of the pelvic cavity, the external organs (vulva) (Fig. 14-2), and the breasts (mammary glands).

Bony pelvis

The Latin word *pelvis* means basin. The pelvis is the part of the trunk below and behind the abdomen. The bony pelvis is composed of the ilium, symphysis pubis, ischium, sacrum, and coccyx. The so-called pelvic brim divides the abdominal false portion from the true portion of the pelvis. The abdominal false pelvis is the part above the arcuate line. The true pelvis is the part below this line. It forms the passageway through which the fetus passes during parturition.

The true pelvis may be considered as having three parts: inlet, cavity, and outlet. The muscles lining the pelvis facilitate movement of the thighs, give form to the pelvic cavity, and provide firm elastic lining to the bony pelvic framework. All organs located in the pelvis are covered by pelvic fascia (Fig. 14-3). The fascia covering some muscles is dense and firm, whereas that covering other

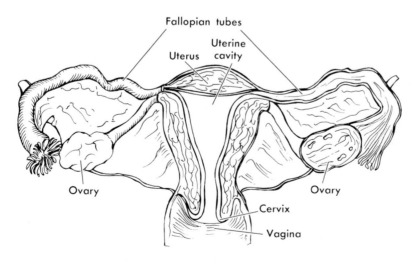

Fig. 14-1. Female reproductive organs.

287

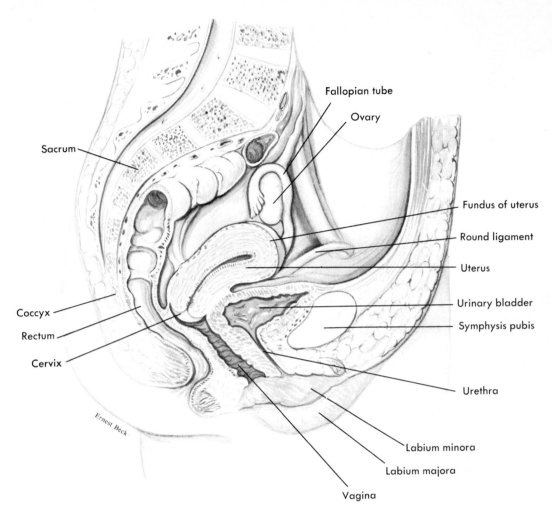

Sacrum

Coccyx

Rectum

Cervix

Ernest Beck

Fallopian tube

Ovary

Fundus of uterus

Round ligament

Uterus

Urinary bladder

Symphysis pubis

Urethra

Labium minora

Labium majora

Vagina

Fig. 14-2. Female pelvic organs as viewed in median sagittal section. (From Anthony, C.P., and Thibodeau, G.A.: Textbook of anatomy and physiology, ed. 12, St. Louis, 1987, The C.V. Mosby Co.)

organs is thin and elastic. The nerves, blood vessels, and ureters coursing through the anatomical structures are closely associated with muscular and fascial structures.

The *pelvic fascia* may be divided into three general groups: parietal, diaphragmatic, and visceral. The parietal pelvic fascia covers the muscles of the true pelvic wall and the perineum. The diaphragmatic fascia covers both sides of the pelvic diaphragm, which is made up of the levator ani and coccygeal muscles (Fig. 14-4). The visceral fascia is thin, flexible fascia that covers the pelvic organs. The *floor of the pelvis,* known as the *pelvic diaphragm,* gives support to the abdominal pelvic viscera in this region. The pelvic diaphragm, consisting of the levator ani and coccygeal muscles with their respective fascial coverings, separates the pelvic cavity from the perineum (Fig. 14-4).

The *levator ani muscles,* varying in thickness and strength, may be divided into three parts, the iliococcygeal, the pubococcygeal, and the puborectal muscles (Fig.

14-4). The fibers of the levator ani muscles blend with the muscle fibers of the rectum and vagina. The fibers (pubovaginal) of the pubococcygeal part of the levator ani muscles, lying directly below the urinary bladder, are involved in the control of micturition. The pubococcygeal fibers of the levator ani muscles control and pull the coccyx forward and assist in the closure of the pelvic outlet. The fibers pull the rectum, vagina, and bladder neck upward toward the symphysis pubis in an effort to close the pelvic outlet and are responsible for the flexure at the anorectal junction. Relaxation of the fibers during defecation permits a straightening at this junction. During parturition the action of the levator ani muscles directs the fetal head into the lower part of the passageway.

The uterus gains much of its support by its direct attachment to the vagina and by indirect attachments to nearby structures such as the rectum and pelvic diaphragm. On each side of the uterus are the broad, round, cardinal, and uterosacral ligaments and levator ani muscles (Fig. 14-5).

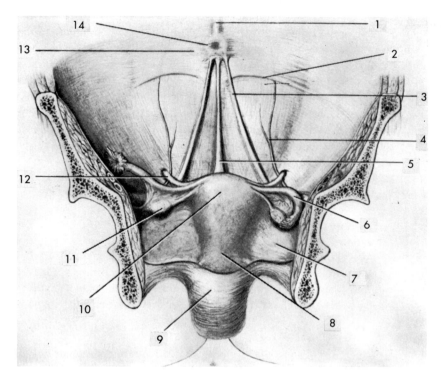

Fig. 14-3. Relationship of female sexual organs to anterior abdominal wall. *1,* Round ligament; *2,* semicircular line of Douglas; *3,* lateral umbilical ligament; *4,* inferior epigastric artery; *5,* medial umbilical ligament; *6,* fallopian tube; *7,* broad ligament; *8,* cervix; *9,* vagina; *10,* uterine corpus; *11,* ovary; *12,* round ligament; *13,* umbilical fascia; *14,* umbilicus. (From Rubin, I.C., and Novak, J.: Integrated gynecology, New York, 1956, McGraw-Hill Book Co.)

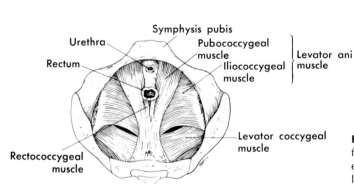

Fig. 14-4. Perineal musculature. (Redrawn from Anthony, C.P., and Thibodeau, G.A.: Textbook of anatomy and physiology, ed. 12, St. Louis, 1987, The C.V. Mosby Co.)

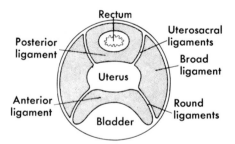

Fig. 14-5. Scheme to show relative positions of eight uterine ligaments formed by folds of peritoneum: two broad ligaments, double folds extending from uterus to side walls of pelvic cavity; two uterosacral ligaments, foldlike extensions of peritoneum from uterus to sacrum; posterior ligament, fold between uterus and rectum; and two round ligaments, folds from uterus to deep inguinal ring. (Redrawn from Anthony, C.P., and Thibodeau, G.A.: Textbook of anatomy and physiology, ed. 12, St. Louis, 1987, The C.V. Mosby Co.)

Pelvic cavity
Uterus

The *uterus* is a pear-shaped organ situated in the pelvic cavity between the bladder anteriorly and the rectum posteriorly. Its upper lateral points, the uterine cornua, receive the fallopian tubes (Fig. 14-1). The fundus of the uterus is the upper rounded portion situated above the level of the tubal openings and just below the pelvic brim. Below, the body of the uterus joins the cervix, from which it is separated by a slight constriction canal called the *isthmus*. The cervix lies at the level of the ischial spines. The body of the uterus communicates with the cervical canal at the internal orifice, called the *internal os*. The constriction (canal) ends at the vaginal portion of the cervix at the external orifice, called the *external os*. This is a small oval aperture situated between two lips.

The Greek word for uterus is *hystera*. The uterine body has three layers: (1) the outer peritoneal, or serous layer, which is a reflection of the pelvic peritoneum; (2) the myometrium, or muscular layer, which houses involuntary muscles, nerves, blood vessels, and lymphatics; and (3) the endometrium, or mucosal layer, which lines the cavity of the uterus.

The *cervix* consists of a supravaginal and a vaginal portion. The supravaginal portion is closely associated with the bladder and the ureters. The vaginal portion of the cervix projects downward and backward into the vaginal vault.

Fallopian tubes or oviducts

The Greek word *salpinx,* meaning trumpet or tube, is used to refer to the fallopian tube (Fig. 14-1). Bilateral tubes, each consisting of a musculomembranous channel about 4 to 5 inches long, form the canals through which the ova from either ovary are conveyed to the uterus. Each fallopian tube leaves the upper portion of the uterus, passes outward toward the sides of the pelvis, and ends in fringe-like projections called *fimbriae*. These fimbriae, or projections, are situated just below the ovaries. How the ova are transported from the ruptured follicles into the uterus is unknown. One theory is that transfer is accomplished through vascular changes, which together with contraction of the smooth muscle fibers of the tube and the peristaltic movements of the tube push the ova toward the uterus. The outer surfaces of the tubes are covered by peritoneum. Each tube receives its blood supply from the branches of the uterine and ovarian arteries.

The right tube and ovary are in close relationship to the cecum and appendix, and the left tube and ovary are near the sigmoid flexure. The close proximity of the fallopian tubes to the ureters should be noted.

Ovaries

The ovaries are situated at the sides of the uterus. Each ovary lies within a depression (ovarian fossa) on the lateral wall of the pelvic cavity and above the broad ligament (Fig. 14-1). The ovary is attached to the posterior surface of the broad ligament by the mesovarium and is suspended by the ovarian ligament.

The ovary, a small, almond-shaped organ, is composed of an outer layer, known as the *cortex,* and an inner vascular layer, known as the *medulla*. The cortex contains ovarian (graafian) follicles in different stages of maturity. After ovulation the corpus luteum arises from the graafian follicle that expelled the ovum. The medulla, lying within the cortex, consists of connective tissue containing nerves, blood, and lymph vessels. The ovary is covered by epithelium, not peritoneum.

The ovaries are homologous with the testes of the male. They produce ova after puberty and also function as endocrine glands, producing hormones. The hormone estrogen is secreted by the ovarian follicles. It controls the development of the secondary sexual characteristics and initiates growth of the lining of the uterus during the menstrual cycle. The hormone progesterone, which is secreted by the corpus luteum, is essential for the implantation of the fertilized ovum and for the development of the embryo.

Ligaments of the uterus

The uterine ligaments are the broad, round, cardinal, and uterosacral (Figs. 14-3 and 14-5).

Broad ligaments

From each side of the uterus the pelvic peritoneum extends laterally, downward, and posteriorly. A double fold of pelvic peritoneum forms the layers of the broad ligament, enclosing the uterus (Fig. 14-3). These layers separate to cover the floor and sides of the pelvis. The uterine tube is situated within the free border of the broad ligament. The part of the broad ligament lying immediately below the uterine tube is termed the *mesosalpinx*. The ovary lies behind the broad ligament.

Round ligaments

Round ligaments are fibromuscular bands attached to the uterus (Figs. 14-2 and 14-3). Each round ligament passes forward and laterally between the layers of the broad ligament to enter the deep inguinal ring.

Cardinal ligaments

Cardinal ligaments are composed of connective tissue with smooth muscle fibers and provide strong support for the uterus.

Uterosacral ligaments

Uterosacral ligaments are a posterior continuation of the peritoneal tissue. The ligaments pass posteriorly to the sacrum on either side of the rectum (Fig. 14-5).

Vagina

The vagina is a collapsed tubelike structure. It functions as the organ for copulation, the excretory duct for products of menstruation, and the birth canal. The anterior wall measures 6 to 8 cm in length and the posterior wall 7 to 10 cm in length (Figs. 14-1 and 14-2). The anterior wall of the vagina is in close contact with the bladder and urethra. The lower posterior wall is anteriorly adjacent to the rectum. The upper portion of the vagina lies above the pelvic floor and is surrounded by visceral pelvic fascia. The lower half is surrounded by the levator ani muscles. The walls of the vagina are lined with mucous membrane.

Fornices

The projection of the cervix into the vaginal vault divides the vault into four regions, called *fornices:* anterior and posterior and right and left lateral.

The posterior fornix is in close contact with the peritoneum of the pouch of Douglas or cul-de-sac. The rectovaginal septum lies between the vagina and rectum. The dense connective tissue separating the anterior wall of the vagina from the distal urethra is termed the *urethrovaginal septum.*

Female external genital organs (vulva)

The external organs, referred to collectively as the *vulva,* include the mons pubis, the labia majora and minora, the clitoris, the vestibule, the urethral orifice, the hymen, and various glandular structures (Fig. 14-6).

The *mons pubis* of the vulva is a rounded elevation of tissue covered by skin and, after puberty, by hair. It is situated over the anterior surface of the symphysis pubis.

The *labia majora* are two folds of skin that extend downward and backward from the mons pubis. They unite below and behind to form the posterior commissure and in front to form the anterior commissure.

The *labia minora* comprise the two delicate folds of skin that lie within the labia majora (Fig. 14-6). Each labium splits into lateral and medial parts. The lateral part forms the *prepuce of clitoris,* and the medial part forms the *frenulum.* The posterior folds of the labia are united by a delicate fold extending between them. This forms the *fossa navicularis.*

The *clitoris* is the homolog of the penis in the male. It hangs free and terminates in a rounded glans (small, sensitive vascular body). Unlike the penis, the clitoris does not contain the urethra.

The *vestibule* is a smooth area surrounded by the labia minora, with the clitoris at its apex and the fossa navicularis at its base. It contains openings for the urethra and the vagina.

The *urethra,* which is about 4 cm long, is close to the anterior vaginal wall and connects the bladder with the urethral meatus. On either side of the urethral meatus lie

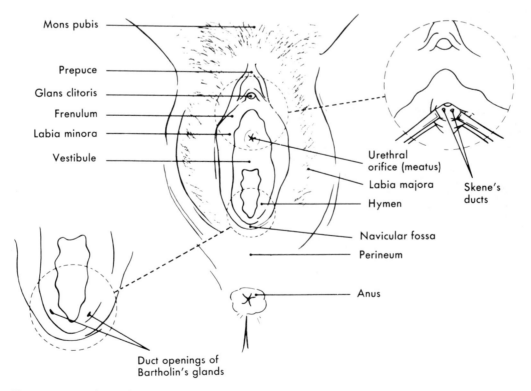

Fig. 14-6. External reproductive organs. (From Jensen, M., Benson, R.C., and Bobak, J.M.: Maternity care: the nurse and the family, ed. 2, St. Louis, 1981, The C.V. Mosby Co.)

two small ducts, termed the *paraurethral ducts,* which are commonly known as *Skene's ducts* (Fig 14-6).

The *vaginal orifice* lies below the urethral meatus. This opening extends through the hymen, which was originally a septum. The configuration and size of the opening vary and cannot be used as a determinant of a virginal state.

Bartholin's glands and ducts lie one on each side of the lower end of the vagina. They are homologs of the bulbourethral glands in the male. These narrow ducts open into the vaginal orifice on the inner aspects of the labia minora.

Vascular, nerve, and lymphatic supplies of the reproductive system

The *blood supply* of the female pelvis is derived from the internal iliac branches of the common iliac artery and is supplemented by the ovarian, superior rectal, and median sacral arteries—branches of the aorta.

The *nerve supply* of the female pelvis comes from the autonomic nerves, which enter the pelvis in the superior hypogastric plexus (presacral nerve).

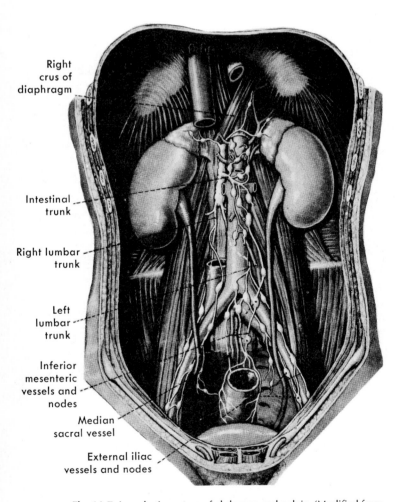

Right crus of diaphragm

Intestinal trunk

Right lumbar trunk

Left lumbar trunk

Inferior mesenteric vessels and nodes

Median sacral vessel

External iliac vessels and nodes

Fig. 14-7. Lymphatic system of abdomen and pelvis. (Modified from Hamilton, W.J., editor: Textbook of human anatomy, ed. 2, St. Louis, 1976, The C.V. Mosby Co.)

The *lymphatics* of the female pelvis either follow the course of the vessels to the iliac and preaortic nodes or empty into the inguinal glands (Fig. 14-7).

PERIOPERATIVE NURSING CONSIDERATIONS
Assessment/nursing diagnosis

The provision of quality perioperative care is dependent on thorough perioperative assessment and care planning. Data are gathered on the gynecologic patient through the review of systems, physical examination, nursing/medical histories, and diagnostic test results located in the patient record.

Initial review of the patient record permits the perioperative nurse to prioritize and validate information upon which the care plan is formulated. Through review of the history and physical, the perioperative nurse interprets and applies information to the plan of care for the individual patient and the surgical interventions to be performed.

Application of interpersonal communication techniques is vital during nursing assessment. The interview may be conducted on the patient care unit or in the holding area of the surgical suite. Open-ended questions, progressing from general to specific, are incorporated throughout this process. For example, the perioperative nurse may initially inquire about the patient's understanding of the surgical intervention to be performed and may then ask questions pertaining to intraoperative positioning, which would include the presence of back pain or limitations in joint mobility.

The assessment includes identification of the gynecologic patient's chief complaint, present problem, social history, and relevant medical and/or surgical histories. A family history includes such information as maternal use of diethylstilbestrol and deaths related to gynecologic disorders, cancer, hypertension, diabetes, and heart disease. Cultural, psychologic, and religious beliefs are identified and incorporated into the care plan. Throughout this process the perioperative nurse must remain open and supportive to assist in establishing a trusting therapeutic relationship. These factors can greatly affect the patient's perception of her intended surgery and play a major role in patient outcomes.

The gynecologic patient's history includes a chronologic listing of each pregnancy with length of gestation, type of delivery, complications during pregnancy, duration of labor, and fetal weight. The menstrual cycle is discussed to include age at onset, length of each cycle, amount of flow, duration of bleeding, and pain or discomfort associated with menses. The amount of flow is described in relationship to the number of sanitary napkins and tampons used. The perioperative nurse should inquire about a history of vaginal infections or discharge. If bleeding is present, the duration, color, and consistency of blood are noted. Questions about use of vaginal douches, creams, and contraceptives are included in the assessment.

A medication history is taken, including use of analgesics, oral contraceptives, estrogen therapy, diuretics, antihypertensives, and cardiac medications. Medication frequency, dosage, and duration of use are noted.

Gynecologic disorders may be associated with urinary problems. Stress incontinence or loss of urine while coughing, sneezing, or laughing should be identified. Pain or burning sensations upon urination are noted. The gynecologic patient may have urologic studies ordered preoperatively, especially in the presence of uterine prolapse.

Results of the physical examination are reviewed by the perioperative nurse. Baseline vital signs, height, weight, and findings from assessment of the thyroid, chest, heart, lungs, breasts, abdomen, pelvis, and rectum are analyzed for their relationship to intraoperative care planning.

The gynecologic patient may undergo numerous diagnostic studies. The studies performed depend on the gynecologic problem or disorder. A *laparoscopy* may be performed for diagnostic or therapeutic reasons. For example, a laparoscopy may be performed for infertility, pelvic pain, pelvic inflammatory disease, ova retrieval for in vitro fertilization, lysis of adhesions, evaluation of pelvic mass, removal of ectopic pregnancy, or tubal sterilization.

Gynecologic surgery is performed in close proximity to the kidneys, ureters, and bladder and may warrant a preoperative urologic exam that would include an *intravenous pyelogram* (IVP) and/or *barium enema* (BE) to establish an anatomic baseline.

Pelvic ultrasound assists in diagnosing ectopic pregnancy, adnexal pathology, and uterine pathology. Uterine fibroids and the presence of blood or fluid in the pelvis may be identified via ultrasound. *Computed tomography* (CT scanning) and *magnetic resonance imaging* (MRI) may be utilized in evaluation of the patient with suspected malignancy in the retroperitoneal lymph nodes or bone.

Preoperatively the gynecologic patient may have a hysterosalpingogram to identify abnormalities in the uterine cavity and occlusions in the tubal folds. This diagnostic tool is useful in detecting potential reasons for infertility.

A *colposcopy,* with colpomicroscopy, is often performed in the physician's office. This examination is indicated for the patient with an abnormal Pap smear suggestive of dysplasia. The diagnostic examination identifies cellular abnormalities that may involve the vulva, vagina, or cervix. It assists with identifying areas of dysplasia and carcinoma in situ. Endocervical curettage may be obtained during the colposcopic procedure to rule out invasive carcinoma or to detect early adenocarcinoma.

Comprehensive perioperative nursing care is a planned process that is implemented to ensure high-quality patient care. The perioperative nursing care plan is formulated after reviewing the patient record and conducting a complete patient assessment. All significant data collected are then incorporated into the perioperative care plan. The gynecologic patient may have multiple nursing diagnoses that warrant perioperative nursing intervention. Nursing

diagnoses for the gynecology patient may include:
- Anxiety related to surgery and surgical outcome
- Potential for urinary retention
- Potential for impaired skin integrity
- Body image disturbance
- Potential for injury related to surgical position

Planning

Planning determines the ability of the perioperative nurse to provide patient care in an organized and individualized manner. Planning involves preparation for both the psychosocial and physiologic needs of the gynecologic patient. Part of the nursing care plan is, therefore, the gathering of the required equipment and supplies and the positioning of accessories, devices, and adjuncts requisite to gynecologic surgical interventions. However, part of planning is also the development of a plan that includes goals derived from the nursing diagnoses. Once these goals are established, nursing interventions are identified that will assist the gynecologic patient to reach the desired goals. Some examples of gynecologic care plans are shown in the Sample Care Plan on pp. 294-295.

Implementation

During implementation of the plan of care, the perioperative nurse performs the identified nursing actions. Part of perioperative care plan implementation includes selecting the appropriate instruments and patient care supplies, patient positioning on the OR bed, antimicrobial skin preparation, draping, creation and maintenance of a sterile field, initiation of safety measures, and patient monitoring. Data continue to be collected, the care plan is documented, and reports are given to relief personnel.

Principles and methods of patient positioning for different types of surgical procedures are described in Chapter 6. The patient is placed in the lithotomy position for most vaginal and vulvar surgery. For abdominal gynecologic surgery, the supine with Trendelenburg's position may be used. Care should be taken to protect the patient from nerve injury and ensure adequate circulatory, renal, and respiratory functions.

Skin preparation and routine draping procedures are described in Chapter 5. A basic vaginal instrument set is required for vaginal and vulvar surgery. A basic abdominal gynecologic instrument set is required for abdominal gynecologic surgery. Surgeons' instrument preferences may vary, and the following instrument sets are not meant to be all-inclusive.

Because pelvic and vaginal procedures involve manipulation of the ureters, bladder, and urethra, indwelling urinary drainage systems are frequently established before or during operations. Either a urethral Foley catheter or a suprapubic cystostomy (Silastic) catheter may be used, depending on the surgeon's preference and the type of procedure. The size of sutures, needles, and drains also varies, depending on surgeon's preference.

Sample Care Plan

NURSING DIAGNOSIS:
Anxiety related to surgery and surgical outcome
GOAL:
Patient will experience reduced anxiety.
INTERVENTIONS:
Introduce self and establish rapport.
Determine signs and symptoms indicating presence of anxiety
  Diaphoresis
  Restlessness
  Hyperventilation
  Tachycardia
  Urinary frequency
  Nausea.
Identify maladaptive and adaptive responses to anxiety.
Encourage use of adaptive coping mechanisms.
Evaluate strengths and resources available to assist patient in coping with anxiety.
Encourage use of relaxation techniques, guided imagery, or music when appropriate for patient.
Identify patient's readiness to learn and provide individualized teaching based on these findings.
Describe sequence of perioperative events to patient in a brief, clear manner.
Use short, simple sentences.
Use calm, firm tone of voice.
Minimize environmental stimuli.
Encourage patient to ventilate feelings and concerns.
Develop therapeutic relationship with patient.
Use active listening skills.
Offer, clarify and further validate information as needed.

NURSING DIAGNOSIS:
Potential for urinary retention
GOAL:
Patient will maintain or regain normal pattern of urinary elimination.
INTERVENTIONS:
Instruct patient on importance of adequate postoperative fluid intake and early ambulation.

Prior to surgery, explain that indwelling urinary catheter will be inserted (as applicable). Review important elements of catheter care, management of drainage system, catheter removal, and signs and symptoms of urinary tract infection.
Encourage patient to verbalize feelings and concerns regarding ability to void postoperatively, presence of indwelling catheter, and catheter removal.
Clarify any misperceptions the patient may have.
Insert indwelling urinary catheter by using aseptic technique.
Obtain urine specimen as required. Connect catheter to closed drainage system.
Document size of catheter inserted and specimens obtained.
Secure tubing to patient to prevent inadvertent stretching or stress on catheter.
Place urine drainage bag where it is readily observable.
Keep drainage bag below level of bladder.
Check patency of catheter and drainage system whenever patient is repositioned.
Observe color and amount of urine; report abnormalities.
Record urinary output.

NURSING DIAGNOSIS:
Potential for impaired skin integrity
GOAL:
The patient's skin will remain intact.
INTERVENTIONS:
Note the presence of any skin rashes, bruises, lacerations, ecchymoses, petechiae, or other alterations. Record them.
Select an appropriate site of placement for electrosurgical dispersive pad (close to the operative site, on area with good muscle mass, free of excessive hair or skin oil).
Verify that patient has no known allergies to antimicrobial skin preparation agents.
Prepare operative site according to the institutional procedure.

Sample Care Plan—cont'd

Keep dependent skin areas around preparation site and electrosurgical pad dry; do not allow solutions to pool.

Keep OR bed surface free of wrinkles.

Place safety and restraining straps so that they are snug but not tight.

Apply dressings to surgical incision line and drain exit sites before surgical drapes are removed to prevent contamination of the incision; use aseptic technique.

After dressing has been applied, cleanse area surrounding incision and drain sites of blood and exudate.

Apply tape gently but firmly to secure dressing in place; allow room for postoperative swelling to prevent tape burns.

Document location of electrosurgical dispersive pad site and ECG leads, antimicrobial skin preparation solution, placement of safety and restraining straps and presence of drains.

NURSING DIAGNOSIS:
Body image disturbance
GOAL:
Patient will effectively cope with disturbance in body image.
INTERVENTIONS:
Encourage patient to express feelings about her diagnosis and surgery and how she believes it will affect her body image.

Clarify any misconceptions.

Maintain the patient's privacy.

Express understanding and assurance to the patient that her feelings and concerns are normal.

Determine patient's readiness to learn, and teach patient information relevant to her body image alteration.

Be nonjudgmental.

Demonstrate empathy and positive regard.

Identify effective coping skills previously used by patient and encourage use of these if appropriate in current situation.

Assist patient to value her present self realistically.

Encourage patient to identify her strengths.

Encourage attendance at self-help groups when appropriate.

NURSING DIAGNOSIS:
Potential for injury related to surgical position
GOAL:
The patient will be free of injury related to the surgical position.
INTERVENTIONS:
Note the presence of any preexisting patient conditions (nutritional status, weight, preoperative chemotherapy, limitations in mobility or range of motion, neurovascular impairments) that place the patient at risk for positional injury. Document them.

Preoperatively, assess and document condition of dependent skin areas.

If possible, have the patient assume the planned surgical position prior to induction of anesthesia. Plan for patient positioning based on any pain or discomfort.

Gather positioning accessories appropriate to the planned position.

Pad OR bed (eggcrate, foam, water or gel-filled mattress) as appropriate to identified patient risk factors.

Pad dependent pressure sites.

Protect vulnerable neurovascular bundles from injury.

Reassess padding and protection on any positional changes.

Maintain body alignment.

Secure patient in position with safety and body straps.

Accomplish all positioning and positional changes slowly, gently, and gradually.

Document position (and positional changes), safety measures, and accessories used.

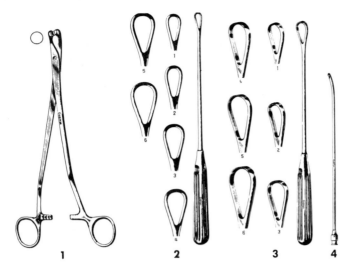

Fig. 14-8. Vaginal instruments: cutting. *1*, Gaylor biopsy forceps; *2*, Thomas uterine curettes (blunt); *3*, Sims uterine curettes (sharp); *4*, endometrial biopsy suction curette. (Courtesy Codman & Shurtleff, Inc., Randolph, Mass.)

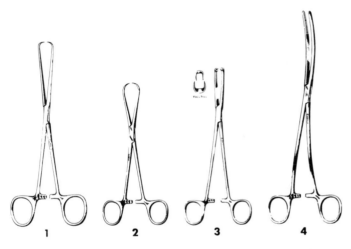

Fig. 14-9. Vaginal instruments: holding. *1*, Uterine tenaculum; *2*, Staude uterine tenaculum; *3*, Jacobs vulsellum forceps; *4*, Bozeman dressing forceps. (Courtesy Codman & Shurtleff, Inc., Randolph, Mass.)

Instrumentation

Vaginal prep set

Disposable preparation sets may be used to prepare the vagina. If they are not available, the perioperative nurse may prepare a basic vaginal prep set that includes the following:

1 Graves vaginal speculum
1 Urethral catheter, 16 or 18 Fr
1 Bozeman dressing forceps
3 Foerster sponge-holding forceps
  Gauze sponges
2 Towels
  Stainless steel cups
  Antimicrobial solutions, as desired

Basic vaginal instrument set

The basic vaginal instrument set includes the following:

Cutting instruments

1 Bard-Parker knife handle, no. 4 with blade no. 20
2 Bard-Parker knife handles, no. 3 with blade no. 10
2 Mayo dissecting scissors, 1 curved and 1 straight, 6¾ inches
1 Metzenbaum scissors, curved, 7 inches
1 Suture scissors
1 Set Sims uterine curettes, sharp (Fig. 14-8)
1 Set Thomas uterine curettes, blunt (Fig. 14-8)
1 Endometrial biopsy suction curette (Fig. 14-8)
1 Gaylor biopsy forceps (Fig. 14-8)

Holding instruments

4 Foerster sponge-holding forceps, 9½ inches
6 Backhaus towel clamps, 5¼ inches
2 Dressing forceps, 5½ inches
2 Tissue forceps with 1 × 2 teeth, 5½ inches
1 Dressing forceps, 10 inches
1 Tissue forceps with 1 × 2 teeth, 10 inches
2 Russian tissue forceps, 8 inches
8 Allis-Adair tissue forceps, 6¼ inches
6 Allis intestinal forceps, 6 inches
2 Babcock intestinal forceps, 6¼ inches
2 Babcock intestinal forceps, 9½ inches
2 Lahey vulsellum forceps, 6 inches

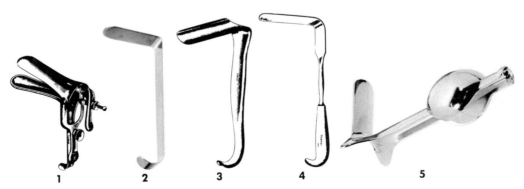

Fig. 14-10. Vaginal instruments: exposing. *1*, Graves self-retaining vaginal speculum; *2*, Heaney hysterectomy retractor; *3*, Doyen vaginal retractor; *4*, Glenner vaginal retractor; *5*, Auvard vaginal speculum (weighted). (Courtesy Codman & Shurtleff, Inc., Randolph, Mass.)

Fig. 14-11. Vaginal instruments: exposing. *1,* Goodell uterine dilator; *2,* Hank uterine dilator; *3,* uterine sound (graduated); *4,* Deschamp ligature carriers (right and left); *5,* Hegar dilators. (Courtesy Codman & Shurtleff, Inc., Randolph, Mass.)

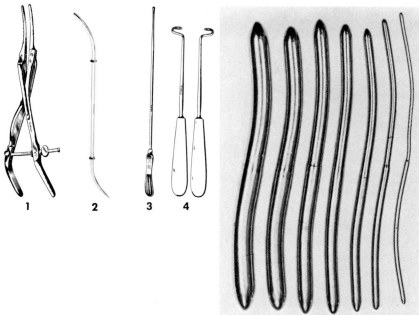

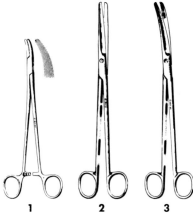

Fig. 14-12. Abdominal gynecologic instruments: cutting and suturing. *1,* Heaney needle holder; *2,* Mayo dissecting scissors (straight, 6¾ inches); *3,* Mayo dissecting scissors (curved, 6¾ inches). (Courtesy Codman & Shurtleff, Inc., Randolph, Mass.)

1 Jacobs vulsellum forceps (Fig. 14-9)
1 Uterine tenaculum (Fig. 14-9)
1 Staude uterine tenaculum (Fig. 14-9)
1 Bozeman dressing forceps (Fig. 14-9)

Clamping instruments

6 Crile hemostats, straight, 6¼ inches
12 Kelly hemostats, curved, 5½ inches
2 Pean forceps, curved, 6¼ inches
2 Ochsner forceps, straight, 6¼ inches
4 Ochsner forceps, straight, 8 inches
4 Heaney hysterectomy forceps, 8¼ inches
6 Rochester-Pean hysterectomy forceps, curved, 9 inches

Exposing instruments

1 Self-retaining vaginal speculum (Fig. 14-10)
1 Jackson vaginal retractor
2 Heaney retractors (Fig. 14-10)
2 Deaver retractors

1 Auvard vaginal speculum, weighted (Fig. 14-10)
1 Doyen vaginal retractor (Fig. 14-10)
1 Uterine sound, graduated (Fig. 14-11)
1 Set Hegar or Hank uterine dilators (Fig. 14-11)
1 Goodell uterine dilator (Fig. 14-11)

Suturing instruments

2 Mayo-Hegar needle holders, 8 inches
2 Heaney needle holders (Fig. 14-12)
2 Crile-Wood needle holders, 6 inches

Accessory items

Suction tubing
Suction tip
Asepto syringe (optional)
Metal tray for surgeon's lap (optional)
Indwelling urinary drainage items: Foley catheter or suprapubic cystostomy (Silastic) catheter
Drain (optional)
Lubricant, water-soluble
Electrosurgical unit, if desired

A basic vaginal prep set is required for abdominal gynecologic surgery. The basic abdominal gynecologic instrument set consists of the basic laparotomy set (Chapter 11), plus the following:

Cutting instruments

1 Jorgenson scissors

Holding instruments

1 Somer uterine elevating forceps (Fig. 14-13)
2 Barrett tenaculum forceps, 7 inches
1 Lahey goiter vulsellum forceps, 6 inches

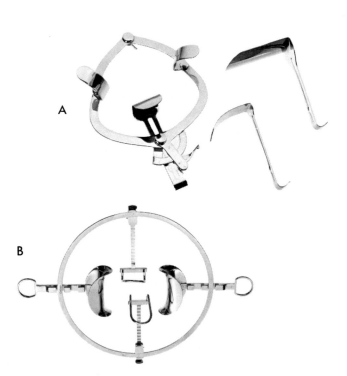

Fig. 14-13. Abdominal gynecologic instruments: clamping. *1,* Rochester-Pean forceps; *2ₐ,* Rochester-Ochsner (straight) forceps; *2ᵦ,* Rochester-Ochsner (curved) forceps; *3,* Heaney hysterectomy forceps; *4,* Somer uterine elevating forceps. (Courtesy Codman & Shurtleff, Inc., Randolph, Mass.)

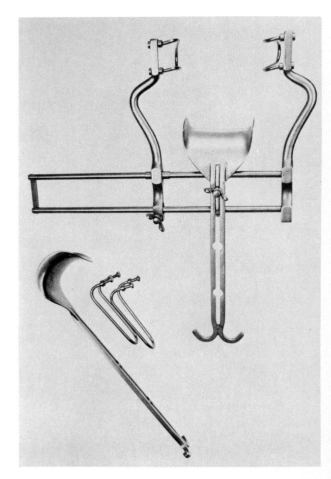

Fig. 14-14. Abdominal gynecologic instruments: exposing. **A,** O'Sullivan-O'Connor self-retaining abdominal retractor; **B,** Martin self-retaining abdominal ring retractor, **C,** Balfour self-retaining retractor with blades. (Courtesy Codman & Shurtleff, Inc., Randolph, Mass.)

Clamping instruments

4 Heaney hysterectomy forceps, 8 inches (Fig. 14-13)

Exposing instruments

1 Martin or O'Sullivan-O'Connor abdominal retractor with blades (Fig. 14-14)
1 Balfour self-retaining retractor with blades (Fig. 14-14)

Suturing instruments

2 Heaney needle holders, 8½ inches
2 Masson needle holders, 10¼ inches

For most abdominal gynecologic procedures, a dilation and curettage set should be available.

Evaluation

During evaluation, the perioperative nurse determines whether the patient met the established goals. Some goals can be reached during the preoperative and intraoperative phases of care; they are evaluated prior to the patient's discharge from the operating room. Others require ongoing monitoring and measurement in the postoperative phase. Part of the perioperative nursing report to the recovery area (PACU, ambulatory recovery) should include the goals of the nursing care plan. They can be phrased as outcome statements, as follows:

- The patient's anxiety was reduced; she verbalized concerns and used personally effective coping strategies.
- Urinary elimination patterns were maintained; urinary output was adequate, and catheter patency was maintained.
- Skin integrity was maintained; there were no reddened areas at dependent pressure sites or at the placement site of the dispersive pad; the incision was aseptically dressed.
- The patient maintained a positive body image; questions were answered and misconceptions clarified.
- There was no evidence of injury related to surgical positioning; range of motion and neurovascular status were consistent with preoperative levels.

SURGICAL INTERVENTIONS
Vulvar surgery

The treatment of early malignant disease of the vulva is accomplished by a skinning technique, local wide excision or, for more multicentric or extensive lesions, simple vulvectomy. These procedures may also be accomplished by use of a laser.

Simple vulvectomy

Simple vulvectomy is removal of the labia majora and labia minora, possibly but not preferably the glans clitoris, and occasionally tissue from the perianal area, with a plastic closure. A simple vulvectomy is usually done for the treatment of carcinoma in situ of the vulva when it is multicentric or for the treatment of Bowen's or Paget's disease. Occasionally a vulvectomy is necessary for the treatment of either leukoplakia or intractable pruritus, especially when a skinning procedure is impractical or has failed.

Procedural considerations. The basic vaginal instrument set is required, plus an electrosurgical unit, if desired.

Operative procedure

1. The affected skin is incised, usually starting anteriorly above the clitoris. The incision is continued laterally to the labia majora, to the midline of the perineum, and around the anus, if it is involved (Fig. 14-15, *A*). A knife, hemostats, gauze sponges on sponge-holding forceps, tissue forceps, and Allis forceps are needed. Bleeding vessels are clamped. Bleeding is also controlled by electrocoagulation or sutures.
2. Periurethral and perivaginal incisions are made. Bleeding of this vascular area can be controlled by means of Kelly or Crile hemostats and electrocoagulation. Ligation of blood vessels should be minimal. Allis-Adair forceps are used for holding diseased tissues.
3. All skin and subcutaneous tissues are undermined and mobilized with curved dissecting scissors, tissue forceps, Allis forceps, and sponges on holding forceps.
4. The wound is closed, usually by simple bilateral Z-plasty or other plastic closure. In some cases skin is excised around the anus to accomplish a sliding skin flap.
5. Closed wound drainage catheters may be placed in the dependent areas, a Foley catheter is inserted, and vaginal gauze packing may be placed in the vagina. Dressings are applied.

Skinning vulvectomy

Skinning vulvectomy is the simple removal of the external skin from the affected area, which has been previously identifed with a stain such as toluidine blue.

The main purpose of this procedure is to preserve the underlying structures of the external genitals. A skinning procedure may be done to treat leukoplakia, intractable pruritus, or other types of skin lesions, such as kraurosis, vitiligo, and chronic venereal granulomas.

Procedural considerations. The instrumentation required is as described for simple vulvectomy.

Operative procedure. The external skin is simply excised from the affected area.

Groin lymphadenectomy and radical vulvectomy

Groin lymphadenectomy and radical vulvectomy are the en bloc dissection of the following structures: a large segment of skin from the abdomen and groin, the labia majora, labia minora, clitoris, mons veneris, and terminal portions of the urethra, vagina, and other vulvar organs, as well as the superficial and deep inguinal nodes, portions of the round ligaments, portions of the saphenous veins, and the

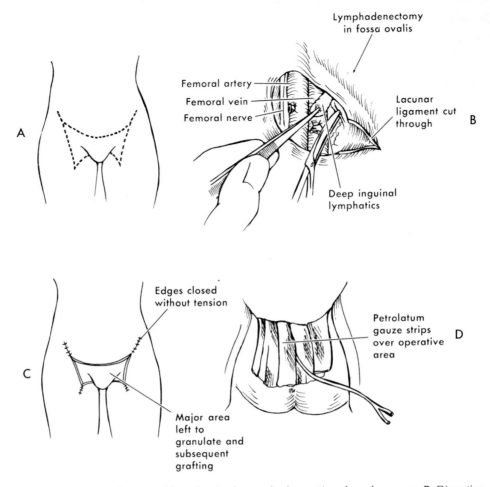

Fig. 14-15. A, Outline of incisional lines for simple or radical operations for vulvar cover. **B,** Dissection is completed, involving nerves, saphenous veins, and muscles, when dissection of distal half of femoral canal has been completed. **C,** Upper edges of abdominal incisions may be partially closed. **D,** With indwelling catheter in bladder, wound is dressed with layers of gauze and held in place with light pressure dressing. (From Ball, T.L.: Gynecologic surgery and urology, ed. 2, St. Louis, 1963, The C.V. Mosby Co.)

lesion itself. It also involves reconstruction of the vaginal walls and pelvic floor and closure of the abdominal wounds (Fig. 14-15). Later, placement of full-thickness pinch or split-thickness grafts (Chapter 24) may be done if the denuded area of the vulva appears too large for normal granulation.

Groin lymphadenectomy and radical vulvectomy involve abdominoperineal dissection and groin dissection, which may be performed as a one- or two-stage operation. When performed as a one-stage operation, it is optimally done by a four-person team.

Procedural considerations. The patient lies supine and may be placed in Trendelenburg's and low lithotomy positions, as required for the various stages. The skin prep includes both the abdomen and vulva, and the skin of the thighs is usually prepped down to the knees. As in other radical surgery, the nursing team should be prepared to measure blood loss and anticipate procedures to combat shock.

For groin lymphadenectomy the basic abdominal gynecologic instrument set is required, plus the following:

Clamping instruments

8 Schmidt tonsil forceps, 7¼ inches
4 Kantrowitz thoracic clamps, 7½ inches
    Ligating clips and appliers

Assessory items (optional)

2 Closed wound drainage systems

For radical vulvectomy the basic vaginal instrument set is required, plus the following:

Exposing instruments

Richardson retractors, assorted sizes
2 Richardson appendectomy retractors, long blade
2 Volkmann rake retractors, three-pronged, dull

Accessory items (optional)

2 Closed wound drainage systems

Operative procedures
Groin lymphadenectomy

1. The first skin incision is made on the side opposite the primary lesion. The end of the incised skin is grasped with Allis forceps. The incision is carried down to the aponeuroses of the external oblique muscle.

2. The fascia over the inguinal ligament and the fascia lata of the upper thigh are exposed, separated, and freed with retractors, knife, scissors, hemostats, and sponges.

3. Bleeding vessels, including the superficial iliac artery and vein, the epigastric artery and vein, and the superficial external pudendal artery and vein, are clamped and ligated. The smaller bleeding vessels are controlled by electrocoagulation.

4. The fibers of the inguinal, hypogastric, and femoral nerves are resected by Metzenbaum scissors, tissue forceps without teeth, and long-bladed retractors.

5. The lymphatic node beds may be identified with silk sutures or metal clips. Fine, long, sharp dissection scissors are needed.

6. The large tissue surfaces are exposed for complete dissection by means of retractors and are protected by warm, moist laparotomy packs. High saphenous vein ligation is performed with scissors, forceps, and hemostats and should be doubly tied with nonreactive suture.

7. The femoral canal is cleaned of its lymphatics; the round ligament is clamped, cut, and ligated.

8. The peritoneum is freed from the muscles; the fascia is dissected free; deep lymphatic nodes and areolar tissue are removed; and vessels and their attachments are clamped, cut, and ligated, using long curved scissors, long tissue forceps, hemostats, and ligatures (Fig. 14-15, B).

9. The lesion is removed. In deep pelvic lymphadenectomy, the ureter may be exposed and the area drained.

10. The inguinal canal is reconstructed, and the wound is partially closed with a nonabsorbable suture (Fig. 14-15, C). A Foley catheter is inserted and the wound is dressed.

Radical vulvectomy

1. The skin incisions of the abdomen and thigh join with those for vulvectomy. The incisions in the vulva encircle the urethra.

2. In the vulvar dissection, terminal portions of the urethra and vagina, the mons veneris, the clitoris, the frenulum, the prepuce of the clitoris, Bartholin's and Skene's glands, and fascial coverings of the vulva are removed with the specimen.

3. Reconstruction of the vaginal walls and the pelvic floor is completed. A Foley catheter is inserted, closed wound drainage catheters are placed in the denuded area, and the wound is dressed with a pressure dressing (Fig. 14-15, D).

Vaginal surgery
Vaginal plastic operation (anterior and posterior repair)

A vaginal plastic operation is reconstruction of the vaginal walls, the pelvic floor, and the muscles and fascia of the urethra, bladder, rectum, and perineum.

A vaginal repair is done to correct a cystocele or a rectocele and to reestablish the support of the anterior and posterior vaginal walls, which will restore the bladder and rectum to their normal positions.

A *cystocele* is a herniation of the bladder that causes the anterior vaginal wall to bulge downward (Fig. 14-16). A defect in the anterior vaginal wall is usually caused by obstetrical or surgical trauma, age, or an inherent weakness. A large protrusion may cause a sensation of pressure in the vagina or present a mass at, or through, the introitus; it may also cause voiding difficulties.

A *rectocele* is formed by a protrusion of the anterior rectal wall (posterior vaginal wall) into the vagina. In general, the anterior rectal wall forms a bulging mass beneath the posterior vaginal mucosa (Fig. 14-16). As the mass pushes downward into the lower vaginal canal, the rectum may be torn from the fascial and muscular attachments of the urogenital diaphragm and the pelvic wall. The levator ani muscles (Fig. 14-4) become stretched or torn. The symptomatic signs are a mass protruding into the vagina, difficulty in evacuating the lower bowel, hemorrhoids, and a feeling of pressure.

An *enterocele* is a herniation of Douglas's cul-de-sac and almost always contains loops of the small intestine. An enterocele herniates into a weakened area between the anterior and posterior vaginal walls.

Procedural considerations. The basic vaginal instrument set is required.

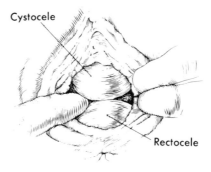

Fig. 14-16. Cystocele and rectocele resulting from unrepaired tears of muscles of pelvic floor and those under bladder, usually resulting from childbirth, surgical trauma, age, or inherent weakness. (From Crossen, R.J.: Diseases of women, ed. 10, St. Louis, 1953, The C.V. Mosby Co.)

Operative procedures

1. Dilatation and curettage may be done.
2. Vaginal retractors are used for exposure. The labia may be sewn back if the exposure is inadequate.

Anterior wall repair

1. The bladder may be drained, or a Foley catheter or suprapubic cystostomy catheter may be inserted (surgeon's preference). Areolar tissue between the bladder and vagina at the bladder reflection is exposed. The full thickness of the vaginal wall is separated up to the bladder neck by a knife, curved scissors, tissue forceps, Allis-Adair or Allis forceps (Fig. 14-17, *A*), and gauze sponges. Bleeding vessels are clamped and tied with ligatures or electrocoagulated.
2. The urethra and bladder neck are mobilized with a knife, gauze sponges, and curved scissors (Fig. 14-17, *B*).
3. Sutures are placed adjacent to the urethra and bladder neck in such a manner that, after they have been tied, a narrowing of the bladder neck and a delineating of the posterior urethrovesical angle occur (Fig. 14-17, *C*).
4. The connective tissue on the lateral aspects of the cervix is sutured into the cervix to shorten the cardinal ligaments.
5. Allis-Adair forceps are applied to the edges of the incision, and the left flap of the vaginal wall is drawn across the midline. Edges are trimmed according to the size of the cystocele (Fig. 14-17, *D*). This process is repeated on the right flap of the vaginal incision.
6. The anterior vaginal wall is closed in a manner resulting in reconstruction of an anterior vaginal fornix (Fig. 14-17, *E*).

Posterior wall repair

1. Allis forceps are placed posteriorly at the mucocutaneous junction on each side, at the hymenal ring, and just above the anus (Fig. 14-18, *A*).
2. Skin and mucosa are incised and dissected from the muscles beneath with a knife, tissue forceps, curved scissors, and gauze sponges.
3. Allis-Adair forceps are placed on the posterior vaginal wall, scar tissue (from obstetrical trauma) is removed, and dissection is continued to the posterior vaginal fornix and laterally, depending on the size of the rectocele (Fig. 14-18, *A* and *B*).
4. The perineum is denuded by sharp dissection, and the trimming of the posterior vaginal wall is carried out with Allis forceps, curved scissors, and gauze sponges.
5. The rectal wall proximal to the puborectal muscle is strengthened by placement of sutures (Fig. 14-18, *C*).
6. Bleeding is controlled, and the vaginal wall is closed from above, downward to the anterior edge of the puborectal muscle. The rectocele is repaired from the posterior fornix to the perineal body (Fig. 14-18, *D* and *E*). Remains of the transverse perineal and bulbocavernous muscles are used to build up the perineum. The anterior edge of the levator ani muscle may be approximated.
7. The mucosa and skin are trimmed, and the remaining closure is effected by interrupted sutures.
8. The vagina may be packed with 2-inch vaginal gauze packing. A Foley catheter or suprapubic cystostomy catheter is inserted, according to the surgeon's preference.

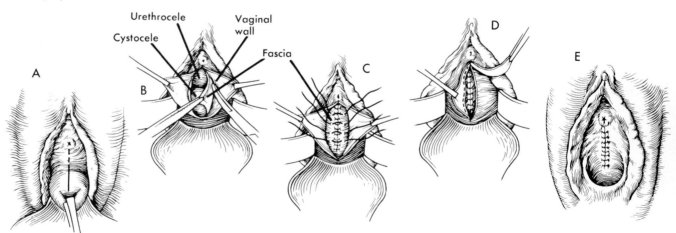

Fig. 14-17. Repair of cystourethrocele. **A,** Cervix pulled down as far as possible with tenaculum. Vertical incision made entirely through to vaginal wall. **B,** Vaginal flaps further dissected upward. Urethral meatus and pubocervical fascia separated from vaginal wall with Mayo scissors. **C,** Fascia brought together with continuous suture, beginning at lowest point and ending near external urethral meatus. A few interrupted sutures placed secondarily. **D,** Excess portion of vaginal wall carefully removed, leaving sufficient amount to be closed with tension. **E,** Completed operation, maintaining bladder and urethra in normal position. (From Counseller, V.S. In Lowrie, R.J., editor: Gynecology: surgical techniques, Springfield, Ill., 1955, Charles C Thomas, Publisher.)

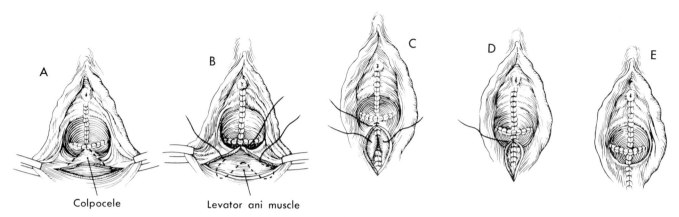

Colpocele

Levator ani muscle

Fig. 14-18. Repair of rectocele. **A,** Exposure of perineum and portion of posterior vaginal wall excised. **B,** Excess skin and excess portion of posterior vaginal wall excised up to vaginal vault. First suture placed in vaginal vault. **C,** Levator ani muscles brought together with interrupted stitches; Colles' fascia brought together over perineum. **D,** Perineum restored and Colles' fascia repaired with interrupted sutures. **E,** Skin of perineum closed. (From Counseller, V.S. In Lowrie, R.J., editor: Gynecology: surgical techniques, Springfield, Ill., 1955, Charles C Thomas, Publishers.)

Enterocele repair. The procedure is illustrated in Fig. 14-19. The peritoneal sac must be carefully dissected from the underlying rectum, the overlying bladder, or both, so that the peritoneal tissues are completely freed from the surrounding structures. The sac is opened to establish true identification and is then closed as high as possible by permanent purse-string sutures. The portion of peritoneal tissue distal to the purse-string ties is then excised, and the area is reinforced locally by transverse suture closures

of whatever supportive tissues may be available. This technique is used to prevent recurrence.

Perineal repair. The procedure is illustrated in Fig. 14-20.

Vesicovaginal fistula repair

A vesicovaginal fistula is repaired by free dissection of the mucosal tissue of the anterior vaginal wall, closing of the fistula tract, and repair of the fascial attachments be-

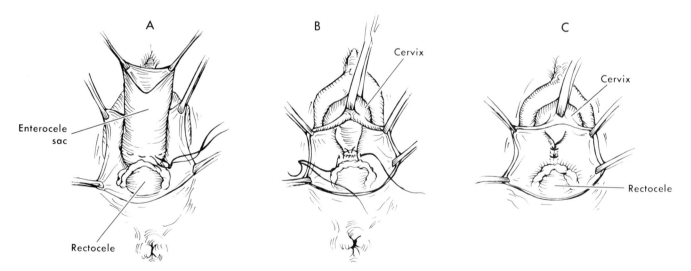

Enterocele sac

Rectocele

Cervix

Cervix

Rectocele

Fig. 14-19. Repair of enterocele. **A,** Transverse incision has been made at mucocutaneous border, as in operation for rectocele. Then posterior vaginal wall mucosa is divided in midline up to cervix. Sac of peritoneum has been excised completely, then opened, and contents pushed into peritoneal cavity. Purse-string suture of no. 1 chromic has been placed about neck of sac. **B,** Uterosacral ligaments that have been exposed are approximated with no. 1 chromic sutures. First suture placed in posterior surface of cervix and retracted remainder of neck of sac. **C,** Two sutures that have been placed in posterior surface of cervix and tied. (Modified from Mattingly, R.F., and Thompson, J.D.: TeLinde's operative gynecology, ed. 6, Philadelphia, 1985, J.B. Lippincott Co.)

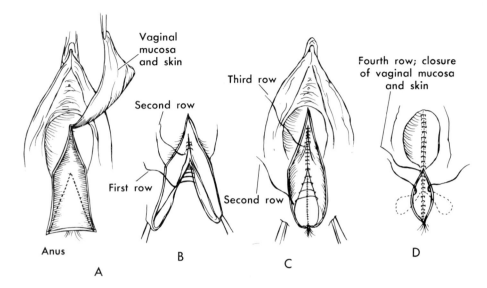

Fig. 14-20. Repair of complete lacerations of the perineum. **A,** Lower margins of incision. **B,** Placement of first and second rows of sutures. **C,** Second and third rows of sutures. **D,** Fourth row of sutures. (Modified from Counseller, V.S. In Lowrie, R.J., editor: Gynecology: surgical techniques, Springfield, Ill., 1955, Charles C Thomas, Publisher.)

tween the bladder and vagina, with establishment of urinary drainage.

Fistulas vary in size from a small opening that permits only slight leakage of urine into the vagina to a large opening that permits all urine to pass into the vagina (Fig. 14-21).

Fistulas may result from radical surgery in the management of pelvic cancer, from radiation therapy without surgery, from chronic ulceration of the vaginal structures, from penetrating wounds, or from obstetric trauma.

A *urethrovaginal fistula* usually causes constant incontinence or difficulty in retaining urine. This condition occurs after damage to the anterior wall and bladder or following radiation therapy or parturition. A *ureterovaginal fistula* develops as a result of injury to the ureter. In some cases, reimplantation of the ureter in the bladder or ureterostomy may be done.

Vaginal approach

Procedural considerations. The basic vaginal instrument set is required, plus the following:

1 Kelly fistula scissors
1 Dressing forceps, 7 inches
2 Probes
2 Skin hooks
  Frazier suction tips, desired sizes
2 Ureteral catheters, desired size
  Sterile water for irrigation

Operative procedure

1. Traction sutures are placed about the fistulous tract; tissues are grasped with Allis-Adair forceps and plain tissue forceps.

2. The scar tissue around the fistula is excised, cleavage between the bladder and vagina is located, and flaps are mobilized with scissors, forceps, and gauze sponges.

3. The bladder mucosa is inverted toward the interior of the bladder with interrupted sutures. The sutures are passed through the muscularis of the bladder down to the mucosa.

4. A second layer of inverting sutures is placed in the bladder and tied, thereby completely inverting the bladder mucosa toward the interior.

5. The vaginal wall is closed with interrupted sutures in a direction opposite the closure of the bladder wall.

6. The bladder is distended with sterile water to determine any leaks. A Foley catheter is left in place; dressing is applied.

Transperitoneal approach

In the presence of a high vesicovaginal fistula, a suprapubic incision is used. The opening from the bladder into the vagina is closed, and the fascial attachments are repaired.

Procedural considerations. The patient is placed in slight Trendelenburg's position. Ureteral catheters may be inserted just before surgery (Chapter 15). The vagina is cleansed and packed with moist gauze saturated with an antibiotic or antimicrobial solution. The abdominal operative site is prepped, and the patient is draped.

The abdominal gynecologic instrument set is required.

Operative procedure

1. A midline abdominal incision is usually made, as described for laparotomy.

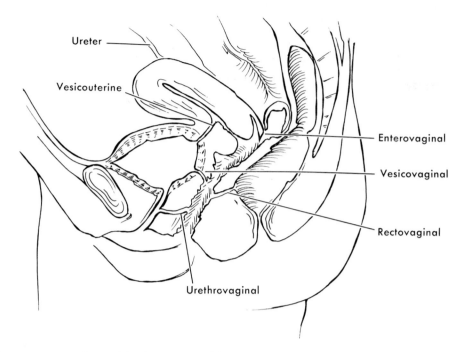

Fig. 14-21. Types of genital fistulas. Urogenital fistula is communication between urethra, bladder, or one of ureters and some part of genital tract. Urethrovaginal, vesicovaginal, or ureterovaginal fistulas, most common types, empty into vaginal canal. (Modified from Huffman, J.W.: Gynecology and obstetrics, Philadelphia, 1962, W.B. Saunders Co.)

2. The fistulous tract is identified; the vaginal vault and the adjacent adherent bladder are separated with scissors, forceps, and sponges.
3. The vesicovaginal septum is dissected down to the healthy tissue beyond the site of the fistula.
4. The fistulous tract is mobilized. The bladder site of the fistula is inverted into the interior of the bladder with two rows of inverting sutures. The muscularis and mucosa layers of the vagina are inverted into the vaginal vault by means of two rows of sutures.
5. The flaps of peritoneum are mobilized, both from the bladder and from the adjacent vaginal vault, and are closed to form a new vesicovaginal reflection of peritoneum below the site of the old fistulous tract.
6. The wound is closed in layers, as for laparotomy. Abdominal dressings are applied. A Foley catheter is left in the bladder.

Rectovaginal fistula repair (vaginal approach)

Rectovaginal fistula repair by the vaginal approach includes repair of the perineum, fascia, and muscle-supporting structures between the rectum and vagina, thereby closing the fistula formed between the rectum and the vagina (Fig. 14-22).

In the presence of a large rectovaginal fistula, as in patients who have incurable cancer, a colostomy may be done (Chapter 11).

Procedural considerations. The basic vaginal instrument set is required for a rectovaginal fistula repair.

Operative procedure

1. The scar tissue and tract between the rectum and vagina are excised (Fig. 14-23); edges of fresh tissue are approximated with absorbable sutures.
2. The rectum and vaginal walls are mobilized; the rectum is closed with inversion of the mucosa into the rectal canal.
3. The vagina is closed transversely or in a sagittal plane different from that of the rectal canal. The vaginal mucosal layer is inverted into the vaginal wall; a Foley catheter is inserted.

Operations for urinary stress incontinence

Surgery for urinary stress incontinence entails repair of the fascial supports and the pubococcygeal muscle (Fig. 14-4) surrounding the urethra and the bladder neck through a vaginal or abdominal approach.

The proper operative approach for the treatment of stress incontinence must be selected specifically for each patient. Normal micturition depends on a finely coordinated group of voluntary and involuntary movements. As a result of volitional impulses, voiding may be inhibited or stopped by the intrinsic muscles of the bladder neck and proximal urethra and the puborectalis division of the levator ani muscle (Chapter 15).

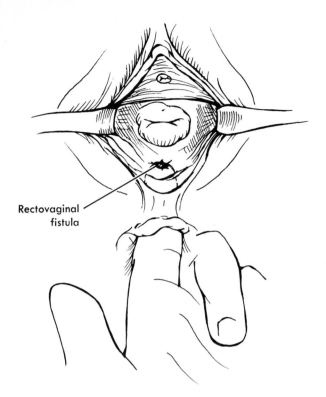

Fig. 14-22. Rectovaginal fistula. Examiner's finger puts tension on rectovaginal septum. (Modified from Huffman, J.W.: Gynecology and obstetrics, Philadelphia, 1962, W.B. Saunders Co.)

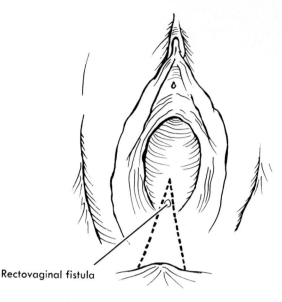

Fig. 14-23. Repair of rectovaginal fistulas of all types essentially same as shown here. Portion of scar tissue to be excised is included within *dotted lines;* repair is as described for complete lacerations of perineum (see Fig. 14-20). (Modified from Counseller, V.S. In Lowrie, R.J., editor: Gynecology: surgical techniques, Springfield, Ill., 1955, Charles C Thomas, Publisher.)

The type of operation selected depends on the severity of stress incontinence, the extent of the condition causing it, the patient's ability to use the anatomical mechanism for voluntary inhibition of urination, and the operations that have previously been performed. States of stress incontinence are classified in relation to frequency and degree of incontinence, the presence of other diseases, and the function of the pubococcygeus muscle (levator ani) (Fig. 14-4).

Previous pelvic operations may have resulted in scarring and distortion, with displacement of the bladder neck to an unfavorable position for proper functioning. Conditions such as uterine prolapse, cystocele, urethrocele, cystourethrocele, or urogenital fistulas following radiation therapy may be associated with stress incontinence.

The aim of any operation for urinary stress incontinence is to improve the performance of a dislodged or dysfunctional vesical neck, to restore normal urethral length, and to tighten and restore the anterior urethral vesical angle.

Operative procedures
Vaginal approach
1. A Foley catheter or suprapubic cystostomy catheter is inserted, according to the surgeon's preference. The posterior vaginal wall is retracted, and an incision is made through the anterior vaginal wall down to the urethra and bladder.

2. The vaginal wall is dissected from the bladder and urethra; the neck of the bladder is sutured together. The wound is closed, as described for vaginal repair.

Vesicourethral suspension. See the Marshall-Marchetti procedure (Chapter 15). Basic steps of the procedure follow.
1. Through a suprapubic abdominal incision, the space of Retzius is entered, and the bladder and urethra are freed from the underlying structures.
2. Mattress sutures are inserted through the perivaginal fascia on either side of the vesicourethral angle area and preferably at right angles to the long axis of the urethra and bladder. These are then passed through the central portion of the undersurface of the symphysis pubis under direct vision. The application of the sutures to the perivaginal connective tissue is done with the surgeon's hand in the vagina to ensure that the suture material is not passed through the vaginal mucosa (Figs. 14-2 and 14-4).
3. The wound is closed and may be drained if the vascularity of the area warrants. An abdominal dressing is applied.

Excision of fibroma of the vagina

Excision of fibroma of the vagina involves the removal of the lesion through a transverse or longitudinal incision of the vaginal wall.

Small cysts or small benign tumors that distort the vagina or those that are ulcerated and infected are treated surgically.

Procedural considerations. A dilatation and curettage set is required, plus six Halsted mosquito hemostats.

Operative procedure

1. The vaginal vault is retracted with lateral retractors. Sutures may be placed on each side of the tumor. The posterior lip of the cervix is grasped with a tenaculum and is drawn anteriorly to expose the operative site.
2. The vaginal wall is incised, and the edges are grasped with traction sutures on curved, taper-point needles or with Allis forceps.
3. The base and its capsule are excised by a knife and curved scissors; bleeding vessels are clamped with Halsted mosquito hemostats and ligated with fine sutures.
4. The vaginal incision is closed with interrupted sutures.

Construction of a vagina

Two basic approaches are used for repairing or overcoming a congenital or surgical defect of the vagina: obtaining a skin graft, which is applied to a mold and placed in the area of vaginal reconstruction, and a simple opening of the area of vaginal reconstruction and the placing of a mold to permit the spontaneous epithelialization of the area.

Procedural considerations. For a skin graft the plastic local instrument set (Chapter 24) is required, plus the following:

Dermatome of choice
Marking pen
Nonadherent gauze dressing

For vaginal construction the basic vaginal instrument set is required, plus the following:

2 Iris scissors, 1 straight and 1 curved, 4½ inches
2 Skin hooks
12 Halsted mosquito hemostats, 6 straight and 6 curved, 5 inches
Ruler
Vaginal mold

Operative procedure

1. The skin graft is taken from the abdomen or anterior thigh. The donor site is dressed in the routine manner with nonadherent gauze and a pressure dressing.
2. The skin graft is kept in a moist gauze sponge until it is ready to be used.
3. A vaginal orifice is created by sharp dissection. Great care must be taken to prevent damage to the rectum or bladder. A mold is used to apply the donor skin or simply to hold the dissected area open to permit spontaneous epithelialization.

Trachelorrhaphy

Trachelorrhaphy is removal of torn surfaces of the anterior and posterior cervical lips and reconstruction of the cervical canal. It is performed to treat deep lacerations of a cervix that is relatively free of infection.

Procedural considerations. The basic vaginal instrument set is required, plus a conization loop electrode, if desired. A Foley catheter may be inserted in the bladder, depending on the surgeon's preference.

Operative procedure

1. The labia are retracted with Allis-Adair tissue forceps or sutures. The cervix is grasped with a tenaculum.
2. The infected tissue of the exocervix is denuded with a knife. The flaps are undermined by means of a knife and curved scissors. Bleeding vessels are clamped and ligated. The mucosa is dissected from the cervix.
3. A small distal portion of the cervical canal is coned with a knife or a loop electrode to remove infected tissue. Bleeding vessels are clamped and ligated.
4. The denuded and coned areas are covered by suturing the mucosal flaps of the exocervix transversely, using interrupted sutures. Tissue forceps, hemostats, and gauze sponges are needed. The sutures are placed in such a manner that the fibromuscular tissue of the cervix is included, thereby eliminating dead space where a hematoma may form and providing a complete reconstructed cervical canal.
5. A vaginal pack may be inserted.

Dilatation of the cervix and curettage

In this procedure, instruments are introduced through the vagina for the purpose of dilating the cervix to permit evacuation of uterine contents. Dilatation of the cervix can also take place by inserting laminaria tents into the cervical os before surgery; these tents are removed immediately before the procedure.

Dilatation and curettage is done either for diagnostic purposes or as a form of therapy for a variety of pelvic conditions such as incomplete abortion, therapeutic abortion, abnormal uterine bleeding, or primary dysmenorrhea. Dilatation and curettage may also be performed when carcinoma of the endometrium is suspected, in the study of infertility, or before amputation of the cervix or an operation for prolapse of the uterus.

Procedural considerations. The dilatation and curettage set includes the following:

Exposing instruments

2 Jackson vaginal retractors
1 Sims vaginal retractor
1 Auvard vaginal speculum, weighted (Fig. 14-10)
2 Deaver retractors
1 Uterine sound, graduated (Fig. 14-11)
1 Set Hegar or Hank uterine dilators (Fig. 14-11)
1 Goodell uterine dilator (Fig. 14-11)

Holding instruments

2 Barrett tenaculum forceps (Fig. 14-9)
1 Jacobs vulsellum forceps (Fig. 14-9)

2 Foerster sponge-holding forceps
1 Bozeman dressing forceps (Fig. 14-9)
1 Fletcher–Van Doren polyp forceps
2 Backhaus towel clamps, 5¼ inches
1 Tissue forceps with 1 × 2 teeth, 5½ inches
1 Russian tissue forceps, 8 inches
1 Dressing forceps, 7¼ inches
2 Allis forceps, 6 inches

Cutting instruments

1 Bard-Parker knife handle, no. 3 with blade no. 10
2 Mayo dissecting scissors, 1 curved and 1 straight, 6¾ inches
1 Set Sims uterine curettes, sharp (Fig. 14-8)
1 Set Thomas uterine curettes, blunt (Fig. 14-8)
1 Heaney uterine curette
1 Gaylor biopsy forceps (Fig. 14-8)

Clamping instruments

2 Crile hemostats, 5½ inches
2 Pean forceps, 6¼ inches

Suturing instruments

1 Mayo-Hegar needle holder, 8 inches
Suture of surgeon's preference, if desired

Accessory items

1 Urethral catheter, 16 or 18 Fr
1 Telfa dressing
1 Ampule oxytocic drug, if desired
Iodoform or plain gauze packing, as desired
Vaginal gauze packing, as desired

Operative procedure

1. A Jackson or Auvard retractor is placed posteriorly in the vagina. A Sims or Deaver retractor is placed anteriorly to expose the cervix. The anterior lip of the cervix is grasped with a tenaculum (Fig. 14-24).
2. The direction of the cervical canal and the depth of the uterine cavity are determined by means of a blunt probe or graduated uterine sound.
3. The cervix is gradually dilated by means of graduated Hegar or Hank dilators and possibly a Goodell uterine dilator.
4. Exploration for pedunculated polyps or myomas may be done with a polyp forceps.
5. The interior of the cervical canal and the cavity of the uterus are curetted to obtain either a fractional or a routine specimen. For specific identification of the site of specimens, the endocervix is scraped with the curette first, and the specimen is separated from the curettings of the uterine endometrium. In a routine curettage, all curettings are sent together for identification of tissue cells.
6. Fragments of endometrium or other dislodged tissues may be removed with warm, moist gauze sponges on sponge-holding forceps or collected on Telfa.
7. Multiple-punch biopsies of the cervical circumference (at the 3, 6, 9, and 12 o'clock positions) may be taken

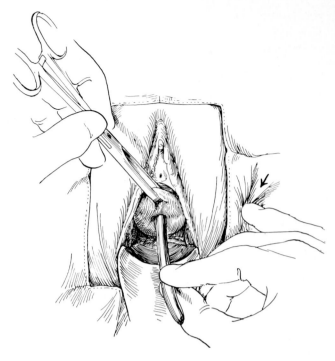

Fig. 14-24. Dilatation of cervix and curettage. Vaginal wall retracted; cervix held by tenaculum; cervix dilated with dilator. Uterine cavity curetted with sharp curettes. (From Ball, T.L.: Gynecologic surgery and urology, ed. 2, St. Louis, 1963, The C.V. Mosby Co.)

with the Gaylor biopsy forceps to supplement the diagnostic studies.

8. Retractors are withdrawn; iodoform or plain gauze packing may be inserted into the uterus, using dressing forceps. The tenaculum is removed from the cervix. A vaginal pack may be inserted.

Suction curettage

Suction curettage is vacuum aspiration of the uterine contents.

Aspiration has proved to be a safe and effective method for early termination of pregnancy and for use in missed and incomplete spontaneous abortions. Advantages are smaller dilatation of the cervix, less damage to the uterus, less blood loss, less chance of uterine perforation, and reduced danger of infection. Laminaria tents may be inserted approximately 4 to 24 hours before suction curettage.

Procedural considerations. The instrumentation required includes the dilatation and curettage set, plus the following:

1 Set of Pratt or Hawkin uterine dilators
1 Placenta forceps, if desired
1 Urethral catheter, 16 or 18 Fr
Sterile cannulas, desired sizes
Aspirator tubing
Vacuum aspirator unit
Oxytocic drugs

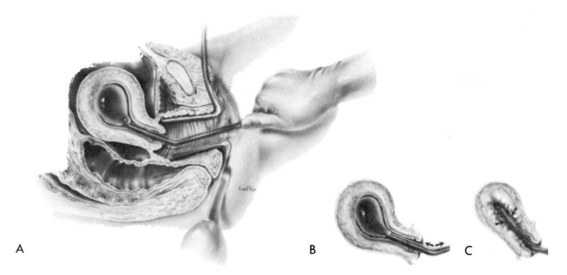

Fig. 14-25. Suction curettage. **A,** Insertion of cannula. **B,** Gentle suction motion to aspirate contents. **C,** Uterine contents evacuated. (From Eaton, C.J.: Technic of uterine aspiration, Berkeley, Calif., Bio-Engineering, Inc.)

Operative procedure

1. The cervix is exposed with an Auvard weighted speculum and an anterior retractor; then the cervix is grasped with a sharp tenaculum and is drawn toward the introitus.
2. The laminaria tents are removed, and the cervix can be further dilated in the routine manner, allowing 1 mm of cannula diameter for each week of pregnancy.
3. The appropriate-sized cannula is inserted into the uterus until the sac is encountered. The suction is turned on with immediate disruption and aspiration of the contents. Continued gentle motion of the cannula removes the uterine contents (Fig. 14-25). Use of uterine curettes may supplement suction in removing the entire uterine contents.
4. Retractors and tenaculum are removed.
5. The specimen, contained in the suction bottle, is removed for pathologic examination.

Removal of pedunculated cervical myoma

Pedunculated lesions may be removed by the snare method or by dissection from the cervical canal with a knife or with cold-knife conization.

Cervical polyps (small pedunculated lesions) stem from the endocervical canal and consist almost entirely of columnar epithelium with or without squamous metaplasia. They may vary in size and are soft, red, and friable. Bleeding may result from the slightest trauma. Usually, the surgeon performs an endometrial and endocervical curettage, and a cytologic smear is taken.

Procedural considerations. A dilatation and curettage set, a tonsil snare with medium snare wire, glass slides, and an electrosurgical unit and a blade electrode are required.

Operative procedure

1. The anterior lip of the cervix is grasped with a Jacobs vulsellum forceps or a tenaculum. The canal is sounded and dilated either to visualize or palpate the base of the pedicle.
2. If the pedicle of the tumor is thin, a tonsil snare may be placed over the body of the tumor, permitting the snare to crush the base of the tumor and to control bleeding. If the tumor is large, its base is dissected out with a knife. Bleeding may be controlled by the use of warm, moist gauze sponges.
3. Iodoform or plain gauze packing may be introduced into the cervical os. The tenaculum is removed from the cervix, and the retractors are withdrawn. A vaginal pack may be inserted for hemostasis.

Shirodkar operation (postconceptional)

The postconceptional Shirodkar operation is placement of a collar-type ligature of Mersilene, Dacron tape, heavy nylon suture, or plastic-covered braided steel suture at the level of the internal os to close it (Fig. 14-26). Incompetence of the cervix is a condition characterized by habitual midtrimester spontaneous abortions. Surgical intervention is designed to prevent cervical dilatation that results in release of uterine contents.

Procedural considerations. Gentle vaginal preparation is carried out. The instrumentation includes the basic vaginal instrument set, plus the following:

2 Deschamps ligature carriers, right and left

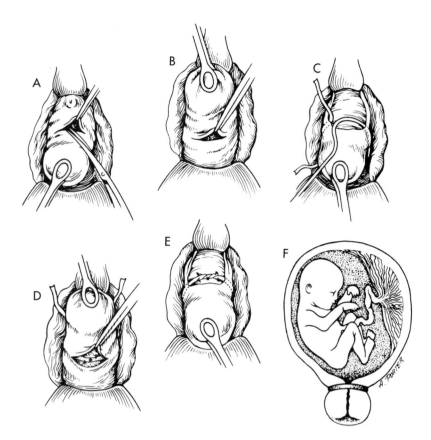

Fig. 14-26. Principles of Shirodkar operation for treatment of incompetent internal cervical os during pregnancy. (From Taylor, E.S.: Essentials of gynecology, ed. 2, Philadelphia, 1962, Lea & Febiger.)

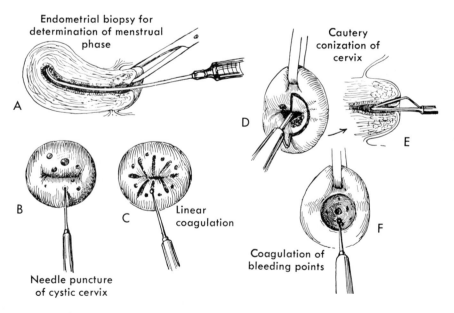

Fig. 14-27. A, Endometrial biopsy technique. **B** to **F,** Methods of treating cervical conditions or obtaining specimens for diagnostic tests. (Modified from Ball, T.L.: Gynecologic surgery and urology, ed. 2, St. Louis, 1963, The C.V. Mosby Co.)

2 Trocar needles
Sutures as noted plus the surgeon's preference for closure of mucosa

Operative procedure

1. Anterior and posterior vaginal retractors are placed, and the cervix is pulled down with smooth ovum or sponge-holding forceps. With smooth tissue forceps and dissecting scissors, the mucosa over the anterior cervix is opened to permit the bladder to be pushed back (Fig. 14-26).
2. The cervix is lifted, and the posterior vaginal mucosa is similarly incised at the level of the peritoneal reflection. The corners of the anterior and posterior incisions are bilaterally approximated in the area of the lateral mucosa with curved tonsil or Allis forceps.
3. The prepared ligature is placed at the desired level by passage of the material through the approximated tissue and is drawn tight posteriorly to close the cervix. The suture material for the ligature is then tied. It is not necessary to suture the ligature to the underlying tissues. The suture material used for this ligation is 5-mm Dacron or Mersilene tape. The anterior and posterior mucosal incisions are usually closed with Dexon or Vicryl no. 2-0 suture to complete the procedure.

Conization and biopsy of the cervix

Diseased cervical tissue is removed to treat strictures of the cervix, chronic cervicitis, epithelial dysplasia, and carcinoma in situ (Fig. 14-27). The conization may be performed by scalpel resection and suturing, by the application of cutting electrosurgical current with an active electrode inserted into the cervical canal, or by use of the laser.

Endometrial biopsy is done to determine the menstrual phase and carry out histologic study of the endometrium. Scalpel conizations are done for diagnostic purposes, such as when a patient has a positive Papanicolaou (Pap) smear. Conization of the cervix, instead of hysterectomy, may be done in some cases to preserve reproductive function. It may also be done for benign or malignant diseases of the cervix and in cases in which total hysterectomy is not feasible.

Procedural considerations. The instruments required include a dilatation and curettage set, an electrosurgical unit, and conization loop and ball-tip electrodes.

Operative procedure (Fig. 14-27)

1. The posterior vaginal wall is retracted by a speculum, and the anterior vaginal wall by lateral retractors. The outer portions of the cervix are grasped with a tenaculum, and the cervix is drawn toward the introitus. Cystic areas of the cervix may be treated with a needle electrode. Endometrial biopsy may be done (Fig. 14-27, A). Bleeding points are coagulated.
2. For cauterization, the electrode is passed into the cervical canal, and the diseased tissue is treated.

3. If a wide conization is performed, the cervix may be sutured and vaginal packing may be used. A Foley catheter may be inserted.

Cesium insertion for cervical and endometrial malignancy

Insertion of cesium into the cervix or endometrium is done for treatment of malignancy. Cesium has generally replaced radium insertions for malignancy of the cervix and endometrium.

Procedural considerations. The patient is brought to the operating room for insertion of the applicators; the cesium is loaded into the applicators later in the radiation department, or in the patient's room under controlled conditions in which all personnel are monitored by use of a dosimeter.

The bladder is drained with a Foley catheter. The Foley balloon is inflated with a radiopaque medium for radiographic visualization after insertion of the cesium. Various cesium applicators may be used according to the surgeon's preference and the area of malignancy.

Interstitial therapy. Cesium needles are available in various lengths with small diameters for insertion into the tissue surrounding the cervix. They are inserted vaginally with a needle applicator and are used as a supplement to intravaginal or intrauterine sources. To facilitate removal, the needles have wires or threads attached to their distal ends.

Culdocentesis and posterior colpotomy (culdotomy)

Needle culdocentesis is insertion of an aspirating needle through the posterior fornix of the vagina. Posterior colpotomy (culdotomy) is incision through the vagina and peritoneum into the cul-de-sac.

Diagnostic needle culdocentesis is done to diagnose ectopic pregnancy and to detect intraperitoneal bleeding or cul-de-sac hematoma. Posterior colpotomy is done to carry out definitive operative procedures: various kinds of tubal ligations, aspiration or the removal of ovarian cysts, the occasional management of an ectopic pregnancy, and exploratory diagnostic operative procedures.

Procedural considerations. The basic vaginal instrument set is required, plus the following:

1 Needle, 15 gauge, 3½ inches
1 Syringe
2 Culture tubes
2 Drains, if desired

An abdominal gynecologic instrument set should be available in case laparotomy is indicated.

Operative procedures

Needle culdocentesis

1. A 15-gauge needle attached to a syringe is inserted through the posterior fornix of the vagina. Suspected

intraperitoneal bleeding is confirmed if dark or red blood flows freely into the syringe. Failure to obtain blood does not rule out the possibility of intraperitoneal bleeding.

2. Bleeding of the vaginal wall is controlled by sutures. Vaginal packing and a Foley catheter may also be used.

Posterior colpotomy

1. A transverse incision is made through the posterior vaginal wall with curved scissors. This incision is carried into the peritoneum, behind the cervix at the superior point of the posterior fornix.
2. Allis forceps are used to facilitate exposure, and hemostasis is obtained by placing a number of sutures in the corners or angles of the wound.
3. The posterior vaginal wall is held open with a weighted retractor.
4. In case of infection in the cul-de-sac, the opening is enlarged enough to permit drainage from the cul-de-sac. The cavity is explored; drains may be inserted.
5. Bleeding of the vaginal wall is controlled by sutures. The peritoneum and the vaginal mucosa are closed with a continuous suture. Vaginal packing and a Foley catheter may also be used.

Marsupialization of Bartholin's duct cyst or abscess

Marsupialization of Bartholin's duct cyst or abscess entails removal or incision of the cyst through the vaginal outlet and drainage of the area. In true marsupialization, the cyst is surgically exteriorized by resecting the anterior wall and suturing the cut edges of the remaining cyst to the adjacent edges of the skin.

A cyst in a Bartholin's gland usually follows acute infection and is treated by marsupialization when it is quiescent. Such cysts are not neoplastic but result from retention of glandular secretions caused by blockage somewhere in the duct system.

Procedural considerations. The basic vaginal instrument set is required, plus the following:

1 Needle, 15 gauge, 3½ inches
1 Syringe
2 Culture tubes
  Iodoform or plain gauze packing
1 Drain, if desired

Operative procedure

1. The labia minora may be sutured to the perineal skin on each side to expose the vaginal introitus.
2. An elliptic incision is made in the mucosa, which is distended over the cyst.
3. The cyst wall is dissected, and, if indicated, removal of the gland is completed with blunt-pointed scissors. The tissue may be everted with sutures and left open. A drain or packing may be inserted, and a dressing is applied.

Hysteroscopy

Hysteroscopy is endoscopic visualization of the uterine cavity and tubal orifices. The common indications for hysteroscopy include evaluation of abnormal uterine bleeding, location and removal of "lost" intrauterine devices, evaluation of infertility, diagnosis and surgical treatment of intrauterine adhesions, verification of submucous leiomyomas or endometrial polyps, resection of uterine septa or submucous leiomyomas, and tubal sterilization. Laparoscopy may be done in association with hysteroscopy to assess the external contour of the uterus.

Procedural considerations. The instrumentation required includes a dilatation and curettage set, plus the following:

1 Hysteroscopy set (Fig. 14-28)
2 Syringes, 50 ml
  Polyethylene tubing
  Fiberoptic light source
  Electrosurgical unit, if desired
  Gas insufflator, if desired

Operative procedure

1. The cervix is exposed with an Auvard weighted speculum and an anterior retractor; the anterior lip of the cervix is grasped with a tenaculum and is drawn toward the introitus.
2. The direction of the cervical canal and the depth of the uterine cavity are determined by means of a graduated uterine sound.
3. The endocervical canal is dilated by means of graduated Hegar or Hank uterine dilators to 6, 7, or 8 mm, depending on the size of the hysteroscope.
4. A self-retaining vacuum cannula with obturator may be placed in contact with the cervix. The cannula is firmly applied to the cervix by vacuum created with a negative pressure.
5. The obturator is withdrawn and the hysteroscope is introduced to the level of the internal cervical os.
6. To achieve satisfactory visualization, the uterine cavity must be distended with one of several media: 32% Dextran 70 in dextrose, dextrose 5% in water (D5W), or carbon dioxide gas insufflation. Injection of 32% Dextran 70 may be under continuous pressure from a 50-ml syringe via polyethylene tubing into the irrigating channel of the hysteroscope. When the syringe is loaded, care must be taken to prevent air bubbles, which distort the view. Uterine distention with D5W may be achieved by inserting a 500-ml plastic bag containing the medium into an intravenous pressure infusor. The fluid runs freely via polyethylene tubing through the channel of the hysteroscope. However, a satisfactory hysteroscopy may not be done if bleeding occurs, because D5W is miscible with blood. Distention with carbon dioxide gas is achieved by a controlled pressure system.
7. Exploration of the uterine cavity is begun.

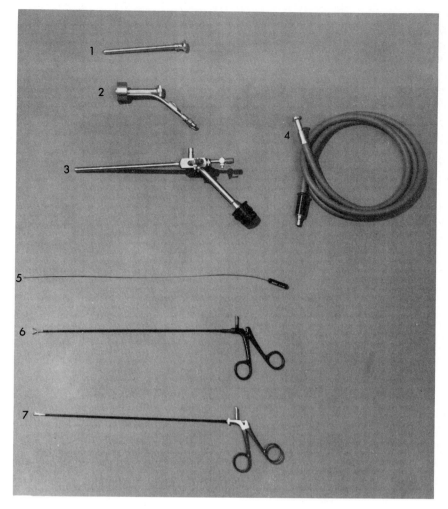

Fig. 14-28. Instruments for hysteroscopy. *1,* Obturator for cannula; *2,* self-retaining vacuum cannula, small; *3,* hysteroscope; *4,* fiberoptic light cord; *5,* coagulation electrode; *6,* grasping forceps; *7,* scissors.

8. Ancillary instruments such as rigid and flexible biopsy forceps, scissors, grasping forceps, insulated coagulation electrodes, or tubal occlusive devices may be introduced for intrauterine manipulation or surgical intervention through the operating channel of the hysteroscope.

9. Upon completion of the procedure, the hysteroscope is withdrawn and the self-retaining vacuum cannula is removed.

10. If 32% Dextran 70 in dextrose is used for uterine distention, the instruments must be rinsed immediately and cleaned in hot water because Dextran has a tendency to harden and is difficult to remove if permitted to dry.

Vaginal hysterectomy

Vaginal hysterectomy is removal of the uterus through an incision made in the vaginal wall and the pelvic cavity. The vaginal approach is contraindicated when a large uterine tumor is present or in pelvic malignancy because of an associated inflammatory process involving the fallopian tubes and ovaries.

Procedural considerations. The instrumentation includes the basic vaginal instrument set; two needles, 22 gauge, 1½ or 3 inches; and two syringes, 10 ml. An abdominal gynecologic instrument set should be available in case laparotomy is indicated.

To facilitate dissection and decrease bleeding, the vaginal walls may be infiltrated with normal saline or a local anesthetic (vasoconstrictors are optional).

Operative procedure

1. The labia may be retracted with sutures. A vaginal retractor is inserted to retract the vaginal wall.

2. Dilatation and curettage may be performed, as previously described (Fig. 14-24).

3. A Jacobs vulsellum forceps, tenaculum, or suture ligature is placed through the cervical lips to permit traction on the cervix (Fig. 14-29).

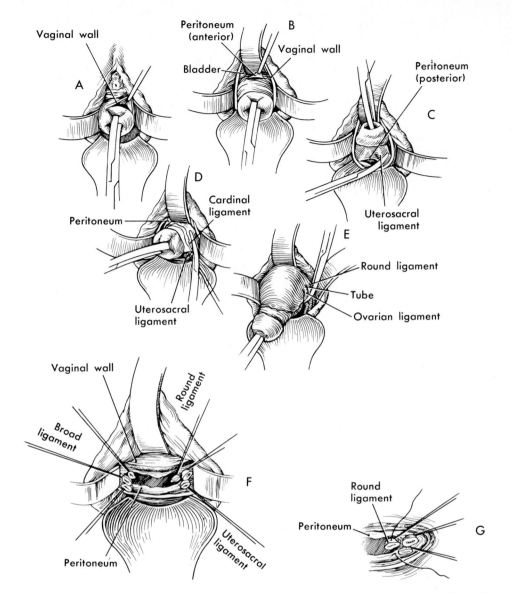

Fig. 14-29. Vaginal hysterectomy. **A,** Incision of vaginal wall around cervix. Anterior vaginal wall slightly elevated. **B,** Deaver retractor on each side; one Deaver retractor under bladder. Peritoneum opened. **C,** Posterior cul-de-sac opened. Heaney clamp applied to left uterosacral ligament. **D,** Left uterosacral ligament cut and tied. Clamp applied to left cardinal ligament. **E,** Clamp applied to ovarian ligament, round ligament, and fallopian tube. **F,** Uterosacral ligament, broad ligament, and round ligament shown in their respective normal positions. **G,** Peritoneum closed and cardinal broad ligament and uterosacral ligaments reattached to angle of vagina. Left uterosacral and broad ligaments anchored. (From Counseller, V.S. in Lowrie, R.J., editor: Gynecology: surgical techniques, Springfield, Ill., 1955, Charles C Thomas, Publisher.)

4. The vaginal wall is incised with a knife anteriorly through the full thickness of the wall. The bladder is freed from the anterior surface of the cervix by sharp and blunt dissection. The bladder is then elevated to expose the peritoneum of the anterior cul-de-sac, which is entered by sharp dissection (Fig. 14-29, *B*).

5. The peritoneum of the posterior cul-de-sac is identified and incised.

6. The uterosacral ligaments containing blood vessels are clamped, cut, and ligated (Fig. 14-29, *C* and *D*). The ends of the ligatures are left long and are tagged with a clamp.

7. The uterus is drawn downward and the bladder held aside with retractors and moist, small laparotomy packs.

8. The cardinal ligament on each side is clamped, cut,

and ligated. The uterine arteries are doubly clamped, cut, and ligated.

9. The fundus is delivered with the aid of a uterine tenaculum.
10. When the ovaries are to be left, the round ligament, the uterovarian ligament, and the fallopian tube on each side are clamped together (Fig. 14-29, *E*) and cut, and the uterus is removed. These pedicles are then ligated.
11. The peritoneum between the rectum and vagina is approximated with a continuous suture. The retroperitoneal obliteration of the cul-de-sac is done by sutures that pass from the vaginal wall through the infundibulopelvic ligament and round ligament, through the cardinal ligament, and out the vaginal wall. The sutures are tied on the vaginal aspect of the new vault (Fig. 14-29, *F* and *G*). The round, cardinal, and ureterosacral ligaments may be individually approximated for additional support.
12. Any existing cystocele and rectocele and the perineum are repaired, as described for vaginal plastic repair (Figs. 14-18 and 14-20). In the presence of prolapse, reconstruction of the pelvic floor may be required.
13. A Foley or suprapubic catheter is usually inserted. The vagina may be packed, and a drain may be inserted.

Abdominal gynecologic surgery
Laparoscopy

Laparoscopy is endoscopic visualization of the peritoneal cavity through the anterior abdominal wall after the establishment of a pneumoperitoneum. It is used in investigating and diagnosing the causes of abdominal and pelvic pain, determining causes of infertility, and evaluating pelvic masses. Ancillary procedures such as adhesiolysis, fulguration of endometriotic implants, aspiration of cysts, biopsy of tissue, aspiration of peritoneal fluid for cytologic study, and tubal sterilization may be performed. Laparoscopy also can be used for oocyte retrieval in in vitro fertilization procedures. Lasers may be used with the laparoscope.

Procedural considerations. A general or local anesthetic is administered. The patient is placed in lithotomy position. The abdomen, perineum, and vagina are prepped. The abdomen and perineum are then draped for a combined procedure. Specially designed drapes with openings for the umbilical and perineal areas may be used. The bladder should be emptied.

A dilatation and curettage may be done with laparoscopic procedures when indicated. After the cervix is exposed and the position and depth of the uterus are confirmed, a Hulka forceps or uterine dilator may be introduced into the cervix to manipulate the uterus during the laparoscopy so that the surgeon has better visibility. If chromotubation to evaluate the patency of the fallopian tubes will be performed during the laparoscopy, an intrauterine cannula is placed in the cervical canal at the time of dilatation and curettage.

The usual instrumentation for the vaginal portion of the procedure includes a dilatation and curettage set, plus the following:

1 Hulka forceps
1 Intrauterine cannula
   Diluted methylene blue or indigo carmine solution, if desired
1 Syringe, 20 ml, if desired

The setup for laparoscopy includes:

1 Laparoscopy set (Fig. 14-30)
1 Syringe, 10 ml
1 Bard-Parker knife handle, no. 3 with blade no. 15 or 11
6 Backhaus towel clamps, 5¼ inches
2 Allis forceps, 6 inches
2 Crile hemostats, 5½ inches
1 Mayo-Hegar needle holder, 6 inches
1 Suture scissors
2 Adson forceps with teeth
2 Skin hooks, if desired
1 Suture for skin closure
   Band-Aid
   Steri-Strip, if desired
   Electrosurgical unit
   Fiberoptic light source
   Gas insufflator for achieving pneumoperitoneum

An abdominal gynecologic instrument set should be available in case laparotomy is indicated.

Operative procedure
1. A small incision (0.7 to 1.2 cm) is made at the inferior margin of the umbilicus.
2. Elevating the skin with a towel clamp on either side of the umbilicus or grasping below the umbilicus with a gauze sponge for traction, the surgeon inserts a Verres needle through the layers of the abdominal wall into the peritoneal cavity.
3. Once the Verres needle is inserted into the peritoneal cavity, a 10-ml syringe partially filled with sterile saline is attached to the Verres needle for aspiration. If the Verres needle has entered a blood vessel, blood is aspirated. If a loop of intestine or the stomach has been entered, aspiration of bowel contents or malodorous gas occurs. If the needle is free in the peritoneal cavity, nothing is aspirated.
4. A plastic or Silastic tubing is attached to the Verres needle and the gas insufflator. Approximately 2 to 3 L of carbon dioxide or nitrous oxide gas are then delivered into the peritoneal cavity to achieve pneumoperitoneum. The intraabdominal pressure must be closely monitored to prevent overdistention of the abdomen and to ensure free passage of gas into the peritoneal cavity.
5. After insufflation is completed, the Verres needle is withdrawn.

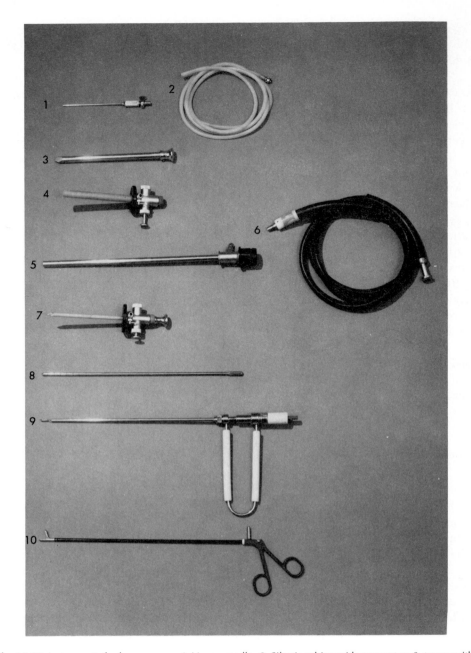

Fig. 14-30. Instruments for laparoscopy. *1*, Verres needle; *2*, Silastic tubing with connector; *3*, trocar with pyramidal tip; *4*, trocar sleeve with trumpet valve; *5*, laparoscope; *6*, fiberoptic light cord; *7*, secondary trocar sleeve and trocar; *8*, calibrated probe; *9*, bipolar forceps; *10*, biopsy forceps.

6. The trocar covered by the trocar sleeve is inserted boldly through the abdominal wall into the peritoneal cavity. The angle taken by the trocar is approximately 45 degrees toward the concavity of the pelvis. The plastic or Silastic tubing is attached to the trocar sleeve and insufflation is resumed. Some surgeons prefer a direct trocar insertion technique or open laparoscopy technique of Hassan to establish the pneumoperitoneum through the valve of the trocar sleeve rather than through a Verres needle.

7. With the trocar sleeve in place, the trocar is withdrawn and the laparoscope is introduced (Fig. 14-31). Visualization of the pelvis and lower abdomen and the visceral contents is begun. If the lens of the laparoscope becomes foggy, touching the lens to a loop of intestine is one method of clearing it.

8. The patient is placed in Trendelenburg's position.

9. If an ancillary instrument such as a biopsy forceps or bipolar forceps is needed, a second trocar with sleeve is inserted under direct laparoscopic visualization through an incision made suprapubically.

10. To test for tubal patency, diluted methylene blue or

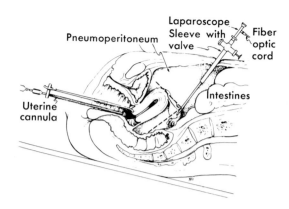

Fig. 14-31. Technique of laparoscopy. (From Cohen, M.R.: J. Obstet. Gynecol. *31*:310, 1968.)

indigo carmine solution is injected through the intrauterine cannula in the cervical canal. If the fallopian tubes are patent, dye can be seen at the fimbriated ends.

11. On completion of the intraabdominal procedure, the laparoscope is withdrawn and the insufflated gas is allowed to escape from the trocar sleeve. The trocar sleeve is removed.

12. Application of skin clips or subcuticular closure of the primary skin incision is followed by placement of a Band-Aid or Steri-Strip.

Pelviscopy

Pelviscopy is an endoscopic approach to pelvic and intraabdominal examination and/or surgery. A curved, 30-degree angle scope is used to visualize the intrapelvic and intraabdominal structures. Accessory instruments used with the pelviscope include: dissecting forceps, grasping forceps, scissors, sponge holders, needle holders, suture forceps, knot tiers, appendix extractors, suction manipulators, and applicators for loop ligature. Endocoagulation and endoligation may be accomplished.

Procedures performed through the pelviscope include: ovarian biopsy, ovarian cyst enucleation and resection, oophorectomy, adnexectomy, enucleation of intramural myomas, appendectomy, fimbrioplasty, and removal of ectopic tubal pregnancy.

Total abdominal hysterectomy

Total abdominal hysterectomy is removal of the entire uterus, including the corpus and the cervix. When total abdominal hysterectomy is combined with bilateral salpingo-oophorectomy, the procedure is commonly termed panhysterectomy or complete hysterectomy.

Total hysterectomy may be performed for symptomatic pelvic relaxation or prolapse, pain associated with pelvic congestion, pelvic inflammatory disease, endometriosis, recurrent ovarian cysts, fibroids (myomas), bleeding with no apparent cause in postmenopausal women, adenomyosis, or dysfunctional uterine bleeding. Total hysterectomy, usually with bilateral salpingo-oophorectomy, is also indicated in anatomic disease, malignancy, premalignant states, and conditions of high risk for development or recurrence of malignancy. Total hysterectomy can also be used to accomplish sterilization.

Procedural considerations. Diagnostic dilatation and curettage usually have already been performed. However, an instrument set should be readily available. Before the abdominal skin prep, an external and internal vaginal prep is done. A Foley catheter is inserted to provide constant bladder drainage during the operation. Supine and Trendelenburg's positions are used. Instrumentation includes the abdominal gynecologic set. Provisions are made to remove from the abdomen and field those instruments used in separating the cervix from the vagina, thereby avoiding vaginal contamination of the pelvis.

Operative procedure

1. In case of an obese patient or for exploration of the upper abdominal cavity, a left rectus or midline incision may be made. For simple hysterectomy a Pfannenstiel incision may be used. The abdominal layers and the peritoneum are opened as described for laparotomy.

2. As the peritoneal cavity is opened, the patient is usually placed in Trendelenburg's position to provide better visualization of the pelvic organs.

3. The round ligament is grasped with forceps, clamped, and ligated with sutures on long needle holders. Pedicles are cut with a knife or Metzenbaum scissors; sutures are tagged with a hemostat to be used as traction later. This procedure is done on both sides (Fig. 14-32, *A*).

4. By use of the surgeon's fingers, the layer of the broad ligament close to the uterus is separated on each side, bleeding vessels are clamped and ligated, and a moist laparotomy pack is inserted behind the flap. The fallopian tube and the utero-ovarian ligaments are double-clamped together, incised, and double-tied with suture ligatures (Fig. 14-32, *B*).

5. The uterus is pulled forward to expose the posterior sheath of the broad ligament, which is incised with a knife or Metzenbaum scissors. Ureters are identified. The uterine vessels and uterosacral ligaments are double-clamped, divided by sharp dissection at the level of the internal os, and ligated with suture ligatures (Fig. 14-32, *C*).

6. The severed uterine vessels are bluntly dissected away from the cervix on each side with the aid of sponges on sponge-holding forceps, scissors, and tissue forceps.

7. The bladder is separated from the cervix and upper vagina with sharp and blunt dissection assisted by sponges on sponge-holding forceps.

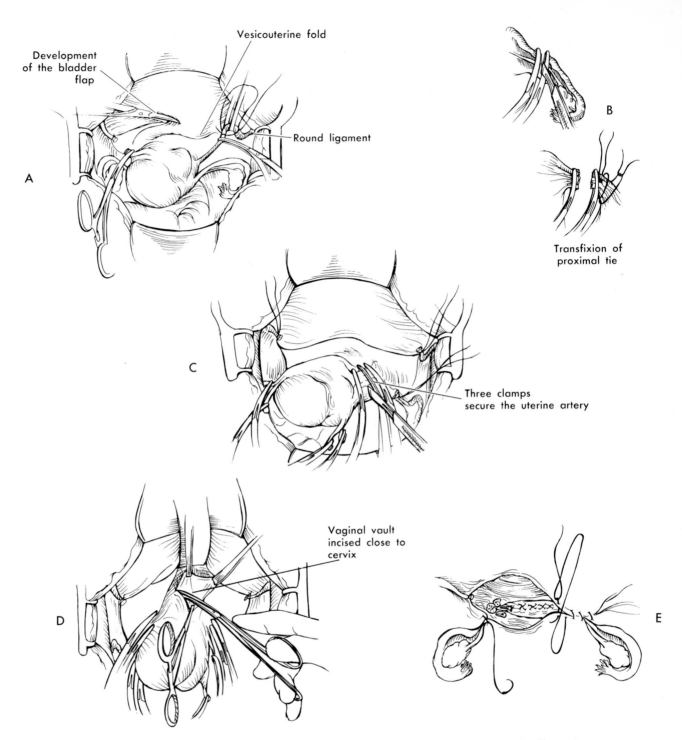

Development
of the bladder
flap

Vesicouterine fold

Round ligament

A

B

Transfixion of
proximal tie

C

Three clamps
secure the uterine artery

D

Vaginal vault
incised close to
cervix

E

Fig. 14-32. Abdominal hysterectomy for single fibroid uterus. **A,** Peritoneum retracted with self-retaining retractors, and organs protected with laparotomy packs saturated in warm normal saline solution. Transverse incision made through uterine peritoneum and carried to each side of uterine attachments of round ligaments. Bleeding vessels clamped and ligated. Round ligament grasped, ligated, and cut. **B,** Tube and ovarian ligaments clamped, cut, and sutured. **C,** Uterus pulled forward, posterior sheath of broad ligaments divided, and uterine artery and veins secured by three heavy curved clamps. Pedicle divided, leaving two hemostats on proximal pedicle. **D,** Bladder separated from cervix and upper vagina. Vaginal vault opened and grasped with Allis forceps. Allis forceps placed on anterior lip of cervix, and dissection of cervix carried out to complete its amputation from vagina. **E,** Three connective tissue thickenings anchored to vaginal vault, vaginal mucosa approximated, and vault closed. As shown, peritoneum closed with continuous suture. (From Ball, T.L.: Operative gynecology and urology, ed. 2, St. Louis, 1963, The C.V. Mosby Co.)

8. The bladder may be retracted with a moist laparotomy pack and a retractor with an angular blade. The vaginal vault is incised close to the cervix with a knife or scissors (Fig. 14-32, *D*).

9. The anterior lip of the cervix is grasped with an Allis, Kocher, or tenaculum forceps. With scissors, the cervix is dissected and amputated from the vagina. The uterus is removed. Potentially contaminated instruments used on the cervix and vagina are placed in a discard basin and removed from the field (including sponge-holding forceps and suction). Bleeding is controlled with hemostats and sutures.

10. The vaginal vault is reconstructed with interrupted sutures. Angle sutures anchor all three connective tissue ligaments to the vaginal vault. The pedicles, fallopian tubes, and ovarian ligaments are left free of the vault.

11. Vaginal mucosa is approximated with a continuous suture on a long needle holder. The muscular coat of the vagina may be closed with figure-of-eight sutures to make the vault of the vagina firm and provide resistance against prolapse. A drain may be placed in the vagina.

12. The peritoneum is closed over the bladder, vaginal vault, and rectum (Fig. 14-32, *E*). The laparotomy packs are removed, and the omentum is drawn over the bowel.

13. The abdominal wound is closed as described for laparotomy closure (Chapter 11).

Abdominal myomectomy

Abdominal myomectomy is removal of fibromyomas, or fibroid tumors, from the uterine wall. Myomectomy is usually done in young women who have symptoms that indicate the presence of tumors and who wish to preserve their potential fertility. Also, tumors may be removed because of infertility, habitual abortion, or distortion of the bladder and other organs. Myomectomy may be performed as a prophylactic measure in conjunction with other abdominopelvic surgery.

Procedural considerations. The basic abdominal gynecologic instrument set is required.

Operative procedure

1. The patient is prepared as described for abdominal hysterectomy. A midline or Pfannenstiel incision is used, and the uterus is exposed.

2. To contract the musculature of the uterine wall, a suitable drug may be injected into the fundus.

3. The fibroid tumor is grasped with a tenaculum. The broad ligament may be opened with curved hemostats and Metzenbaum scissors to determine the course of the ureter or to free the bladder.

4. Each tumor is shelled out of its bed, using blunt and sharp instruments. Bleeding vessels are clamped and ligated or electrocoagulated.

5. The uterus is reconstructed with interrupted or continuous sutures.

6. The perimetrium is closed over the operative site. The abdominal wound is closed.

Radical hysterectomy (Wertheim)

Radical hysterectomy is en bloc dissection with careful removal of all recognizable lymph nodes in the pelvis, together with wide removal of the uterus, tubes, ovaries, supporting ligaments, and upper vagina. Extensive dissection of the ureters and of the bladder is also involved.

Radical abdominal hysterectomy is performed in the presence of cervical carcinoma, with or without attendant radiation therapy. Abdominal exploration determines lymph node involvement. With no lymph node involvement, a wide-cuff hysterectomy is performed. The uterus, tubes, and ovaries, together with most of the parametrial tissues and the upper portion of the vagina, are dissected en bloc. Dissection of the ureters from the paracervical structures takes place so that the ligaments supporting the uterus and vagina can be removed. Radical abdominal hysterectomy can also be used in certain cases of endometrial carcinoma.

Procedural considerations. Careful estimation of blood loss and calculation of urinary output are needed throughout the operative procedure.

The patient is prepped as described for total abdominal hysterectomy. Ureteral catheters may be inserted before the procedure. The basic abdominal gynecologic instrument set is required, plus the following:

8 Schmidt tonsil forceps, 7¼ inches
6 Mixter forceps, 9 inches
1 Bard-Parker knife handle, no. 4 long with blade no. 20
2 Cushing vein retractors
2 DeBakey tissue forceps, 12 inches
  Ligating clips and appliers
  Kitner sponges
2 Closed wound drainage systems

Operative procedure

1. The skin is incised, and the abdominal layers are opened, as described for laparotomy.

2. The peritoneum is cut at its reflection on the anterior surface of the uterus between the round ligaments (Fig. 14-33, *A*). By blunt dissection, the bladder surface is freed from the cervix and vagina.

3. The right round and infundibulopelvic ligaments are clamped, cut with a knife or Metzenbaum scissors, and ligated with sutures to expose the external iliac artery. The ureter is identified and retracted with a vein retractor (Fig. 14-33, *B*).

4. The lymph and areolar tissues are dissected from the iliac artery, obturator fossa, and ureter with Lahey forceps, Kitner sponges, and Metzenbaum scissors. A complete lymph gland dissection removes the tissue from Cloquet's node to the bifurcation of the iliac ar-

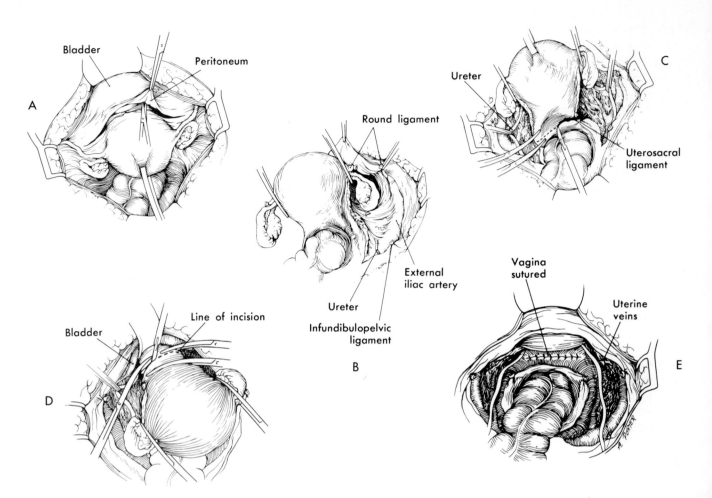

Fig. 14-33. Wertheim radical hysterectomy. **A,** With upward traction applied on uterus, peritoneum is incised from round ligament to round ligament. **B,** Right round and infundibulopelvic ligaments are ligated and cut, thus exposing right external iliac artery. **C,** Uterus is held upward and forward, exposing cul-de-sac, which is incised as shown by *dotted line* **D,** After dissection is completed, vagina is doubly clamped preparatory to transection, after which entire specimen is lifted out en masse. **E,** Vagina is closed. Peritoneum remains to be reperitonealized. (Redrawn from Mattingly, R.F., and Thompson, J.D.: TeLinde's operative gynecology, ed. 6, Philadelphia, 1985, J.B. Lippincott Co.)

teries bilaterally. The uterine artery and vein are clamped, cut, and doubly ligated.

5. The uterus is elevated, the cul-de-sac is opened (Fig. 14-33, *C*), and the uterosacral and cardinal ligaments are clamped, cut with scissors, and doubly ligated with suture ligatures. The pararectal and paravesical areolar tissues are dissected free to skeletonize the upper vagina, and the paraurethral tissues are removed as near to the pelvic walls as possible.

6. The upper third of the vagina is cross-clamped with Heaney forceps (Fig. 14-33, *D*) and divided with a long no. 4 knife handle and no. 20 blade. The uterus and surrounding tissues are removed. Electrocoagulation is useful in minimizing venous oozing from small venules and capillaries. Lowering the head of the operating bed 15 degrees is also helpful in reducing the oozing of blood and serum. Careful apposition of the skin edges with interrupted mattress sutures must take

place to prevent overlapping of the skin edges and a resulting delay in healing.

7. The vagina is sutured open with a running locked stitch, and closed wound drainage is provided from above (Fig. 14-33, *E*). The pelvis is peritonealized with a continuous suture.

8. The abdominal wound is closed (retention sutures may be used) and dressed in the usual manner. Vaginal packing and drains may be used.

Pelvic exenteration

Pelvic exenteration is en bloc removal of the rectum, distal sigmoid colon, the urinary bladder and the distal ureters, the internal iliac vessels and their lateral branches, all pelvic reproductive organs and lymph nodes, and the entire pelvic floor with the accompanying pelvic peritoneum, levator muscles, and perineum. A partial exenteration, either anterior or posterior, may be performed, depending on the origin of the carcinoma and the extent of local tissue invasion.

The success of modern deep pelvic surgery for malignant abdominoperineal lesions is attributable to increased knowledge regarding aseptic and surgical techniques, anesthesia, transfusions, intravenous antibiotic therapy, and the pathophysiology of involved organs. Current therapeutic techniques evolved after determination of the modes of metastasis, resective possibilities, and means of reestablishing modified physiologic function.

Pelvic exenteration is the preferred treatment for recurrent or persistent carcinoma of the cervix after radiation therapy; it is also applicable to carcinomas of the endometrium or rectum. Exenteration is considered only after a thorough investigation of the patient and disease status to determine if there is a reasonable chance of cure and of return to a productive life. The surgeon can determine with finality the chance of resectability with cure at the time of abdominal exploration.

The need for creation of urinary and bowel diversions must also be considered, together with the patient's ability to cope with these diversions postoperatively. Total pelvic exenteration has been advocated as the definitive procedure of choice in a critical clinical situation.

Psychologic preparation of the patient and family by the nurse and physician is a prime requisite. Nursing care should be directed toward supporting the patient during therapy and helping the patient maintain personal dignity.

Procedural considerations. The bowel is cleansed preoperatively with antibiotics and enemas. A nasogastric tube, Foley catheter, and rectal tube are inserted before or during surgery. Antiembolic stockings are placed on both legs. Cardiac and central venous pressure monitoring is maintained throughout the procedure.

The patient is placed in the supine position with legs abducted in the "ski" position or elevated in a modified lithotomy position to allow access to the perineum without disruptive position changes. Skin prepping includes the abdomen, thighs, perineum, and the internal vaginal vault.

The circulating and scrub nurses must be alert to fluid and blood loss, irrigation solutions must be accurately measured, laparotomy packs must be weighed to assess blood volume loss, and the anesthesiologist and surgical team must be apprised of the measurements.

When the colon is transected or ureteral drainage is diverted into an ileosegment, the gastrointestinal technique as described in Chapter 11 should be followed.

Separate instrument setups are required for the abdominal and perineal approaches. Extra drapes, gowns, and gloves should be available. For the abdominal approach, the basic abdominal gynecologic instrument set and instrumentation described previously for abdominoperineal resection (Chapter 11) are required, plus the following:

1 Bard-Parker knife handle, no. 4 long, with blade no. 20
1 Nelson dissecting scissors, 11 inches

8 Schnidt tonsil forceps, 7¼ inches
6 Mixter forceps, 9 inches
6 Allis forceps, 9¼ inches
8 Rochester-Pean hysterectomy forceps, 9 inches
4 Right-angled clamps, 12 inches
2 Stille kidney clamps, 9 inches
2 Cushing vein retractors
2 DeBakey tissue forceps, 12 inches
2 Mayo-Hegar needle holders, 12 inches
Ligating clips and appliers
Red rubber catheters, assorted sizes
Colostomy bag
Ileostomy bag

For the perineal approach, the basic vaginal instrument set is required. To prevent contamination, the anus may be closed with a purse-string suture.

Operative procedure

1. A long midline incision from the symphysis pubis to the umbilicus is made, and the abdomen is opened in the usual manner. A second incision within the perineum encircling the vestibule and anus is also made.

2. The peritoneal cavity is explored for metastasis to the liver, the nodes of the celiac axis, the superior mesenteric artery, and the paraaortic tissues.

3. The pelvis is explored, and the peritoneum along the brim of the pelvis examined for lymph node involvement. Frozen sections may be indicated. The obturator fossa and the region of the uterosacral ligaments are explored. When findings at exploration are negative, retractors are placed and the small bowel is packed off with moist laparotomy packs (Fig. 14-34).

4. The sigmoid mesocolon is freed and sectioned by means of intestinal clamps and a scalpel or a stapling device. The proximal end is exteriorized through an opening in the left side of the abdomen; an intestinal clamp is left across the lumen until later, when the permanent colostomy will be secured to the skin.

5. The remaining sigmoid mesentery is clamped with Rochester-Pean forceps, cut, and ligated down to and including the superior hemorrhoidal vessels. Long instruments and sutures are used to facilitate reaching the deep pelvic structures.

6. The distal sigmoid colon is closed with an inverting

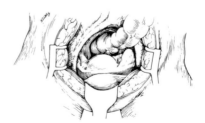

Fig. 14-34. Pelvic exenteration. Pelvic viscera in situ as viewed from operating surgeon's vantage point after retractors are placed and small bowel is packed off. (Redrawn from Lindenauer, S.M., and others: Arch. Surg. 96:493, 1968.)

suture. The sigmoid colon and rectum are freed from the sacrococcygeal area by blunt and sharp dissection.

7. The lateral pelvic peritoneum is cut along the iliac vessels; the ovarian vessels and round ligaments on each side are clamped with Rochester-Pean forceps, cut, and doubly ligated.

8. The peritoneum is incised over the dome of the bladder with a long knife and Metzenbaum scissors, and the bladder is separated from the symphysis pubis down to the urethra.

9. The ureters are identified and divided 2 to 3 cm below the brim of the pelvis. The proximal end is left open to allow urinary drainage while the distal end is ligated.

10. The hypogastric artery, the internal iliac vein, and the superior and inferior gluteal vessels are exposed, clamped with hemostats, doubly ligated, and cut. The external iliac vein is retracted to allow evacuation of the contents of the obturator fossa, leaving the obturator nerve intact. Care must be taken in dissection not to damage the sacral plexus and sciatic nerve.

11. The internal pudendal vessels are isolated, ligated with transfixion sutures, and cut. The remaining soft tissue attachments of the pelvis are clamped and cut. Steps 10 and 11 are then performed on the opposite side.

12. The perineum is incised by an elliptic incision that includes the clitoris and anus. The ischiorectal fat is incised up to the area of the levator muscle.

13. The coccygeal attachment of the rectum is severed. The levator muscles are severed at their lateral attachments by means of a long no. 4 knife handle with no. 20 blade; hemostasis is maintained by pressure and traction.

14. The paravesical and paravaginal tissues are resected from the periosteum of the symphysis pubis and superior pubic rami by means of a knife. The specimen

is completely freed and removed from the pelvis (Fig. 14-35).

15. After residual bleeding vessels are identified and controlled by transfixing ligatures, the subcutaneous tissue is closed by interrupted sutures. A drain is placed in the wound, and the skin is closed.

16. In the abdomen, further residual bleeding vessels are controlled. Packs may be left in the pelvis to be removed through the perineum after 48 hours.

17. The ileosegment is then fashioned and the ureters anastomosed to it in the manner described in Chapter 15. The external stoma of the ileosegment is placed on the right side of the abdomen.

18. A red rubber, multieyed tube, size 16 Fr, is inserted into the proximal jejunum for the length of the jejunum and the ileum to aid in postoperative bowel decompression. It is sutured to the bowel with a purse-string suture and brought out to the skin, where it is sutured in place.

19. A gastrostomy tube is placed in the stomach in the same manner.

20. Hemostasis is checked. The small intestines are carefully repositioned into the pelvis. Packs and retractors are removed (Fig. 14-36).

21. The peritoneum, rectus muscles, and fascial sheaths are closed with interrupted figure-of-eight sutures. The skin is closed with interrupted sutures.

22. The colostomy stoma is prepared by removing the intestinal clamp from the sigmoid colon, opening the colon, and suturing the stoma to the skin edges (Fig. 14-37).

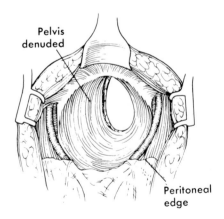

Fig. 14-35. Pelvic exenteration, continued. Empty pelvis after dissection of paravesical and paravaginal tissues and removal of specimen en bloc. (Redrawn from Lindenauer, S.M., and others: Arch. Surg. 96:493, 1968.)

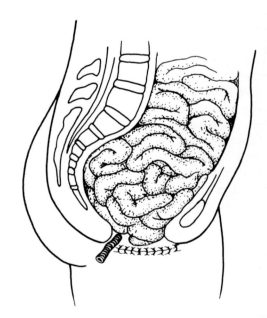

Fig. 14-36. Pelvic exenteration, continued. Sagittal view of small bowel above pelvic defect. Perineal packing and/or drain may be used. (Redrawn from Lindenauer, S.M., and others: Arch. Surg. 96:493, 1968.)

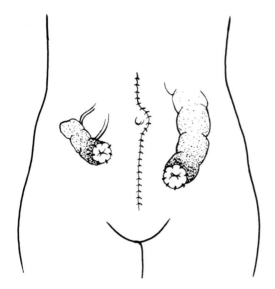

Fig. 14-37. Pelvic exenteration, continued. After closure of abdominal wall, colostomy and ileostomy stomas are sutured to skin edges. (Redrawn from Lindenauer, S.M., and others: Arch. Surg. 96:493, 1968.)

23. The abdominal wound and tube sites are dressed in the usual manner. Drainage bags are applied to the colostomy and ileostomy stomas. A perineal dressing may be secured by means of a T binder.

Surgery for conditions that affect fertility
Uterine suspension

Uterine suspension is shortening of the ligaments of the uterus and positioning them retroperitoneally. The ligaments are then sutured bilaterally to the undersurface of the abdominal fascia in the corners of the transverse incision to ensure the maintenance of an anterior position of the uterus. This prevents the fallopian tubes and ovaries from entrapment in the cul-de-sac.

Uterine suspension is done as part of a conservative surgical treatment of pelvic inflammatory disease or endometriosis. It is also indicated in patients who require lysis of extensive pelvic adhesions, for the correction of the symptoms of uterine retroversion, and for uterine prolapse in young women.

Procedural considerations. The basic abdominal gynecologic instrument set is required.

Operative procedure

1. The abdomen is opened as described for myomectomy.
2. The suspension is accomplished. If it is being done to correct uterine prolapse, a strip of Mersilene material is placed retroperitoneally to elevate the uterus at the level of the internal os posteriorly and to correct the prolapse into the vagina.
3. The wound is closed in layers, as described for laparotomy.

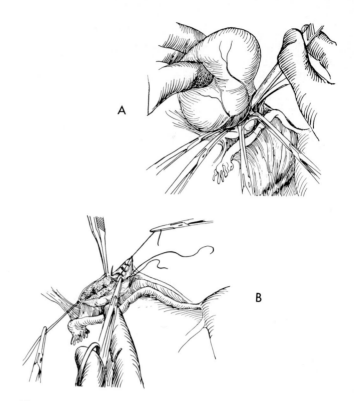

Fig. 14-38. Resection of small cyst from ovary. **A,** Incision made around ovary near junction of cyst wall and normal ovarian tissue. Knife handle is convenient instrument for shelling out cyst. **B,** Wound in ovary closed. (From Ball, T.L.: Operative gynecology and urology, ed. 2, St. Louis, 1963, The C.V. Mosby Co.)

Oophorectomy and oophorocystectomy

Oophorectomy is removal of an ovary. Oophorocystectomy is removal of an ovarian cyst (Fig. 14-38). Functional cysts comprise the majority of ovarian enlargements; follicular cysts are the most common. Functional cysts develop in the corpus luteum. Corpus luteum cysts are usually larger than other functional cysts. The true ovarian epithelial tumors, serous cystadenomas and pseudomucinous cystadenomas, are prone to malignant change.

The choice of operation depends on the patient's age and symptoms, findings during physical examination, and direct examination of the adnexa during exploration. If the ovarian tumor is recognized as benign, only the visibly diseased portions of the adnexa are removed. In the presence of dermoid, follicular, and corpus luteum cysts, the cyst is usually enucleated, and most of the ovarian parenchyma is preserved. In tubal pregnancy the pregnant fallopian tube is usually removed and in some cases the ovary also.

Procedural considerations. The basic abdominal gynecologic instrument set is required, plus the following:

1 Trocar and cannula
Suction tubing

1 Syringe, 10 ml
1 Needle, 21 gauge, 1½ inches

Operative procedure

1. The abdominal cavity is opened, as described for laparotomy.
2A. *For removal of a large ovarian cyst,* a purse-string suture may be placed in the cyst wall, and a trocar is introduced in its center; the suture is tightened around the trocar as the fluid is aspirated. The trocar is removed, and the purse-string suture is tied. All normal ovarian tissue is preserved.
2B. *For removal of a dermoid cyst,* the field is protected with laparotomy packs because the contents of such cysts produce irritation if they are spilled into the peritoneal cavity. An incision is made along the base of the cyst between the wall and normal ovarian tissue. The cystic wall is dissected away. The ovary is closed with interrupted or continuous sutures.
2C. *For decortication of the enlarged ovary and wedge resection,* a large segment of the ovarian cortex opposite the hilum is removed. The cysts are punctured with a needlepoint and collapsed. A wedge of ovarian stroma, extending deep in the hilum, is resected with a small knife; the cortex of the ovary is closed with interrupted or continuous sutures.
3. To prevent prolapse of the tube into the cul-de-sac, it may be sutured to the posterior sheath of the broad ligament.
4. The abdominal wound is closed as described for laparotomy.

Salpingo-oophorectomy

Salpingo-oophorectomy is removal of a fallopian tube and all or part of the associated ovary. Unilateral salpingo-oophorectomy may be done in some young women who are anxious to have children after all other methods of treatment have failed to cure chronic salpingo-oophoritis, in patients with ectopic tubal gestation, or in those with certain disease conditions of the adnexa or large adnexal cysts. If both tubes and ovaries are diseased, they are removed with total hysterectomy.

Procedural considerations. The basic abdominal gynecologic instrument set is required.

Operative procedure

1. The abdominal cavity is opened, as described for laparotomy.
2. The affected tube is grasped with Allis or Babcock forceps. The infundibulopelvic ligament is clamped with hemostats, cut, and ligated.
3. The mesosalpinx is grasped with hemostats and divided with the suspensory ligament of the ovary.
4. The cornual attachment of the tube is excised with a knife or curved scissors. Bleeding vessels are clamped and ligated.
5. The edges of the broad ligament are peritonealized from the uterine horn to the infundibulopelvic ligament, as described for total hysterectomy.
6. The wound is closed, as described for laparotomy; dressings are applied.

Microscopic reconstructive surgery of the fallopian tube

The obstructed portion of a fallopian tube may be removed and the tube reconstructed to create patency of the remaining portion of the tube in order to promote the possibility of fertilization. Reconstructive surgery of the tube, categorically called *tuboplasty,* includes reanastomosis, salpingoneostomy, fimbrioplasty, and lysis of adhesions.

Microsurgical correction of tubal pathology is the most successful way to perform tuboplasties and may be employed in all previously mentioned methods. The laser may be adapted to the operating microscope for use in tubal reconstructive surgery (Chapter 10).

Procedural considerations. The patient is placed in the supine position. The vagina is prepped as described previously. A Foley catheter is inserted into the bladder. A Kahn, Calvin, Rubin, Hui, or Humi cannula or a pediatric Foley catheter may be placed in the uterine cavity for intraoperative chromotubation with diluted methylene blue or indigo carmine solution. Intraoperative chromotubation can also be achieved by applying a Buxton uterine clamp around the lower segment of the uterus and inserting an Angiocath catheter through the fundus into the cavity. A vaginal pack may be placed in the vagina to help elevate the uterus.

The basic abdominal gynecologic instrument set is required, plus the following:

2 Iris scissors, 1 curved and 1 straight
2 Adson forceps without teeth
8 Halsted mosquito hemostats, 4 curved and 4 straight
1 Set Bowman lacrimal probes
2 Webster needle holders
1 Frazier suction tip, no. 2
1 Kirschner retractor, if desired
1 Buxton uterine clamp, if desired

Basic microsurgical instruments

2 Micro scissors, 1 curved and 1 straight
1 Microbayonet scissors, curved
2 Jeweler's forceps, no. 5
2 Jeweler's forceps, no. 7
1 Micro forceps with platform
1 Micro forceps with platform and very fine teeth
1 Fallopian tube forceps
1 Petit point mosquito hemostat
2 Micro needle holders, 1 curved and 1 straight
1 Ball tip nerve hook
2 Serrefines
3 Glass or Teflon rods

Accessory items

2 Micro needle electrodes

1 Electrosurgical pencil with fingertip control
1 Swolin electrosurgical handpiece, if desired
1 Bipolar forceps with cord
1 Irrigator for microsurgery with 2 irrigator cannulas, if desired
  Syringes and blunted needles for irrigation of the tissues
  Plastic or Silastic tubing and connectors
  Diluted methylene blue or indigo carmine solution
  Diluted heparinized lactated Ringer's solution
  Microscope drape
  Microscope or operative loupes
  Electrosurgical unit with monopolar and bipolar capabilities
  Video monitoring system, if desired

Operative procedure. Operative procedures for correction of postsurgical tubal occlusion are usually performed under the operating microscope. Other reconstructive procedures vary according to the nature of the pathological condition of the tube and may be done under the operating microscope or by use of operative loupes.

In microsurgery the surgeon must make sure that virtually no instruments are used in contact with the fallopian tube except those necessary to carry out the surgical technique. Microsurgery for infertility requires the use of specialized and delicate instruments. Each of these instruments is designed to permit gentle, atraumatic handling of tissues and prevent abrasions, lacerations, and vascular damage.

The tissues must be continually irrigated to prevent drying of the serosal surfaces. Ringer's lactate solution alone or with heparin added may be used as the irrigating solution.

Meticulous hemostasis is required in microsurgery. Irrigation is used to identify the bleeders. Hemostasis can be achieved by electrocoagulation with a microneedle electrode or very fine bipolar forceps.

When a carbon dioxide laser beam is used, the smoke from laser vaporization should be evacuated through suction to prevent carbon deposits on the tissue.

Tubal ligation. Tubal ligation is interruption of fallopian tube continuity, resulting in sterilization of the patient. In general, the indication for sterilization depends entirely on the desire of the patient. Certain medical indications and concern for the psychosocial needs of the patient are factors, and occasionally an obstetric indication exists, such as inherited fetal deformity. However, at least in the United States, sterilization is entirely a voluntary procedure. In many of the states, a sterilization permit does not have to be signed by the husband. Good presurgical counseling is needed for the patient and her husband or significant other because this procedure is not predictably reversible. Patients may elect to have the procedure performed on an ambulatory surgery basis at a time that is convenient for them.

The optimal time for sterilization is approximately 24 hours after vaginal delivery. This method does not delay the normal discharge time for the patient. An objection to this practice is that the danger of hemorrhage still exists soon after delivery. With a normal delivery, tubal ligation is done on the first or second postpartum day. If a cesarean section is done, the tubes may be ligated at that time.

Operative procedures. Many new surgical methods and techniques are available for tubal ligation. The objective of each method is to achieve complete closure of the fallopian tube so that conception is prevented. When a segment of each fallopian tube is excised, it is preserved for pathologic examination. General surgical considerations are directed to excising a section of each fallopian tube, ligating the severed ends, achieving hemostasis, and incorporating the proximal stump within layers of the mesosalpinx.

Laparoscopic tubal occlusion
1. Operative procedure is the same as for laparoscopy.
2. An accessory suprapubic incision may be made for the occluding instrument.
3. Sterilization takes place by the use of electrocoagulation or thermal coagulation or by the placement of a tubal clip or plastic ring after the tube has been identified and isolated in the grasping forceps.

Vaginal approach (posterior colpotomy)
1. Operative procedure is the same as for posterior colpotomy.
2. Sterilization can take place by the placement of a tubal clip or plastic ring, by fimbriectomy, or by ligation of the proximal portion of the fallopian tubes with a permanent suture.

Minilaparotomy approach
1. A 2-cm transverse incision is made above the pubic hairline.
2. A large bivalved speculum may be placed through the incision and into the peritoneal cavity. The large Graves bivalve speculum serves as a small abdominal retractor and permits easy access to the tubes.
3. Tubal clips or plastic rings can be applied, or the original Pomeroy method of ligation can be carried out.

In vitro fertilization and embryo transfer

Fertilization may be achieved by retrieval of oocytes from the ovary, followed by in vitro fertilization with sperm and implantation of the fertilized oocytes (embryos) into the uterine cavity.

In vitro fertilization and embryo transfer are indicated for women who have had bilateral absence or irreparable obstruction of the fallopian tubes, for women who have undergone tubal reconstructive surgery and have not conceived within 1 year after surgery, for women who have cervical or immunologic factors and have not conceived following treatment or for whom no treatment is available, for women who have failed to conceive following conservative surgery and hormonal suppressive therapy for endometriosis, for couples who have unexplained infertility, and for oligospermia as a cause of infertility. This procedure has raised many legal and ethical issues in its early stage of development.

To be a candidate for in vitro fertilization and embryo transfer, a woman must have at least one functioning ovary. The ovaries must be physically accessible for laparoscopic follicular aspiration unless aspiration is done under ultrasound-guided transabdominal or transvaginal puncture. The uterus must be normal and have functioning endometrium. The husband's semen must have sufficient motile sperm for insemination.

The treatment cycle for in vitro fertilization and embryo transfer can be divided into five stages: follicular development, aspiration of the mature preovulatory follicles, sperm preparation, in vitro fertilization, and embryo transfer. Laparoscopic aspiration of the follicles is the only stage that must occur in the operating room. Embryo transfer may or may not take place in the operating room. The treatment cycle is extremely stressful for the wife and the husband; both need emotional support from all members of the in vitro fertilization team.

Follicular development

Although a spontaneous ovulatory cycle was used for recovery of the oocyte in the early development of in vitro fertilization, all programs at present use a stimulated cycle to obtain multiple oocytes.

With a stimulated cycle, induction of ovulation is achieved by one of three regimens. The first regimen is clomiphene citrate (Clomid) and human chorionic gonadotropin (HCG). The patient receives 50 to 150 mg/day of Clomid for 5 days starting at a specified point in her menstrual cycle. On the day following the last dose of Clomid, the patient begins daily ultrasonic scanning and determination of serum level of estrogen to monitor follicular growth. The timing for HCG administration is based on the size and rate of growth of the follicles and the level of serum estradiol. To ensure follicular maturation, 4000 to 10,000 units of HCG is then administered to the patient.

The second regimen is human menopausal gonadotropin (HMG) and HCG. The patient receives 1 to 3 ampules of HMG daily starting on day 3 or day 5 of her menstrual cycle, depending on the protocol. Monitoring methods and timing of the HCG are similar to the Clomid regimen.

The third regimen is a combination of Clomid, HMG, and HCG. The patient receives Clomid for 5 days, followed by daily administration of HMG. In all three regimens, oocyte retrieval is performed 34 to 36 hours after the administration of HCG.

Aspiration of the mature preovulatory follicles

Follicular aspiration may be performed via an ultrasound-guided transabdominal or transvaginal puncture or via laparoscopic technique. In most in vitro fertilization programs, the laparoscopic follicular aspiration technique is used. In addition to the regular laparoscopic instruments,

a grasping forceps, an aspirating needle with needle sleeve, a trap to collect the follicular fluid and ovum, and a suctioning device are needed. A closed-circuit television monitoring system may be used.

The laparoscopy is performed with the patient in the supine or modified lithotomy position. Normally, instruments are not placed in the cervix or vagina. The pneumoperitoneum may be achieved with 100% carbon dioxide or a gas mixture of 90% nitrogen, 5% oxygen, and 5% carbon dioixide.

1. Follicular aspiration may be performed using a double-puncture or a triple-puncture technique.
2. The ovary is stabilized against the pelvic side wall by grasping the utero-ovarian ligament with grasping forceps.
3. The aspirating needle is placed in contact with the surface of the follicle.
4. Suction is applied as the follicle is punctured. The needle tip is moved within the follicle in an attempt to dislodge the cumulus mass from the follicle wall.
5. After the follicle has collapsed, suction is disconnected before the needle is removed from the follicle; this disconnection prevents aspiration of carbon dioxide.
6. After the needle is outside the peritoneal cavity, suction is reapplied to empty the fluid contained within the tubing into the ovum trap.
7. The ovum trap is changed, and culture medium is aspirated into another ovum trap to rinse the needle and ensure that the oocyte is not retained within the tubing.
8. The follicular aspirate is transferred immediately to the embryo laboratory where it is inspected microscopically for the presence of an oocyte. If an oocyte is not identified, the aspirating needle is reintroduced into the follicle. The follicle is redistended with culture media and is reaspirated.
9. The laparoscopic procedure is completed after all available follicles are aspirated.

Sperm preparation

A semen sample is obtained from the husband. After liquefaction, the semen is washed of seminal plasma by centrifugation twice in culture medium and incubated at 37° C until the time of insemination.

In vitro fertilization

The oocytes and surrounding cumulus are transferred to culture medium to complete maturation. The oocytes are incubated for different periods of time, depending on the degree of maturation of the oocytes before insemination. Oocytes may be inseminated with 50,000 to 200,000 motile sperm to each oocyte.

Evaluation of fertilization in the tissue culture dish requires visualization of the oocyte approximately 18 hours after insemination. The presence of two pronuclei is taken as presumptive evidence of fertilization, and the oocyte is transferred to growth medium. The embryo should be at the four-cell stage by 32 to 40 hours after insemination.

Embryo transfer

No anesthesia is required. The patient may be placed in the knee-chest or lithotomy position. A Graves vaginal speculum is inserted into the vagina. A single-tooth tenaculum may be used to grasp the cervix.

As soon as the patient is ready, the embryos are loaded into the transfer catheter with a minute amount of transfer medium and two small air bubbles. The catheter is carefully introduced into the uterine cavity, and the embryos are expelled. The catheter is withdrawn and returned to the laboratory, where is it examined for retained embryos. If the embryos have not been retained in the catheter, the speculum is removed.

Following embryo transfer, the patient is placed in the supine or modified jackknife position, depending on the position of the uterus, for 4 to 24 hours.

A new approach to in vitro fertilization called the *gamete intrafallopian transfer* (GIFT) has recently been introduced. It has been proven successful for women with long-standing infertility who have at least one patent fallopian tube. Oocyte retrieval for the GIFT approach may be accomplished by laparoscope, minilaparotomy, or vaginal aspiration using ultrasound guidance. Egg fertilization occurs within fallopian tube.

In the future, in vitro fertilization program development may include cryopreservation of embryos, donor eggs, donor sperm, and embryo sitters (implantation of embryos into surrogate mothers). As technical problems are overcome and moral and ethical issues resolved, these advances are becoming a reality.

Cesarean birth

Cesarean birth is delivery of the fetus or fetuses through an abdominal incision. In general, cesarean birth is employed whenever further delay in delivery may seriously compromise the fetus, the mother, or both, yet vaginal delivery cannot be safely accomplished. In recent years the use of cesarean birth has increased as a result of fetal monitoring, fetal scalp blood sampling for pH determination, and the widespread emphasis on recognition of actual or suspected impairment of fetal well-being if delivery were delayed or vaginal delivery attempted. Reasons for cesarean birth include malposition and malpresentation, cephalopelvic disproportion, abruptio placentae, toxemia, fetal distress, uterine dysfunction, placenta previa, prolapsed cord, previous pelvic surgery, cervical dystocia, active herpes, progenitalis, and diabetes.

Patients about to undergo cesarean birth need careful assessment and emotional support. Because cesarean birth frequently involve emergency situations, the patient may express grave concern for the infant's well-being. If the patient has participated in childbirth classes, she may feel that she has failed in some way. When the mother chooses regional anesthesia, the father may be permitted to enter the operating room and witness the birth. This should occur only if the father has had adequate preparation during the pregnancy and if hospital policy permits. The father provides emotional support and can be included in the bonding that takes place at birth. The mother, if awake, is shown and allowed to hold the infant. The nurse is caring for two patients: the mother and the infant.

Procedural considerations. The patient should be in a supine position with elevation of the right side to ensure adequate venous return during preparation and surgery. If a general anesthetic is to be employed, *all* preparations, including skin prepping, bladder drainage, draping, suction connection, counts, and gowning and gloving of all scrubbed personnel, must be done before induction. In many hospitals, personnel from the nursery are notified when the cesarean birth is scheduled so they are in attendance for the delivery. The nursery personnel generally provide a radiant warmer (Fig. 14-39) and usually perform

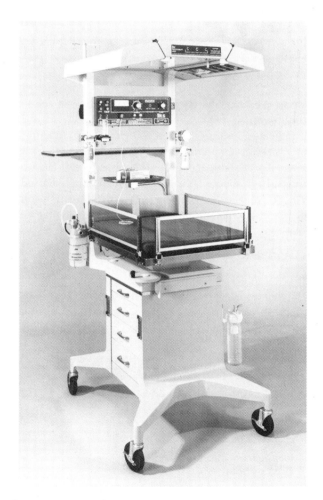

Fig. 14-39. Neonatal intensive care unit. (Courtesy Ohio Medical Products, Madison, Wis.)

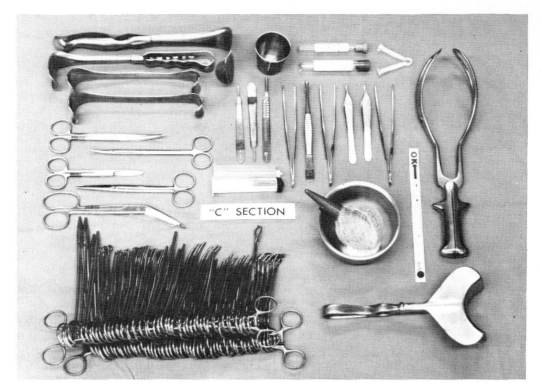

Fig. 14-40. Instrument setup for cesarean birth. (Courtesy Edward Weck & Co., Research Triangle Park, N.C.)

the immediate postdelivery care of the infant in the operating room.

If indicated, hair is clipped or shaved from the abdomen from above the umbilicus to the level of the mons pubis and laterally to above the level of the iliac crests. The skin is prepped for abdominal surgery. The vagina is not prepared. A Foley catheter is inserted. Instrumentation includes the basic abdominal gynecologic set, plus the following (Fig. 14-40):

Cutting instrument

1 Lister bandage scissors

Holding instruments

4 Foerster sponge-holding (ring) forceps, 7 inches
6 Pennington forceps

Clamping instruments

2 Cord clamps

Exposing instruments

1 DeLee retractor

Obstetrical instruments

1 Pair delivery forceps, if desired
1 Head extractor, if desired

Accessory items

2 Laboratory tubes for cord blood
1 Drain (optional)
1 Bulb syringe

Operative procedure

1. An infraumbilical vertical incision or lower transverse Pfannenstiel incision is made. The incision should be long enough to allow the infant to be delivered without difficulty, but no longer. Therefore, the length of the incision varies with the estimated size of the fetus.

2. The abdominal wall is opened in layers. The rectus and pyramidalis muscles are separated in the midline by sharp and blunt dissection to expose the underlying transversalis fascia and peritoneum.

3. The peritoneum is elevated with two Crile hemostats about 2 cm apart. The peritoneum between the two clamps is palpated to rule out the inclusion of bowel, omentum, or bladder. The peritoneum is opened, and the abdominal cavity entered.

4. Bleeding sites anywhere in the abdominal incision may be clamped but not ligated until later unless the clamps obstruct exposure.

5. The uterus is quickly but carefully palpated to determine the size and presenting part of the fetus as well as the direction and degree of rotation of the uterus.

6. The reflection of peritoneum (serosa) above the upper margin of the bladder and overlying the anterior lower uterine segment is gently separated by sharp and blunt dissection.

7. The developed bladder flap is held downward beneath the symphysis with a bladder retractor such as the DeLee.

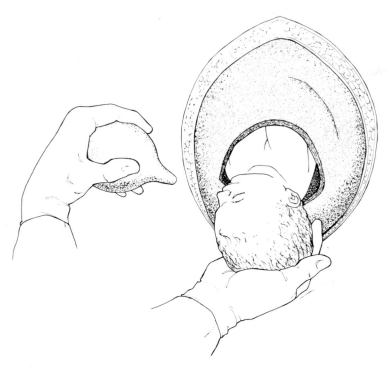

Fig. 14-41. Cesarean birth. Delivery of head; bulb syringe used to clear nares and mouth of amniotic fluid.

8. The uterus is opened with a knife through the lower uterine segment about 2 cm above the detached bladder. Once the uterus is opened, the incision can be extended by cutting laterally with a large bandage scissors or by simply spreading the incision by means of lateral pressure applied with each index finger when the lower uterine segment is thin.

9. The presenting membranes are incised. Suction is imperative here, and many surgeons prefer no suction tip (only the large open end of the suction tubing) during the expulsion and suctioning of amniotic fluid.

10. All retractors are removed. The fetal head is gently elevated, either manually or by use of obstetrical forceps, through the incision, aided by transabdominal fundal pressure. The pressure helps expel the fetus.

11. As soon as the head is delivered, a bulb syringe is used to aspirate the exposed nares and mouth to minimize aspiration of amniotic fluid and its contents (Fig. 14-41).

12. As soon as the shoulders are delivered, about 20 units of oxytocin per liter of fluid is administered intravenously so that the uterus contracts; this minimizes blood loss and aids expulsion of the placenta and membranes.

13. On delivery of the entire infant, the cord is clamped and cut and the infant given to the member of the team who is responsible for resuscitation efforts as needed. A sterile gown or sheet should be provided to the individual receiving the infant to avoid any break in aseptic technique during transfer of the infant.

14. The edges of the uterine incision are promptly clamped with Pean forceps, ring forceps, or Pennington clamps.

15. The placenta is delivered and placed in a large receptacle provided from the back table. Fundal massage or manual removal may be employed to hasten delivery of the placenta and reduce bleeding.

16. One or two separate layers of suture may be used to close the uterine incision.

17. Following determination that there is no further bleeding after closure of the uterine incision, the cut edges of the serosa overlying the uterus and bladder are approximated with a continuous suture.

18. Any blood, blood clots, vernix, and amniotic fluid in the pelvis and peritoneal cavity are removed. The fallopian tubes and ovaries are also inspected. Tubal ligation may be carried out at this point.

19. The peritoneum and each abdominal layer are closed.

BIBLIOGRAPHY

Baggish, M.S., and Dorsey, J.H.: Carbon dioxide laser for combination excisional-vaporization conization, Am. J. Obstet. Gynecol. *151:*23, 1985.

Baggish, M.S., and Dorsey, J.H.: CO_2 laser for treatment of vulvar carcinoma in situ, Obstet. Gynecol. *57:*371, 1981.

Berek, J.S., Hacker, N.F., and Lagasse, L.D.: Vaginal reconstruction performed simultaneously with pelvic exenteration, Obstet. Gynecol. *63:*318, 1984.

Bhiwandiwala, P.P., Mumford, S.D., and Feldblum, P.J.: A comparison of different laparoscopic sterilization occlusion techniques in 24,439 procedures, Am. J. Obstet. Gynecol. *144:*319, 1982.

Bobak, I.M., Jenson, M.D., and Zaler, M.K.: Maternity and gynecologic care: The nurse and the family, ed. 4, St. Louis, 1989, The C.V. Mosby Co.

Brown, N.L.: Carbon dioxide lasers: advantages and disadvantages in gyn surgery, AORN J. *42:*53, 1985.

Copeland, C., Wing, R., and Hulka, J.F.: Direct trocar insertion at laparoscopy: an evaluation, Obstet. Gynecol. *62:*655, 1983.

Creighton, H.: In vitro fertilization, Nurs. Management *16:*12, 1985.

Dugan, K.K.: The bleak outlook of ovarian carcinoma, Am. J. Nurs. *85:*144, 1985.

Fleming, C., and Jenks, A.D.: Microscopic tubal reversal, AORN J. *37:*199, 1983.

Fogel, C.I., and Woods, N.F.: Health care of women: a nursing perspective, St. Louis, 1981, The C.V. Mosby Co.

Friberg, J., and Gleicher, N., editors: Journal of In Vitro Fertilization and Embryo Transfer *1:*1, 1984.

Gomel, V.: Microsurgery in female infertility, Boston, 1983, Little, Brown & Co.

Gray, H.: Anatomy of the human body, ed. 37, Philadelphia, 1989, Lea & Febiger.

Griffin, M.E.: Resolving infertility: an emotional crisis, AORN J. *38:*597, 1983.

Grimes, E.M.: Open laparoscopy with conventional instrumentation, Obstet. Gynecol. *57:*375, 1981.

Hacker, N.F., and others: Radical vulvectomy and bilateral inguinal lymphadenectomy through separate groin incisions, Obstet. Gynecol. *58:*574, 1981.

Hallmark, G., and Findlay, M.: Cesarean birth in the operating room, AORN J. *36:*978, 1982.

Hawkins, J.W., and Higgins, L.P.: Maternity and gynecological nursing: women's health care, Philadelphia, 1989, J.B. Lippincott Co.

Keye, W.R., Jr.: Laser surgery in gynecology and obstetrics, Boston, 1985, G.K. Hall Medical Publishers.

Kistner, R.W.: Gynecology principles and practice, ed. 4, Chicago, 1980. Year Book Medical Publishers.

Matthews, K.: Pelviscopy: An endoscopic alternative, AORN J. *47:*1218, 1988.

Mattingly, R.F., and Thompson, J.D.: TeLinde's operative gynecology, ed. 6, Philadelphia, 1985, J.B. Lippincott Co.

Menning, B.E.: The emotional needs of infertile couples, Fertil. Steril. *34:*313, 1980.

Neuwirth, R.S., and others: Hysteroscopic resection of intrauterine scars using a new technique, Obstet. Gynecol. *60:*111, 1982.

Petersen, N.F., and Rhoe, J.: Endometriosis: Obtaining relief via "Near Contact" laparoscopy, AORN J. *48:*700, 1988.

Pitkin, R.M., and Zlatnik, F.J.: Year book of obstetrics and gynecology, Chicago, 1985, Year Book Medical Publishers.

Pritchard, J.A., MacDonald, P.C., and Grant, N.F.: Williams obstetrics, ed. 17, Norwalk, Conn., 1985, Appleton-Century-Crofts.

Rothrock, J.C.: Perioperative Care Planning, St. Louis, 1990, The C.V. Mosby Co.

Silber, S.J., and Cohen, R.: Microsurgical reversal of tubal sterilization: factors affecting pregnancy rate, with long-term follow-up, Obstet. Gynecol. *64:*679, 1984.

Thibodeau, G.A.: Anthony's textbook of anatomy and physiology, ed. 13, St. Louis, 1990, The C.V. Mosby Co.

Thompson, J.M., and others: Mosby's manual of clinical nursing, ed. 2, Philadelphia, 1989, The C.V. Mosby Co.

Wallach, E.E., and Kempers, R.D., editors: Modern trends in infertility and conception control, vol. 2, Philadelphia, 1988, Harper & Row.

Wells, M.P.: In vitro fertilization: hope for childless couples, AORN J. *38:*591, 1983.

Wells, M.P., and Villano, K.: Total abdominal hysterectomy: perioperative patient care, AORN J. *42:*368, 1985.

White, L.D., and White, P.F.: Midtrimester abortion patients, AORN J. *34:*756, 1981.

Wolf, D.P., and Quigley, M.M., editors: Human in vitro fertilization and embryo transfer, New York, 1984, Plenum Press.

15 Genitourinary surgery

GRATIA M. NAGLE

Over the past decade major changes in genitourinary surgery have occurred. The influences of the Nd:YAG and CO_2 lasers, ultrasound, and sonic lithotripsy, as well as those of other new and innovative diagnostic procedures, have made treatment far more precise.

The perioperative urology nurse has new challenges to face with these advancements. For the perioperative urology nurse to function optimally, up-to-date knowledge and peak technical skills are priorities. Increasing health care costs and the pressures to contain them are resulting in more procedures being done on an outpatient or short-stay basis, and in limited time being allowed for preoperative teaching and discharge planning. Frequently, this important task falls to the perioperative nursing team. The success of surgical intervention depends greatly on the perioperative nurse's ability and knowledge in developing a perioperative plan of care.

SURGICAL ANATOMY

A comprehensive understanding of the anatomic structures involved in genitourinary surgery is required to facilitate proper selection of instrumentation, equipment, and patient position. Collaboration with the urologist's plan of care is necessary in preparing the patient for surgery.

The normal urinary tract comprises a pair of kidneys, two ureters, the urinary bladder, and the urethra. Urine is excreted by the kidneys and conveyed to the bladder through the ureters, muscular tubes 25 cm long. Urine is stored in the bladder, which serves as a reservoir until its full capacity is reached, and is eliminated from the body by way of the urethra (Fig. 15-1).

Kidneys

The kidneys are located in the retroperitoneal space along the lateral borders of the psoas muscle, one on each side of the vertebral column at the level of the twelfth thoracic to the third lumbar vertebra. Usually the right kidney is several centimeters lower than the left because the liver rests above and anterior to the right kidney (Fig. 15-1).

Each kidney is surrounded by a mass of fatty and loose areolar tissue known as *perirenal fat*. A capsule enclosing the renal space is known as *fascia renalis* or *Gerota's fascia*. These structures help keep the kidneys in their normal position. The anterior and posterior relationships of the kidneys are shown in Fig. 15-2.

On the medial side of each kidney is a concave area known as the *hilum* through which the renal artery and vein enter and leave. The *renal pelvis,* a funnel-shaped structure that lies posterior to the renal vascular pedicle, divides into several branches within the kidney called *calyces* (Fig. 15-3). When surgery is indicated in these structures, a posterior flank approach is preferred. When surgery for removal of a mass is anticipated, a transabdominal or thoracoabdominal incision is often chosen.

The kidneys are highly vascular organs that process approximately one fifth of the entire volume of blood at any one time. The blood supply of the kidney is conveyed through the renal artery, a large branch of the aorta (Fig. 15-4), and leaves the kidney through the renal vein. On entering the kidney the renal artery divides into anterior and posterior sections that undergo further division into lobular arteries. Renal arteriography is performed before several types of surgical procedures to help identify the patient's renal vascular anatomy.

The renal lymphatic supply originates beneath the capsule of the kidney and empties into the lumbar lymph nodes at the junction of the renal vascular pedicle and aorta. The nerves of the autonomic (involuntary) nervous system come from the lumbar sympathetic trunk and from the vagus. Removal of the nerve pathways disrupts the ability to feel pain without impairing renal function. The renal artery and vein with their accompanying nerves and lymphatics are referred to as the *pedicle* of the kidney.

Adrenal glands

The adrenal glands lie retroperitoneally beneath the diaphragm at the medial aspects of the superior pole of each kidney. On the right side the gland is adjacent to the inferior vena cava; on the left side it is posterior to the stomach and pancreas. Each adrenal gland has a medulla, which secretes adrenalin (epinephrine), and a cortex, which secretes steroids and other hormones. The glands are liberally supplied with arterial branches from the phrenic and renal arteries and from the aorta. The venous

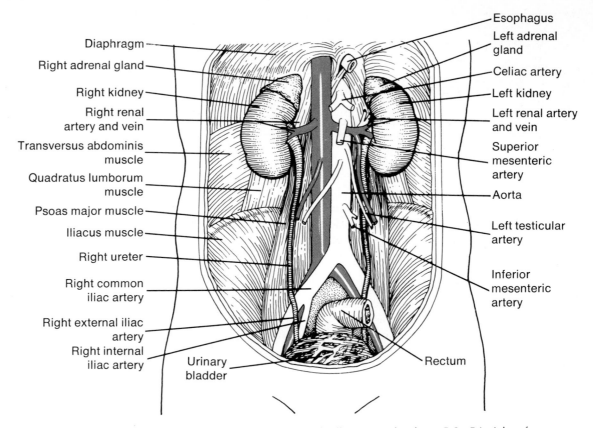

Esophagus

Left adrenal gland

Celiac artery

Left kidney

Left renal artery and vein

Superior mesenteric artery

Aorta

Left testicular artery

Inferior mesenteric artery

Diaphragm

Right adrenal gland

Right kidney

Right renal artery and vein

Transversus abdominis muscle

Quadratus lumborum muscle

Psoas major muscle

Iliacus muscle

Right ureter

Right common iliac artery

Right external iliac artery

Right internal iliac artery

Urinary bladder

Rectum

Fig. 15-1. Location of urinary system organs. (From Broadwell, D.C., and Jackson, B.S.: Principles of ostomy care, St. Louis, 1982, The C.V. Mosby Co.)

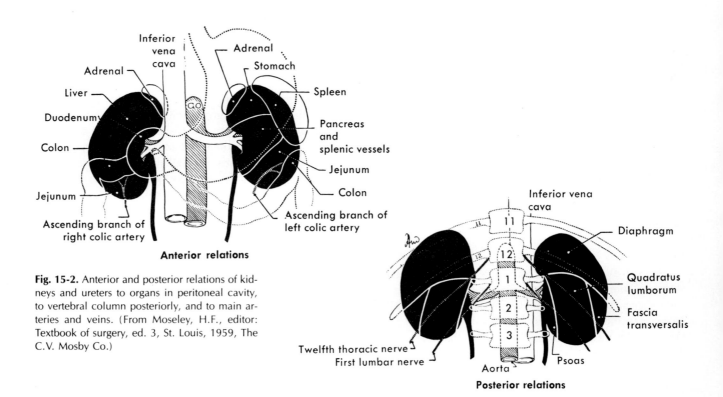

Anterior relations

Inferior vena cava

Adrenal

Stomach

Spleen

Pancreas and splenic vessels

Jejunum

Colon

Ascending branch of left colic artery

Adrenal

Liver

Duodenum

Colon

Jejunum

Ascending branch of right colic artery

Posterior relations

Inferior vena cava

Diaphragm

Quadratus lumborum

Fascia transversalis

Psoas

Aorta

Twelfth thoracic nerve

First lumbar nerve

Fig. 15-2. Anterior and posterior relations of kidneys and ureters to organs in peritoneal cavity, to vertebral column posteriorly, and to main arteries and veins. (From Moseley, H.F., editor: Textbook of surgery, ed. 3, St. Louis, 1959, The C.V. Mosby Co.)

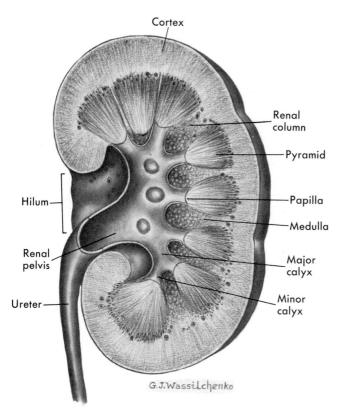

Fig. 15-3. Normal kidney. (Modified from Thompson, J.M., and others: Clinical nursing, St. Louis, 1986, The C.V. Mosby Co.)

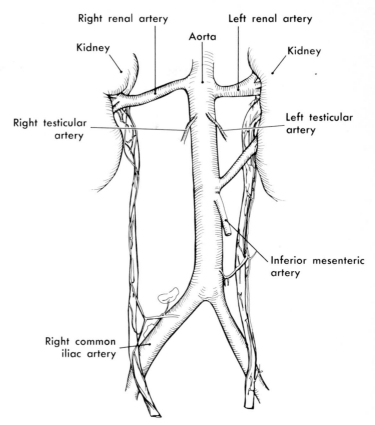

Fig. 15-4. Blood supply of kidneys. (Adapted by permission from J.C.B. Grant's Atlas of anatomy, 6th ed. Copyright ©1972, The Williams & Wilkins Co.)

drainage is accomplished on the right by the inferior vena cava and on the left by the left renal vein.

Ureters

Each ureter is a continuation of the renal pelvis. In an adult the ureter extends from the renal pelvis to the base of the bladder and is approximately 25 to 30 cm long and 4 to 5 mm in diameter (Fig. 15-5). It is a fibromuscular cylindrical tube lined by transitional epithelium (urothelium). As urine accumulates in the renal pelvis, slight distention initiates a wave of muscular contractions. This peristaltic activity continues down the ureter, propelling urine into the bladder.

The ureter has three areas of narrowing where calculi may become lodged and pose a potential problem with pain and obstruction: (1) the ureteropelvic junction, (2) the crossing of the ureter over the iliac vessels, and (3) the ureterovesical junction (Fig. 15-5). Urine may sometimes cause calculi to be washed down the ureter to produce severe ureteral colic. Of all renal calculi, 90% are spontaneously passed into the bladder. However, if they become lodged in the ureter, a ureteroscopy, stone manipulation, or ureterolithotomy may be indicated. During pelvic or intestinal surgery, ureteral catheters or stents are

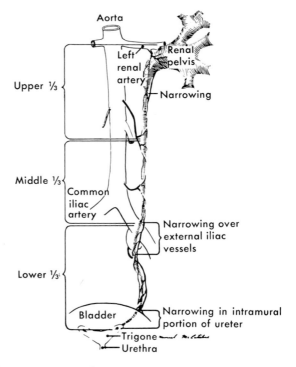

Fig. 15-5. Anatomy of ureter. (From Colby, F.H.: Essential urology, ed. 4, Baltimore, The Williams & Wilkins Co.)

often inserted to facilitate positive identification of the ureters and reduce the potential for severing or ligating them.

Urinary bladder

The adult urinary bladder is a hollow muscular viscus that acts as a reservoir for urine until micturition occurs. It has an outer adventitial and inner urothelial layer. The trigone, a triangular area, forms the base of the bladder. The three corners of the trigone correspond to the orifices of the ureters and the bladder neck (opening of the urethra) (Fig. 15-6).

Physiologically, the bladder fills with urine and expands into the abdominal cavity. The extraperitoneal location is advantageous because a suprapubic incision may be performed without violating the peritoneum and potentially causing intraperitoneal complications.

The main arterial supply of the bladder is derived from the branches of the internal iliac artery.

The bladder's size, position, and relation to the bowel, rectum, and reproductive organs vary according to the bladder's distention. In a female the vagina lies dorsal to the base of the bladder and parallel to the urethra (Fig. 15-7). In a male the prostate gland is interposed between the bladder neck and the urethra (Fig. 15-8). These anatomic relationships are important during pelvic surgery.

The process of bladder evacuation appears to be initiated by nerve cells from the sacral division of the autonomic nervous system. These sacral reflex centers are controlled by higher voluntary centers in the brain. Stimulation of the sacral centers results in contraction of the bladder muscles and relaxation of the bladder outlet sphincters. Muscle tone maintains closure of the sphincters when the bladder is at rest, thus enabling continence.

Urethra

The *male urethra,* normally 20 to 25 cm long, extends from the bladder neck to the tip of the penis and varies in diameter from 7 to 10 mm. It is subdivided into three portions: the prostatic, membranous, and penile urethra.

The prostatic urethra is approximately 2 to 4 cm long and is the widest portion of the urethra. On the floor of

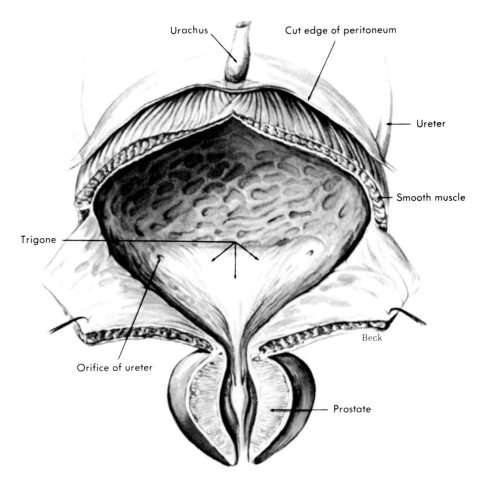

Fig. 15-6. Male urinary bladder cut to show interior. (From Anthony, C.P., and Kolthoff, N.J.: Anatomy and physiology, ed. 9, St. Louis, 1975, The C.V Mosby Co.)

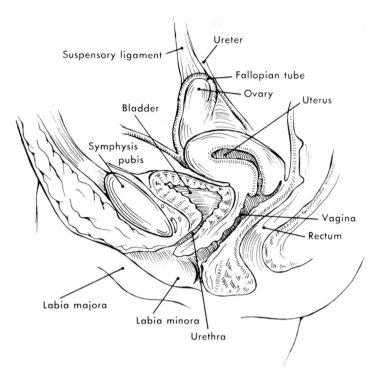

Fig. 15-7. Female genitourinary and reproductive anatomy. (Modified from Keuhnelian, J., and Sanders, V.: Urologic nursing, New York, 1970, Macmillan, Inc.)

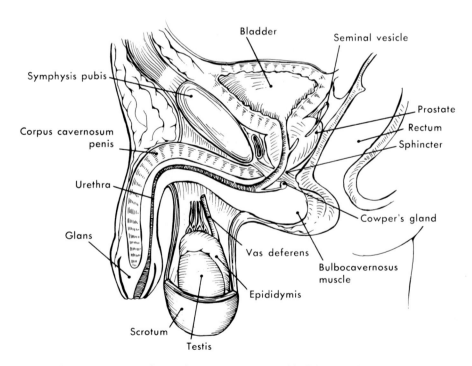

Fig. 15-8. Male genitourinary and reproductive anatomy. (Modified from Keuhnelian, J., and Sanders, V.: Urologic nursing, New York, 1970, Macmillan, Inc.)

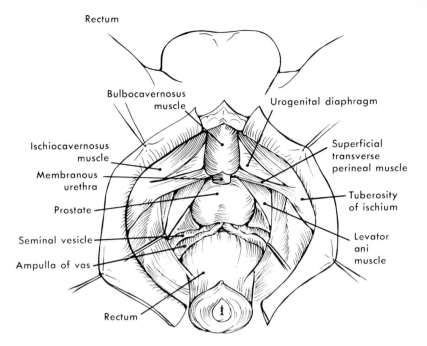

Rectum

Bulbocavernosus
muscle

Urogenital diaphragm

Ischiocavernosus
muscle

Superficial
transverse
perineal muscle

Membranous
urethra

Prostate

Tuberosity
of ischium

Seminal vesicle

Levator
ani
muscle

Ampulla of vas

Rectum

Fig. 15-9. Anatomy of male perineum and contiguous structures. (Modified from Campbell, M.F., and Harrison, J.H., editors: Urology, vols. 1 to 3, ed. 3, Philadelphia, 1970, W.B. Saunders Co.)

the prostatic urethra is the verumontanum, which contains the openings of the ejaculatory ducts.

The membranous urethra is the shortest portion, measuring approximately 2 cm long and extending from the external sphincter to the apex of the prostate (Fig. 15-9).

The penile or pendulous urethra lies within the corpus spongiosum. The urothelium of the urethra is continuous with that of the bladder.

The *female urethra* is a narrow, membranous tube about 4 cm in length and 6 mm in diameter. The urethra lies behind and beneath the symphysis pubis. It passes through the internal and external sphincter and the urogenital diaphragm. Because the female urethra is short, microorganisms find easy access to the bladder and subsequently cause infection.

Male reproductive organs

The male reproductive organs include several paired structures: the testes, epididymides, seminal ducts (vas deferens), seminal vesicles, ejaculatory ducts, and bulbourethral glands. Other organs of the reproductive tract are the penis, prostate gland, and urethra.

The *scrotum* is located behind and below the base of the penis and in front of the anus. Each loose sac contains and supports the testis, the epididymis, and some of the spermatic cord. The two sides of the scrotum are separated from each other by a median raphe. Within the scrotum are two cavities or sacs that are lined with smooth and glistening tissue, the *tunica vaginalis*. Normally, a small amount of clear fluid is contained in the tunica vaginalis.

The condition known as *hydrocele* is an abnormal accumulation of this fluid.

The *testes* manufacture the spermatozoa and also contain specialized cells (Leydig's) that produce the male hormone, testosterone. Each testis consists of many tubules in which the sperm are formed, surrounded by dense capsules of connective tissue. The tubules coalesce and continue into the adjacent epididymis, where the sperm mature and are stored.

The *epididymis* is a long, convoluted duct located along the posterolateral surface of the testis. It is closely attached to the testicle by fibrous tissue and secretes seminal fluid, which gives the sperm a fluid medium in which to migrate. The *vas deferens* (ductus deferens, or seminal duct) is a distal continuation of the epididymis as it enters the prostate gland and conveys the sperm to the seminal vesicle.

The vas deferens lies within the *spermatic cord* in the inguinal region. The spermatic cord also contains veins, arteries, lymphatics, nerves, and surrounding connective tissue (cremaster muscle), which give support to the testes. The terminal portion of each vas deferens is called the *ejaculatory duct;* it passes between the lobes of the prostate gland and opens into the posterior urethra.

The accessory reproductive glands include the seminal vesicles, prostate gland, and bulbourethral gland. The seminal vesicles unite with the vas deferens on either side, are situated behind the bladder, and produce protein and fructose for the nutrition of the sperm cell. Sperm and prostatic fluid are discharged at the time of ejaculation.

The *prostate gland* is a fibromuscular organ located at

the base of the bladder neck and the triangular ligament completely surrounding the urethra. The gland is about 4 cm at its base and about 2 cm in depth and weighs approximately 20 g (Fig. 15-8).

The prostate consists essentially of six lobes: anterior, posterior, median (middle), subcervical, and right and left lateral. The posterior lobe is readily palpable during rectal examination and prone to cancerous degeneration.

Behind the prostatic capsule is a fibrous sheath known as the true prostatic capsule, which separates the prostate gland and the seminal vesicles from the rectum. This fascia is of importance when perineal prostatectomy is contemplated.

The lobes of the prostate gland secrete highly alkaline fluid that dilutes the testicular secretion as it is excreted from the ejaculatory ducts. These secretions are believed essential to the passage of spermatozoa and helpful in keeping them alive. The arterial supply to the prostate is derived from the pudendal, inferior vesical, and hemorrhoidal arteries.

Cowper's glands (bulbourethral glands) are located on either side of the membranous portion of the urethra. Each gland, by way of its duct, empties mucous secretions into the urethra.

The *penis* is suspended from the pubic symphysis by the suspensory ligaments. The penis contains three distinct vascular spongelike bodies: the two upper bodies are called the *right* and *left corpus cavernosum*, and the lower body, the *corpus spongiosum urethrae*. The tissue contains a network of vascular channels that fill with blood during erection. At the distal end of the penis, the skin is doubly folded to form the so-called prepuce, or foreskin, which serves as a covering for the glans penis (Fig. 15-8). The glans penis contains the urethral orifice.

PERIOPERATIVE NURSING CONSIDERATIONS
Assessment/nursing diagnosis

Patients entering a hospital or ambulatory surgery unit for genitourinary surgery exhibit many emotions and reactions. These feelings encompass fear, embarrassment, helplessness, hostility, anger, and grief. To most, a successful surgical outcome is of prime importance. The urology patient population varies from infants with congenital anomalies to the elderly with physiologic impairments. Owing to the dramatic increase in oupatient surgery, the nursing staff must prepare to meet patients' specific needs, from preoperative teaching to postoperative home care. The families of patients need to be involved in this preparation process. Patient education begins in the urologist's office. Communication between the office and perioperative nursing staff facilitates continuity of care and increases the efficiency and effectiveness of surgical procedures.

In addition to routine admission information, urologic and cardiac histories are usually obtained. This information, which includes vital signs, the patient's primary problem, history of the present illness, nature of symptoms, and limitations imposed by the disease condition, should be reviewed. Nursing observation should include the patient's general physical appearance, as well as nonverbal behaviors such as restlessness, which may indicate discomfort or anxiety. Any limitations in mobility or sensory deficits should be noted. Urologic procedures frequently require positions that create unusual stress for the patient, both anatomic and physiologic. Assessment must provide the perioperative nurse with data adequate to support planning and facilitate postoperative evaluation.

Many urologic surgical interventions require the patient to be in a flank position, causing compression on the vena cava. Additionally, large amounts of irrigating fluids are frequently used intraoperatively. For these reasons, a current cardiac and electrolyte status should be available for review. Laboratory studies that have been done preoperatively may include serum and urine electrolytes, blood sugar, BUN, urinalysis and urine cultures, cardiac enzymes, CBC, PT and PTT, blood chemistry profiles, ECG, and chest x-rays. The medical history, including a list of medications and any history of an infectious process, should be reviewed. Specific genitourinary studies can also be found in the patient's medical record. They may encompass all or some of the following: CT scans, IVPs and KUBs, urinary flow studies, fluoroscopic exams (angiography, cavernosography), prostatic specific antigen, and ultrasounds. After the medical record is reviewed, assessment information compiled, and perioperative nursing diagnoses identified, the perioperative plan of care is formulated. For patients undergoing genitourinary surgery, the following nursing diagnoses are usually applicable:

- Impaired gas exchange related to surgical position and consequent alteration in respiratory ventilation/perfusion
- Potential for fluid and electrolyte imbalance related to intraoperative irrigation and fluid loss
- Potential for urinary tract infection (or alteration in urinary elimination) related to instrumentation of the urinary tract and placement of urinary catheter
- Potential for injury related to surgical position
- Anxiety and/or embarrassment related to exposure of and surgery on external genitalia and surgical outcome

Planning

Care plans are the organization framework for perioperative nursing activities. Frequently, the urology patient presents a complex medical picture. Any alterations in the patient's physical status may impact both the surgical and postoperative course. A review of the patient record, communication with the patient and/or family, and knowledge gained from other members of the patient care team should be used to formulate the nursing data base. A Sample Care Plan for the genitourinary surgery patient is shown on p. 338.

Sample Care Plan

NURSING DIAGNOSIS:

Impaired gas exchange related to surgical position and consequent alteration in respiratory ventilation/perfusion

GOAL:

Patient will maintain adequate gas exchange.

INTERVENTIONS:

Position patient to provide maximum lung perfusion.

Monitor for and report signs of impaired gas exchange.

Administer oxygen as ordered; assist with intubation and maintenance of airway during positioning.

Assist with collection of arterial blood gases and report results promptly.

Apply cardiac monitor, blood pressure cuff, and pulse oximeter.

NURSING DIAGNOSIS:

Potential for fluid volume and electrolyte imbalance related to intraoperative irrigation and fluid loss

GOAL:

Patient will evidence no signs of fluid or electrolyte imbalance.

INTERVENTIONS:

Monitor patency of intravenous lines.

Monitor ECG, vital signs, and pulmonary status as appropriate.

Monitor blood loss.

Monitor urine output and note color of urine; report output less than 30 cc/hour and changes in the color of urine.

Provide intravenous fluids as requested, and assist with administration as necessary.

Maintain an accurate record of intake and output.

NURSING DIAGNOSIS:

Potential for urinary tract infection (or alteration in urinary elimination) related to instrumentation of the urinary tract and placement of urinary catheter

GOAL:

Patient will be free of urinary tract infection or altered patterns of urinary elimination.

INTERVENTIONS:

Follow aseptic technique during catheter insertion and connection to drainage device.

Maintain closed gravity drainage system.

Note color and character of urine; report abnormalities.

Keep drainage tubing and collection device below the level of the patient's bladder.

Keep urine draining freely; avoid kinks in tubing.

Check patency of catheter following all positional changes.

Anchor drainage tubing to patient to prevent pulling and/or retraction of tubing.

Assess bladder for distention.

Include catheter care and measures to facilitate voiding following catheter removal as part of preoperative teaching to patient and/or family.

NURSING DIAGNOSIS:

Potential for injury related to surgical position

GOAL:

Patient will exhibit no signs of improper positioning following surgery.

INTERVENTIONS:

Maintain proper body alignment.

Pad all bony prominences.

Avoid compression of vulnerable nerves and neurovascular bundles.

Secure patient to operating room bed without friction or pressure.

Provide support stockings or antiembolism device as indicated.

NURSING DIAGNOSIS:

Anxiety and/or embarrassment related to exposure of and surgery on external genitalia and surgical outcome

GOAL:

Patient will verbalize feelings to perioperative nurse.

INTERVENTIONS:

Provide an accepting and supportive atmosphere.

Use touch (as appropriate) to convey caring and support.

Encourage expression of feelings.

Promote feelings of self-worth.

Offer suggestions to cope with anxieties.

Facilitate or assist patient in using coping strategies (relaxation, music, guided imagery).

Maintain patient privacy.

Implementation

Care plan implementation begins during the patient interview. Patient education that is concise and simply explained enhances the final surgical outcome. Meeting the patient's emotional needs is a nursing priority. A calm patient absorbs more and is more receptive to perioperative teaching. Explanations of what to expect throughout the operative period allays fears and nurtures confidence in the nursing care provided. Perioperative nursing care requires the collection and provision of numerous supplies and equipment to support the smooth implementation of the care plan.

Positioning

Thorough understanding of the urologic OR bed and its functions is essential to provide optimum patient positioning for each operative procedure. The position in which the patient is placed for surgery is determined by the particular operation to be performed. For urologic operative procedures, the patient is placed in the lateral, supine, or lithotomy position, which may be exaggerated to give optimum access to the organ involved, particularly in radical surgery of the prostate and bladder. Considerable care must be taken to ensure that the patient's position does not interfere with respiration or circulation. It is essential to avoid displacement of the joints and undue tension on neurovascular bundles or ligaments, particularly in an aged or debilitated patient.

A patient positioned laterally (flank position) for renal surgery has the spine extended for greater access to the retroperitoneal space. Padding and stabilized support with pillows, sandbags, and straps should be available for precise anatomic positioning and safety. If an electrosurgical unit is to be used, care must be taken that no part of the patient touches metal equipment other than the indifferent electrode (dispersive or "ground pad") attached to the unit.

In some procedures involving stones of the kidneys or ureters, intraoperative x-ray examinations or fluoroscopy may be required. If x-ray films are to be taken, the patient must be on an operating room bed with an x-ray cassette holder. If the OR bed design does not accommodate x-ray cassettes, an x-ray cassette holder must be placed under the patient who is in the supine, prone, or lithotomy position before the procedure begins. If the patient is in the lateral position with the bed flexed and kidney rest up, the x-ray cassette is placed under the patient at the time of x-ray exposure.

Aseptic techniques and safety measures

Aseptic techniques must be carefully maintained. Skin preparation and draping procedures (Chapter 5) vary, depending on the surgery to be performed and individual hospital policy. Special care must be taken when cleansing the perineal area.

Transurethral passage of instruments and catheters requires meticulous technique to prevent retrograde infections of the urinary tract. Visualization of the bladder during transurethral procedures is enhanced by darkening the room. Provision should be made for proper adjustments to lighting.

Electrosurgical units and fiberoptic light systems are frequent adjuncts in urologic surgery. The staff must be familiar with safety precautions during their use.

Use of irrigating fluids

When the bladder is to be opened or manipulated, a continuous flow of sterile distilled irrigating fluid is administered to distend the bladder for effective visualization. Commercially prepared sterile irrigation solutions with appropriate closed administration sets are highly recommended. Such closed systems prevent the inherent risks of cross-contamination.

For simple observation cystoscopy, retrograde pyelography, and simple bladder tumor fulgurations, sterile distilled water may be used without complication. However, during transurethral resection of the prostate, venous sinuses may be opened, and varying amounts of irrigant are invariably absorbed into the bloodstream. Studies indicate that the use of distilled water for transurethral resection of the prostate may result in hemolysis of erythrocytes and possible renal failure. Other important complications include dilutional hyponatremia and cardiac decompensation.

Ideally, a clear, nonelectrolytic, and isosmotic solution should be used. The most widely used urologic irrigating fluids are 3.3% sorbitol, an isomer of mannitol, and 1.5% glycine, an aminoacetic solution. Other recommended solutions include 5% mannitol, 1.8% urea, and 4% glucose. In dilute solutions, sorbitol and glycine have many properties that make them particularly useful for irrigation during transurethral prostatectomy. At their slightly hypotonic concentrations, they do not produce hemolysis. Because the solutions are nonelectrolytic, they do not cause dispersion of high-frequency current with consequent loss of electrosurgical cutting capacity, as occurs with normal saline.

Commercially prepared sterile irrigation solutions are available in collapsible bags and rigid plastic containers. The newer rigid containers have the same advantage as collapsible bags. Neither is dependent on air, and each may be hung in series, thus providing continuous irrigation without interruption. Air bubbles, a problem that distorts visibility during the procedure, are eliminated with these systems.

Thorough knowledge of the potential hazards encountered intraoperatively during transurethral surgery is extremely important. Although complications are more prevalent in the postoperative stage, close observation during the intraoperative period may prove lifesaving. Symptoms such as sudden restlessness, apprehension, irritability,

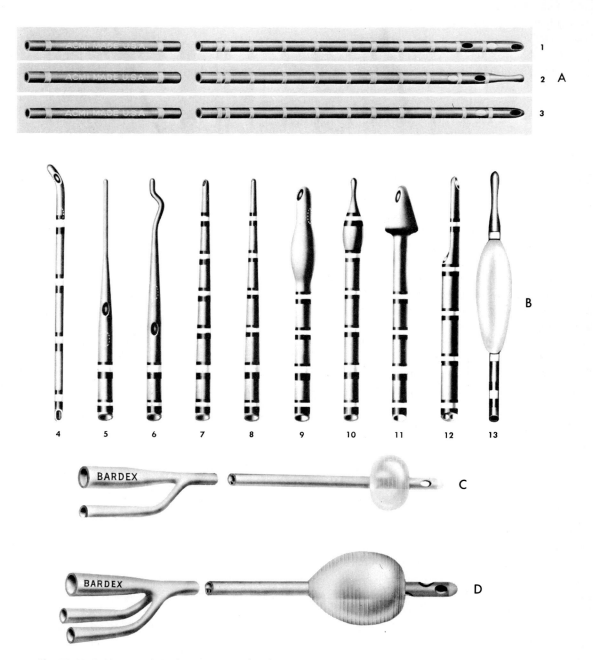

Fig. 15-10. A, X-ray graduated woven ureteral catheters are made of nylon or plastic material and have outer surfacing to provide flexibility, for easy entry without kinking. Eyes provide adequate high-flow rate. Catheter tips constructed for specific procedures as shown. *1,* Whistle tip; *2,* olive tip; *3,* round tip. **B,** X-ray graduated woven ureteral catheters and bougies. *4,* Wishard catheter, flat, coude tip; *5,* Blasucci catheter, flexible filiform tip; *6,* Blasucci catheter, flexible spiral filiform tip; *7,* Garceau catheter, tapered for dilatation, whistle tip; *8,* Garceau bougie, tapered for dilatation, conical tip; *9,* Braasch bulb catheter, whistle tip; *10,* Braasch bougie, bulb tip; *11,* Cone tip catheter (for ureteropyelography); *12,* Hyams double-lumen catheter; *13,* Dourmashkin dilator with inflation balloon, olive tip. **C,** Foley retention catheter. **D,** Bard three-way hemostatic catheter. (Courtesy American ACMI, Stamford, Conn.)

slow pulse, and rising blood pressure may suggest the transurethral resection syndrome, a shift of body fluids and electrolytes caused by a decrease of extracellular sodium. Serum electrolyte laboratory studies should be obtained without delay. Minimum amounts of fluids should be given. Irrigation fluid should be under as little pressure as possible, and the bladder emptied before it reaches full capacity to prevent intravesical pressure. Occasionally an operating room has the capacity to perform these crucial laboratory tests intraoperatively so results are available for interpretation in a short time. If a low serum sodium value is reported, hypertonic sodium chloride is added to the intravenous line, or intravenous diuretics such as furosemide (Lasix) may be used. If the patient's reaction is severe, surgery may have to be terminated.

Endoscopic and ancillary equipment

Cystoscopic and ancillary equipment may vary from one institution to another. Therefore, it is valuable to have a reference manual or Kardex system that illustrates and describes in detail the required instrumentation for each specific procedure.

The basic cystoscopy tray should include instruments and accessory items that are routinely used for all cystoscopy procedures. If ureteral catheterization is planned, catheterizing telescopes or an Albarran bridge of the appropriate size, which can be packaged and gas sterilized separately, may be easily added to the basic cystoscopy setup. Instruments for transurethral surgery and other special procedures may be wrapped and gas sterilized on separate trays and available on request. This concept minimizes handling of the delicate lensed instruments and ultimately reduces costly repairs.

In some instances during cystoscopic procedures, additional instrumentation is required. Instruments of various types and sizes, for example, a visual obturator, biopsy forceps, urethral sounds, Philips filiforms and followers, and Ellik evacuators may be packaged separately, sterilized, and available when needed.

Urethral and ureteral catheters

A variety of urethral and ureteral catheters are necessary in the management of urologic disease. Catheters are designed for specific procedures to meet the individualized needs of particular patients. Ureteral catheters are manufactured of polyvinyl or polyurethane material and are graduated so that the urologist may determine the exact distance the catheter has been inserted into the ureter. Most manufacturers provide disposable catheters double-wrapped in peel-open packages to allow aseptic handling during ureteral insertion. Some indications for the use of ureteral catheters are to (1) perform retrograde pyelography, (2) identify the ureters during pelvic or intestinal surgery, and (3) bypass partial or complete obstruction that may be present as a result of ureteral tumors, calculi, or strictures.

Frequently used ureteral catheters include the whistle tip, round, Braasch bulb, spiral, cone, and olive tip (Fig. 15-10). The spiral Blasucci is useful when difficulty occurs in introducing a ureteral catheter past the ureterovesical junction. When a retrograde ureterogram is indicated, a Braasch bulb or cone-tip ureteral catheter may be helpful in occluding the ureteral orifice to accomplish the x-ray study effectively. When a ureteral catheter is left indwelling, a special adapter (Fig. 15-11) can be connected to the end of the ureteral catheter to facilitate connection to a closed urinary drainage system.

Indwelling double-pigtail or double-J stents are now available (Fig. 15-12). These catheters are passed cystoscopically to reside within the ureter. When the guidewire is removed from the core of the stent, a proximal and distal J or pigtail forms in the tubing to retain the stents. Some surgeons opt to tie a nonabsorbable suture to the distal end, which then extends through the urethra. They can then remove the stent in the office setting postoperatively.

Urethral catheters have a multitude of functions as stents, drainage tubes, and in diagnostic studies in the operating room. Urethral catheters are generally divided into two categories, plain and indwelling, and range in different French sizes, most commonly from 12 through 30. The Foley catheter is the most frequently used indwelling (retention) catheter and is manufactured with a

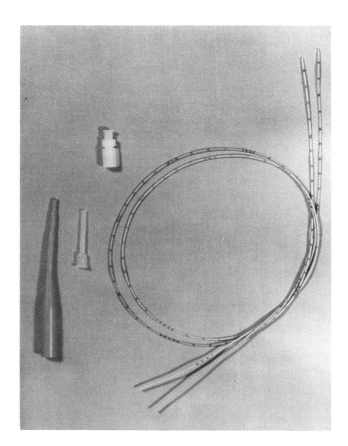

Fig. 15-11. Ureteral catheters and adapters.

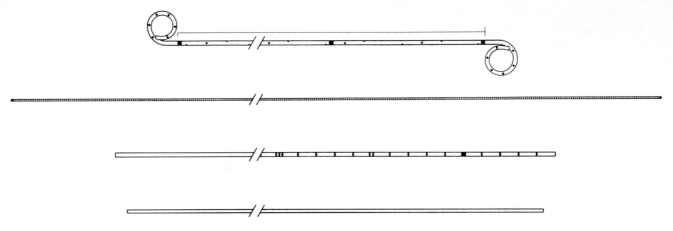

Fig. 15-12. Double-pigtail stent set. (Courtesy Cook Urological, Spencer, Indiana.)

variety of balloon sizes, tip styles, lengths, and eye arrangements (Fig. 15-10, *C*).

After prostatic surgery, a three-way Foley catheter with a 30-cc balloon capacity may be left indwelling (Fig. 15-10, *D*). This type of catheter is preferred because it facilitates continuous bladder irrigation and the large balloon aids in achieving hemostasis in the prostatic bed. At times the urologist may apply light traction on the Foley catheter, which causes pressure against the bladder neck and aids in hemostasis.

Diagnostic studies are also performed in the cystoscopy suite and require special catheters for specific studies. For example, the Davis double-balloon urethrographic catheter (Fig. 15-13, *A*) is used to diagnose lesions of the female urethra, such as urethral strictures, diverticula, or fistulas. To accomplish female urethrography, the catheter is inserted through the urethra into the bladder; the two balloons on the catheter are inflated, effectively isolating the urethra, and contrast is injected to visualize the entire urethra (Fig. 15-13, *B*).

Another type of self-retaining catheter frequently used in the operating room is a Pezzer, also known as a "mushroom" catheter. It may be straight or angulated with a large single channel and preformed tip in the shape of a mushroom. The flexible mushroom tip helps keep the catheter in place. This catheter is used primarily to drain the bladder suprapubically, often for poor-risk patients who have uremia, neurogenic bladder syndrome, or possibly long-standing urinary retention. The catheter is inserted in the bladder through a midline or small transverse abdominal wall incision and secured to the abdomen with tape. The Malecot four-winged catheter is often used as a nephrostomy tube to provide temporary, and in some cases permanent, diversion of urine after kidney surgery and when renal tissue needs to be restored (Fig. 15-14). A Foley catheter of preferred size may also be used for this purpose. Nephrostomy tube replacement is accomplished by introducing the

catheter into the surgical tract with a straight catheter guide and securing it in place with a nephrostomy retention disk, one size smaller than the nephrostomy tube being used. The flanges of the disk are then taped to the skin. The use of other variations of urethral catheters will be described later in the text.

Photography in urology

The use of photographic and video imaging equipment in urologic surgery serves to document the patient's disease, the progress of a disease process, and long-term follow-up. It is also an important teaching resource. Video equipment adapts to endoscopic instrumentation and has the capability of projecting an enhanced image on a television monitor and permitting members of the surgical team to observe and learn during the actual surgical procedure (Figs. 15-15 and 15-16).

Other forms of visual aids, such as slides and photographs, are used in teaching, as visual references in publication, and as documentation in patient records.

When any form of photography or video imaging is used, the patient's privacy must be ensured and an informed consent should be obtained. Special release forms should also be signed by the patient for any video tapes or photographs to be used in teaching or publications.

Evaluation

Before the patient is taken to the postanesthesia care unit (PACU) or observation unit, his or her general condition is evaluated. The general appearance of the skin is assessed. Bony prominences, prepped and draped areas, and areas contacted by the attachment of ancillary equipment (ESU pad, ECG leads) are noted for signs of pressure, irritation, or other changes from the preoperative status.

Many urology patients are discharged to PACU with drains inserted, including urethral, ureteral, suprapubic,

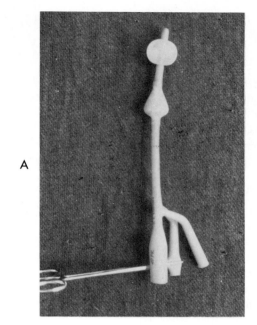

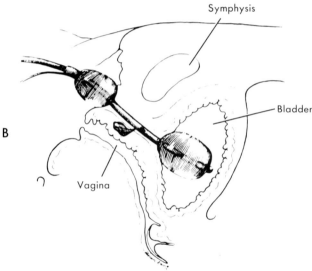

Fig. 15-13. A, Double-balloon Davis urethrographic catheter. **B,** Diagrammatic drawing of Davis urethrographic catheter in female bladder. One balloon is inflated in bladder, and the other is inflated externally at urethral orifice.

and wound drains. Local anesthesia may have been used for either primary analgesia or postoperative pain management. A complete report to the PACU nurse should include intraoperative position, problems specific to the patient, and preoperative comprehension and anxiety levels. Documentation of medications administered from the sterile field or by the perioperative nurse should include time of administration, medication, dosage, site of administration, route of administration, and who performed the application and/or injection. Drains should be labeled and documented as to insertion site and time and date of insertion; labeling is preferable on the collection device. Documentation of drains should also include type of drain and collection device, who performed the insertion, and character of drainage. Any postoperative observations prior to or during transport should be recorded. Evaluation should also address whether the patient met the identified goals related to specific nursing diagnoses in the perioperative nursing care plan. These goals, included in the documentation and report to the PACU, may be phrased as follows:

- The patient maintained adequate gas exchange; lung expansion and O_2 saturation were satisfactory.
- The patient evidenced no signs of fluid or electrolyte imbalance; vital signs were stable, arterial blood gases were within normal limits, and urinary output was adequate.
- The patient maintained patency of the urinary catheter with no signs of infection or retention. The patient should void without difficulty following catheter removal.
- The patient had no evidence of positional injury; neurovascular status was consistent with preoperative level, and skin integrity was intact.
- The patient verbalized concerns to the perioperative nurse.

ALTERNATIVES TO SURGERY: CURRENT DRUG THERAPIES

Patients with various types of cancer may be treated in the urology office setting with new therapeutic modalities.

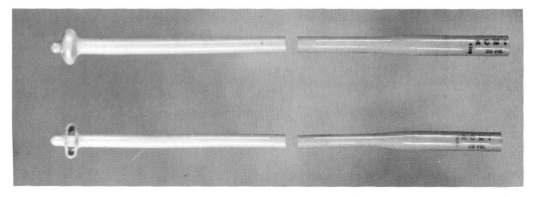

Fig. 15-14. Pezzer (mushroom) catheter and Malecot (bat-wing) four-winged catheter.

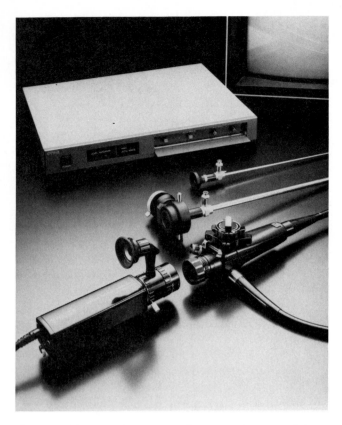

Fig. 15-15. Olympus video system, indicating attachment capabilities of both rigid and flexible instruments. (Courtesy Olympus Corp., Lake Success, N.Y.)

These measures may be initiated instead of surgery or as an adjunct to surgery.

Superficial bladder cancer

Patients with bladder cancer that has been staged as Ta, CIS, and T_1 (stage A or carcinoma in situ) are being treated with intravesical chemotherapy agents such as thiotepa, mitomycin, Adriamycin, and BCG (Soloway, 1987). These medications are proving effective in both the eradication of obvious tumor and the prevention of recurrence.

Prostatic cancer

In an attempt to provide cost-effective, curative treatment with a low morbidity, recent trials have initiated a treatment protocol that may prove superior to the open surgery approach. Following a thorough workup, including serum prostatic-specific antigen and acid phosphatase as well as bone scans, CT or MRI scans of the pelvis, transrectal guided ultrasound biopsies, and histologic grading of the malignancy, select patients with well or moderately differentiated lesions may be candidates for transperineal ultrasound-guided implantation of radium seeds. The seeds are inserted in the operating room during a short-stay patient admission. The radiation dose is doubled or tripled from that delivered by standard radiation techniques. There is decreased risk to the surrounding tissue because of the limited 1-cm penetration range of the seeds. The radium employed is iodine-125 or palladium-103.

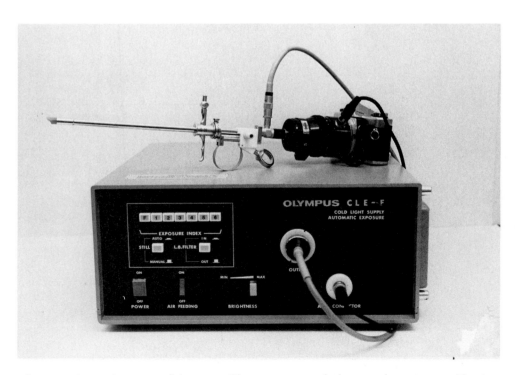

Fig. 15-16. Automatic exposure light source, Olympus camera and adapter, and resectoscope. (Courtesy Olympus Corp., Lake Success, N.Y.)

Penile cancer

Options are now available to avoid the disfiguring surgery previously indicated for penile cancer. Bleomycin, usually combined with irradiation, is showing great success in patients with known metastasis. Methotrexate is another relatively new and effective agent. A third therapy involves the use of cis-platinum. All these modalities are showing favorable results for patients with selected stages of penile carcinoma.

SURGICAL INTERVENTIONS
Diagnostic and endoscopic procedures
Cystoscopy

Cystoscopy is an endoscopic examination of the lower urinary tract, including visual inspection of the interior of the urethra, the bladder, and the ureteral orifices using the cystoscope, a versatile optical instrument with a variety of telescopic lenses. In a male patient special attention is given to the examination of the verumontanum (which contains the ejaculatory ducts), the bladder neck, and the median and lateral lobes of the prostate. In a female patient, the urethra, bladder neck, and bladder are examined.

Cystoscopy is an important diagnostic tool that provides the urologist with valuable information concerning the patient's urologic condition. Indications for cystoscopy include hematuria, urinary retention, urinary incontinence, urinary tract infection, tumors, fistulas, and vesical calculus disease.

Procedural considerations. Once in the cystoscopy suite, the patient should be greeted by name and identified by hospital number. The nurse should check the chart for operative consent and pertinent laboratory reports. Intravenous pyelograms, any diagnostic studies, and chest x-ray films should also be available for review.

Customarily, the patient voids immediately before the procedure. This practice is of particular importance in ruling out residual urine in the bladder. The patient is then placed on the cystoscopy bed. Correct positioning of the patient requires optimum relaxation of muscles of the legs and perineum. Proper positioning of the knee crutches on the cystoscopy bed is a vital consideration for patient safety and comfort. When knee crutches are properly positioned, the curve of the yoke suspension should flow outward from the perineum, as do the patient's legs. Padding the knee crutches is beneficial in reducing pressure on the popliteal areas. If sling stirrups that support only the feet are employed, the post should be padded and positioned to prevent pressure on the peroneal nerve. After the patient is properly positioned, the bed is tilted so that the patient's head is slightly higher than the buttocks to allow the prep solution to drain into the collecting pan. The pooling of solutions beneath the patient may cause skin reaction and severe irritation.

If the cystoscopic procedure requires the use of an electrosurgical unit, the dispersive pad is placed on the patient

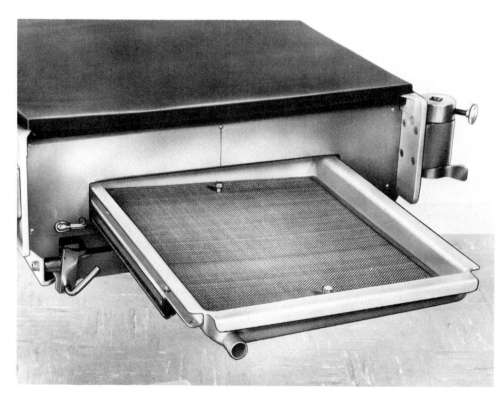

Fig. 15-17. Sterile screen placed over drainage drawer on cystoscopy table.

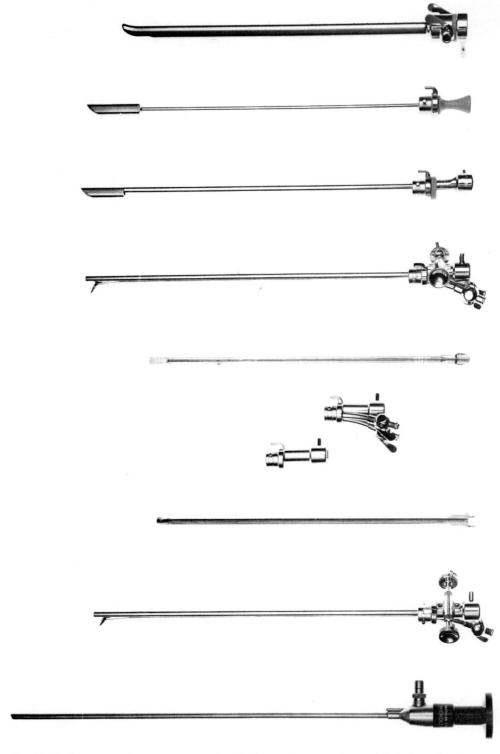

Fig. 15-18. Instruments for cystoscopy, catheterization, and retrograde ureteral pyelography. *Top to bottom,* Cystoscope sheath, obturator, visual obturator, double-catheterizing Albarran bridge, double-catheterizing fin, double-catheterizing bridge, examining bridge, stationary deflector, operating Albarran bridge, telescope. (Courtesy American ACMI, Stamford, Conn.)

in direct contact with the skin as close to the operative site as practical, usually on the upper thigh.

After proper positioning of the patient, the nurse or urologist dons gloves and preps the entire pubic area, including the scrotum and perineum, with an antimicrobial solution. A screen is placed over the drainage pan on the cystoscopy bed (Fig. 15-17). Disposable draping systems with a sterile screen material incorporated into them are available. The patient is then draped according to hospital procedure. Adequate draping is important to ensure that aseptic technique is maintained during the urologic procedure. If a general anesthetic is required, it is administered before prepping and draping. If a topical anesthetic is preferred, it is instilled into the urethra of the male patient after prepping and draping but before instrumentation. For a female patient, a cotton applicator that has been dipped into the anesthetic solution is placed in the urethral meatus. Lidocaine, 1% (Xylocaine) or 2% (Anestacon), is usually used. If the patient is allergic to lidocaine, instillation of 50 to 60 cc of lubricant accompanied by anesthesia monitored sedation is often adequate to afford painless access to the urethra and bladder. The patient should be informed that a sensation of pressure is to be expected.

The cystoscopy setup should include the following:

Prep set and solutions
Cystourethroscope (Fig. 15-18)
1 Short bridge
1 Fiberoptic light cord
1 Lateral telescope
1 Foroblique telescope
1 Luer-Lok stopcock and irrigation tubing
Lubricant, water-soluble
1 Calibrated container to measure residual urine
2 Test tubes, screwtop, for urine specimens
Gauze sponges
1 Albarran bridge
2 Rubber catheter "nipples" or adapters

Local or topical anesthetic supplies

Medicine glass for anesthetic solution or gel
Syringe, disposable 10 ml, to instill dye
Penile clamp (to occlude male urethra after local anesthetic is instilled)
Urethral syringe for anesthetic

Accessory items

Cystoscopy drape pack
Irrigation system
Gown and gloves
Fiberoptic light source
Electrosurgical unit

Several devices are available to support the cystourethroscope during the injection of radiopaque dye or while x-ray films are developed. One such device is a "tite grip" towel holder, commonly used by dentists, which consists of a chrome chain with a clip on each end. These clips are attached to the cystoscopy drape, one on each side of the scope, with the chain below the scope, supporting it. The device can be decontaminated after use, packaged, sterilized, and reused.

The flexible cystoscope (Fig. 15-19) is used for patients with obstructive symptoms resulting from prostatic hyperplasia and rigid prostatic urethra. In addition, the flexible cystoscope can be used for patients who cannot assume a lithotomy position, such as those with spinal cord injuries or severe arthritis. Flexible cystoscopy may be accomplished with the use of a local anesthetic, although it is not usually necessary. It affords the patient a higher degree of comfort, is less traumatic to the urethra, and can be performed in the patient's bed on the nursing unit.

Cleaning, sterilization, disinfection, and maintenance of endoscopic equipment are important procedures in the care of fiberoptic lensed instruments. Ultimately, this process reduces costly repairs and ensures the availability of properly functioning instruments.

Protective padding should be placed on the countertop and on the bottom of the sink in the instrument decontamination area to prevent possible damage to lensed telescopes. After each surgical procedure, components of each cystoscopic set should be disassembled and soaked in a solution of warm water and germicidal detergent. All stopcocks and sheaths should be cleaned thoroughly with a soft brush to remove blood, dried lubricant jelly, or other debris. Instruments should then be thoroughly rinsed in warm water, placed on protective padding, and allowed to dry. All moving parts must be individually evaluated for mobility. An instrument milk may be applied as required. The patency of all outlets must be maintained to ensure proper sterilization or disinfection. Fiberoptic light cords must not be tangled, twisted, or sharply angulated; otherwise, the fibers break inside the instrument.

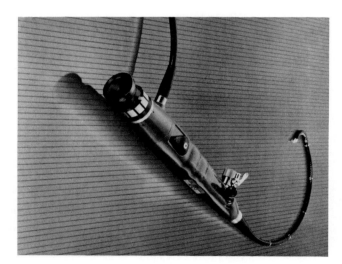

Fig. 15-19. Flexible cystoscope. (Courtesy American ACMI, Stamford, Conn.)

Sterilization of instruments with steam or ethylene oxide provides the greatest assurance of eliminating the risk of infections transmitted by contaminated instruments (Chapter 5). According to the Centers for Disease Control (CDC), however, sterilization is not essential for items classified as semicritical, for example, cystoscopes. High-level disinfection with an agent, such as activated glutaraldehyde or dialdehyde, that can destroy vegetative microorganisms, most fungal spores, tubercle bacilli, and small nonlipid viruses is recommended. In most situations, meticulous cleaning of endoscopic instruments followed by appropriate high-level disinfection provides reasonable assurance that the items are safe to use. The level of disinfection is based on the contact time, temperature, and concentration of the active ingredients of the disinfectant, as well as the nature of microbial contamination.

For sterilization or disinfection, instruments should be assembled on a covered tray and protected with padding. Because the lens system is delicate and costly, a plastic covering available from some manufacturers may be used to protect the lens.

Various instrument manufacturers provide sterilization containers for endoscopy equipment and have written recommendations for the cleaning, sterilization, and disinfection of their equipment.

Operative procedure

1. After the urologist has scrubbed, gowned, and gloved, the fiberoptic light cord is connected to the light source and tested for proper intensity. The irrigating system is set up, and, if required, the high-frequency cord is connected to an electrosurgical unit.

2. The cystourethroscope is lubricated and introduced into the urethra, the obturator withdrawn, and residual urine obtained, provided the patient voided before the examination. The specimen may be saved for culture studies or cytologic studies. The cystourethroscope is connected to the irrigating system, and the telescope inserted and locked in place. The urologist controls the flow and volume of fluid by adjusting the stopcock on the scope. If difficulty is encountered during insertion, the visual obturator may be used to introduce the scope under direct vision. This accessory is constructed to smooth the fenestral edges of the cystourethroscope. It requires the use of the telescope for direct vision and permits irrigation during introduction.

3. Stone removal, bladder biopsy, or bladder fulguration

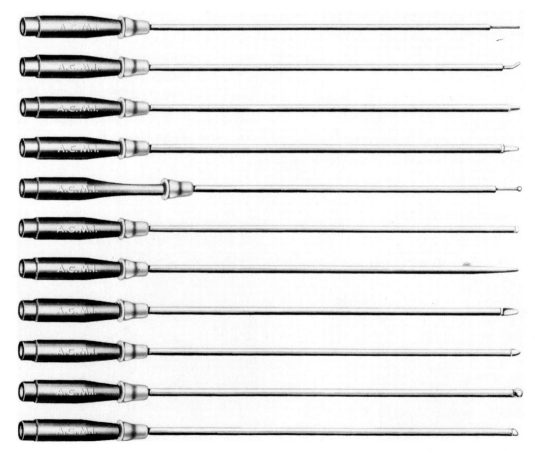

Fig. 15-20. Cystoscopic fulgurating electrodes with various types of tips. (Courtesy American ACMI, Stamford, Conn.; from Morel, A., and Wise, G.J.: Urologic endoscopic procedures, ed. 2, St. Louis, 1979, The C.V. Mosby Co.)

may be performed by using special cystoscopic accessories such as the Hendrickson-Bigelow lithotrite, which is used to crush large bladder calculi. This procedure is called a *litholapaxy*. Lowsley forceps, Wappler rigid cup forceps, and flexible foreign body forceps may also be employed. Bladder fulguration requires the use of flexible stem electrodes available in various French sizes and tip configurations such as the ball, cone, dome, and bayonet tip (Fig. 15-20).

4. For retrograde ureteral catheterization and pyelography, ureteral catheters are passed through the cystoscope sheath and directed by the Albarran bridge deflector through the ureteral orifice and into the ureter. A radiopaque substance, such as 30% Renografin or 50% Hypaque, is then injected, and an x-ray film taken to outline the entire upper urinary collecting system.

Pediatric cystoscopy

Pediatric cystoscopy is the endoscopic examination of the lower urinary tract of pediatric patients. The major difference between adult and pediatric cystoscopy is the size of the instruments used and consideration of the small, delicate orifices of the pediatric patient. Indications for pediatric cystoscopy include urinary tract infection, en-

uresis, urethral valves, diverticula, bladder neck contractures, bladder tumors, and urinary tract obstructions.

Procedural considerations. The pediatric patient should be greeted by name and identified by hospital number. The patient's chart is checked for operative consent and pertinent laboratory reports. Intravenous pyelograms and chest x-ray films should also be available for review. The cystoscopy setup will have the same type of components as that for the adult cystoscopy patient except that the size of the cystourethroscope system will be specific to the pediatric patient's needs (Fig. 15-21).

Each pediatric cystourethroscope is designed to fit specific component parts and is very delicate. Therefore, the perioperative nurse must be familiar with the proper use of the system and handle the components carefully. The resectoscope component is commonly used to resect urethral valves and occasionally bladder tumors, using the resectoscope loop. The cold knife may be used with the resectoscope to cut urethral strictures and occasionally to resect a urethral valve.

The most common anesthesia used for the pediatric patient is general anesthesia. Following induction of anesthesia, the child is placed in a lithotomy position and prepped and draped according to hospital procedure.

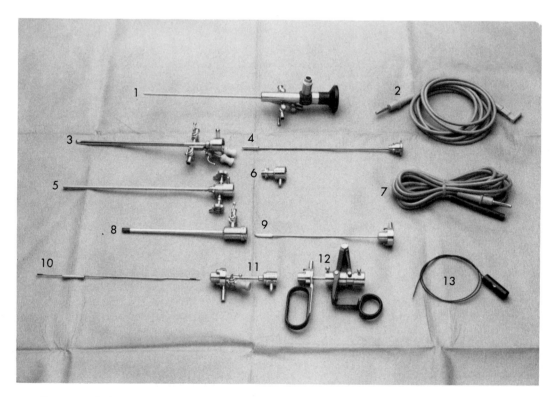

Fig. 15-21. Pediatric cystoscopy instrumentation. *1,* 8 Fr cystoscope; *2,* fiberoptic light cord; *3* and *4,* 13 Fr cystoscope sheath and obturator; *5,* deflector; *6,* bridge; *7,* high-frequency cable; *8* and *9,* 13 Fr resectoscope sheath and obturator; *10,* resectoscope loop; *11,* bridge; *12,* working element; and *13,* ball tip electrode. (Courtesy Karl Storz Endoscopy—America, Inc., Culver City, Calif.)

Maintenance of body temperature is of special concern in children. Every effort should be made to limit exposure of the body surface. Chapter 29 provides a thorough discussion of important perioperative nursing considerations for pediatric patients.

Operative procedure. The pediatric cystourethroscope is lubricated and inserted through the urethra into the bladder. The light cord and irrigation tubing are attached to the telescope and cystoscope, and the examination is performed.

Transurethral ureteropyeloscopy

Transurethral ureteropyeloscopy is an endoscopic examination of the ureters and renal pelvis. The use of rigid or flexible ureteroscopes or ureteropyeloscopes provides the opportunity to diagnose filling defects in the ureter and renal pelvis, congenital anomalies, hematuria, ureteral obstruction, and damage from trauma. Manipulation, fragmentation, basketing of ureteral and renal calculi, and retrieval of foreign bodies are possible with transurethral ureteropyeloscopy. It may also be used to manage residual sludge (steinstrasse) following extracorporeal shock wave lithotripsy. Ureteral strictures may also be treated transurethrally, and biopsies of tumors of the ureter and renal pelvis may be performed under direct visualization. Internal ureteral stents may also be inserted for ureteral patency. These range in size from 3 to 8.5 Fr and are available in single and double J and pigtail configurations.

Procedural considerations. The setup is similar to that for a cystoscopy with the addition of a flexible or rigid ureteroscope system (Fig. 15-22). A critical factor in this procedure is allowing enough time for careful dilation of the ureter under C-Arm fluoroscopy. The flexible ureteroscope has gained popularity because of the inherent tip mobility, which provides a more panoramic view of the entire circumference of the ureter. The nurse must be able to tilt the radiolucent operative bed at head and foot and laterally, as well as raise the bed height.

In addition to the standard cystoscopy setup, the following equipment should be available:

1 Ureteroscope, flexible or rigid (or both)
  Ureteral dilators, graduated sizes and styles
  Ureteral stone baskets, 3–5 Fr, of various styles
1 Ureteral grasping forceps
1 Ureteral biopsy forceps
1 Ureteral snare
1 Ureteral scissors
  Ureteral catheters, various styles and sizes
  Ureteral stents
  Radiographic dye

Operations on the penis and the urethra
Laser ablation of condylomata and penile carcinoma

Laser ablation of condylomata or penile cancer is the eradication of diseased tissue by means of a laser beam. Laser therapy has been determined, through clinical trials, to be effective therapy for condylomata and penile cancers that are refractive to other treatments. One of the major advantages of the laser is that heat is distributed evenly to the tissue underlying the lesion. The recurrence rate following laser ablation has been extremely low, with cure rates ranging from 88% to 95%. When any laser is being

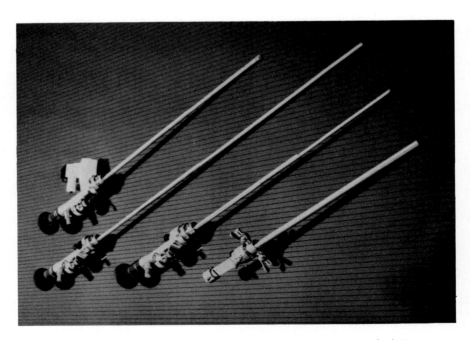

Fig. 15-22. Rigid ureteroscope system. (Courtesy American ACMI, Stamford, Conn.)

used, guidelines appropriate to that system must be initiated (see Chapter 10).

Procedural considerations. Laser treatment may be performed successfully with a local infiltration of anesthetic. A U-shaped craterlike lesion of predetermined depth with a 2-mm radius can be created. A power setting ranging from 2 to 20 W on continuous or superpulse mode is generally used. With laser ablation, less edema and necrosis occur, fibrosis is minimized, and rapid healing is facilitated. The argon, CO_2, and Nd:YAG lasers are all suitable for this therapeutic application.

Operative procedure. The operator moves the beam transversely across the tissue and then in a crosshatch matrix, thereby treating all perimeters of the lesion. Periodically the area should be wiped with a sponge moistened in acetic acid (3% to 5% vinegar). This treatment causes diseased tissue to stand out and allows therapy to deeper layers.

The affected areas may be coated with Polymyxin ointment or a similar antibiotic. Wounds are generally left uncovered. Postoperatively a mild oral pain medication is usually adequate.

Circumcision

Circumcision is the excision of the foreskin (prepuce) of the glans penis. Circumcision may be done prophylactically in infancy. The surgery may be performed for religious reasons, for example, as is required in specific faiths. Provision should be made in a hospital to observe the religious needs and preferences of the parents.

Circumcision is also performed for the relief of phimosis, a condition in which the orifice of the prepuce is stenosed or too narrow to permit easy retraction behind the glans. Another condition, balanoposthitis, results in an inflamed glans and mucous membrane with purulent discharge and may require circumcision. In addition, circumcision may be done to prevent recurrent paraphimosis, a condition in which the prepuce cannot be reduced easily from a retracted position.

Procedural considerations. Newborns are generally positioned on a specially constructed board that facilitates restraint by immobilizing the limbs and exposing the genitals. Frequently, no anesthesia is used in this age group. Older children require anesthesia. Adults may be offered the option of local or general anesthesia.

For infants, the setup includes fine plastic instruments. A Gomco clamp of the appropriate size, a Plastibell, or the Hollister disposable circumcision device may be preferred. The Hollister device includes sutures that are sealed in a sterile packet ready for use. For older patients a plastic instrument set is used. Petrolatum gauze for dressing should be available.

Operative procedure

1. If the prepuce is adherent, a probe or hemostat may be used to break up adhesions. The prepuce is clamped

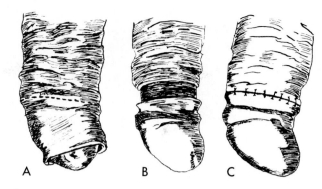

Fig. 15-23. Circumcision. **A,** Prepuce is incised toward coronal margin. **B,** Prepuce is completely separated from glans. **C,** Raw edges of skin incision are approximated to coronal cuff of mucosal prepuce.

in the dorsal midline and incised toward the coronal margin (Fig. 15-23, *A*), leaving about 5 cm of coronal mucosa intact. A similar procedure is performed ventrally. The two incisions are then joined circumferentially. Alternatively, a superficial, circumferential incision is made in the skin with a scalpel at the level of the coronal sulcus and the mucosa at the base of the glans. The redundant skin is undermined between the circumferential incisions and removed as a complete cuff (Fig. 15-23, *B*). Bleeding vessels are coagulated or clamped with mosquito hemostats and tied with fine absorbable ligatures.

2. The raw edges of the skin incision are approximated to a coronal cuff of mucosal prepuce with no. 4-0 or 5-0 absorbable sutures on atraumatic needles (Fig. 15-23, *C*). The wound is usually dressed with petrolatum gauze.

Excision of urethral caruncle

Excision of an urethral caruncle entails the removal of papillary or sessile tumors from the urethra. A urethral caruncle is a benign lesion or inflammatory prolapse of the external urinary meatus in the female.

Procedural considerations. The patient is placed in the lithotomy position. A minor or plastic set, an electrosurgical unit, and a local anesthetic are used. A urethral catheter of an appropriate size may be required if the distal urethral prolapse is severe.

Operative procedure. With a small Metzenbaum scissors, the tumor is exposed and excised within a wedge of ventral urethral tissue. Figure-of-eight no. 4-0 absorbable sutures at the edge of the incision are usually sufficient to achieve good hemostasis (Fig. 15-24).

Urethral meatotomy

Urethral meatotomy is an incisional enlargement of the external urethral meatus to relieve stenosis or stricture at the external meatus that may be congenital or acquired.

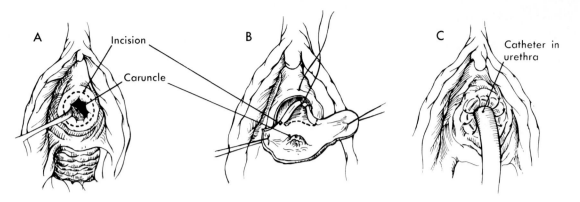

Fig. 15-24. Excision of sessile growth. **A,** Incision around urethral meatus and caruncle. **B,** Urethra freed from caruncle, meatus dissected back to healthy tissue, and caruncle excised. **C,** Reanastomosis of mucocutaneous junction, and catheter inserted. (From Flocks, R.H., and Clup, D.A.: Surgical urology, 4th ed. Copyright © 1975 by Year Book Medical Publishers, Inc., Chicago. Used by permission.)

Procedural considerations. A male patient is placed in the supine position. Prepping and draping are as described for urethral catheterization. For a female patient the lithotomy position is used. Local anesthesia is generally employed. A plastic instrument set is needed. A petrolatum gauze dressing is usually applied.

Operative procedure. A straight hemostat is placed on the ventral surface of the meatus. An incision is made along the frenum to enlarge the opening and overcome the stricture. Bleeding vessels are clamped and ligated with fine plain surgical gut sutures. The mucosal layer is sutured to the skin with fine absorbable sutures. A dressing of petrolatum gauze may be applied.

Urethral dilatation and internal urethrotomy

Urethral dilatation and internal urethrotomy entail the gradual dilatation and lysis of a urethral stricture to provide relief of distal lower urinary tract obstruction. Urethral strictures or narrowing of the urethra may be caused by a congenital malformation that is usually found at the external urinary meatus. Infection or trauma may also contribute to stricture of the membranous and pendulous urethra. One method of treating urethral stricture disease is by periodic dilatation with Philips filiforms and followers or Van Buren sounds.

Procedural considerations. The male patient may be placed in a supine position for routine urethral dilatation and in lithotomy position for other procedures. Prepping and draping are as required for male catheterization. A local anesthetic such as lidocaine (Xylocaine gel or Anestacon) should be used. The female patient is placed in the lithotomy position. A cotton-tipped applicator dipped in the local anesthetic or a urethral syringe filled with anesthetic is placed in the urethral opening. Female urethral dilatation is performed with short, straight metal dilators or with hollow McCarthy dilators, through which a catheterized urine specimen can also be obtained.

The setup includes the following:

Urethrotomes (Fig. 15-25)
Direct viewing telescope and bridge for ureteral catheters
Resectoscope working element, sheath, obturator, and cold knives
Urethral dilators

Accessory items

Philips filiforms and followers
Van Buren sounds
Irrigation system
Prep set and solutions
Silicone Foley catheter
Syringe, 20 ml
Lubricant, water-soluble
Fiberoptic light cord
Luer-Lok water adapter
Cystoscopy drape pack
Sterile gown and gloves
Cystoscopy setup, if required

Operative procedures

Gradual dilatation. In a male patient the urethra is lubricated and anesthetized with a viscous anesthetic that is instilled into the urethra with a 10-ml syringe. A penile clamp occludes the penile urethra at the coronal sulcus and keeps the anesthetic within the urethra. Philips filiforms of various tips and sizes are introduced first in an attempt to pass an instrument beyond the urethral stricture. Followers of increasing size are attached to the filiforms and passed through the strictured area of the urethra, stretching the scarred area (Fig. 15-26). Slow dilatation is also achieved with a small catheter or filiform left in the urethra. It leads to softening of the stricture over the course of several days. Before use or sterilization, the filiforms and followers should be carefully inspected for damaged or weak points, particularly around the screw thread end. Van Buren sounds may also be used for urethral dilatation.

Internal urethrotomy. Under direct vision, the assem-

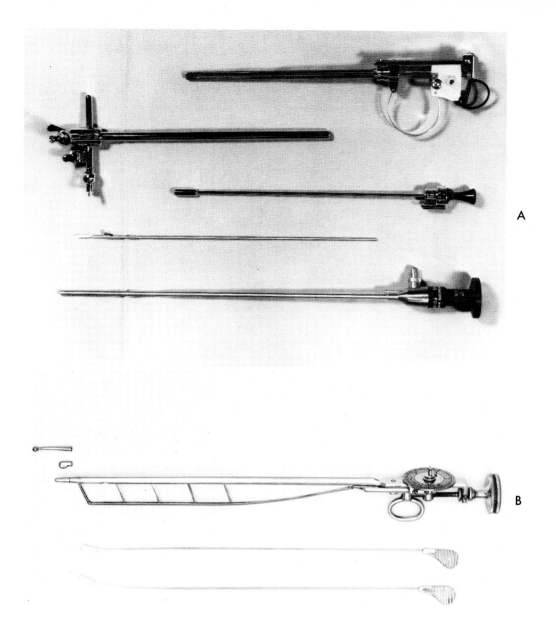

Fig. 15-25. A, American ACMI internal urethrotome components. **B,** Otis urethrotome components.

bled visualizing urethrotome is inserted into the urethra. When necessary, a filiform or ureteral catheter is fed into the catheterizing channel to help identify the patent portion of the urethra. The urethrotome is advanced to the desired position, and the blade is used to incise the urethral scar. The normal urethra must be increased 1 cm proximally and distally beyond the stricture to achieve good results. A silicone Foley catheter is usually left in place for 3 to 5 days after surgery.

Hypospadias repair

Hypospadias repair is repair of a urethral meatus that is proximal to its normal glandular position at the tip of the penis. There are varying degrees of hypospadias. The meatus may be on the ventral surface of the glans, on the corona, anywhere along the shaft, in the scrotum, or even in the perineum. The more proximal the opening, the greater the degree of chordee (ventral curvature of the penis). Chordee are fibrous bands that extend from the hypospadiac urethral meatus to the tip of the glans and represent the abnormally developed urethra and its investing layer of Buck's fascia, dartos, and skin.

Principles of hypospadias repair consist of release of chordee, thereby straightening the penis, and reconstruction of the urethra. Surgeons prefer to do a one-stage hypospadias repair in cases of distal penile hypospadias with minimal chordee. Recently there has been a resurgence of interest in one-stage repairs.

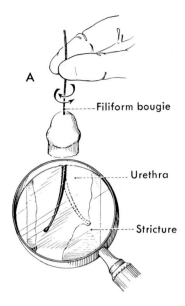

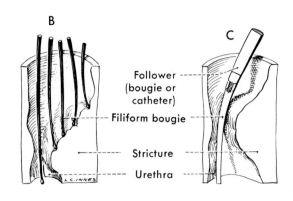

Fig. 15-26. Method of using coude-tipped bougie for passing stricture. **A,** Bougie is withdrawn 1 to 2 cm each time obstruction is met; bougie is rotated and then is passed inward again. **B,** Method of using multiple bougies to pass through urethral stricture. Pocket is filled with bougie tips; this displaces one to opening through stricture. **C,** Philips filiform and follower. Follower is screwed onto end of filiform. Filiform passed through stricture guides follower through. (From Barnes, R.W., and Hadley, H.L.: Urological practice, St. Louis, 1954, The C.V. Mosby Co.)

One complication of hypospadias repair is urethral fistula formation, which can be repaired without much difficulty. Correction of strictures is more troublesome.

Procedural considerations. The patient is placed in the supine position with legs apart. The urine is diverted with a urethral catheter. The instrument setup varies according to the surgeon's preference. However, a minor set with fine plastic instruments is generally required, and sutures, polyethylene infant feeding tubes, silicone tubing or silicone Foley catheters, and drains may be desired. Owens gauze, Elastomull, Coban, and Elastoplast, as well as adhesive tape, are generally required for the dressing, which is an important part of the hypospadias repair.

Operative procedures

Chordee repair

1. An incision is made around the penis. The skin is stripped back from the phallus by subcutaneous dissection (Fig. 15-27, *A* and *B*).
2. Fibrous tissue on the ventral surface is removed, correcting the ventral curvature of the penis.
3. A buttonhole incision is made in the dorsal skin flap, and the glans penis is brought through the opening (Fig. 15-27, *C* and *D*).
4. The edges of the buttonhole incision are sutured to the skin adjacent to the corona. If skin is excessive at the extremities of the transverse suture, it may be trimmed (Fig. 15-27, *E*).
5. The skin flap distal to the buttonhole incision covers the denuded ventral surface of the penis and is sutured to the retracted skin margin (Fig. 15-27, *F*).
6. An indwelling catheter is placed, and the wound is dressed.

Urethral reconstruction. Many procedures are described for construction of a urethra. They may be divided into three general groups: (1) buried skin tube (Fig. 15-28), (2) buried skin flap (Fig. 15-29), and (3) free graft (Fig. 15-30). There are also many combinations of these procedures. In all the procedures some type of temporary urinary diversion, such as a perineal urethrostomy, is used.

Epispadias repair

An epispadias repair is the correction of the absence of the dorsal wall of the urethra and the position of the corpora cavernosa, ventral to the urethra. The surgical procedures employed in the correction of epispadias depend on the extent of the deformity. In mild incomplete defects, the repair is the same as a simple hypospadias repair. Complete deformity is always associated with urinary incontinence because of little or no development of the bladder neck; thus, the operation is much more involved. The least severe form of the exstrophy epispadias complex is balanitic epispadias, in which the urethra opens on the dorsum of the glans, or penile epispadias, in which the urethra opens on the shaft of the penis. The more severe variety, which occurs when the urethra opens on the proximal shaft or in the penopubic position, is generally associated with severe dorsal chordee and urinary incontinence.

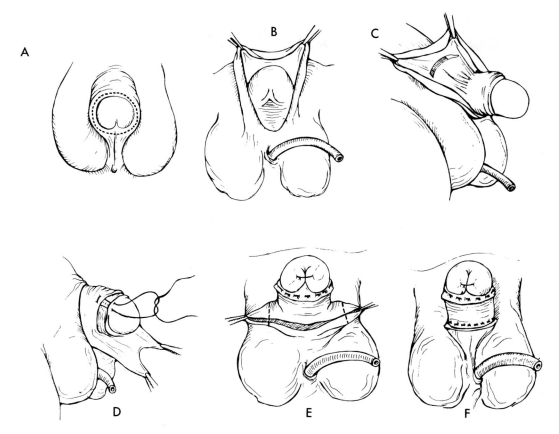

Fig. 15-27. Chordee procedure in hypospadias repair. (Modified from Dodson, A.I.: Urological surgery, ed. 4, St. Louis, 1970, The C.V. Mosby Co.)

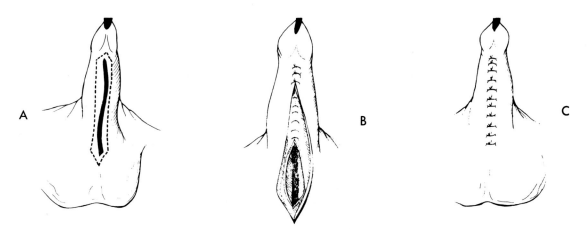

Fig. 15-28. Urethral reconstruction—buried skin tube. **A,** Parallel incisions, which meet as they encircle meatus proximally, made on ventral surface of shaft of penis. **B,** Medial edges of incision undermined so longitudinal skin flap can be sutured around catheter. **C,** Lateral edges undermined until sufficient relaxation and mobilization are obtained to suture them over catheter. (From Flocks, R.H., and Clup, D.A.: Surgical urology, 4th ed. Copyright © 1975 by Year Book Medical Publishers, Inc., Chicago. Used by permission.)

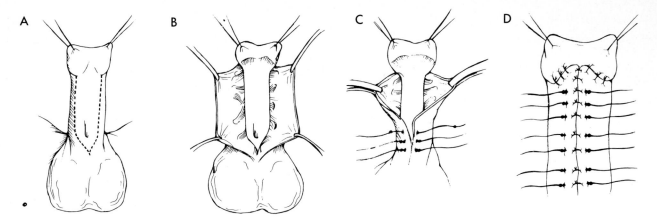

Fig. 15-29. Urethral reconstruction—buried skin flap. **A,** Incision made on ventral surface of penile shaft. **B,** Lateral edges of incision undermined. **C,** Lateral edges brought over rectangular flap of skin and sutured. No tube is formed. **D,** Sutures reinforced with wire tension sutures held in place with small lead shot. When healing, buried skin flap epithelializes in circular manner to form epithelial cyst that can be used as distal urethra. (From Flocks, R.H., and Clup, D.A.: Surgical urology, 4th ed. Copyright © 1975 by Year Book Medical Publishers, Inc., Chicago. Used by permission.)

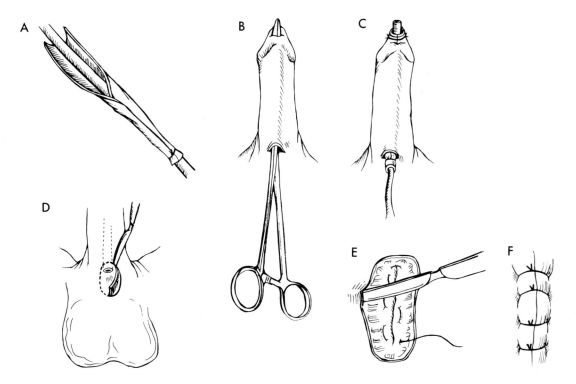

Fig. 15-30. Urethral reconstruction—free graft. **A,** Skin graft, which is taken from non-hairbearing area such as inner aspect of upper arm, is wrapped around stiff catheter and anchored at each end. **B,** Bed for graft is prepared by making transverse incision in front of urethral meatus and bluntly dissecting to tip of glans penis. **C,** Catheter with graft pulled through channel with forceps. When graft is in place, both catheter and graft are anchored with sutures at both ends. **D,** Final closure of urethra is accomplished by incising skin around fistulous openings. **E,** Inner margins of incision are closed over catheter. **F,** Lateral margins of incision are undermined and closed in several layers. Catheter is then removed wth diversion of urine flow through perineal urethrostomy or suprapubic cystostomy. (From Flocks, R.H., and Clup, D.A.: Surgical urology, 4th ed. Copyright © 1975 by Year Book Medical Publishers, Inc., Chicago. Used by permission.)

Procedural considerations. The setup for an epispadias repair is as described for hypospadias repair.

Operative procedure

First-stage epispadias repair. A vertical incision is made distal to the epispadiac meatus and carried circumferentially to the dorsal coronal margin. The foreshortened dorsal urethral strip is lifted off the corpora cavernosa, and the ventral prepuce (foreskin) is rotated dorsally to cover the dorsal skin defect created by penile straightening.

Second-stage epispadias repair

1. A vertical suprapubic incision is made, exposing the anterior bladder wall and widened vesical neck. A wedge section of the anterolateral prostatic urethra is removed on either side, so that when it is reconstructed a more normal caliber prostatic urethra is formed (Fig. 15-31, *A*).
2. The roof of the membranous urethra is removed (Fig. 15-31, *B*).
3. The prostatic urethra is closed, including muscle that is sutured together in the midline, with absorbable sutures. The bladder is closed, leaving a suprapubic catheter indwelling. The abdomen is closed in layers (Fig. 15-31, *C*).

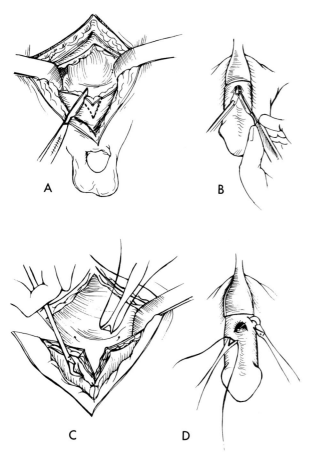

Fig. 15-31. Epispadias repair. (From Flocks, R.H., and Clup, D.A.: Surgical urology, 4th ed. Copyright © 1975 by Year Book Medical Publishers, Inc., Chicago. Used by permission.)

4. The anterior urethra is closed after outlining an appropriate-sized octagonal strip or dorsal penile skin (Fig. 15-31, *D*).
5. The remainder of the repair, that is, the creation of the urethra and its coverage with lateral penile skin, is the reverse procedure of a second-stage hypospadias repair.

Urethroplasty

Urethroplasty is reconstructive surgery of the urethra. Strictures, urethral fractures, or narrowing of the urethral lumen are congenital, inflammatory, or traumatic in origin. Various surgical techniques are described in the surgical treatment of stricture disease.

Procedural considerations. The patient is placed in the exaggerated lithotomy position. Routine prepping and draping procedures are employed with precautions for protecting the anus (that is, the use of an impervious plastic adherent drape). The instrument setup includes a minor instrument set with fine plastic instruments for dissection and plastic repair. Strictures may be located deep, requiring special instruments such as Turner-Warwick needles and retractors (Fig. 15-32). A Denis-Browne ring retractor is also helpful (Fig. 15-33). Fiberoptic lighting is desirable, and an electrosurgical unit may be required.

Operative procedure

First-stage Johanson urethroplasty

1. An inverted U incision is made in the perineum from the inner borders of the ischial tuberosities up to and including the base of the scrotum. A Van Buren sound is passed into the urethra up to the stricture. The bulbocavernosus muscle is dissected and retracted laterally.
2. An incision is made in the urethra over the strictured area and is extended at least 1 cm beyond the diseased area of the urethra in each direction (Fig. 15-34, *A*).
3. The abnormal scar tissue is excised or simply incised, because scrotal skin ultimately increases the lumen (Fig. 15-34, *B*). A no. 28 sound is passed through the proximal and the distal urethral lumina to rule out further stricture. The remaining urethral mucosa is sutured with fine absorbable suture to the scrotal skin (Fig. 15-34, *C*). A cystotomy tube to divert the urinary stream may be left indwelling and removed in 5 to 7 days.

Approximately 3 months after the first stage, if the operative site is healing and the patient is voiding adequately, a second-stage procedure is performed.

Second-stage Johanson urethroplasty

1. A Robinson catheter is temporarily inserted into the bladder through the proximal urethral stoma. The skin is incised along prolongitudinal lines, and flaps of skin are developed to construct a new urethra.
2. The flaps are brought together in the midline and closed with a continuous or interrupted fine absorbable suture to a predetermined caliber.

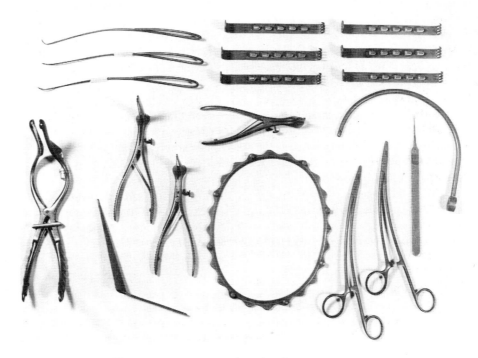

Fig. 15-32. Turner-Warwick urethroplasty instruments.

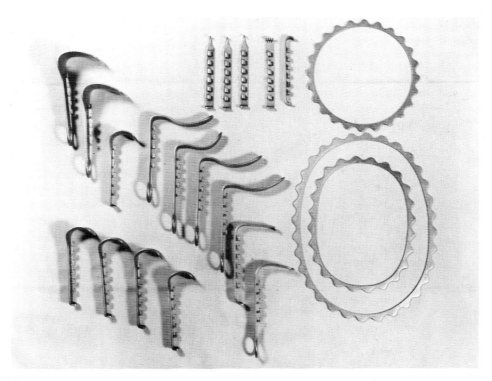

Fig. 15-33. Denis-Browne self-retaining ring retractor.

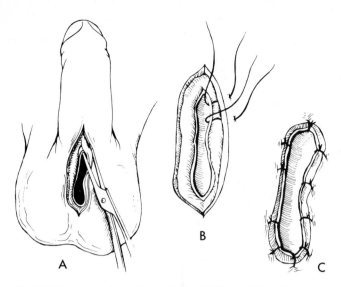

Fig. 15-34. Urethroplasty. (From Flocks, R.H., and Clup, D.A.: Surgical urology, 4th ed. Copyright © 1975 by Year Book Medical Publishers, Inc., Chicago. Used by permission.)

7. The apex is sutured into position at the verumontanum end of the stricture and then at the distal ends, with the epidermal side toward the urethral lumen.
8. Interrupted absorbable sutures of 4-0 are placed to hold the graft in position.
9. The cystoscope is again inserted and the urethra irrigated to check for suture line leaks.
10. A Foley or fenestrated catheter is inserted to serve as a stent.
11. The corpora spongiosa is approximated and closed over the patched area as a separate layer with interrupted 3-0 absorbable sutures.
12. Subcutaneous 4-0 absorbable sutures are placed.
13. The skin and the graft site are closed with interrupted 4-0 sutures.
14. A suprapubic catheter is inserted to divert urine for healing.
15. Petrolatum gauze is wrapped around the penis and covered with gauze sponges and fluffed dressings. A scrotal supporter is applied to provide support and pressure.

Penectomy

Penectomy is the partial or total removal of a cancerous penis. The procedure selected is dependent on the extent of involvement and disease stage. Invasive penile cancer not suited for irradiation owing to its size, depth, or location is best dealt with by penectomy. Excision of a 2-cm gross tumor margin is adequate for local management. Partial penectomy may afford a sufficient length for directable and upright urination. At least 3 cm of viable proximal shaft is necessary for considering a partial penectomy. If the residual stump is inadequate in length, detachment and mobilization of the suspensory ligaments may be an option in selected patients. A total penectomy is generally required when tumor margins are beyond a 2-cm retrievable length from the penoscrotal junction.

Reconstruction is possible following penectomy. Evaluation must take into account sexual, urinary, and cosmetic factors. Extensive or proximally invasive lesions that include the scrotum, perineum, abdominal wall, and/or pubis necessitate emasculation as well as expanded resection of involved tissues.

Procedural considerations. The setup necessary is similar to that for any inguinal surgery, with the addition of a medium drain for use as a tourniquet.

Operative procedure

Partial penectomy

1. The lesion is excluded by a towel attached to the planned amputation line. A penile tourniquet is applied at the base.
2. Following circumferential skin incision, the cavernous bodies are divided to the urethra (Fig. 15-35).
3. Dorsal vessels are ligated, and the urethra is dissected proximally and distally to obtain a 1-cm redundant flap.

3. Layers of subcutaneous tissue are dissected free, then sutured over the newly constructed urethra with interrupted absorbable sutures.
4. A bulky pressure dressing is applied. Suprapubic cystostomy drainage is an option, but a urethral catheter usually suffices.

Horton-Devine urethroplasty (urethral patch graft)

Urethral patch graft is a one-stage operative procedure for the correction of a urethral stricture, similar to the Johanson urethroplasty.

Procedural considerations. Those points of importance that apply for the Johanson urethroplasty also apply here.

Operative procedure

1. The patient is placed in the lithotomy position.
2. A no. 17 cystoscope is passed into the posterior urethra.
3. A no. 20 urethral dilator is passed into the posterior urethra. A vertical incision in the midline of the perineum is made into the urethral lumen. The cystoscope is reinserted, and whether the incision traversed the stricture is determined.
4. The defect is measured.
5. A circumferential incision on the posterior penile shaft is made to harvest an oval piece of skin the size of the defect.
6. The epidermal side of the graft is defatted, and absorbable sutures of 4-0 are placed at the apex and base.

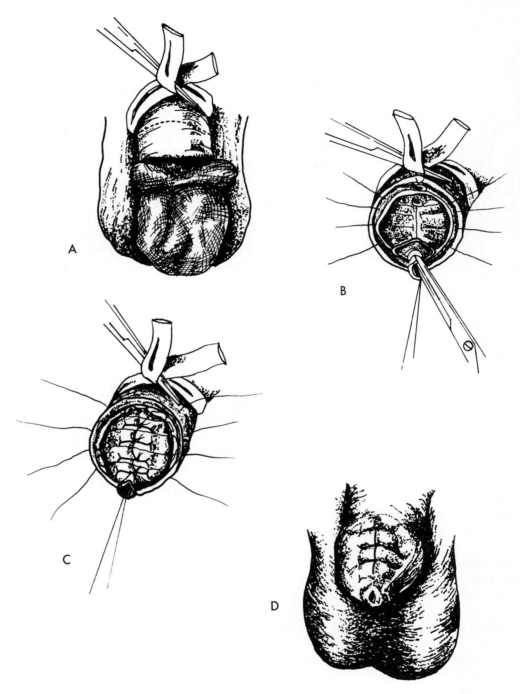

Fig. 15-35. Partial penectomy. **A,** Exclusion of the lesion from the field. **B,** The corpora are divided with a 2-cm gross margin. **C,** The dorsal vessels are ligated, margins of the tunica albuginea approximated, and the urethra spatulated. **D,** Simple skin closure and urethral meatus formation complete the procedure.

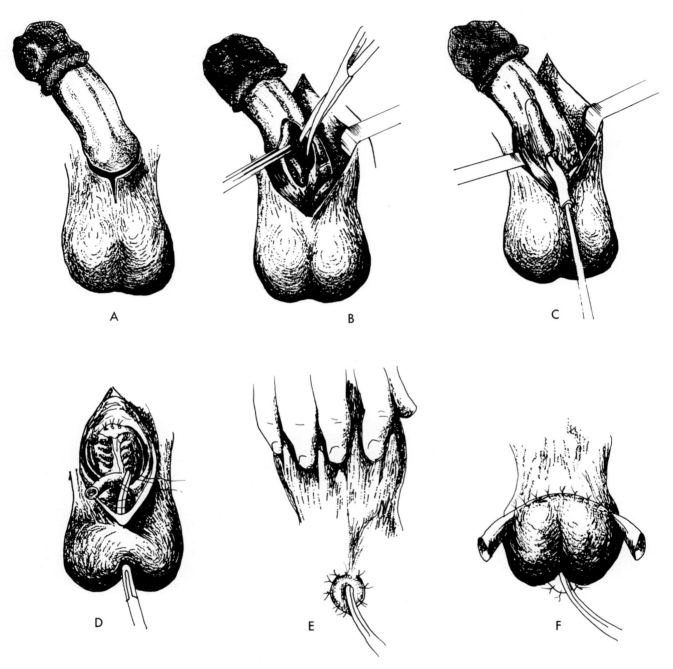

Fig. 15-36. Total penectomy. **A,** Circumferential incision around penile base. **B,** Urethra mobilized through incision in Buck's fascia. **C,** Following division of the suspensory ligament, the urethra is transected from the corpora. **D,** Traction suture through tunnel at penile base aids urethral dissection for transposition of urethra to perineum. **E,** Urethra is spatulated and sutured to skin through button hole in perineum. **F,** Amputation line is closed horizontally, elevating scrotum away from urethral opening.

4. Without sacrificing the tumor margin, the urethra is then divided. Interrupted sutures are placed on the opposite margins of the tunica albuginea to secure the corpora.
5. The tourniquet is removed, and hemostasis is achieved.
6. Following the dorsal urethrotomy, a skin-to-urethra anastomosis is performed. The redundant skin flap is then dorsally approximated.
7. A small urinary catheter is inserted, and a nonadherent dressing applied. They are generally removed in 3 or 4 days.

Total penectomy

1. A vertical elliptic incision is made around the penile base (Fig. 15-36).
2. The suspensory ligaments and dorsal vessels are divided as corporal dissection is carried out.
3. The distal urethra and its ventral traction are divided, aiding the urethral dissection, which extends from the corpora to the bulbar region. Then the corpora are separated and ligated.
4. An ellipse of skin approximately 1 cm in size is taken from the perineal area. A tunnel is fashioned in the perineal subcutaneous layer of tissue.
5. The urethra is grasped with a forceps and transferred to the perineum.
6. The urethra is spatulated and a skin-to-urethra anastomosis is performed.
7. The primary incision is closed.

8. A urinary catheter is inserted, and the wound covered with a nonadherent dressing.

Penile implant

A penile prosthesis is implanted for treatment of organic sexual impotence. Sexual impotence may be caused by (1) diabetes mellitus, (2) priapism, (3) Peyronie's disease, (4) penile trauma, (5) pelvic surgery, (6) neurologic disease (in selected cases), and (7) idiopathic impotence (in carefully screened patients). The penile implant serves as a stent to enable vaginal penetration for sexual intercourse.

Procedural considerations. Regional or general anesthesia is required. The patient is placed in either the supine or lithotomy position. Routine skin prepping and draping are carried out. To prevent urethral injury and potential urinary retention, a no. 14 or 16 Fr Foley catheter may be inserted to identify the urethra intraoperatively. Electrosurgery may be required.

The instrument setup includes a minor set with fine instruments, plus the following:

Hegar dilators
Penile prosthesis of urologist's choice (Fig. 15-37)
Furlow inserter (Fig. 15-38, *A* and *B*)
Closing tool (see Fig. 15-38 *C*)
Denis-Browne retractor
Assembly tool (Fig. 15-39)
Connectors of choice

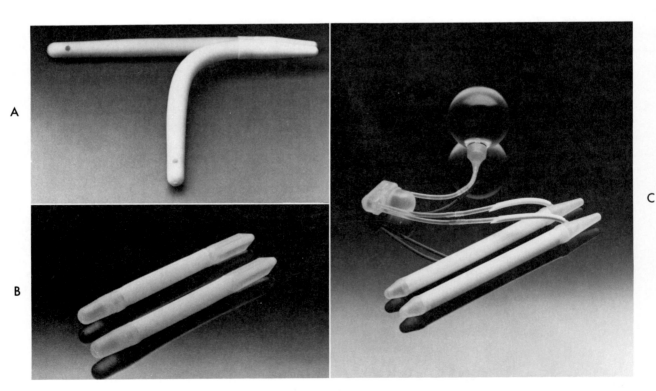

Fig. 15-37. A, AMS malleable 600 penile prosthesis. **B,** AMS Hydroflex penile prosthesis. **C,** AMS 700CX inflatable penile prosthesis. (Courtesy American Medical Systems, Minnetonka, Minn.)

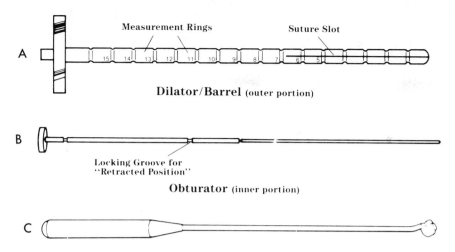

Measurement Rings   Suture Slot

A   Dilator/Barrel (outer portion)

B   Locking Groove for "Retracted Position"

Obturator (inner portion)

C

Fig. 15-38. Furlow insertion device. **A,** Dilator/barrel (outer portion). **B,** Obturator (inner portion). **C,** Closing tool. (Courtesy American Medical Systems, Minnetonka, Minn.)

A disastrous complication to a penile implant is infection of the prosthesis. Meticulous aseptic technique and careful draping are essential. The anus should be isolated in the perineal approach. An antibiotic irrigant and systemic antibiotics may be required.

Operative procedures

Implantation of noninflatable (semirigid) prosthesis

1. A hemicircular incision is made on the dorsal surface of the penis (Fig. 15-40, *A*). Some surgeons may choose a suprapubic or penoscrotal approach.
2. The tunica albuginea is incised over the corpus in a longitudinal manner (Fig. 15-40, *B*) and the corpus is dilated proximally and distally (Fig. 15-40, *C* and *D*) with Hegar dilators. Care must be taken not to perforate the urethra. Measurements are taken with the Furlow inserter.
3. The prosthesis is inserted in the corpus (Fig. 15-40, *E* and *F*). Proper placement is evident immediately by change in the configuration of the penis with no buck-

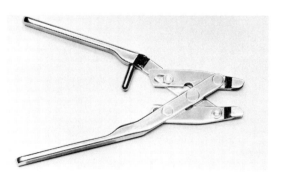

Fig. 15-39. Assembly tool. (Courtesy American Medical Systems, Minnetonka, Minn.)

ling of the glans (Fig. 15-40, *G*). The tunica albuginea is then closed with a no. 2-0 absorbable continuous suture: no. 3-0 absorbable interrupted sutures are used for skin closure.

4. Petrolatum gauze or 2-inch Kling tube gauze may be used for the dressing.
5. A Foley catheter is inserted, and the amount and color of urine are noted. Some surgeons divert the urine intraoperatively.

Implantation of inflatable prosthesis

1. A transverse suprapubic incision is made. The prosthetic reservoir is placed in the prevesical space.
2. Following exposure of the corpora cavernosa at the basis of the penis, the corpora are dilated distally and proximally. The Furlow inserter is used for measuring corporal length.
3. Inflatable silicone rods of the appropriate size are inserted into the corpora.
4. The pump is then placed in the most dependent portion of the scrotum.
5. The rods and reservoir are connected with the connectors of choice (Fig. 15-41), using the assembly tool, to the pump and tested for inflation and deflation (Fig. 15-42).
6. The prosthetic device is left in a partially inflated position to reduce bleeding and promote healing.
7. The incision is closed and a dressing applied.

Deep dorsal and emissary vein ligation

This procedure entails the ligation and/or elimination of the penile deep dorsal vein and its tributaries. It is a treatment undertaken for vascular-related impotence. Care is taken to avoid damage to the arteries and nerves lying alongside the deep dorsal vein.

A common cause of erectile dysfunction in patients with organic impotence is vascular compromise. Prior to un-

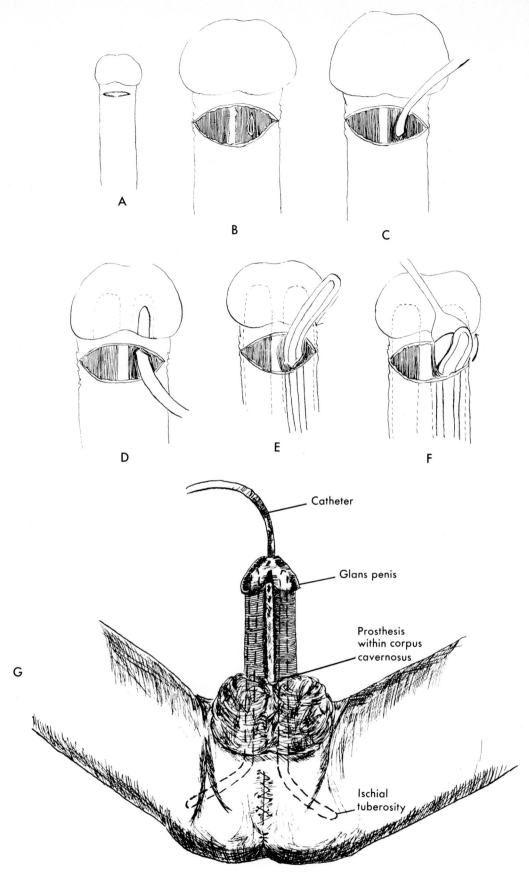

Fig. 15-40. Penile implant. **A,** Hemicircular incision on dorsal surface of penis. **B,** Opening of tunica albuginea. **C,** Dilatation of corpus down to crura. **D,** Dilatation down glans. **E,** Prosthesis being inserted. **F,** Distal prosthesis tip inserted with eyelid retractor to lift corpus. **G,** Penile prosthesis in place.

Catheter

Glans penis

Prosthesis within corpus cavernosus

Ischial tuberosity

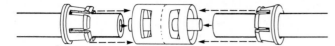

Fig. 15-41. Quik-connectors. (Courtesy American Medical Systems, Minnetonka, MN.)

dergoing surgical intervention, a definitive diagnosis of a corporal leak is made through dynamic infusion cavernosometry and cavernosography. Diagnostic results may indicate failure-to-store or failure-to-fill impotence. Patients with vascular compromise in a given anatomic region tend be compromised elsewhere as well. Many are diabetic or hypertensive. Because of this, the perioperative nurse must exercise great care in positioning the patient to prevent further damage to the patient's altered tissue perfusion.

Procedural considerations. In addition to a standard herniorrhaphy setup (Chap. 13), the perioperative nurse needs to have the following supplies and equipment available for the procedure:

Denis-Browne retractor
Right-angle retractors
Short, narrow Deaver retractors
Gemini clamps
Delicate, curved mosquito hemostats
Schnidt hemostats
Blunt delicate dissecting scissors
Sharp delicate dissecting scissors
5-inch angled vascular scissors
Debakey forceps
Bipolar coagulator with microtip
Kittner dissectors
Doppler probe and unit (probe must be sterile)
4-0 Vicryl on a microvascular needle
3-0 Dexon or vicryl on a T-16 or RB-1 needle
Vascular ties

Optional medications

Papaverine
Prostaglandin
Methylene blue
1% Lidocaine
0.9% Normal saline
0.5% Marcaine
Thrombin, topical

Miscellaneous supplies

Doppler gel, sterile packet
No. 16 5-cc balloon Foley catheter and attached drainage bag
Butterfly needle, 21-gauge, and 60-cc syringe
Medium drain
Hypodermic needle, 27-gauge

The patient is placed in the supine position with the legs separated. Draping is carried out as for a herniorrhaphy with the genitalia exposed. The operative area is squared off with five towels, one under the scrotum, and the remainder placed at the iliac crests and umbilicus and under the penis. The Foley catheter is inserted before the incision is made.

Operative procedure

1. An infrapubic incision is made at the base of the penis and deepened until the neurovascular bundle is identified.
2. The penis is degloved, and dissection is carried out toward the glans penis through Colles' fascia and Buck's fascia to the deep dorsal vein.
3. The deep dorsal vein is separated from the surrounding tissue and ligated at the suspensory level and at the glans penis. It is then excised from the corporal base, extending from the distal to the proximal ligatures.
4. The cavernous and crural veins are suture ligated.
5. All circumflex and emissary branches are ligated or coagulated.
6. The suspensory ligament is detached, and the entire deep and accessory dorsal vein is removed.
7. Hemostasis is established, and the suspensory ligaments are reattached with 2-0 nonabsorbable suture in an interrupted figure-of-eight pattern. The fascial layers are approximated and closed in an interrupted fashion with 4-0 absorbable suture.
8. The penis is returned to its normal position, and the closure is carried out in three layers.
9. Marcaine is injected during wound closure to afford a more comfortable recovery period.
10. The wound is covered with gauze sponges. Fluffs are placed over the scrotal area, and an athletic supporter is applied.

Revascularization of the penile arteries

The relationship of focal arterial occlusive disease to sexual dysfunction has led to efforts to rectify the resulting impotence. Investigational reconstructive surgery is taking place in patients who demonstrate correctable vascular disease in the large arteries. The most widely attempted repairs are end-to-end and end-to-side microscopic anastomosis of the distal inferior epigastric artery to the proximal deep dorsal artery near the pubic level, below the rectus muscle and Buck's fascia. Paramedian and infrapubic incisions are made, and the arteries freed and tunneled. This procedure requires both a urologist and a vascular surgeon. Currently the success rate stands at 60% to 65%.

Bladder exstrophy repair

Bladder exstrophy repair corrects a more severe form of epispadias, in which the anterior bladder wall as well as the roof of the urethra is absent. Bladder exstrophy is always accompanied by wide separation of the rectus muscles of the lower abdominal wall and by diastasis of the pubic bone with anterior displacement of the anus. Repair of bladder exstrophy requires an adequate-sized bladder for ultimate continence to be achieved. This procedure is preferably performed in the neonatal period.

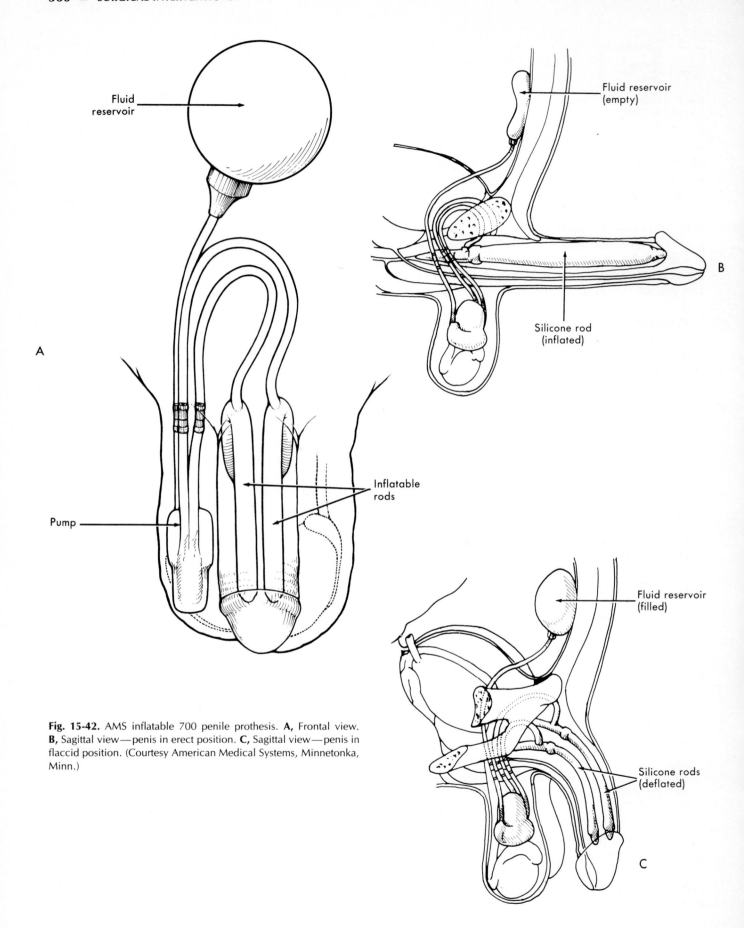

Fluid
reservoir

Fluid reservoir
(empty)

Silicone rod
(inflated)

B

A

Inflatable
rods

Pump

Fluid reservoir
(filled)

Silicone rods
(deflated)

C

Fig. 15-42. AMS inflatable 700 penile prothesis. **A,** Frontal view. **B,** Sagittal view—penis in erect position. **C,** Sagittal view—penis in flaccid position. (Courtesy American Medical Systems, Minnetonka, Minn.)

Procedural considerations. The infant is placed in a supine position, and the abdomen and thighs are prepped and draped. Instruments are as required for hypospadias repair (see p. 353).

Operative procedure

1. An incision is made around the exposed bladder medial to the paravesical neck mucosa. The incision is carried distally across the epispadiac urethra distal to the verumontanum. The paravesical mucosa is preserved for urethral lengthening. The bladder is then freed from the rectus fascia and the peritoneum. The dorsal chordee is released, and the mobilized paravesical mucosa is apposed in the midline and sutured to the proximal urethra just distal to the verumontanum.

2. The bladder wall is closed vertically in two layers with no. 3-0 absorbable sutures; a suprapubic tube is inserted for drainage.

3. The bladder neck is loosely reconstructed by approximating the interpubic ligament, which extends between the proximal end of the phallus and the pubic bone.

4. The symphysis pubis is approximated with a heavy no. 2 nonabsorbable suture. During this step the assistant rotates the iliac bones anteriorly.

Iliac osteotomy

When closure of the bladder exstrophy is delayed beyond the neonatal period, bilateral iliac osteotomies are required to bring the symphysis pubis together in the midline. A vesical neck plasty is performed at a later date with bilateral ureteral reimplantation. The penis may be closed before, during, or some time after the vesical neck plasty.

Procedural considerations. The infant is placed in the prone position with a folded towel under the pelvis.

Operative procedure. A vertical incision is made 0.5 cm lateral to the sacroiliac joints. The iliac bone is exposed, and osteotomy is performed through both tables to bring the pubic bones together in the midline after reconstruction of the bladder.

Operations on the scrotum and testicles
Hydrocelectomy

A hydrocele is an abnormal accumulation of fluid within the scrotum. The fluid is contained within the tunica vaginalis. Excessive secretion or accumulation of hydrocele fluid may be the result of infection or trauma. A hydrocelectomy is the excision of the tunica vaginalis of the testis to remove the enlarged, fluid-filled sac.

Procedural considerations. The patient is placed in the supine position. Preparation and draping of the patient include routine cleansing of the external genitals and draping of the patient with a fenestrated sheet. A minor instrument set is required, including a small drain, 30-ml syringe, 20-gauge 2-inch aspirating needle, and suspensory dressing.

Operative procedure

1. An anterolateral incision is made in the skin of the scrotum over the hydrocele mass by a scalpel with a no. 20 blade (Fig. 15-43, *A*). Bleeding is controlled with Crile hemostats, and vessels are ligated with no. 3-0 absorbable ligatures.

2. Small retractors may be placed, after which the fascial layers are incised to expose the tunica vaginalis (Fig. 15-43, *B*). With fine scissors, forceps, and blunt dissection, the hydrocele is dissected free and delivered (Fig. 15-43, *C*). The sac is opened, and the fluid contents are aspirated.

3. The sac is inverted so that it surrounds the testis, epididymis, and distal cord. Excess tunica vaginalis is excised, and the edges of the remaining tunica are sutured with a continuous no. 4-0 absorbable suture. The testicle is "bottled" by the inverted tunica vaginalis, and the testis may then be returned to the sac (Fig. 15-43, *D*, and *E*).

4. A drain is placed within the scrotum and brought out through a stab wound in the most dependent portion of the scrotum. The scrotal incision is closed in layers with no. 3-0 absorbable sutures. The skin is closed with interrupted no. 4-0 absorbable sutures. A fluff compression dressing contained in a scrotal support (suspensory) aids in reducing postoperative scrotal edema.

Vasectomy

A vasectomy is the excision of a section of the vas deferens (Fig. 15-44).

The operation is performed electively as a permanent method of sterilization and also before prostatectomy to prevent possible postoperative epididymitis. Because of the serious implications of permanent sterilization, particular attention must be paid to acquiring informed consent.

Procedural considerations. The patient usually lies in the supine position, although the patient can be in the lithotomy position if vasectomy is performed prior to transurethral prostatectomy. The patient may be under local or general anesthesia for this procedure. A minor instrument set, collodion dressing, and scrotal suspensory are needed.

Operative procedure

1. The vas is located by digital palpation of the upper part of the scrotum. A small incision is made in the skin over the vas (Fig. 15-44, *A*).

2. An Allis forceps or small towel clamp is inserted into the scrotal incision to grasp the vas and deliver it to the surface of the wound (Fig. 15-44, *B*). The vas is denuded of surrounding tissues, and straight hemostats are placed on either side of the Allis forceps to crush the vas.

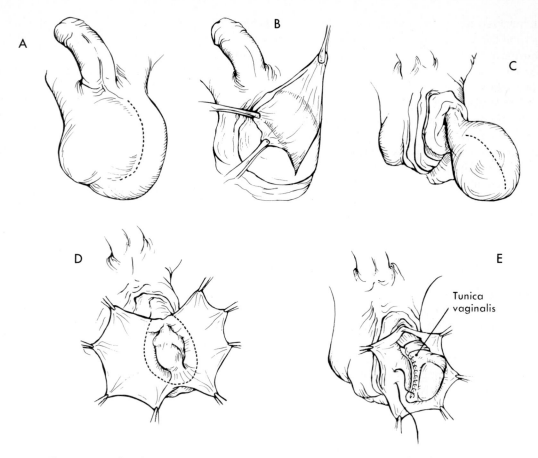

Fig. 15-43. Hydrocelectomy. (From Dodson, A.I.: Urological surgery, ed. 4, St. Louis, 1970, The C.V. Mosby Co.)

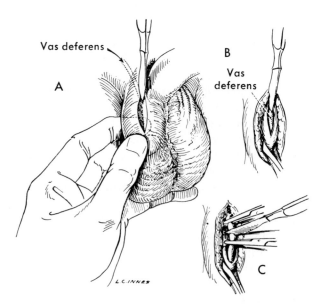

Fig. 15-44. Vasectomy (vas ligation). **A,** Vas grasped between surgeon's thumb in front and first and second fingers behind. Incision 2 cm long made over vas. **B,** Vas grasped with Allis forceps and denuded of surrounding tissues. **C,** Vas clamped with two hemostats and incised between them. (From Barnes, R.W., and Hadley, H.L.: Urological practice, St. Louis, 1954, The C.V. Mosby Co.)

3. The vas is cut between the clamps (Fig. 15-44, *C*), and a section is removed. The cut ends are ligated with no. 0 absorbable ties. The cut ends of the vas may also be electrocoagulated, and the severed ends of the vas allowed to return to the scrotum. Some surgeons bury the vasal ends in the perivasal sheath or seal them with hemoclips.

4. The skin incision is closed with no. 4-0 absorbable interrupted sutures. The patient is instructed to wear a scrotal support of the appropriate size for approximately 3 to 4 days.

Vasovasostomy

Vasovasostomy is the surgical reanastomosis of the vas deferens, utilizing the operative microscope. The number of vasal reanastomosis procedures has increased dramatically; a significant number of men who have had a vasectomy want to regain their fertility. A precise reconnection can be performed with the use of a microscope and a modified two-layer anastomosis. Success rates vary from 40% to 70%.

Procedural considerations. A minor instrument set is required, with the addition of selected microsurgical instruments and sutures:

Castroviejo needle holders
Westcott scissors, sharp and blunt
2 Straight Bishop-Harmon forceps
2 Straight tying forceps
Jeweler's forceps, straight and J-shaped
Lacrimal probes, 0000-0
Vasectomy clamps
Micro bulldogs
Nylon 10-0 on a GS16 needle
Nylon, 8-0, 9-0
Zoom microscope with foot pedals for focus, magnification, and position
Bipolar coagulator with micropoint
Blunt irrigating needle, no. 27
Bulb syringe

Operative procedure

1. After the vas deferens has been located by external manipulation, a vertical scrotal incision is made.
2. The testicle, epididymis, and vas are displaced from the scrotum.
3. The vasectomy site is identified and the scarred area excised.
4. The proximal end of the vas deferens is cut back until fluid is expressed.
5. Fluid is collected on a glass slide and examined for the presence of live sperm. Surgery continues if results for sperm are negative unless an epididymal obstruction exists.
6. The distal end of the vas is resected until a normal lumen is visible. The distal and proximal lumina are then dilated.
7. The two portions of the vas are placed in an approximator clip with background material placed underneath.
8. Six stitches of 10-0 nylon are placed in the inner layer. The proximal end is sutured through the serosa to the mucosa, and the distal end through the mucosa to the serosa.
9. A second layer of eight to ten stitches of 9-0 nylon is placed without penetrating the lumen of the vas.
10. The incision is closed in two layers with interrupted 3-0 and 4-0 absorbable sutures.
11. Gauze sponges and an athletic supporter are placed on the patient to provide a pressure dressing.
12. Postoperative precautions include no lifting or ejaculation for a minimum of 2 weeks. The sperm count and viability of sperm are rechecked at 3- and 6-month intervals.

Epididymectomy

An epididymectomy is the excision of the epididymis from the testis. Epididymectomy is rarely performed today but may be indicated to treat degenerative cystic disease or infection of the epididymis.

Procedural considerations. The patient is placed in the supine position with the legs slightly abducted. A general anesthetic is required. Setup is as described for hydrocelectomy, plus an electrosurgical unit, if desired.

Operative procedure

1. An anterolateral incision is made over the testis in the scrotum to expose the tunica vaginalis.
2. The tunica is incised to expose the testis and overlying epididymis.
3. An incision is made along the superior head of the epididymis, which is then sharply dissected from the testis. A portion of the vas deferens may also be excised.
4. Bleeding is controlled by electrocoagulation and chromic ties. The skin wound is closed with no. 4-0 absorbable sutures. A small drain may be left intrascrotally for 24 to 48 hours.

Spermatocelectomy

Spermatocelectomy is removal of a spermatocele. A spermatocele, a lobulated intrascrotal cystic mass attached to the superior head of the epididymis, is usually caused by an obstruction of the tubular system that conveys the sperm. Epididymovasostomies (end-to-side anastomoses between the vas deferens and the epididymis) have been attempted after excision of the surgical mass to maintain continuity of the ductal system. Usually this type of procedure requires the operative microscope for an accurate anastomosis.

Procedural considerations. The setup for a spermatocelectomy is as described for a hydrocelectomy, plus the following:

1 Syringe, 10 ml
1 Needle, blunt, 20 gauge
Methylene blue solution
Hydrogen peroxide
Polyethylene tubing, 20 Fr or other size, as desired
Silk sutures or fine wire
Absorbable sutures, no. 4-0 or 5-0, on fine plastic curved needles
Lead shot
Isotonic saline solution
Microscope and slides, if desired

Operative procedure

1. The mass is approached through a scrotal incision as described for hydrocelectomy (Fig. 15-43).
2. The structures of the testis and spermatic cord are identified, and the cystic structure is dissected free. Bleeding is controlled with electrocoagulation.
3. The wound is closed and dressed as described for hydrocelectomy.

Varicocelectomy

A varicocelectomy is the high ligation of the gonadal veins of the testes. Varicocelectomy is done to reduce venous backflow of blood into the venous plexus around the testes and to improve spermatogenesis. When surgery for this condition was devised 70 years ago, the veins of the pampiniform plexus were ligated and divided individually.

This condition occurs more frequently on the left side because the gonadal vein of the left testis unites retroperitoneally with the renal vein at a 90-degree angle and is consequently under greater back-pressure. As a result of this unusual back-pressure, the pampiniform plexus of the spermatic cord becomes tortuous and engorged, resembling a bag of worms.

Procedural considerations. The setup is as described for hydrocelectomy.

Operative procedure
1. The incision may be made low in the inguinal canal or in the upper portion of the scrotum. The structures of the spermatic cord are identified, and the vessels dissected free from the vas deferens (Fig. 15-45, *A*).
2. The abnormal dilated veins in the inguinal canal are clamped and ligated (Fig. 15-45, *B*). The redundant portions are excised.
3. A drain may be placed. The incision is closed in layers.

Testicular biopsy

A biopsy of the testicle is a wedge excision of suspicious tissue for diagnostic confirmation, often prior to treatment for testicular carcinoma. In some situations, a needle biopsy of the testicle may be adequate and appropriate.

Procedural considerations. If required, hair may be removed from the scrotum, which is then aseptically cleansed. General, regional, or local anesthesia may be selected. A minor instrument set is used. Special fixatives, such as Bouin's or Zenker's solution, must be available. Formalin destroys the germinal epithelium and should not be used.

Operative procedure
1. The scrotum is held firmly on its posterior aspect. This causes the skin on the anterior aspect to stretch tightly over the incisional site, forcing the epididymis to remain posterior and allowing the scrotal skin to part without retraction.
2. A 1- to 2-cm vertical incision is made, with care taken to avoid injury to the epididymis.
3. The incision is continued to the tunica vaginalis. As the tunica is incised, there should be a normal efflux of clear fluid.
4. Absorbable stay sutures (4-0) are placed in the tunica vaginalis. Two more are placed in the tunica albuginea.
5. A small ellipse of tunica with its tubules is resected with a scalpel in a shaving action, with no-touch technique.
6. The specimen is placed in the fixative and the wound closed in three layers with 3-0 and 4-0 absorbable suture.
7. Gauze sponges and fluffed dressings are placed over and around the scrotum. An athletic supporter is applied to provide pressure and support.

Orchiectomy

An orchiectomy is the removal of the testis or testes. Removal of both testes is castration and renders the patient sterile and deficient of the hormone testosterone, which is responsible for development of secondary sexual characteristics and potency. This operation, like vasectomy, has legal implications that require particular attention to acquiring informed consent for surgery. Bilateral orchiectomy is usually performed to control symptomatic metastatic carcinoma of the prostate gland. A unilateral orchiectomy may be indicated because of testicular cancer,

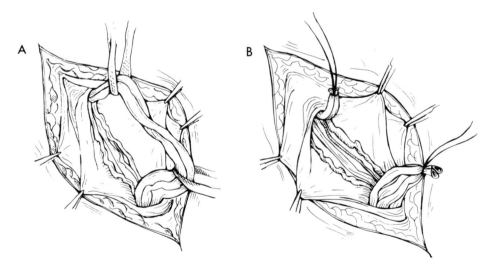

Fig. 15-45. Varicocelectomy. (Modified from Dodson, A.I.: Urological surgery, ed. 4, St. Louis, 1970, The C.V. Mosby Co.)

trauma, or infection. In many situations a prosthesis may be implanted for cosmetic or psychologic reasons. Prostheses are usually made of silicone gel to approximate normal testicular consistency.

Procedural considerations. The patient is placed in the supine position and draped according to hospital procedure. A minor instrument setup is required, plus a testicular prosthesis, if specified.

Operative procedure

1A. For benign conditions the incision is made over the anterolateral surface of the midportion of the scrotum. The skin incision is carried through the subcutaneous and fascial layers through the tunica vaginalis, exposing the testicle. Retractors are placed, and bleeding vessels are clamped and tied. The spermatic cord is divided into two or three vascular bundles. Each vascular bundle is doubly clamped, cut, and ligated—first with no. 0 absorbable suture ligature and then with a proximal free no. 0 absorbable tie. The vas is separately ligated with a no. 0 absorbable tie. The testis is removed.

1B. For malignant conditions the incision is begun just above the internal ring, extending downward and inward over the inguinal canal to the external inguinal ring. The inguinal canal is exposed, and the spermatic cord is dissected free, cross-clamped, and divided into vascular bundles at the internal ring. Gentle forward traction is applied to the cord, which is dissected from its bed. The testis is everted into the wound from the scrotum and excised.

2. Bleeding is controlled with electrocoagulation. A small drain may be placed in the empty hemiscrotum if desired. The external oblique fascia is reapproximated with no. 2-0 absorbable interrupted sutures. Subcutaneous tissue, including Scarpa's fascia, is closed with no. 4-0 absorbable sutures. The skin is reapproximated with surgical staples or 4-0 subcuticular suture.

Radical lymphadenectomy

Radical lymphadenectomy is a bilateral resection of retroperitoneal lymph nodes. Dissection usually includes lymph nodes, channels, and fat around both renal pedicles, the vena cava, and the aorta, including the bifurcation of the aorta. Lymph node dissection is performed for treatment of nonseminomatous testicular tumors. The procedure is performed after radical inguinal orchiectomy.

Procedural considerations. The patient is placed in the supine position. If the dissection is unilateral, the patient is supine with the operative side tilted upward. Routine skin preparation from nipples to midthigh and draping procedures are carried out. Long fine dissection instruments along with basic laparotomy instruments are required.

Operative procedure

1. A midline abdominal incision is made from the xiphoid process to the symphysis pubis. The abdominal contents are explored to determine the degree of gross nodal involvement. The colon is either packed within the abdominal cavity or mobilized and kept moist outside the abdomen.

2. The posterior peritoneum is opened between the aorta and the vena cava.

3. By blunt and sharp dissection, the lymphatic structures and fat are removed en bloc from around both renal pedicles, the vena cava, and the aorta from above the renal hilum to beyond the bifurcation of the iliac vessels on the side of the original testicular neoplasm.

4. The spermatic vessels of the affected side are removed down to and including the stump of the previous orchiectomy.

5. The inferior mesenteric artery may be sacrificed if technically necessary, but the superior mesenteric artery is not disturbed. The ureter on the affected side is skeletonized to remove any perilymphatic tissue.

6. If reperitonealization is desired, the posterior peritoneum is closed with a no. 2-0 absorbable continuous suture. The viscera are repositioned into the abdominal cavity, and the wound is closed, usually without placement of a drain.

Orchiopexy

An orchiopexy is the surgical placement and fixation of the testicle in a normal anatomic position in the scrotal sac. If the testis fails to descend into the scrotum during gestation, then it is considered undescended. An undescended testis becomes arrested somewhere along its normal path of descent. If it is palpable in a position other than its normal path of descent, its position is considered to be ectopic.

A retractile testis is one in which the testis has fully descended into the scrotum but retracts out of the scrotum as a result of contraction of the cremaster muscle. Gentle manipulation allows replacement of the testis in the most dependent portion of the scrotum. Retractile testes require no surgical or hormonal treatment.

All testes that are undescended after 1 year, including those that are unresponsive to hormone injections, require surgical placement in the scrotum for optimum maturation.

Procedural considerations. The setup is as described for hydrocelectomy. General anesthesia is required. Preparation and draping include the lower abdomen, genitals, and thighs. Because this operation is usually performed on children, a setup containing small, delicate instruments and sutures is required.

Operative procedure

1. An inguinal incision is generally employed for exploration of undescended testes (Fig. 15-46, *A*). Most

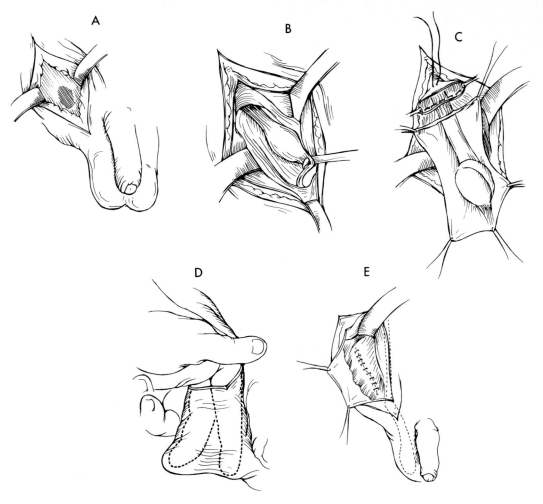

Fig. 15-46. Orchiopexy. **A,** Inguinal incision exposing inguinal canal. **B,** Identification and liberation of testis and spermatic cord. Dissection of spermatic vessels should be carried as high as internal inguinal ring or into abdominal cavity, so that needed length to bring testis into scrotum is available. **C,** Accompanying hernia repaired. **D,** Pocket created in scrotum with fingers by stretching and pulling fascia. **E,** Testis anchored in scrotum with chromic gut sutures. (From Flocks, R.H., and Clup, D.A.: Surgical urology, 4th ed. Copyright © 1975 by Year Book Medical Publishers, Inc., Chicago. Used by permission.)

undescended testes are located in the superficial inguinal pouch or inguinal canal.

2. The external oblique aponeurosis is opened through the external inguinal ring, exposing the inguinal canal; the gubernacular attachments of the undescended testis are freed (Fig. 15-46, *B*).

3. All adhesions and the associated inguinal hernial sac are freed to lengthen the cord. The hernia sac is transected, twisted, and ligated with sutures (Fig. 15-46, *C*).

4. A scrotal pocket is created (Fig. 15-46, *D*), and the testis is anchored in a normal anatomic position within the scrotum (Fig. 15-46, *E*).

Orchiopexy may be accomplished by several surgical methods. The dependent portion of the undescended testis may be sutured to the base of the scrotum with absorbable or nonabsorbable sutures brought out through the scrotal wall and tied over a peanut dissector or pledget. The most popular method used is anchoring the testis into a dissected subdartos pouch. In this procedure a small midtransverse scrotal incision is made, and space between the skin and the dartos muscle dissected. The testis is then brought through a small hole in the dartos into the subdartos pouch and anchored in position by the traction suture. The overlying skin of the subdartos pouch is closed with fine absorbable suture material. The inguinal incision is repaired in layers with no. 3-0 absorbable sutures. The skin is closed with a subcuticular suture; Steri-Strips are used for dressing.

Testicular detorsion

Torsion of the testicle, spermatic cord, appendix testis, or testis epididymis may be extravaginal or intravaginal in presentation. Intravaginal torsion is generally due to the absence of the usual attachment of the posterior aspect of the testes to the scrotal wall. In this instance, the tunica covers the epididymis and testis. Twisting of the vascular pedicle can result, causing extreme pain. It is more commonly found in pubescent boys and young adults.

Procedural considerations. These patients generally present on an emergency basis. Surgery must occur as soon as possible to prevent death of the affected testicle. Emotional support is important, as the patient may fear loss of sexuality and/or disturbances in body image. Instrumentation required includes a setup as described for hydrocelectomy.

Operative procedure

1. A scrotal incision is made through the tunica vaginalis, and the spermatic cord is untwisted.
2. If normal color returns to the testis, it is anchored with three nonabsorbable sutures through the tunica to the scrotal wall or median septum.
3. The contralateral scrotal compartment is usually opened, and the other testicle and spermatic cord examined. To prevent a future torsion on the unaffected side, the testis is often anchored to its surrounding structures.
4. Closure may be done in two or three layers with 3-0 and 4-0 absorbable interrupted sutures.
5. A support dressing of gauze sponges, fluffs, and a scrotal supporter is applied.

Operations on the prostate gland

Glandular hyperplasia of the prostatic urethra usually manifests itself after the age of 55. Prostatic enlargement may occur in one or more lobes of the prostate but most frequently occurs in the lateral or median lobes. Progressive growth of the hyperplastic gland compresses the remaining normal prostatic tissue, forming what is called a "surgical capsule." The growth of adenomatous tissue slowly encroaches on the prostatic urethral lumen, causing obstruction to urinary outflow.

Prostatic enlargement may be benign or malignant. In benign prostatic hypertrophy, only the periurethral adenomatous portion of the gland is removed (see Fig. 15-8). Operable prostatic malignancy requires radical prostatectomy, which includes removal of the entire prostate gland and the seminal vesicles. Before prostatic surgery, it is necessary to determine the prostatic serum acid phosphatase level. If the prostatic fraction of this test is elevated, the patient probably has metastatic carcinoma of the prostate. In such instances a bone scan and skeletal survey are necessary for confirmation. If these tests are negative, however, the possibility of hemolytic anemia, Gaucher's disease, or Paget's disease of the bone must be considered. If these tests are positive, a transrectal needle biopsy or Franzen transrectal aspiration biopsy may be performed to confirm the diagnosis.

Three open surgical approaches are possible in removing the benign hyperplastic obstructive prostate gland: re-

tropubic prostatectomy, suprapubic prostatectomy, and perineal prostatectomy. Transurethral prostatectomy is an endoscopic (closed) surgical approach that may be performed on some patients. If the prostate gland is cancerous, a radical retropubic or radical perineal prostatectomy is performed.

Several factors must be taken into account to determine the best route for removal of the prostatic obstruction: the age and medical condition of the patient, the size of the gland and location of the pathologic condition, and the presence of associated medical disease.

Prostatic needle biopsy

Needle biopsy of the prostate is indicated for patients in whom prostatic cancer is clinically suspected. It may be accomplished transperineally or transrectally with a needle designed for this purpose.

Procedural considerations. Needle biopsy of the prostate has the risk of both intraoperative and postoperative bleeding. Many surgeons prefer to incise the puncture site with a no. 11 or no. 15 scalpel blade and suture the site with 4-0 absorbable suture following the biopsy. Electrosurgery may also be utilized. A cystoscopic examination often accompanies a needle biopsy. Unlike many diagnostic procedures, a needle biopsy often requires the assistance of a scrub nurse.

Operative procedure

Core needle biopsy

Transrectal approach. The Tru-Cut or Vim-Silverman biopsy needle is inserted into the rectum along the volar aspect of the surgeon's index finger. The needle is advanced to abut against the nodule. The obturator is removed, and the cutting blades are inserted and/or advanced. When the blades are in position, the outer sheath is advanced over them and twisted to receive a slender thread of prostate tissue. This technique is believed to be easier to accomplish than transperineal biopsy.

Transperineal approach. The examining finger is inserted in the rectum and the induration identified. The needle is inserted through the perineal skin and guided ahead until the tip abuts the lesion. The biopsy is taken in the same fashion as described for the transrectal approach. Transperineal biopsy is thought to hold less risk of infection and postoperative bleeding.

Fine needle aspiration biopsy. A finger is inserted in the rectum and the nodule identified. The Franzen biopsy needle is inserted, with the index finger of the free hand guiding it into the rectum. A finger cot may be slipped over both the finger and the needle. A 22 gauge needle is passed into the guide needle and advanced. Suction is applied with an aspiration syringe while the tip is moved back and forth within the lesion. The suction is then released and the needle withdrawn. The aspirate is placed on a glass slide and smeared, or expressed into a sterile glass jar.

Prostatic ultrasonography. A transrectal transducer is covered with a sleeve and used to provide linear and radial scans on an imaging screen. The patient is in a lateral position, and the probe is introduced into the rectum to about 10 cm above the anal verge. The needle penetrates the rectal mucosa with the Bard (spring-loaded) Biobty gun. This technique is practically painless and is frequently performed in the office setting if ultrasound is available there. Lesions as small as 2 to 3 cm are visible with this procedure. Transurethral ultrasound with biopsy is twice as sensitive as standard techniques in diagnosing carcinoma of the prostate.

Transurethral resection of the prostate gland

By means of a resectoscope passed into the bladder through the urethra, successive pieces of tissue are removed from around the bladder neck and the lobes of the prostate gland are resected, leaving the capsule intact. The resectoscope uses a stabilized cutting loop to resect tissue and coagulate blood vessels by means of electric current. The electric current that powers the electrode is supplied by a high-frequency electrosurgical unit. The current settings are as specified by the urologist, who activates the cutting or coagulating current with a foot pedal during the course of the procedure.

Transurethral resection of the prostate (TURP) is one of four acceptable surgical methods of treating obstructive enlargement of the prostate gland. Several factors influence the surgical approach: size of the gland and location of the pathological condition, age and condition of the patient, and presence of associated diseases.

Controversy continues in regard to the efficacy of prophylactic vasectomy to prevent the postoperative complication of epididymo-orchitis. If vasectomy is to be done, it should be performed immediately before the transurethral procedure. The patient must be well informed and have full understanding of the implications of the procedure. Operative consent is mandatory.

Nd:YAG laser application to the prostatic bed may be performed following evacuation of tissue in an effort to eradicate residual tumor. It is investigational at this time, but results are promising, with a low recurrence rate in patients with T_1 and T_2 stages of carcinoma of the prostate.

Procedural considerations. The instrument setup for transurethral resection of the prostate is as described for cystoscopy with additional necessary instruments. The four principal types of resectoscopes are McCarthy, Nesbit, Iglesias, and Baumrucker (Fig. 15-47). Adult resectoscopes range in size from 24 to 28 Fr and have the following components: Foroblique telescope, operating

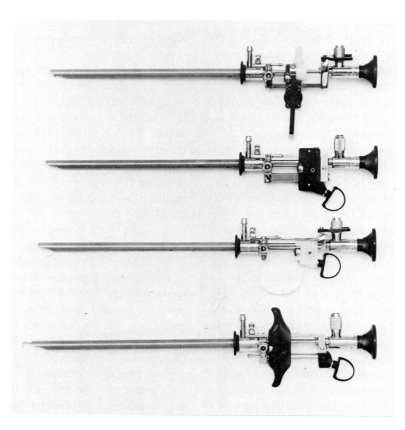

Fig. 15-47. Adult resectoscopes. *Top to bottom,* McCarthy, Nesbit, Iglesias, and Baumrucker.

element, postresectoscope sheaths and obturators, and cutting loops (Fig. 15-48). Supplementary instruments include a resectoscope adapter and a lateral telescope.

A transurethral resection of the prostate requires the following instrument setup:

Resectoscope (multiple working elements)
Foroblique telescope as well as a backup telescope
Stabilized or unstabilized cutting loops
Postresectoscope sheath with corresponding Timberlake obturator
Cystourethroscope
Fiberoptic light cord
Stopcock water adapter
High-frequency cord
Resectoscope adapter
Short bridge

Accessory items (may be sterilized on tray or added)

Brush (to clean tissue from cutting loops)
Towel clamps (optional)
Plain forceps
Prep set and solutions
Toomey syringe
Syringe, 20 ml
Ellik evacuator
Van Buren sounds
Strainer and small basin
Lubricant, water-soluble
Foley catheter (no. 22 or no. 24, 30 cc, 3 way)
Disposable urologic drape with rectal sheath (Fig. 15-49)
Cystoscopy drape pack
Sterile gowns and gloves as required

Items ready in cystoscopy room

Irrigation system
Fiberoptic light source
Electrosurgical unit
Urinary drainage system

A continuous flow of isotonic and nonelectrolytic irrigating fluid is necessary to ensure transmission of electrical current and clear visualization throughout surgery. Irrigating solution such as 1.5% glycine or 3.3% sorbitol, 3 to 6 L, may be connected in tandem to provide a constant flow. At all times nursing personnel must be alert to replace the irrigation solution as required.

During transurethral prostatic surgery, return of irrigation fluid must be monitored because bladder perforation may occur. The nurse should be aware of the early symptoms and measures employed to remedy this complication. The patient usually experiences significant respiratory changes and abdominal discomfort. Other important observations are rigidity and swelling of the lower abdomen, coupled with changes in sensorium.

If bladder perforation with extravasation of irrigating fluid is evident, the surgical procedure is discontinued and a cystogram is obtained immediately. The site of the perforation is radiographically determined, and surgical closure is accomplished through a cystotomy incision.

Operative procedure

1. The urologist checks the endoscopic instruments before performing the transurethral procedure. In transurethral prostatic surgery the urethra is usually first dilated with sounds from 20 to 30 Fr.

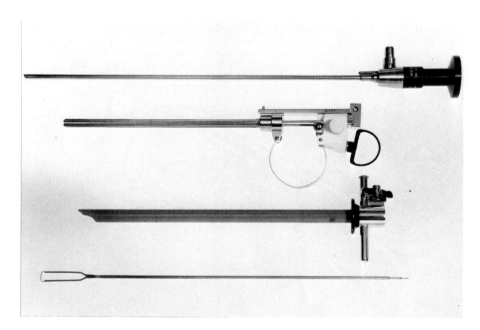

Fig. 15-48. Resectoscope components: Foroblique telescope, Iglesias operating element, postresectoscope sheath, and cutting loop. (Courtesy American ACMI, Stamford, Conn.; from Morel, A., and Wise, G.J.: Urologic endoscopic procedures, ed. 2, St. Louis, 1979, The C.V. Mosby Co.)

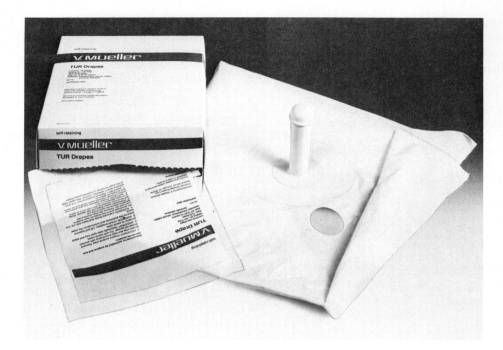

Fig. 15-49. Disposable urologic drape with rectal sheath. (Courtesy American V. Mueller, Chicago, Ill.; from Morel, A., and Wise, G.J.: Urologic endoscopic procedures, ed. 2, St. Louis, 1979, The C.V. Mosby Co.)

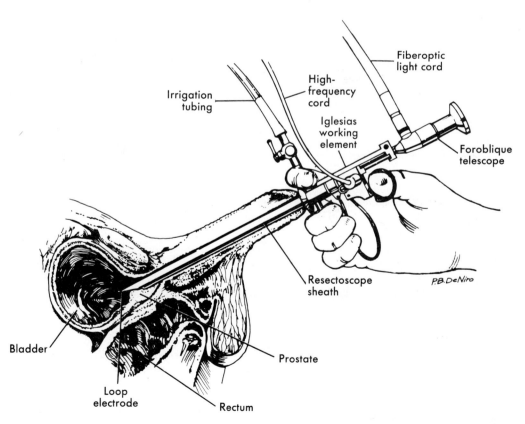

Fig. 15-50. Sectional view illustrating removal of portion of hypertrophied middle lobe of prostate gland with Iglesias resectoscope.

2. Cystourethroscopy is performed to assess the degree of prostatic obstruction, as well as to inspect the bladder. Some urologists perform this diagnostic procedure several days before surgery, whereas others perform the examination in the operating room immediately before surgery.

3. A well-lubricated postresectoscope sheath with its fitted Timberlake obturator is passed into the urethra. The Timberlake obturator is removed, and the working element (resectoscope), assembled with the Foroblique telescope and cutting loop, is inserted through the sheath. The irrigation tubing, light cord, and high-frequency cord are appropriately connected. Irrigation fluid is allowed to fill the bladder. Initial inspection of the prostatic urethra and bladder trigone is carried out. After determining the location of the ureteral orifice, the urologist initiates electrodissection, alternating cutting and coagulating currents as required (Fig. 15-50). At intervals the bladder is drained, washing out prostatic tissue and small blood clots. At times it is necessary to employ the Ellik evacuator to remove resected prostatic tissue. To do this, the urologist must remove the working element of the resectoscope. The nozzle of the evacuator is fitted onto the resectoscope sheath, and by manual pulsatile pressure the bladder contents are removed. A basin of glycine solution with an Ellik evacuator and Toomey syringe should be readily available for manual irrigation.

4. When the prostatic resection is completed, the prostatic fossa is inspected to ensure that all bleeding points have been coagulated. The resectoscope is then removed and a Foley catheter (22 or 24 Fr, two- or three-way, 30-cc balloon) is inserted into the bladder for urinary drainage. The balloon is inflated (Fig. 15-51, A) and pulled gently in traction against the bladder neck to help control venous bleeding (Fig. 15-51, B). The Foley balloon must not be inflated within the prostatic fossa (Fig. 15-51, C), where it may cause excessive bleeding from the resected prostatic capsule.

5. If desired, continuous irrigation with gravity drainage is initiated with normal saline as the bladder irrigant, instead of sorbitol or glycine. A 2000-ml urinary drainage system is suggested to avoid frequent emptying of the drainage bag.

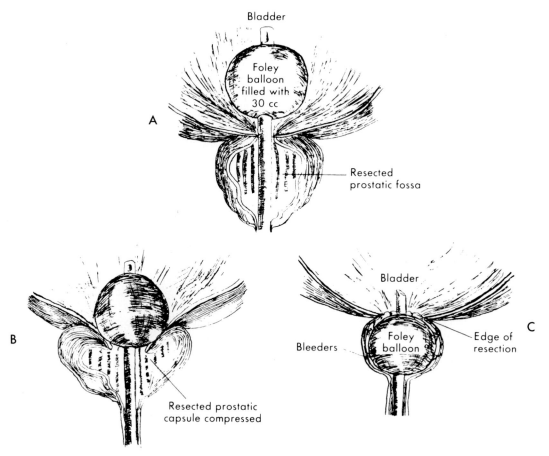

Fig. 15-51. A, Proper position for Foley catheter with inflated balloon beyond prostatic capsule. **B,** Foley catheter inflated balloon is pulled gently in traction at bladder neck. **C,** Foley balloon should not be inflated within prostatic fossa.

Transurethral resection with a continuous flow resectoscope

Prostatic tissue or bladder tumors are resected via a transurethral approach, using a continuous flow resectoscope (CFR) (Fig. 15-52). Unique components of the CFR include an outlet stopcock to which a suction tube is attached, an inflow tube on the inner sheath, and outflow holes on the outer sheath. These features enable the urologist to resect tissue without interruption to empty the bladder, as must be done with the standard resectoscope.

The continuous flow technique decreases intravesical pressure on the bladder during the procedure, provides a clearer field of vision owing to the constant inflow and outflow of irrigant, reduces the operating time because the resection process must not be interrupted to evacuate the bladder, and provides a "still" bladder for the resection of bladder tumors.

Procedural considerations. The setup is as described for the standard transurethral resection of the prostate, with the addition of the CFR, a thick-walled Silastic suction tubing, and possibly a continuous flow pump.

Operating procedure. The procedure for transurethral resection with a CFR is as described previously for transurethral resection of prostate. The manufacturer's recommendations relating to the height of irrigation fluids and placement of the CFR pump should be followed.

Balloon dilatation of the prostatic urethra (Transcystoscopic urethroplasty)

Balloon dilatation is an alternative approach to surgical TURP, resulting from advances in radiologic techniques and balloon catheter technology. In many patients with urinary outlet obstruction, the prostatic urethra can be stretched to promote a more acceptable urinary flow. Other standard methods of treatment may easily be employed if the patient does not respond to balloon dilatation. The 5-year success rate is 60%.

Procedural considerations. In addition to a standard cystoscopy setup, the uroplasty TCU dilatation catheter system is needed (Fig. 15-53). It includes the following equipment:

Dilatation catheter (a triple-lumen catheter with a 15-cc capacity)
Calibration catheter
Sheath and obturator, 26 Fr
Inflation device

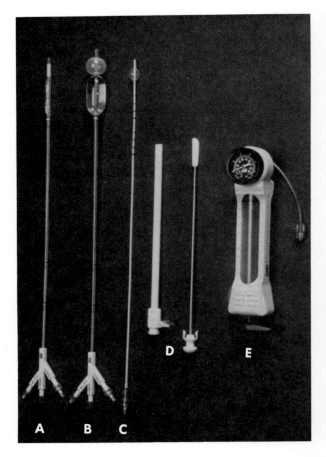

Fig. 15-53. Uroplasty TCU dilatation catheter system. **A,** Urethral dilatation catheter, deflated. **B,** Urethral dilatation catheter, inflated. **C,** Urethral calibration catheter. **D,** Disposable 26 Fr sheath obturator. **E,** Inflation device. (Courtesy Advanced Surgical Intervention, San Clemente, Calif.)

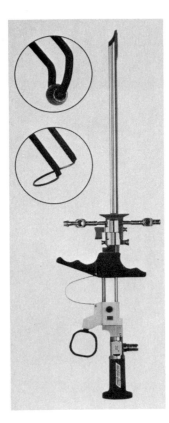

Fig. 15-52. CFR resectoscope. (Courtesy Circon-ACMI, Stamford, Conn.)

Operative procedure

1. A routine cystoscopy is carried out.
2. The length of the prostatic urethra is calibrated by manual exam, direct vision, and measurements with the calibration catheter (Fig. 15-54, *A*).
3. The urologist selects the balloon catheter of the appropriate size (Fig. 15-54, *B*).
4. The dilatation catheter is placed through the 26 Fr sheath so that the proximal end of the balloon is beyond the external sphincter (Fig. 15-54, *C*), and the Foley balloon is inflated (Fig. 15-54, *D*).
5. The balloon is inflated with the inflation device for 10 minutes at a pressure of 3 to 4 atmospheres while under direct endoscopic control (Fig. 15-54, *E*).
6. A Foley catheter is inserted following the procedure to control bleeding and swelling of tissue. The catheter remains in place for 48 hours.

Retropubic prostatectomy

Retropubic prostatectomy is the enucleation of hypertrophic prostatic tissue through an incision in the anterior prostatic capsule by an extravesical approach. The retropubic approach is the most frequently used technique for open prostatectomy. It offers ideal exposure of the prostate bed and vesical neck; excellent hemostasis is obtained, and intraoperative and postoperative bleeding is minimized.

Procedural considerations. The patient is placed in a slight Trendelenburg's position with a bolster under the pelvis and the legs slightly abducted. Routine skin prep-

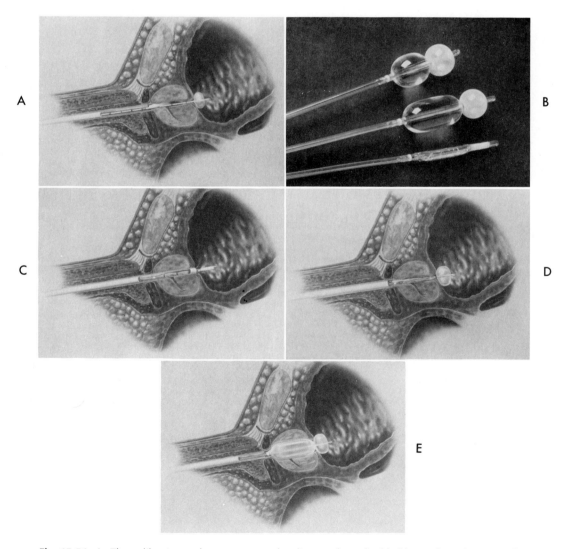

Fig. 15-54. A, The calibration catheter measures the distance from the bladder neck to the external sphincter. This measurement is used to select the proper length dilatation catheter. **B,** Inflated and deflated. **C,** The dilatation catheter is inserted, **D,** and Foley balloon inflated (using syringe and sterile fluid). **E,** Dilatation balloon inflated using inflation device to 3 atm pressure for 10 minutes. (Courtesy Advanced Surgical Intervention, San Clemente, Calif.)

aration is carried out. Electrosurgery is usually employed.

The draping procedure conforms to individual operating room policy, and the procedure listed below is a suggested method for draping the patient.

1. The first towel, with a cuff, is placed under the scrotum.
2. The next three towels are placed around the lower abdominal incision site, followed by a sterile laparotomy sheet.
3. A fifth towel, folded in half, is placed over the penis

and scrotum below the retropubic incision site and secured with two towel clamps.

The instrument setup includes a basic laparotomy set and bladder and prostatic instruments (Figs. 15-55 and 15-56). The following supplies should be readily available:

Jackson-Pratt drains
Lubricant, water-soluble
Syringe, 30 ml
Urinary drainage system
Foley catheter, 20 Fr, 5-cc balloon
Foley catheter, 22 or 24 Fr, 30-cc balloon

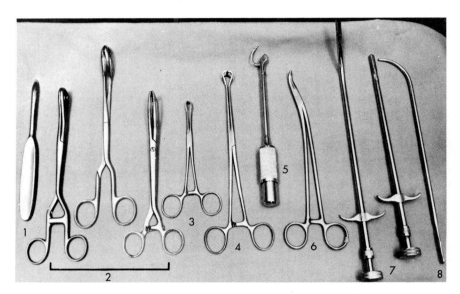

Fig. 15-55. Prostatic instruments. *1,* Prostatic enucleator; *2,* three prostatic lobe forceps; *3,* Lahey forceps; *4,* long Babcock forceps; *5,* boomerang; *6,* Heaney needle holder; *7,* two Lowsley prostatic tractors; *8,* urethral sound.

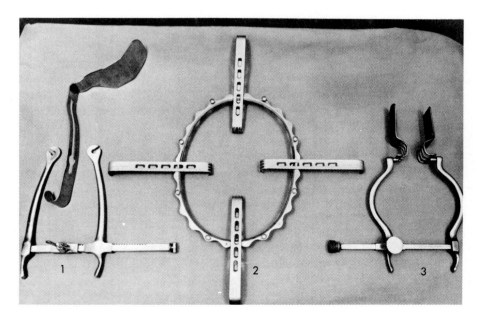

Fig. 15-56. Retractors for prostatectomy. *1,* Millin retropubic bladder retractor; *2,* Denis-Browne ring retractor (perineal); *3,* Masson-Judd bladder retractor (suprapubic).

Operative procedure

1. Through a Pfannenstiel incision, the anterior rectus sheath is incised along with portions of the internal and external oblique muscles. The rectus abdominis muscles are retracted laterally to expose the space of Retzius.
2. The anterior portion of the prostatic capsule is incised transversely (Fig. 15-57, *A*), and the prostatic adenoma may be dissected or finger enucleated from the "surgical capsule" (Fig. 15-57, *B*).
3. To decrease the chance of postoperative impotence, an attempt is made to spare the neurovascular bundle that abuts the prostate.
4. Care is taken to place hemostatic sutures at the 5 and 7 o'clock positions, encompassing the vesical neck and prostatic capsule in order to ligate the primary blood supply to the prostate (Fig. 15-57, *C*). Other bleeding points within the capsule may be suture ligated with no. 2-0 absorbable sutures.
5. A Foley catheter is inserted in the urethra and through the bladder neck and inflated within the bladder. Frequently a three-way catheter is used to afford continuous bladder irrigation.
6. The prostatic capsule incision is closed with either a continuous or an interrupted no. 0 absorbable suture (Fig. 15-57, *D*). A drain is placed in the space of Retzius and brought out through the fascia and skin through a separate stab incision. The abdominal incision is then closed in layers, and the wound is dressed.
7. If continuous bladder irrigation is to be used, normal saline solution irrigation is initiated through a 4000-ml closed irrigation system.

Suprapubic prostatectomy

Suprapubic prostatectomy is the removal, through a suprapubic incision, of benign periurethral glandular tissue obstructing the outlet of the urinary tract. One advantage of the suprapubic approach is that it allows access for surgical correction of any existing bladder condition such as vesical calculi or vesical diverticula.

Control of bleeding is a major consideration in any prostatectomy and is one disadvantage of the suprapubic approach. Because the prostate is located beneath the symphysis pubis, ligation of bleeding capsular vessels is exceedingly difficult. However, control of hemorrhage and replacement of blood loss, coupled with skilled nursing

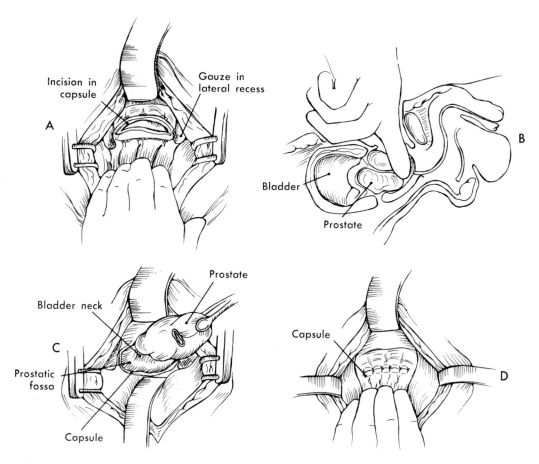

Fig. 15-57. Retropubic prostatectomy. (Modified from Dodson, A.I.: Urological surgery, ed. 4, St. Louis, 1970, The C.V. Mosby Co.)

care and early mobilization of the patient, have greatly minimized complications.

Procedural considerations. Spinal, epidural, and general anesthesia may be equally acceptable types of anesthesia for patients having a suprapubic prostatectomy, depending on the medical condition of the patient. The patient is placed in a slight Trendelenburg's position with a bolster under the buttocks and the legs abducted. Skin preparation, draping, and instrumentation are as described for retropubic prostatectomy.

Operative procedure

1. Bilateral vasectomy may be performed to decrease the postoperative incidence of epididymitis and orchitis. A meatotomy may also be required if the penile meatus is too small to accommodate a Foley catheter.
2. A Foley catheter is inserted through the urethra into the bladder, and the bladder inflated with a preferred irrigating fluid. This maneuver facilitates identification of the bladder.
3. A transverse lower abdominal incision is made through the skin and the two layers of superficial fascia (Fig. 15-58, *A*). The external and internal oblique muscles are cut along the lines of the original incision. Bleeding vessels are clamped, coagulated, or tied with fine absorbable ties.
4. The rectus muscles are separated in the midline and retracted laterally.
5. The bladder is opened at the dome with a scalpel. Liquid contents are aspirated, and the bladder incision is enlarged. The bladder is visually and manually explored for calculi, a tumor, or diverticula.
6. The tip of the index finger of the operating hand is inserted through the vesical neck into the prostatic urethra, and the adenomatous tissue is enucleated. If difficulty is experienced with the enucleation, a finger may be placed in the rectum to elevate the prostate gland (Fig. 15-58, *B*). Aseptic technique is maintained during enucleation with the use of a sterile rectal sheath on the finger placed in the rectum.

7. After enucleation is completed, attention is directed to maintaining good hemostasis by suture ligation of the vesical neck at the 5 and 7 o'clock positions. Other significant bleeding points may also be ligated.
8. A suprapubic catheter of the urologist's choice is placed into the bladder lumen through a small stab incision. A 22 or 24 Fr three-way Foley catheter with a 30-cc balloon is inserted into the urethra, and the balloon is inflated to a size that prevents the catheter from falling or being pulled into the prostatic fossa (Fig. 15-59). The cystotomy incision is then closed with interrupted no. 0 absorbable sutures. A drain is left along the cystotomy incision, brought out through a separate stab wound, and secured to the skin with a silk suture. The muscles, fascia, and subcutaneous tissues are closed in layers, and a dressing is applied.
9. Normal saline irrigation solution is connected to the Foley catheter to provide continuous irrigation to the bladder to reduce clot formation and maintain catheter patency. Continuous irrigation may be initiated during closure.

Perineal prostatectomy

Perineal prostatectomy is the removal of a prostatic adenoma through a perineal approach. Radical perineal excision for prostatic carcinoma may also be performed by the perineal approach and involves removal of the entire gland, its capsule, and seminal vesicles. A perineal approach to the prostate gland is most suitable when open prostatic biopsy is desired and, after receiving pathological confirmation, radical excision is to follow. Other advantages include preservation of the bladder neck, improved urethrovesical anastomosis, and easier control of bleeding. Several surgical disadvantages are listed below:

1. Inability to perform biopsy of the iliac and obturator nodes for determining extension of disease
2. Incidence of urinary incontinence compatible with other radical prostatic procedures

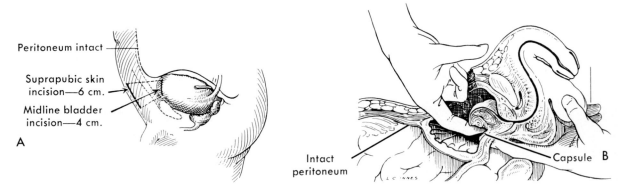

Fig. 15-58. A, Anatomic delineation. **B,** Enucleation of prostate by suprapubic approach. (From Barnes, R.W., and Hadley, H.L.: Urological practice, St. Louis, 1954, The C.V. Mosby Co.)

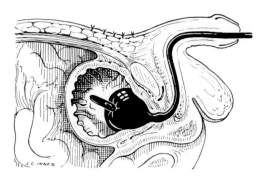

Fig. 15-59. Balloon of Foley catheter inflated to size that prevents catheter from being pulled into prostatic fossa. (From Barnes, R.W., and Hadley, H.L.: Urological practice, St. Louis, 1954, The C.V. Mosby Co.)

3. Loss of sexual potency
4. Urethrorectal fistulas

Procedural considerations. The patient is placed in an exaggerated lithotomy position with a bolster beneath the sacrum, placing the perineum as parallel to the operating room bed as possible. Stirrups should be well padded to protect the popliteal fossa. Routine skin preparation is carried out. Special draping is as follows:

1. A towel folded in half is placed over the pubic area.
2. Two leggings, with points down, are placed over the legs.

3. One towel folded in half (lengthwise) is placed below the anus.
4. A large sheet fully opened with a large cuff is placed across from one stirrup to the other and secured by towel clamps.
5. A laparotomy sheet follows, with the short end to the floor.
6. A large sheet is placed over each leg.

The instrument setup is as described for suprapubic prostatectomy, omitting abdominal self-retaining retractors and adding the following:

Straight and curved Lowsley tractors (Fig. 15-60)
Roux retractors
Jackson retractors, short and long blades
Doyen vaginal retractors
Perineal prostatic retractors (Fig. 15-61)
Sauerbruch retractors, narrow and wide

Operative procedure

1. A curved Lowsley tractor (Fig. 15-55) is placed through the urethra into the bladder and held back by the second assistant, causing the prostate to be pushed down toward the perineum.
2. An inverted U-shaped incision is made from one ischial tuberosity to another, curving just anterior to the anus (Fig. 15-62, *A*).
3. The posterior drapes are clipped to the posterior lip

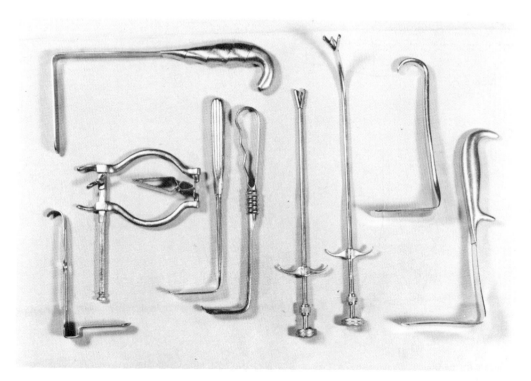

Fig. 15-60. Perineal and suprapubic prostatectomy instruments, including straight and curved Lowsley tractors.

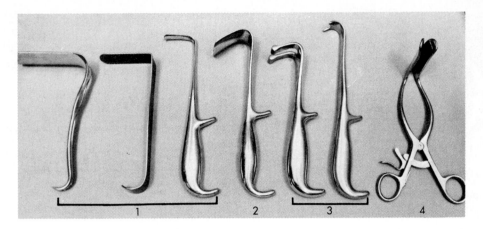

Fig. 15-61. Perineal prostatectomy retractors. *1,* Three prostatic lateral retractors; *2,* prostatic anterior retractor; *3,* two prostatic bifurcated retractors; *4,* self-retaining retractor.

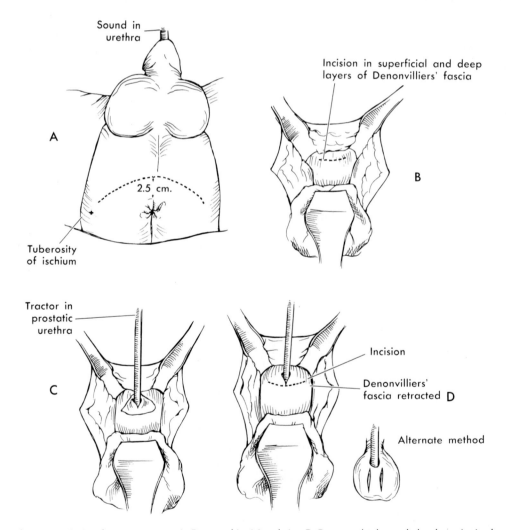

Fig. 15-62. Perineal prostatectomy. **A,** Proposed incisional site. **B,** Rectourethral muscle has been incised and pushed downward from central tendon, and levator ani muscles on each side have been divided; incision in superficial and deep layers of Denonvilliers' fascia is shown. **C,** Urethrotomy in prostatic urethra. **D,** Incision in prostatic capsule.

of the incision, draping the anus out of the sterile field.

4. Subcutaneous bleeders are clamped with straight mosquitoes and coagulated or tied with no. 3-0 absorbable ligatures.

5. The central tendon is isolated, clamped, and cut, and the levator ani muscle exposed and retracted superiorly (Fig. 15-62, *B*). The prostate gland is then exposed.

6. Biopsy of the prostate may be performed for pathologic confirmation. If the results are negative, the prostatic adenoma is removed. If the frozen section reveals malignancy, the urologist may choose to do a radical prostatectomy at this time.

7. If simple enucleation is to be performed, the curved Lowsley tractor is removed from the urethra, and the straight Lowsley inserted into the incision (Fig. 15-62, *C* and *D*).

8. Two ring forceps are used to grasp the prostatic lobes. The straight Lowsley tractor is removed, and the adenoma is manually enucleated from the "surgical capsule" (Fig. 15-62, *E*).

9. A 22 Fr Foley catheter with a 30-cc balloon is inserted through the urethra into the bladder (Fig. 15-62, *F*).

10. The capsulotomy incision is repaired with a continuous no. 0 absorbable suture (Fig. 15-62, *G*). A drain is left in place at the level of the capsulotomy incision.

11. The subcutaneous tissue is reapproximated with no. 3-0 absorbable suture. The skin incision is reapproximated with no. 2-0 nonabsorbable mattress sutures (Fig. 15-62, *H*).

12. The wound is dressed with Telfa, 4 × 8 inch gauze pads, and tape.

13. A vasectomy may be performed.

Operations on the bladder

Operations on the urinary bladder may be performed through an open abdominal incision or a transurethral route. Special transurethral instruments such as the lithotrite may be used to crush vesical calculi manually (Fig. 15-63). An electrohydraulic cystolithotriptor may be used

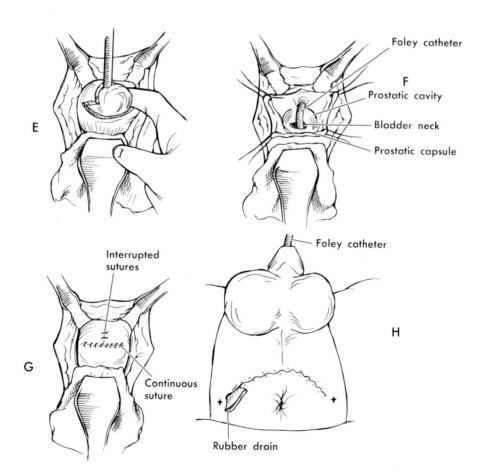

Fig. 15-62, cont'd. E, Enucleating entire prostate with aid of finger. **F,** Catheter in urethra and bladder; exposure of prostatic bed. **G,** Closure of inverted-T incision. **H,** Closure of perineal wound. (Modified from Dodson, A.I.: Urological surgery, ed. 4, St. Louis, 1970, The C.V. Mosby Co.)

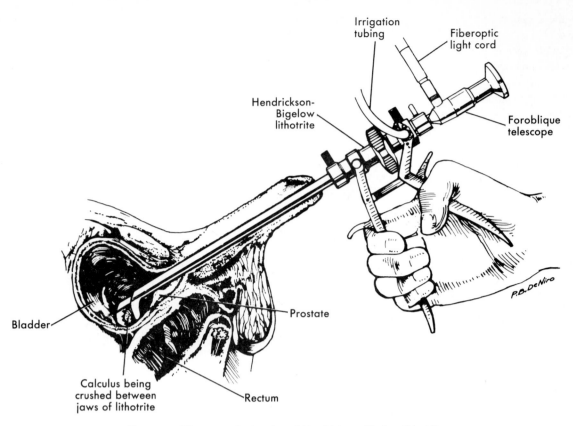

Irrigation
tubing

Fiberoptic
light cord

Hendrickson-
Bigelow
lithotrite

Foroblique
telescope

P.B.DeNiro

Bladder

Prostate

Calculus being
crushed between
jaws of lithotrite

Rectum

Fig. 15-63. Diagrammatic drawing of Hendrickson-Bigelow lithotrite.

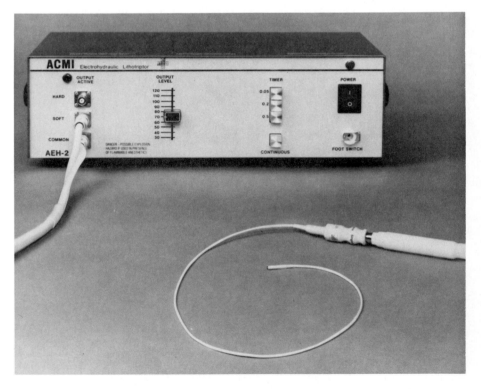

Fig. 15-64. ACMI electrohydraulic lithotriptor. (Courtesy American ACMI, Stamford, Conn.)

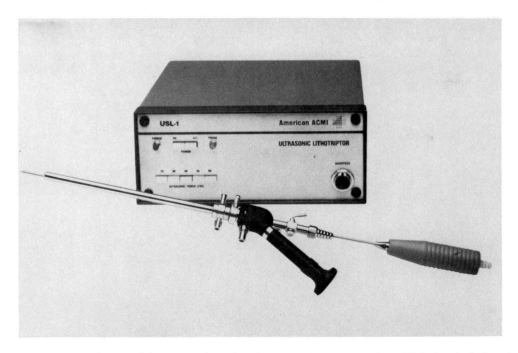

Fig. 15-65. Ultrasonic lithotriptor with rigid nephroscope. (Courtesy American ACMI, Stamford, Conn.)

to fragment the stone within the bladder by using shock waves initiated by electric current (Fig. 15-64).

Ultrasonic lithotripsy is another procedure used in the management of vesical calculi. Ultrasound waves are transmitted through a hollow metal probe (sonotrode), which creates vibration at the tip. When applied to the surface of a calculus, the vibrating tip drills and fragments the calculus. This mechanical disintegration is continued until the stone is reduced to small fragments that are evacuated by suction through the hollow center of the probe (Fig. 15-65).

Stones may also be removed from the bladder through a suprapubic incision (cystolithotomy). Bladder tumors, diverticula, congenital defects, or trauma may necessitate an open abdominal approach. A thorough diagnostic workup and endoscopic examination can help to determine the appropriate surgical approach to be employed. Radical procedures, such as total cystectomy, are performed for the treatment of invasive carcinoma of the bladder and require permanent urinary diversion.

For most open bladder surgery the patient is placed in the supine position with a bolster under the pelvis. Trendelenburg's position may be desired, because this position tilts the head down and allows the viscera to fall cephalad. This allows excellent exposure of the pelvic organs, including the bladder. The patient is draped as described for routine suprapubic prostatectomy, using a disposable impermeable drape that is placed immediately below the bladder incision. A catheter of choice may be inserted into the urethra and the bladder distended with sterile saline at the start of surgery for easy identification. Electrosurgery may be desired. The instrument setup for open bladder operations requires a basic laparotomy set, plus the following:

2 Masson-Judd bladder retractors (Fig. 15-56)
3 Thyroid traction forceps, long
3 Thyroid traction forceps, short
2 Retropubic needle holders or other long needle holders as desired
1 Trocar (optional)
  Closed wound suction drains
  Assorted Foley, Pezzer, and Malecot catheters in available sizes
  Vessel loops
  Catheter stylet
  Electrosurgical unit

Suprapubic cystotomy (cystostomy)

Cystotomy is an opening made into the urinary bladder through a low abdominal incision. When a drainage tube is inserted into the bladder through an abdominal incision, the procedure is a cystostomy.

Operative procedure

1. A vertical or Pfannenstiel incision (transverse) is used (Fig. 15-66, *A*). The surgical approach is as described for suprapubic prostatectomy.
2. The bladder is distended with saline solution that is instilled with an Asepto syringe through a catheter. The dome of the bladder is then dissected free with Metzenbaum scissors. The wall of the bladder is grasped on either side of the midline with Allis forceps. Two traction sutures may be placed through the bladder wall

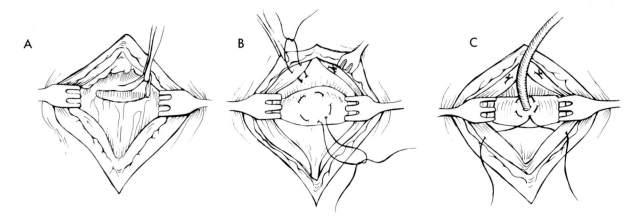

Fig. 15-66. Suprapubic cystostomy. **A,** Incision. **B,** Purse-string and traction sutures in preparation for stab wound in bladder. **C,** Cystostomy tube in bladder. (Modified from Dodson, A.I.: Urological surgery, ed. 4, St. Louis, 1970, The C.V. Mosby Co.)

and held with straight hemostats (Fig. 15-66, *B*). The bladder is then incised downward with a scalpel. Bleeding vessels in the bladder wall are clamped and ligated. The bladder contents are aspirated with a Poole suction.

3. The bladder opening may be extended if the bladder is to be explored for diverticula or calculi. A large-sized Malecot or Pezzer catheter is introduced into the bladder.

4. The incision is closed snugly about the catheter with absorbable sutures to render the closure watertight about the cystostomy tube (Fig. 15-66, *C*). The muscle, fascia, and subcutaneous tissue are closed with chromic or Dexon suture, and the skin with staples or nonabsorbable material. The cystostomy tube is further secured to the skin with a heavy black silk suture to prevent it from being inadvertently dislodged from the bladder. A drain such as a Jackson-Pratt may be left in the prevesical space.

5. The wound is dressed, and the cystostomy tube connected to a straight urinary drainage system.

Transurethral resection of bladder tumors

Bladder lesions may be removed using a standard resectoscope, working element, loop, and a Foroblique telescope, which is passed through the urethra into the bladder. A 24 Fr cystoscope sheath with a catheterizing bridge and biopsy forceps may be used to remove bladder tumors located at the very top or dome of the bladder (Fig. 15-67).

Transitional cell carcinoma of the bladder is one of the most difficult lesions to track because it can occur wherever there is transitional cell lining of the urinary tract. Bladder cancer has a tendency to recur in other areas of the bladder even after complete resection of the original lesions.

Usually the surgeon removes not only the bladder lesion but also a portion of the muscle of the bladder underlying the lesion so the pathologist can determine if any tumor has invaded the muscle. Also, random biopsies of the normal bladder lining are taken because transitional cell carcinoma in situ may be found on microscopic examination.

Lesions that deeply invade the muscle must be treated with an open surgical procedure, such as a partial cystectomy or total cystectomy.

Procedural considerations. The resection technique, setup, and preparation of the patient are similar to those for transurethral resection of the prostate with a few exceptions. A general or a spinal anesthetic is administered. If the surgeon has any questions about lesions existing in the upper urinary tract, a retrograde pyelogram is done.

Sterile water is recommended as an irrigating solution in transurethral resection of bladder tumors. As few vessels are uncovered during this short resection procedure, water absorption with hemolysis and systemic complications such as hyponatremia do not occur. In addition, there is a tendency for cancer cells released during the procedure to absorb water, causing them to rupture and lyse rather than remain viable and capable of implanting in the raw surface of the bladder created by the surgery.

On completion of the procedure, a large catheter, usually a 24 Fr, is passed into the bladder and connected to drainage.

Transurethral laser treatment of bladder tumors

The neodymium:yttrium-aluminum-garnet (Nd:YAG) laser is used to destroy small bladder tumors and may be used to coagulate the tumor bed of larger bladder tumors resected with an electrosurgical loop. It produces a powerful, highly focused beam of light in the near infrared range that is transmitted to the tumor site through a flexible glass fiber. This laser fiber is passed through the catheter channel of a cystoscope, and the fiber is directed by a deflecting laser bridge (Fig. 15-68).

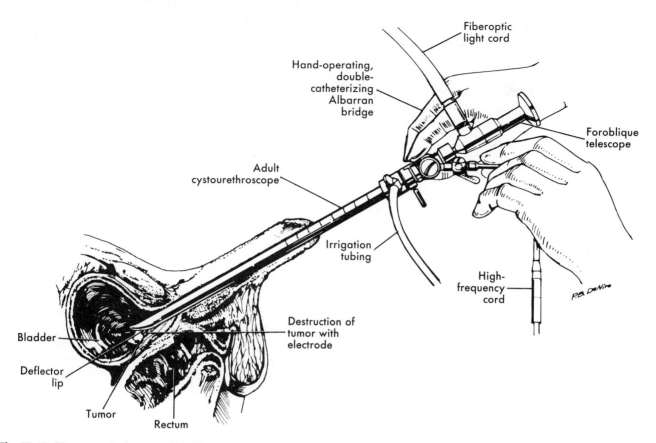

Fig. 15-67. Diagrammatic drawing of bladder fulguration.

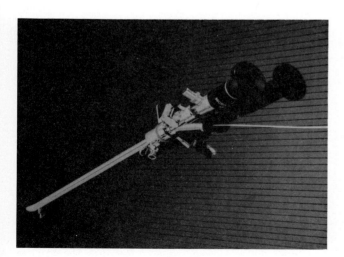

Fig. 15-68. Laser bridge, laser fiber deflected, Foroblique telescope, 21 Fr cystoscope sheath. (Courtesy American ACMI, Stamford, Conn.)

The advantages of the Nd:YAG laser in the irradiation of bladder tumors are that bleeding is minimized, only sedation is required, operating time is short, there is minimal damage to healthy tissue, and there is no need for postoperative drainage of the bladder by a urethral catheter.

Trocar cystostomy

Trocar cystostomy requires opening the bladder, draining by puncture with a needle or trocar, and inserting a catheter.

Procedural considerations. A minor set of instruments is required, along with the following accessory items:

1 Silver probe
1 Grooved director
1 Anthony suction tube and tubing
1 Trocar
  Catheters, as required

A local anesthesia setup may be used.

Operative procedure. The skin at the site of the puncture is nicked with a scalpel, and the trocar is inserted into the bladder. The trocar obturator is withdrawn, the bladder is drained through the trocar by suction, and a catheter is passed through the trocar cannula into the bladder. The cannula is carefully withdrawn, and the catheter is sutured to the wound edges. The wound is dressed.

Suprapubic cystolithotomy

Suprapubic cystolithotomy is the removal of calculi from the bladder. Obstructions, such as prostatic enlargement or foreign bodies, are common causes of bladder calculi and may be corrected at the time of surgery.

Procedural considerations. The instrument setup for open bladder operations is used, plus the following:

2 Millin T-shaped stone forceps
2 Millin capsule forceps
1 Lewkowitz lithotomy forceps

Operative procedure. The surgical approach is similar to that described for subrapubic cystotomy. When the bladder is opened, calculi are identified and extracted. If indicated, bladder outlet obstruction is repaired.

Repair of vesical fistulas

Vesical fistulas occurring between the bladder and the intestines or vagina may be repaired surgically. Vesicointestinal fistula may be caused by ulcerative colitis, diverticulitis, or neoplasms of the colon or rectum.

Vesicovaginal fistula may also be a complication of radiotherapy for cervical cancer or endoscopic procedures involving surgery of the trigone or vesical neck. Such fistulas are also caused by obstetrical injuries and hysterectomies.

Procedural considerations. The instrument setup is as described for open bladder operations. An intestinal resection setup (Chapter 11) is also necessary for vesicointestinal fistulas. For vesicovaginal fistulas, vaginal preparation and a colporrhaphy set (Chapter 14) with colostomy or ileostomy instruments are used.

Operative procedure. A colostomy proximal to the fistula may be performed to protect the repaired segment of bowel. The communicating area of bladder and bowel is totally resected. Generally, an end-to-end bowel resection is performed after excision of the involved intestinal segment. The bladder is then repaired in three layers.

If the fistula is at the dome of the bladder, the approach will be extraperitoneal. A suprapubic tube is usually left in the bladder in these cases. If the fistula is in the trigone of the bladder, a vaginal approach may be employed.

Bladder neck operation (Y-V–plasty)

A bladder neck operation is an open plastic revision of a strictured bladder neck. A Y-V–plasty is performed to overcome contracture of the bladder neck caused by primary or secondary stricture.

Procedural considerations. The patient is placed in a modified Trendelenburg's position. Epidural, spinal, or general anesthesia may be used. Instrumentation is as for open bladder operations.

Operative procedure
1. The bladder is approached through a transverse Pfan-
nenstiel incision in the same manner as in retropubic prostatectomy. A self-retaining retractor is employed to achieve exposure.
2. Fine traction sutures on small, fine, cutting-edge needles (cleft palate type) are placed at the base and on either side of the urethra to start the pattern for the plastic dissection.
3. With the aid of the traction sutures and an Allis forceps, the anterior bladder wall, bladder neck, and urethra are visualized. A Y incision is made in the anterior bladder wall with its distal end extending through the vesical neck and prostate at the 12 o'clock position (Fig. 15-69, A). Bleeding vessels in the wall of the bladder and bladder neck are ligated. The broad-based V flap is developed, and the length of the Y arm is determined by how far the stricture extends beyond the vesical neck.
4. The apex of the V is mobilized so it fits into the leg of the Y incision (Fig. 15-69, B). In this manner the vesical outlet is greatly increased in diameter. A catheter is placed in the urethra as a guide. A suture is taken through the apex of the V and into the prostatic urethra to the base of the Y and tied. The closure of the plastic repair is completed with mattress sutures on atraumatic needles (Fig. 15-69, C).
5. A cystostomy tube is placed in the bladder, and the bladder and abdominal wall are closed in the usual manner for cystostomy.

Vesicourethral suspension (Marshall-Marchetti operation)

The Marshall-Marchetti operation requires elevation of the pubococcygeal muscle surrounding the urethra and bladder neck for the correction of stress incontinence caused by an abnormal urethrovesical angle.

Procedural considerations. The patient is usually placed in a moderate Trendelenburg's position. Legs are placed in frog-leg position, with supports under each knee, to allow for intraoperative vaginal manipulation. Abdominal and vaginal preps are required. A Foley catheter is inserted into the urethra at the beginning of surgery.

The basic laparotomy set is used, and the following instruments are added:

1 Masson-Judd bladder retractor
2 Extra-long needle holders, retropubic needle holders, or Heaney needle holders
 Nonabsorbable sutures, no. 0 or 1, swaged to ⅝-circle needles

Operative procedure
1. A Foley catheter is inserted in the bladder through the urethra. A suprapubic transverse incision is made to expose the prevesical space of Retzius. The bladder retractor is positioned with small, moist laparotomy pads in place.

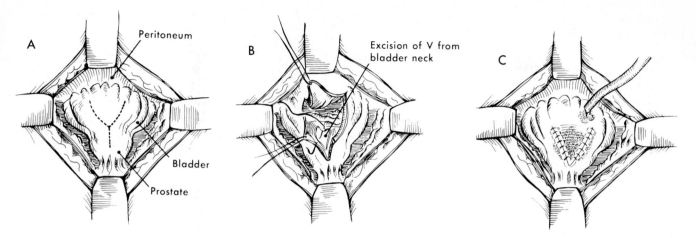

Fig. 15-69. Bladder neck operation. **A,** Y incision. **B,** Conversion of Y incision to V closure. **C,** V closure. (From Flocks, R.H. and Clup, D.A.: Surgical urology, 4th ed. Copyright © 1975 by Year Book Medical Publishers, Inc., Chicago. Used by permission.)

2. The bladder and urethra are freed from the posterior surface of the rectus muscle and symphysis pubis by gentle blunt manipulation.
3. The assistant places two fingers into the vagina and lifts the urethra upward against the symphysis pubis so that the periurethral musculofascial structures are more easily repaired by the surgeon.
4. A heavy, nonabsorbable atraumatic suture on a Heaney needle holder is placed through the supporting fascia of the vaginal wall on each side of the urethra. The suture is then passed through the symphysis pubis, providing support to the urethra and bladder neck.
5. Generally, a row of three heavy, nonabsorbable sutures is placed on each side of the urethra, the most proximal being located just at the vesical neck.
6. The area is drained, and the wound is closed in layers and dressed.
7. The vagina may be packed with 2-inch packing, which should be removed after 24 to 36 hours. The Foley catheter is connected to a closed urinary drainage system.

Endoscopic bladder neck suspension (Stamey procedure)

Endoscopic suspension of the vesical neck for stress incontinence, developed by Stamey, has distinct advantages over open retropubic urethrovesical suspensions. The incision is superficial, the bladder and bladder neck are not dissected, and the paraurethral tissues that suspend the vesical neck are buttressed vaginally. This operation was the first to use the cystoscope to place sutures exactly at the vesical neck. A similar procedure, the Pereyra procedure, involves urethrovesical suspension with vagino-urethroplasty.

Procedural considerations. The patient is placed in the lithotomy position. Although the procedure is not lengthy, care must be taken to ensure proper body alignment and avoid pressure areas when positioning the patient. The legs, positioned in stirrups, are extended to promote a flat lower abdomen. The buttocks must be at the edge of the lower hinge of the operating room bed for placement of the weighted vaginal retractor. A lumbar support may assist to alleviate undue stress on the lower back and sacrum. After preoperative hair removal, the entire perineum, vagina, and suprapubic area are prepped. A drape is placed across the rectum to isolate it from the surgical field.

Instrumentation includes:

Vaginal instrument set
Cystoscopy setup
Stamey needles—straight, 15-degree, and 30-degree (Fig. 15-70)

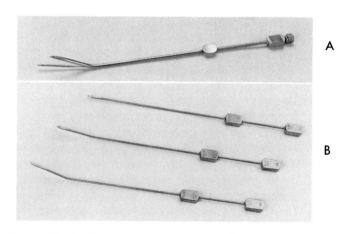

Fig. 15-70. A, Litvak Pereyra ligature needle, 28 cm long. **B,** Stamey needles. Used in conjunction with the treatment of urinary incontinence in the female. (Courtesy Pilling Co., Fort Washington, PA.)

Martin needles, no. 7 (optional)
Foley catheter, 14 Fr, 5 cc
Cystocath, no. 12
Asepto syringe
Vaginal packing
Nylon or Prolene suture ties, no. 2
Gore-Tex bolsters, 4-mm

Medications

Antibiotic irrigation (often Gentamicin)
Indigo carmine (for IV administration)
Triple Sulfa vaginal cream

Operative procedure

1. The labia minora are sutured laterally to expose the vaginal introitus.
2. Two symmetrical transverse incisions are made to the left and right of the midline at the upper border of the symphysis pubis.
3. The tissue is spread bluntly to the anterior rectus muscle.
4. Gauze is then packed into each incision while the vaginal portion of the procedure is carried out.
5. The urethral length is measured with a Foley catheter by placing the inflated balloon at the internal vesical neck. The point of the urethral meatus is marked on the catheter, and the Foley is deflated and withdrawn. The catheter is then reinflated, and the length from meatal mark to the balloon is measured.
6. The Foley is reinserted and inflated. The weighted speculum is placed in the vagina, and the anterior vaginal mucosa is incised in a T shape about 2 to 2.5 cm in length.
7. The vaginal tissue is separated from the urethra by spreading the scissors in the plane between the tissues. The vertical portion of the T is made following the mucosal separation from the urethra. Incision is complete when the tip of the index finger can rest against the bladder neck.
8. The Stamey needle of choice (Fig. 15-70) is inserted into the medial edge of one of the suprapubic incisions and through the rectus fascia just above the symphysis pubis.
9. The superior edge of the symphysis is probed with the needle tip, and the needle is passed 1 to 2 cm parallel to the posterior symphysis.
10. One index finger is inserted into the vagina at the bladder neck as the other maneuvers the needle along the bladder neck and through the fascia and periurethral tissues.
11. The Foley is removed and the cystoscope inserted to check the needle position.
12. Heavy no. 2 suture material is threaded into the needle eye and the needle pulled suprapubically. Hemostats are placed on each suture end.
13. The needle is then passed a second time about 1 cm

lateral to the first puncture with the suture placed on tension. Position is again checked cystoscopically.
14. The vaginal end of the suture is buttressed with the Gore-Tex material and placed through the needle's eye. The Gore-Tex is guided into the urethrovesical junction.
15. The entire procedure is repeated on the other side.
16. The cystoscope is reinserted and the bladder filled. Under direct visualization, the sutures are pulled upward so that the flow of fluid is alternately released and stopped.
17. The Foley is reinserted and the sutures are tied into position in the suprapubic incisions. The incisions are then closed with absorbable sutures.
18. The vaginal mucosa is closed with 3-0 absorbable suture and the sulfa cream–coated vaginal pack inserted. The Foley may be removed.
19. A stab wound can be made in the lower abdomen for placement of a cystocath while the bladder is still full.
20. A small gauze dressing is placed over the abdominal wounds and the cystocath secured and connected to drainage.

Implantation of a prosthetic urethral sphincter

This procedure is usually done as a last measure in patients with stress incontinence where other modalities have failed. Problems with the device have included foreign body reaction, persistent urethral pressure, and fluid hydraulic failure.

Procedural considerations. The artificial sphincter unit has an abdominally placed, pressure-regulated reservoir that maintains a constant, predetermined pressure on the periurethral cuff. Because of the connection between the reservoir and cuff, any increase in intraabdominal pressure transmits more fluid into the cuff. This connection allows for a compensatory increase in urethral resistance during coughing or straining.

The scrotal or labial pump shifts the fluid in the cuff to the reservoir to allow bladder emptying. The fluid reenters the cuff through a resistor in about 60 to 120 seconds. The locking button in the AMS 800 artificial sphincter unit traps fluid in the reservoir to allow activation of the cuff.

A standard laparotomy setup is required as well as the sphincter components, 12.5% Hypaque, and an antibiotic solution, as used with the penile implant. The patient may be placed in a modified lithotomy position.

Operative procedure

1. Inguinal and perineal incisions are made.
2. The bulbar urethra is mobilized through a transverse incision above the inguinal ligament and lateral to the pubic tubercle. The reservoir is placed in the prevesical space.
3. If the cuff is to be around the bladder neck, the patient is supine and a lower abdominal incision is made to expose the bladder neck.

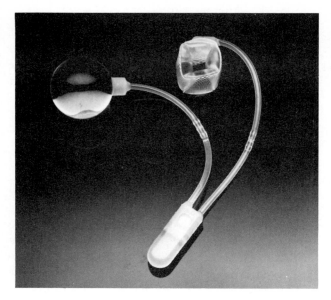

Fig. 15-71. AMS Sphincter 800. (Courtesy American Medical Systems, Minnetonka, Minn.)

4. The pump is introduced through the abdominal incision and transferred to the scrotum or labia through a subcutaneous tunnel.
5. The reservoir, cuff, and pump are filled with 12.5% Hypaque to the appropriate volume (Fig. 15-71).
6. The wound is closed and dressed with gauze sponges. A urethral catheter is usually not inserted.

Cystectomy

Cystectomy is the total excision of the urinary bladder and adjacent structures. Cystectomy is a surgical consideration when a vesical malignancy has not invaded the muscular wall of the entire bladder or when frequent recurrences of widespread papillary tumors do not respond to endoscopic or chemotherapeutic management. The patient should be medically able to withstand surgery with the expectation of reasonable longevity. Total cystectomy necessitates permanent urinary diversion into an ileal or colonic conduit. Conservative measures such as radiotherapy or chemotherapy may be used when the neoplasm is far advanced.

In a male patient the prostate gland, seminal vesicles, and distal ureters are removed with the bladder and its peritoneal surface. In a woman the bladder, urethra, distal ureters, uterus, cervix, and proximal third of the vagina are removed.

Procedural considerations. The patient is placed in the supine position. Instruments are as described for major abdominal procedures. For a male patient, if the prostate and seminal vesicles are to be removed, prostatectomy instruments should be added. For a woman, vaginal and abdominal hysterectomy instruments should be added (Chapter 14).

Operative procedure

1. A midline incision from the epigastrium to the symphysis pubis, curving to the left of the umbilicus, is generally preferred.
2. The incision is deepened, the rectus muscles retracted laterally, and the peritoneum opened. At this point, long instruments are necessary.
3. In a male patient the bladder dome is lifted at its peritoneal surface. Dissection proceeds laterally on either side with ligation of the major vesical arteries. The bladder is then retracted to expose the prostate and seminal vesicles, which are dissected free in continuity with the bladder. The vas deferens is divided, and the urethra cut at the level of the pelvic diaphragm.
4. The surgical specimen consisting of the bladder, distal ureters, prostate, seminal vesicles, and distal vas is removed en bloc. The urethra is ligated with absorbable suture.
5. Lap pads are placed in the denuded pelvis, and pressure is applied to reduce blood loss from oozing.
6. Urinary diversion by isolated ileal or colonic conduit may be performed. Direct anastomosis of the ureters to the colon may be performed by ureterosigmoidostomy.
7. The surgical approach for total cystectomy in the female patient is as described for the male patient, but the urethra is removed in continuity with the bladder and internal reproductive organs.

Radical cystectomy and lymphadenectomy

Radical cystectomy and lymphadenectomy require total excision of the urinary bladder and contiguous organs as well as pelvic lymph nodes (iliac and obturator). Radical cystectomy and lymphadenectomy are indicated when larger tumors penetrate the full thickness of the bladder wall and invade perivesical fat. Urinary diversion is also performed in this slightly more extensive surgery.

Procedural considerations. The setup and operative procedures are described on p. 371 and above.

Bladder replacement
Right colocystoplasty

This procedure has become more functionally effective with the use of intermittent self-catheterization and selective implantation of a prosthetic urinary sphincter. Depending on the extent of involvement, the right colon may be used to replace the bladder, the bladder and prostatic urethra, or the bladder and prostate with a direct enteric-to-proximal bulbar urethral anastomosis.

The ideal candidate for a right colocystoplasty following cystectomy for carcinoma is a male with a normal urethra, a proximally located, well-differentiated bladder tumor, absence of carcinoma in situ, and proof that the prostatic urethra is free of disease. High-dose radiation offers appreciable risks for postoperative complications and is contraindicated with enterourethral anastomosis.

Ileocecal bladder substitution

Over the last 30 years, attempts at bladder replacement with an ileal segment of bowel have yielded disappointing results. There has been a high incidence of recurrence, renal damage, incontinence, and postoperative strictures and fistulas. The ileum has been used as a reservoir to restore urinary continuity because it possesses a low intraluminal pressure. However, the short mesentery does not always permit the bowel to reach the urethra. The results with the current antireflux techniques are not consistently successful.

Although most patients have attained daytime urinary control, the majority still have problems with enuresis. Deterioration of the upper urinary tract is a known risk with this procedure, and therefore ileocecal substitution is met with mixed reactions and recommendations.

Sigmoidocystoplasty

Because of its ease of construction, bladder proximity, decreased obstruction from mucus, and large capacity, the sigmoid colon has been more appealing to many surgeons in their attempt to create a new bladder. More efficient emptying with a larger reservoir capacity seems to occur with a sigmoid replacement. Results yield higher intraluminal pressures, more effective urinary flow rates, and less nocturnal incontinence than with ileal segments.

Ileoascending cystoplasty

In an effort to improve the intestinal reservoir's capacity and antirefluxing effectiveness, the use of the ascending colon as a continent reservoir was introduced in 1965. This technique has a number of anatomic advantages over other methods of bladder replacement. The segment used can include the hepatic flexure and proximal transverse colon. A large-capacity reservoir is obtained, and colonic incision or tailoring is not required to achieve an appropriate shape. It easily reaches any site within the pelvis and can be anastomosed directly to the urethra without tension.

Ileal conduit

The ileal conduit is one method by which the urine flow is diverted to an isolated loop of bowel. One end of the isolated loop is brought out through the skin so the urine can be collected in a pouch, which is intermittently emptied. The stoma site should be carefully selected preoperatively by the surgeon and enterostomal therapist. The selected site, usually in the right lower quadrant of the abdomen (Fig. 15-72, *A*), is marked with a fine needle dipped in methylene blue to prevent erasure during skin preparation. The surgeon's goal is to create a round, protruding stoma without wrinkles in the skin to prevent urine leakage under the collecting device. Puckering around the stoma is minimized by using a subcuticular technique when suturing the stoma in place.

Procedural considerations. The patient is placed in the supine position. A prostatectomy or hysterectomy may also be done at the time of surgery.

Operative procedure

1. The bladder is decompressed with a catheter. The

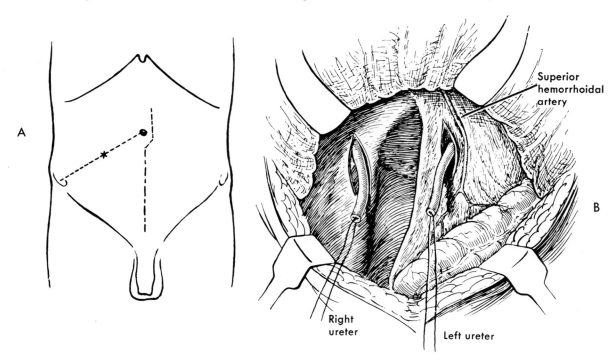

Fig. 15-72. Major steps of operation for ileal conduit, urinary diversion. **A,** Site of ileal stoma. **B,** Ureters freed. Left ureter brought under base of mesosigmoid colon.

abdomen is entered through a midline abdominal incision. A self-retaining abdominal retractor is placed so the viscera are excluded from the region of dissection.

2. The ureters are identified and mobilized by severing them 1 to 1½ inches from the bladder (Fig. 15-72, *B*). A retroperitoneal tunnel is made so that the left ureter lies close to the right ureter.

3. The distal ileum and mesentery are inspected to identify the bowel's blood supply. A drain is passed through the mesentery, midway between the two main arterial arcades adjacent to the ileum at the proximal and distal ends of the selected segment. This segment usually comprises 15 to 20 cm of the terminal ileum, a few centimeters from the ileocecal valve (Fig. 15-72, *C*).

4. Care is exercised to preserve the ileocecal artery and adequate circulation to the isolated ileal segment. The peritoneum is incised over the proposed line of division

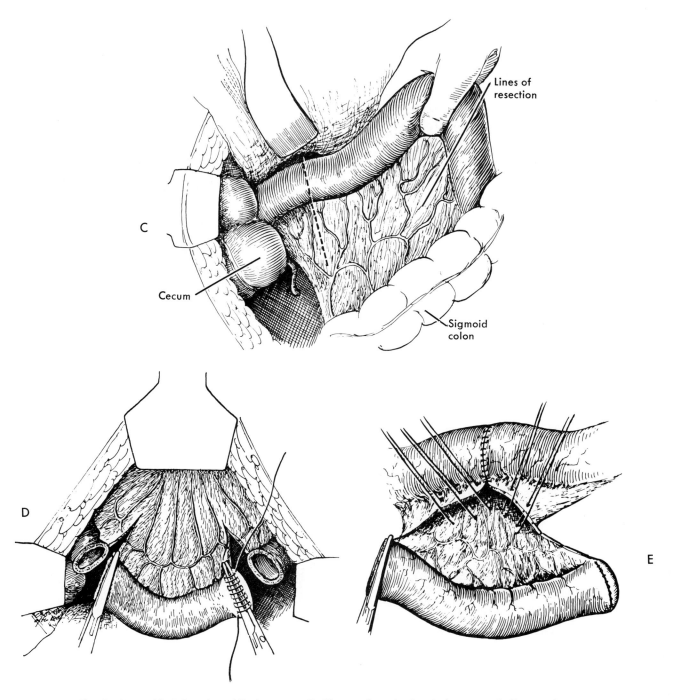

Fig. 15-72, cont'd. C, Location of ileal segment. **D,** Closure of proximal end of segment. **E,** Closure of opening at base of mesentery of segment showing transverse approximation.

Continued.

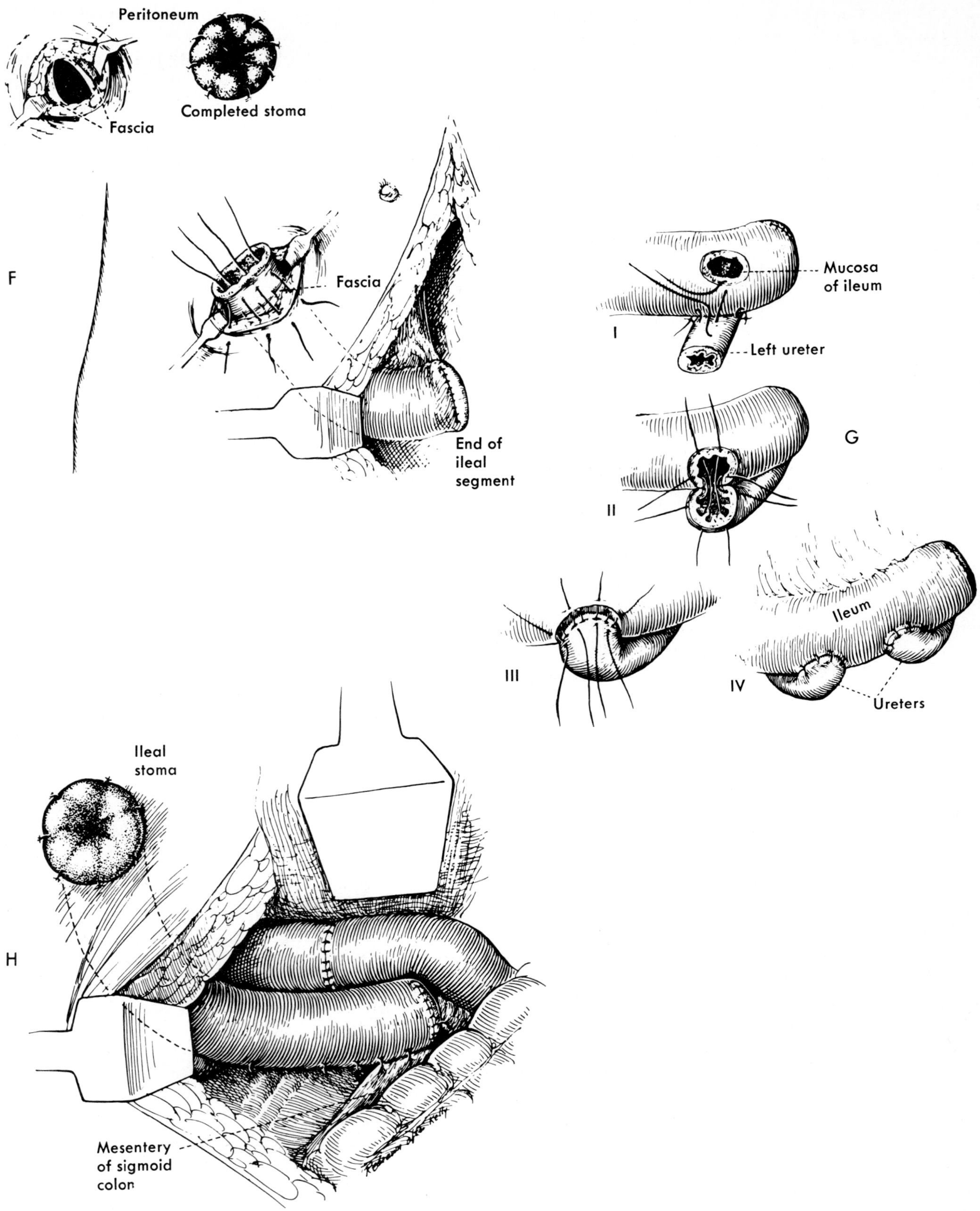

Peritoneum

Completed stoma

Fascia

F

Fascia

End of
ileal
segment

Mucosa
of ileum

Left ureter

I

G

II

III

IV

Ileum

Ureters

Ileal
stoma

H

Mesentery
of sigmoid
colon

Fig. 15-72, cont'd. F, Preparation of stoma. **G,** Ureteroilal anastomosis. **H,** Completed segment. (From Cordonnier, J.J.: Surgery of the ureter and urinary conduits. In Campbell, F.M., and Harrison, J.H., editors: Urology, ed. 3, Philadelphia, 1970, W.B. Saunders Co.)

of the mesentery. Dennis or Gavin-Miller intestinal clamps are placed across the ileum, and the bowel is divided flush with the clamps (Fig. 15-72, *D*). By gastrointestinal technique (Chapter 11), the proximal end of the isolated ileal segment is closed first with a layer of absorbable sutures and then with a second layer of interrupted no. 2-0 nonabsorbable sutures. The proximal and distal segments of ileum are reanastomosed end to end in two layers.

5. The mesenteric incision is closed with interrupted nonabsorbable sutures (Fig. 15-72, *E*).
6. The closed proximal end of the conduit segment is fixed to the posterior peritoneum. The ureters are implanted in the ileal segment by fine instruments and no. 4-0 absorbable ureteral sutures on atraumatic needles (Fig. 15-72, *F* and *G*). The peritoneum and muscle of the abdominal wall lateral to the original incision are separated by blunt dissection. The abdominal opening for the stoma is made. The distal opening of the ileal conduit is then drawn through a fenestration in the muscle, fascia, and skin. The ileum is fixed to the fascia with quadrant sutures of no. 2-0. A rosebud stoma is constructed at the same time the ileum is sutured to the skin with subcuticular suture (Fig. 15-72, *H*). Ureteral stents are usually left in the stoma, and a urinary collecting pouch is placed over the rosebud stoma to collect urine. The wound is drained with two Jackson-Pratt drains. The abdominal incision is closed with no. 0 nonabsorbable suture. The skin is reapproximated with skin staples.

Cystectomy may be performed before or after this procedure, depending on the patient's condition and diagnosis. In some cases the surgeon may choose not to remove the bladder rather than to subject a debilitated patient to further surgery. In cases of bladder carcinoma, the surgeon may elect to treat the patient with radiation in an attempt to decrease the size of the tumor and "sterilize" the regional lymph nodes before performing a cystectomy.

Operations on the ureters and the kidneys

Stones, infections, and tumors are the most common causes of urinary tract obstruction necessitating surgery to prevent renal obstruction and subsequent failure. Obstruction may also result from congenital malformations or previous operations on the urinary tract (Fig. 15-73).

Although the causes of many kidney stones are obscure, certain conditions such as obstruction, stasis, or imbalance of metabolism predispose to their formation. Stones may form from various elements: calcium oxalate, calcium phosphate, magnesium ammonium phosphate, uric acid, calcium carbonate, or cystine. Stones removed during surgery are usually subjected to chemical analysis. Stones obtained as surgical specimens should be submitted in a dry jar. Fixative agents such as formalin invalidate the results of the analysis.

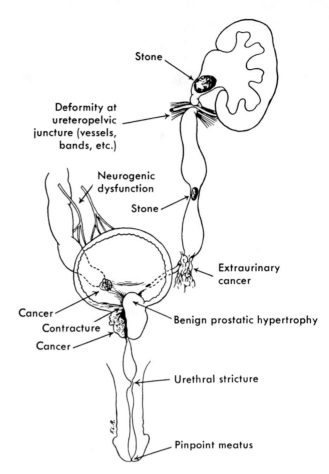

Fig. 15-73. Some common causes of urinary tract obstruction vary in location and nature, but all can destroy renal function, usually in presence of infection. (From Marshall, V.F.: Textbook of urology, ed. 2, New York, 1964, Harper & Row, Publishers.)

Stones in the renal pelvis may fall into the ureteropelvic junction and obstruct the flow of urine. However, calculi less than 1 cm in diameter may pass down the ureter and lodge at a more distal location, such as where the ureter crosses the iliac vessels or at the ureterovesical junction. A stone may remain in a renal calyx and continue to enlarge, eventually filling the entire renal collecting system (staghorn calculus).

Hydroureteronephrosis, infection, and destruction of renal parenchyma frequently result from unrelieved obstruction.

Hypothermia is useful in renal stone surgery as a means of prolonging the safe period of renal ischemia during extensive parenchymal manipulation. This method is also employed for surgery of the renal artery. Several methods enable renal cooling: ice slush or cold saline solution, surface cooling coils, perfusion of cold solutions through the renal artery, or a variation of these basic techniques, for example, perfusion of the renal pelvis with saline that has been cooled by a coil immersed in ice slush.

Procedural considerations. Saline slush for renal surgery may be prepared in several ways:

1. Sterile Mason jars are filled with sterile normal saline solution and double-wrapped in sterile plastic bags. Each bag should be individually wrapped and secured with a twist tie. The Mason jars are placed for 2 to 3 hours in a bucket of ice to which 2 pints of isopropyl alcohol and two boxes of salt are added and mixed. When the saline is ready for use, the circulating nurse removes the wrapped Mason jar from the ice, opens the plastic bags by sterile technique, and presents the Mason jar to the scrub nurse. The scrub nurse shakes the contents of the Mason jar to cause crystallization of the saline. The slush is removed from the Mason jar with a sterile spoon.

2. A rigid plastic container of 1000 ml of normal saline irrigation solution may be placed on its side in a freezer several hours before surgery. To prevent the solution from solidifying, the container should be rotated one-half turn every 20 to 30 minutes. Sterile "slush" may then be poured directly into a sterile basin as required.

3. A refrigeration unit that produces sterile slush provides a cost-effective, time-saving alternative to the other methods of slush preparation.

Surgical approach in renal surgery is predicated on the patient's somatotype, the need for exposure to a part or all of the kidney, and the surgical procedure to be performed. In the case of renal masses, attention is directed toward control of the vascular pedicle. For this reason

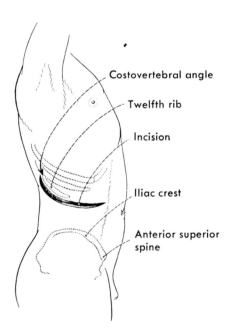

Fig. 15-74. Incision for lumbar approach to kidney. It is made parallel to twelfth rib and 1 cm below it, and extends from costovertebral angle to point 3 cm above anterosuperior iliac spine. (From Barnes, R.W., and Hadley, H.L.: Urological practice, St. Louis, 1954, The C.V. Mosby Co.)

patient position and surgical exposure are of prime consideration. There are three principal surgical approaches to the kidney:

1. The lumbar or simple flank incision is most frequently used and may include removal of the eleventh or twelfth rib. The incision begins at the posterior axillary line and parallels the course of the twelfth rib. It extends forward and slightly downward between the iliac crest and the thorax (Fig. 15-74).

2. The transthoracic, transdiaphragmatic exposure is employed primarily for large upper pole renal neoplasms. The tenth and eleventh ribs are usually removed, and the chest cavity is opened, collapsing the lung. The leaves of the diaphragm are separated to expose the kidney. A large retractor, such as a Finochietto, and chest drains are required.

3. For the transabdominal transperitoneal incision, the patient is placed in a supine position with bolsters under the flank and lower thorax. This effectively places the flank in an oblique position, causing the abdominal viscera to fall away from the operative incision. This approach is used for renal neoplasms and affords an excellent approach to the renal pedicle.

Diversionary surgery on the ureter

Ureterostomy (ureterotomy) is opening the ureter for continued drainage from it into another body part.

Cutaneous ureterostomy is diversion of the flow of urine from the kidney, through the ureter, away from the bladder, and onto the skin of the lower abdomen (Fig. 15-75). A suitable urinary collecting device is placed over the ureteral stoma to keep the patient dry.

Ureterectomy is complete removal of the ureter. This procedure is generally employed in collecting system tumors and includes nephrectomy and the excision of a cuff of bladder.

Ureterolithotomy is incision into the ureter and removal of an obstructing calculus.

Ureteroureterostomy is segmental resection of a diseased portion of the ureter and reconstruction in continuity of the two normal segments.

Ureteroenterostomy is diversion of the ureter into a segment of the ileum (ureteroileostomy) or into the sigmoid colon (ureterosigmoidostomy). The common terms used in describing these procedures are *ileal urinary conduit* and *ureterosigmoidostomy* (Fig. 15-75).

Ureteroneocystostomy (ureterovesical anastomosis) is division of the distal ureter from the bladder and reimplantation of the ureter into the bladder with a submucosal tunnel.

Reconstructive operations may be indicated because of a pathologic condition of the bladder or lower ureter that interferes with normal drainage. Conditions requiring urinary diversion or reconstruction of the urinary tract include malignancy, cystitis, stricture, trauma, and congenital ure-

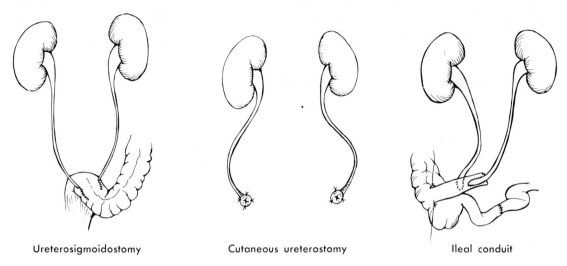

Ureterosigmoidostomy   Cutaneous ureterostomy   Ileal conduit

Fig. 15-75. Methods of permanent urinary diversion. (From Keuhnelian, J.G., and Sanders, V.E.: Urologic nursing, New York, 1970, Macmillan, Inc.)

terovesical reflux. Invasive vesical malignancy requiring surgical removal of the bladder necessitates urinary diversion.

Procedural considerations. The site of the incision and position of the patient depend on the nature of the proposed surgery. The patient may be placed in the supine position for abdominal surgery, in modified Trendelenburg's position for low abdominal or pelvic surgery, or in the lateral position for high or midureteral obstructing calculi.

Instruments include the nephrectomy set, plus plastic instrumentation for pyeloplasty. Additional instruments may be required, depending on the type of operation and the surgical approach used.

Operative procedures

Ureteral anastomosis

1. The ureter is exposed through the desired incision, which is determined by the location of the ureteral reimplantation. A ureteral catheter, passed retrograde, may be used to facilitate identification and isolation of the ureter. The ureter is identified and dissected free with long forceps and scissors.
2. The ureter is picked up with fine traction sutures, freed from the surrounding tissues, and severed at the desired level.
3. The distal end of the ureter is ligated, and the proximal stoma is transferred to the site of anastomosis. The anastomosis is accomplished with fine dissection instruments and fine atraumatic sutures.
4. A soft splinting catheter is usually left in place until healing has taken place and free drainage is ensured.
5. The wound is closed in layers and dressed in the routine manner.

Ureterolithotomy. A kidney, ureter, and bladder x-ray film should be taken immediately before surgery to deter-

mine the exact location of the stone. The surgeon may also schedule a cystoscopic examination preoperatively and may attempt to remove the calculus endoscopically if the stone is in the most distal portion of the ureter.

The location of the calculus determines the surgical approach. A calculus high in the ureter requires a flank incision with possible removal of the twelfth rib; a more distal ureteral calculus requires a lower abdominal incision. Both of these have been described previously in some detail. After exposure of the ureter, the calculus may be kept stationary with Babcock clamps or vessel loops applied above and below the calculus. With a no. 15 blade, the incision in the ureter is made directly over the calculus. The calculus may then be easily removed with a Randall stone forceps. A 10 Fr catheter is passed proximally up and distally down the ureter while irrigating with saline to check for ureteral patency and to dislodge any remaining fragments of calculus. The ureter is closed with no. 4-0 or 5-0 absorbable sutures. All urologic stones should be placed in dry receptacles and sent to the chemistry laboratory for analysis. Either of the approaches described requires routine layer surgical closure.

Ureterocutaneous transplant, ureterosigmoid anastomosis, and ileal conduit are urinary diversionary procedures performed when the bladder is no longer functional as a proper urine reservoir. Following are etiologic factors in causing irreparable vesical dysfunction: chronic inflammation, interstitial cystitis, neurogenic bladder, exstrophy, trauma, tumor, or infiltrative disease (amyloidosis).

Ureterocutaneous transplant (anastomosis). The surgical approach is the same as for a low ureterolithotomy, and the ureter is divided as far distally as possible. The severed ureter is passed retroperitoneally through the lower abdominal wall and is sutured to the skin with an absorbable, everting suture of no. 4-0 on an atraumatic needle to form a stoma. The ureter is handled gently with plastic instruments, fixation forceps, and iris scissors. A small Silastic stenting catheter is passed up into the ureter and is left in situ for 48 to 72 hours, during which time ureteral edema subsides. The patient will require a urine-collecting device after surgery.

Ureterosigmoid anastomosis

1. The peritoneal cavity is entered in the routine manner through a lower left paramedian incision. The major portion of the large bowel is protected with moist packs. Deep retractors are placed in position, and with long forceps and scissors the posterior peritoneum is incised.
2. The ureters are identified and divided close to the bladder. The ureters are mobilized and brought through the posterior peritoneal incision to lie near the sigmoid. Traction sutures and smooth tissue forceps are used to handle the ureters.
3. The sigmoid colon is mobilized to prevent tension on the ureteroenteric anastomosis. The sigmoid colon is sutured with no. 3-0 nonabsorbable material to the pelvic peritoneum at a point where the ureter falls easily on the bowel. Using a scalpel with a no. 15 blade, an incision is made into the tenia of the sigmoid down to

the mucosal layer. The edges of the tenia are undermined to create two parallel flaps.
4. The ureter is laid on the bowel mucosa, and a small slit is made through the mucosa into the lumen of the colon.
5. With fixation forceps and iris scissors, the ureter is beveled to lie flat in the tunical incision. The distal ureter is anchored to the bowel mucosa with no. 4-0 absorbable ureteral sutures on atraumatic needles. The other ureter is anastomosed in the same manner in a position slightly above the first.
6. The tunicae are then loosely reapproximated over the ureter with no. 4-0 absorbable sutures, creating an antireflux anastomosis.
7. The posterior peritoneum is closed with fine, nonabsorbable sutures. Drains are brought out retroperitoneally. The incision is closed, and the wound is dressed.

Procedures for opening the kidney

Nephrotomy is incision into the kidney, usually over a collecting system containing a calculus. *Pyelotomy* is incision into the renal pelvis used as an access to stones in the renal pelvis or collecting system. *Pyelostomy* is an

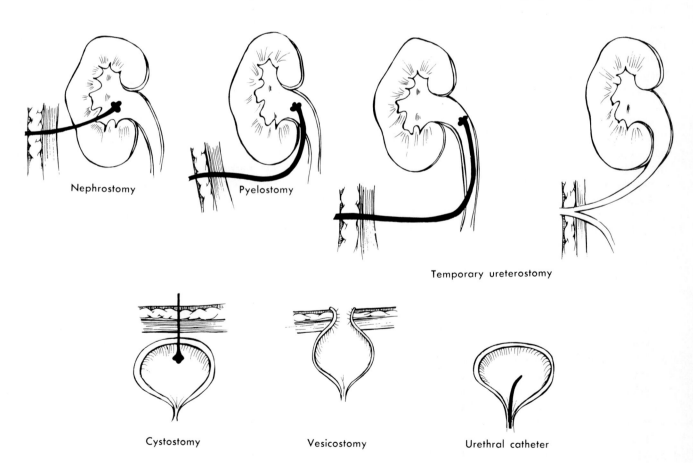

Nephrostomy   Pyelostomy

Temporary ureterostomy

Cystostomy   Vesicostomy   Urethral catheter

Fig. 15-76. Types of urinary diversions. (From Sabiston, D.C., Jr., editor: Davis-Christopher textbook of surgery: the biological basis of modern surgical practice, ed. 12, Philadelphia, 1981, W.B. Saunders Co.)

opening made in the renal pelvis for temporarily or permanently diverting the flow of urine (Fig. 15-76). *Pyelolithotomy* is removal of a calculus through an opening in the renal pelvis. *Nephrostomy* is creation of an opening into the kidney to maintain temporary or permanent urinary drainage (Fig. 15-76). A nephrostomy is used to correct an obstruction of the urinary tract and to conserve and permit physiologic functioning of renal tissue. It is also used to provide permanent urinary drainage when a ureter is obstructed or temporary urinary drainage immediately following a plastic repair on the kidney or renal pelvis.

Operative procedures

Pyelotomy or pyelostomy. The pelvis of the kidney is incised with a small scalpel blade. Fine traction sutures may be placed at the edges of the incision for gentle retraction while the pelvis and calyces are explored. In pyelostomy a small Malecot catheter is placed through the incision into the renal pelvis. Pyelotomy should be used only for very short periods of renal drainage, because tubes tend to dislodge easily from the renal pelvis.

Nephrostomy. A curved clamp or stone forceps is passed through a pyelotomy incision into the renal pelvis and then out through the substance of the renal parenchyma via a lower pole minor calyx. The tip of a Malecot or Pezzer catheter is drawn into the renal pelvis, and the pyelotomy incision is sutured closed. The distal end of the nephrostomy tube is brought out through a separate stab incision in the flank. A two-way Foley catheter is frequently used for this purpose. A drain is placed at the level of the pyelotomy incision, and all layers are closed in the regular manner.

Pyelolithotomy and nephrolithotomy. The renal pelvis is opened (Fig. 15-77), and the pelvic calculus gently removed. The pelvis and collecting systems are thoroughly irrigated with saline using an Asepto syringe to dislodge the small remaining calculi and remove them from the kidney. Nephrolithotomy is employed when calculi are locked in the calyceal system and cannot be removed through a pyelotomy incision. In such cases the renal parenchyma above the calculus is incised and the calculus removed. In many instances such a situation is associated with a calyceal diverticulum. After removal of the calculus, the collecting system is closed and the renal cortex reapproximated with deep hemostatic no. 2-0 absorbable sutures.

A nephroscope is sometimes used to localize and remove calyceal calculi (Fig. 15-78). It is also useful in staghorn calculi nephroscopy to remove residual fragments in the pelvic portion of the calculus.

Closure. An incision in the renal pelvis may be closed with no. 4-0 absorbable atraumatic sutures. The renal fossa is drained and closed, as for nephrectomy. Reinforced absorbent dressings are useful, because generally some urinary leakage occurs for 3 to 4 days after surgery.

Nephroureterectomy

Nephroureterectomy is removal of a kidney and its entire ureter. This procedure is indicated for hydroureteronephrosis of such a degree that reconstructive repair is impossible. It is also employed for collecting system tumors of the kidney and ureter.

Procedural considerations. This procedure usually requires two separate incisions: a flank incision to facilitate exposure and delivery of the kidney, and a lower hemi-suprapubic incision to free the lower portion of the ureter from the bladder. Only one instrument set is required, but

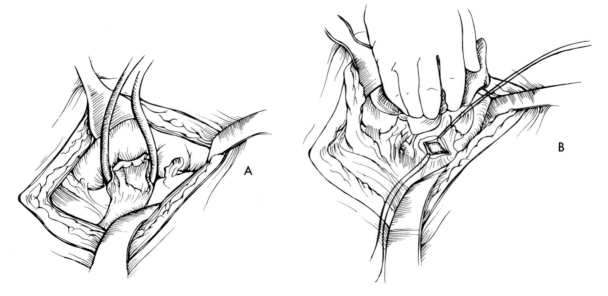

Fig. 15-77. Pyelolithotomy. **A,** Exposing renal pelvis. **B,** Incision into renal pelvis. (Modified from Dodson, A.I.: Urological surgery, ed. 4, St. Louis, 1970, The C.V. Mosby Co.)

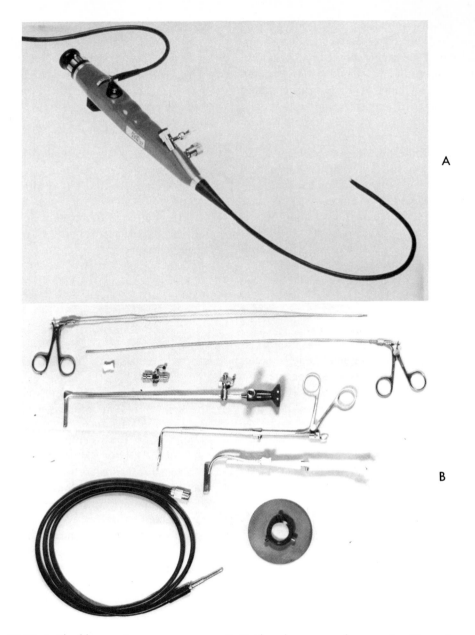

Fig. 15-78. A, Flexible percutaneous neproscope. **B,** Rigid nephroscope and accessories. (**A** courtesy American ACMI, Stamford, Conn.)

a second skin preparation setup and set of sterile drapes are necessary.

Operative procedure

1. The patient is placed in a lateral position. The kidney and upper ureter are exposed, as described for nephrectomy. Simple nephrectomy is performed as previously described. The kidney is placed in a plastic bag to prevent possible spillage of tumor cells. The ureter is not cut at this time but is mobilized as far distally as possible.

2. The operating room bed is adjusted so surgery on the lower ureter may proceed. The abdomen is prepped,

sterile drapes are applied, and an abdominal incision is made to expose the lower ureter and bladder on the operative side. These structures are identified and mobilized. The ureter and a small cuff of the bladder are removed in continuity, and the bladder is repaired with a single layer of no. 2-0 absorbable interrupted sutures.

3. The ureter and cuff of bladder may be pulled superiorly into the flank incision, where the intact kidney and ureter may be removed from the surgical field.

4. A 18 or 20 Fr Foley catheter is left in the bladder, and a drain is placed behind the bladder. Both incisions are closed in sequence in the usual manner.

Reconstructive operations on the kidney

Pyeloplasty is revision or plastic reconstruction of the renal pelvis. *Ureteroplasty* is reconstruction of the ureter distal to the ureteropelvic junction. *Foley Y-V pyeloureteroplasty* is combined correction of a redundant renal pelvis and resection of a stenotic portion of the ureteropelvic junction (Fig. 15-79). Pyeloplasty is done to create a better anatomic relationship between the renal pelvis and the proximal ureter and to allow proper urinary drainage from the kidney to the bladder. A temporary nephrostomy is usually included in such surgery to protect the plastic reconstruction of the ureteropelvic junction. Usually, tissue healing has occurred in 10 to 12 days, and the nephrostomy tube is removed once ureteral patency is demonstrated.

Procedural considerations. The instrument setup is as described for nephrectomy, plus the following:

1 Schnidt gall duct forceps, small
1 Metzenbaum dissecting scissors, small, straight, and fine
1 Metzenbaum dissecting scissors, small, curved, and fine
1 Iris scissors, curved
2 Vascular tissue forceps, plain, 7 inches
2 Vascular tissue forceps with teeth, 7 inches
2 Vascular needle holders, 7 inches
12 Mosquito hemostats, straight and curved, 5 inches
Ureteral catheter for splinting
Red rubber catheters, 8 and 10 Fr
5 Randall stone forceps
Chromic sutures, fine, on atraumatic needles

Operative procedure

1. The kidney and upper ureter are exposed, as described for nephrectomy, by the desired surgical approach.

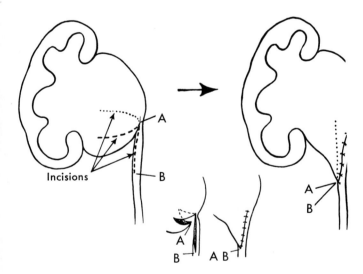

Fig. 15-79. Plastic Y-V repair (Foley type) for ureteropelvic obstruction at outlet of renal pelvis. This is actually conversion of Y incision in three dimensions into two-dimensional V incision. Nephrostomy and splinting catheter through anastomosis are usually employed. (From Marshall, V.F.: Textbook of urology, ed. 2, New York, 1964, Harper & Row, Publishers.)

2. The renal pelvis and ureter are incised, trimmed, and shaped to the desired contour with fine forceps and scissors. A caliper and a ruler may be used for establishing more precise relationships when plastic repair is undertaken. Anchoring sutures or soft rubber drains may be used for traction during reconstruction of the renal pelvis. All suture material used in such repairs is absorbable.

The Foley Y-V–plasty technique may be followed as shown in Fig. 15-79. It converts a Y-shaped surgical incision of the renal pelvis into a V as described in the illustrations. This provides a larger funnel-shaped uretero-pelvic junction. Interrupted no. 4-0 or 5-0 absorbable sutures are used in the repair.

3. A Silastic tubing may be used to stent the repaired pelvis until adequate healing has occurred. A nephrostomy tube is also placed within the pelvis to divert urine safely while the edema in the area of the plastic repair resolves.

4. A drain is placed where the pelvis was reconstructed, and the surgical incision is closed in layers.

Percutaneous nephrolithotomy and litholapaxy

Percutaneous nephrolithotomy and litholapaxy facilitate the removal or disintegration of renal stones using a rigid or flexible nephroscope (Fig. 15-78) passed through a percutaneous nephrostomy tract. Accessory instrumentation, such as the ultrasound wand (sonotrode), electrohydraulic lithotriptor probe, stone basket, or stone grasper, is passed through the lumen of the nephroscope to achieve the desired result.

The uroradiologic team develops criteria for patient selection. Ideally the patient is in good health and nonobese, and the calculus is no larger than 1 cm in diameter, free floating, radiopaque, and solitary. The patient may have had previous renal surgery or stone recurrence and may have an established nephrostomy tract. However, this technique may also be used for patients who have not had previous surgery. With advances in technology complemented by the experience gained by the uroradiology team, patients with more complex problems are being managed.

Creation of the nephrostomy tract and removal of the stone can be accomplished by three different methods.

In the one-step procedure, creation of the nephrostomy tract, tract dilatation, and stone removal are completed in a single session. The radiologist and urologist are both present, and the patient is managed with intravenous sedation.

In the immediate two-step procedure, the radiologist places the nephrostomy tube under radiographic guidance and the urologist removes the stone later the same day or the next morning. The second step is usually done in the operating room with the patient under general anesthesia.

In the delayed two-step procedure, the nephrostomy tract is established with the patient under local anesthesia.

The patient is discharged the following day with a 22 or 24 Fr nephrostomy tube connected to drainage. The patient is readmitted to the hospital 5 to 7 days later for the percutaneous removal of the calculus under general anesthesia.

Of basic concern during the operative phase are the patient's position, the type of anesthesia to be given, medications required during surgery, and catheter management during and after the procedure. The patient's position, which may be prone or up to 30 degrees prone-oblique, and the draping procedure depend on whether the surgical procedure is done in the radiology department or the operating room and the type of x-ray equipment that will be used.

Extracorporeal shock wave lithotripsy

A noninvasive approach to urolithiasis management is the use of the extracorporeal shock wave lithotriptor (ESWL). This device disintegrates kidney stones by introducing shock waves through a liquid medium into the body. Immediately before the procedure, an x-ray examination is made to pinpoint the position of the kidney stones. The anesthetized patient, often under epidural anesthesia, is then positioned and strapped to a gantry and lowered into a lithotriptor tub filled with specially treated water. Precise adjustments of the gantry are made to position the patient so the kidney stone is in the external focus of the ellipsoidal reflector. Alternatively, second-generation ESWL units use water-filled cushions adjacent to the kidney area. An x-ray image intensifier with two monitors is used to visualize the kidney stone at the focal point of the shock wave. After every 100 shocks, fluo-roscopy is used to locate remaining stone particles. Adjustments are made, and the patient is repositioned before further treatments. An x-ray examination is also made immediately after the procedure to determine the size and location of stone fragments ("gravel").

ESWL is often used in conjunction with percutaneous nephrolithotomy, surgery, and transurethral ureteropyeloscopy if the patient does not pass the gravel.

Nephrectomy

Nephrectomy is the surgical removal of a kidney. It is performed as a means of definitive therapy for a number of renal problems, such as congenital ureteropelvic junction obstruction with severe hydronephrosis, renal tumors, renal trauma, calculous disease with infection, cortical abscess, pyelonephrosis, and renovascular hypertension.

Procedural considerations. In routine renal surgery the patient is placed in the lateral position with the loin directly over the kidney rest. The operative flank is uppermost, with the patient's back brought to the edge of the operating room bed. The upper arm is supported on an overhead arm support, and the lower arm flexed at the elbow so that the hand rests on or under the head pillow. The patient's legs are positioned by placing a pillow between them and flexing the lower leg at the knee. The upper leg remains extended. The kidney rest is then raised, and when the desired bed flexion is achieved, 3-inch adhesive tape is used to stabilize the patient throughout surgery. Routine skin preparation and draping procedures are carried out.

The nephrectomy setup includes routine laparotomy setup, kidney instruments (Fig. 15-80), and the following:

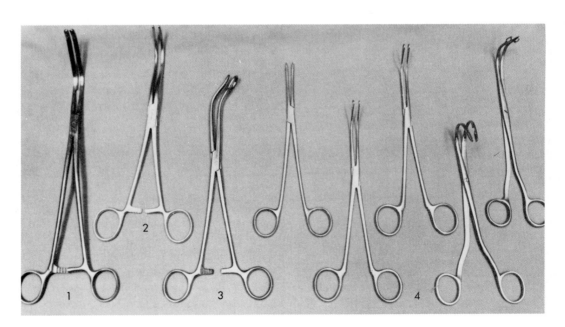

Fig. 15-80. Kidney instruments. *1,* Satinsky pedicle clamp; *2,* Mayo pedicle clamp; *3,* Lewkowitz lithotomy forceps; *4,* set of five Randall stone forceps.

2 Satinsky, Herrick, or Mayo pedicle clamps
1 Lewkowitz lithotomy forceps
5 Randall stone forceps, varied sizes
1 Silver probe (Bakes dilators may be used)
  Rubber catheter, 8 or 10 Fr
  Asepto syringe
  Pezzer or Malecot catheter
  Closed wound drainage system
  Vessel loops

In certain nephrectomies, the chest or the gastrointestinal tract may be opened. If the chest is opened, appropriate instruments and suction are needed. When the gastrointestinal tract is opened, precautions must be taken in the anastomosis and closure techniques. For rib resection, the following instruments are added to the nephrectomy setup:

1 Finochietto rib retractor, large
1 Matson costal periosteotome
1 Alexander costal periosteotome
2 Doyen rib raspatories, right and left

1 Bethune rib cutter
1 Double-action duckbill rongeur
1 Bailey rib approximator
1 Langenbeck periosteal elevator

Operative procedure (lumbar approach)

1. The incision is carried through the skin, fat, and fascia (Fig. 15-81, *A*). Bleeding vessels are clamped with hemostats and ligated.
2. The external oblique, internal oblique, and transversalis muscles are sequentially exposed and incised in the direction of the initial skin incision.
3. If necessary, a rib or ribs (eleventh or twelfth) may be resected to provide better access to the kidney. The periosteum is stripped with an Alexander costal periosteotome and Doyen rib raspatory.
4. A scalpel and heavy scissors may be used to cut through the lumbocostal ligaments. The rib is grasped with an Ochsner clamp and cut with rib shears, removing the portion necessary to expose the kidney.

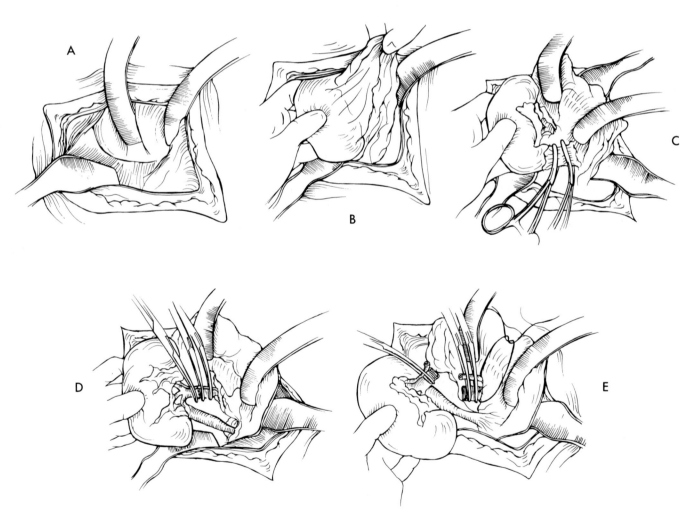

Fig. 15-81. Nephrectomy. **A,** Incision. **B,** Gerota's fascia. **C,** Clamping of ureter. **D,** Clamping of renal vein and artery. **E,** Excision of kidney. (From Dodson, A.I.: Urological surgery, ed. 4, St. Louis, 1970, The C.V. Mosby Co.)

5. Gerota's fascia is identified and incised with Metzenbaum scissors (Fig. 15-81, *B*). The incision is extended, and the kidney and perirenal fat are exposed by blunt and sharp dissection. *Note:* All perirenal fat that is removed during surgery may be saved in a small basin of normal saline. Perirenal fat may be used later as a bolster to stop bleeding.

6. The ureter is identified, separated from its adjacent structures, doubly clamped, divided, and ligated with absorbable no. 0 material (Fig. 15-81, *C*).

7. The kidney pedicle containing the major blood vessels is isolated and doubly clamped; each vessel is triply ligated with heavy ties (Fig. 15-81, *D*). Each vessel is then severed, leaving two ligatures remaining on the pedicle, and the kidney is removed (Fig. 15-81, *E*).

8. The renal fossa is explored for bleeding, and necessary hemostasis achieved. The fossa is then irrigated with normal saline, and the irrigant removed by suction. A drain is placed in the empty fossa and brought out through a separate stab incision in the skin.

9. The fascia and muscles are closed in layers with interrupted, absorbable sutures. If necessary, retention sutures may be used in obese or chronically ill individuals in whom wound healing may be a problem. The skin edges are approximated with interrupted sutures or with skin staples.

10. The drain is secured, and the wound dressed.

Heminephrectomy

Heminephrectomy is removal of a portion of the kidney. It is usually indicated for conditions involving the lower or upper pole of the kidney, such as calculous disease, or trauma limited to one pole of a kidney. In rare instances in which a patient has only one kidney, such surgery may be used for renal neoplasms to avoid the need for dialysis and subsequent renal transplantation.

Procedural considerations. The setup is as described for nephrectomy.

Operative procedure

1. The kidney and its pedicle should be completely mobilized as described for nephrectomy.

2. The main vessels may be temporarily occluded for only 20 to 30 minutes, after which progressive renal damage may occur. Local hypothermia may be indicated to prolong ischemic operating time.

3. The renal capsule is incised and stripped back. A wedge of kidney tissue containing the diseased or damaged cortex is excised (Fig. 15-82, *A*). Interlobar fat or arcuate and interlobular arteries are clamped with Hopkins' clamps and suture ligated with no. 4-0 absorbable suture on urologic needles.

4. The open collecting system is reapproximated with a continuous no. 4-0 suture.

5. Perirenal fat is placed in the area in which tissue was excised, and the renal parenchyma is reapproximated with horizontal mattress sutures (Fig. 15-82, *B*). If possible, the renal capsule is reapproximated with a continuous no. 2-0 suture.

Radical nephrectomy

Radical nephrectomy is excision of kidney, perirenal fat, adrenal gland, Gerota's capsule (fascia), and contiguous periaortic lymph nodes. This procedure is performed for parenchymal renal neoplasms. A lumbar, transthoracic, or transabdominal approach to the kidney is performed, depending on the size and location of the lesion. The transthoracic or transabdominal approach is preferred be-

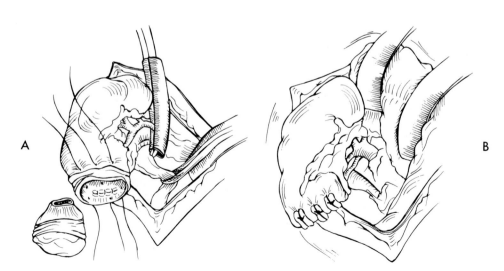

Fig. 15-82. Heminephrectomy. **A,** Resection of diseased kidney tissue. **B,** Suture line. (From Dodson, A.I.: Urological surgery, ed. 4, St. Louis, 1970, The C.V. Mosby Co.)

cause the blood vessels of the kidney can be more easily reached and ligated before the tumor is mobilized, thus decreasing the possibility of tumor embolization into the bloodstream.

Procedural considerations. The setup is as described for nephrectomy.

Operative procedure

1. In general, the procedure is as described for nephrectomy with two exceptions: (a) the renal pedicle is ligated before the kidney is mobilized, and (b) Gerota's capsule is not incised but is removed en bloc with the kidney.
2. Involved lymph nodes surrounding the renal pedicle are excised.
3. A chest tube is inserted if the transthoracic approach is used.

Kidney transplant

Kidney transplant entails transplantation of a living related or cadaveric donor kidney into the recipient's iliac fossa (Fig. 15-83).

A kidney transplant is performed in an effort to restore renal function and thus maintain life in a patient who has end-stage renal disease.

Transplant from a living donor

The kidney donor must be in perfect health. A complete workup verifies the presence of two normal kidneys. Blood

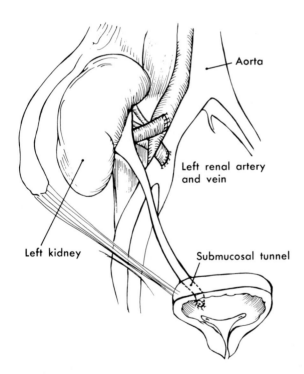

Fig. 15-83. Transplanted kidney in recipient's iliac fossa. (From Flocks, R.H., and Clup, D.A.: Surgical urology, 4th ed. Copyright © 1975 by Year Book Medical Publishers, Inc., Chicago. Used by permission.)

type, tissue type, and lymphocyte cross-matching determine donor-recipient compatibility. An arteriogram visualizes the renal arterial status and rules out the presence of renal lesions. A kidney with a single renal artery is preferred, but kidneys with double and triple arteries may be used if necessary.

The ideal living donor is an identical twin, although any immediate family member (usually a sibling or parent) may be a donor if the person is medically acceptable.

Procedural considerations. Two adjacent operating rooms are prepared for the procedures; surgery on the donor and recipient proceeds simultaneously.

A Foley catheter is inserted and left in the donor's bladder to measure urinary output and prevent bladder distention from the increased urine production induced by diuretics. The donor is placed in the lateral position, prepared from midchest to midthigh, and draped in the usual manner, exposing the flank area.

Required instruments and equipment are identical to the nephrectomy setup plus the following for the sterile perfusion table (Fig. 15-84):

    1 IV pole
      Electrolyte solution (in iced basin until needed)
    2 Intravenous extension tubes, sterile
    1 Kidney basin with cold (4° C) intravenous saline solution
    1 Stopcock, three-way
    1 Needle catheter (Medicut), 18-gauge
    6 Mosquito hemostats
    2 Vascular forceps, fine, 3 inches
    1 Metzenbaum scissors, fine
    1 Suture scissors
    1 Kelly hemostat

An electrolyte solution of Ringer's lactate, Solu-Medrol, and lidocaine 1% is commonly used to perfuse the harvested kidney. Collins' or Sachs' solution may be used to perfuse cadaveric kidneys following harvest but should never be used to perfuse a kidney from a living donor because of the potential effect of elevated potassium in the recipient owing to residual perfusate in the kidney.

Operative procedure

1. The donor nephrectomy procedure is as described for nephrectomy; however, the ureter and renal vein and artery require meticulous dissection.
2. Maximum length of the ureter is achieved by dividing it at or below the pelvic rim if possible. To preserve adequate ureteral vascularization, the surgeon is cautious not to skeletonize the ureter.
3. Particular care must be taken to remove the maximum length of the renal vein and artery. To obtain the maximum length of the right renal vein sometimes requires partial occlusion of the inferior vena cava with a Satinsky clamp and dissection of a portion of the inferior vena cava. Repair of the inferior vena cava is made with a continuous no. 4-0 or 5-0 vascular suture.
4. Five minutes before the surgeon clamps the renal vessels, 5000 units of heparin sodium is systemically ad-

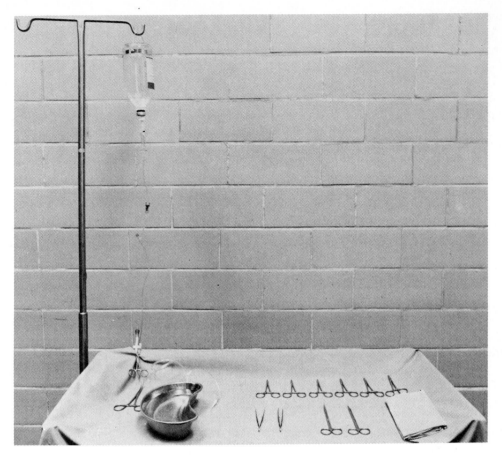

Fig. 15-84. Kidney perfusion table setup.

ministered to the patient to prevent intravascular clotting. Immediately after the kidney is removed from the donor, 50 mg of protamine sulfate is given intravenously to reverse the heparinization. Furosemide, mannitol, and intravenous fluids are administered to the donor to maintain adequate urinary output from the donor's remaining kidney.

5. Gentle handling of the kidney is essential. Team members must prevent undue traction on the vascular pedicle, which may induce vasospasm and reduce perfusion of the kidney.

6. To reduce warm ischemia time, the surgeon double-clamps the vein and the artery, excises the kidney, and immediately places it in cold saline solution on a sterile back table where the kidney is flushed with the designated electrolyte solution. Warm ischemia time (from the clamping of renal vessels to a point at which the kidney is perfused with cold electrolyte solution) should be kept to a minimum to prevent acute tubular necrosis and to maintain maximum renal function after transplantation. Mosquito clamps and fine vascular forceps are used to expose the renal artery to permit insertion of a needle catheter, for example, a Medicut. The cold electrolyte solution passes through the intra-

venous tubing and the needle catheter, flushing any remaining donor's blood from the kidney. This also decreases the kidney's metabolic rate by lowering its temperature. Flushing time is usually 2 to 5 minutes. After flushing, trimming the vessels of adventitia may be necessary to facilitate the vascular anastomosis to the recipient's iliac vessels.

7. The kidney, in cold saline solution, is covered with sterile drapes and taken by the surgeon to the room in which the recipient's iliac vessels have been exposed.

8. Wound closure for the donor is as described for nephrectomy.

Transplant from a cadaveric donor

The ideal cadaveric donor is young, free of infection and cancer, normotensive until a short time before death, and under hospital observation several hours before death. Permission to harvest the donor kidney must be obtained from the family and the medical examiner after brain death has been unequivocally established. Awareness of existing state legislation in this complex area is advisable.

Procedural considerations. After brain death has been established, the donor is taken to the surgical suite with respiratory and cardiac function maintained mechanically.

The donor is placed in the supine position and is prepared for a laparotomy. Anticoagulant and alpha-adrenergic blocking agents are administered systemically during the procedure. Adequate renal perfusion and function are maintained with intravenous fluids and diuretics.

Instruments and equipment are the same as for the nephrectomy setup, excluding the rib instruments and adding the following:

Cutting instruments

1 Metzenbaum scissors, 9¼ inches
1 Suture scissors, 9¼ inches
1 Metzenbaum scissors, fine
1 Suture scissors

Holding instruments

2 Vascular forceps, fine
3 DeBakey forceps, 4, 7, and 10 inches

Clamping instruments

12 Dean hemostatic forceps
12 Mosquito hemostats
 6 DeBakey clamps, angled
   Clip appliers with medium and large clips
 6 Bulldog clamps
 4 Vascular clamps, angled, large

Exposing instruments

2 Deaver retractors, extrawide
2 Harrington splanchnic retractors, small and large

Suturing instruments

4 Vascular needle holders, 2 short and 2 long

Accessory items

 Electrolyte solution (Sachs or Collins, cold (in iced basin
   until needed)
1 IV pole
2 Intravenous extension tubes, sterile
1 Kidney basin with cold (4° C) intravenous saline solution
1 Stopcock, three-way
1 Needle catheter (Medicut), 18-gauge
1 Centimeter ruler
1 Electrosurgical unit
 Perfusion machine or kidney transplant equipment and ice

Operative procedure

1. A midline incision is made from the xiphoid process to the symphysis pubis with bilateral supraumbilical transverse extensions through the skin, subcutaneous layer, fascia, and muscle.
2. Hemostasis is obtained with clamps, ties, suture ligatures, and electrocoagulation.
3. The kidney, renal vessels, and ureter are carefully dissected with Metzenbaum scissors, DeBakey forceps, and Dean hemostatic forceps.
4. Heparin sodium, 15,000 units, is given intravenously 5 to 10 minutes before clamping the renal vessels.

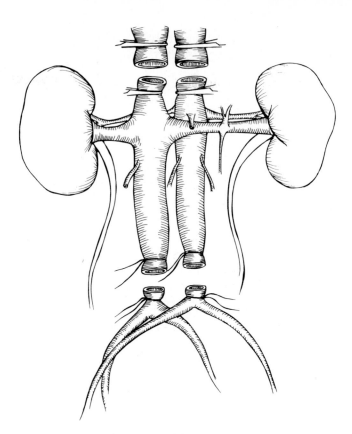

Fig. 15-85. En bloc resection.

5. One method of resection is en bloc resection (harvesting of donor kidneys) (Fig. 15-85), which involves the removal of sections of the inferior vena cava and aorta with both kidneys in continuity. An incision is made along the route of the small bowel mesentery up to the esophageal hiatus. The entire gastrointestinal tract, spleen, and inferior portion of the pancreas are mobilized by dividing the celiac axis and the superior mesenteric artery, exposing the entire retroperitoneal region. The inferior vena cava and aorta are clamped below the renal vessels with vascular clamps, and the vessels are divided. Lumbar tributaries are secured with metal clips and are divided. The kidneys and ureters are freed from their surrounding soft tissues. The ureters are divided distally at the pelvic brim. The suprarenal aorta and inferior vena cava are clamped and divided at the level of the diaphragm. The vessels and kidneys are severed from the surgical field, and the aorta and vena cava are ligated.
6. After removal of the kidneys, immediate perfusion with cold (4° C) electrolyte solution is carried out as in step 5 for a donor kidney.
7. The kidneys are placed in a container of cold saline solution and surrounded by saline slush in an insulated carrier or placed on a hypothermic pulsatile perfusion machine for transport (Fig. 15-86).

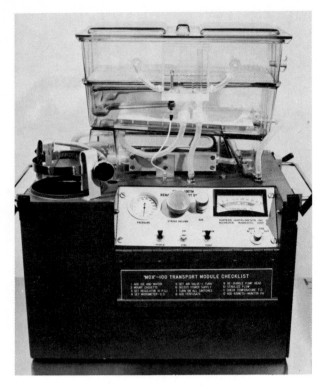

Fig. 15-86. Waters hypothermic, pulsatile perfusion machine for transport of donor organs.

8. While kidney perfusion is begun, the abdominal lymph nodes and spleen are removed for use in tissue typing.
9. The incision is closed with interrupted sutures.
10. Artificial life-support systems are terminated.

Transplant recipient

Each potential recipient is judged individually in regard to kidney transplantation. Most persons below the age of 55 years are acceptable; older patients are less tolerant of postoperative complications. Transplantation in infants is still experimental. Contraindications for renal transplantation include (1) systemic disease that precludes major surgery, (2) oxalosis, (3) active cancer, and (4) Fabry's disease. If required, a patient may need to undergo bilateral nephrectomy before renal transplantation for the following reasons: (1) to control hypertension; (2) to remove infected, bleeding, or polycystic kidneys; and (3) to remove the ureters if vesicoureteral reflux exists. A splenectomy may also be performed at this time to decrease the leukopenic and thrombocytopenic effects of immunosuppressive drugs.

Procedural considerations. The patient is placed in the supine position. A Foley catheter with an attached Silastic stenting catheter is inserted in the bladder by sterile technique. From 50 to 75 ml of antibiotic solution is instilled in the bladder through a sterile catheter tip syringe,

allowed to remain for 20 minutes, and drained. The patient is prepped from nipples to knees and is draped in the routine manner.

Instruments and equipment required are the routine laparotomy setup, plus the following:

Cutting instruments

1 Metzenbaum scissors, 9¼ inches
1 Suture scissors, 9¼ inches
1 Metzenbaum scissors, fine
1 Suture scissors, fine
1 Potts scissors, angled

Holding instruments

3 DeBakey forceps, 4, 7, and 10 inches
2 Vascular forceps, fine, 3 inches

Clamping instruments

12 Dean hemostatic forceps
12 Mosquito hemostats, straight
 6 Mosquito hemostats, curved
 6 DeBakey clamps, angled
 2 Clip appliers with medium and large clips
 3 Bulldog clamps, curved
 3 Bulldog clamps, straight

Exposing instruments

2 Harrington splanchnic retractors, small and large

Suturing instruments

4 Vascular needle holders, 2 long and 2 short

Accessory items

2 Asepto syringes
1 Centimeter ruler
1 Needle catheter (Medicut), 18-gauge on 10-ml syringe
1 Closed wound drainage system
 Electrosurgical unit
1 Pediatric feeding tube, 5 Fr
1 Stockinette, 3 × 10 inches
 Heparin sodium solution (1:1000)
 Intravenous saline solution, cold (4° C)

Operative procedure

1. A curved, lower quadrant incision is made through the skin, subcutaneous layer, fascia, and muscle. Bleeding is controlled with clamps, ties, and electrocoagulation.
2. The inferior epigastric vessels are divided between suture ligatures. A retroperitoneal dissection is performed by mobilizing the peritoneum superiorly and medially. A Balfour self-retaining retractor is placed in the wound for exposure, and a wide Deaver retractor is inserted to reflect the peritoneum superiorly and medially.
3. With the use of the 9½-inch Metzenbaum scissors and the DeBakey forceps, dissection is made along the entire length of the external and common iliac arteries to the bifurcation of the aorta and continuing down

the internal iliac artery. The internal iliac artery is ligated distally and divided, with proximal control maintained by a vascular clamp. The iliac vein is dissected free by ligating and dividing the internal iliac venous branches with no. 3-0 nonabsorbable sutures or ligating clips.

4. The donor kidney is brought into the operative field and placed in cold (4° C) intravenous saline solution.

5. Mosquito hemostats, 4-inch DeBakey forceps, and curved and straight fine scissors are used to make the necessary alterations on the donor kidney vessels to facilitate the anastomoses.

6. The donor kidney is returned to the cold intravenous saline solution until the time of the anastomosis.

7. Two angled DeBakey vascular clamps are placed on the internal iliac vein. A no. 11 blade is used to make a 1-cm incision in the iliac vein between the clamps. The vessel is rinsed with heparin sodium solution (10 units/ml) in the Asepto syringe. An angled Potts scissors is used to extend the incision to accommodate the donor renal vein.

8. The donor kidney is placed in the 3 × 10 inch, cold saline–soaked stockinette, with the renal vessels exiting from a hole in the side. Use of the stockinette prevents direct contact with the kidney and therefore trauma. The renal vein is anastomosed to the side of the recipient's iliac vein with no. 5-0, double-armed, vascular sutures. In like manner, the renal artery is anastomosed end to end with the proximal portion of the internal iliac artery using no. 5-0 vascular sutures. The vessels are irrigated proximally and distally with heparin sodium solution by using the 10-ml syringe attached to the Medicut catheter before placing the final sutures.

9. The stockinette is removed for adequate visualization of the entire kidney.

10. The angled DeBakey clamps are removed from the venous vessels, and the anastomosis is checked for leakage. Immediately afterward, the clamps on the internal iliac artery are released, and the anastomosis is checked. Meticulous inspection is made of the hilum and surface of the kidney for bleeding and infarction. Diuretics are given intravenously as needed.

11. Attention is now directed to the ureter and bladder. Two long Allis forceps are used to grasp the anterior bladder wall. Using a scalpel with a no. 10 knife blade, a 4-cm incision is made anteriorly. Two narrow Harrington retractors and one narrow Deaver retractor are inserted in the bladder for exposure. The ureter is passed through the bladder wall and tunneled suburothelially for 2 to 2.5 cm. The spatulated end of the ureter is then sutured into the bladder urothelium with four to six no. 4-0 or 5-0 atraumatic absorbable sutures, creating a ureteroneocystostomy.

12. A 5 Fr pediatric infant feeding tube is passed through the ureteroneocystostomy, up to the renal pelvis, and out through the urethra with the Foley catheter. This stenting catheter will remain in place for 36 to 48 hours to ensure ureteral patency during a period in which ureteral edema may occur.

13. Retractors are removed, and the bladder is closed in three layers:
   a. Continuous no. 4-0 absorbable suture for urothelial closure
   b. Interrupted no. 2-0 absorbable suture for closure of bladder muscles
   c. An imbricating layer of no. 2-0 nonabsorbable material to bury the suture line

14. The bladder is irrigated with normal saline to check for leaks.

15. The renal anastomoses are again checked for bleeding.

16. Three metal clips are placed on the superior, inferior, and lateral aspects of the kidney to radiographically measure renal size and determine postoperative swelling.

17. Retractors are removed from the incision.

18. Closed wound suction drains are inserted into the wound, brought through the skin laterally, and secured with no. 2-0 nonabsorbable suture on a cutting needle.

19. Muscle and fascial layers are closed with a single layer of no. 0 nonabsorbable sutures on a large atraumatic needle. The subcutaneous layer is closed with no. 3-0 absorbable sutures on an atraumatic needle. Skin closure is accomplished with skin staples.

20. Dressings are applied.

21. The bladder is irrigated with 50 to 75 ml of antibiotic solution to prevent infection and free any blood clots.

Operations on the adrenal glands
Adrenalectomy

Adrenalectomy is partial or total excision of one or both adrenal glands. It may be performed for several reasons: hypersecretion of adrenal hormones, neoplasms of the adrenal gland, or secondary treatment of neoplasms elsewhere in the body that are dependent on adrenal hormonal secretions, such as carcinoma of the prostate and breast.

Procedural considerations. For unilateral adrenalectomy the patient may be placed in the lateral or supine position (Chapter 6). More often, however, both glands are explored, and the supine or prone position is selected. The prone position is especially useful for debilitated patients with an advanced neoplasm.

Lateral approach. The setup for a lateral approach is as described for nephrectomy, including rib resection instruments, vascular instruments, and vessel clips and appliers.

Abdominal approach. The setup for an abdominal approach is as described for laparotomy, including vascular instruments, extra long scissors, tissue forceps, Rochester-Pean forceps, Mixter forceps, and needle holders. Penrose tubing is needed for retraction. Vessel clips and appliers may also be needed, as well as various sizes of silk sutures.

Operative procedures
Lateral approach

1. A flank incision is performed as described for nephrectomy. The twelfth and sometimes the eleventh ribs are resected for optimum exposure of the upper pole of the kidney.
2. An opening is made through the transverse fascia with scissors. The pleura and diaphragm are protected with moist packs, and Gerota's capsule is incised to expose the kidney and adrenal gland.
3. The gland is identified and dissected free from the upper pole of the kidney by scissors and Babcock forceps. The blood supply of the gland is identified, clamped or clipped, and divided. Bleeding vessels are ligated. To release the glands, the left adrenal vein, a branch of the left renal vein, is separated by clamping and cutting. The right adrenal vein, a tributary of the vena cava, is also divided. Fine vascular sutures may be required to repair inadvertent injury to the vena cava.
4. When hemostasis has been ensured, the wound is closed sequentially in layers: muscle, fascia, subcutaneous tissue, and skin.

Abdominal approach

1. The abdominal wall is incised with an upper abdominal incision, and the peritoneal cavity is opened and explored. Bleeding vessels are clamped and ligated.
2. The abdominal wound is retracted, and the surrounding organs are protected with moist laparotomy packs, using instruments and sutures as described for routine laparotomy.
3. The retroperitoneal area near the diaphragm is opened on the left side, exposing the renal fascia.
4. The renal fascia is opened to reveal the left kidney and adrenal gland.
5. The adrenal gland is freed from the kidney by sharp and blunt dissection, clamping and ligating all bleeding vessels with no. 3-0 nonabsorbable sutures.
6. After all bleeding is controlled, the kidney is gently replaced in the renal fascia, which is closed with interrupted no. 0 absorbable sutures.
7. The peritoneum is closed over the left kidney and renal fascia.
8. The abdominal retractors are rearranged to give access to the peritoneum over the right kidney and adrenal gland. Care must be taken to prevent trauma to the liver.
9. The same procedure is repeated on the right side, taking care to clamp and ligate the short adrenal vein.
10. The abdomen is inspected for bleeding vessels, which are clamped and ligated.
11. The wound is closed as in laparotomy.

REFERENCE

Soloway, M.S.: Evaluation and management of patient's superficial bladder cancer, Urol. Clin. North Am., 14:4, 1987, Philadelphia.

BIBLIOGRAPHY

Blasko, J.C., and others: Abstract—Transperineal ultrasound-guided implants of the prostate, Seattle, Wash., 1989.

Bush, I.M., Guinan, P., and Lanners, J.: Ureterenoscopy, Urol. Clin. North Am. 9:131, 1982.

Cawood, C.D.: Urologic endoscopy and instrumentation, Stamford, Conn., 1980, American Cystoscope Makers, Division of American Hospital Supply Corp.

Claymen, R.V., and Castaneda-Zuniga, W.R.: Techniques in endourology: a guide to the percutaneous removal of renal and ureteral calculi, Minneapolis, Minn., 1984.

Clayman, R.V., and others: Nephroscopy: advances and adjuncts, Urol. Clin. North Am. 9:51, 1982.

Cleaning, disinfecting and sterilizing patient care equipment: guidelines for handwashing and hospital environment, Atlanta, 1985, Centers for Disease Control.

Cooner, W.H., Eggers, G.W., and Lichtenstein, P.: Prostate cancer: new hope for early diagnosis, Ultrasonography in Urology, NYU Medical Center, 1988.

Ehrlich, R.: Modern techniques in surgery, Mt. Kisco, NY, 1980, Futura Publishing.

Expand extracorporeal shockwave lithotripsy, Urol. Times, July, 1983.

Furlow, W.L.: Implantation of a new semiautomatic artificial genitourinary sphincter: experience with primary activation and deactivation in 47 patients, J. Urol. 126:741, 1981.

Glenn, J.F., editor: Urologic surgery, ed. 2, New York, 1975, Harper & Row.

Goldstein, I.: Penile revascularization, Urol. Clin. North Am. 14:4, 1987.

Hofstetter, A., and others: Endoscopic neodymium-YAG laser application for destroying bladder tumors, Dept. of Urology, Municipal Hospital; Messerschmitt-Bolkow-Blohm; Institute of Pathology, Municipal Hospital Schwabing, Munich, Eur. Urol. 7:278, 1981.

Huffman, J.L., Bagley, D.H., and Lyon, E.S.: Ureteroscopy, Philadelphia, 1988, W.B. Saunders Co.

Jonas, U., and Jacobi, G.H.: Silicone-silver penile prosthesis: description, operative approach and results, J. Urol. 123:865, 1980.

Lerner, J., and Kahn, Z.: Mosby's manual of urologic nursing, St. Louis, 1982, The C.V. Mosby Co.

Malloy, T.R., Wein, A.J., and Carpiniello, V.L.: Surgical results with artificial urinary sphincter, Urology 19:6, 1982.

Montague, D.K., and others: Disorders of male sexual dysfunction, Chicago, 1988, Year Book Medical Publishers.

Phipps, W.J., Long, B.C., and Woods, N.F.: Medical-surgical nursing, ed. 4, St. Louis, 1991, The C.V. Mosby Co.

Reddy, P.K., and others: Balloon dilatation of the prostate for treatment of benign hyperplasia, Urol. Clin. North Am. 15:3, 1988.

Resnick, M.I., and others: The use of large and small bowel in urologic surgery, Urol. Clin. North Am. 13:2, 1986.

Skinner, D.G., and Lieskovsky, G.: Diagnosis and management of genitourinary cancer, Philadelphia, 1987, W.B. Saunders Co.

Shockwave lithotripsy cited, Urol. Times, Dec., 1984.

Smith, J.A., and others: Lasers and other technologic advances in urology, Urol. Clin. North Am. 13:3, 1986.

Thibodeau, G.A.: Anthony's textbook of anatomy and physiology, ed. 13, St. Louis, 1990, The C.V. Mosby Co.

Uroplasty TCU dilatation catheter: Clinical evaluator's manual, San Clemente, CA, 1989, Advanced Surgical Intervention.

Walsh, P.C., and others: Campbell's urology, ed. 5, 3 vols., Philadelphia, 1986, W.B. Saunders Co.

Wickham, J.E.A., and Miller, R.A.: Percutaneous renal surgery, Edinburgh, 1983, Churchill Livingstone.

16 Thyroid and parathyroid surgery

BILLIE FERNSEBNER

The thyroid gland functions primarily to secrete thyroxine, a hormone essential to metabolism. Surgery for goiter, long a part of modern surgery, has been reduced since the introduction of iodine therapy in 1923. Since 1941, indications for surgery on the thyroid gland have changed because of the use of radioactive iodine and antithyroid drugs that decrease the activity of the gland. Diseases of the thyroid gland that require surgical intervention are primarily nodules of the thyroid and diffuse toxic goiters associated with hyperthyroidism. Benign nodules are classified as adenomas, colloid nodules, thyroiditis, and cysts. Malignant lesions of the thyroid are rare and usually present in patients who received low-dose external radiation to the head and neck area or who have a family history of medullary cancer of the thyroid.

Diseases of the thyroid are usually manifested by alterations in hormonal secretion, enlargement of the thyroid, or both. Three forms of treatment are available: antithyroid drugs, radioactive iodine, and surgery. Prior to undergoing surgery, patients usually have their hyperthyroid state controlled with antithyroid drugs and potassium iodide. Patients thus treated are restored to a euthyroid state and do not exhibit the common symptoms of rapid pulse, tremors, and nervous symptoms often associated with hyperactivity of the thyroid gland.

The function of the parathyroid gland in body metabolism is most important. The endocrine secretion of parathormone regulates and maintains the metabolism and homeostasis of blood calcium concentrations. Removal of all parathyroid tissue results in severe tetany or death. The primary disease attributed to the parathyroid glands is hyperparathyroidism, which results in elevation of calcium in the blood. Disturbances of the parathyroid glands have been linked to tetany, bone disease, renal calculi, and many other systemic abnormalities. Surgical interest is focused on definitive treatment of hyperparathyroidism.

The diagnosis of hyperparathyroidism is being made more frequently with the increased use of diagnostic tests that include multiphasic screening of blood calcium. Manifestations may be quite subtle; many patients in whom hypercalcemia is determined are without any apparent symptoms.

SURGICAL ANATOMY
Thyroid gland

The thyroid gland is a highly vascular organ situated at the front of the neck. It consists of right and left lobes united by a middle portion, the isthmus. The isthmus is situated near the base of the neck, and the lobes lie below the larynx and beside the trachea. The upper pole of the gland is hidden beneath the upper end of the sternothyroid muscle. The lower pole extends to the sixth tracheal ring. The posterior surface of the isthmus is adherent to the anterior surface of the tracheal rings, and the gland is enclosed by the pretracheal fascia (Fig. 16-1).

Blood supply to the thyroid is from the external carotid arteries via the superior thyroid arteries and from the subclavian arteries via the inferior thyroid arteries. The thyroid gland is drained by three pairs of veins that extend from a plexus formed on the surface of the gland and on the front of the trachea. The capillaries form a dense plexus in the connective tissue around the follicles.

On each side the superior laryngeal nerve lies in proximity to the superior thyroid artery. The recurrent laryngeal nerve that supplies the vocal cord ascends from the mediastinum and is in close association with the tracheoesophageal sulcus and the inferior thyroid artery. Sympathetic and parasympathetic nerves enter the gland, probably exerting their influence primarily on blood flow. Numerous lymphatics of the pretracheal fascia and carotid sheath drain the gland.

The thyroid gland is important in maintaining the metabolic rate at a level compatible with health and efficiency. It is not, however, essential to life. Removal of the thyroid results in reduction of the oxidative processes of the body. Supplemental drugs help maintain a more normal metabolic rate for body processes.

The primary function of the thyroid gland is iodine metabolism. Ingested iodides are absorbed from the gastrointestinal tract into the circulatory system, from which they are sequestered by the thyroid gland. Iodides are converted into thyroid hormones, some of which are stored in the gland as thyroglobulin or are secreted into the blood as thyroid hormone.

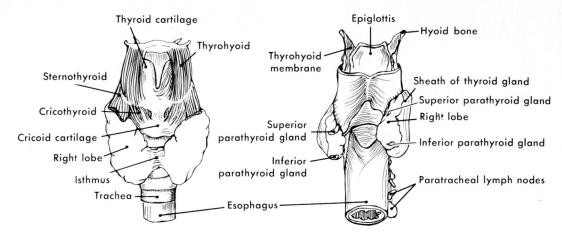

Fig. 16-1. Thyroid and parathyroid glands. Note their relation to each other and to trachea. *Left,* Anterior view; *right,* posterior view.

Parathyroid gland

The parathyroid glands consist of at least four small masses of tissue lying behind or, rarely, within the thyroid gland inside the pretracheal fascia. The upper pair of glands lies behind the superior pole of the thyroid; the lower pair lies near the lower pole of the thyroid (Fig. 16-1). Aberrant nodules of parathyroid tissue may be found outside the pretracheal fascia as low as the superior mediastinum, especially within the thymus. The glands are reddish to yellowish tan. Each normally measures 3 to 5 mm in diameter and weighs an average of 35 to 40 mg.

The parathyroid gland located dorsal to the upper pole of the thyroid receives its blood from the superior thyroid artery, and the venous blood returns via tributaries of the middle and inferior thyroid veins. The parathyroid gland located in the lower pole receives blood from the branches of the descending inferior thyroid artery and the intrathymic artery. A mediastinal parathyroid receives blood from the thymic branch of the internal mammary artery.

PERIOPERATIVE NURSING CONSIDERATIONS
Assessment/nursing diagnosis

Preoperatively, the patient with hyperthyroidism most likely has undergone appropriate drug therapy that has returned the thyroid hormone levels and metabolic state to normal. Nonetheless, the perioperative nurse should assess the patient for the presence of any symptoms that may relate to accelerated metabolism. They include irritability, hyperexcitability and exaggerated emotional responses, an abnormally elevated resting pulse, weight loss with fatigue and weakness, elevated systolic blood pressure, and cardiac symptoms such as congestive heart failure or atrial fibrillation, especially in the elderly patient. The patient's cardiac and respiratory rate, muscle strength, elimination patterns, history of weight loss and heat intolerance, and emotional status should be noted. The patient may be anxious about the disease state and the success of surgery and

may express concern regarding surgery in the area of the head and neck and its cosmetic results. Patients who are concerned about body image should have the opportunity to discuss these issues with the perioperative nurse. Skin integrity should be determined; patients with hyperthyroidism may have finely textured skin and edema in the lower extremities, placing them at risk for skin breakdown.

In addition to clinical signs and symptoms, results of diagnostic tests should be reviewed in the medical record. Tests performed most commonly prior to thyroid surgery include measurements of T_3 (triiodothyronine) and T_4 (thyroxine) and radioisotope or ultrasonic scans. Common laboratory and diagnostic tests and their normal ranges follow:

Direct and indirect measures of T_4 and T_3

Thyroid function tests are interpreted in light of the patient's clinical presentation. They complement the findings of physical examination.

Serum T_4 (T_4)
 Normal 4.9–12.0
Free thyroxine (FT_4)
 Normal 2.8 ± 0.5 ng/100 ml
Resin T_3 uptake (RT_3U)
 Normal 25–35%*
Free thyroxine index (FTI)
 Normal 6.4–10.5*
Radioactive iodine uptake (RAIU)
 Normal <25%*
Serum TSH (TSH)
 Normal 0–6 µU/ml*
Thyroxine-binding globulin capacity (TBG)
 Normal 15–25 µg T_4/100 ml ± 1.8 µg

*Variations with labs used

Assessment of thyroid anatomy

In addition to palpating the thyroid gland for size, contour, consistency, nodes, and fixation, scans yield evidence of thyroid anatomy.

Thyroid isotope scan
   Normal: Even distribution, normal size, shape and position
Ultrasonic scan
   Normal: Uniform tissue density

Tests used in the diagnosis of hyperparathyroidism are serum parathormone (reference value less than 25 pg/ml) and high-resolution real time ultrasonography.

Preoperative patient education should include an explanation of perioperative events, discussion and demonstration of the collar type of dressing to be used, and explanation of the closed wound suction drainage system, if its use is anticipated. The patient should also be instructed in ways to support the neck postoperatively to prevent strain on the incision line.

Hyperparathyroidism causes an imbalance in the level of serum calcium and a decrease in the level of serum phosphate. Nursing diagnoses and care planning will be based on these imbalances and the severity of the associated symptoms. Some patients are asymptomatic. Other patients have symptoms that manifest themselves as disturbances in the renal, gastrointestinal, cardiovascular, skeletal, or central nervous system.

Assessment should include determining whether the patient is apathetic or emotionally irritable; whether there is muscle weakness and fatigue; skeletal pain or tenderness; nausea; vomiting; constipation; peptic ulcer disease; cardiac dysrhythmias; or renal damage, stones, or disease. If any of these signs or symptoms are present, the plan of care should be adjusted. Otherwise, perioperative nursing management of the patient undergoing parathyroidectomy is essentially the same as for thyroidectomy. In the early postoperative period, the patient should be closely observed for any signs of tetany.

Assessment concludes with the formulation of nursing diagnoses. In addition to nursing diagnoses such as the potential for injury from positioning and the potential for impaired skin integrity, additional nursing diagnoses that are potential areas of concern for the patient undergoing thyroid or parathyroid surgery should be considered. These may include the following:

- Swallowing, impaired, related to mechanical obstruction (enlarged thyroid preoperatively; edema postoperatively)
- Body temperature, altered, due to altered metabolic rate
- Body image disturbance related to surgical scar in prominent location
- Potential for ineffective airway clearance related to obstruction (enlarged thyroid preoperatively; edema postoperatively)
- Potential for impaired gas exchange related to postoperative bleeding or swelling or inability to move secretions

Planning

During planning, specific goals and interventions are set to meet the patient's individual needs and to expedite the surgical intervention. In addition to goals of providing safe, effective, injury-free perioperative nursing care, additional goals based on nursing diagnoses for the patient undergoing thyroid or parathyroid surgery are developed. Part of all care planning involves the identification and anticipation of potential patient problems. Perioperative nurses act interdependently with the members of the anesthesia and surgical team in identifying and treating some of these potential problems.

A potential problem for patients with hyperthyroidism is thyroid storm (thyrotoxic crisis). It can occur in patients who are partially controlled or who are untreated for their hyperthyroidism. It rarely occurs with patients who are in a euthyroid state. Thyrotoxic crisis can be precipitated by a stressful event such as surgery. Collaborating with the surgical and anesthesia team, the perioperative nurse engages in interventions that are aimed at reducing body temperature and heart rate, prepares oxygen and intravenous solutions, and administers medications as prescribed.

A Sample Care Plan for the patient undergoing thyroid or parathyroid surgery is shown on p. 416. As in many perioperative care situations, nursing diagnoses and interventions extend through the preoperative, intraoperative, and postoperative phases. They have been identified as to phase of care where appropriate.

Implementation
Positioning

The patient is placed in a modified dorsal recumbent position, with an inflatable pillow or rolled sheet placed between the scapulae to extend the neck and raise the shoulders. The head is stabilized by placement on a doughnut or a foam headrest. Some surgeons prefer a doughnut placed inside a molded plastic "doggie" dish for more stability. If an inflatable pillow is used, it should be placed (uninflated) before the patient is anesthetized and then inflated. Some surgeons prefer to flex the OR bed and then level the legs and elevate the back until distended neck veins disappear. Others position the patient with the bed slanted downward in the reverse Trendelenburg's position. The latter necessitates the use of a padded footboard to keep the feet in proper alignment and prevent the patient from sliding down on the bed. The arms are positioned at the sides or placed on the abdomen with the elbows adequately protected by the lift sheet or elbow guards. The safety strap is placed snugly but not tightly across the thighs (see Chapter 6).

Skin preparation

The operative area, including the anterior neck region, lateral surfaces of the neck down to the outer aspects of the shoulder, and the upper anterior chest region, is pre-

Sample Care Plan

NURSING DIAGNOSIS:
Swallowing, impaired, related to mechanical obstruction (enlarged thyroid preoperatively; edema postoperatively)
GOAL:
Swallowing will be unimpaired; the patient will not aspirate secretions.
INTERVENTIONS:
Keep suction line and catheter ready until patient is discharged from OR.
Monitor for and report difficulty in swallowing.
Gently suction oropharyngeal secretions as required.
Keep vein open postoperatively until patient can swallow without difficulty.

NURSING DIAGNOSIS:
Body temperature, alterated, due to altered metabolic rate
GOAL:
Patient's body temperature will be maintained within normal range.
INTERVENTIONS:
Monitor patient's temperature; report abnormalities.
Provide light covers if temperature elevated or patient states he or she is warm.
Change linens preoperatively and postoperatively if wet from perspiration.
Avoid using plasticized drapes.

NURSING DIAGNOSIS:
Body image disturbance related to surgical scar
GOAL:
Patient will verbalize decreased disturbance in feelings related to body image.
INTERVENTIONS:
Explain that incision is made in natural fold of skin.
Explain how techniques used for surgical closure minimize scarring.
Suggest that jewelry, scarves, and certain necklines can be used to cover scar until normal fading occurs.

Instruct patient in postoperative turning measures that decrease strain on suture line.

NURSING DIAGNOSIS:
Potential for ineffective airway clearance related to obstruction secondary to enlarged thyroid (preoperatively) or edema (postoperatively)
GOAL:
Patient's airway will remain patent.
INTERVENTIONS:
Position patient so that enlarged gland does not obstruct airway. Head of transport vehicle may need to be elevated preoperatively.
Assist anesthesia personnel during induction.
Monitor respiratory rate and signs of respiratory distress (stridor, wheezing, dyspnea, labored respirations).
Observe dressing and neck area (front, sides, and back) for signs of edema or bleeding (postoperatively).

NURSING DIAGNOSIS:
Potential for impaired gas exchange related to postoperative bleeding/swelling or inability to move secretions
GOAL:
Patient's gas exchange will remain effective.
INTERVENTIONS:
Monitor respiratory status and results of pulse oximetry.
If patient is extubated in OR, be prepared to assist anesthesia personnel; closely observe for respiratory stridor or respiratory obstruction (recurrent laryngeal nerve injury). Tracheostomy may be required.
Assess color of nailbeds.
Monitor surgical site for swelling and/or bleeding.
Suction patient as required to remove secretions (trach tray should be available).

pared with an antimicrobial solution. Appropriate precautions must be taken to prevent solution from pooling under the neck or in the axillary spaces. The patient is draped with sterile towels and a fenestrated sheet.

The surgeon marks the incision site with a "scratch" of a scalpel in the normal neck creases and skin lines, which helps to ensure a wound line that blends with the patient's neck anatomy.

Instrumentation

A standard instrument setup for thyroid surgery includes the following:

Soft tissue/plastic surgery instruments

2 Knife handles, 1 each no. 3 and no. 7
2 Tissue forceps, Brown Adson
10 Straight mosquito hemostats
10 Curved mosquito hemostats
4 Allis forceps
2 Baby Moynihans
4 Kochers
1 Jacobson forceps
2 Plastic needle holders, 5 inch
2 Vascular needle holders, 7 inch
2 Steven's scissors (curved and straight)
2 Mayo scissors (curved and straight)
2 Suction tips (Frazier and tonsil)
2 Skin hooks
2 Tracheal hooks
2 Senn retractors
2 Thyroid pole retractors
2 Small dull Weitlaners
2 Richardson retractors, shallow

Additional instruments

2 Smooth neuro forceps
2 Diamond jaw forceps
4 Schnidt forceps
2 Judd Allis forceps
2 Double hooks
2 Small right angle clamps
2 Regular right angle clamps
2 Vascular needle holders, 5 inch
2 Medium dull rake retractors
2 Gelpi retractors
2 Vein retractors
Clip applier and clips

Evaluation

Evaluation of interventions determines effectiveness of positioning aids and pressure-relief devices, "drip" towels to collect excess prep solutions, and other interventions based on the patient's special needs.

The report to PACU personnel includes the surgical procedure, anesthesia given, location of drain, if any, dressing used, condition of skin postoperatively, and any other information specific to the patient's nursing diagnoses. Documentation is according to hospital protocol. It should reflect achievement of patient goals related to planned interventions; these should also be included in the nursing report to PACU personnel. Achievement of goals may be stated as patient outcomes.

For the nursing diagnoses selected for this patient, the following outcomes would be communicated:
- Swallowing was unimpaired.
- Body temperature was maintained within a normal range.
- The patient verbalized decreased negative feelings about body image.
- The airway remained patent; there was no edema at the surgical site or signs of respiratory distress.
- Gas exchange was adequate; O_2 saturation remained normal. The patient was extubated without incident (as applicable).

SURGICAL INTERVENTIONS

Total thyroidectomy, subtotal thyroidectomy, and thyroid lobectomy

Thyroidectomy is removal of the entire thyroid gland; subtotal thyroidectomy leaves the posterior portions of each lobe intact in order to protect the recurrent laryngeal nerves and the integrity of the parathyroid glands; thyroid lobectomy is removal of a lobe of the thyroid gland. The purpose of surgical intervention relates to the patient's medical diagnoses.

Hyperthyroidism (Graves' disease) is associated with diffuse, bilateral enlargement of the thyroid gland. In Hashimoto's thyroiditis, thought to be an autoimmune disease, nontender enlargement of the gland occurs. Surgery is performed to relieve tracheal obstruction. Nontoxic nodular goiter does not produce an excess of hormones and is noninflammatory in character. In this condition, thyroid tissue proliferates in an attempt to produce the minimal hormonal requirement. Surgery may be indicated to relieve tracheal or esophageal obstruction or rule out a malignant nodule of the thyroid gland. Total thyroidectomy is done for malignant tumors.

Procedural considerations. The patient is positioned as previously described (see p. 415). The skin is antiseptically prepared. A thyroid instrument set is required. The incision site is "scratched" with a scalpel in the normal neck creases to mark the incision line.

Operative procedure

1. A transverse incision is made through the skin and first layer of the cervical fascia and platysma muscle, approximately 2 cm above the sternoclavicular junction or in the normal skin crease that was previously scratched (Fig. 16-2).
2. Flaps may be held away from the wound with stay sutures inserted through the cervical fascia and platysma muscle, or the skin edges of flaps may be inverted and covered with skin towels by means of heavy sutures or small towel clamps.
3. The upper skin flap is undermined to the level of the

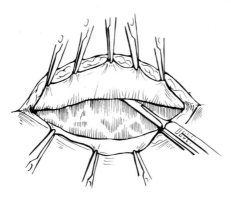

Fig. 16-2. Beginning of throidectomy. Skin flaps are created by dissection deep to platysma muscle and cervical fascia.

cricoid cartilage; the lower flap is then undermined to the sternoclavicular joint with a knife, fine curved scissors, tissue forceps, and gauze sponges. Bleeding vessels are clamped with hemostats and ligated with fine, nonabsorbable sutures.

4. The fascia in the midline is incised between the strap (sternohyoid) muscles with a knife (Fig. 16-3, *A*); the sternocleidomastoid muscle may be retracted with a loop retractor; the strap muscles may be divided between clamps, using Ochsner or Crile hemostats and a knife. The divided muscles are retracted from the operative site with retractors, thereby exposing the diseased lobe. This maneuver is necessary only for markedly enlarged lobes. Usually the strap muscles may be retracted to provide adequate exposure.

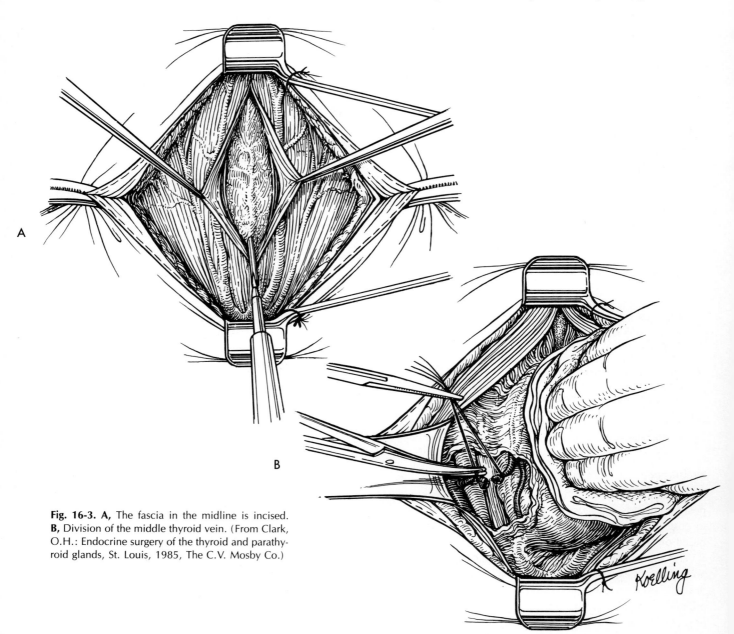

Fig. 16-3. A, The fascia in the midline is incised. **B,** Division of the middle thyroid vein. (From Clark, O.H.: Endocrine surgery of the thyroid and parathyroid glands, St. Louis, 1985, The C.V. Mosby Co.)

5. The inferior and middle thyroid veins are clamped, divided with Metzenbaum scissors, and ligated with fine nonabsorbable sutures (Fig. 16-3, *B*).
6. The lobe is rotated medially, and the loose areolar tissue is divided posteriorly and medially toward the tracheoesophageal sulcus with hemostats and Metzenbaum scissors. Small sponges are used for blunt dissection. Bleeding is controlled by hemostats and ligatures, as well as by electrocoagulation. The recurrent laryngeal nerve is identified and carefully preserved (Fig. 16-4, *A*).
7. The thyroid lobe is pulled downward, and the avascular tissue between the trachea and upper pole of the thyroid is dissected by means of Metzenbaum scissors.

8. The superior thyroid artery is secured with two or three curved hemostats; the artery is ligated and divided and then is transfixed with nonabsorbable sutures.
9. The inferior thyroid artery is identified and ligated by means of fine forceps, sutures, and scissors (Fig. 16-4, *A*). The thyroid lobe is then dissected away from the recurrent nerve with Metzenbaum scissors and hemostats. Bleeding vessels are clamped with hemostats and ligated with fine nonabsorbable sutures.
10. The lobe is elevated with Lahey vulsellum clamps; it is freed from the trachea with fine scissors, forceps, knife, and hemostats. The fibrous bands attached to the trachea and cricoid cartilage are divided.
11. The isthmus of the gland is elevated with fine forceps

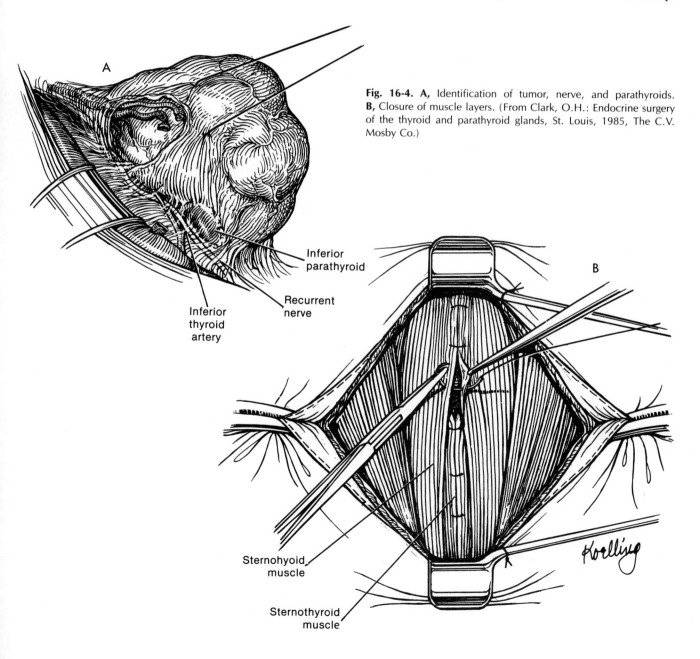

Fig. 16-4. A, Identification of tumor, nerve, and parathyroids. **B,** Closure of muscle layers. (From Clark, O.H.: Endocrine surgery of the thyroid and parathyroid glands, St. Louis, 1985, The C.V. Mosby Co.)

and divided between Crile hemostats with scissors. The resection of the lobe is completed, and the lobe is removed. Care is taken throughout the procedure to identify and preserve the parathyroid glands and other critical structures.

12. The cut surface of the opposite lobe requires careful hemostasis.

13. The strap muscles, if severed, are approximated with interrupted absorbable or nonabsorbable sutures. A drain may be inserted in the thyroid bed and brought out between the strap muscles and sternocleidomastoid muscle. Many surgeons prefer to drain the wound laterally through the sternocleidomastoid muscle and the lateral extremity of the incision in the belief that this will produce better healing and cosmetic results. However, drainage is usually unnecessary.

14. The edges of the platysma muscle are approximated (Fig. 16-4, *B*). The skin edges are then approximated with interrupted, fine nonabsorbable sutures or skin clips.

15. Gauze dressings are applied to the wound; a thyroid collar type of dressing may be applied. This dressing consists of strips of adhesive tape (Fig. 16-5) or Elastoplast, 2 inches wide and 28 inches long, with a folded gauze covering its center portion. The gauze prevents the patient's hair from coming in contact with the tape. The dressing is brought from the back of the neck to the front, and the free ends of the collar are crossed and secured over the chest. The dressing is further secured by additional strips of tape.

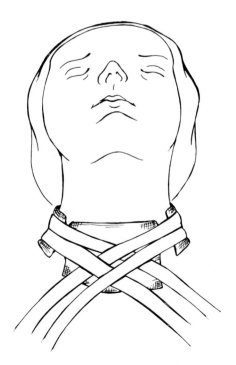

Fig. 16-5. Thyroid collar type of dressing.

Substernal or intrathoracic thyroidectomy

Extensions of enlarging goiters into the substernal and intrathoracic regions are frequently seen. They may cause tracheal and esophageal obstruction, in which case they are usually excised surgically. Longer instruments are usually required. Splitting the sternum is rarely necessary.

Thyroglossal duct cystectomy

Thyroglossal duct cystectomy is complete excision of all portions of the cyst and duct, as well as a portion of the hyoid bone, which contains the duct, to avoid recurrent cystic formation and to prevent infections. The thyroglossal duct is an embryological structure present during the descent of the thyroid gland into the anterior neck. When present in an adult, it exists as a pretracheal cystic pouch attached to the hyoid bone, with or without a sinus tract to the base of the tongue at the foramen cecum.

Procedural considerations. The perioperative nursing assessment should be appropriate to the patient's age, as the patient is frequently a child or teenager (see Chapter 30). Reassurance and information regarding the procedure should be given.

A thyroidectomy setup, plus the following instruments, is used:

1 Periosteal elevator, small
1 Duckbill rongeur, small
1 Bone cutter, small
1 Syringe, 5 ml, with appropriate needle
  Methylene blue dye for injection

Operative procedure

1. After the head is extended and the chin is elevated, an incision is made between the hyoid bone and the thyroid cartilage through the subcutaneous tissue.

2. The platysma muscle is incised, and the flaps are raised as described previously.

3. The strap (sternohyoid) muscles are separated in the midline.

4. Sharp and blunt dissections are used to mobilize the cyst and duct, up to the attachment to the hyoid bone. The hyoid bone is transected twice with bone-cutting forceps, and the segment of bone and cyst is freed from adjacent structures.

5. The cephalic part of the duct is identified, a transfixion suture no. 3-0 is passed through it, and the duct is transected. (Methylene blue dye injection is used occasionally to visualize the whole tract.)

6. The cyst is removed. The strap muscles are closed with interrupted, fine silk sutures. A drain may be placed. The skin is closed with interrupted no. 5-0 nonabsorbable sutures or skin clips.

Parathyroidectomy

Parathyroidectomy is excision of one or more parathyroid glands. Normal or atrophic glands are not removed. The presence of adenomas (hypersecreting neoplasms), hyperplasia, or carcinomas requires surgical excision. In the last case, resection of lymph nodes is essential, although metastasis may also occur by way of the bloodstream. After local excision, a metastasis may cause hypersecretion of parathormone.

Procedural considerations. The instrument setup is identical to that for thyroid operations, with the addition of numerous specimen containers that are necessary for the multiple biopsies used to determine the presence or absence of parathyroid tissue.

Operative procedure

1. See approach to the thyroid gland, described previously.
2. With the thyroid gland visible, a thorough exploration of the "normal" locations of the four parathyroid glands is conducted. Meticulous hemostasis by means of mosquito hemostats and fine ligatures is a prerequisite to location and identification of these small glands.
3. The thyroid gland is gently rotated anteriorly to provide access to the posterior thyroid sulcus, where the parathyroid glands are almost always found. Indentification of the parathyroid vascular pedicle as it leaves the superior thyroid artery is an excellent means of locating the upper gland. Metzenbaum scissors, mosquito hemostats, and Kitner sponges are used in the dissection.
4. Attention is directed toward the posterior lateral surface of the thyroid lobe or just beneath the lower thyroid pole, where the lower parathyroid gland is frequently found. Again, finding the vascular pedicle from the inferior thyroid artery may aid in identification. Occasionally the lower pair is found in the thymic capsule or tissue, in which case a portion of the thymus is resected.
5. Should one of the parathyroid glands evidence disease, it is resected by clamping the vascular pedicle with mosquito hemostats, dividing with small scissors or knife, and ligating with a fine nonabsorbable suture. The question of how much parathyroid tissue to remove is controversial and relates to whether single or multiple glands are involved, regardless of their size and appearance. A portion of one gland must remain to prevent complications.
6. The neck region is explored for aberrant parathyroid tissue, which is also resected.
7. The remainder of the operation is the same as that described for the thyroid gland.
8. A dressing is applied as described for thyroid surgery.

BIBLIOGRAPHY

Bradley, E.L., DiGirolamo, M., and Tarcan, Y.: Modified subtotal thyroidectomy in the management of Graves' disease, Surgery 87:623, 1980.

Corbett, J.V.: Laboratory tests and diagnostic procedures with nursing diagnoses, ed. 2, Norwalk, Conn., 1987, Appleton-Century-Crofts.

Edis, A.J., Ayala, L.A., and Egdahl, R.H.: Manual of endocrine surgery, ed. 2, New York, 1984, Springer-Verlag Co.

Farrar, W.B.: Complications of thyroidectomy, Surg. Clin. North Am. 63:1353, 1983.

Kaplan, E.L.: Surgical endocrinology. In Polk, H.C., and others: Basic surgery, ed. 3, Norwalk, Conn., 1986, Appleton-Century-Crofts.

Kneedler, J.A., and Dodge, G.H.: Perioperative patient care, the nursing perspective, ed. 2, Boston, 1987, Blackwell Scientific Publications.

Saxe, A.W., and others: Parathyroid autotransplantation: indications and techniques, AORN J. 44:396, 1986.

Thibodeau, G.A.: Anthony's textbook of anatomy and physiology, ed. 13, St. Louis, 1990, The C.V. Mosby Co.

17 Breast surgery

ROSEMARY ANN ROTH

Pathologic breast conditions, indicated by benign or malignant tumors and infections, are some of the most common and emotionally upsetting health problems confronting women. They occasionally occur in men. In women particularly, changing hormone levels from puberty throughout the remainder of life affect breast tissue in its physical and microscopic characteristics. In association with these changes, numerous dysfunctions, malformations, and tumors may occur.

Operative procedures on the mammary glands may be indicated in the presence of disease or as a result of other physical or psychologic patient considerations. Reconstructive surgery of the breast is discussed in Chapter 24.

SURGICAL ANATOMY

The breasts are bilateral mammary glands that lie on the pectoralis major fascia of the anterior chest wall. They are surrounded by a layer of fat and are encased in an envelope of skin. The breasts extend from the second to the sixth rib and horizontally from the lateral edge of the sternum to the anterior axillary line. The largest part of the mammary gland rests on the connective tissue of the pectoralis major muscle and laterally on the serratus anterior, with a normal global contour occurring as a result of the fascial support (Cooper's ligaments). An elongation of mammary tissue normally extends on the pectoralis major toward the axilla and is known as the tail of Spence (Fig. 17-1).

Each breast is made up of 12 to 20 glandular lobes that are separated by connective tissue and adipose tissue deposits. Each lobe is subdivided into lobules in which are embedded the secreting cells (alveoli) arranged in grapelike clusters around minute ducts. The lobes are positioned in a spiral fashion around the nipple. Each lobe is drained by a single lactiferous duct that opens on the nipple (Fig. 17-2). The nipple, located in the fourth intercostal space, forms a conical projection into which the ducts open independent of each other on the surface. A pigmented circular area called the areola surrounds the nipple. Smooth contractile muscle fibers of the areola allow for nipple contraction.

Three major arterial systems generously supply the mammary glands with blood. The main sources are branches of the internal mammary and the lateral branches of the anterior aortic intercostal arteries, all of which form an extensive network of anastomoses over the breast. A third source is the pectoral branch deriving from a branch of the axillary artery.

The veins that mainly drain the breasts follow the course of the arteries. The superficial veins frequently become dilated during pregnancy. They are also often dilated over an area that contains disease. One route of venous drainage from the breast is significant in that it forms an anastomosis with the intercostal veins that in turn joins with the vertebral veins.

The lymph drainage system generally follows the course of the vessels. The lymphatics drain into two main areas represented by the axillary nodes and the internal mammary chain of nodes (Fig. 17-3). An average of 53 lymph nodes occurs in the axillary area. The internal mammary nodes are few in number but are responsible for most of the lymph drainage from the upper and lower inner quadrants of the breast. Thus one can see how the lymph system could be a channel for the spread of malignant disease from the breast to associated areas of the chest wall or to the axilla.

The nerve supply is mainly from the anterior cutaneous branches of the upper intercostal nerves, the third and fourth branches of the cervical plexus, and the lateral cutaneous branches of the intercostal nerves.

Occasionally, developmental errors of the breast occur. Additional nipples or extramammary tissue in the axilla or over the upper abdomen may be present. The preferred treatment of these supernumerary structures often is excision. Absence of one or both nipples may also occur and may be associated with absence of the underlying pectoral muscle and chest wall.

The mammary glands are affected by three types of physiologic changes: (1) those related to growth and development, (2) those related to the menstrual cycle, and (3) those related to pregnancy and lactation. The mammary glands are present at birth in both males and females. Hormonal stimulation, however, produces the development and function of these glands in females. Estrogen promotes growth of the ductal structures, whereas progesterone promotes development of the alveoli. Both of these hormones act synergistically with the pituitary growth hormones, prolactin and corticotropin, to produce the structure and function of the glands.

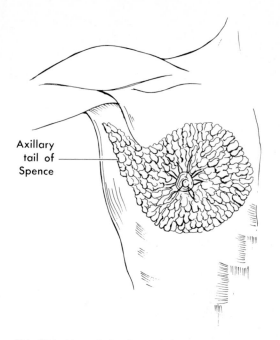

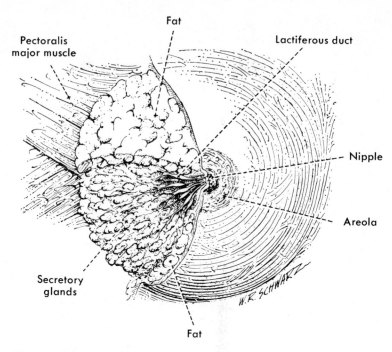

Fig. 17-1. Normal distribution of mammary tissue of adult female breast. Note long tail of Spence extending into axilla. (Modified from Schwartz, S.I., and others: Principles of surgery, ed. 5, New York, 1989, McGraw-Hill Book Co.)

Fig. 17-2. Diagrammatic cross-section of mammary gland showing relationship of various anatomic structures. (From Jorstad, L.H.: Surgery of the breast, St. Louis, 1964, The C.V. Mosby Co.; drawing by W.R. Schwarz.)

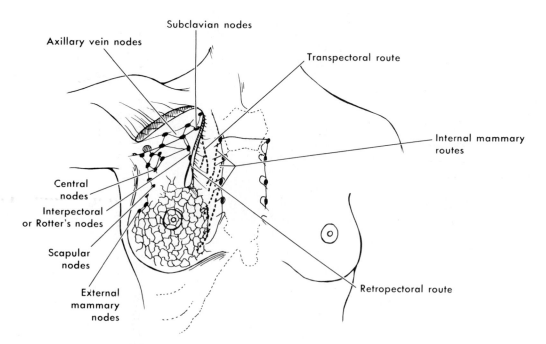

Fig. 17-3. Normal distribution of mammary tissue and lymphatic system of adult female breast. (Modified from Southwick, H.W., Slaughter, D.P., and Humphrey, L.J.: Surgery of the breast. Copyright 1968 by Year Book Medical Publishers, Inc., Chicago. Used by permission.)

Breast cancer

Breast cancer primarily affects women. Until it can be prevented, early detection is the greatest hope for its control. All women should practice monthly self-examination and immediately report any changes or masses to a physician.

Benign breast lesions, such as fibrocystic disease and fibroadenomas, are the most common lesions excised. The older the patient, the more likely that a mass is malignant. The most common form of breast cancer is infiltrating ductal carcinoma.

The cause of breast cancer is still unknown. Many factors, including environmental, dietary, and familial influences, have been suggested as contributors to its development. Whatever the cause of breast cancer, its incidence is definitely increasing. The previously held belief that breast cancer spreads by direct extension from the initial site in the breast to adjacent lymph nodes is probably incorrect. Breast cancer is now thought to be a systemic condition. Distant body metastases may have already occurred without adjacent lymph node involvement at the time of its palpable detection. This theory could explain why the radical breast surgery of the past, which involved removal of all axillary and intramammary lymph nodes, did not greatly lower mortality. Less radical surgery is the treatment of choice today. Surgical excision of the tumor, the use of radiation therapy alone, and a combination of surgery and radiation therapy have become viable alternatives. The use of chemotherapy with stage I cancer (Table 17-2) is not recommended due to the low mortality

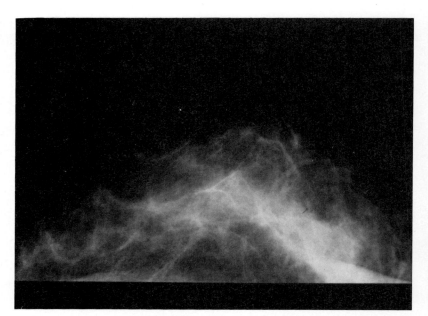

Fig. 17-4. Mammogram. Craniocaudad view of normal breast. (Courtesy Wende W. Logan, M.D., Rochester, N.Y., and the Breast Clinic of Rochester.)

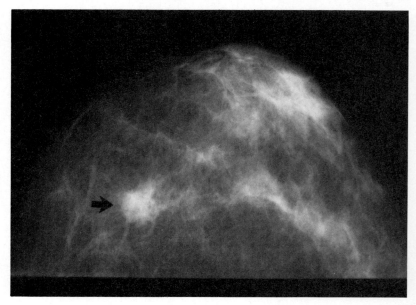

Fig. 17-5. Mammogram. Craniocaudad view of breast. *Arrow* indicates unpalpable lesion of about 1.5 cm. (Courtesy Wende W. Logan, M.D., Rochester, N.Y., and the Breast Clinic of Rochester.)

of this stage and the long-term effects of chemotherapeutic agents. Chemotherapy is valuable for cancers with high probability of recurrence.

Detection of a breast mass can occur during a routine physical examination or self-examination. External physical changes, such as discharge from the nipple or dimpling of the skin, can also indicate the presence of a pathologic process.

Imaging methodologies, such as mammography, thermography, and ultrasonography, have helped in the detection of breast masses too small for clinical detection. Thermography displays a pictorial representation of the heat patterns on the surface of the breast that may demonstrate signs of abnormality through asymmetry in the pictures. Ultrasonography differentiates between solid versus cystic lesions. Computed tomography (CT) and magnetic resonance imaging (MRI) can also be used in the differentiation of small, dense breast lesions. Survival from breast cancer is best when detected early, reducing axillary lymph node involvement and improving long-term survival. Tumor size can usually be correlated with involvement of lymph nodes. The larger the tumor, the more likely that lymph nodes are involved.

The best available screening mechanism for occult and palpable lesions is x-ray mammography (Fig. 17-4). Mammograms can detect abnormal-appearing densities and clusters of calcium deposits that are clinically nonpalpable (Fig. 17-5). These masses may be only 3 to 10 mm in diameter.

In mammography the entire breast is visualized by directing x-ray beams in several planes through the breast, yielding craniocaudad and other views (Fig. 17-4). Mammograms should be analyzed by a trained radiologist, who sends the report to the referring physician. In some in-

stances, such as when the lesion is too small to palpate, mammograms are done immediately before surgery. The lesions, previously detected by mammogram, are localized by the insertion of a needle(s) or a wire that is inserted through the needle. The needle(s) may be left in place or removed after insertion of the wire (Fig. 17-6). Once the suspect area is identified, the needle or wire is taped in place, and the patient is sent to the operating room for surgical biopsy. After biopsy, the specimen can be sent back for mammography validation of the correct surgical excision of the questionable breast tissue prior to the pathologic examination.

The accuracy of mammography depends on careful x-ray technique and breast size, structure, and density. Radiation dosage varies with individuals and techniques. As a result of improvement in radiologic techniques, the radiation exposure in a mammogram is very low. The benefits of this screening mechanism far outweigh the minute risks of radiation exposure.

Surgical treatment ranges from removal of only the tumor to radical mastectomy involving the breast, pectoral muscles, axillary lymph nodes, and all fat, fascia, and adjacent tissues. The choice of operation depends on the size, site, and the stage of the disease. Radiation therapy, chemotherapy, or hormonal therapy may be used in conjunction with surgery or as alternative treatment methods.

Techniques have been developed that determine the ability of breast cancer to bind with estrogen and progestins. This positive binding capability identifies the patient with a hormone-dependent tumor. About two thirds of all breast cancers are positive for estrogen binding, and the majority of these tumors are also positive for progestins. The presence of receptor sites is conducive to hormone manipulation. The use of antiestrogen Tamoxifen, in ad-

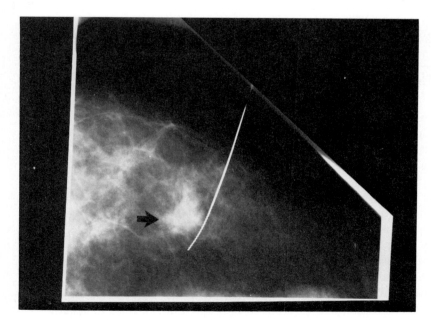

Fig. 17-6. Mammogram section. Craniocaudad view of breast. *Arrow* indicates lesion localized by wire before surgical excision. (Courtesy Wende W. Logan, M.D., Rochester, N.Y., and the Breast Clinic of Rochester.)

Table 17-1. TNM classification of breast cancer*

	Class	Description
Tumor (at greatest dimension)	T_1	≤2 cm
	T_2	>2≤5 cm
	T_3	>5 cm
	T_4	Any size with extension to chest wall or skin
Nodes	N_0	No palpable nodes
	N_1	Movable nodes
	N_2	Fixed nodes
	N_3	Supraclavicular or infraclavicular nodes
Metastasis	M_0	No distant metastasis
	M_1	Distant metastasis

Modified from Tish Knobf, M.K.: Am. J. Nurs. 9:1110, 1984. Copyright © 1984, American Journal of Nursing Company. Reprinted with permission.
*T refers to the gross palpable size and skin fixation of the local tumor; N to the number, size, and location of regional nodes involved; and M to the presence of distant metastases. Prognosis is poorer when four or more nodes are involved. Distant metastases are a grave prognosis.

Table 17-2. Clinical staging for breast cancer*

Stage	Tumor	Nodes	Metastasis
I	T_1	N_0N_1	M_0
II	T_2	N_0N_1	M_0
III	T_3	N_0N_1	M_0
	T_1	N_2	M_0
	T_2	N_3	M_0
IV	Any T	Any N	M_1

Modified from Tish Knobf, M.K.: Am. J. Nurs. 9:1110, 1984. Copyright © 1984, American Journal of Nursing Company. Reprinted with permission.
*See Table 17-1 for description of TNM classification.

dition to surgery and chemotherapy, increases the disease-free state in premenopausal and postmenopausal women with positive binding for estrogen. Tumors excised at surgery are evaluated for their estrogen and progestin-binding abilities.

Breast cancer is usually staged to measure the extent of the disease and to classify patients for possible treatment modalities. The TNM classification has been adopted as a mechanism to clinically stage this disease (Tables 17-1 and 17-2). The results of staging are used in designing the treatment plan.

PERIOPERATIVE NURSING CONSIDERATIONS
Assessment/nursing diagnosis

A patient undergoing breast surgery can be extremely apprehensive about the possibilities of having a malignancy, losing a body part, facing a negative reaction from the spouse and/or family, and experiencing a change in self-image. During a preoperative interview, the perioperative nurse should assess the patient's level of anxiety and possible causes. Identification of the patient's fears and concerns helps the nurse in planning appropriate nursing interventions. The patient should identify the breast that is affected and, if possible, the quadrant of the breast mass. The nurse should assess the patient's understanding of the proposed surgical procedure. Reinforcement of knowledge or correction of misunderstandings is possible

only if the nurse identifies the patient's current level of knowledge.

Discharge planning should begin as soon as the patient is informed of the necessity for surgery or when the nurse first meets the patient. Information about appropriate exercises, prosthetic devices, reconstructive techniques, and available community support groups should be given to the patient. The perioperative nurse provides or reinforces information based on clinical nursing judgment; the patient's desire for information, readiness to learn, and anxiety level are all considered.

Based on the nursing assessment, the perioperative nurse constructs nursing diagnoses to be used in developing a plan of care. Possible nursing diagnoses for a patient undergoing breast surgery would include:

- Anxiety related to the fear of cancer
- Body image disturbance related to loss of body part
- Anticipatory grieving related to potential loss of body part
- Potential for injury related to use of electrosurgery
- Knowledge deficit related to unfamiliarity with perioperative routines

Planning

Utilizing nursing diagnoses, the perioperative nurse can individualize the plan of care for each patient and allow for communication with other colleagues on the patient care team. The care plan for a patient undergoing breast surgery can include nursing interventions that allow the patient freedom to express concerns, that answer specific questions, and that discuss prosthetic or breast reconstruction, as appropriate. The Sample Care Plan shows some examples.

Implementation

Before surgery, the perioperative nurse should procure the necessary medical and surgical supplies and equipment

Sample Care Plan

NURSING DIAGNOSIS:
Anxiety related to fear of cancer
GOAL:
Patient will verbalize decreased anxiety.
INTERVENTIONS:
Allow time for patient's questions.
Assess verbal and nonverbal signs of anxiety.
Encourage ventilation of concerns and fears.
Provide emotional support and comfort measures (warm blankets, touch as appropriate).
Maintain quiet environment.
Demonstrate warmth, calmness, and acceptance of the patient's anxiety.
Instruct the patient in relaxation techniques such as rhythmic breathing or guided imagery.
Record patient's reactions.

NURSING DIAGNOSIS:
Body image disturbance related to loss of body part
GOAL:
Patient will discuss feelings regarding outcome of the surgical procedure.
INTERVENTIONS:
Allow patient to discuss concerns about her sexual attractiveness and perceived loss of femininity.
Discuss available resources and options (external prosthesis, alternatives in garments and dress, reconstructive surgery, as appropriate). Make referrals to nurse on discharge unit as indicated.
Maintain the patient's privacy.

NURSING DIAGNOSIS:
Anticipatory grieving related to loss of body part
GOAL:
Patient will discuss feelings regarding the proposed outcome of the surgical procedure.
INTERVENTIONS:
Allow ventilation of feelings.
Clarify misconceptions.
Promote an environment of support, respect, and comfort.

Refer to other professionals as appropriate.
Explore realistic alternatives and breast reconstruction.

NURSING DIAGNOSIS:
Potential for injury related to use of electrosurgery
GOAL:
Patient will experience no untoward injury from electrosurgery.
INTERVENTIONS:
Position the dispersive pad as close to the operative site as possible.
Select a site that is clean and dry, with good muscle mass; note the condition of the skin.
Protect pad from fluids and contact with metal objects.
Turn electrosurgical unit on after dispersive pad and active electrode are connected.
Set power setting as low as possible to achieve desired effect.
Use holster for active electrode on the sterile field.
Check dispersive pad contact and all connections after changes in position or requests to increase power.
Evaluate the condition of the skin upon removal of the dispersive pad.

NURSING DIAGNOSIS:
Knowledge deficit related to unfamiliarity with perioperative routines
GOAL:
Patient will verbalize understanding of the perioperative routines.
INTERVENTIONS:
Assess the patient's experience with previous surgical procedures.
Provide clear and concise explanations of all nursing interventions.
Explain roles of the health care team members.
Encourage questions.

for the intended operation. Mammogram results should be available in the OR for the surgeon's review. A breast biopsy under local anesthesia will require local anesthetics, adjunct sedation, and monitoring equipment (ECG, pulse oximeter, blood pressure apparatus). Patient allergies should be again reviewed and the patient closely observed for allergic or toxic reactions to local anesthetics. For a mastectomy, extra sponges are often needed. An electrosurgical unit is used to provide both hemostasis and tissue dissection. The incision site is usually drained postoperatively with a closed wound suction device. Ensuring the availability of supplies before the procedure allows the nurse to remain with, monitor, and observe the patient.

During the intraoperative phase, the patient is placed on the OR bed in a *supine position* with the operative side near the edge of the bed. The arm on the involved side is extended on a padded armboard. Depending on the location of the lesion and the planned surgery, a small pad can be placed under the operative side to facilitate exposure of the incision area. Positioning the OR bed in slight Fowler's with a lateral tilt away from the surgeon can facilitate exposure.

Skin preparation depends on the location of the lesion and the surgery intended. Skin preparation solutions vary, depending on the surgeon's preference. For a breast biopsy, the area prepared is usually the affected breast and the immediate surrounding skin. For a mastectomy, the area prepared can extend from above the clavicle to the umbilicus and from the opposite nipple to the bedline of the operative side, including the axilla, and possibly the upper arm on the operative side.

Surgical draping should allow exposure of the affected breast. For a mastectomy, the arm on the operative side should be draped free using a stockinette and drapes that allow free movement of the arm to facilitate access to the axilla. If a breast biopsy is to be immediately followed by a modified radical mastectomy, the surgeon may prefer to repeat the skin preparation and surgical draping before proceeding with the definitive surgery. Breast biopsy *instruments* include:

Cutting instruments

2 Knife handles, no. 3, with no. 10 and no. 15 blades
2 Mayo scissors, 1 straight and 1 curved
1 Tissue scissors

Holding instruments

6 Hemostats
4 Kelly hemostats
4 Allis forceps
4 Towel clamps
2 Tissue forceps with teeth

Exposing instruments

2 Muscle retractors, small
2 Rake retractors, small

1 Set of intraductal probes
2 Skin hooks

Suturing items

1 Needle holder
2 Packages of sutures, 1 absorbable and 1 nonabsorbable, usually on atraumatic cutting needles

Instruments and supplies for a modified radical mastectomy include:

Cutting instruments

2 Knife handles, no. 3, with no. 10 and no. 15 blades
2 Mayo scissors, 1 straight and 1 curved
2 Tissue scissors, regular and long

Holding instruments

16 Hemostats (number will vary with size of breast)
6 Kelly hemostats
12 Allis forceps
8 Lahey clamps
6 Kocher hemostatic forceps
8 Towel clamps
2 Tissue forceps with teeth
2 Tissue forceps without teeth
2 Adson forceps with teeth

Exposing instruments

2 U.S. Army retractors
4 Richardson retractors, 2 small and 2 medium
4 Rakes, four-prong, 2 small and 2 medium
2 Skin hooks
3 Berens skin-flap retractors

Suturing items

4 Needle holders
Suture material, usually atraumatic on cutting needles

Accessory items

Closed wound suction device
Electrosurgical unit
Marking pen
Suction tip and tubing

During implementation of the care plan, the perioperative nurse continues to collect data, continuously reassesses the patient's needs and the needs of the surgical team, provides nursing interventions, and documents care delivered. Formats for care plan documentation vary from institution to institution. However, documentation of patient problems and nursing interventions addressing these problems is important for any surgical patient. For the patient undergoing breast surgery, consideration should be given to documenting the patient's level of anxiety, the surgical position and accessory positioning devices used, the location of the electrosurgical dispersive pad, unit settings and identification number, results of perioperative monitoring, medications administered by the perioperative nurse or from the sterile field, and any drains incorporated in the surgical dressing.

Evaluation

Evaluation of the patient prior to discharge from the operating room includes both general observation parameters important for every surgical patient as well as specific evaluation of the goals of the care plan. The patient's skin at dependent pressure sites, skin preparation sites, and the dispersive pad placement site should be assessed. Whether the dressing is intact and the wound suction device is properly functioning should be noted. The report to the nurse in the PACU should include any unusual events or patient problems during surgery, the incorporation of any drains in the wound, and the results of care plan goal achievement. These goals, based on the nursing diagnoses selected, may be a part of documentation as well as the nursing report. They may be communicated as patient outcomes as follows:

- The patient's anxiety was reduced.
- The patient discussed feelings about the surgery and its outcome.
- There was no injury related to use of electrosurgery.
- The patient verbalized an understanding of perioperative routines.

SURGICAL INTERVENTIONS

Biopsy of breast tissue

Biopsy of breast tissue is removal of suspicious tissue for pathologic examination. In a *needle biopsy*, a Vim-Silverman or disposable cutting type of needle is introduced and advanced into the breast mass to entrap a core or plug of tissue. The needle is withdrawn, and the tissue specimen is sent for diagnostic examination (Fig. 17-7). In an *incisional biopsy*, a portion of the mass is surgically excised using a curved incision line. The tissue is sent for pathologic examination. In an *excisional biopsy*, the entire tumor mass is excised from adjacent tissue for examination as with incisional biopsy. Biopsy is indicated in the presence of a tumor mass detected by palpation, mammography, nipple discharge, or skin changes. Fibroadenoma, an isolated cyst, or intraductal papilloma may be encountered. Definitive surgical treatment is contraindicated in the absence of a formal biopsy.

Procedural considerations. The biopsy procedure has little risk and is usually done under local anesthesia. The short delay between biopsy and further treatment does not adversely affect survival. However, when an extensive surgical procedure is anticipated, general anesthesia is preferred. In this instance the patient has given consent to proceed with the more definitive surgery.

Operative procedure

1. An incision in the direction of the skin lines or along the border of the areola is made over the tumor mass. The circumareolar incision gives the best cosmetic effect.
2. Gentle traction is applied to the mass with holding forceps. If the lesion is small, the entire mass and an

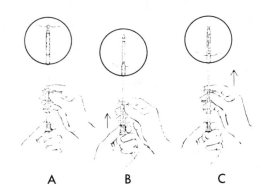

Fig. 17-7. Technique for needle biopsy of breast.
1. Site is prepared as required. For percutaneous procedures, adequate anesthesia is ensured and skin incised with scalpel. If distance measurement is desired, tissue depth spacer is slipped on needle before procedure.
2. With obturator fully retracted to cover specimen notch, cannula hub is held and needle assembly inserted *up* to tissue from which specimen is to be secured as shown in **A.**
3. Larger H-shaped cannula handle is held firmly to stabilize assembly, and obturator hub is quickly advanced as far as permitted, which will position specimen notch in tissue for biopsy as shown in **B.**
4. To cut tissue that has prolapsed into specimen notch, H-shaped cannula handle is quickly advanced as shown in **C.**
5. Needle assembly is withdrawn with cannula still advanced over obturator.
6. Obturator is advanced to remove biopsy specimen from specimen notch. (Courtesy Travenol Laboratories, Inc., Deerfield, Ill.)

edge of normal tissue are removed by sharp dissection. If a large lesion is present, a small incisional biopsy of the main mass is done. The tissue specimen is examined by a frozen section to determine immediate diagnosis while the patient is still anesthetized. If a 48-hour permanent section is required, the patient will be scheduled at a later time for any further surgery that may be necessary.

3A. If the lesion is benign, the subcutaneous breast tissue of the wound is approximated with an absorbable suture. The skin is closed with fine sutures or skin staples, and a firm pressure dressing is applied.

3B. If the lesion is malignant, the incision is tightly closed with a continuous locking suture on a cutting needle.

4. If a more extensive operation is required, it may be performed immediately. The team members regown and glove; the operative site is again prepped and draped. A separate sterile setup and set of instruments for a more radical procedure are then used.

Incision and drainage for abscess

Incision of an inflamed and suppurative area of the breast is performed for drainage of abscess. Abscesses occur most frequently as a result of infections in a lactating breast. Staphylococcal or streptococcal organisms enter the breast through abraded or lacerated nipple surfaces or through the lactiferous ducts. Chronic abscesses are rare. Free drainage is required with the association of an abscess around the nipple or in breast tissue.

Procedural considerations. Instruments are the same as for a biopsy.

Operative procedure

1. Generally, a radial incision extending outward from the nipple or a circumareolar incision is preferred. A short incision in the thoracomammary fold may be used for deep breast abscesses in the lower or outer quadrant.
2. After skin incision, the wound is deepened until pus is encountered.
3. A curved hemostat is directed into the cavity to determine the extent of the abscess cavity. Cultures for aerobic and anaerobic organisms are usually taken.
4. Loculations are broken up by exploring the cavity with the index finger.
5. The opening is enlarged to ensure adequate drainage, the cavity is irrigated with warm saline solution, and bleeding vessels are ligated with absorbable sutures or coagulated.
6. The wound is drained or loosely packed with gauze. Healing occurs by granulation.

Segmental resection (lumpectomy, quadrant resection, wedge resection)

Segmental resection is removal of the tumor mass with at least a 1-inch margin of surrounding tissue. A segmental resection combined with an axillary node dissection and irradiation in stage I and II breast cancer appears to provide results equal to a more radical procedure. If one or more axillary nodes are involved, chemotherapy is also recommended.

Procedural considerations. Instruments required are as described for a modified radical mastectomy. In patients with large breasts, increased bleeding may occur, requiring additional hemostatic clamps.

Operative procedure. The procedure is as described for excisional biopsy.

Axillary node dissection

Axillary node dissection is the removal of the axillary nodes through an incision in the axilla. An axillary dissection is usually done through a separate incision from other breast operations. The removal and examination of the axillary nodes allows staging (Tables 17-1 and 17-2) of the disease. Adjunct treatment can be more accurately planned when the pathologic stage is known.

Procedural considerations. The patient is placed supine on the operating room bed with the operative side near the bed edge. The arm on the operative side is extended to less than 90 degrees on an armboard. The skin is prepared and draped as previously described.

Operative procedure

1. An incision is made slightly posterior and parallel to the upper lateral border of the pectoralis major muscle, or transversely across the axilla.
2. The fascia is incised over the pectoralis muscle. The pectoralis minor muscle is exposed. Major blood and lymphatic vessels are clamped and ligated. The use of electrosurgery is avoided around the axillary vessels and nerves.
3. The tissue over the axillary vein is incised.
4. The lymph nodes between the pectoralis major and pectoralis minor muscles are removed. Care is taken not to injure the medial and lateral nerves of the pectoralis major muscle.
5. The axillary fat and lymph nodes are freed from the axillary vein and chest wall. The long thoracic nerve is identified along the chest wall near the axillary vein, and the thoracodorsal nerve posteriorly is dissected free from the specimen. The nerves are spared to preserve muscle function.
6. The fat and nodes are removed. The incision is closed with sutures and staples, and a dressing is applied. A suction drain is usually placed through a separate stab incision for lymphatic drainage.

Subcutaneous mastectomy (adenomammectomy)

Subcutaneous mastectomy is removal of all breast tissue with the overlying skin and nipple left intact. Subcutaneous mastectomy is recommended for patients who have central tumors of noninvasive origin, chronic cystic mastitis, hyperplastic duct changes, or multiple fibroadenomas, or who have undergone a number of previous biopsies. A prosthesis may be inserted at the time of mastectomy or at a later date. Marked bleeding at the time of surgery is a contraindication to the insertion of a prosthesis.

Procedural considerations. The patient is positioned as for a biopsy. A modified radical mastectomy instrument set is required. If a prosthesis is to be inserted, equipment listed for augmentation mammoplasty (Chapter 24) is also required.

Operative procedure

1. An incision is usually begun in the inframammary crease and may be made on the medial or the lateral aspect of the breast. Some surgeons initially remove and preserve the nipple areola complex by employing lateral extensions of wide periareolar incisions.
2. Blunt dissection is performed to elevate the breast from the pectoral fascia.
3. The breast tissue is removed from the skin with an attempt made to remain in a plane between the subcutaneous tissue and the breast. Dissection is carried out toward the axilla; with care, 90% or more of the breast tissue can be removed, including the tail of Spence. Some lymph nodes in the axillary area also

may be removed. Bleeding vessels are clamped and ligated.

4. A decision is made at this time as to whether a prosthesis can be inserted (augmentation mammoplasty). If the subareolar tissue shows no signs of tumor, as verified by a pathologist, the areolar complex is placed on a de-epithelialized dermal bed.

5. A closed wound suction catheter may be inserted. The wound is closed, and a light pressure dressing is applied.

Simple mastectomy (total mastectomy)

Simple mastectomy is removal of the entire involved breast without lymph node dissection. A simple mastectomy is performed to remove extensive benign disease, if malignancy is believed to be confined only to the breast tissue, or as a palliative measure to remove an ulcerated advanced malignancy.

Procedural considerations. The patient is positioned as for a biopsy. A modified radical mastectomy instrument set is required.

Operative procedure

1. Through a transverse elliptical incision (Fig. 17-8, *A*), using a knife and curved scissors, the skin edges are freed from the fascia. Bleeding vessels are clamped with hemostats and ligated with sutures or coagulated.

2. The skin edges of the wound can be protected with warm, moist laparotomy pads; the breast tissue is grasped with Allis forceps and is dissected free from the underlying pectoral fascia with curved scissors and knife.

3. The tumor and all breast tissue are removed. Bleeding vessels are clamped and ligated or coagulated.

4. A closed wound drainage catheter may be inserted and anchored to the skin with a fine suture. The wound is closed with fine sutures or staples, and a dressing is applied.

Modified radical mastectomy

Modified radical mastectomy is performed following a tissue biopsy with a positive diagnosis of malignancy and involves removal of the involved breast and all axillary contents (all three levels of nodes—axillary, pectoral, and superior apical). The underlying pectoral muscles are not removed before or after removal of axillary nodes. A modified radical mastectomy is done to remove the involved area with the hope of decreasing the spread of the malignancy. This surgery's elliptic incision with lateral extension toward the axilla gives a good cosmetic result for plastic surgery reconstruction (Chapter 24), provides good arm movement because the pectoralis muscles are not removed, and usually does not require a skin graft.

Procedural considerations. The patient is placed supine on the operating room bed with the operative side near the bed edge. The arm on the operative side is extended to less than 90 degrees on a padded armboard. The skin is prepared and draped as previously described. Instruments and supplies for a modified radical mastectomy are required (p. 428).

Operative procedure

1. An oblique elliptic incision with a lateral extension toward the axilla is made through the subcutaneous tissue (Fig. 17-8, *A*). The bleeding points are controlled with hemostats and ligatures or electrocoagulation.

2. The skin is undercut in all directions to the limits of the dissection by means of a no. 3 knife handle with a no. 10 blade, curved scissors, or retractors. Knife blades need to be changed frequently to ensure precise dissection.

3. The margins of the skin flaps are covered with warm, moist laparotomy pads and held away with retractors. The fascia and breast are resected from the pectoralis major muscle (Fig. 17-8, *B*) starting near the clavicle down to the midportion of the sternum. The pectoralis muscle is left intact.

4. The intercostal arteries and veins are clamped and ligated.

5. The axillary flap is retracted for a complete dissection of the axilla. Careful attention is directed to preventing injury to the axillary vein and medial and lateral nerves of the pectoralis major muscle.

6. The fascia is dissected from the lateral edge of the pectoralis muscle (Fig. 17-8, *C*). Ligation of the vessels is preferred in the axilla and adjacent to the sternum. The fascia is then dissected from the serratus anterior muscle. The thoracic and thoracodorsal nerves are preserved (Fig. 17-8, *D*).

7. The breast and axillary fascia are freed from the latissimus dorsi muscle and suspensory ligaments (Fig. 17-8, *E*). The specimen is then passed off the field.

8. The surgical area is inspected for bleeding sites, which are ligated and coagulated. The wound is irrigated with normal saline. Closed wound suction catheters are inserted into the wound through stab wounds and secured to the skin with a nonabsorbable suture on a cutting needle (Fig. 17-8, *F*).

9. A few absorbable sutures may be used in the subcutaneous tissue to approximate the skin flaps. The incision is closed with interrupted nonabsorbable sutures or staples.

10. The dressing can be a simple gauze dressing, a bulky dressing held in place by a Surgi-Bra, or a gauze or elastic bandage wrap.

Radical mastectomy

Radical mastectomy entails en bloc removal of the entire involved breast, the pectoral muscles, the axillary lymph nodes, and all fat, fascia, and adjacent muscles. A radical mastectomy is done to remove the total involved

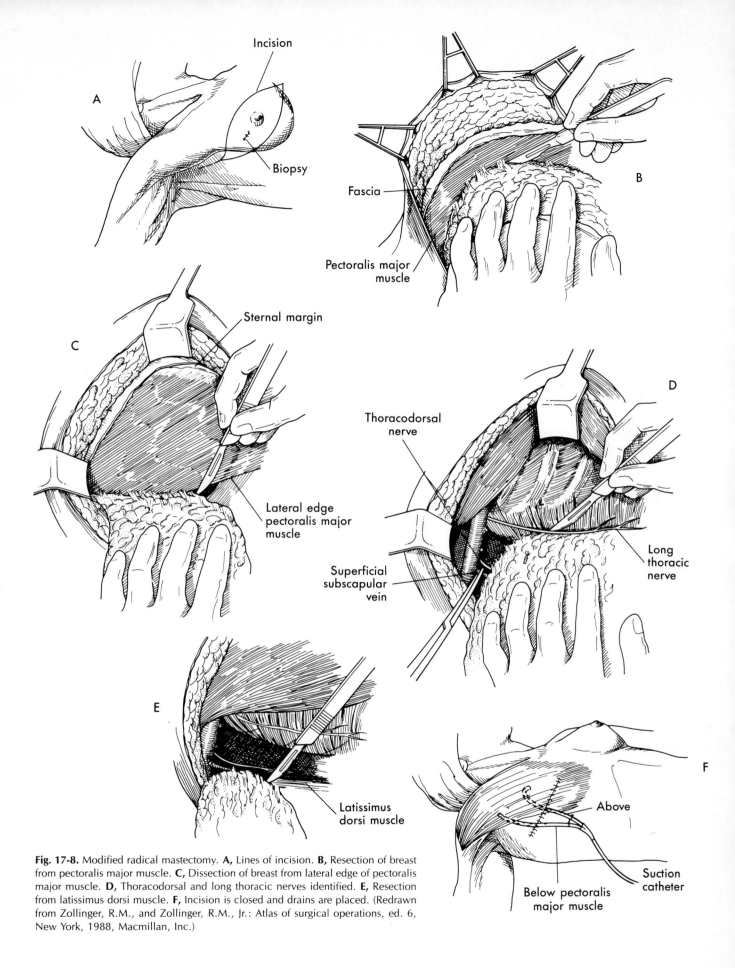

Fig. 17-8. Modified radical mastectomy. **A,** Lines of incision. **B,** Resection of breast from pectoralis major muscle. **C,** Dissection of breast from lateral edge of pectoralis major muscle. **D,** Thoracodorsal and long thoracic nerves identified. **E,** Resection from latissimus dorsi muscle. **F,** Incision is closed and drains are placed. (Redrawn from Zollinger, R.M., and Zollinger, R.M., Jr.: Atlas of surgical operations, ed. 6, New York, 1988, Macmillan, Inc.)

Labels within figure:

- Incision
- Biopsy
- Fascia
- Pectoralis major muscle
- Sternal margin
- Lateral edge pectoralis major muscle
- Thoracodorsal nerve
- Superficial subscapular vein
- Long thoracic nerve
- Latissimus dorsi muscle
- Above
- Below pectoralis major muscle
- Suction catheter

area with the hope of decreasing the spread of the malignancy, especially when the cancer has spread to the pectoralis muscles.

Procedural considerations. Preoperatively, the surgeon may prepare the skin of the anterior surface of the thigh in the event that a skin graft is needed. When a skin graft is to be performed, a separate setup is needed for taking the graft from the donor site (Chapter 24).

Operative procedure. The operative procedure is as described for a modified radical mastectomy except for dissection, division, ligation, and removal of the major and minor pectoralis muscles.

BIBLIOGRAPHY

Bland, D.S.: Pulse oximetry: monitoring hemoglobin oxygen saturation. AORN J. 45:964, 1987.

Cooperman, A., and others: Breast cancer, Surg. Clin. North Am. 64:6, 1984.

Gray, H.: Anatomy of the human body, ed. 30, Philadelphia, 1989, Lea & Febiger.

Greiner, L., and Weiler, C.: What do women know about treatment choices? Am. J. Nurs. 11:1570, 1983.

Hardy, J.: Hardy's textbook of surgery, ed. 2, Philadelphia, 1988, J.B. Lippincott Co.

Hassey, K.M., and others: Radiation alternative to mastectomy, Am. J. Nurs. 11:1567, 1983.

Ivey, D.F.: Local anesthesia: implications for the perioperative nurse. AORN J. 45:682, 1987.

Mauldin, B.: Breast reconstruction after mastectomy. AORN J. 31:612, 1980.

Leuze, M., and McKenzie, J.: Preoperative assessment: using the Roy adaptation model. AORN J. 46:1122, 1987.

Nora, P.F.: Operative surgery, ed. 3, Philadelphia, 1990, W.B. Saunders.

Nyamathi, A., and Kashiwabara, A.: Preoperative anxiety: its effect on cognitive thinking. AORN J. 47:164, 1988.

Osborne, M.P.: The biologic basis for breast cancer treatment options, Bull. Am. Coll. Surg. 71:4, 1986.

Sabiston, D.C., Jr., editor: Davis-Christopher textbook of surgery: the biological basis of modern surgical practice, ed. 13, Philadelphia, 1986, W.B. Saunders Co.

Schwartz, S., and others: Principles of surgery, ed. 5, New York, 1989, McGraw-Hill Book Co.

Stanfied, V.: Perioperative documentation: integrating nursing diagnoses on the patient record. AORN J. 46:699, 1987.

Thibodeau, G.A.: Anthony's textbook of anatomy and physiology, ed. 13, St. Louis, 1990, The C.V. Mosby Co.

Tish Knobf, M.K.: Breast cancer, Am. J. Nurs. 9:1110, 1984.

U.S. Department of Health and Human Services: The breast cancer digest, Washington, D.C., 1980, National Institutes of Health.

Way, L.W., editor: Current surgical diagnosis and treatment, ed. 8, Norwalk, Conn., 1988, Appleton & Lange.

Winchester, D.P.: The relationship of fibrocystic disease to breast cancer, Bull. Am. Coll. Surg. 71:29, 1986.

Zollinger, R.M., and Zollinger, R.M., Jr.: Atlas of surgical operations, ed. 6, New York, 1988, Macmillan.

18 Ophthalmic surgery

ELAINE THOMSON-KEITH

In the time of Hippocrates, eye surgery was confined to operations on the eyelid. Until the early twentieth century, little progress was made. Since then, significant advances have taken place in ophthalmology and anesthesia. With the implementation of aseptic technique, introduction of antibiotics, and improvements in management of the surgical patient, ophthalmic surgery, like other surgical specialties, has expanded its horizons dramatically.

Innovative developments in laser applications and microsurgical technology challenge the nurse who assists in the care of the ophthalmic patient. The perioperative nurse who practices in ophthalmologic surgery must combine the art and science of nursing with up-to-date knowledge and finely tuned, highly technologic skills.

In the last decade, advances in surgical techniques and improved anesthetics, along with increasing pressures to contain health care costs, have created another major change in the management of patients who undergo ophthalmologic surgery. Except for a small percentage of patients who have complex procedures or medical problems that contraindicate early discharge, patients today who have eye surgery do so on an outpatient basis. Only patients with the most difficult procedures require hospitalization postoperatively, and many of those patients have operations on the day of admission. Therefore, preoperative preparation, and in most cases discharge teaching, occurs in a limited time period and is often the responsibility of the perioperative nursing team. The success of the surgical intervention depends, to a degree, on the knowledge and skill of that team as they develop and implement a perioperative plan of care.

SURGICAL ANATOMY

A working knowledge of the anatomic structures involved in ophthalmic surgery is necessary to facilitate selection of instrumentation and equipment for the procedure. The surgical team must also use this knowledge to understand the surgeon's plan of treatment and prepare the patient appropriately.

Bony orbit

The two orbital cavities are situated on either side of the midvertical line of the skull between the cranium and the skeleton of the face. Above each orbit are the anterior cranial fossa and the frontal sinus; medially, the nasal cavity; below, the maxillary sinus; and laterally, from behind forward, the middle cranial and temporal fossa (Fig. 18-1).

The seven bones that form the orbit are the maxilla, palatine, frontal, sphenoidal, zygomatic, ethmoid, and lacrimal bones. The margins of the bony orbit may be divided into four continuous parts: supraorbital, lateral, infraorbital, and medial.

The orbit may be considered as a four-sided pyramid, with its base directed forward, laterally, and slightly downward and its apex facing posteriorly. The periosteum of the orbital walls is continuous with the dura mater.

The orbit is essentially a socket for the eyeball and the muscles, nerves, and vessels necessary for proper functioning of the eye (Fig. 18-2). The orbit is also a distribution center for certain vessels and nerves that supply the facial areas around the orbital aperture.

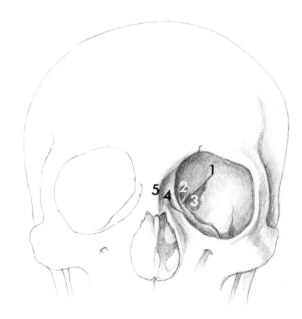

Fig. 18-1. Bony orbital cavity, *1*, communicates with brain through optic foramen; *2*, transmits optic nerve through superior orbital fissure; *3*, transmits most of other nerves and vessels entering orbit (lacrimal fossa); *4*, contains lacrimal sac; and, *5*, is bounded medially by nasal bone.

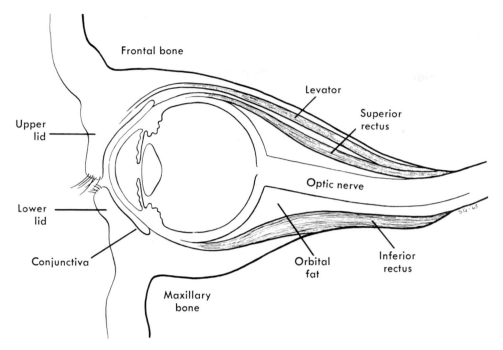

Fig. 18-2. Diagrammatic section of orbit. (From Saunders, W.H., and others: Nursing care in eye, ear, nose, and throat disorders, ed. 4, St. Louis, 1979, The C.V. Mosby Co.)

Conjunctiva and lacrimal apparatus

The conjunctiva is a thin, transparent mucous membrane that lines the back surface of the eyelids and the front surface of the globe. The conjunctiva forms a sac (conjunctival sac) that is open in front. The opening is called the *palpebral fissure*. When the eye is closed, the fissure becomes a mere slit.

The conjunctiva is divided into a palpebral and a bulbar part. The palpebral portion lines the back of the eyelids and contains the openings (puncta) of the lacrimal canaliculi, which establish a passageway between the conjunctival sac and the inferior meatus of the nose. The bulbar part of the conjunctiva is transparent, allowing the sclera, or "white of the eye," to show through. The central portion of the bulbar conjunctiva is continuous at the limbus with the anterior epithelium of the cornea.

The *lacrimal apparatus* consists of the lacrimal gland and its ducts, the lacrimal passages, the lacrimal canaliculi and sac, and the nasal lacrimal duct. The lacrimal gland produces tears and secretes them through a series of ducts into the conjunctival sac. The tears then make their way inward to the puncta, from which they are conducted by the canaliculi to the lacrimal sac and finally pass into the nasal duct. When the lacrimal glands secrete too profusely, the normal drainage process becomes insufficient and overflow tearing results (Fig. 18-3).

Eyelids

The eyelids are two movable musculofibrous folds in front of each orbit that protect the globe and the eye from light.

The upper eyelid is more mobile and larger than the lower. The upper and lower lids meet at the medial and lateral angles *(canthi)* of the eye. The palpebral fissure, as previously mentioned, is located between the margins of the two eyelids. When the eye is closed, the cornea is completely covered by the upper eyelid. The eyelids are closed by the orbicular muscle of the eye, which is a circular muscle that acts as a sphincter. When the fibers contract, the eyes close. The upper lid is opened by the levator muscle, which is innervated by the third cranial nerve, as well as by relaxation of the orbicular muscle.

The eyelid consists of several layers. From front to back these are the skin, subcutaneous tissue that contains lymphatics, and muscles. Dense fibrous tissue, called *tarsal cartilage,* forms the framework of the lids. The tarsus is anchored to the walls of the orbit by the medial and lateral palpebral ligaments.

The free margins of each eyelid possess two or three rows of hairs called *cilia,* or eyelashes. Posterior to the lashes is a row of glandular orifices of the meibomian glands. Near the medial edges the free margin of each eyelid presents an opening called the *punctum lacrimale.* The eyelids distribute all adnexal secretions, thereby keeping the cornea moist and washing away any dust.

Muscles

The extrinsic ocular muscles of the eyeball are the four rectus and two oblique muscles. These six striated muscles are inserted into the sclera by tendons. These muscles,

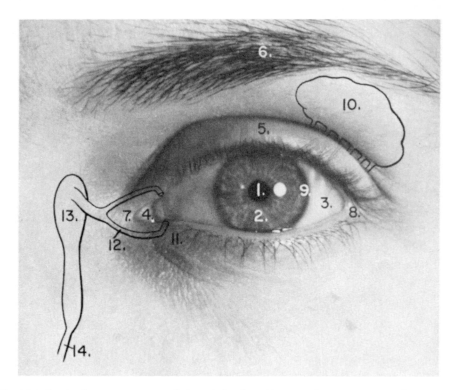

Fig. 18-3. Lacrimal apparatus, external view. *1*, Pupil; *2*, iris; *3*, conjunctiva; *4*, caruncle; *5*, upper lid; *6*, brow; *7*, inner canthus; *8*, outer canthus; *9*, limbus; *10*, lacrimal gland; *11*, near lower lacrimal punctum; *12*, lower lacrimal canaliculus *13*, lacrimal sac; *14*, nasolacrimal duct. (From Saunders, W.H., and others: Nursing care in eye, ear, nose and throat disorders, ed. 4, St. Louis, 1979, The C.V. Mosby Co.)

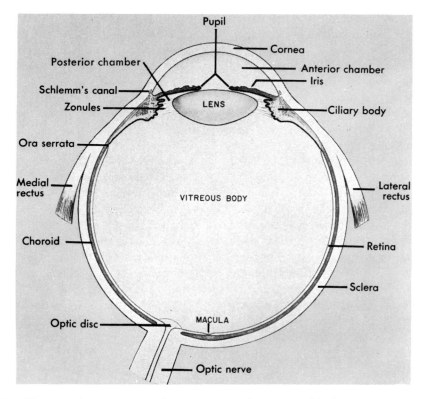

Fig. 18-4. Diagrammatic cross-section of eye. (From Saunders, W.H., and others: Nursing care in eye, ear, nose, and throat disorders, ed. 4, St. Louis, 1979, The C.V. Mosby Co.)

except for the interior oblique muscles, arise from the back of the orbit. All the muscles are supplied by cranial nerves: third (oculomotor), fourth (trochlear), and sixth (abducens). The muscles work in pairs. Movements of the eyes are brought about by an increase in the tone of one set of muscles and a decrease in the tone of the antagonistic muscles. According to the position of the recti muscles in the eyes, they are referred to as the superior rectus, inferior rectus, medial rectus, and lateral rectus muscles. The oblique muscles insert on the back of the eye and are designated the superior oblique and inferior oblique muscles.

Globe

The eyeball (globe) is supported in the orbital cavity on a cushion of fat and fascia. It is composed of three layers surrounding a fluid-filled center and occupies less than one third of the orbit. The external, corneal-scleral layer is fibrous and protects the other two. The middle, vascular, pigmented layer is comprised of the iris, ciliary body, and choroid, and the internal layer is the sensory retina. The fluid contents, which give the eye its globular shape, are aqueous humor, anteriorly, and vitreous humor, posterior to the lens. The lens, suspended behind the pupillary opening of the iris, and the cornea, combined with the aqueous and vitreous, form the refractive media of the eye (Fig. 18-4)

External layer (corneal-scleral)

The *cornea* is the anterior, transparent, avascular part of the external layer. It is crescent shaped and joins the sclera at a transitional zone called the *limbus*. The cornea is composed of five layers: the epithelium, Bowman's membrane, stroma (substantia propria), Descemet's membrane, and endothelium (Fig. 18-5). The epithelium consists of five or six constantly renewing cell layers and many nerve endings, which account for corneal sensitivity. Bowman's membrane is composed of connective tissue fibers and forms a barrier to trauma and infection. If damaged, it does not regenerate, and a permanent scar is left. The stroma accounts for 90% of the corneal thickness and is composed of multiple lamellar fibers. The endothelium is a single layer of hexagonal cells that do not regenerate. These cells are responsible for the proper state of dehydration (deturgescence) that keeps the cornea clear. Damage to these cells causes corneal edema and loss of transparency (Fig. 18-6). The cornea serves as a window through which light rays pass to the retina. The branches of the ophthalmic division of the fifth cranial nerve supply the cornea. Descemet's membrane is a thin layer between the endothelial layer of the cornea and the substantia propria. This membrane may become inflamed (descemetitis) or protude (descemetocele).

The *sclera* is the posterior opaque part of the external layer. A portion of the sclera can be seen through the

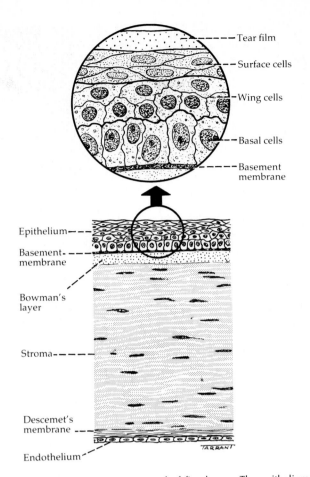

Fig. 18-5. The cornea is composed of five layers: The epithelium, Bowman's membrane, stroma (substantia propria), Descemet's membrane, endothelium. (From Kanski, J.J.: Clinical ophthalmology, London, 1984, Butterworth & Co.)

conjunctiva as the white of the eye. The sclera is made up of collagenous fibers loosely connected with fascia, which receives the tendons of the muscles of the globe. The sclera is pierced by the ciliary arteries and nerves and posteriorly by the optic nerve (Fig. 18-4).

Middle layer

The middle covering of the eye comprises the choroid, ciliary body, and iris from behind forward. The *choroid* contains many blood vessels and is the main source of nourishment of the receptor cell and pigment epithelial layer of the retina (Fig. 18-4).

The *ciliary body* consists of an extension of the choroidal blood vessels, a mass of muscle tissue, and an extension of the neuroepithelium of the retina. It extends 6 to 6.5 mm from the root of the iris to the ora serrata (Fig. 18-7). The anterior 2 mm of the ciliary body is called the pars plicata, and the posterior 4 to 5 mm is the pars plana (Fig. 18-8). The ciliary muscle effects accommodation. The neuroepithelium is secretory in nature and is responsible for the formation of the aqueous humor.

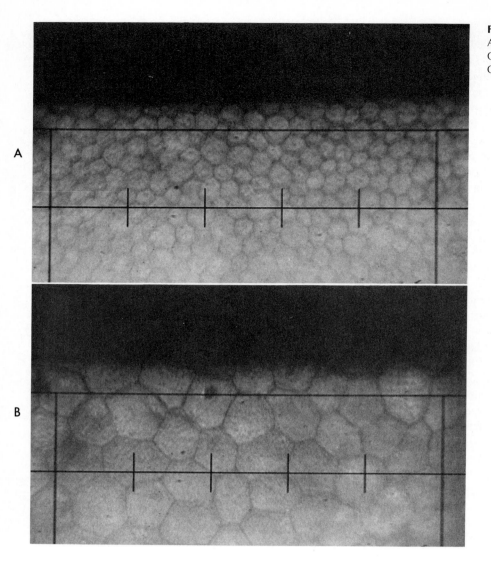

A

B

Fig. 18-6. Endothelial cells. **A,** Normal. **B,** Abnormal. (Courtesy Lorraine Koury, Argon Ophthalmic Laboratory, Inc., Portland, Ore.)

Fig. 18-7. Diagrammatic section of the anterior eye and the aqueous circulation. (From Saunders, W.H., and others: Nursing care in eye, ear, nose, and throat disorders, ed. 4, St. Louis, 1979, The C.V. Mosby Co.)

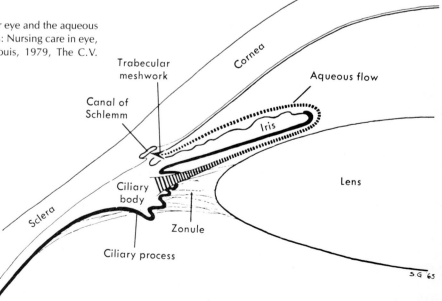

Trabecular meshwork

Canal of Schlemm

Cornea

Aqueous flow

Iris

Lens

Sclera

Ciliary body

Zonule

Ciliary process

SG 65

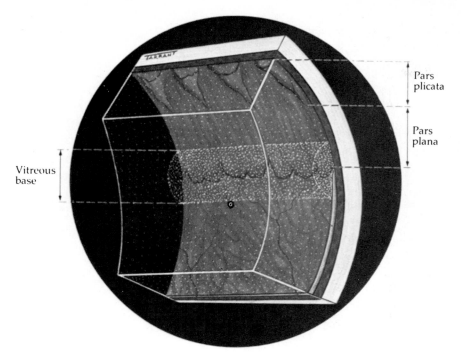

Fig. 18-8. Anatomy of pars plana. (From Kanski, J.J.: Clinical ophthalmology, London, 1984, Butterworth & Co.)

The *iris,* a thin membrane, is the anterior portion of the middle-layer and is situated in front of the lens. The peripheral border of the iris is attached to the ciliary body, whereas its central border is free. The iris aperture is located slightly nasal to its center, known as the *pupil* (Fig. 18-4). The iris divides the space between the cornea and the lens into an anterior and a posterior chamber. Both chambers are filled with aqueous humor.

The iris with its many striations regulates the amount of light entering the eye and assists in obtaining clear images. The iris moves by means of smooth muscle fibers within the connective tissue. The sphincter pupillae muscle contracts the pupil, and the dilator pupillae dilates it. As more light strikes the eye, the sphincter constricts the pupil.

Internal layer

The innermost layer, sometimes called the nervous covering, is the *retina.* The retina is a thin, transparent membrane extending from the ora serrata to the optic disc (Figs. 18-4 and 18-9). This network of nerve cells and fibers receives images of external objects and transfers the impression via the optic nerve, optic tracts, lateral geniculate body, and optic radiations to the occipital lobe of the cerebrum. The nerve fibers from the retina converge to become the optic nerve, which enters the eyeball almost at its posterior point, slightly to the inner side. The point at which the nerve enters the eyeball is called the *optic disc* (Fig. 18-9). In field testing, this is the anatomical blind spot.

The retina is composed of many layers. The pigment epithelium is a single layer of epithelial cells on the external side of the retina through which oxygen and other nutrients are diffused from the choroid. The other nine layers of the retina consist of photoreceptor cells (rods and cones) and sensory neurons (bipolar cells and ganglion

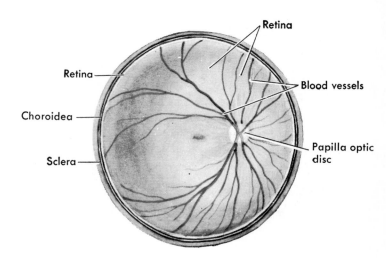

Fig. 18-9. Normal fundus of eye: view of eye seen through ophthalmoscope. (From Anthony, C.P., and Kolthoff, N.J.: Textbook of anatomy and physiology, ed. 9, St. Louis, 1975, The C.V. Mosby Co.)

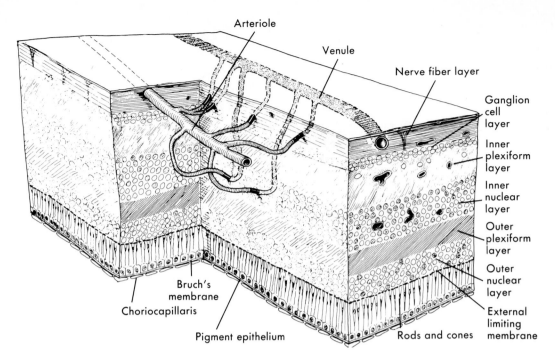

Arteriole

Venule

Nerve fiber layer

Ganglion cell layer

Inner plexiform layer

Inner nuclear layer

Outer plexiform layer

Outer nuclear layer

External limiting membrane

Bruch's membrane

Choriocapillaris

Pigment epithelium

Rods and cones

Fig. 18-10. Retinal arterioles provide two major capillary layers in the retina: one in the nerve fiber layer and one in the inner nuclear layer. In general, diseases affecting primarily the arteries, such as vascular hypertension, involve the capillary network in the nerve fiber layer, whereas predominantly venous diseases, such as diabetes mellitus, involve the layer of capillaries in the inner nuclear layer. The outer receptors together with their cell bodies in the outer nuclear layer and a portion of the outer plexiform layer are nurtured by the choriocapillaris of the choroid. Both systems are necessary to the function of the retina. (From Newell, F.W.: Ophthalmology: principles and concepts, ed. 5, St. Louis, 1982, The C.V. Mosby Co.)

cells) (Fig. 18-10). The photoreceptors within the retina respond to light energy and initiate the neural response, which is eventually interpreted in the occipital cortex. The point of highest resolution is the foveal pit, which exists in the center of the area that takes on a yellow hue after death (macula lutea).

An inverted image of the object being viewed is focused on the retina. The nerve fibers leaving the retina by the way of the optic nerve travel to the lateral geniculate body of the thalamus. The fibers nasal to the foveal pit cross in the optic chiasma to go to the contralateral geniculate body. Thus all fibers composing the same half of the visual field project to the same geniculate body, from which fibers project to the ipsi lateral occipital cortex for interpretation.

Refractive apparatus

The refractive apparatus consists of the cornea, the aqueous humor, the lens, and the vitreous body (Fig. 18-4).

The cornea has the greatest refractive power of the ocular structures. Variations in the curvature of the cornea change its refractive power (Fig. 18-11).

The *lens* of the eye is biconvex and has a diameter of

1 cm (Figs. 18-4 and 18-7). It is suspended behind the iris and connected to the ciliary body by zonular fibers. Its anterior and posterior surfaces are separated by a rounded border, the *equator*. The crystalline lens does not shed cells. As it grows, the cells are compressed and harden. The lens can expand and retract by means of the zonular fibers (accommodation); this accommodative power is lost with the aging process, as the lens loses its elasticity when the cells harden. This is the reason many older persons need bifocals. Eventually the hardening causes opacity of the lens, termed a *cataract*.

The *vitreous body* is a glasslike, transparent, gelatinous mass composed of 99% water and 1% collagen and hyaluronic acid. It fills the posterior four fifths of the eyeball and is adherent to the retina at the vitreous base.

The central components of a light wave enter the eyes perpendicularly, and a light wave enters at the sides obliquely. For clear vision the oblique rays must converge and come to a focus with the central rays on the retina. Light rays from an object pass through the system of refractory devices—the cornea, aqueous humor, lens, and vitreous—and are refracted so that the rays strike the macular area.

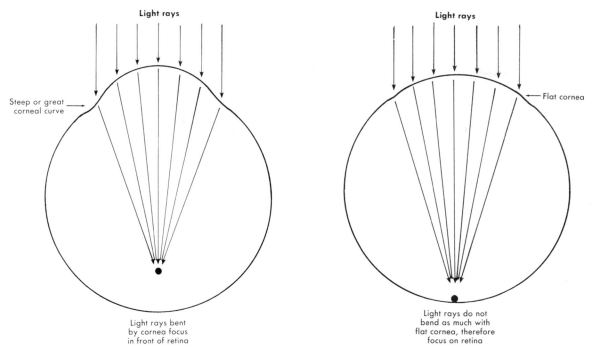

Fig. 18-11. Variations in the curvature of the cornea change its refractive power.

Nerve and blood supply

The optic nerve (second cranial nerve) extends between the posterior eyeball and the optic chiasma (Fig. 18-12). This nerve carries visual impulses, as well as the sensations of pain, touch, and temperature, from the eye and its surrounding structures to the brain. The third cranial nerve (oculomotor) is the primary motor nerve to all rectus muscles except the lateral rectus, which is innervated by the sixth cranial nerve (abducens). The fourth cranial nerve (trochlear) innervates the superior oblique muscle.

The ophthalmic artery, the main arterial supply to the orbit and globe, is a branch of the internal carotid artery. It divides into branches supplying the globe, muscles, and eyelids. The central retinal artery and central retinal vein travel through the optic nerve and provide an independent circulation for the inner retina.

PERIOPERATIVE NURSING CONSIDERATIONS
Assessment/nursing diagnosis

Patients entering the hospital or ambulatory unit for eye surgery exhibit many emotions and reactions, such as hostility, anger, fear, grief, and helplessness. Of prime concern to most is the success of the surgical procedure. Patients undergoing eye surgery vary from infants with congenital conditions to geriatric patients whose conditions are a result of the aging process. With the increase in outpatient surgery, the staff must not only be prepared to meet the specific needs of each patient when providing care but also prepare the patient for home care.

Preparation is begun in the physician's office or clinic. Communication with the physician's office to coordinate patient preparation and teaching increases the efficiency and effectiveness of preoperative procedures.

Admission assessment

On the patient's admission to the unit, a staff member should fully orient the patient to the physical surroundings. It may be helpful to walk with the patient to familiarize him or her with areas of the room and nursing unit. Constant description and reinforcement are important to the visually impaired. Subtle changes such as approaching the patient from the nonaffected side increase the patient's independence, facilitate care, and decrease the possibility of startling the patient. Consistency in nursing personnel helps the patient recognize familiar voices and faces. It is preferable to have all ophthalmic patients in one area to decrease the risk of cross-contamination and to provide specialized care.

In addition to routine admission information and review of medications the patient is currently taking, an ocular history must be obtained. It should include the patient's primary problem, history of the present illness, nature of symptoms, and limitations imposed on the patient by the disease or condition. A medical history, including other body systems, should also be obtained because ocular problems may be directly related to other diseases. An external examination of the eye, including lids, lashes, conjunctiva, and lacrimal apparatus, should be performed

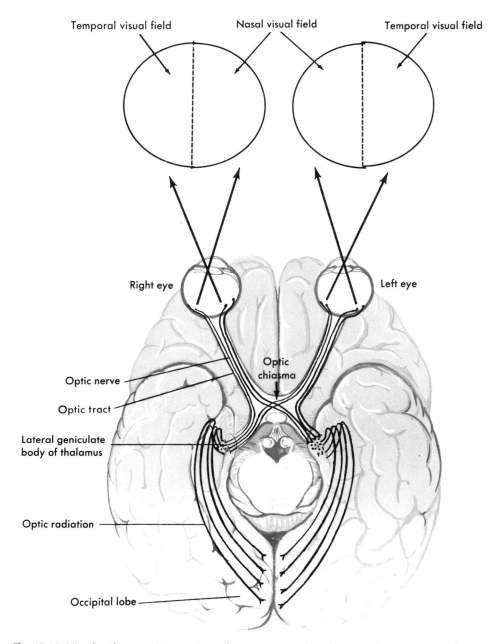

Temporal visual field   Nasal visual field   Temporal visual field

Right eye   Left eye

Optic
chiasma

Optic nerve

Optic tract

Lateral geniculate
body of thalamus

Optic radiation

Occipital lobe

Fig. 18-12. Visual pathways. Note structures that compose each pathway: optic nerve, optic chiasma, lateral geniculate body of thalamus, optic radiations, and visual cortex of occipital lobe. Fibers from nasal portion of each retina cross over to opposite side at optic chiasma, hence terminating in lateral geniculate body of opposite side. Location of lesion in visual pathway determines resulting visual defect. For example, destruction of an optic nerve produces permanent blindness in same eye, and pressure on optic chiasma (by pituitary tumor, for instance) produces bitemporal hemianopsia, or more simply, blindness in both temporal visual fields because it destroys fibers from nasal sides of both retinas. (Modified from Thibodeau, G.A.: Anthony's textbook of anatomy and physiology, ed. 13, St. Louis, 1990, The C.V. Mosby Co.)

to detect any deviations from normal. The corneal reflex should be tested, and the cornea inspected for superficial irregularities. Pupil size and contour should be noted, as well as pupillary reaction, both direct and consensual. Anterior chamber depth should be checked with oblique illumination to alert staff members to the potential for angle closure with dilation of the pupil (Fig. 18-13).

Function of the extraocular muscles should be determined. Movement should be synchronous, and visual lines should meet on a fixed object. Documentation of this examination must be descriptive, accurate, and concise. It is of value later in assessing the outcome of the procedure.

After the assessment information has been compiled, nursing diagnoses are identified and the plan of care for the entire perioperative period is developed. Nursing di-

agnoses related to the care of patients having ophthalmic procedures might include:

- Knowledge deficit related to diagnosis, surgical intervention, and home care management
- Visual sensory or perceptual alteration related to surgical intervention
- Anxiety related to surgical intervention and its outcome
- Potential for injury related to increased intraocular pressure
- Potential for infection related to surgical intervention

Assessment overview
Observations/findings

These should be obtained and/or confirmed during perioperative nursing assessment.

- General appearance of the eye (swelling, redness, skin condition around eyes)
- Observe for irritation (itching, burning)
- Position of eyelids, condition of upper and lower lid surfaces, eyelid spasm
- Visual acuity, pupillary dilation (note whether pupils are equal, round, reactive to light and accommodative), visual fields
- Extraocular muscle movement
- Note any drainage from eye (type and amount)
- Vital signs (obtain and record)
- Observe for and note any restlessness, discomfort, anxiety
- Limitations in mobility, if any, should be noted
- Current and significant past medical problems (eye disease, diabetes, cardiovascular disease, hypertension, allergies)
- Current medication history

Laboratory studies

The results of these studies, as applicable to the individual patient, should be reviewed during perioperative nursing assessment. Deviations from normal should be noted and recorded.

- Blood sugar
- Serum potassium and other electrolytes
- Electrocardiogram and/or chest x-ray
- Serum enzymes and other blood work (CBC, coagulation studies)

Planning

Care plans are the framework for organizing activities in the perioperative period. Although ophthalmic surgery is often perceived as minor due to the small incision site and because many procedures generally are not lengthy, the perioperative nurse must be fully prepared for potential complications or emergencies. Patients who are admitted to the ophthalmic surgical unit often have complex medical histories. Following a review of the patient record, sup-

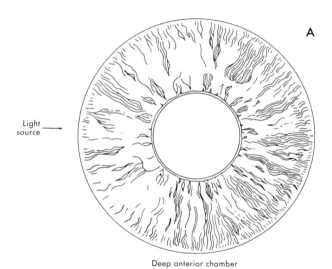

A

Light source →

Deep anterior chamber

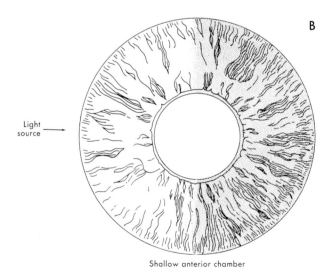

B

Light source →

Shallow anterior chamber

Fig. 18-13. Oblique illumination of cornea. **A,** Normal anterior chamber depth (entire iris illuminated). **B,** Shallow anterior chamber (half of the iris is in shadow).

Sample Care Plan

NURSING DIAGNOSIS:
Knowledge deficit related to diagnosis, surgical intervention, and home care management
GOAL:
Patient and/or significant other will verbalize knowledge of the diagnosis, planned intervention, and requirements for home care maintenance.
INTERVENTIONS:
Determine the patient's understanding of the diagnosis, the planned surgical intervention, and the type of anesthesia to be administered.
Clarify misconceptions and provide additional explanations (or refer to appropriate member of health care team).
Explain sequence of perioperative events and what to expect in the operating room in terms that the patient can understand.
Review postoperative limitations to self-care activities.
Provide and review written instructions (in large letters) regarding medications, including specific techniques for instilling eye drops and ophthalmic medications, application of compresses (as applicable), and application of appropriate eye dressing or protective shield.
Supervise patient practice with prescribed self-care activities (for example, instillation of medications).

NURSING DIAGNOSIS:
Visual sensory/perceptual alteration related to surgical intervention
GOAL:
Patient will cope with visual sensory/perceptual alteration safely.
INTERVENTIONS:
Introduce self and other team members so that patient can recognize voices.
Familiarize and orient patient to immediate surroundings; continuously reorient patient.
Approach patient from unaffected side.
Offer reassurance, explanations, and understanding.
Prior to discharge, review and have patient list safety measures to prevent falls and other injuries.
Refer patient to appropriate agency if home assistance is required.

NURSING DIAGNOSIS:
Anxiety related to surgical intervention and its outcome
GOAL:
Patient will verbalize concerns and fears and utilize coping mechanisms.
INTERVENTIONS:
Allow patient time to verbalize concerns.
Assist the patient to identify the source of anxiety.

plemented by a patient and/or family interview or collaboration with colleagues, data collected are incorporated into a perioperative plan for patient care. The Sample Care Plan demonstrates how data may be organized.

Implementation

Implementation of the care plan actually begins during the patient interview. Planning to meet the patient's educational needs should play an equal role with meeting other needs. Review and reinforcement of information initially provided in the physician's office ensure consistency in teaching. Written material and audiovisual media (television, films, pictures, and slides) may be used to enhance patient education programs but do not eliminate the need for direct interchange with patients or feedback from them. Family members or friends should be included to add support and increase understanding of the planned surgery. The ophthalmic patient should be informed of the purpose and desired results of preoperative eyedrops and sedation. An explanation of what to expect from the anesthetic decreases the patient's anxiety level and enables the patient to cooperate better. The perioperative nurse should discuss

Sample Care Plan—cont'd

Help the patient identify existing personal strengths and external resources.

Encourage independence by allowing patient to assist with plan of care; involve patient in identifying diversional activities.

Observe the patient's facial expressions, body posture, and vital signs.

Broadly classify the patient's level of anxiety based on nursing observation (low, moderate, high).

Offer comfort measures (for example, warm blankets).

Provide emotional support; reinforce information the patient has been previously given.

Use touch (as appropriate) to communicate reassurance.

Control environmental stimuli in the OR.

NURSING DIAGNOSIS:

Potential for injury related to increased intraocular pressure

GOAL:

Patient will identify activities that increase intraocular pressure.

INTERVENTIONS:

Monitor for the presence of, or an increase in, eye pain, pain around orbit, blurred vision, reddened eye, abdominal pain, nausea, vomiting, neurological changes, and changes in visual fields; initiate appropriate nursing action.

Instruct the patient to refrain from excessive exertion, such as crying, coughing, straining, rapid movements, bending over, lifting, rubbing the eyes, and blowing the nose.

Discuss methods to facilitate bowel elimination (diet, appropriate exercise, stool softeners if prescribed).

NURSING DIAGNOSIS:

Potential for infection related to surgical intervention

GOAL:

Patient will be free of signs and symptoms of postoperative infection.

INTERVENTIONS:

Preoperatively, note whether the patient has a preexisting infection, is immunocompromised, or has other conditions that compromise resistance to infection.

Maintain an aseptic perioperative environment.

Adhere to good handwashing practices.

Determine and record the wound classification.

Postoperatively, monitor vital signs, fluid balance, and presence of pain.

Instruct the patient in self-care, including postoperative antibiotic therapy, if prescribed.

Teach the patient to wash her or his hands prior to the instillation of any ophthalmic medications.

Instruct the patient to watch for redness, pain, swelling, drainage, and changes in visual acuity postoperatively, and report these problems promptly to the physician.

---

the activities and routines of the intraoperative period. A brief description of the operating room and its equipment, on the patient's arrival in the surgical suite, helps allay the patient's fears.

The patient should be informed of what to expect immediately after surgery so that the postoperative recovery period is less stressful. Reassurance is especially important for patients whose eyes will be patched postoperatively.

Thorough preoperative preparation plays a vital role in the successful outcome of the surgical procedure.

General duties of the perioperative nursing team are

discussed in the previous chapters. However, some considerations are specific to the ophthalmic patient. Because many ophthalmic procedures are performed under local anesthesia, the circulating nurse or an additional monitor nurse, if available, must be prepared to monitor the patient and provide supportive care. Ophthalmic patients, like other surgical patients, have increased sensitivity to noise and activities within the room. The room should be kept quiet and peaceful to decrease the patient's anxiety and increase cooperation.

The scrub nurse has additional responsibilities. Foreign

substances must not be introduced intraocularly. Lint-free barriers should be used to create the sterile field on the instrument table; gloved hands must be wiped with moistened towels to remove powder particles before the procedure begins. The portion of an instrument used in an intraocular wound should not be touched by gloved hands, and debris should be cleansed from instruments with cellulose sponges. All solutions on the sterile field must be clearly labeled, and intraocular solutions must be separated from those not used intraocularly.

The entire surgical team must be knowledgeable about their roles and be prepared to function quickly in the event of a complication.

Ophthalmic pharmacology

Medications used in the perioperative period are extremely important to the outcome of the procedure and the safety of the patient.

Drugs for diagnosing and treating eye disorders are extremely potent. One error could result in total, irreversible blindness.

The patient's medical and ocular histories determine the selection of an appropriate ophthalmic agent. This information should be included in the patient's initial nursing assessment.

The following established protocols for each medication administration greatly reduce the possibility of medication errors:

1. The nurse must be knowledgeable about the specific medication ordered, including purpose, strength, action, duration, adverse reactions, route of administration, and contraindications.
2. Expiration dates should be checked prior to medication administration.
3. The medication label must be checked during preparation and again immediately before administration. This precaution is especially important because many ophthalmic drugs are distributed in single-dose units that closely resemble one another.
4. The patient must be positively identified, and the site of the administration must be clearly translated from the physician's orders. The abbreviations OD, OS, and OU indicate right eye, left eye, and both eyes, respectively.
5. Ensuring that the precise dose of medication is given at its scheduled time greatly enhances its effectiveness.

The patient should be made aware of the expected effect of each medication to be able to evaluate its effectiveness, detect signs and symptoms of adverse reactions, and know when to notify the physician concerning problems. The patient should also be well informed of the special considerations associated with specific medications so that appropriate safety precautions can be taken. An example is protection of the cornea after application of a topical anesthetic.

Selection of specific medication is influenced by the physician's education and experience and the patient's disease condition. Following is a classification of ophthalmic medications and specific examples of use.

Dilating drops

Dilating drops (mydriatics and cycloplegics) are used to dilate the pupil for objective examination of the retina, testing of refraction, or easier removal of the lens. Mydriatic drugs dilate the pupil but permit the patient to focus. The most commonly used mydriatic is phenylephrine 2%, 5%, or 10% (Neo-Synephrine).

A cycloplegic drug dilates the pupil and also inhibits focusing of the eye. This type of drug aids refraction procedures. Commonly used cycloplegics are tropicamide (Mydriacyl) 1%, atropine 1%, and cyclopentolate 1% (Cyclogyl). Atropine has a long-lasting effect.

Constricting drops

Miotic drugs increase contraction of the sphincter of the iris, thus causing the pupil to contract and constrict. Commonly used miotics are pilocarpine 1% to 4% and phospholine iodide 0.012% to 0.25%. In addition to their action on the pupil, miotics improve the ease with which the aqueous fluid escapes from the eye, thereby resulting in a decrease in intraocular pressure. Miotics are used in the treatment of glaucoma.

Phospholine iodide is usually discontinued before intraocular surgery is performed. Phospholine iodide, isoflurophate (DFP, Floropryl), and demecarium bromide (Humorsol) are irreversible anticholinesterase drugs and may cause prolonged apnea when used in conjunction with succinylcholine (Anectine).

Pilocarpine is often used after the extraction of a cataractous lens to cause sustained pupillary contraction and prevent vitreous rupture.

Acetylcholine is the natural cholinergic transmitter released by the parasympathetic nerves to the iris sphincter. It is relatively unstable in solution. Acetylcholine (Miochol) is often used intraocularly to produce rapid pupillary contraction (constriction), especially after the insertion of an artificial lens, or pseudophakia. Acetylcholine is prepared immediately before use.

Carbochol (Isoptocarbochol) is used to manage narrow- and wide-angle glaucoma. Recent studies (Silverstone, Hufnagle & Miller, 1989) indicate significantly less elevation in intraocular pressure postoperatively when carbochol (Miostat) 0.01% is used in place of acetylcholine intraoperatively.

Corticosteroids

A great number of corticosteroid preparations exist. Corticosteroids are used to inhibit the normal inflammatory response to noxious stimuli. Corticosteroids reduce the resistance of the eye to invasion by bacteria, viruses, and fungi. Presence of active infection is therefore an important contraindication to therapy with cortisone and its derivatives in the treatment of allergic eye conditions and chronic inflammations.

Hyperosmotic agents

Hyperosmotic drugs increase the osmolarity of the serum and, by the effect of the induced osmotic pressure gradient, shrink the vitreous body and reduce the intraocular pressure. These drugs are used routinely in the preoperative medication of patients undergoing ophthalmic surgery, as well as therapeutically in cases of uncontrolled glaucoma (usually angle-closure glaucoma).

The commonly used agents may be divided into those given orally (glycerol and isosorbide) and those given parenterally (mannitol and urea). Hyperosmotic drugs by their nature induce diuresis; nursing personnel must be aware of this and have urinals, bedpans, and sterile urethral catheters available.

Antibiotics, lubricants, and stains

The method or route of administration of an antibiotic agent depends on the location of the problem. Selection of the drug is based on the nature and sensitivity of the organism isolated, the physicians's clinical experience, the sensitivity and response of the patient, and the disease. Topical antibiotics are used in the treatment of lid and surface infections and often employed prophylactically to prevent infection. Bacitracin and neomycin sulfate are commonly used antibiotic ointments.

Systemic administration of an antibiotic is prescribed for an infection in the posterior portion of the eye or orbit. An infection of this nature can threaten sight. Selection of the specific antibiotic follows the previously mentioned criteria.

Ophthalmic lubricants are used for corneal protection in situations such as faulty lid closure, complications of lacrimal gland disease, and prominence of the corneal surface in thyroid disease. Methylcellulose 0.5% is considered an excellent ophthalmic lubricant.

Fluorescein sodium is a dye and topical stain commonly used for diagnostic purposes. An intravenous preparation of the dye is used in fluorescein angiography to diagnose retinal pathology. Fluorescein strips or solution is used to stain the cornea in evaluating disruption of the corneal epithelium. The use of fluorescein strips is preferred to the use of solution because the solution can easily become contaminated. In its dilute form, fluorescein is yellow-green and temporarily stains the areas of denuded corneal epithelium.

Sodium hyaluronate (Healon, Amvisc, Viscot) functions as a lubricant and as a viscoelastic support, maintaining a separation between tissues. It is used in intra-ocular procedures to protect the corneal endothelium and as a tamponade and vitreous substitute during surgery of the retina and vitreous.

Sedation, when indicated, may be ordered and managed by either the surgeon or the anesthesiologist. The nurse, however, is often accountable for managing the patient's response to the sedation and the local anesthetic in the perioperative period.

Anesthesia

Local or local standby (monitored anesthesia care) anesthesia is preferred for most eye surgery. Consideration must be given to the patient's age, systemic condition, and discharge plan in determining whether to use preoperative sedation.

The circulating nurse assembles the sterile local anesthesia setup as ordered by the surgeon before the patient enters the operating room. The nurse checks the drugs to ensure correct medications and proper concentrations and dosages. Needles and syringes of proper sizes and gauges are necessary.

Drugs

Tetracaine (Pontocaine) in a 0.5% solution and proparacaine hydrochloride (Ophthaine) in a 0.5% solution are two commonly used topical anesthetics. They have a rapid onset (5 to 20 seconds) and a moderate duration of action (10 to 20 minutes).

Cocaine 1% to 4% has a rapid onset and a moderate duration. It must never be injected. Cocaine produces excellent surface anesthesia but induces loosening of the corneal epithelium.

Epinephrine 1:1000 solution is a vasoconstrictor that may be applied topically to mucous membranes to decrease bleeding.

Lidocaine 1% to 2% is the most commonly used medication for infiltration anesthesia or nerve blocks. It has rapid onset, a fairly long duration of action, and good diffusion properties. Allergic reactions are rare, and cross-sensitivity with other local anesthetic agents is unusual. Marcaine in a 0.25% to 0.5% solution is used in certain cases because of its long duration.

Epinephrine in a 1:50,000 to 1:200,000 solution may be combined with injectable local anesthetics such as lidocaine to prolong anesthesia and reduce bleeding. Epinephrine in a 1:1000 solution is not used with local anesthetics because it can cause cardiac dysrhythmias.

Hyaluronidase (Wydase) is an enzyme that is commonly mixed with anesthetic solutions (75 units/10 ml) to increase diffusion of the anesthetic through the tissue and thus improve the effectiveness of the nerve block.

Methods used for administration of local anesthetics

The three methods of administration are instillation of eyedrops, infiltration, and block or regional anesthesia.

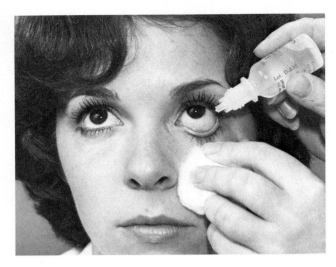

Fig. 18-14. Proper position of head for instillation of eyedrops. Gentle retraction of lower lid is necessary for drop to be placed in lower cul-de-sac.

Instillation of eyedrops (Fig. 18-14). With the patient's face tilted upward, the first drop is placed in the lower cul-de-sac, and the succeeding drops (number depends on the type of operation to be performed) may be placed from above, with the patient looking downward and the upper lid raised. Gentle retraction of the lower lid is necessary for placing eyedrops in the lower cul-de-sac. Care should be taken to avoid placing eyedrops directly onto the cornea. The natural blinking of the lids distributes the drug evenly on the eye surface, regardless of where the drop is placed. When a toxic drug is instilled, the inner corner of the eyelids should be dried of excessive fluid with a tissue or clean cotton ball after each drop to minimize systemic absorption of the drug. The tip of any drug applicator must not touch the patient's skin or any part of the eye.

Infiltration method. The surgeon injects the anesthetic solution beneath the skin, beneath the conjunctiva, or into Tenon's capsule, depending on the type of surgery.

Block or regional anesthesia. Retrobulbar anesthesia is injection of anesthetic solution into the base of the eyelids at the level of the orbital margins or behind the eyeball to block the ciliary ganglion and nerves (Fig. 18-15). For eyelid repairs the solution is injected through the lower lid. For operations on the lacrimal apparatus, the anesthetic is injected at the level of the anterior ethmoidal foramen to anesthetize the internal and external nasal nerves. Retrobulbar injection is usually performed 10 to 15 minutes before surgery to produce temporary paralysis of the extraocular muscles.

In the Van Lint block method, procaine or another local anesthetic is injected into the orbicular muscle where it reaches the ends of the facial nerve (Fig. 18-16, *A*). The O'Brien akinesia technique requires blocking of the facial

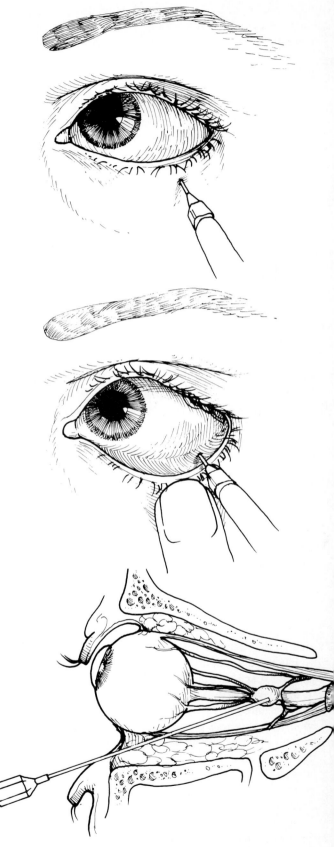

Fig. 18-15. Retrobulbar block for regional anesthesia.

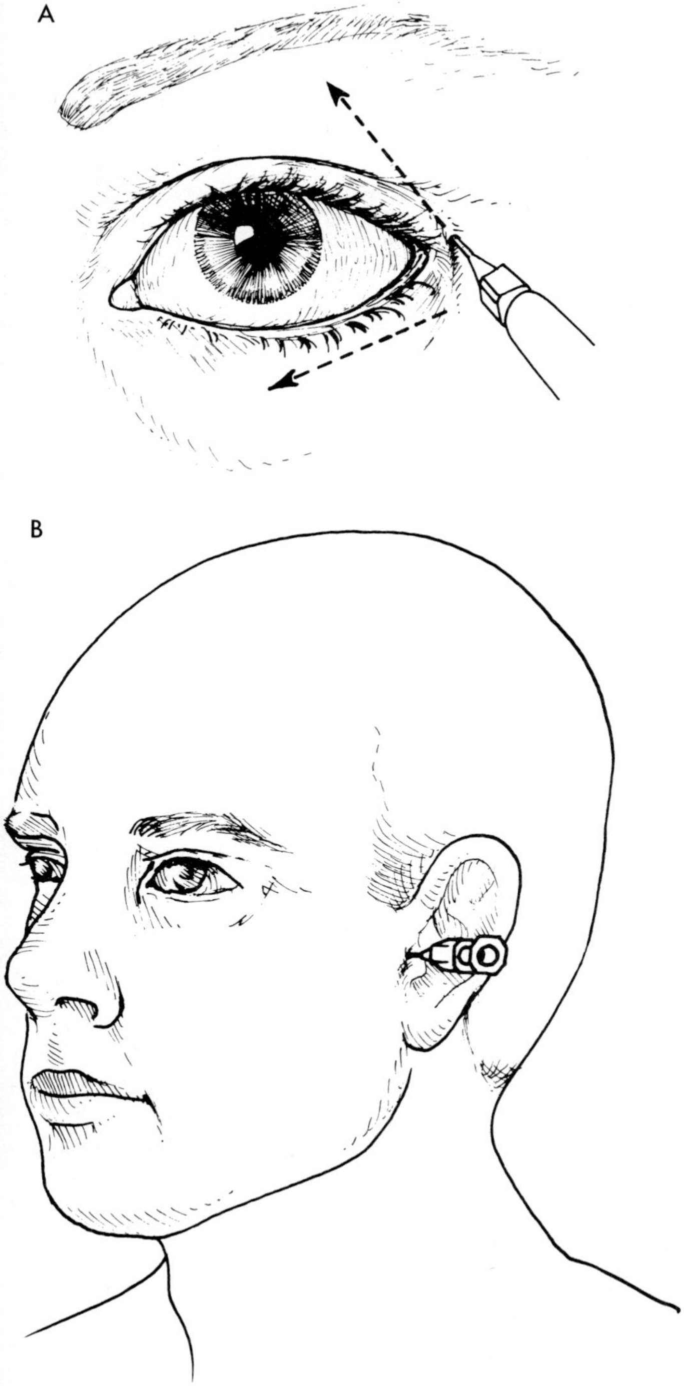

nerve just anterior to the tragus of the ear (Fig. 18-16, *B*). These blocks are used to prevent "squeezing" of the lids during ocular procedures.

General anesthesia

Youth, dementia, severe anxiety, specific systemic diseases, and long duration of the operative procedure are among the conditions that may dictate use of general anesthesia.

Patient preparation

Members of the nursing team have several important responsibilities in the admission of the patient to the operating room and in the preparation of the room and the equipment. Technologic advances in ophthalmic surgery require that nurses have familiarity with equipment and check each piece carefully before the patient arrives in the operating room.

Scrupulous attention to aseptic technique and nursing measures designed for safety and comfort of the patient are of prime importance. The duties of the nursing team include the following:

1. Identifying the patient by name if awake; seeking patient cooperation and confidence by speaking softly, distinctly, and confidently; and endeavoring to keep the patient quiet and relaxed by staying close by and establishing contact by touch
2. Checking the patient's name on the wristband with the name on the chart and on the surgical schedule
3. Reviewing the surgeon's preoperative orders and nurses' notes to determine if the correct operative eye has been prepared properly and other procedures have been carried out according to hospital policies
4. Reaffirming preoperative orders with the surgeon if necessary
5. Preparing the operating room bed, making sure all the necessary attachments are in readiness
6. Starting an intravenous drip, placing the blood pressure cuff and pulse oximeter, recording the baseline blood pressure and heart rate, and attaching the cardiac monitor

Preparation of the face

The operative site is prepared under aseptic conditions. Topical anesthetic drops are administered first, if the patient is to be given a local anesthetic. A sterile prep tray containing sterile normal saline solution, irrigation bulb, basins, cotton sponges, cotton-tipped applicators, towels, and antimicrobial skin disinfectant is prepared.

The clipping of eyelashes or shaving of eyebrows is not routinely done. When eyelashes are clipped, it is done before the skin preparation. A thin film of water-soluble lubricant is smoothed over the cutting surfaces of a curved eyelash scissors so the free lashes adhere to the blades rather than fall into the eyes or onto the face.

Fig. 18-16. A, Van Lint block. **B,** O'Brien akinesia blocking of the facial nerve.

Eye preparation includes cleansing the eyelids of both eyes, lid margins, lashes, eyebrows, and surrounding skin with an appropriate antimicrobial solution (Fig. 18-17). Care is taken to prevent the solution from entering the patient's eyes and ears. The eyes are then irrigated with normal saline solution using an irrigation bulb (Fig. 18-18). To properly clean the lid margins, the lids should be everted and cleaned with cotton-tipped applicators moistened with antimicrobial skin disinfectant (Fig. 18-19).

When toxic chemicals or small particles of foreign matter must be removed, the eyes are irrigated with tepid sterile physiologic saline solution. The conjunctival sac is thoroughly flushed, using an irrigation bulb or an Asepto syringe.

Draping

The local anesthetic may be injected before completion of the draping procedure. Aseptic principles for draping a patient for an operation are discussed in Chapter 5.

Special concerns for eye surgery draping include eliminating lint and fiber particles and providing adequate air exchange for patients receiving local anesthetics. A method of draping is shown in Fig. 18-20. This method eliminates the need to lift the patient's head while draping and facilitates drape removal at the end of the procedure.

Another method of draping is shown in Fig. 18-21. In this method:

1. The head is draped with a double-thickness half sheet and two towels.
2. A large folded sheet is used to cover the patient and operating room bed.
3. A fenestrated plastic eye sheet is placed over the operative site.

Instrumentation

Rapid progress in ophthalmic surgical techniques and instrumentation has contributed to almost unbelievable results for eye patients. Exacting performance of eye instruments is crucial to the success of operations.

Basic eye instruments are shown in Fig. 18-22. An ophthalmic forceps, called a fixation forceps, is used to hold tissue firmly in place or provide traction before incision. It has an angled tooth that overlaps for secure fixation (Fig. 18-23). Several styles are available, and selection depends on the surgeon's preference. A suturing forceps is used to pick up wound edges for dissection or suturing. It is a single-toothed forceps with the teeth at right angles to the shank of the forceps (Fig. 18-24). Suturing forceps are available in many styles with varying sizes of teeth, such as a Castroviejo 0.12 mm or 0.5 mm. A utility or dressing forceps is used for gentle handling of delicate tissue. It has fine serrations on its straight shank and is commonly called a fine serrated forceps (Fig. 18-25).

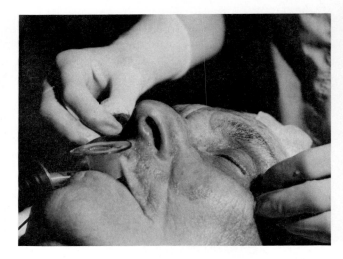

Fig. 18-17. Prepping procedure for eye surgery.

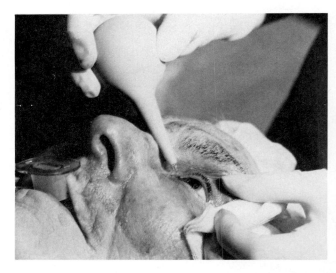

Fig. 18-18. Bulb syringe and normal saline solution are used to irrigate eye during prepping procedure. Direction of solution flow is always to outer, lateral side of face.

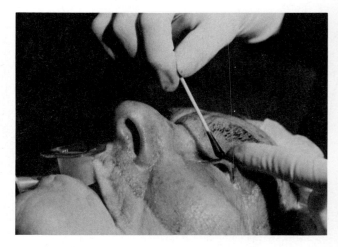

Fig. 18-19. Eyelid is everted when cleaning lid margins.

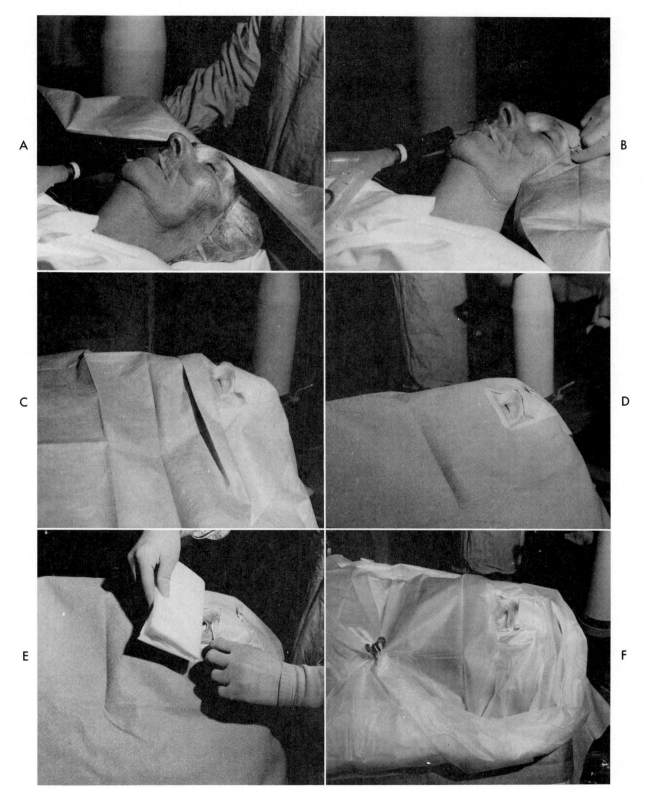

Fig. 18-20. Method of draping. **A,** With both hands under cuff of head drape, scrub nurse places adhesive strip above brow line. **B,** Adhesive strip is secured along side of patient's head anterior to ears. **C,** Adhesive towel drape is placed over patient's nose for general anesthesia. **D,** Split sheet is used to cover operating room bed and to isolate operative eye. **E,** Clear plastic adhesive drape is placed over operative eye. **F,** Drape is secured to collect irrigation fluid.

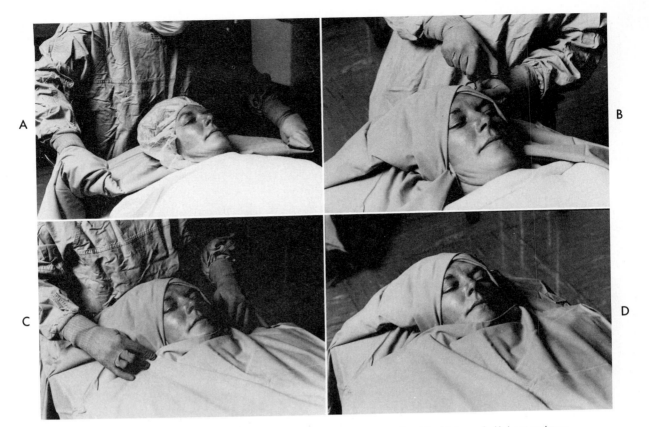

Fig. 18-21. Alternative method of draping of eye surgery patient. **A,** Double-thickness half sheet and two towels are placed under head. **B,** Towel is secured around head covering ears and hair. **C,** Patient and operating room bed are covered with large folded sheet. **D,** Patient under local anesthetic is now ready for fenestrated plastic drape, completing procedure.

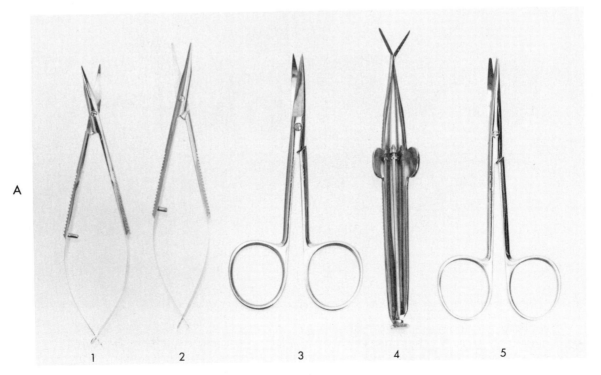

Fig. 18-22. For legend see opposite page.

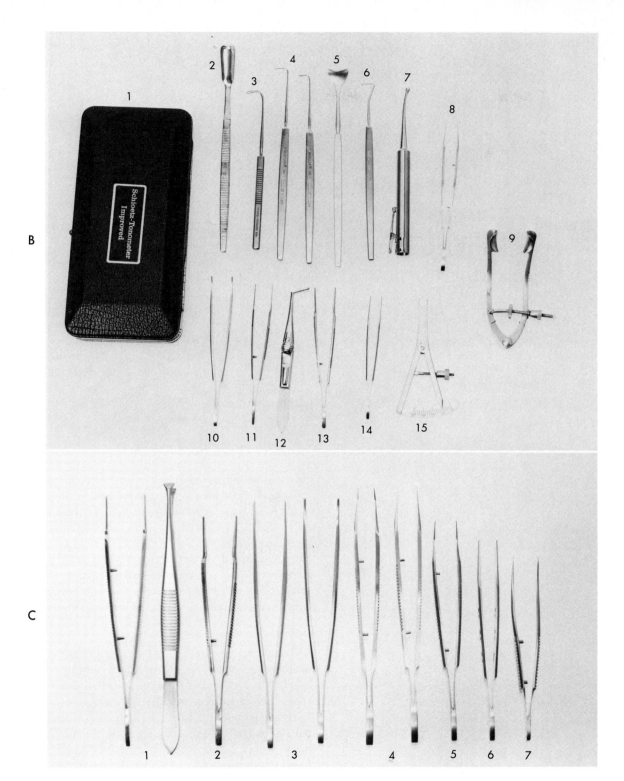

Fig. 18-22. Basic eye instruments. **A,** *1,* Westcott stitch scissors; *2,* Westcott tenotomy scissors; *3,* Knapp iris scissors; *4,* deWecker iris scissors; *5,* Stevens tenotomy scissors. **B,** *1,* Schiotz tonometer; *2,* Arruga retractor; *3,* Gass retinal detachment hook; *4,* muscle hooks; *5,* DeMarres lid retractor; *6,* Green muscle hook; *7,* scleral depressor; *8,* Castroviejo suturing forceps; *9,* Lancaster eye speculum; *10,* curved serrated utility forceps; *11,* fixation forceps; *12,* Jameson recession forceps; *13,* Alabama tying forceps; *14,* Bishop-Harman suturing forceps; *15,* Castroviejo caliper. **C,** *1,* Fixation forceps (Lester and von Graefe); *2,* Alabama tying forceps; *3,* straight and curved serrated utility dressing forceps; *4,* Castroviejo suturing forceps; 0.12 and 0.5 mm; *5,* angled McPherson suturing forceps; *6,* Bishop-Harman suturing forceps; *7,* Colibri corneal forceps.

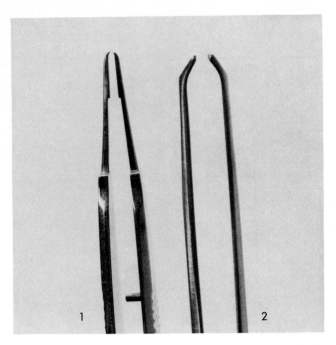

Fig. 18-23. Fixation forceps. *1,* Lester fixation forceps; *2,* von Graefe fixation forceps.

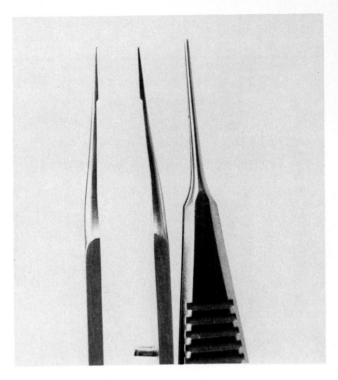

Fig. 18-24. Suturing forceps.

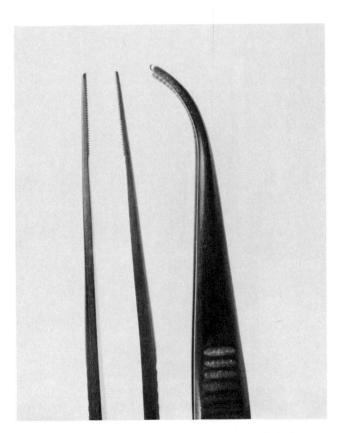

Fig. 18-25. Utility or dressing forceps, commonly called "fine serrated" forceps.

A variety of ophthalmic forceps are designed for specific use with different tissues of the eye. Some of those most commonly used are illustrated in Fig. 18-26.

Increased use of the microscope has brought changes in the design of ophthalmic instruments. Many microsurgical instruments were shortened to fit within a surgeon's hand web-space because of preference and facility of movement. Special surface finishes are used to reduce light reflection. Instruments are designed with round handles for smoother motion and rotation under the microscope.

Care and handling

To maintain the quality and precision of all ophthalmic instruments, including microsurgical instruments, strict criteria for care and handling must be followed. Storage cases protect instrument tips and cutting surfaces. The instruments should be inspected under magnification when purchased and before and after each use, observing for burrs on tips, nicks on cutting surfaces, and alignment of jaws. Eye instruments should be cleaned during use with nonfibrous sponges to avoid damaging delicate instrument tips. Personnel handling instruments should know the name and purpose of each instrument. Tissue can be damaged by the use of an inappropriate instrument, and instruments can be damaged by inappropriate use. After use, the instruments should be cleaned and thoroughly dried before storage.

It is recommended that microsurgical instruments undergo ultrasonic cleaning with distilled water and an appropriate cleansing agent. They can be individually hand-held or immersed together in the ultrasonic cleaner as long as they are not touching each other. Instruments should be rinsed with distilled water and thoroughly dried. A hot air blower (never a towel) should be used for drying instruments. Instrument lubricant should not be used on irri-

gating cannulas because residue can be introduced into the eye and cause damage.

In addition to basic care and handling, a routine preventive maintenance program should be established for sharpening, realigning, and adjusting the precision eye instruments. Keeping an instrument in good repair is much less expensive than buying a new one.

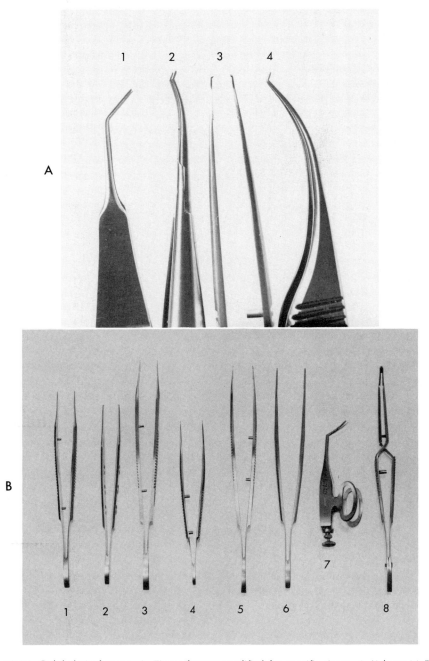

Fig. 18-26. Ophthalmic forceps. **A,** Tissue forceps modified for specific tissue. *1,* Kelman-McPherson angled tissue forceps with teeth; *2,* Corneoscleral forceps; *3,* Castroviejo corneal forceps; *4,* Colibri corneal forceps, 0.12 mm (may be used for iris). **B,** *1,* Lester fixation forceps; *2,* Bishop-Harman suturing forceps; *3,* Castroviejo suturing forceps; *4,* Colibri corneal forceps; *5,* Castroviejo-Colibri corneal forceps; *6,* Castroviejo tying forceps; *7,* VonMandach capsule fragment and clot forceps; *8,* Castroviejo cross action capsule forceps.

Basic setup

Each ophthalmic operating room should have a sufficient number of basic, standard eye surgery setups, which can be supplemented to meet specific needs (Figs. 18-27 and 18-28). Instruments routinely needed for a type of operation and each surgeon's preferences should be kept on file.

Ophthalmic sutures

Sutures used in ophthalmic surgery are very fine, and range in size from nos. 4-0 to 10-0. Fine eye sutures produce minimum reaction and discomfort for the patient. They should be handled as little as possible to avoid weakening and fraying. Surgical gut and collagen suture, which is packaged in solution, should be rinsed before use to

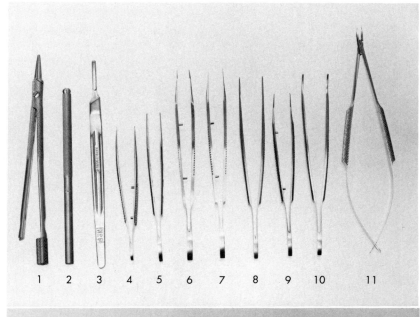

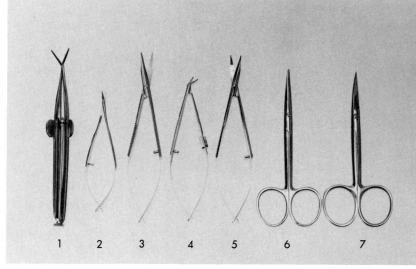

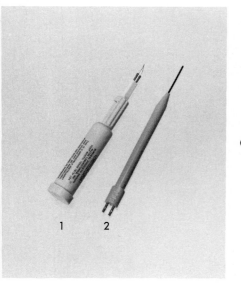

BASIC EYE INSTRUMENT SET
Self-retaining eye speculum (Fig. 18-22)
Lid retractor (Fig. 18-22)
Muscle hooks (Fig. 18-22)
Knife handle
Scissors (tenotomy, stitch, corneal, iris)
Forceps (suturing fine and heavy, iris, fixation, tying)
Caliper
Needle holders (micro and heavy)
Irrigating cannula (19- and 27-gauge)
Iris spatula

Fig. 18-27. Basic eye instrument setup. **A,** *1,* Blade breaker and handle; *2,* Beaver knife handle; *3,*no. 9 Bard-Parker knife handle; *4,* Colibri corneal forceps; *5,* Bishop-Harman suturing forceps; *6,* Castroviejo 0.5-mm suturing forceps; *7,* Castroviejo 0.12-mm suturing forceps; *8,* Castroviejo tying forceps; *9,* Kelman-McPherson suturing forceps; *10,* serrated utility dressing forceps; *11,* curved microsurgical needle holder. **B,** *1,* deWecker scissors; *2,* Vannas iridocapsulotomy scissors; *3,* Westcott tenotomy scissors; *4,* Troutman-Castroviejo corneal scissors; *5,* Westcott stitch scissors; *6,* Knapp strabismus scissors; *7,* Knapp iris scissors. **C,***1,* Disposable eye cautery; *2,* disposable bipolar erasertip eye cautery.

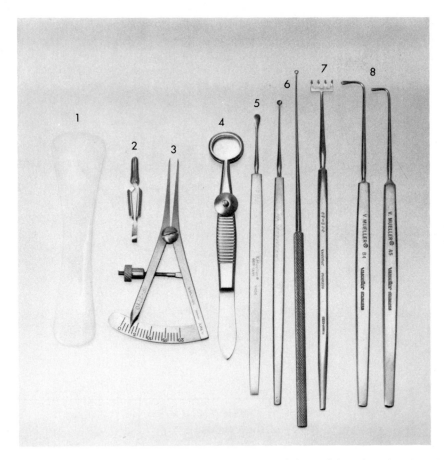

BASIC INSTRUMENTS FOR SURGERY
OF THE EYELIDS AND CONJUNCTIVA
WITH ALTERNATIVES
Eye speculum (Lancaster [Fig. 18-22],
Guyton-Park, Barraquer)
Scissors: tenotomy (Westcott, Stevens);
sharp (Westcott, Stevens); blunt
(Westcott, Stevens); suture (Stevens,
Wilmer utility) (Fig. 18-22)
Tissue forceps: delicate tissue; fixation
(Lester, O'Brien); suturing (Castro-
viejo, Bishop-Harman) (Fig. 18-22)
No. 9 Bard-Parker knife handle with no.
11 and no. 15 blades (Fig. 18-27)
Gill corneal knife
Muscle hooks (von Graefe, Jameson)
Chalazion curette (Heath, Skeele)
Chalazion clamp (DeMarres, Green,
Heath)
Ptosis forceps (Berke, Berens), not
shown
Entropion forceps (Snellen), not shown
Lid forceps (Erhardt [Fig. 18-36], Green)
Lid plate (Jaeger)
Retractor (Fink, Knapp)
Caliper (Castroviejo)
Serrefine

Fig. 18-28. Instruments for surgery of the eyelids and conjunctiva. *1,* Jaeger lid plate; *2,* serrefine; *3,* caliper; *4,* Green chalazion clamp; *5,* Gill corneal knife; *6,* chalazion curettes; *7,* retractor; *8,* muscle hooks.

prevent introducing irritants into the eye. Ophthalmic needles are also very delicate and must be handled with extreme care. Before use, needles must be inspected for evidence of burrs.

Ophthalmic dressings

At the completion of the operation, the operative eye area is cleansed with saline sponges.

Antibiotic ointment may be thinly spread over the skin and eyelashes to prevent adhesion of the bandage. This is frequently done after plastic procedures on the lids or lacrimal ducts.

Dressings are applied to prevent palpebral movements, protect the operative wound from dust and external contaminants, and absorb any blood and tears produced.

The initial dressing, usually an eye pad, is commercially prepared and sterilized. The eye dressing is held in place with plastic, paper, or cellophane strips (Fig. 18-29, *A*).

After intraocular operations, when external pressure on the eyes might be harmful, the initial dressing is covered with a protector such as a perforated aluminum plate, con-

vex flexible celluloid plate, or another variety of shield (Fig. 18-29, *B*).

A pressure bandage may be used when a compression effect is desired. A gauze roller bandage is applied over the initial dressing, encircling the head.

Evaluation

Before the patient is transported to the PACU or observation unit, his or her general condition is evaluated. The general appearance of the skin is assessed, with areas around the face and bony prominences noted for redness and other changes from the preoperative condition.

If the procedure was lengthy and osmotics were given, the patient may be catheterized while still anesthetized. A report to the receiving nurse in the PACU or observation area should include postoperative positioning requirements, potential problems specific to the patient, and preoperative anxiety level and utilization of coping mechanisms. Most patients have one or both eyes patched, and the sensory deficit should be noted. Documentation of all postoperative observations is important.

Evaluation should address whether the patient met the

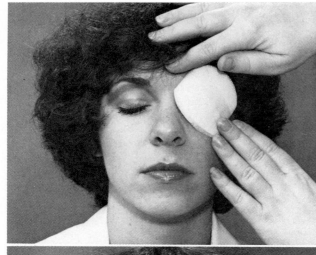

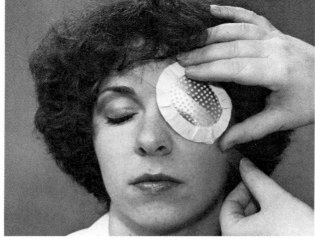

Fig. 18-29. A, Eye dressing is held in place by plastic, paper, or cellophane strips. Lids are gently closed before patch is applied. **B,** Protection of wound is provided by application of metal shield over dressing.

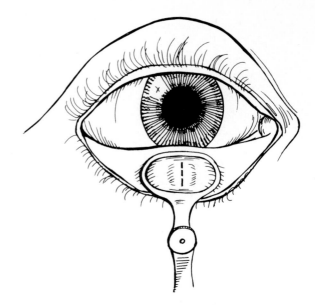

Fig. 18-30. Clamp everts eyelid during surgery for chalazion. Incision has been made on inner lid surface to avoid scarring. Viscous contents of chalazion will be removed with curette.

identified perioperative nursing goals; the patient's responses may be documented as outcome statements. The following examples are based on the nursing diagnoses identified in the care plan on pp. 444-445.

- The patient and/or significant other verbalized knowledge regarding the diagnosis, planned intervention, and requirements for home care maintenance.
- The patient safely coped with visual sensory and perceptual alterations.
- The patient verbalized concerns and fears and utilized coping mechanisms.
- The patient identified activities that may increase intraocular pressure.
- The patient will remain free of signs and symptoms of postoperative infection.

SURGICAL INTERVENTIONS
Surgery of the eyelids

The procedures most commonly performed on the eyelids are for treatment of chalazion, entropion, and ectropion, excisional biopsy, and repair of traumatic injuries.

Removal of chalazion

Removal of a chalazion is the incision and curettage of a chronic granulomatous inflammation of one or more of the meibomian glands in the tarsal plate of the eyelid.

Procedural considerations. The patient is prepared as described for general ophthalmic surgery. This procedure is most commonly done with local anesthesia.

Operative procedure

1. The affected lid is everted with a chalazion clamp (Fig. 18-30) to expose the chalazion.
2. A cruciate incision is made on the inner lid surface, using a sharp knife; corners of the tarsal plate are resected (Fig. 18-30).
3. The contents of the chalazion are removed with a chalazion curette. The eye is dressed and patched.

Canthotomy

Canthotomy is lengthening the opening (slit) between the eyelids before cataract surgery when exposure of the globe is inadequate or when correction of ankyloblepharon or blepharochalasis is necessary.

Procedural considerations. The patient is prepared as described for general ophthalmic surgery. This procedure is most commonly done with local anesthesia.

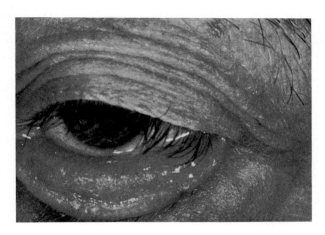

Fig. 18-31. Ectropion, or turning out of lid, is most commonly caused by senile relaxation of eyelid framework. (From Saunders, W.H., and others: Nursing care in eye, ear, nose and throat disorders, ed. 4, St. Louis, 1979, The C.V. Mosby Co.)

Operative procedure

1. A hemostat is clamped over the full thickness of the outer canthus and left in place for 60 seconds.
2. The skin and conjunctiva are incised. For canthoplasty, the adjacent bulbar conjunctiva is dissected, and its borders and those of the skin are sutured together with fine silk sutures.
3. The affected eye is dressed and patched.

Surgery for positional defects of the eyelids

Several techniques are available to treat faulty position of the eyelids. Plastic surgery is effective in the treatment of entropion, ectropion (Fig. 18-31), and blepharochalasis of the eyelids.

Plastic repair of entropion

Plastic repair of entropion is surgical correction of muscular fibers of the lid, everting the lid margins and eyelashes. Entropion (turning inward of the lid) usually affects the lower lid but may affect the upper lid. It seldom occurs in persons under 40 years of age. The two types are spastic and cicatricial. Spastic entropion results from degeneration of facial attachments between the pretarsal muscle and the tarsus, which permits the pretarsal muscle to override the lid margin during contraction. Cicatricial entropion is a complication of either the upper or lower tarsus and its conjunctiva, turning in the lashes (trichiasis) so they rub on the cornea.

Procedural considerations. A local or general anesthetic may be used, and usually a pressure dressing is required.

Operative procedure. Entropion treatment involves either removing a base-down triangle of skin, muscle, and tarsus and suturing the edges together to evert the lid margin, or exposing the orbicular muscle, dividing it, and suturing it to the lower border of the tarsus.

Plastic repair of ectropion

Plastic repair of ectropion is an operation to shorten the lower lid in a horizontal direction. Ectropion (sagging and eversion of the lower lid), usually bilateral, is common in older persons. Ectropion may be caused by the relaxation of the orbicular muscle. Symptoms are tearing, conjunctival infection, and irritation. Minor ectropion may be treated by electrosurgical penetrations through the conjunctiva. Surgery is indicated when facial paralysis is permanent or when scarring follows lacerations, lesions, or penetrating injuries and the cornea becomes exposed, resulting in ulceration and photophobia.

Operative procedure. Correction of cicatricial ectropion is accomplished either by mobilization of the surrounding skin or by free grafting. Many procedures have been devised, such as the *Wharton Jones V-Y procedure*, free whole skin graft, or epidermis graft. The operation includes removal of scar tissue and approximation of layers, small sliding grafts from the immediate area by means of Z-plasty or V-Y incision if loss is minimal, and free graft from the upper lid for the lower lid by means of tarsorrhaphy.

The *Kuhnt-Szymanowski procedure* is performed to treat senile or complete atonic ectropion. The external two thirds or the entire lid is split, the tarsoconjunctival triangle is resected, and the wound is closed by means of sutures in such a manner that a new canthus is produced (Fig. 18-32).

Plastic repair for blepharochalasis

Plastic repair for blepharochalasis is removal of redundant skin of the upper eyelids. Blepharochalasis causes the upper lids to hang down over the eyes, sometimes obscuring vision. It may occur in older persons who have lost normal elasticity of the skin of the upper lids or in persons who have suffered from persistent angioneurotic edema with stretching of the skin of the eyelids.

Operative procedure. An elliptic segment of skin of the upper lid is removed by a plastic surgical technique.

Surgery for unilateral or bilateral ptosis. Drooping of the upper lid may be congenital, acquired, or senile. In congenital ptosis, there usually is weakness of the superior rectus muscle. Acquired ptosis is generally caused by laceration of the third cranial nerve, the levator muscle, or both. Tumors may cause ptosis. Senile ptosis is the result of poor muscle tone of the levator.

The objective of ptosis surgery is to achieve a perfect cosmetic result by creating a good upper lid fold with elevation of the lid. The many surgical procedures that have been devised are based on the advancement of the levator muscle, the frontalis muscles, or the superior rectus muscle. These muscles are the elevating forces of the upper lids. Some of the techniques involve resection of the levator (Iliff method), use of the superior rectus muscle (Berke method), or modification of other methods such as

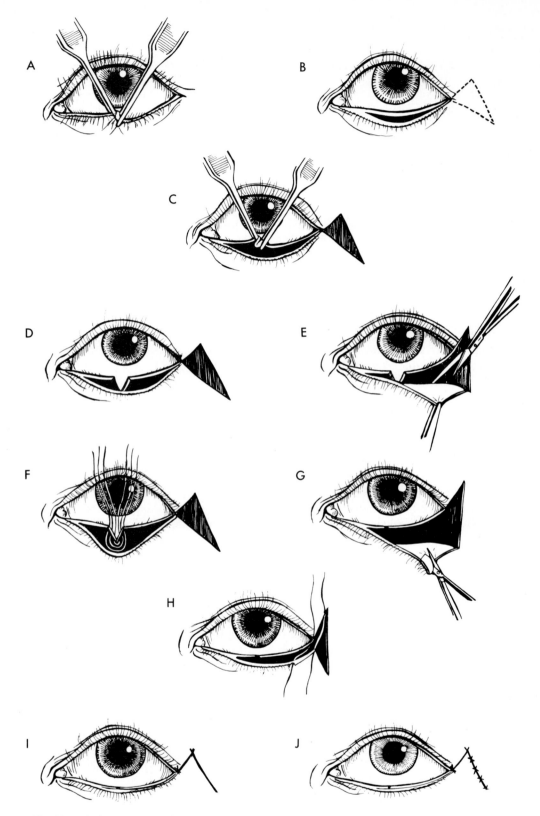

Fig. 18-32. Kuhnt-Szymanowski operation for atonic ectropion. **A,** Lower lid picked up with two smooth forceps, and amount of lengthening needed gauged. **B,** Lateral skin triangle marked, and lid split. **C,** Lateral triangle resected, and amount of tarsoconjunctiva to be excised gauged. **D,** Tarsoconjunctival triangle receded. **E,** Skin-muscle lamina dissected free. **F,** Tarsal wound closed. **G,** Excess cilia resected. **H,** Sutures placed to form a new canthus. **I,** Sutures tied. **J,** Final closure done. (Modified from Fox, S.A.: Ophthalmic plastic surgery, ed. 3, New York, 1963, Grune & Stratton, Inc.)

the Motais, Crawford frontalis collagen sling procedure, or Silver-Hildreth method.

Iliff method (resection of the levator)

The Iliff method is creation of an effective upper lid by shortening the levator muscle and reapproximating the conjunctiva and muscles to reestablish the correct relationship of the involved structures. General anesthesia is preferred.

Operative procedure

1. The upper lid is everted over the lid clamp. With a sharp-pointed scissors, two buttonhole incisions are made through the conjunctiva, medial and lateral to the superior edge of the tarsus.
2. A blunt scissors is directed through the buttonhole incisions and spread open to enlarge the incisional opening. As the scissors is withdrawn, the angular, rubber-shod, jawed ptosis clamps are positioned to contain the conjunctiva, superior edge of the tarsus, superior arcuate artery, aponeurosis of the levator, and orbital septum.
3. Another incision is made with scissors distal to the clamp and through all structures held by the clamp.
4. The orbital septum is freed from the clamp. Structures between the orbital septum and the levator are dissected by means of blunt instruments.
5. Traction is applied to the clamp. Double-armed chromic sutures no. 4-0 are inserted from the cut tarsal edge through all structures held by the clamp. The tissues distal to the suture line are excised.
6. The free end of each of the double-armed sutures is passed through the orbital septum, between the skin and tarsus, and brought out through the skin at the cilia margin.
7. Sutures are tied over a silicone strip or small beads. Redundant skin is invaginated with a peg to form a good lid fold.
8. The eye is closed by fastening a single suture that is passed through the skin of the lower lid to the forehead by means of an adhesive strip. Bland eye ointment is applied, and eye pads are secured by means of non-allergenic adhesive tape.

Silver-Hildreth Supramid suspension

The Silver-Hildreth method is attachment of the lid to the frontalis muscle by Supramid sutures anchored in the periosteum. This procedure may be done in the total absence of levator and superior rectus action.

Operative procedure

1. An incision is made in the lid fold, exposing the tarsus. An incision is made over the eyebrow centrally to the frontalis muscle.
2. A double-armed 4-0 Supramid suture is woven through the tarsus.

3. The needles are removed from the suture, and the suture is threaded on a Wright fascia needle.
4. The fascia needle is passed under the skin of the lid through the periosteum of the orbital rim and out through the brow incision. This is repeated so both ends of the suture are in the brow incision.
5. The suture is tied as it lies on the frontalis muscle.
6. The skin is closed with a nylon, subcuticular, continuous suture no. 6-0.
7. The conjunctival sac is filled with antibiotic ointment. A double-armed, silk suture no. 4-0 is passed through the center of the lower lid margin and fastened to the brow with adhesive tape, thus covering the exposed cornea. A pressure dressing is applied.

Excisional biopsy

Excisional biopsy is removal of lesions, either neoplastic (benign or malignant) or viral in nature, for diagnostic examination. Basal cell carcinomas account for 95% of neoplastic lesions of the lid; the treatment of choice is excisional biopsy. Viral lesions such as papilloma and molluscum contagiosum are also treated in this way.

Operative procedure. Through-and-through excision of skin, muscle, tarsus, and conjunctiva is followed by careful structural closure of anatomic spaces.

Surgery for traumatic injuries

Lacerations of the lids, including damage to the inferior canaliculus, are repaired surgically.

Procedural considerations. Tantamount to success is the careful approximation of the borders of the lid margin and the ends of a torn canaliculus.

Lacerations of the lid margin are closed with a silk suture no. 5-0 to align the gray line of the lid that lies between the lash follicles and the orifices of the meibomian glands. Once this anatomic line has been approximated, all other sutures are placed, maintaining the approximation.

If the canaliculus has been lacerated, a pigtail probe is passed through the uninvolved punctum, through the sac, and carefully through the proximal and distal ends of the lacerated structure to emerge from the involved punctum. A Supramid suture no. 4-0 is hooked onto the probe and, by reversing the previous procedure, is pulled out of the uninvolved punctum, thus establishing continuity of the system. Accurate plastic closure of the lid defect is then carried out.

Blepharopigmentation and eyebrow enhancement

In a microsurgical procedure, neutral pigments are permanently implanted intradermally between the eyelashes (blepharopigmentation) or in the eyebrows (eyebrow enhancement) to improve their appearance.

This is a cosmetic procedure performed in an ambulatory surgery facility or physician's office. It was devel-

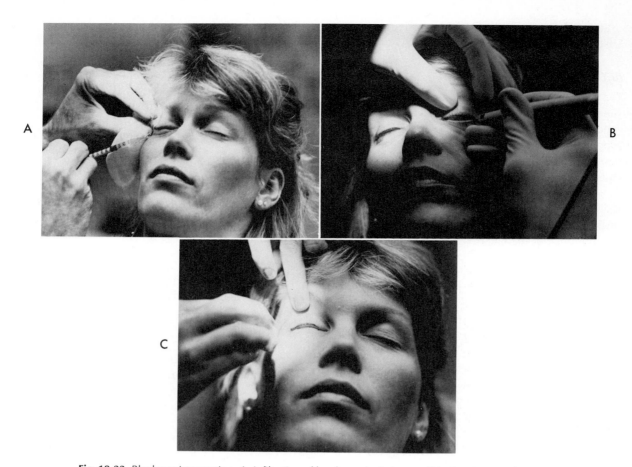

Fig. 18-33. Blepharopigmentation. **A,** Infiltration of local anesthetic into eyelids. **B,** Injection of pigment with electric needle in dermis of eyelid along eyelash margins. **C,** Completion of blepharopigmentation to upper eyelash margin.

oped as an enhancement for scant eyebrows or in some cases replacement for eyeliner, particularly for individuals with allergies to cosmetics, contact lens wearers, visually impaired persons, or patients with limited dexterity.

Procedural considerations. Patients may need ice packs or sedation before infiltration of local anesthetic to reduce discomfort. The eyelids and brows are prepared as described for eye surgery, ensuring that the lid margins and lashes are cleaned thoroughly. A thin film of clear antibiotic ointment is placed on the lids to prevent staining of the superficial layers of the eyelid skin. Postoperatively, cold compresses or ice packs are applied to reduce edema and ecchymosis.

Operative procedure (Fig. 18-33)

1. A slow regional injection with a 1½-inch, 27- to 30-gauge needle is used to introduce the local anesthetic.
2. Sterile pigment is injected within the dermis of the lid at a depth no less than 0.5 mm and no greater than 1.5 mm, using a disposable electric needle.
3. At the completion of the procedure, the skin is cleansed with saline to remove superficial pigment. Antibiotic ointment is placed in each eye.

Surgery of the conjunctiva

The conjunctiva of the eye is transparent, elastic, and abundant. Traumatic lacerations caused by injury as well as deficits resulting from excision of tumors, cysts, nevi, or pterygiums can usually be repaired by simple undermining and suturing.

Pterygium excision

A pterygium is a fleshy, triangular encroachment onto the cornea. Pterygiums tend to be bilateral. When a pterygium encroaches on the visual axis, it is removed surgically.

Operative procedure. The major steps in the McReynolds technique are illustrated in Fig. 18-34.

A pterygium can also be excised totally, and the limbus treated with an eye cautery or electrocoagulation. The conjunctiva can then be closed, or the sclera can be left bare.

Excisional biopsy

Any suspect lesion of the conjunctiva can be removed by simple elliptical excision and sent for pathological ex-

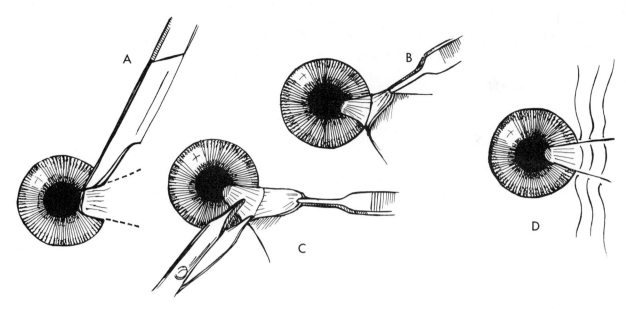

Fig. 18-34. McReynolds technique for pterygium repair. **A,** Cornea around head of pterygium is incised. **B,** Pterygium flap is dissected upward, leaving clear cornea. **C,** Lower margin of pterygium is dissected, and whole pterygium is freed from sclera. **D,** Sutures are placed for closure of conjunctiva.

amination. The conjunctiva may or may not be closed, depending on the surgeon's particular technique.

Reformation of the cul-de-sac (mucous membrane graft)

Reformation of the cul-de-sac involves the application of a mucous membrane graft to the conjunctiva to correct motility or exposure problems.

Various conditions and injuries, such as infections, trachoma, or chemical burns, may cause severe scarring and contractures of the conjunctiva and the underlying tissues, which may lead to problems with motility or exposure. Simple dissection is usually unsatisfactory. The patient generally requires extra mucous membrane, which may be obtained from excess conjunctiva from the opposite eye, if available, or as a mucous membrane graft from the oral cavity.

Operative procedure

1. A local anesthetic solution is injected into the mucous membrane of the lower lid or the lateral wall of the mouth with a separate set of instruments.
2. An elliptical incision is made with a no. 15 knife blade. (If the incision is made into the lateral wall, the opening of the parotid duct must be avoided.)
3. A thin, full-thickness layer of the mucous membrane is removed by sharp dissection. A second method is the use of an electric Castroviejo dermatome. The mucous membrane is then obtained from the lower lip.
4. The wound is approximated with silk suture no. 4-0.

5. The mucous membrane graft is placed in a Neosporin solution, the surgeon regowns and regloves, and another set of sterile instruments is used for reconstruction of the cul-de-sac.

Surgery of the lacrimal gland and apparatus

Surgery of the lacrimal gland and apparatus is usually performed for treatment or diagnosis of tumors of the lacrimal fossa or to correct deficient drainage with overflow of tears. Chronic dacryocystitis in adults (Fig. 18-35) requires dacryocystorhinostomy because of resistant obstruction of the nasolacrimal duct. Dacryocystorhinostomy is also performed when the lower canaliculus is patent but the tear duct is blocked, causing epiphora that the patient

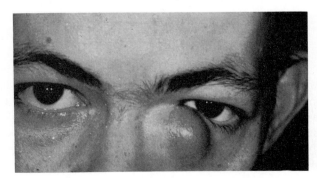

Fig. 18-35. Chronic infection of lacrimal sac (dacryocystitis) causes swelling of inner lower corner of eye socket. (From Saunders, W.H., and others: Nursing care in eye, ear, nose, and throat disorders, ed. 4, St. Louis, 1979, The C.V. Mosby Co.)

INSTRUMENTS FOR LACRIMAL SURGERY
   WITH ALTERNATIVES
Eye speculum (Lancaster [Fig. 18-22],
   Barraquer)
Scissors: tenotomy (Westcott, Stevens) sharp;
   tenotomy (Westcott, Stevens) blunt; suture
   (Stevens, Wilmer); utility (Knapp) (Fig.
   18-22)
Tissue forceps: delicate; fixation (von Graefe,
   O'Brien); suturing (Castroviejo, Bishop-
   Harman) (Fig. 18-22)
Needle holder (Castroviejo, Kalt, Barraquer)
   (Fig. 18-27)
Berens lid everter, not shown
No. 9 Bard-Parker knife handle with no. 11
   and no. 15 blades (Fig. 18-27)
von Graefe cataract knife, not shown
Lacrimal probes (Bowman, Williams)
Worst pigtail probe
Lacrimal trephine (Arruga, Stryker) and
   Stryker-Iliff saw
Lacrimal chisel (Fig. 18-37)
Lacrimal dilators (Wilder, Castroviejo)
Freer elevator
Bone curette, not shown
Lacrimal sac retractor, self-retaining and
   Knapp
Cautery
Lacrimal cannulas, Veirs dacryocysto-
   rhinostomy set
Kerrison rongeur

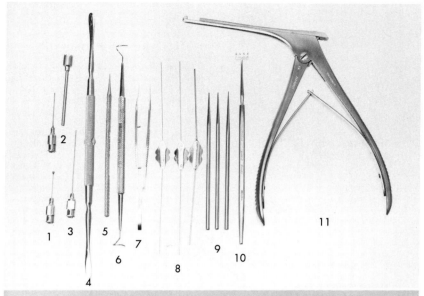

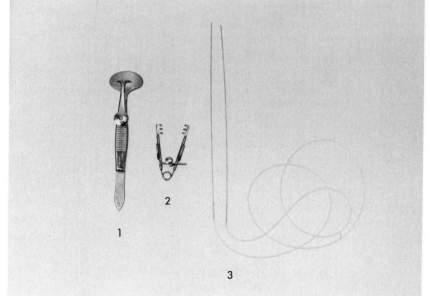

Fig. 18-36. Instruments for surgery of the lacrimal system. **A,** *1,* Lacrimal cannulas, bulbous tip and straight; *2,* Arruga trephine; *3,* McIntyre lacrimal irrigating cannula; *4,* Freer elevator; *5,* Muldoon dilator; *6,* Worst pigtail probe; *7,* Castroviejo suturing forceps; *8,* Bowman lacrimal probes; *9,* Nettleship-Wilder lacrimal dilators; *10,* lacrimal sac retractor; *11,* small Kerrison rongeur. **B,** *1,* Erhardt lid clamp; *2,* lacrimal sac retractor; *3,* Quickert canaliculus probe.

cannot tolerate. This deformity frequently follows a malunited fracture of the medial wall of the orbit. Dacryocystorhinostomy creates a new, large opening between the lacrimal sac and the nose.

Instrumentation for surgery of the lacrimal system is shown in Fig. 18-36.

Surgery of the lacrimal fossa

Surgery of the lacrimal fossa is performed for biopsy of any structure in the lacrimal fossa and possible removal of the lacrimal gland (extirpation) to eliminate excessive tearing.

Operative procedure

1. The lacrimal fossa, which is in the upper temporal quadrant of the orbit, may be approached directly through the lid or through the conjunctiva by everting the upper lid. The lacrimal gland is divided into a palpebral and an orbital part by the orbital septum. All drainage ducts go through the palpebral portion; surgery on this part alone affects tearing because, although

the orbital part is intact, no access to the eye is available.

2. Routine surgical closure procedures are followed.

Probing

The opening of the lacrimal drainage system posterior and inferior to the inferior nasal conchae is closed in approximately 35% of newborns. In most cases this closure opens spontaneously within the first 2 or 3 months of life. When the lacrimal drainage system does not open spontaneously, an acute infectious process involving the lacrimal drainage system becomes obvious. The infectious process is treated with antibiotics, followed by probing.

In a child under 6 months of age, the probing procedure may be done with mummification, using topical anesthesia. After this age the procedure is done with general anesthesia.

Operative procedure

1. Manipulation is done through the upper punctum and canaliculus to prevent trauma to the inferior part of the system, which carries 90% to 95% of the total secretions.

2. The upper punctum is dilated first with a sterile safety pin and then with a punctum dilator. A lacrimal probe is then passed through the upper punctum and canalic-

ulus into the sac, where resistance is met from the lacrimal bone. The probe is rotated 90 degrees, passed through the bony canal, and forced through the imperforate opening into the nose. A small amount of blood may be regurgitated at this time. The procedure may be repeated with a larger probe.

3. With a blunt lacrimal needle, a fluorescein solution is irrigated through the punctum to ensure the patency of the system.

Dacryocystorhinostomy

Dacryocystorhinostomy is the establishment of a new tear passageway for drainage directly into the nasal cavity.

Procedural considerations. The nasal cavity is anesthetized topically with cocaine just before surgery, and a general anesthetic is administered in the operating room. The patient is prepared as described for eye surgery.

Operative procedure (Fig. 18-37)

1. An incision is made on the nasal side of the orbital rim. With blunt-pointed, curved, or flat scissors, a knife, retractors, and forceps, dissection is carried down to the periosteum, which is separated from the bone with elevators.

2. Through the lower canaliculus, the sac is probed, identified, and displaced laterally.

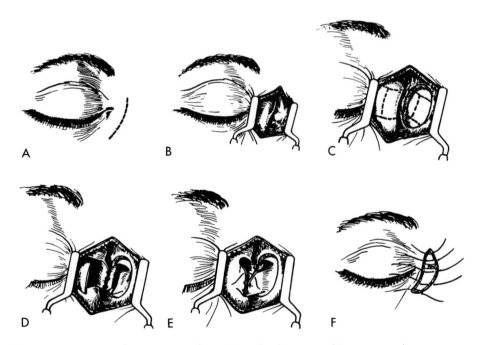

Fig. 18-37. Dacryocystorhinostomy. **A,** Skin incision for dacryocystorhinostomy or dacryocystectomy. **B,** Lacrimal sac and lacrimal bone exposed. **C,** Opening made in lacrimal bone and lacrimal crest, with *dotted lines* indicating incision to be made in wall of sac and in nasal periosteum and mucosa. **D,** Posterior flap of wall of sac sutured to posterior flap of nasal mucosa. **E,** Anterior flap of wall of sac sutured to anterior flap of nasal mucosa. (Drawing is somewhat distorted for visualization of relative positions.) **F,** Reattachment of medial canthal ligament, and wire sutures in position for closure of skin incision. (From Allen, J.H., editor: May's manual of the diseases of the eye, ed. 23, Baltimore, 1963, The Williams & Wilkins Co.)

3. The anterior lacrimal crest is perforated with a power saw, dental drill, or mallet and chisel. The hole is enlarged with rongeurs. During this time the cornea is protected by a metal retractor or plastic contact lens.

4. Irregular fragments of bone and fibrous tissue are removed, and hemostasis is obtained with bone wax if necessary.

5. The lacrimal sac and nasal mucosa are incised with H incisions with the long line vertical.

6. The mucous membrane of the nose is sutured to that of the lacrimal sac with no. 4-0 chromic sutures. A probe is passed through the nostril into the base of the wound to test the opening from the sac into the nose. A French catheter may be passed from the nose and sutured into the roof of the sac with no. 4-0 chromic sutures. It remains in place until the sutures absorb, thereby acting as a stent about which epithelial union between the lacrimal and nasal mucosa can occur.

7. The interior flap of mucous membrane from the nose and sac is sutured with interrupted, chromic no. 4-0 sutures. Skin margins are approximated and closed with silk sutures no. 6-0. Interpalpebral sutures are placed to maintain position of the eyelids under the dressing. The wound is dressed.

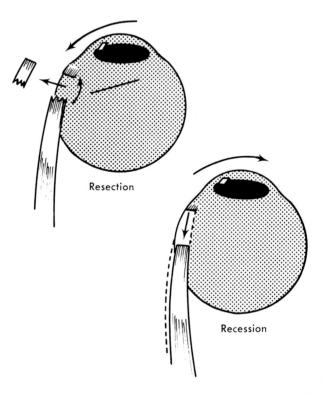

Fig. 18-38. In surgery for strabismus, *resection* of part of ocular muscle tendon rotates eye toward operated muscle, whereas *recession* moves muscle tendon backward on eye, permitting eye to rotate away from operated muscle. (Modified from Havener, W.H.: Synopsis of ophthalmology, ed. 5, St. Louis, 1979, The C.V. Mosby Co.)

Surgery for strabismus

Strabismus (squint) is the inability to direct the two eyes at the same object because of lack of coordination of the extraocular muscles. Corrective surgery is performed to change the relative strength of individual muscles and therefore improve coordination (Fig. 18-38).

The deviation of the eye may be inward, outward, upward, or downward. The amount of deviation is a measurement of the angle formed by the visual axis of the two eyes. The lateral rectus muscle abducts the eye, the medial rectus muscle adducts it, and the other ocular muscles have both primary and secondary functions in elevation, depression, intorsion, and extorsion, according to the position of the eye.

Basically, two surgical approaches are used to correct strabismus: strengthening is usually accomplished by a resection procedure, and weakening is usually done with a recession procedure. Operating on three or more muscles, in two stages, may be necessary. To some extent the type of strabismus influences the type of surgery. Instrumentation for strabismus surgery is illustrated in Fig. 18-39.

Resection

Resection is removal of a portion of muscle and attachment of cut ends (Fig. 18-38).

Procedural considerations. Suture material varies according to the surgeon's preference, but usually the suture is on a spatula needle. The patient is prepared as described previously for eye surgery; local or general anesthesia is used. Perioperative nurses should be aware that tension or traction on ocular muscles can precipitate bradycardia.

Operative procedure

1. A speculum is inserted, and the conjunctiva is incised at one border of the muscle to be resected.

2. The muscle insertion is hooked with a muscle hook, and the conjunctiva over the insertion is opened.

3. Double-armed sutures are passed through the muscle belly at the desired position of shortening, and the muscle is incised anterior to this suture.

4. The stump of the muscle is excised from the insertion, and the muscle is then sutured to the insertion using the double-armed suture.

5. The conjunctiva is closed with an absorbable suture.

Recession

Recession is severance of the muscle from its original insertion with reattachment more posteriorly on the sclera (Fig. 18-38).

Operative procedure

1. The insertion of the muscle is exposed as described previously.

2. Sutures are passed through the muscle tendon at its insertion into the globe, and the tendon is severed distal to the suture.

INSTRUMENTS FOR SURGERY OF EYE
MUSCLES WITH ALTERNATIVES
Eye speculum (Maumenee-Park, Weiss, Lancaster)
Scissors: suture (Stevens, Knapp); tenotomy (Westcott) sharp and blunt; Stevens curved and straight
Tissue forceps: delicate, fixation (Lester, von Graefe), suturing (Castroviejo)
Needle holder (Barraquer, Kalt)
Irrigating cannula, 19-gauge
No. 9 Bard-Parker knife handle with no. 15 blade
Muscle forceps (Jameson, Berens)
Muscle hooks (Jameson, von Graefe)
Caliper (Castroviejo)
Tissue retractor (Fink, Costenbader), lacrimal sac retractor
Tendon tucker (Fink), not shown
Biprong marker (Fink), not shown
Serrefine
Mosquito hemostat

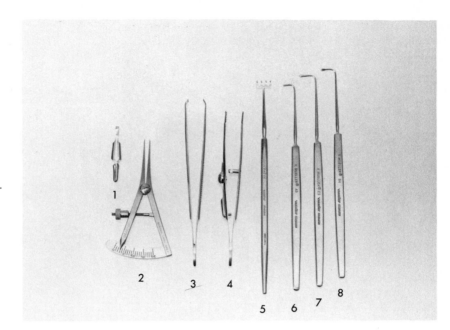

Fig. 18-39. Instruments for surgery of eye muscles. *1,* Serrefine; *2,* Castroviejo caliper; *3,* von Graefe fixation forceps; *4,* Jameson recession forceps; *5,* lacrimal sac retractor; *6* to *8,* von Graefe strabismus hooks, small, medium, and large.

3. With calipers, marks are made on the globe at the desired distance behind the insertion, and the muscle is anchored to the globe at that point.
4. The conjunctiva is closed with absorbable suture.

Myectomy

Myectomy is a method of weakening the action of a muscle. This may be done as a lengthening procedure such as a Z marginal tenotomy or myectomy or an intersheath tenotomy of the superior oblique tendon, or it may be a complete severance of a muscle, such as an inferior oblique myectomy procedure.

Operative procedure
1. The involved muscle is isolated.
2. Cuts from opposite sides of the muscle are made through approximately three fourths of the width of the muscle, effectively lengthening the muscle.
3A. In the case of the superior oblique muscle, the tendon sheath is opened and graded sections of tendon are excised, according to the needs of the patient.
3B. Myectomy of the inferior oblique muscle is done in a graded manner by placing two Kelly hemostats across the muscle belly lateral to the inferior rectus muscle and excising the isolated strip muscle. The ends of the muscle are cauterized and released. Because of the peculiar anatomy of this muscle, lateral discontinuity weakens the muscle but does not paralyze it.

Tuck

A tuck is a method of shortening a muscle and thus strengthening it. Tucking is performed primarily on the superior oblique muscle.

Operative procedure
1. An incision is made in the conjunctiva, medial to the superior rectus muscle.
2. The Fink-Scobie hook is passed posteriorly into the orbit, and the superior oblique muscle is hooked and brought into the incision.
3. The Fink tucker is placed over the tendon, and a graded doubling of the tendon, like looping a rope, is completed.
4. A double-armed Supramid suture is passed through the base of the loop, effectively shortening the muscle.
5. The tip of the loop is sutured to the sclera. (Surgeons commonly attempt to tuck the muscle lateral to the superior rectus muscle.)
6. The conjunctiva is closed with absorbable sutures.

Surgery of the globe and orbit

Rupture of the eyeball may be direct at the site of injury or, more frequently, indirect from an increase in intraocular pressure that causes the wall of the eyeball to tear at weaker points such as the limbus. When the intraocular contents have become so deranged that useful function is prohibited, removal of the eye contents (evisceration procedure) or of the entire eyeball (enucleation) is indicated. If either

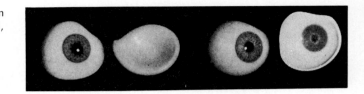

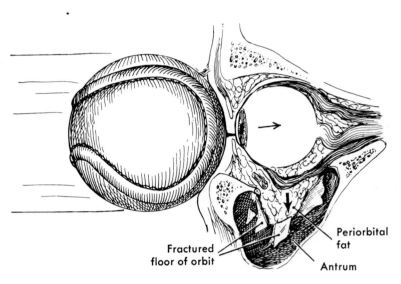

Fig. 18-41. Ball has struck rim of orbit and has pressed orbital contents backward, displacing fragments of bone into maxillary sinus. Inferior rectus muscle is incarcerated in fracture. Inferior oblique muscle may also be involved. (From Paton, R.T., and Katzin, H.M.: Atlas of eye surgery, ed. 2, New York, 1962, McGraw-Hill Book Co.)

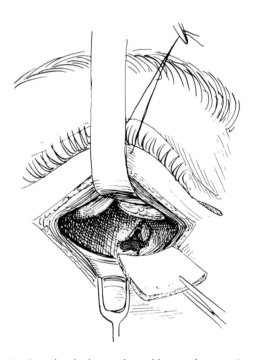

Fig. 18-42. Cross-hatched area shows blowout fracture site. Autogenous graft from iliac crest is held by forceps ready to be placed over fractured site. Graft usually does not require suturing. (From Paton, R.T., and Katzin, H.M.: Atlas of eye surgery, ed. 2, New York, 1962, McGraw-Hill Book Co.)

procedure is required, an inert globe may be implanted as a space filler and to aid in the movement of a prosthesis (artificial eye) (Fig. 18-40).

Fractures of the walls of the orbit (Fig. 18-41) may be caused by direct blows or by extension of a fracture line from adjacent bones (Figs. 18-41 and 18-42). Isolated orbital floor, or blowout, fractures usually follow injury to the region of the eye by an object the size of an apple or an adult's fist. Orbital contents herniate into the maxillary sinus, and the inferior rectus or inferior oblique muscle may become incarcerated at the fracture site. A Caldwell-Luc antrostomy (Chapter 20) may be done with reduction of the fracture from below, or the fracture site may be approached directly through the lower lid along the orbital floor and the prolapsed tissue reduced, the orbital floor reduced, and the orbital floor defect bridged with a graft of bone, cartilage, or plastic material. Instrumentation for surgery of the globe and orbit is illustrated in Fig. 18-43.

Repair of lacerations

The preferred method of closing corneal lacerations is with direct appositional suturing viewed through an operating microscope. No. 10-0 suture is generally used.

Tissue adhesives, that is, cyanoacrylate monomers, are

being used experimentally. The tissue adhesive is applied to well-dried tissue that has been properly oriented anatomically. It polymerizes and seals the wound on contact with the tissue. The tissue adhesive is supplied in packaged sterile vials (Co-Apt).

Cultures are usually obtained at the time of surgery. Antibiotics are injected subconjunctivally before the dressings are applied.

Enucleation

Enucleation is removal of the entire eyeball.

Operative procedure

1. A speculum retractor is introduced into the palpebral fissure.
2. The conjunctiva is divided around the cornea with sharp and blunt dissection.
3. The medial, lateral, inferior, and superior rectus muscles are divided, leaving a stump of medial rectus muscle. The globe is separated from Tenon's capsule with blunt-pointed, curved scissors, retractors, hemostats, and forceps.
4. The eye is rotated laterally by grasping the stump of the medial rectus muscle.

INSTRUMENTS FOR SURGERY OF THE
GLOBE OR ORBIT WITH ALTERNATIVES
Eye speculum (Guyton-Park, Lancaster) (Fig. 18-22)
Mosquito hemostat (Hartman, Halsted), not shown
Needle holder (Barraquer, Alabama-Green)
Scissors: suture (Stevens, Wilmer utility); Westcott right and left; tenotomy (Stevens curved and straight)
Forceps: tissue (Bishop-Harman, jewelers'); fixation (Lester, von Graefe); suturing (Castroviejo, Bonaccolto)
No. 9 Bard-Parker knife handle with no. 11 and no. 15 blades
Blade breaker and holder
Muscle forceps (Jameson, King-Pierce)
Muscle hooks (Jameson, von Graefe)
Fink lacrimal sac retractor
Lacrimal sac chisel (West) and Freer periosteum elevator
Evisceration spoon (Bunge) and enucleation spoon (Wells)
Enucleation scissors (Bunge)
Sphere introducer and holder with implant of surgeon's choice
Serrefine and irrigation cannula no. 19
Kerrison rongeur
Power saw, tonsil snare, mallet, bone curette, dermatome, eye cautery available

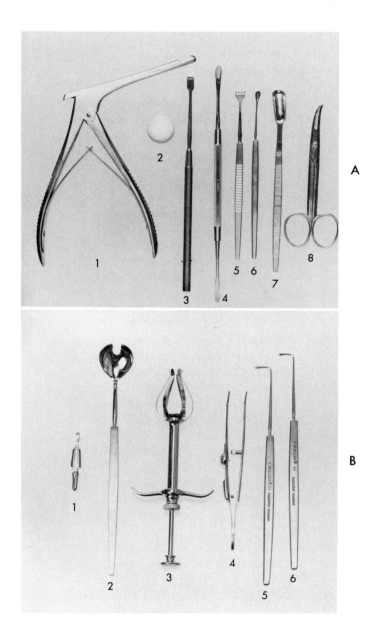

Fig. 18-43. Instruments for surgery of globe or orbit. **A,** *1,* Kerrison rongeur; *2,* orbital implant or sphere; *3,* lacrimal chisel; *4,* Freer elevator; *5,* lacrimal sac retractor; *6,* exenteration spoon; *7,* Arruga orbital retractor; *8,* enucleation scissors. **B,** *1,* Serrefine; *2,* Wells evisceration spoon; *3,* sphere introducer and holder; *4,* Jameson recession forceps; *5 and 6,* von Graefe muscle hooks.

5. A large, curved hemostat is passed behind the globe, and the optic nerve is clamped for 60 seconds. The hemostat is removed, the enucleation scissors is passed posteriorly, and the optic nerve is transected. The oblique muscles are severed as the eye is lifted out of the socket by the stump of the medial rectus muscle.
6. The muscle cone is packed with saline sponges to obtain hemostasis.
7. The muscle cone is filled with an implant, and Tenon's capsule and conjunctiva are carefully closed.
8. A socket conformer is placed in the cul-de-sac.
9. A pressure dressing is applied.

Evisceration

Evisceration is removal of the contents of the eye, leaving intact the sclera and the attached muscles.
Operative procedure
1. The conjunctiva is not separated from the sclera as it is for enucleation. A sharp-pointed knife is inserted through the limbus anterior to the iris.
2. The contents of the eye (iris, vitreous, lens) are removed.
3. The choroid adhering to the sclera is removed with curettes.
4. Bleeding is controlled with delicate hemostatic forceps, electrocoagulation, and sutures.
5. A plastic implant is placed within the empty shell.
6. The conjunctival and scleral edges are brought together with silk sutures no. 4-0 or 5-0, and a pressure dressing is applied.

Repair of fracture of the orbit (blowout)

A fractured orbit (see Fig. 18-42) is repaired by means of graft or realignment of contents of the orbit.
Procedural considerations. The setup is as for dacryocystorhinostomy, plus a graft set (for implantation of an autogenous graft or synthetic graft materials of various sizes and thicknesses) and a flexible, narrow-width retractor. The patient is prepared as described for eye surgery. A general anesthetic is usually administered.
Operative procedure
1. The maximum ocular rotation is tested by exerting traction with a forceps on the tendon of the inferior rectus muscle to determine if the inferior muscle sling is trapped in the fracture.
2. To distribute tension over the lower lid and stretch the orbicular muscle, a traction suture is inserted through the lower lid margin.
3. With a no. 3 knife handle and no. 15 blade, the lower lid is incised in the lid fold above the orbital rim.
4. The skin is separated from the orbicular muscle, and the orbital septum is identified by blunt dissection. Dissection is continued down to the periosteum of the orbital rim by means of scissors, loop retractors, elevators, and forceps.

5. The periosteum of the orbital rim is incised with a no. 15 blade. With periosteal elevators, the floor of the orbit is exposed and explored. When the fracture site is identified, bone spicules are removed, and the herniated contents are freed from the maxillary antrum. The contents of the orbit are elevated by means of narrow-width, flexible retractors. A traction suture of no. 4-0 silk is placed around the tendon of the inferior rectus muscle.
6. An autogenous graft is taken from the iliac crest, or an alloplastic material of proper size is used to repair the bony defect. The material may or may not be anchored to the orbital rim by wire sutures.
7. The periosteum is carefully closed with no. 4-0 chromic sutures.
8. The skin is closed with no. 6-0 silk, and a pressure dressing is applied.

Exenteration

Exenteration is removal of the entire orbital contents, including periosteum, for certain malignancies of the glove or orbit.
Procedural considerations. Considerations are as described for fracture of the orbit. General anesthesia is usually administered.
Operative procedure
1. Depending on circumstances, exenteration of the eye may or may not include the removal of the lids. An incision is made down to the orbital rim, through the periosteum, and around the entire orbit.
2. With periosteal elevators, the periosteum is freed from the orbital walls and the apex of the orbit.
3. The optic nerve is clamped, and the entire contents of the orbit are removed en bloc.
4. Hemostasis is obtained by the use of electrocoagulation and bone wax.
5. A skin graft or temporal muscle implant may be used to fill the orbital cavity, but this is not usually done. In most cases iodoform gauze is used to fill the cavity, a pressure dressing is put in place, and the cavity is allowed to granulate.

Surgery of the cornea

Surgery of the cornea is indicated for a variety of conditions in which cosmetic, therapeutic, restorative, and refractive outcomes are desired. New technology has been responsible for the introduction of procedures that offer more choices for restoration of vision.

Instrumentation for corneal transplants (lamellar and penetrating), as well as for repair of lacerations and removal of foreign bodies of the cornea, is shown in Fig. 18-44.

Corneal transplant (keratoplasty)

A corneal transplant is grafting of corneal tissue from one human eye to another (Figs. 18-45 and 18-46). Ker-

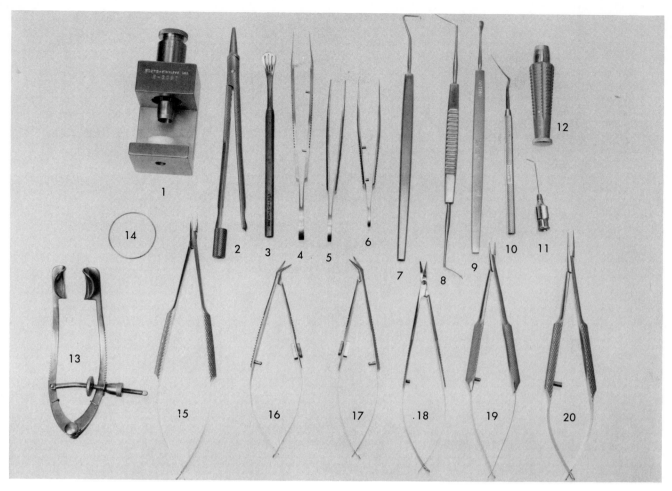

Fig. 18-44. Instruments for corneal transplant and other procedures on the cornea. *1,* Universal trephine handle with Cottingham punch; *2,* blade breaker; *3,* Paton spatula; *4,* Castroviejo suturing forceps, 0.12 mm; *5,* Bishop-Harman forceps; *6,* Colibri corneal forceps; *7,* Green strabismus hook; *8,* Castroviejo cyclodialysis spatula; *9,* Gill corneal knife; *10,* Troutman corneal dissector; *11,* air cannula, 27-gauge; *12,* Castroviejo trephine; *13,* Lancaster eye speculum; *14,* Flieringa ring; *15,* Barraquer curved micro needleholder; *16* and *17,* Troutman-Castroviejo corneal scissors, right and left; *18,* Castroviejo corneal scissors; *19,* straight micro needle holder; *20,* corneal scleral forceps.

atoplasty may be classified as (1) lamellar (partial-thickness) graft, (2) penetrating (whole-thickness) graft, (3) keratectomy (peeling of the cornea), and (4) tatooing (simulation of a pupil), which is rarely done. A corneal transplant is performed when the patient's cornea is thickened and opacified. The transparency of the cornea may be impaired as a result of infection, thermal or chemical burns, or certain diseases of unknown cause. A corneal transplant is done to improve vision when the basic visual structures of the eye, that is, the retina and optic nerve, are functioning properly.

Corneas are obtained from recently deceased persons. Eye banks help coordinate services for such operations.

Operative procedures

Penetrating keratoplasty (performed with operating microscope)

1. The eye speculum is put in place, and superior rectus

and inferior rectus bridle sutures are placed if a Flieringa ring is not to be used. If a ring is used, it is sutured in place with four Dacron sutures no. 5-0.

2. The eye from the eye bank is removed from its container and may be washed in Neosporin solution, or a corneoscleral button that has been stored in tissue culture medium or that has been frozen (and is thawed) is removed from its container.

3. The donor eye from the eye bank is then wrapped in a surgical dressing for stabilization. The cornea is excised from the donor eye by means of a corneal trephine cataract knife, corneal scissors, and forceps after the epithelium is removed with a sponge. The graft is placed, epithelial side down, in a Petri dish containing a saline-moistened gauze (Fig. 18-45). Some surgeons preplace sutures in the graft. Others place the corneoscleral button epithelial (outside) surface down on

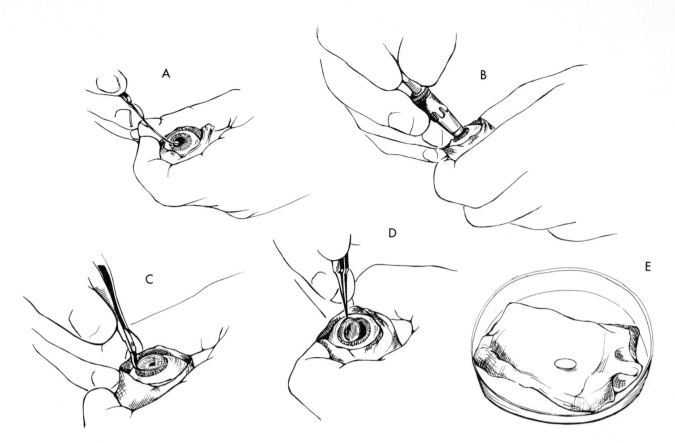

Fig. 18-45. A, Epithelium from donor cornea is being removed by abrading with iris spatula. Donor eye is wrapped in smooth gauze dressing. **B,** Donor eye is firmly grasped in surgeon's left hand, and corneal trephine is centered on donor eye. With twisting motion, cornea is cut through its entire thickness. **C,** Corneal scissors are used to cut any areas of corneal tissue that have not been penetrated by trephine. **D,** Corneal button is removed with fine forceps, with care taken not to touch endothelial surface. **E,** Donor corneal button is stored on moistened gauze pad, endothelial side up in covered Petri dish to preserve moisture.

a sterile Teflon block. The corneal trephine is then used as a punch, and the donor button is pressed out centrally.

4. The section of cornea removed from the recipient's eye may be the same size as the graft taken from the donor's eye or may be up to 0.5 mm smaller. The anterior chamber is entered with one of the variety of cataract knives, and the button is excised with corneal scissors. (Care must be taken to close the guard on the trephine after use to prevent damage to the cutting surface.)

5. Peripheral iridectomies or iridotomies may be performed at this time at the surgeon's discretion, or a cataract extraction may be completed if the lens is opaque.

6. The graft is placed into the opening of the recipient's eye and anchored in place by means of four single-armed sutures placed at the four cardinal meridians, viewed through an operating microscope. The graft is sutured to the host with either continuous or interrupted nylon sutures no. 10-0 (Fig. 18-46).

7. Air or sodium hyaluronic acid (Healon) may be injected into the anterior chamber of the recipient's eye to keep the iris from adhering to the suture line. Mydriatic or miotic solutions are used at the surgeon's discretion.

8. A subconjunctival injection of antibiotic solution or a topical application of antibiotic drops may be used at the completion of the procedure. An eye patch and a metal guard are applied.

Lamellar keratoplasty

1. The eye speculum and superior rectus and inferior rectus bridle sutures are placed if needed.

2. The eye from the eye bank is removed from its container and washed in Neosporin solution.

3. The eye is wrapped in a surgical dressing. A groove is made at the desired depth in the cornea with the trephine. The Castroviejo keratome is set at the desired depth, and the lamellar sheet of cornea is removed and placed in a Petri dish.

4. The recipient cornea is grooved with the same trephine to the appropriate depth. Using the operating microscope, the surgeon performs a lamellar resection, that is, removes the anterior part of the cornea at a prede-

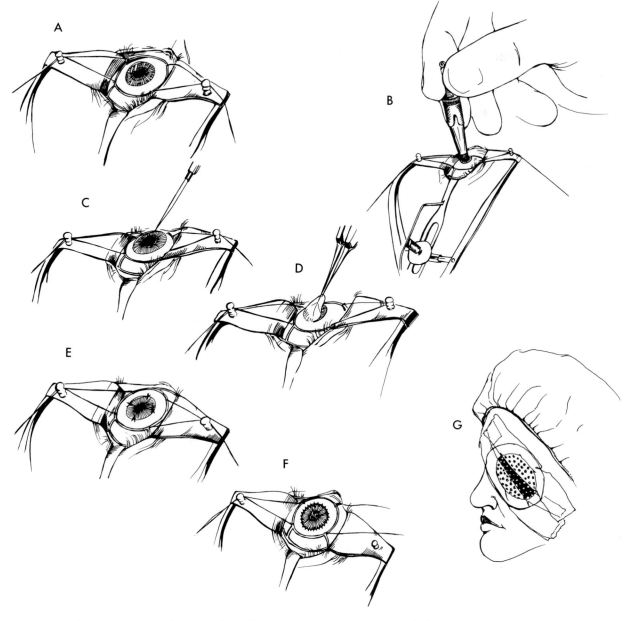

Fig. 18-46. A, Eye of patient who will undergo combined procedure including corneal transplantation and cataract extraction. Double Bonaccolto-Flieringa fixation ring is sutured in place with no. 5-0 Dacron sutures posted over solid bladed eye speculum. **B,** Corneal trephine is placed on recipient cornea, and partial penetration is made approximately three fourths through stroma. **C,** Anterior chamber is entered through groove with Wheeler knife. Remainder of button is excised with right and left micro-Katzin corneal scissors. **D,** Corneal button is removed. **E,** Donor button sutured in place with four no. 8-0 black silk sutures. **F,** Cornea sutured in place with continuous no. 10-0 suture, with air in anterior chamber. **G,** Patient postoperatively with Fox shield properly applied on bony margins.

termined depth with a Gill knife, Beaver knife blade no. 64, or other corneal splitter.

5. The donor tissue is sutured in place with a continuous 10-0 nylon suture.
6. A mydriatic agent and subconjunctival or topical antibiotics may be used.
7. The eye is patched.

Eye bank procedure

Donor eyes are removed immediately after death in accordance with legal regulations. The eye bank may be a central community agency or may be owned and operated by a hospital. The bank generally supplies the containers for eyes and sets forth regulations for the procedure. The enucleations are usually done in the hospital morgue under aseptic conditions.

A special consent form is required and should be signed by the authorized next of kin and by a hospital representative designated by hospital policy.

Procedural considerations. The eyes are washed and irrigated in the routine manner of preparation for eye surgery. The sterile field, drapes, and instruments are essentially the same as those for an enucleation on a living patient.

Operative procedure

1. Eye specimen bottles are labeled for right and left eyes. The speculum is inserted, and after routine enucleation the donated eye is placed in the sterile specimen bottle with the cornea up. The eye is supported on a sponge that has been soaked in saline solution. An antibiotic solution may be placed on the cornea. The eye sockets are packed with cotton, and the lids are closed.
2. Specimen bottles are sealed with tape and labeled with the donor's name, time and cause of death, time of enucleation, and date.
3. Appropriate specimens may be placed in tissue culture medium for short-term storage (72 hours) or frozen for long-term storage after the necessary manipulation.

Keratorefractive procedures

Keratorefractive procedures are corneal procedures designed to correct myopia, astigmatism, and aphakia. Many of these procedures are still in the developmental stages and are considered investigational. They include radial keratotomy, keratomileusis, epikeratophakia, and keratophakia. These procedures require reshaping the cornea with relaxing incisions or cryolathing corneal tissue to change the refractive power of the cornea.

Radial keratotomy

Radial keratotomy is a series of precise, partial-thickness radial incisions in the cornea from a 3-mm or larger central optical zone to the limbus. These incisions result in a flattening of the cornea, which reduces the refractive error.

Radial keratotomy was first performed by Sato in Japan in 1953. In 1972 the procedure was studied and modified by the Russian physicians Fyodorov and Durnev, who in 1974 began investigation of the procedure in humans, using anterior radial corneal incisions. In 1978, after review of the 4 years of data collected in Russia, Bores introduced radial keratotomy in the United States. Since then, modifications in the procedure have improved the predictability of results. Studies to ascertain the long-term results continue.

Radial keratotomy is a procedure for an adult who has at least −2 diopters of myopia and whose eye is otherwise healthy. Preoperative measurement of corneal curvature (keratometry), corneal thickness (ultrasonic pachymetry), and refractive error is required to assist in the determination of optical zone diameter and depth of incisions.

Procedural considerations. The surgery is performed as an outpatient procedure with local and topical anesthetics. The patient is prepared as for routine ophthalmic surgery.

Operative procedure

1. As the patient focuses on the fixation device attached to the objective lens of the operating microscope (Fig. 18-47, *A*), the visual axis is marked.
2. The blade depth is set on the micrometer of the surgical knife (diamond, sapphire, or steel) and double-checked against a micrometer gauge (Fig. 18-47, *B*).
3. The surgeon fixates the glove with a double-toothed Bores fixation forceps to decrease rotation.
4. Radial incisions are made from the margin of the optical zone to the limbus (Fig. 18-48). The numbers and depth are determined by the amount of correction desired.
5. The depth of the incisions is checked to verify uniformity.
6. The incisions are irrigated with balanced salt solution (BSS). An antibiotic solution is instilled, and an eye patch applied.

Epikeratophakia

Epikeratophakia is a form of refractive keratoplasty for the correction of aphakia, myopia, and keratoconus. A piece of donor corneal tissue is shaped to a specific diopter power on a cryolathe. This tissue is sutured to the recipient cornea to change the corneal curvature and thus the refractive power of the cornea. The patient's central cornea is not surgically invaded, and the donor tissue can be removed with no residual visual effects. Epikeratophakia is therefore reversible. Lyophilized (freeze-dried) tissue lenticles are available from a few sources.

Operative procedure

1. The preshaped donor tissue (lenticle) is rehydrated in BSS containing 100 μg/ml of IV gentamicin for 20 minutes before application onto the recipient's eye.
2. The lenticle is placed on a Teflon block and kept moist with BSS.
3. Anesthesia is administered.
4. The lid speculum is placed between the lids.
5. A topical anesthetic (cocaine 4%) is instilled in the operative eye.
6. The visual axis of the recipient eye is marked by the surgeon.
7. A cellulose sponge is used to scrape off the patient's corneal epithelium. The debris is thoroughly removed by irrigation and aspiration. (All epithelial cells must be removed to prevent them from growing in the interface between the lenticle and the recipient cornea in the postoperative period.)
8. A circular keratotomy of 0.25- to 0.30-mm depth is made with a trephine. Again the wound is irrigated and aspirated to remove debris thoroughly.
9. A wedge-shaped anulus of the anterior stroma for 360 degrees on the inner aspect of trephine mark is removed with scissors and forceps.

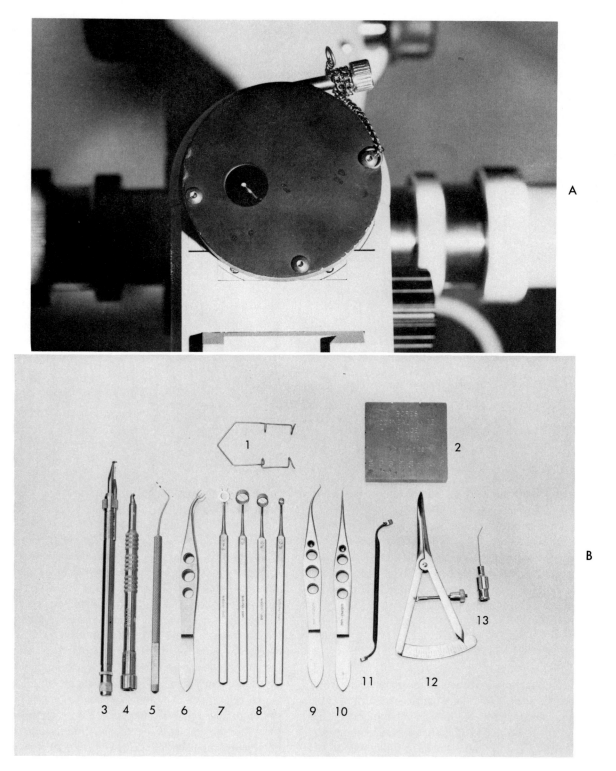

Fig. 18-47. Radial keratotomy instrumentation. **A,** Fixation device attached to microscope for patient to focus to mark optical zone (as viewed by patient). **B,** *1,* Barraquer wire speculum; *2,* Bores corneal knife gauge; *3,* Katena micrometer XTAL sapphire knife; *4,* Storz micrometer diamond knife; *5,* incision depth gauge; *6,* Rubman-Bores corneal fixation forceps; *7,* Bores corneal marker for eight radial incisions; *8,* Hoffer corneal markers with cross-hairs; *9,* 0.12-mm Castroviejo-Colibri very delicate forceps; *10,* Bores incision spreading forceps; *11,* elliptical optic center marker; *12,* Castroviejo caliper; *13,* 27-gauge air cannula.

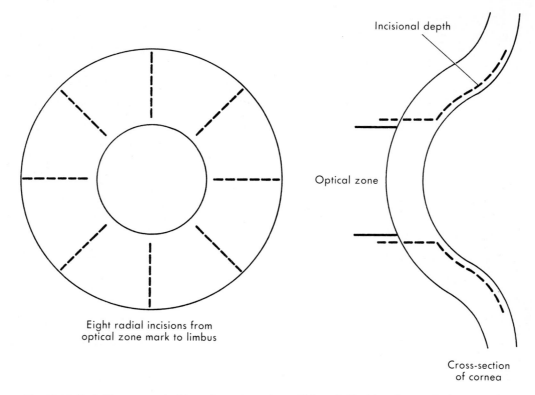

Incisional depth

Optical zone

Cross-section
of cornea

Eight radial incisions from
optical zone mark to limbus

Fig. 18-48. Radial keratotomy incisions shown from above. Eight radial incisions from optical zone mark to limbus. Cross-section of cornea indicates cuts perpendicular to optical zone through partial thickness of cornea (usually 80% to 95%).

10. The lenticle is positioned and sutured into place with no. 10-0 nylon interrupted sutures.
11. Suture knots are rotated and buried under the surface of the recipient side of the trephine cut.
12. A bandage contact lens is positioned on the eye. The prescribed drugs (usually an antiinflammatory agent and an antibiotic) are injected or instilled. The eye is patched; a shield is secured in place.

Surgery of the lens
Cataract extraction, generally with operating microscope

A cataract extraction is removal of the opaque lens from the interior of the eye. The lens consists of 65% water, 35% protein, and a trace of other body minerals. The disorders of the lens are opacification and dislocation, resulting in blurred vision without pain or inflammation.

Cataracts (opacification) vary in degree of density, size, and location and are usually caused by aging or trauma.

Two basic methods, intracapsular and extracapsular extraction, are usually employed to remove the lens.

The *intracapsular* method of cataract removal consists of removing the lens within its capsule.

In the *extracapsular* method, the anterior portion of the capsule is first ruptured and removed, and the lens cortex and nucleus are expressed from the eye, leaving the posterior capsule behind.

Restoration of functional vision is necessary after removal of the crystalline lens. At present four options are available for correction of aphakia (absence of the lens). A patient can be fitted with aphakic spectacles 4 to 8 weeks after lens extraction. These corrective lenses are acceptable only for binocular aphakia. They distort peripheral vision and produce a significant change in image size. Contact lenses are also used to correct aphakia. They offer an excellent option for visual correction and can be used for monocular aphakia. A third option is epikeratophakia. This procedure can be considered for patients with low endothelial cell counts. The fourth option for visual correction following lens removal, and the one most commonly used today, is the implantation of an artificial lens made of polymethyl methacrylate (PMMA). New designs and new implant materials challenge nursing personnel to keep abreast of constant changes in techniques for intraocular lens (IOL) implantations.

The IOLs offer many advantages to patients. They are used for monocular aphakic correction. Rehabilitation times for patients are shortened. The IOLs may be placed in the anterior chamber, iris plane, or posterior chamber. Iris plane or iris-fixated lenses are seldom used today.

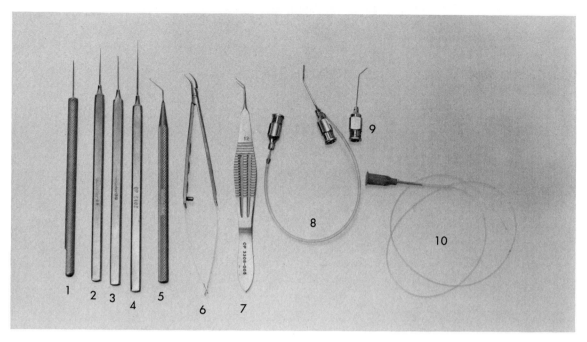

Fig. 18-49. Instrumentation for intraocular lens implantation. *1,* Round-handled Sinsky micro lens hook; *2,* Sinsky micro lens hook; *3,* Kugler cloverleaf lens manipulator; *4,* Bonn iris hook; *5,* Fenzl lens hook; *6,* Shepard lens holding forceps; *7,* Castroviejo corneoscleral suturing forceps with angled tip; *8,* Morrison irrigation and aspiration cannula; *9,* air or Healon cannula; *10,* disposable Kelman anterior chamber maintainer.

Posterior lenses can be implanted only when the cataract was removed by extracapsular lens extraction (ECCE). This is the most physiologic position for an artificial lens and has led to a return to ECCE, which is now the most common method of lens extraction. Anterior chamber lenses are used after intracapsular lens extraction (ICCE) and for secondary lens implantation.

The IOLs are available in various powers at 0.5 diopter steps. The necessary power is determined by measuring the curvature of the patient's cornea (keratometry) and the axial length (length from cornea to retina). A mathematical formula is then used to calculate the correct lens power.

Procedural considerations. Instrumentation varies with surgeon's preference (Fig. 18-49) but usually includes forceps to insert the lens and lens haptics and a hook to aid in rotating and positioning the lens. Instrumentation for lens procedures is shown in Fig. 18-50, and IOLs are shown in Fig. 18-51. Nursing personnel must be familiar with hospital policies pertaining to IOLs and their use.

Operative procedure

Intracapsular method (Fig. 18-52)

1. A speculum is placed in the eye to hold the lids apart.
2. The globe is held by transfixion with a silk suture no. 4-0, which is inserted under the tendon of the superior rectus muscle and clamped to the drape. A conjunctival flap, either limbal or fornix based, may be prepared with the use of the scissors. Some surgeons do not dissect a flap.
3. Bleeding points are coagulated by means of a bipolar unit which provides maximum coagulation with minimum tissue necrosis. Partially penetrating incisions (grooves) are made at the limbus or in the cornea.
4. Corneoscleral or corneocorneal sutures are passed through the lips of the wounds. These sutures are looped out of the groove and set in an orderly manner around the margins of the incision.
5. With the keratome, or knife, the anterior chamber is entered, and the limbal wound is enlarged with corneal scissors.
6. A peripheral iridectomy or sector iridectomy is performed. Alpha-chymotrypsin (Zolyse) is injected through the iridectomy. The lens is grasped, in most cases with a cryoextractor, and extracted slowly from the eye.
7. The pupil is usually constricted with acetylcholine (Miochol) if an IOL is inserted.
8. The corneoscleral sutures are tied, and the conjunctival flap is reapproximated with either absorbable or nonabsorbable sutures of the desired size.
9. Pilocarpine 2% or atropine 1% may be applied topically. Antibiotics may be used topically or subconjunctivally. The eye is dressed and patched.
10. If, at any time during the operation, vitreous gel is extruded from the eye, a partial vitrectomy is performed to prevent vitreous from becoming incorpo-

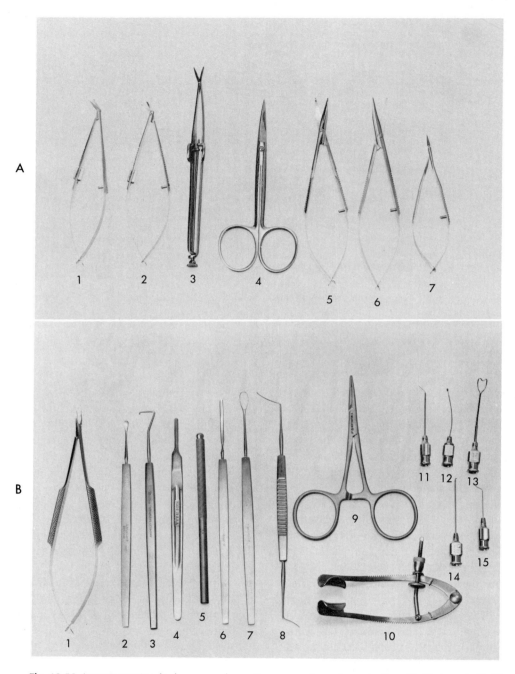

Fig. 18-50. Instrumentation for lens procedures. Forceps used are shown in Figs. 18-22 through 18-27. **A,** *1* and *2,* Troutman-Castroviejo corneal scissors; *3,* deWecker iris scissors; *4,* Knapp straight iris scissors; *5,* Westcott stitch scissors; *6,* Westcott tenotomy scissors; *7,* Vannas iridocapsulotomy scissors. **B,** *1,* Curved Barraquer needleholder; *2,* Gill corneal knife; *3,* Green strabismus hook; *4,* no. 9 Bard-Parker knife handle; *5,* Beaver knife handle; *6,* Wheeler iris spatula; *7,* lens loop; *8,* Castroviejo cyclodialysis spatula; *9,* Hartman mosquito hemostat; *10,* Lancaster eye speculum; *11,* Healon cannula; *12,* olive-tip irrigating cannula; *13,* irrigating vectis loop; *14,* lacrimal irrigator; *15,* air cannula.

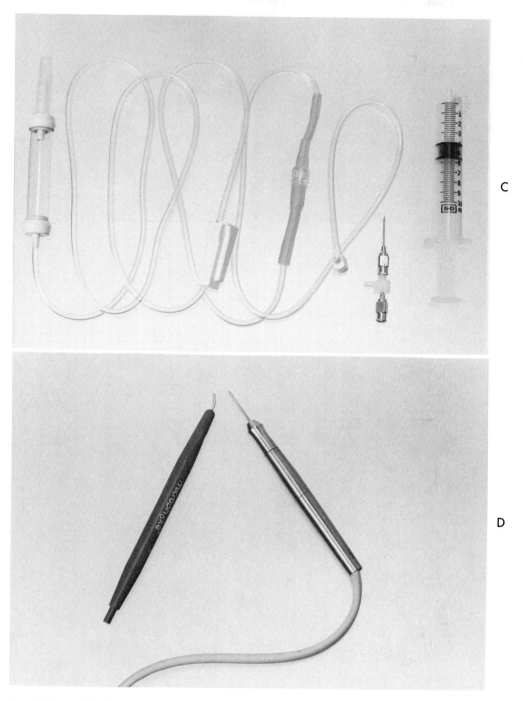

Fig. 18-50, cont'd. C, McIntyre infusion set with connector and coaxial irrigation-aspiration system. **D,** Disposable microphake cryoextractor; curved Frigitronics cataract cryoextractor (control console shown in Fig. 18-66, *D*).

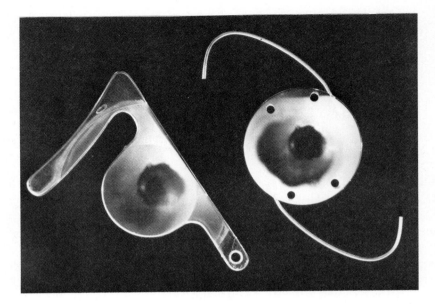

Fig. 18-51. *Left,* Kelman type II anterior chamber intraocular lens; *right,* Kratz variation posterior chamber intraocular lens, elliptical open loop.

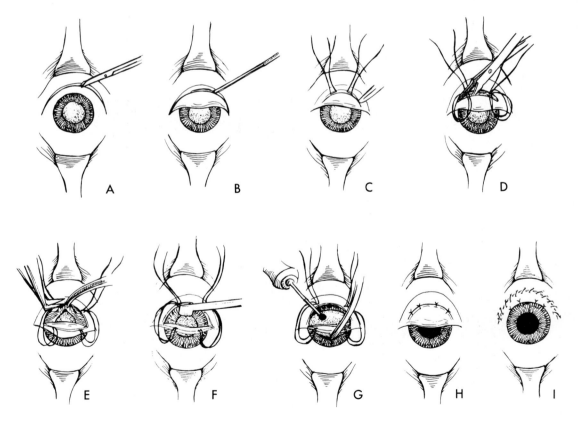

Fig. 18-52. Intracapsular lens extraction. **A,** Preparation of conjunctival flap with scissors. **B,** Nonpenetrating (partial-thickness) incision made at limbus or in cornea. **C,** Corneoscleral sutures are placed. **D,** Limbal incision completed with scissors. **E,** Peripheral iridectomy is performed. **F,** Iris retractor in place for delivery of lens. **G,** Lens grasped and pulled slowly from eye with cryostat unit. **H,** Corneoscleral sutures tied. **I,** Conjunctival flap reapproximated and sutured. (Modified from King, J.H., and Wadsworth, J.A.C.: An atlas of ophthalmic surgery, ed. 2, Philadelphia, 1970, J.B. Lippincott Co.)

rated into the wound, which can lead to various postoperative complications. The first step usually involves an attempt to aspirate liquefied vitreous from the eye with a 19-gauge blunt needle on a 2-ml syringe. Once this is accomplished, solid vitreous may be removed by the use of Weck-Cel sponges and scissors (Westcott) or by using any of the various vitrectomy instruments available.

Extracapsular method. The standard procedure for extracapsular lens extraction (ECCE) is similar to an intracapsular extraction up to step 6, removal of the lens. At this point the capsule of the lens is opened by means of a cystotome or capsule forceps; the lens nucleus is removed by expression and a lens loop; the lens cortex is removed by irrigation and aspiration using a coaxial cannula system. Cycloplegic agents are generally used. The remainder of the procedure is as outlined previously for intracapsular extraction. If a posterior chamber IOL is used, the pupil is constricted with acetylcholine after the lens insertion.

Phacoemulsification. Over the past years a number of microsurgical techniques have been developed for lens removal through a small incision. Basically, each technique involves opening the lens capsule and using ultrasonic energy to fragment the hard lens material, which can then be aspirated from the eye.

The subsequent description and illustrations relate to the use of the Cavitron phacoemulsification unit (Fig. 18-53). All personnel using specialized instruments and equipment must have thorough knowledge of their operation, as well as possible problems and actions to correct them.

1. After a superior rectus bridle suture is placed, a small limbal-based flap is dissected superiorly.
2. The surgical limbus is cleaned by sharp dissection with a Beaver knife blade. Hemostasis is obtained with a disposable eye cautery.
3. A 3-mm incision is made into the eye with either a keratome or a micro sharp knife.
4. The lens capsule is opened with a cystotome or capsule forceps. The anterior chamber may be kept formed with air or irrigating solution.
5. The lens nucleus is loosened from the cortex with the cystotome or a blunt cyclodialysis spatula.
6. The ultrasonic handpiece is checked by the physician for appropriate vacuum control. *This check should be made before any handpiece is introduced into the eye.*
7. The ultrasonic handpiece is introduced into the eye. Three positions are possible for the operation of the foot pedal under the surgeon's control: (1) irrigation alone; (2) irrigation and aspiration; and (3) irrigation, aspiration, and ultrasonic power. As the surgeon manipulates the handpiece and operates the footpedal to emulsify the lens nucleus, the nurse is responsible for operating the other controls and monitoring the function of the instrument.

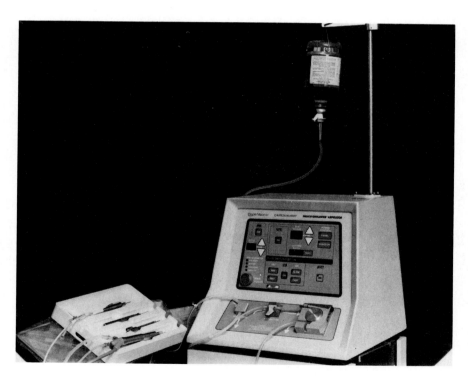

Fig. 18-53. Coopervision Cavitron/Kelman Phaco Emulsifier Aspirator Model 9000. Instrument tray shows AVIT handpiece, irrigation cystotome, irrigation-aspiration (IA) handpiece, and ultrasonic handpiece. (Courtesy Coopervision Surgical Co., Irvine, Calif.)

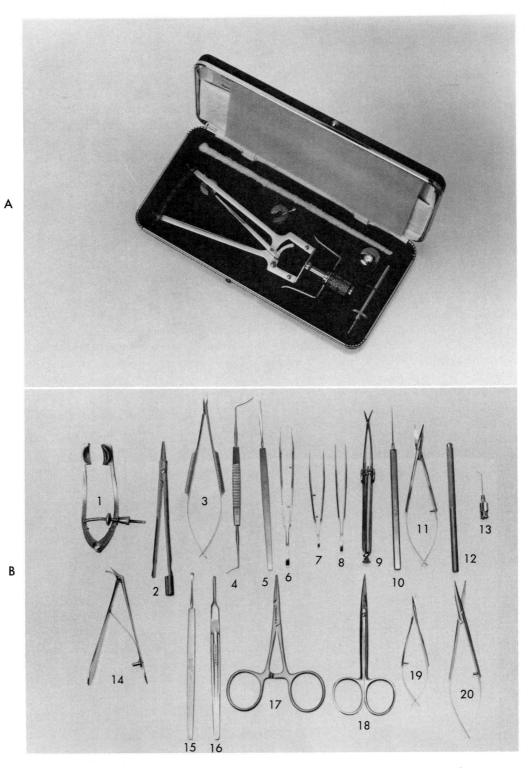

Fig. 18-54. Instrumentation for glaucoma surgery. **A,** Schiotz tonometer to measure intraocular pressure (may be autoclaved). **B,** *1,* Lancaster eye speculum; *2,* blade breaker; *3,* Barraquer curved needle holder; *4,* Castroviejo cyclodialysis spatula; *5,* Wheeler iris spatula; *6,* Castroviejo 0.12-mm suturing forceps; *7,* Colibri corneal forceps; *8,* Bishop-Harman tissue forceps; *9,* deWecker iris scissors; *10,* Bonn iris hook; *11,* Westcott stitch scissors; *12,* Beaver knife handle; *13,* air injection cannula; *14,* Holth scleral punch; *15,* Gill corneal knife; *16,* no. 9 Bard-Parker knife handle; *17,* Hartman mosquito hemostat; *18,* Knapp strabismus scissors; *19,* Vannas iridocapsulotomy scissors; *20,* Westcott tenotomy scissors.

8. When the lens nucleus has been emulsified and removed, the lens cortex is removed with the 0.3-mm aspiration-irrigation handpiece.

9. If an IOL is to be implanted, the wound is extended to accommodate the lens diameter, the IOL is inserted, and acetylcholine may be introduced to constrict the pupil.

10. A peripheral iridectomy may be performed.

11. The corneoscleral wound is closed with 7-0 or 8-0 absorbable suture, a 10-0 nonabsorbable suture, or a combination of both.

12. The conjunctival flap is closed.

13. The eye is appropriately dressed.

Surgical procedures for glaucoma
Iridectomy

Iridectomy is removal of a section of iris tissue. Peripheral iridectomy is done in the treatment of acute, subacute, or chronic angle-closure glaucoma when extensive peripheral anterior synechiae have not formed. This operation is performed to reestablish communication between the posterior and anterior chambers, thus relieving pupillary block and permitting the iris root to drop away from the trabecular meshwork to reestablish the outflow of aqueous fluid through Schlemm's canal.

Procedural considerations. Instrumentation for glaucoma surgery is shown in Fig. 18-54.

Operative procedure

1. The speculum is introduced. The globe is fixed with a no. 4-0 silk suture passed under the superior rectus tendon with a fixation forceps and needle holder. The suture is fastened to the drape with a hemostat.

2. A small peritomy is performed at the superior limbus. The corneoscleral junction is scraped clean of epithelium. With a Beaver knife handle and no. 64 blade, a limbal groove is made down to Descemet's membrane.

3. The anterior chamber is entered with a no. 15 blade. Pressure is placed on the posterior lip of the wound to prolapse the iris. The iris is grasped, and either a peripheral or sector iridectomy is performed. The iris is stroked back into position by external manipulation with a spatula over the cornea.

4. The wound is closed with absorbable suture. Subconjunctival antibiotics may be administered, and an eye dressing applied.

Elliot trephination

Elliot trephination is the formation of a drainage channel to the subconjunctival space in the treatment of chronic glaucoma. The object of Elliot trephination is to establish a route of aqueous drainage to subconjunctival space for absorption. The operation is done primarily for open-angle glaucoma. Postoperatively, the aqueous matter escapes through the scleral hole into the subconjunctival space, where it is absorbed into the bloodstream.

Operative procedure

1. A superior rectus bridle suture of no. 4-0 silk is placed and clamped to the drape.

2. Two milliliters of saline (with the possible addition of 1 drop of 1:1000 epinephrine) are injected superiorly beneath Tenon's capsule to dissect a flap from the underlying sclera.

3. The conjunctiva is incised to the sclera. The flap is dissected anteriorly into clear cornea.

4. With the conjunctival flap raised by means of forceps, the trephine is applied at the corneal limbus.

5. After completion of trephination, the scleral disc is cut at its hinge if it is not free.

6. An iridectomy is performed with iris forceps and deWecker scissors.

7. The operative area is cleansed of blood, and the conjunctival flap is resutured with a no. 6-0 or 7-0 silk suture. Cycloplegic agents are administered. The eye is dressed with a patch and a metal guard.

Anterior and posterior lid sclerectomies

Anterior and posterior lid sclerectomies are performed to provide a drainage channel to the subconjunctival space in the treatment of chronic glaucoma.

Operative procedure

1. The procedure is as described for Elliot trephination through the dissection of the conjunctival flap (steps 1 to 3).

2A. For *thermal sclerectomy* a scleral flap is made approximately 3 mm from the limbus with a Beaver no. 64 blade. The disposable eye cautery with a transilluminating head is used to outline the anterior chamber. The eye cautery is used to apply heat energy to the posterior wound edge under the scleral flap. The anterior chamber is entered with a clean sweep of the cautery. The iris usually prolapses spontaneously, or an iris forceps is used to grasp the iris, and a peripheral or radial iridectomy is performed.

2B. For *punch sclerectomy* an incision is made into the anterior chamber at the anterior or posterior margin of the limbus after the anterior chamber has been outlined with a transilluminator. A punch is introduced, and sections of either the anterior or posterior lip are removed, depending on which incision has been made. An iridectomy is performed.

3. A careful closure of conjunctiva and Tenon's capsule is accomplished with no. 6-0 silk suture, leaving both ends free.

4. Air is introduced under the flap with a blunt 30-gauge needle on a 2-ml syringe.

5. The conjunctival flap is closed with a continuous suture. The free ends may be used to delimit the bleb. Atropine sulfate 1% is dropped on the eye, and an eye dressing is applied.

Cyclodialysis

Cyclodialysis is the formation of a communication between the anterior chamber and the space located between the sclera and the choroid. This reduces aqueous secretion and thus induces lower pressure. In this surgical procedure, aqueous secretion is reduced and absorption into the suprachoroidal space is increased. Cyclodialysis is usually reserved for treatment of glaucoma associated with peripheral anterior synechiae.

Operative procedure

1. A superior rectus bridle suture of no. 4-0 silk is put in place and clamped to the drape.
2. In one of the superior quadrants between the rectus muscles, the conjunctiva is incised and dissected from the sclera. An incision is made through the sclera to the suprachoroidal space with the use of a Beaver no. 64 blade.
3. A cyclodialysis spatula is introduced through the scleral opening, and the anterior chamber is entered in the region of the iris root; the ciliary body is thus detached from the sclera by means of the spatula. The scleral incision is closed.
4. The conjunctiva is closed with fine sutures. A dressing is applied.

Trabeculectomy

The term *trabeculectomy* is a misnomer because it implies that part of the trabecular meshwork is removed during surgery. Any of the previously described operations for glaucoma may be called a trabeculectomy, with the addition of the dissection of a partial-thickness, limbal-based scleral flap before the anterior chamber is entered. This scleral limbal flap may or may not be loosely sutured before the conjunctival flap is closed.

Goniotomy

Goniotomy is the opening of a congenital membrane from the iris surface to Schwalbe's line, allowing aqueous humor to reach the trabecular meshwork in cases of congenital glaucoma.

Operative procedure

1. The patient is anesthetized without intubation.
2. An examination is performed. Corneal clarity and size, intraocular pressure, microscopic examination of the anterior segment (including gonioscopy), and examination of the posterior pole of the eye (especially the optic disc) are recorded.
3. The patient is intubated, if indicated, and prepped and draped.
4. A pediatric eye speculum and superior and inferior rectus bridle sutures are placed.
5. Under microscopic control with an appropriate gonioprism in place, the Maumenee irrigating knife is introduced through the temporal limbus. The anterior chamber is kept formed by constant irrigation through the knife. The anterior chamber is crossed, and the membrane covering the iris and angle structures is cut without damaging the trabecular meshwork. The knife is removed.
6. Air may be introduced into the eye, and a suture may be used.
7. A cycloplegic agent may be used topically.
8. The eye is dressed.

Laser therapy

Argon or Nd-YAG laser therapy is being used to treat acute (angle-closure) glaucoma and open-angle glaucoma. Laser therapy is a fairly uncomplicated outpatient procedure in which a slit lamp is used for delivery of the laser beam. Laser treatment of glaucoma is a noninvasive procedure and, if successful, may eliminate the need for more invasive surgical procedures.

Laser trabeculoplasty

Laser trabeculoplasty is treatment for open-angle glaucoma by the placement of laser burns in the posterior part of the trabeculum, anterior to the scleral spur, to cause the surface of the trabecular meshwork to contract. This theoretically pulls open the adjacent intertrabecular spaces, resulting in increased aqueous outflow.

Procedural considerations. Preoperative sedation is usually unnecessary. A topical anesthetic such as proparacaine is used. Intraocular pressure is measured preoperatively. Laser precautions are initiated (see Chapter 10).

Operative procedure for argon laser trabeculoplasty

1. One or two proparacaine (for example, Ophthaine) drops are instilled in the operative eye.
2. The patient is positioned at the laser slit lamp (Fig. 18-55).
3. A three-mirror Goldmann lens is placed, allowing visualization of the chamber angle and retraction of the eye lid. The nurse assists in this placement.
4. A landmark is selected as a starting point and laser treatment is begun, using a 50-μm spot size for 0.1 second at 850 milliwatts power. The laser "burns" are placed in the midtrabecular meshwork, pigmented zone, to yield about 20 burns in each quadrant for a total of 70 to 90 burns. The power should be titrated to the threshold of whitening or tiny bubble formation.
5. One hour after completion of the treatment, the intraocular pressure should be measured, and topical prednisolone or dexamethasone drops should be instilled.
6. The procedure may be performed in two treatment segments rather than completed in one.

Argon laser iridotomy

Argon laser iridotomy is the placement of penetrating argon laser burns in the peripheral iris to create an opening,

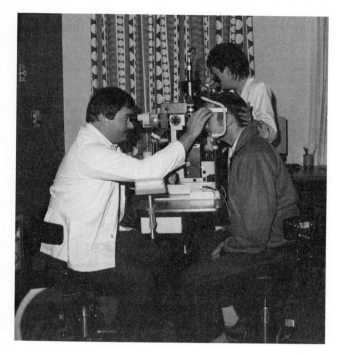

Fig. 18-55. Patient positioned at argon laser slit lamp for treatment of glaucoma.

allowing aqueous humor to flow from the posterior chamber into the anterior chamber and out through Schlemm's canal to treat angle-closure glaucoma.

Procedural considerations. The operative considerations are as for laser trabeculoplasty.

Operative procedure
1. Topical anesthetic drops of proparacaine or an equivalent are instilled.
2. The patient is positioned at the laser slit lamp.
3. The Abraham lens is placed in the operative eye.
4. An iris crypt or "thin" area of iris is selected.
5. Initial burns are placed in a circle to put the iris on a stretch using 200-μm spot size for 0.1 second at 200 to 300 milliwatts power. (Usually six to eight burns accomplish this.)
6. Penetrating burns are placed as needed to make an adequate opening (usually 10 to 30 applications) using 50-μm spot size for 0.1 to 0.2 second at 600 to 1000 milliwatts power.
7. Prednisolone or dexamethasone eye drops are instilled into the operative eye.

Cyclocryotherapy

Cyclocryotherapy is a procedure used in the treatment of glaucoma. The procedure decreases aqueous secretions by ablation of the secretory ciliary epithelium by employing a retinal cryoprobe to freeze a portion of the ciliary body.

Procedural considerations. The procedure is usually performed with topical anesthesia and retrobulbar injection. The patient is prepared as for ophthalmic surgery.

Operative procedure
1. A topical anesthestic is applied, and retrobulbar injection of a local anesthetic drug is done.
2. A lid speculum is placed in the operative eye.
3. The glove is fixed with a forceps, and the retinal cryoprobe is placed about 5 mm from the limbus to prevent freezing the cornea and damaging the trabecular meshwork.
4. The upper half of the ciliary body is treated with six applications of the cryoprobe for 60 seconds each at $-70°$ C.
5. Lid closure is verified. The corneal surface is protected with an eye patch.

Surgery for retinal detachment

Retinal detachment is a separation of the neural retinal layer from the pigmented epithelium layer of the retina. Retinal detachment may occur because of the presence of intraocular neoplasms originating in the retina or choroid (exudative type) or, more commonly, as a result of retinal tears or holes associated with injury, degeneration, or rhegmatogenous detachment.

Retinal detachment usually causes the sudden onset of the appearance of floating spots before the eye, resulting from freeing of pigment or blood cells in the vitreous. The vitreous humor of the eye is a gelatinous liquid possessing an ultrastructure of fine protein fibers in a network arrangement, with some attachment to the retina. Fluid from the vitreous cavity may seep through the retinal tears and separate the retinal components. The detachment progresses as the liquid seeps behind the retina. The part of the retina that has become separated from its nutritional source becomes damaged and relatively nonfunctional.

Prompt treatment of retinal detachment is aimed at preventing permanent loss of central vision. Reattachment of the retina can be accomplished only by surgery. Repair is done from outside the globe. The surgery involves sealing off the area in which the tear or hole is located and may include drainage of the subretinal fluid (Fig. 18-56).

Surgical procedures performed in the treatment of retinal detachment include scleral buckling using episcleral and intrascleral techniques with diathermy or cryotherapy. Cryosurgery or light coagulation may be used alone or in combination with a buckling procedure. Instrumentation for retinal surgery is shown in Fig. 18-57 (pp. 488-489).

In the treatment of retinal detachment, the aim is to return the retina to its normal anatomic position. The purpose of surgery for retinal detachment is to cause an intrusion or push into the eye at the site of the pathologic cause. Treatment by diathermy or cryotherapy causes an inflammatory reaction that leads to a permanent adhesion between the detached retina and underlying structures.

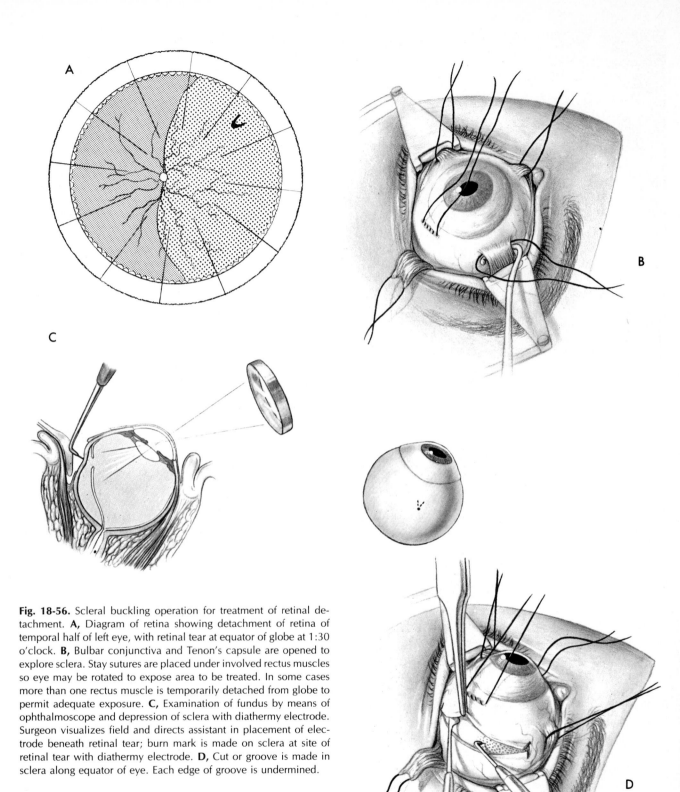

Fig. 18-56. Scleral buckling operation for treatment of retinal detachment. **A,** Diagram of retina showing detachment of retina of temporal half of left eye, with retinal tear at equator of globe at 1:30 o'clock. **B,** Bulbar conjunctiva and Tenon's capsule are opened to explore sclera. Stay sutures are placed under involved rectus muscles so eye may be rotated to expose area to be treated. In some cases more than one rectus muscle is temporarily detached from globe to permit adequate exposure. **C,** Examination of fundus by means of ophthalmoscope and depression of sclera with diathermy electrode. Surgeon visualizes field and directs assistant in placement of electrode beneath retinal tear; burn mark is made on sclera at site of retinal tear with diathermy electrode. **D,** Cut or groove is made in sclera along equator of eye. Each edge of groove is undermined.

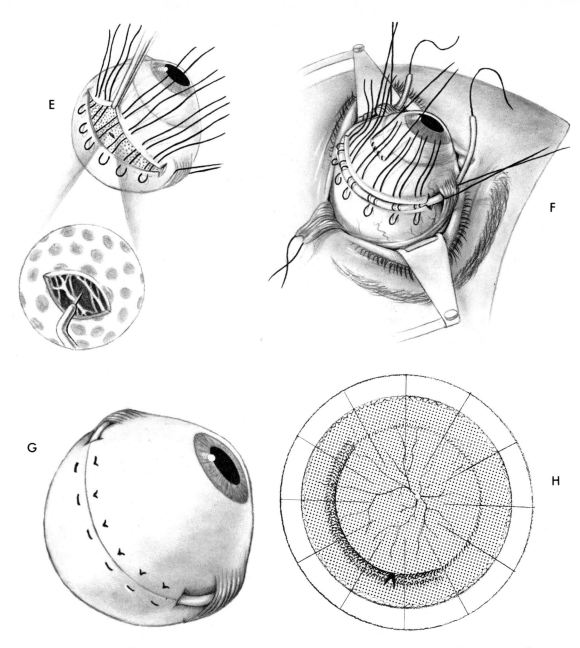

Fig. 18-56, cont'd. E, Mattress sutures of surgeon's preference are placed across scleral groove. Small incision is made through remaining layer of sclera down to choroid. Choroid is punctured with fine electrode to allow subretinal fluid to drain. **F,** A no. 40 Silastic band is laid in bed of scleral groove under mattress sutures. When retinal tears are large, a silicone patch may be placed under band. **G,** Edges of scleral groove are closed over Silastic band. **H,** Diagram of fundus with retina in place and 1:30 o'clock retinal tear on buckle. Diathermy reaction is seen on buckle from 12 to 5:30 o'clock. (From Advancing with surgery, Somerville, N.J., Ethicon, Inc.)

Procedural considerations. The patient is prepared as for general ophthalmic surgery.

Operative procedures. A detailed drawing of the retina is made before surgery and is displayed in the operating suite. On the basis of this drawing, the conjunctiva is opened to a previously determined extent, that is, 90 degrees for a simple horseshoe tear or 360 degrees for an aphakic detachment. With the indirect ophthalmoscope, the abnormality is localized under direct visualization, and nonpenetrating diathermy marks are made over the site by indentation.

Episcleral technique

1. Cryotherapy is applied to the pathologic areas under direct visualization (an iceball is seen to form in the proper areas until all of the lesion has been treated).
2. If a localized plombage (push) is to be used, Dacron

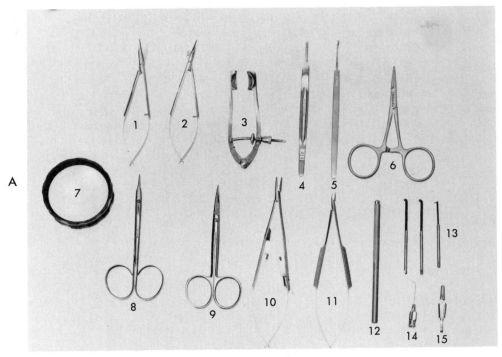

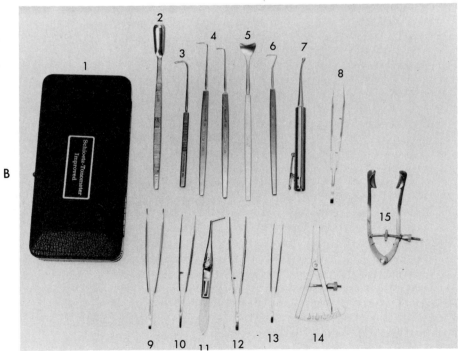

Fig. 18-57. Instruments for retinal surgery. **A,** *1,* Westcott tenotomy scissors; *2,* Westcott stitch scissors; *3,* Lancaster eye speculum; *4,* no. 9 Bard-Parker knife handle; *5,* Gill knife; *6,* Hartman mosquito hemostat; *7,* Nikon 20 D lens; *8,* straight Stevens scissors; *9,* Knapp strabismus scissors; *10,* Snowden-Pencer plastic needle holder; *11,* Barraquer fine needle holder; *12,* Beaver knife handle; *13,* diathermy tips; *14,* air cannula; *15,* serrefine. **B,** *1,* Schiotz tonometer; *2,* Arruga orbital retractor; *3,* Gass retinal detachment hook; *4,* muscle hooks; *5,* DeMarres lid retractor; *6,* Green strabismus hook; *7,* Wilder scleral depressor; *8,* 0.12-mm Castroviejo suturing forceps; *9,* curved serrated utility forceps; *10,* Lester fixation forceps; *11,* Jameson recession forceps; *12,* Alabama tying forceps; *13,* Bishop-Harman tissue forceps; *14,* Castroviejo caliper; *15,* Lancaster eye speculum.

sutures are set in the sclera surrounding the lesion and tied over Silastic sponges, causing the outer shell of the eye to be pushed toward the elevated retina. If an encircling band is to be used, belt loops are made in the sclera in four quadrants with no. 64 and 66 Beaver blades. A no. 40 Silastic band is passed 360 degrees around the eye through the belt loops, and a self-holding Watzke sleeve or sutures are applied to the band to maintain a predetermined circumference. This causes a 360-degree constriction of the outer coats into the eye.

3. If drainage of subretinal fluid is desired, under direct visualization an area is chosen in which a significant fluid level exists under the retina, and a diathermy mark is made on the sclera. The sclera is split to the choroid, and a preplaced suture is inserted. A small amount of diathermy is applied to the choroid bed. A needle is then used to puncture the choroid into the subretinal space to permit drainage of fluid. The preplaced suture is tied.

Scleral resection. An incision is made into the sclera, and a scleral flap is dissected both anteriorly and posteriorly from the original incision. Diathermy can be used in this bed, or cryotherapy can be used under direct visualization. Preserved eye bank sclera or a groove piece no. 20 may be sutured into the bed, using a Supramid suture no. 4-0 or Dacron sutures no. 5-0 with or without an encircling band as previously described. Drainage of subretinal fluid may be accomplished as previously de-

scribed. Air or other replacement or ballast fluids may be introduced into the eye after the drainage of subretinal fluid. This is usually done through the pars plana under direct visualization.

A culture may be taken at the end of the surgery, and a subconjunctival injection of an antibiotic, steroid, or both may be given unless contraindicated. The conjunctiva is closed with a selected suture material, and the eye is patched.

Vitrectomy

Vitrectomy is narrowly defined as removal of all or part of the vitreous gel (body). In the broader clinical sense of the term, it also includes the cutting and removal of fibrotic membranes, removal of epiretinal membranes, and electrocoagulation of bleeding vessels. In its normal state the vitreous gel of the eye is transparent. In certain disease states, bleeding from damaged or newly formed vessels may cause the vitreous to become opaque, which may severely decrease vision. In addition to the patient's inability to see, the ophthalmologist is unable to visualize the retina and therefore treat the underlying pathologic condition before permanent damage can occur. In these cases vitrectomy is indicated to allow the patient to see and the surgeon to institute treatment if indicated.

Certain ophthalmic diseases are associated with the formation of membranes, which may block the visual axis and cause decreased vision. Contraction of these membranes may produce traction-type or rhegmatogenous retinal detachment. In these cases vitrectomy is indicated to relieve the underlying pathologic processes leading to decreased vision.

The main indications for vitrectomy in the anterior segment are:

1. Vitreous loss during cataract extraction
2. Opacities in the anterior segment
3. Complications associated with vitreous in the anterior chamber
4. Miscellaneous causes, such as hyphema, pupillary membranes, and residual soft lens material

The main indications for posterior segment vitrectomy via the pars plana are:

1. Vitreous opacities, long-standing
2. Advanced diabetic eye disease
3. Severe intraocular trauma
4. Retained foreign bodies
5. Proliferative vitreoretinopathy
6. Retinal detachment from giant tears
7. Endophthalmitis
8. Diagnostic vitreous biopsy

Procedural considerations. The procedure varies according to the location of the pathologic condition (anterior or posterior segments), the instrumentation available, and

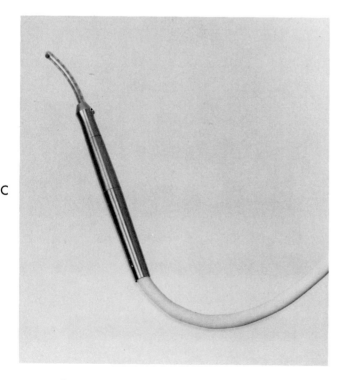

C

Fig. 18-57, cont'd. C, Frigitronics retinal cryoprobe.

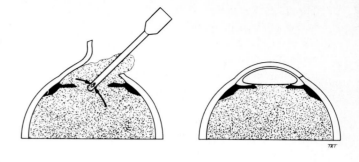

Fig. 18-58. Diagram of management of vitreous loss at the time of cataract extraction. (From Kanski, J.J.: Clinical ophthalmology, London, 1984, Butterworth & Co.)

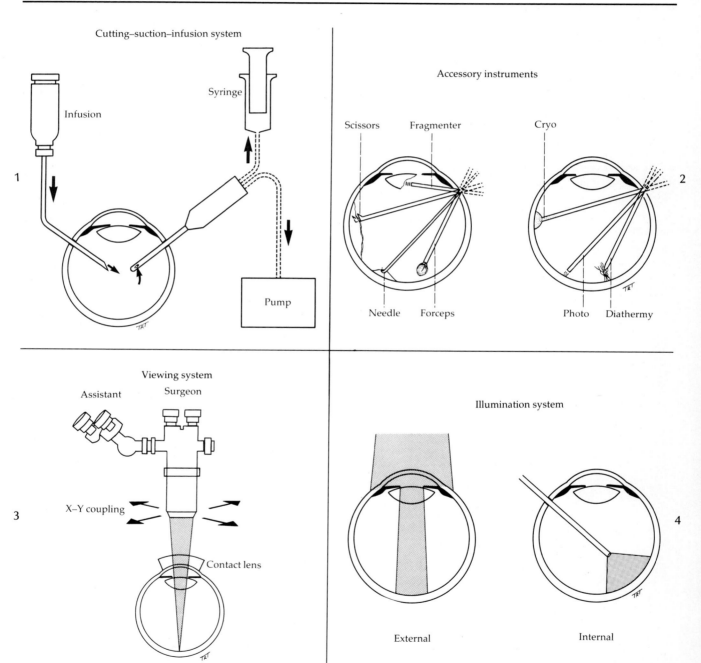

Fig. 18-59. Vitrectomy procedures require, *1*, cutting-suction-infusion system; *2*, accessory instruments; *3*, viewing system with X-Y coupling; and *4*, illumination system. (From Kanski, J.J.: Clinical ophthalmology, London, 1984, Butterworth & Co.)

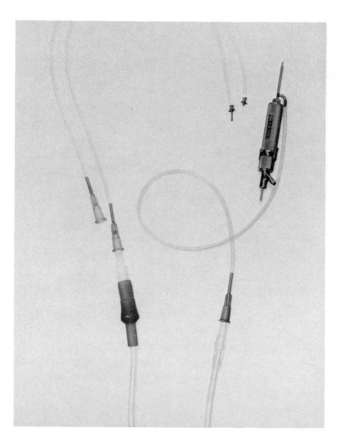

Fig. 18-60. Infusion systems for vitrectomy. Infusion cannulas; Ocutome probe with Charles infusion sleeve attached.

the surgeon's preference. A pathologic condition in the anterior segment can be approached through a limbal incision, as in lens extraction with vitreous loss (Fig. 18-58); through "open sky," after trephine incision for penetrating keratoplasty; or through the pars plana. A pathologic condition in the posterior segment is usually approached through the pars plana.

Vitrectomy is a microsurgical procedure requiring a viewing system (operating microscope with an X-Y coupling, zoom lens, and fine focus), an illumination system, a cutting-suction-infusion system, and accessory instruments (Fig. 18-59).

The infusion system consists of a 500-ml bottle of buffered balanced salt solution, such as BSS Plus, a standard intravenous administration set, and an infusion needle or sleeve (Fig. 18-60), or it may be part of a single multifunction handpiece (Fig. 18-61). The level of intraocular pressure can be varied by elevating or lowering the infusion bottle in relation to the patient's eye.

The suction and cutting systems vary in sophistication from the battery-powered, manual-aspirating, guillotine cutter of the disposable Kaufman II vitrector (Fig. 18-62) to the pneumatically driven, vacuum suction, guillotine cutter of the Octome II (Fig. 18-63). A variety of instruments are available, but all cutters engage tissue into a port and then cut it by shearing action between the edges of a moving and a nonmoving part. Guillotine cutters have a linear, to-and-fro action, whereas reciprocating or oscillating cutters rotate in a clockwise-counterclockwise

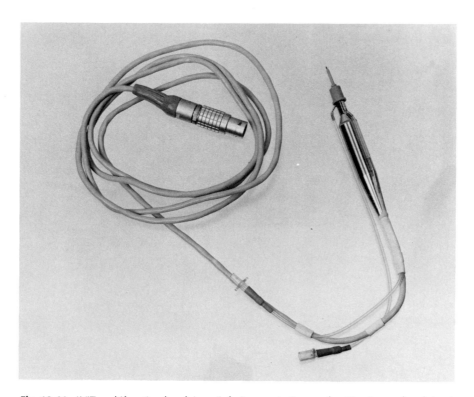

Fig. 18-61. AVIT multifunction handpiece (infusion, aspiration, and cutting in one handpiece).

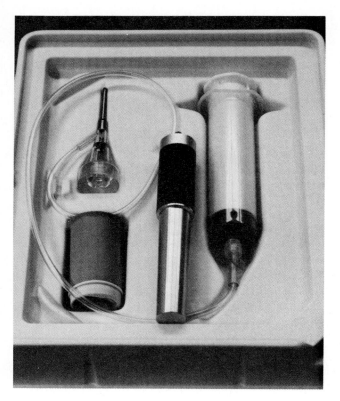

Fig. 18-62. Disposable Kaufman vitrector with motor.

fashion (Fig. 18-64). Suction can be operated manually with a syringe (Kaufman II Vitrector) or mechanically using a pump controlled by a foot switch to maintain the level of aspiration.

Illumination for vitrectomy is external, using the operating microscope for anterior segment vitrectomy, and internal, using a fiberoptic light pipe (endoillumination), shown in Fig. 18-65.

Accessory instruments (Fig. 18-66) usually have a 20-gauge diameter so they can be interchanged throughout the procedure. Accessory instruments include:

Hooks, picks, and scissors for dissection of membranes
Micro foreign body forceps
Flute needles for evacuating pools of blood or for fluid gas exchange
Endocoagulators, either xenon or argon, for intraocular photocoagulation
Intraocular cryoprobe for cryocoagulation

To prepare for a vitrectomy procedure, the nurse must know the location of the problem, how the surgeon plans to address the problem (route of entry into the eye—anterior or posterior, open sky or closed), instrumentation to be used, and anticipated extent and length of the procedure.

Instrument and equipment functioning should be thoroughly checked before bringing the patient into the operating room. When a lens extraction procedure is planned, vitrectomy instrumentation should be ready in the event of accidental vitreous loss. When preparing for pars plana vitrectomy in the posterior segment, the nurse must be

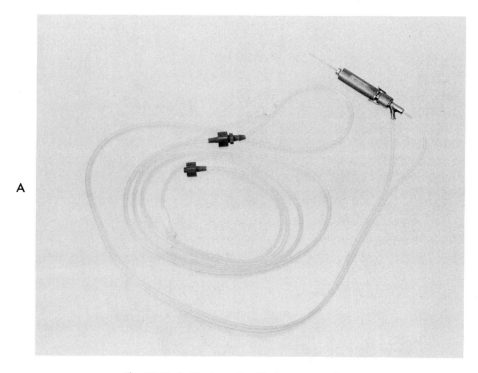

A

Fig. 18-63. A, Ocutome II guillotine-type suction cutter.

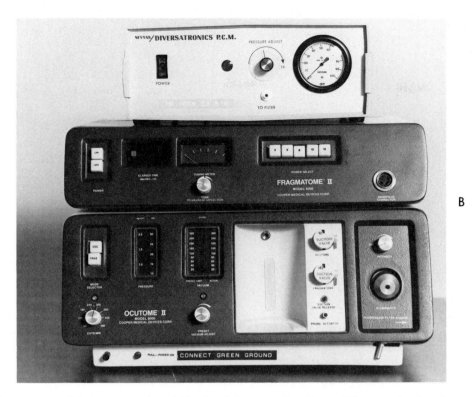

B

Fig. 18-63, cont'd. B, Power consoles used for closed vitrectomy. *Top,* Nevvas/Diversatronics air exchange unit; *middle,* Fragmatome console for lens fragmenting during closed vitrectomy; *bottom,* Ocutome II console for suction cutting with fiberoptic light source.

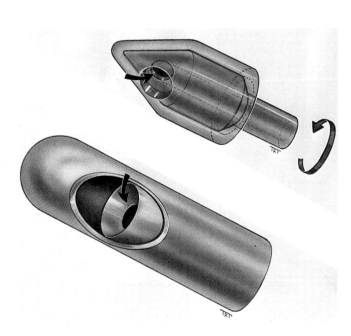

Fig. 18-64. Two types of suction cutters. *Above right,* Rotary cutter. *Below left,* Guillotine cutter. (From Kanski, J.J.: Clinical ophthalmology, London, 1984, Butterworth & Co.)

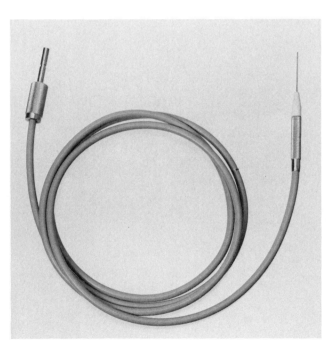

Fig. 18-65. Fiberoptic light pipe (Endoilluminator).

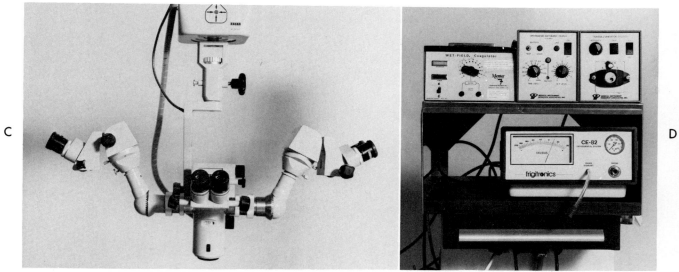

Fig. 18-66. Accessory instruments for vitrectomy. **A,** *1,* Endocoagulator; *2,* Rappazio foreign body forceps; *3,* Sutherlund membrane pick; *4,* handle for Charles flute needle; *5,* irrigating contact lens; *6,* Charles flute needles. **B,** Accessory instruments are extremely delicate, as shown in the Grishaber vitreous scissors, and require careful handling. **C,** Microscope with X-Y coupling and stereo binocular observation tubes, essential for vitreous surgery. **D,** Power sources for accessory instruments: Wetfield bipolar coagulator, ophthalmic diathermy, and Frigitronics cryosurgical system.

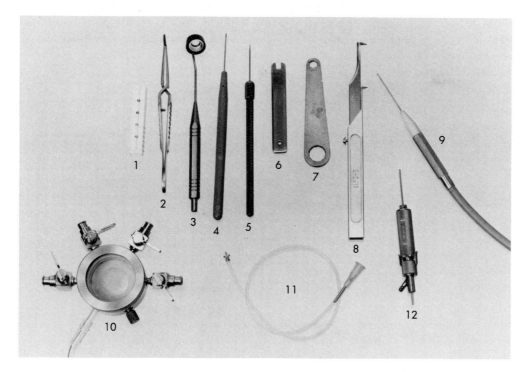

Fig. 18-67. Vitrectomy instrumentation (used with instrumentation for retinal detachment; see Fig. 18-57 C). *1,* Scleral plugs, 19- or 20-gauge; *2,* scleral plug forceps; *3,* irrigating contact lens; *4,* disposable MVR knife; *5,* Girard handle with MVR blade; *6,* Fragmatome wrench; *7,* Ocutome wrench; *8,* caliper; *9,* Endoilluminator; *10,* manifold; *11,* infusion cannula; *12,* Ocutome cutter.

aware that a combined scleral buckling procedure may be necessary.

For repair of a giant retinal tear, a special operating room bed may be used, allowing the patient to be turned to a prone position after the vitrectomy procedure for exchange of fluid and air or a special gas to tamponade the retina.

Vitrectomy procedures vary in length from less than 1 hour to over 6 hours. When a long procedure is anticipated, care must be taken to protect the patient's skin and reduce pressure areas. A foam mattress pad, heel and elbow protectors, and elasticized stockings may be used. When positioned for vitrectomy, the patient's head should be higher than the heart, the cheeks higher than the forehead, and the neck extended. A wrist support may be placed around the patient's head to support the surgeon's wrist during manipulation of the intraocular instruments.

While draping, the nurse should provide for removal of infusion fluid from the operative field and take care to protect electrical foot switches from fluid damage. Instrumentation for vitrectomy is shown in Fig. 18-67.

Operative procedures

Anterior vitrectomy for accidental vitreous loss (Fig. 18-68)

1. A vitreous cutter is placed in the eye through the cataract wound. This can be either a multifunction hand-

piece, such as the AVIT handpiece (Fig. 18-69), or the Kaufman II Vitrector (Fig. 18-62), which has only suction and cutting functions. Infusion is not needed for this procedure.

2. The cutter is placed in the middle of the pupil, posterior to the iris, and enough vitreous is removed to ensure

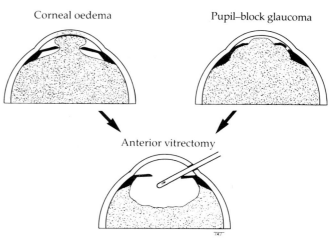

Fig. 18-68. Diagram of anterior vitrectomy procedure for complications of vitreous in anterior chamber. (From Kanski, J.J.: Clinical ophthalmology, London, 1984, Butterworth & Co.)

that no vitreous remains in the anterior chamber and that the iris has fallen back into normal position.

3. The pupil is constricted with acetylcholine. The anterior chamber may be filled with air.
4. The procedure is completed as for lens extraction.

Anterior vitrectomy (Fig. 18-68)

1. Appropriate fixation sutures or a lid speculum is placed.
2. An incision is made at the limbus either through clear cornea or under a conjunctival flap. One to three incisions are made, depending on the vitreous cutter chosen and the technique.
3. If a multifunction probe is not used, an infusion cannula is placed in one incision and the vitreous cutter in another. A third incision may be used for an accessory instrument. The vitreous is removed.
4. The incisions are closed.
5. The eye is patched.

Pars plana vitrectomy (Fig. 18-69)

1. A lid speculum and appropriate fixation sutures are placed.
2. Three incisions are made through the pars plana; one for infusion, one for endoillumination, and one for a vitreous cutter.
3. The infusion line is sutured in place with a purse-string suture of no. 5-0 Dacron. The line is checked to ensure proper placement.
4. The operating microscope is aligned, and a fundus lens is fixed on the anterior surface of the cornea.
5. The infusion rate, cutting rate, and aspiration rate are set on the machine console. The vitreous is removed under direct visualization.
6. Once the medium has been removed and the retinal condition visualized, the necessary treatment is completed with vitrectomy instruments or accessories, or a scleral buckling procedure may be performed.
7. The pars plana incisions are closed, and the conjunc-

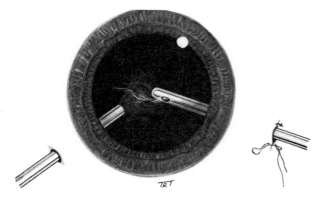

Fig. 18-69. Introduction of cutter and fiberoptic light pipe through pars plana for posterior vitrectomy. (From Kanski, J.J.: Clinical ophthalmology, London, 1984, Butterworth & Co.)

tival incision is sutured. Cultures from the vitreous washings are taken, if necessary.

8. Subconjunctival injections of steroids or antibiotics are given if necessary, the eye is patched, and an eye shield is secured in place.

Laser photocoagulation and cryotherapy treatments

In addition to the intraocular photocoagulation with argon laser or cryocoagulation used during vitrectomy procedures, argon laser photocoagulation can be delivered through a slit lamp to the retina as a noninvasive, outpatient procedure. Argon laser photocoagulation is used to treat flat retinal holes or tears, sites of potential pathologic conditions, and vascular proliferative diseases, such as diabetic retinopathy.

Laser treatment
Operative procedure

1. The patient's pupil is dilated, and a retrobulbar anesthetic may be used.
2. Proparacaine drops are instilled into the operative eye.
3. A three-mirror Goldmann lens is placed on the cornea, and the patient is positioned at the laser slit lamp.
4. The proper spot size, power setting, and duration of exposure are set.
5. Laser burns are placed in the prescribed areas.
6. The patient's eye is irrigated with physiologic saline solution to remove the viscous lens lubricant.
7. The eye is patched as necessary.

An Nd:YAG laser is also used for lysis of vitreous strands or bands and to open opaque posterior capsules. The procedure is similar to argon laser treatment in its delivery through a slit lamp. A Peyman lens for a specific depth is selected and used in place of the Goldmann lens when cutting vitreous strands. No lens or anesthetic is needed to open posterior capsules. The patient is positioned at the laser slit lamp, and pulsed laser applications using 1 to 3 millijoules of power are used to open the posterior capsule.

Cryocoagulation

Cryocoagulation through the conjunctiva may be used to treat some pathologic conditions of the retina when a more invasive procedure is unnecessary or the area is not accessible with laser.

Operative procedure

1. The operative eye is anesthetized with local anesthetic injections and topical drops.
2. A lid speculum is placed in the operative eye.
3. The globe is positioned with a fixation forceps, and the pathologic area is localized with the indirect ophthalmoscope.
4. The retinal cryoprobe is applied to the external surface

of the globe in the area of the pathologic condition, and the area is treated.

5. The eye is patched.

Operating microscope

During the past 10 years there has been a dramatic increase in the number of microsurgical procedures in various surgical disciplines. Although the operating microscope is employed in many types of surgical procedures, its major use is in ophthalmology. Because of the demand for use of the operating microscope and its special adaptations, nurses must understand the basic principles of operation and care of this important piece of surgical equipment.

Basic principles

To facilitate understanding of the functions of the operating microscope, a few basic optical principles are defined and explained. A microscope is a monocular or binocular instrument with a close-up lens for magnification. Binoculars are two telescopes mounted side by side that give stereoscopic vision. The length of the binoculars is condensed by the use of prisms.

Magnification is the process by which the apparent size of an image is increased. Magnification of an image is increased by moving the object closer to the eye or by using optical aids such as telescopes, binoculars, or microscopes that increase image size on the retina without reducing the eye-to-object distance. The amount of image increase becomes the *magnification value* of the optical aid.

Illumination is the source of light used to view an object. The microscope illuminator is the light source used to throw light downward to illuminate the surgical area. The most common type of microscope illumination used today is *coaxial illumination*. Light from the illuminator bulb is routed near the viewing axis of the microscope and projected down through the objective lens (Fig. 18-70). Coaxial illumination can be transferred through a fiberoptic cable or from an incandescent bulb housed near the objective lens of the microscope. This type of shadow-free illumination provides a bright circular spot that is uniformly illuminated even in deep and narrow wounds. Fiberoptic illumination increases the diameter of the illuminated field and the light intensity.

Principal parts of the microscope are the eyepieces, binocular tubes, magnification changer, objective lens, illumination cord, beam splitter, and X-Y coupling (Fig. 18-71).

The *eyepieces* or *oculars* are the lenses through which a surgeon views the microsurgical field. Eyepieces are interchangeable and are available in four magnifying

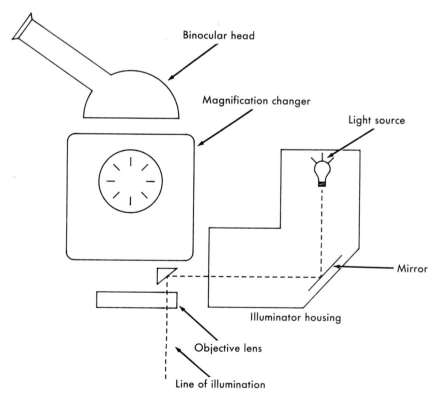

Fig. 18-70. Illumination system of operating microscope. Light from illuminator bulb is routed near viewing axis of microscope and projected down through objective lens.

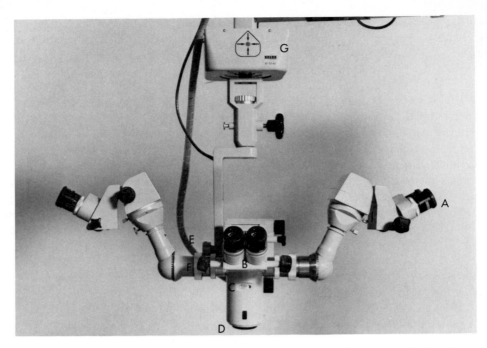

Fig. 18-71. Operating microscope. *A,* Oculars or eyepieces; *B,* binocular tubes; *C,* magnification changer; *D,* objective lens; *E,* illumination cord; *F,* beam splitter; *G,* X-Y coupling.

powers: 10×, 12.5×, 16×, and 20×. The working distance and the size of the surgical field determine the powers of the objective and the ocular lens, respectively. The objective lens is the lens attached to the bottom of the microscope, and the working distance is the distance between the objective lens and the operative field. For instance, in a procedure with long working distances and small surgical fields, a 20× ocular lens and a 300-mm objective lens might be used. This combination is commonly employed in neurosurgery. A procedure with shorter working distance and needing less magnification for a relatively large surgical field, such as an ophthalmic procedure, might require a 12.5× ocular lens and a 150- or 175-mm objective lens.

To focus the microscope, the user sets the spherical diopter adjustment on the oculars to correspond to his or her individual eyeglass correction and works without eyeglasses. The oculars can be adjusted to accommodate corrections of −9 to +9 diopters. Users who have astigmatism should wear their eyeglasses and set the oculars at zero.

The oculars or eyepieces fit into *binocular tubes* containing prisms that reduce the focal length of the microscope. The binocular tubes permit the distance between the eyepieces to be adjusted to fit the pupillary distance of the user (the distance between the pupils of the user's eyes), ensuring stereoscopic vision.

The *magnification changer* allows change in the mag-

nification of a basic optical system. Two types of changers used on microscopes are the revolving telescope type, in which miniature telescopes of differing powers are rotated into position via knobs on the microscope body, and the zoom type, which is a motorized system of shifting lens elements to vary magnification, operated with a hand switch or foot control.

The magnification changer is a part of the *microscope body,* which is attached to a support that allows the instrument to be tilted. The lower end of the microscope body has a threaded mount for the *objective lens.* The diopter power of the objective lens determines the focal length and therefore the working distance of the microscope.

On the upper portion of the microscope body is a dovetail receptacle for attaching accessories. A *beam splitter* fits into the receptacle, permitting the attachment of binocular and monocular observation tubes and documentation accessories such as cameras and video equipment. A beam splitter has two-way mirrors or prisms that divert or split the optical image in several directions. This allows for attachment of binocular observation tubes, necessary for surgical assistants, and cameras or video equipment. With use of a beam splitter at least 50% of available light is diverted away from the surgeon's oculars. However, the human eye is usually versatile enough to adjust to lower light levels. Adequate lighting is essential for photographic systems, which may in some instances require a beam splitter that diverts as much as 70% of the available light. The *X-Y coupling* enables the operator to move the microscope head diagonally and accurately over the operative field. The choice of microscope accessories varies according to requirements of the procedure and the surgeon's preferences.

Many methods of mounting the operating microscope are used, including manually operated floor stands, motorized floor stands, and ceiling- or wall-mounted suspension systems with either manual or electromechanical height adjustment.

Care and maintenance

Proper care and maintenance of the operating microscope are essential to ensure optimal function and durability of this sophisticated, expensive piece of equipment.

Procedures include (1) inspection and cleaning of all external lens surfaces before use; (2) checking all power controls including illumination intensity, magnification changer, focus, and X-Y coupling to ensure proper functioning before use; (3) checking the needed accessories such as objective lens and power, beam splitter, cameras, observer tubes, and filters; and (4) cleaning and covering after use.

Care of optics

Before and after each procedure, all external lens surfaces should be cleaned and inspected. Internal surfaces are checked for cleanliness and damage. Scratched or damaged optical systems must be repaired or replaced.

The following procedure is used for cleaning lens surfaces:

1. Loose particles (lint or dust) are removed with a soft, clean brush used to clean camera lenses or with a rubber bulb (ear syringe). When a bulb syringe is used, the bulb is held about 1 cm from the surface and squeezed briskly, directing the air toward the lens surface.
2. Blood, water, and irrigating solutions are removed with a cotton-tipped applicator or cotton ball moistened with distilled water. A circular motion is used, beginning at the center of the optic and working toward the outer edge (lens paper may also be used). The surface is dried with a cotton-tipped applicator or cotton ball in the same manner.
3. Oil or fingerprints are removed with a cleaning solvent of commercially prepared lens cleaning solution or with 50% denatured alcohol. The lens is wiped with a lightly moistened cotton-tipped applicator or cotton ball in a circular motion. The process is repeated until the surface is clean and free of streaks.

Solvents should be used sparingly. Excessive fluid may destroy the cemented surfaces of the lens.

Cleaning

The external surfaces of the microscope should be cleansed after use and before storage. The cleaning procedures are as follows:

1. The external surfaces are washed with a clean, damp cloth moistened with a mild soap or disinfecting solution.
2. The surfaces are wiped dry with a lint-free cloth.
3. The function of each moving part is inspected during the cleaning process. The coupling joints can be greased with petrolatum jelly if necessary. The lamp cables should be free of kinks. A new bulb should be used for each procedure expected to be over 4 hours in duration. Fiberoptic cables should not be bent or kinked. Tips of the fiberoptic cables are cleaned with cotton-tipped applicators.
4. The carriage is moved to its lowest position. The locks on the arm are loosened, and the ocular systems are moved toward the base.
5. Dust caps are placed over the eyepieces, and a dust cover over the microscope head. The microscope is ready for storage.

Proper care and preventive maintenance add years of service to an operating microscope. Checking the microscope before use and being knowledgeable about proper function of the microscope and its accessories are responsibilities of the perioperative nurse.

REFERENCE

Silverstone, D.E., Hufnagle, T., and Miller, J.M.: Effect of carbochol and acetylcholine on the corneal endothelium and IOP in cataract surgery, Free paper presented at the American Academy of Ophthalmology, New Orleans, 1989.

BIBLIOGRAPHY

Atkinson, L.J., and Kohn, M.L.: Berry and Kohn's introduction to operating room technique, ed. 6, New York, 1986, McGraw-Hill Book Co.

Barnhart, E.R.: Physicians' desk reference for ophthalmology, ed. 14, Oradell, N.J., 1986, Medical Economics Company.

Boyd-Monk, H.: Surgical intervention to stop glaucoma, J. Ophthalmic Nurs. Technol. 4:12, 1985.

Boyd-Monk, H.: Symposia on ophthalmic nursing, Nurs. Clin. North Am. *16*:3, 1981.

Boyd-Monk, H., and Steinmetz, C.: Nursing care of the eye. Norwalk, Conn., 1987, Appleton & Lange.

Butler, M., and Thomson, E.: Care of the eye patient, Proceedings from World Conference of Operating Room Nurses III, Denver, 1983, Association of Operating Room Nurses.

Care and handling of surgical instruments, Randolph, Mass., 1981, Codman & Shurtleff, Inc.

Crawford, F.: Ambulatory surgery: the elderly patient, AORN J. 41:356, 1985.

Dobbie, J.G.: What's new in surgery: ophthalmic surgery, Am. Coll. Surg. Bull. 71:22, 1986.

Easterlin, M., and Schneider, H.: Calculating intraocular lens power, J. Ophthalmic Nurs. Technol. 4:6, 1985.

Gaston, N.C.: Keratorefractive surgery: new horizons, AORN J. 33:1068, 1981.

Hahn, A.B., Barkin, R.L. and Oestreich, S.J.K.: Pharmacology in nursing, ed. 15, St. Louis, 1982, The C.V. Mosby Co.

Hamrick, S., and Meredith, L.L.: Therapeutic ultrasound: a precise non-invasive therapy for glaucoma, AORN J. 47:10, 1988.

Haper, M.: Training manual for surgical microscopes, St. Louis, 1981, Storz Instrument Co.

Hoerenz, P.: The operating microscope, IV., J. Microsurg. 1:364, 2:22, 1980: 2:179, 1981.

Holden, J.: Don't just tell your patients—teach them, RN 48:29, July 1985.

Hollwich, F.: Ophthalmology, ed. 2, New York, 1985, Thieme-Stratton.

Hollwich, F.: Pocket atlas of ophthalmology, ed. 2, New York, 1986, Thieme-Stratton.

Hursey, L.C.T.: Intraocular lens implant: a clear way to correct cloudy vision, AORN J. 39:880, 1984.

Jennings, B.: The Nd:YAG: a knife without a blade, J. Ophthalmic Nurs. Technol. 4:16, 1985.

Kanski, J.: Clinical ophthalmology, London, 1984, Butterworth & Co.

King, J., and Wadsworth, J.: An atlas of ophthalmic surgery, ed. 3, Philadelphia, 1981, J.B. Lippincott Co.

Kunkel, J.: Teaching: getting your message through, Nurs. Life 1:36, 1981.

Lambrix, K.K.: Epikeratophakia, AORN J. 46:2, 1987.

Langseth, F.: Transscleral cyclophotocoagulation: a laser treatment for glaucoma. AORN J. 48:6, 1988.

Luckmann, J., and Sorensen, K.C.: Medical-surgical nursing: a psychophysiologic approach, ed. 3, Philadelphia, 1987, W.B. Saunders Co.

McClurg, E.: Developing an effective patient teaching program, AORN J. 34:474, 1981.

MacFadyen, J.S.: Caring for the patient with a primary retinal detachment, Am. J. Nurs. 80:920, 1980.

Mackety, C.: Posterior capsulotomy with the Nd:YAG laser, J. Ophthalmic Nurs. Technol. 4:16, 1985.

Moore, C.: Scleral buckling for retinal detachment, AORN J. 36:495, 1982.

Murray-Lipshutz, C.: Good nursing care wards off disaster, J. Ophthalmic Nurs. Technol. 4:16, 1985.

Nelson, L.B.: Pediatric ophthalmology, Philadelphia, 1984, W.B. Saunders Co.

Nimmo, M., and Sturgis, M.: A comprehensive look at the operating microscope, Periop. Nurs. Q. 1:1, 1985.

Perrin, E.D.: Laser therapy for diabetic retinopathy, Am. J. Nurs. 80:664, 1980.

Powell, K.: Radial keratotomy: a continuing controversy, J. Ophthalmic Nurs. Technol. 4:6, 1985.

Redman, B.: The process of patient education, ed. 5, St. Louis, 1984, The C.V. Mosby Co.

Saunders, W.H., and others: Nursing care in eye, ear, nose, and throat disorders, ed. 4, St. Louis, 1979, The C.V. Mosby Co.

Schneeman, Y.T., and Taylor, J.A.: A technical look at vitrectomy, AORN J. 33:876, 1981.

Schrader, E.S.: Surgeons summarize progress, AORN J. 33:73, 1981.

Schremp, P.: Discharge instructions: providing continuing care for ophthalmic patients, J. Ophthalmic Nurs. Technol. 4:30, 1985.

Smith, J.F., and Nachazel, D.P., Jr.: Ophthalmologic nursing, Boston, 1980, Little, Brown & Co.

Spadoni, D., and Cain, C.L.: Laser blepharoplasty: The transconjunctival method, AORN J. 47:11, 1988.

Smith, S.: Standards of ophthalmic nursing practice. San Francisco, 1985, American Society of Ophthalmic R.N.'s (ASORN) in conjunction with American Academy of Ophthalmology.

Stein, H., and Slatt, B.: The ophthalmic assistant: fundamentals and clinical practice, ed. 4, St. Louis, 1983, The C.V. Mosby Co.

Taylor, J.: Are you missing what your patients can teach you? RN 47:63, June 1984.

Thomson-Keith, E.: Care of the ophthalmology patient. Denver, 1986, The Association of Operating Room Nurses, Inc.

Tumulty, G., and Resler, M.: Managing glaucoma using argon laser therapy, J. Ophthalmic Nurs. Technol. 4:9, 1985.

Vaughan, D., and Asbury, T.: General ophthalmology, ed. 10, Los Altos, Calif., 1983, Lange Medical Publications.

Waring, G.: Shaping the eye for better vision: refractive corneal surgery, Journal for Blindness Prevention Professionals and Volunteers 53:20, 1984.

Wong, E.K., Wang, S., and Leopold, I.H.: How ophthalmic drugs can fool you, RN 43:36, Mar. 1980.

19 Otologic surgery

MYRNA GRAVES

New concepts and procedures related to otologic surgery are being introduced, and older procedures are constantly being refined. Antibiotics, the operating microscope, delicate instruments, improvements in implantable prosthetic devices, and better understanding of the anatomy and physiology of the ear enable the otologic surgeon to perform procedures that improve patients' hearing and to have greater control over diseases of the middle ear and mastoid. Surgical treatment for sensorineural hearing loss, or Ménière's disease, can be offered to patients who are afflicted by intolerable tinnitus or vertigo severe enough to be disabling. Surgical treatment aimed at correcting hearing losses resulting from conduction apparatus abnormalities includes stapedectomy and ossicular replacement procedures. New hope for deaf patients has been found in the area of cochlear implantation. Technologic advancements have contributed significantly to improved outcomes for patients with otologic problems.

The Latin word *audire* means to hear; thus, the word *auditory* refers to the sense of hearing. The physical nature of sound results from the compression and rarefaction of pressure waves and moving molecules, but the sensations humans actually experience are the product of complex mechanical, electrical, and psychologic interactions in the ear and central nervous system. The study of the ear and its diseases is known as *otology*, derived from the Greek word *otos*, meaning ear.

The ear is a complex mechanism that receives sound waves, discriminates their frequencies, and then transmits this information to the central nervous system for interpretation. When a person falls asleep, hearing is the last sense to disappear; when a person awakens, it is the first sense to return. An additional function of the human ear is the maintenance of body equilibrium.

In order for a person to hear:

1. The sound waves collect in the auricle.
2. The waves pass into the external canal and cause the eardrum to vibrate.
3. The ossicles, arranged in a lever system, respond to the vibration and thus amplify the sound. First the malleus moves, and then this movement is transmitted to the incus, which in turn transmits it to the stapes.
4. The small footplate of the stapes delivers the sound to the inner ear by rocking the oval window.
5. Sound pressure, delivered through the oval window into the cochlea, agitates the perilymph and endolymph.
6. Relief of pressure is provided by shielding of the round window from sound.
7. The receptors of hearing (hair cells) are distorted, causing the mechanical waves to be transformed into electrochemical impulses.
8. These impulses are sent by way of the acoustic nerve to the brainstem (pons) and then are relayed to the temporal cortex of the brain, where they are interpreted as meaningful sound.

The amplitude of the air waves that strike the tympanic membrane determines the loudness or intensity of the sound. In dealing with hearing loss, the loudness is measured in decibels (dB). It is a logarithmic method of dealing with large numbers; the decibel is a ratio, not an absolute value, that compares the relationship between two sound intensities and the smallest perceptible change in loudness that the human ear can hear. Hearing loss is expressed by recording auditory acuity for each frequency in decibels.

SURGICAL ANATOMY

The ear is comprised of three distinct divisions: the external ear, the middle ear, and the inner ear (Fig. 19-1). The middle and inner ear structures are situated within the temporal bone, which forms a part of the skull base.

External ear

The external ear consists of an *auricle*, or *pinna*, and an external *auditory canal* (Fig. 19-2) that ends at the *tympanic membrane*, or eardrums. In humans the auricle is motionless and has little function in collecting sound. It is covered with skin and consists of an elastic cartilaginous plate and minimal subcutaneous tissue. The unique form is a result of various elevations and depressions in the cartilaginous framework.

The external ear has an abundant blood and lymphatic supply. The nerve supply to the external ear is derived primarily from the auriculotemporal branch of the trigeminal nerve (fifth cranial nerve) and from the cervical

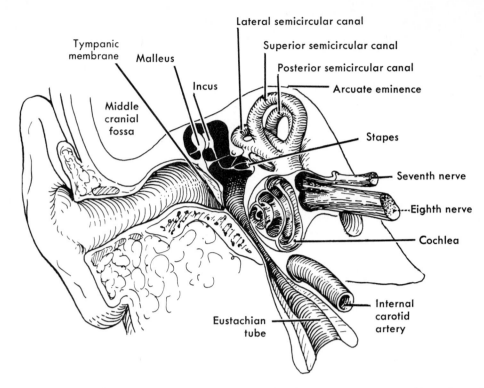

Fig. 19-1. Schematic drawing of external ear, middle ear, and inner ear. It is not possible to show all structures in a single plane; therefore, there are distortions from actual anatomy in this schema. (Modified from DeWeese, D.D., and Saunders, W.H.: Textbook of otolaryngology, ed. 3, St. Louis, 1968, The C.V. Mosby Co.)

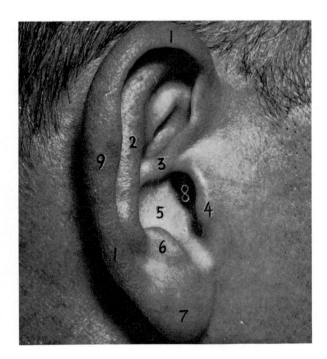

Fig. 19-2. Auricle. *1*, Helix; *2*, antihelix; *3*, crus of helix; *4*, tragus; *5*, concha; *6*, antitragus; *7*, lobule; *8*, external auditory meatus; *9*, Darwin's tubercle. (From DeWeese, D.D., and Saunders, W.H.: Textbook of otolaryngology, ed. 6, St. Louis, 1982, The C.V. Mosby Co.)

nerves, C1 and C2. A branch of the vagus nerve (tenth cranial nerve) enters the posterior part of the ear canal and, together with the trigeminal nerve, supplies sensation to the ear canal.

The external auditory canal collects sound waves and serves as a protector and a pressure amplifier. This canal is a twisting passageway about one-half inch long, directed inward and forward, lying between the concha and the tympanic membrane. It terminates medially at the sulcus (depression) of the tympanic membrane. The walls of the outer third of the canal are fibrocartilaginous, and those of the inner two thirds are bony. The physician inspects the eardrum in adults by drawing the auricle upward and backward and in children by drawing the auricle downward and backward. This straightens the cartilaginous portion of the canal to improve visibility. Lying within the cartilaginous portion of the external canal are fine hairs, sebaceous glands, and special glands that produce cerumen. The skin overlying the bony canal lacks these dermal appendages. The tympanic membrane, or eardrum, stretches across the deepest part of the ear canal and serves as a partition between the external canal and the tympanic cavity (Fig. 19-1).

Tympanic membrane

The *tympanic membrane* is composed of three layers: the external layer, which is continuous with the epidermal

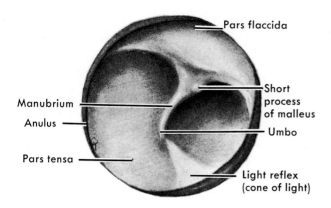

Fig. 19-3. Landmarks of right tympanic membrane. Size of pars flaccida is exaggerated in this drawing. (From DeWeese, D.D., and Saunders, W.H.: Textbook of otolaryngology, ed. 6, St. Louis, 1982, The C.V. Mosby Co.)

lining of the canal; the middle fibrous layer; and the inner layer, which is a continuation of the mucous membrane of the middle ear. The small upper portion of the tympanic membrane, known as the *pars flaccida,* is devoid of the fibrous layer (Fig. 19-3). The larger, vibrating part of the tympanic membrane, which has a fibrous layer, is called the *pars tensa* (Fig. 19-3). At the edge of the tympanic membrane, the thickened fibrous layer forms a thickened incomplete band called the *anulus,* which anchors the eardrum to the end of the external canal.

Middle ear

The middle ear is a narrow, irregular, air-containing cavity in the tympanic portion of the temporal bone behind the eardrum. In this oblong air-filled space are three small bones or ossicles—the malleus, incus, and stapes (Figs. 19-1 and 19-4)—as well as the facial nerve, which controls movements of the face. The *chorda tympani nerve,* a branch of the facial nerve that provides taste from the anterior two thirds of the tongue (Fig. 19-5) is also included in this space. Sensation inside the middle ear is provided by the *glossopharyngeal nerve.* The temporal lobe of the brain and its meninges are separated from the middle ear and mastoid by a thin plate of bone, the *tegmen tympani.* The tympanic cavity communicates anteriorly, via the eustachian tube, with the nasopharynx and posteriorly, via the aditus, with the mastoid air cells. The middle ear is lined with mucous membrane, which extends into the mastoid and down the eustachian tube (Fig. 19-1). The inner ear forms the medial wall of the tympanic cavity. The promontory on the medial wall marks the first turn of the cochlea in the internal ear (Fig. 19-6). Above and slightly behind the promontory is an opening, called the *oval window* (Fig. 19-5), to which the stapes is connected. Below the promontory, covered by mucous membrane, is the round window of the cochlea.

The ossicles in the middle ear cavity form a chain that conducts vibrations from the eardrum across the middle ear into the oval window, the opening in the inner ear. The *malleus,* resembling a hammer, consists of a head, neck, handle, and short process (Fig. 19-4). The handle and short process of the malleus are attached to the undersurface of the eardrum and join the eardrum to the second bone in series, the *incus.* The incus, which resembles an anvil, consists of a body and long and short processes (Fig. 19-4). The long crus of the incus is in contact

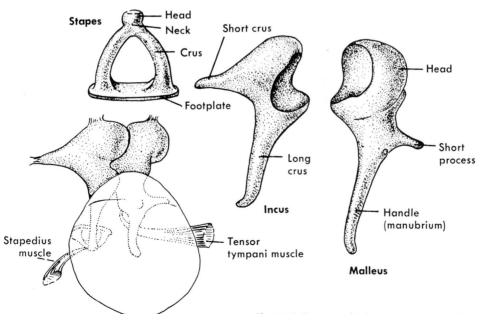

Fig. 19-4. Drawing of right ear showing articulated ossicles of middle ear. (From DeWeese, D.D., and Saunders, W.H.: Textbook of otolaryngology, ed. 6, St. Louis, 1982, The C.V. Mosby Co.)

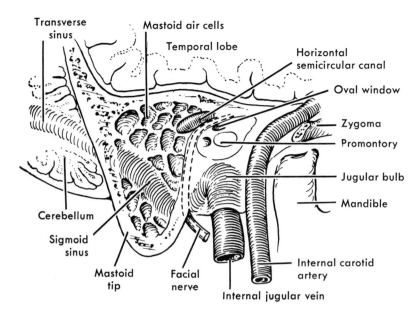

Fig. 19-5. Composite drawing of right ear showing relationship between middle ear, mastoid, and surrounding structures. (From DeWeese, D.D., and Saunders, W.H.: Textbook of otolaryngology, ed. 6, St. Louis, 1982, The C.V. Mosby Co.)

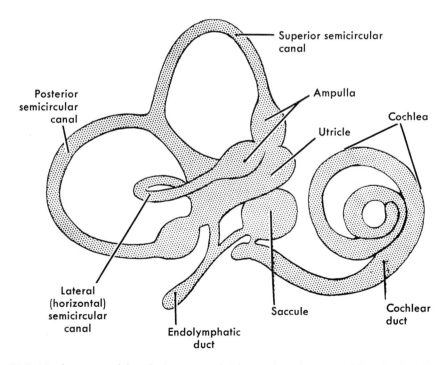

Fig. 19-6. Membranous endolymphatic system of right ear, lateral view. Endolymph of cochlea and labyrinth is continuous. Bony capsule of internal ear surrounds endolymphatic system and is separated from it by perilymphatic space. (From DeWeese, D.D., and Saunders, W.H.: Textbook of otolaryngology, ed. 3, St. Louis, 1968, The C.V. Mosby Co.)

with the third and innermost bone, the *stapes*. Resembling a stirrup, the stapes consists of a head, neck, anterior and posterior crura, and footplate that fits into the oval window (Fig. 19-4). The tensor tympani and stapedius muscles attach to the ossicles. The tensor tympani muscle acts to draw the drum inward to increase tension of the drum, whereas the stapedius muscle acts to draw the stapes away from the oval window to dampen intense and potentially damaging vibrations passing through the ossicles into the inner ear. The middle ear and mastoid are supplied with blood from the branches of the internal and external carotid artery systems (Fig. 19-5). The stylomastoid, tympanic, petrosal, and caroticotympanic arteries form numerous anastomoses with one another.

Inner ear

The inner ear is a complex structure located in the petrous or rocklike portion of the temporal bone. It has two distinct parts, each with specific functions that are delicately coordinated. One partition, the cochlea, is concerned with the special sense of hearing, and the other, the vestibular labyrinth, with the maintenance of equilibrium. The two major parts of the inner ear, the cochlea and the vestibular labyrinth, have various compartments.

The bony cochlea and vestibular labyrinth lie in the petrous portion of the temporal bone. In the small channels of these two structures are two distinct fluids: the perilymph and endolymph. The *perilymph*, lying in the bony canals, surrounds the membranous inner ear and thus serves as a protective cushion to the end organ receptors for hearing. The perilymph is continuous with the subarachnoid space and its cerebrospinal fluid through the aqueduct of the cochlea (cochlear duct). The *endolymph*, which is contained in a fragile membranous tube, bathes and nourishes the sensory cells and their supporting structures. The endolymph in the cochlea and labyrinth is contained in a continuous closed array of membranes, sacs, and channels referred to as the *endolymphatic system* (Fig. 19-6).

Cochlea

The *cochlea* has a tubular configuration that winds as a spiral around the modiolus or central part. Within the cochlea are three compartments (Fig. 19-7): the scala vestibuli, which is associated with the oval window; the scala tympani, which is associated with the round window; and the cochlear duct. The scala vestibuli and scala tympani are filled with perilymph, whereas the cochlear duct contains endolymph.

On the vestibular surface of the basilar membrane of the cochlea is the delicate neural end organ for hearing, the *organ of Corti*. From its neuroepithelium project thousands of fragile *hair cells* that are set in motion by vibrations passing from the ossicles to the perilymph via the oval window. The organ of Corti extends along the entire

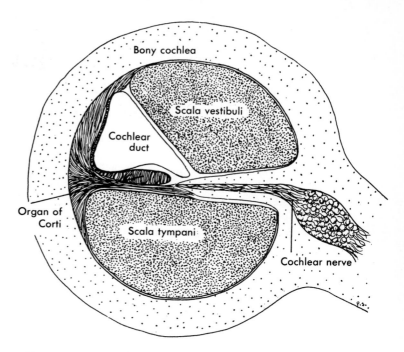

Fig. 19-7. Diagram of cross-section of cochlea. (From DeWeese, D.D., and Saunders, W.H.: Textbook of otolaryngology, ed. 3, St. Louis, 1968, The C.V. Mosby Co.)

length of the cochlea, except at the apex of the modiolus, where the scala tympani and the scala vestibuli join.

The cochlea converts the mechanical energy of wave movement from vibrations in the perilymph into electrochemical impulses by means of the hair cells of the organ of Corti.

The inner ear is connected with the brain through the acoustic nerve, which enters the temporal cortex of the cerebrum, where the impulses are then interpreted as meaningful sound. This connecting fiber system is located on both sides of the brain.

Vestibular labyrinth

The *vestibular labyrinth* of the inner ear is composed of the utricle, saccule, and three semicircular canals known as the lateral, superior, and posterior canals (Fig. 19-6). In each ear the canals are arranged at right angles to one another so that any movement of the head excites at least one of the semicircular canals. Each canal is enlarged at a point near the utricle. In this enlargement, called the *ampulla* of the canal, resides the specialized neuroepithelium to detect movement in the endolymph within the semicircular canal (Fig. 19-6).

The maculae of the utricle and saccule of the vestibular labyrinth are gravity oriented and concerned with static equilibrium. The neural fibers from the maculae and ampullae of the semicircular canals join to form the vestibular portion of the eighth cranial nerve.

The blood supply of the internal ear is derived from the

internal auditory branches of the basilar artery. The internal auditory artery enters the internal meatus and divides into the cochlea and vestibular labyrinthine branches. The veins from the cochlea and labyrinth exit the temporal bone with the vestibular and cochlear aqueducts and empty into the sigmoid sinus and jugular bulb.

Temporal bone

The temporal bone is composed of five separate parts, which are joined by suture lines. Only the tympanic and petrous portions contain structures directly related to hearing. The *squamous* portion is a large piece of bone that is frequently pneumatized. On its external surface is a groove for the middle temporal artery; on its internal surface are grooves for the middle meningeal vessels.

The *mastoid* portion of the temporal bone lies behind the osseous canal below the squamous portion. The sternocleidomastoid and digastric muscles attach to the mastoid tip. The cortex of the mastoid covers a system of intercommunicating air cells. The mastoid antrum is the largest of these air-containing cavities and connects directly with the middle ear through the aditus. The air cells are lined with a thin mucous membrane that is continuous with the mucous membrane of the middle ear.

The *petrous* portion of the temporal bone fuses with the base of the skull and contains the structures of the inner ear, including the sensory end organs of hearing and equilibrium. In the petrous portion are openings for the trigeminal ganglion and the facial and cochleovestibular nerves.

The *zygomatic* portion of the temporal bone extends anteriorly and joins the zygoma or malar bone of the cheek.

The *tympanic* portion of the temporal bone contains the middle ear and forms part of the ear canal.

PERIOPERATIVE NURSING CONSIDERATIONS
Assessment/nursing diagnosis

The preoperative assessment of the patient undergoing otologic surgery should include all elements of an assessment done for any other type of surgery: chart review, conferring with appropriate unit personnel responsible for the care of the patient, and, of prime importance, the patient interview. Chart review should include close attention to blood pressure and patient allergies, especially if drug related, because some otologic procedures are performed under local anesthesia. Any antibiotic sensitivities should also be carefully noted. Physical limitations such as arthritis and back or neck problems should be identified to provide for optimum patient comfort during the surgical procedure. The perioperative nurse should be able to answer patient questions related to the procedure in a clear and concise manner. All information gained should be documented to facilitate care of the patient intraoperatively and postoperatively. Some assessment factors to be considered include: history of ear disorders, trauma, or surgery; position, size, and symmetry of the ear; skin color, texture, and lesions; patient's age and communication status; use of hearing aid; level of comprehension and adaptive responses (for example, signing, lip reading, gestures); speech pattern; environmental factors; patient's willingness to cooperate with treatment; and coping mechanisms used by patient.

Examples of nursing diagnoses that pertain to many patients having otologic surgery include:

- Sensory/perceptual alteration (auditory)
- Anxiety related to surgical procedure
- Powerlessness due to hearing deficit
- Potential for injury, related to sensory deficit

Planning

Plans for patient teaching should be implemented preoperatively and should include the following:

1. The patient should be advised that the ear canal should be kept dry for 10 days to 2 weeks after surgery. The patient should also be told that some hair may be shaved from around the ear, depending upon the procedure. This may cause some concern for black patients, whose hair regrowth may be slow.
2. The patient should be cautioned not to lie on the operated ear for the first 24 hours after surgery. The head of the bed should be elevated during this period.
3. The patient should be told that vertigo may occur for a day or so after surgery and that in that case the patient should obtain assistance to get out of bed. Moving slowly and smoothly may alleviate these unpleasant sensations. If the symptoms persist or are severe, antimotion drugs may be necessary.
4. The patient should be cautioned against deep coughing or nose blowing. If sneezing is unavoidable, both the nose and the mouth should be kept open. These points are important and should be reinforced; strict adherence may prevent dislodgment of a graft or prosthesis.
5. The patient should be made aware that hearing may be diminished during the immediate postoperative period. The nurse should emphasize that this condition is temporary and that the hearing will improve gradually.
6. The patient should be reminded not to swim or dive during the first several months after surgery. In addition, the patient should be cautioned not to drive during the first postoperative week. Air travel is also not advised during the first postoperative week; after that, it may be allowed only in a commercial airliner or other airplane with a pressurized cabin.
7. If an upper respiratory infection or any other change in physical status occurs, the patient should consult the physician immediately.

8. Other special preoperative instructions may be needed, depending on the patient's physical status or the surgeon's requests. The surgeon usually discusses these points with the patient when the decision for surgery is made. Nursing personnel can explain the principles to the patient and clarify any questions that the patient may have.

A smooth intraoperative phase depends on effective planning to meet the patient's care needs based on a thorough preoperative assessment of the patient and proper application of information gained from the assessment process. A well-defined plan enables the circulating nurse to provide appropriate care for the awake patient as soon as the patient enters the operating room. Necessary equipment, such as a cardiac monitor, pulse oximeter, blood pressure apparatus, oxygen setup, suction equipment, and emergency drugs, should be available for use by the nurse monitoring the patient during surgery.

The Sample Care Plan shows a generic care plan addressing the needs of the patient undergoing otologic surgery.

Sample Care Plan

NURSING DIAGNOSIS:
Sensory/perceptual alteration (auditory)
GOAL:
Patient will demonstrate improved self-expression and decreased frustration with communication.
INTERVENTIONS:
Identify a method by which patient can communicate basic needs.
Promote continuity of care to reduce frustration.
Identify factors that promote communication.
Allow patient to wear hearing aid to the OR.
Speak slowly and deliberately into the dominant ear.

NURSING DIAGNOSIS:
Anxiety related to surgical procedure
GOAL:
Patient will demonstrate reduced anxiety and effective coping mechanisms.
INTERVENTIONS:
Explain all activities performed by the nursing staff and provide additional explanations as necessary.
Assure patient that he or she will be informed before any procedure is performed.
Provide time for patient to express fears and concerns.
Provide emotional support and frequent patient contact (for example, touch).
Maintain quiet environment and minimize stimuli.
Assess patient's coping mechanisms; assist patient to initiate them.

NURSING DIAGNOSIS:
Powerlessness due to hearing deficit
GOAL:
Patient will be able to identify factors that can be controlled by her or him, family, nursing staff, or surgical team.
INTERVENTIONS:
Increase effective communication between patient and health care personnel regarding the surgical intervention.
Allow patient to assume position of comfort.
Offer emotional support.
Ensure privacy.
Provide patient and family opportunities to express their feelings.
Provide and reinforce information given to patient.
Keep needed items within reach during postoperative period.

NURSING DIAGNOSIS:
Injury, potential for, related to sensory deficit
GOAL:
Patient will be free from injury at completion of perioperative experience.
INTERVENTIONS:
Speak clearly and deliberately to patient and confirm that patient has heard and understood communications.
Provide adequate assistance during movement onto OR bed and positioning.
Complete all transfer and positioning maneuvers slowly.
Identify physical limitations and position or support patient accordingly to provide optimal comfort during the procedure.

Implementation

Depending on the departmental policy related to care of patients receiving local anesthesia, an intravenous infusion may be started to supply the patient with fluids during surgery and provide a pathway for additional medications. Drug allergies can be handled more effectively intraoperatively if known before the day of surgery. Appropriate alternative drugs should be available in accordance with the surgeon's preference.

The surgeon may begin the local anesthetic administration in the preoperative holding area or in the operating room proper before surgical preparation. With this in mind, the circulating nurse must assist in starting the procedure as efficiently as possible and at the same time observe the patient for signs of any reaction to the local anesthetic, such as restlessness, apprehension, skin pallor, sweating, palpitations (if epinephrine is added to the local anesthetic), tremors, weakness, or fainting. As with other patient complications, these should be reported to the surgeon immediately.

The patient's visual and hearing perception may be somewhat altered by the preoperative sedation. The circulating nurse is responsible for providing a quiet atmosphere during the surgery; a gentle reminder to those in the room to speak quietly and a sign posted outside the operating room indicating that a local anesthetic has been administered to the patient are helpful. A radio playing softly in the background may be soothing to the patient. If departmental policy permits use of radios in the operating room, they must be inspected and approved by electrical safety personnel before use. For infection control, radios should be kept within the surgical suite.

During the course of surgery, the circulating nurse or a monitor nurse should continually monitor vital signs, the rate of fluid infusion, and the patient's general condition. The nurse should try to make a restless patient more comfortable. Just seeing the nurse is often enough to reassure the patient. If the patient becomes extremely restless and uncooperative, the surgeon may order additional medication. Medication should be administered in accordance with department standards, and the patient should be observed closely for adverse reactions.

Positioning

Depending on the type of microscope and operating room bed used, the patient may be placed on the bed in the opposite direction from the normal supine position, with the patient's head at the foot of the bed. This positioning facilitates proper placement of the microscope. The patient should be placed on the operating room bed with the operative side as close to the edge of the bed as possible. This positioning gives the surgeon access in viewing all areas of the middle ear and mastoid. The patient is secured on the operating room bed to ensure safety if the bed is laterally rotated during the procedure. If the patient

has neck or back problems caused by arthritis or other conditions, special padding or supports should be provided.

Quietness and immobility of the patient are necessary in otological surgery. In some procedures, such as myringotomy with the patient under local anesthesia, an attendant should hold the patient's head firmly in position. For other operations such as stapedectomy, the patient's head may be immobilized and supported in a foam headrest. Several types of commercial foam headrests are available for this use. The patient's comfort and proper body alignment are important, especially in long procedures such as tympanoplasty.

Preparation of the operative site

For most otologic procedures, the hair is removed and skin shaved at least 1 inch from the site of the proposed incision. The hair is removed primarily from the area above the ear for an endaural approach and behind the ear for a postauricular approach. Petrolatum may be rubbed into the hair along the hairline or a commercial adhesive spray may be used, and the hair is then brushed away from the operative field.

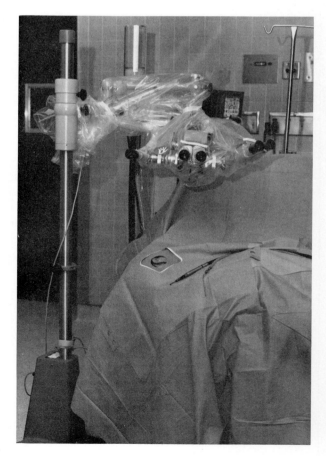

Fig. 19-8. Draped microscope in place over patient in preparation for stapedectomy. Suction, tubing, and drill are assembled in position ready for use.

A povidone-iodine solution is used to prep the exposed auricle and the periauricular skin. The meatus is cleansed with cotton applicators. The surgeon should determine if the external ear canal is to be filled with the prepping solution. A skin degreaser, such as Freon, may be used to dry the ear canal. The face may be prepped on the operative side to permit observation of facial nerve stimulation; alcohol is used to prevent discoloration of the face in the immediate postoperative period.

Draping

The draping procedure is usually based on the surgeon's preference. Typically, for major otologic procedures, the towels and drapes are placed on the patient as follows: Three or four towels, folded lengthwise, are placed around the operative site. (The surgeon may choose to expose a portion of the face on the affected side to observe facial nerve movement.) A disposable, antistatic, adhesive drape may be applied under the drape towels or over the towels and body drape.

A fenestrated drape is unfolded over the patient and the head of the bed, with the operative site in view through the opening. Sterile tape may then be applied to secure the sheet to the patient.

The draped Mayo stand with sterile instruments and the draped operating microscope are positioned over the patient (Fig. 19-8). The scrub nurse usually stands near the instrument table and passes the instruments in such a manner that the surgeon does not have to turn away from the microscope.

Instrumentation

Standard ear surgery setup

A basic setup for otologic procedures (excluding myringotomy) includes an ear, nose, and throat (ENT) drape pack, a basin set, a skin prep set, instruments, ear prostheses if needed, and OR bed accessories. A microscope (Fig. 19-9) and a variety of drills should be available, based on the type of surgical procedure being performed.

A universal set of ear surgery instruments can be used for all middle ear procedures. When an endaural approach is required, only endaural retractors must be added to the universal set. The set includes the following items:

2 Towel clamps, nonperforating, 5¼ inches.
6 Towel clamps, nonperforating, 3 inches
2 Knife handles, no. 3, with no. 15 blades
8 Mosquito hemostats, curved, 5 inches
2 Rochester-Pean forceps, curved, 6¼ inches
1 Metzenbaum scissors, short, curved
1 Metzenbaum scissors, short, straight
1 Plastic scissors, sharp, curved
1 Plastic scissors, dull, curved
1 Foman upper lateral scissors
1 Bellucci scissors
1 Mayo scissors, straight

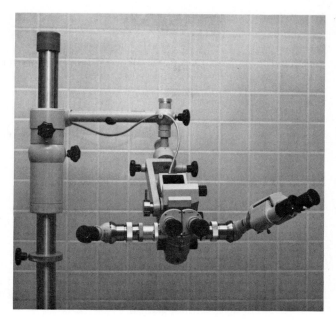

Fig. 19-9. Operating microscope used during various otologic procedures. Lens system allows magnification of 6 to 40 times without change in distance between microscope and ear. Halogen light provides excellent visualization.

2 Brown needle holders
1 Malleus nipper (Fig. 19-10)
1 House-Dieter malleus nipper
1 Bayonet tissue forceps, short (Fig. 19-10)
2 Adson tissue forceps with teeth
2 Frazier suction tips (Fig. 19-10)
4 Baron suction tips, nos. 5 and 7 Fr, 2 each (Fig. 19-10)
2 House suction tips
4 Rosen suction tips
1 Dean elevator
1 Endaural speculum (Fig. 19-10)
6 Ear specula, assorted sizes (Fig. 19-10)
1 Shea speculum holder (Fig. 19-10)
2 Senn retractors
2 Rake retractors, dull
2 Saunders-Paparella self-retaining retractors, two-pronged (Fig. 19-10)
2 Schuknecht self-retaining retractors, three-pronged (Fig. 19-10)
2 Wullstein self-retaining retractors, three-pronged (Fig. 19-10)
1 Small Richardson retractor
1 Ruler
2 Lempert mastoid curettes (Fig. 19-10)
8 Medicine cups
2 Rubber ear syringes
1 Cutting block

Microsurgical middle ear forceps (Fig. 19-11)

Cup forceps, large
Cup forceps, standard
Cup forceps, miniature
House alligator forceps, smooth
Alligator forceps, miniature
Alligator forceps, large

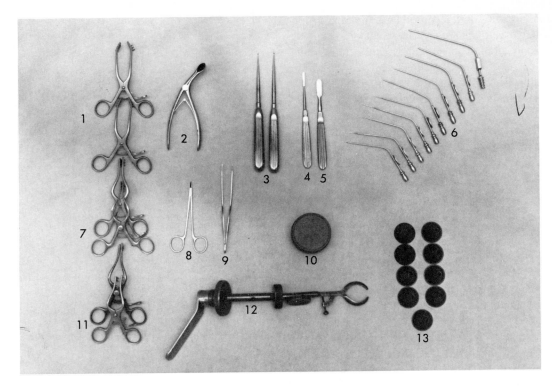

Fig. 19-10. Otologic instruments used for middle ear procedures. *1,* Schuknecht self-retaining retractors; *2,* endaural speculum; *3,* Lempert mastoid curettes; *4,* Joseph elevator; *5,* Dean elevator; *6,* suction tips of assorted sizes; *7,* Wullstein self-retaining retractors; *8,* malleus nipper; *9,* bayonet tissue forceps; *10,* cutting block; *11,* Saunders-Paparella self-retaining retractors; *12,* Shea speculum holders; *13,* ear specula of assorted sizes.

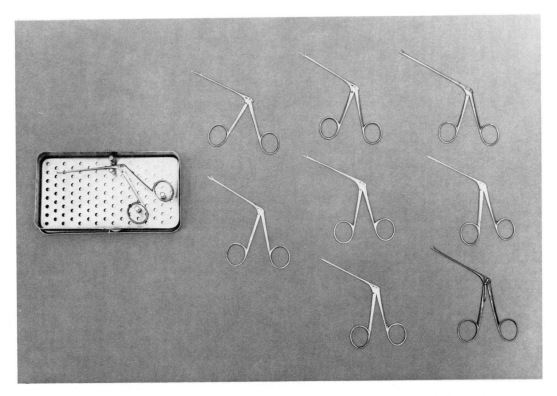

Fig. 19-11. Microsurgical middle ear forceps, including various sizes of cup forceps and alligator forceps.

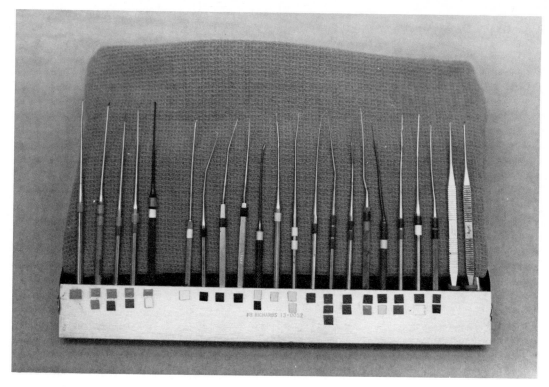

Fig. 19-12. Microsurgical middle ear instruments in protective rack, including various types of knives, hoes, needles, and hooks. The delicacy of these instruments requires protection of the tips.

Microsurgical middle ear instruments (usually in protective rack) (Fig. 19-12)

Myers-Schlosser canal knife
Lancet-Bellucci canal knife
House sickle knife
House incal stapedial knife
Austin right-angle elevator
Hough drum scraper
Oval window rasp
Billeau earloop
Gilford duckbill
Hough hoe, 90-degree
Hough excavator hoe
Paparella curette
House-Barbara straight needle
Rosen needle
Fisch excavators
McGee footplate hooks, assorted lengths
House crura hooks, assorted lengths
Saunders stapes hooks, assorted lengths
Schuknecht hooks, assorted lengths
Wire closure forceps, as needed for specific prostheses
Strut introducer, as needed for specific prostheses

Accessory items

Suction tubing
Antibiotic ointment
Gauze packing
Closure suture
Drill (Fig. 19-13)
Operating microscope with sterile cover (Fig. 19-8)

Electrosurgical unit
Headlight (if microscope not used)

Care and handling of otologic instruments

The basic principles of care, handling, and sterilization of instruments are discussed in Chapter 5. Delicate instruments should be handled individually. To prevent damage, they should not be put into a large basin of cleaning solution or allowed to come into contact with each other. They should be washed, rinsed, and dried individually. A soft-bristled toothbrush can be used to clean the instruments, and care should be used to prevent damage to their tips. Fine, delicate instruments for tympanoplasty and stapedectomy procedures should be kept in a special instrument rack. This type of metal tray separates instruments from one another, protects them from damage, and facilitates handling during surgery. The instruments should be arranged in the rack from left to right or from right to left, in the order of use.

Operating microscope

The operative site is viewed by means of a microscope, which illuminates and magnifies the small, delicate anatomic structures encountered in otologic surgery. Several kinds of operating microscopes (Fig. 19-9) with different attachments are available for otologic surgery. The microscope may be a floor or ceiling-mounted model. For op-

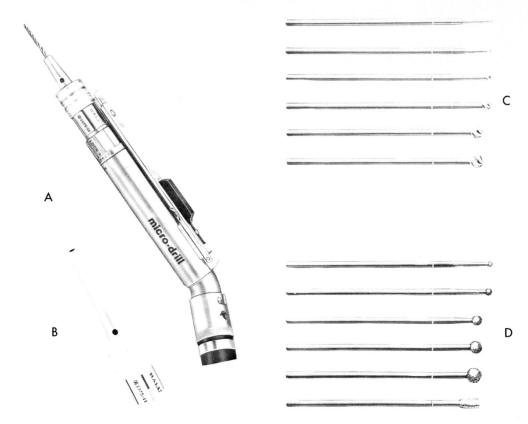

Fig. 19-13. Hall micro-ototome. **A,** Angled handpiece. **B,** Long burr guard. **C** and **D,** Sampling of various, **C,** cutting and, **D,** polishing burrs used during middle ear surgery. (Courtesy Zimmer, Inc., Warsaw, Ind.)

erations through an ear speculum the microscope provides direct light and permits the surgeon to work effectively at a distance by using selected magnification of 6, 10, 16, 25, or 40 times.

Numerous types of heads are available for the microscope, along with teaching attachments through which other team members may view the surgery. The surgeon selects the lens, type of head used, and eyepiece angulation.

The lenses used in the microscope come in various powers of magnification and are interchangeable. Before lenses are put into the microscope, they should be checked to ensure that they are free of lint, dust, fingerprints, and soil.

The surgeon adjusts the microscope before it is draped for surgery and manipulates it during the procedure. The microscope is draped with a sterile cover (Fig. 19-8).

Care should be taken when removing the drapes from the microscope to avoid discarding the eyepieces with the drapes or dropping them on the floor. Eyepieces have been lost or damaged in this manner, necessitating costly repair or replacement.

When the microscope is not in use, it should be kept in a storage area that is away from traffic, free of dust, and properly ventilated. Ideally, a set of eyepieces should be left in the scope to prevent the inside of the scope from becoming dusty. The microscope may also be covered with either a protective cover or a plastic bag.

Specula

Varying sizes of specula are needed to fit the different sizes and shapes of the ear canals encountered.

Needles and syringes for local anesthesia

Local anesthesia is preferred for some operations and is given by block injections (Chapter 9).

For stapes surgery the initial local anesthetic, such as a solution of lidocaine with epinephrine, is injected with a 27-gauge, 1½-inch needle attached to a 5-ml syringe. If a secondary injection is needed, a heavier-gauged (26-gauge, 1½-inch) needle is generally used.

Knives

For myringotomy a sharp knife in perfect condition is needed. Disposable myringotomy knives are used only once. Nondisposable myringotomy knives should be sharpened after each use. Prepackaged, sterile, disposable myringotomy sets are available from several manufacturers and are now widely used. They are relatively inexpensive and provide good instrumentation for the surgeon. For stapes surgery the circumferential knives with blades facing to the right and others to the left are designed for various purposes: (1) to make the primary incision, (2) to elevate the periosteum, (3) to enucleate the fibrous anulus, (4) to separate the incudostapedial joint, and (5) to dissect or resect the scar tissue or the stapedial tendon.

Scissors

Mayo and Metzenbaum scissors are used in otologic surgery, depending on the tissue to be excised. Delicate scissors with angular blades (Bellucci type) are used in middle ear operations to incise and divide the stapedial tendon or scar tissue bands.

Drills and burrs

Electric or air-driven drills or ototomes and burrs are used to remove bone. Cortical and hard cellular bone may be removed by means of an electric drill with a rotating type of burr. For stapes procedures, several microburrs are needed.

A mini-Stryker or Hall micro-ototome drill fitted with either the straight or angled handpiece may be the drill of choice in this circumstance. A complete selection of bits, from round cutting burrs to diamond polishing burrs (Fig. 19-13), should be available. The purpose of cutting burrs is to remove the bone quickly from areas not close to vital structures. Conversely, diamond or polishing burrs are used on bone around vital structures because these burrs remove the bone more slowly and transfer less heat to surrounding bone.

The scrub nurse must be familiar with the various drill systems available. Some surgeons believe that the air-powered systems offer more speed and torque. Others think that the electric-powered drills offer equal torque yet better control of the drill tip. Knowledge of the method of burr seating, cleaning, maintenance, and sterilization of the drill system is imperative to ensure maximum use of the drill system.

During surgery the surgeon holds the handpiece in the same manner as a pen and uses the sides of the burr as the cutting edge. A wire brush may be sterilized and used by the scrub nurse to keep the burrs clean and free of bone bits during the procedure. At the end of the procedure, the burrs should be thoroughly cleaned, inspected for nicks or other damage, and discarded if necessary. Because of the speed and torque of the drill, continuous irrigation is necessary to minimize the transfer of heat from the burr to surrounding bone and structures. Some surgeons prefer to have the scrub nurse irrigate as they suction and drill; others choose a suction irrigator that allows them to control the amount and direction of the irrigation as they drill and suction away debris.

Bone curettes

Various types of bone curettes are used to remove soft bone or substance on the dura, on the sinus wall, or in the vicinity of the facial nerve. Curettes must be sharp. For stapes surgery, strong shank curettes are needed to remove the anulus and posterior canal wall bone or bridge.

Dissecting forceps

In radical mastoidectomy and tympanoplasty, several types of grasping and cutting alligator forceps are needed for manipulation within the canal and the middle ear (Fig. 19-11).

Suction tips

For mastoidectomy and tympanoplasty procedures, several patent suction cannulae are needed. Adequate suctioning must be available at all times.

For stapes surgery the tips of the suction apparatus must be available in various gauges (18, 22, and 24) and equipped with finger valves to vary the degree of suction (Fig. 19-10). These fine needle suction tips must be flushed frequently during the procedure with either saline or sterile water to prevent clogging.

Coagulation tips

In radical mastoidectomy, tympanoplasty, and stapes procedures, electrocoagulation is used to control oozing. In stapes surgery a monopolar or bipolar insulated suction tip may be used to coagulate small bleeding vessels at the margin of the incision. This tip is attached to the active electrode of a delicate coagulating machine. The objective is to control oozing and prevent blood from entering the middle ear during suctioning.

Continuous irrigation equipment

Irrigation of the operative field is done frequently with sterile warm saline, Tis-U-Sol, or Ringer's solution, suctioning apparatus, and bulb syringes to prevent clogging of the burr and to remove bone dust in areas where osteogenesis is to be avoided.

Synthetic materials to control bleeding

Absorbable gelatin sponge (Gelfoam) plugs or pledgets may be placed against the bone. Bone wax may be used in some cases; however, it is a foreign body, and absorbable substances are preferred.

Anesthesia

Ear procedures in children are done with general anesthesia; adults may receive local or general anesthetics. For procedures such as endaural radical mastoidectomy and tympanoplasty, a general anesthetic with endotracheal intubation is used. A local block anesthetic such as lidocaine with epinephrine or occasionally a general anesthetic may be administered for stapes surgery.

Lasers

The role of the carbon dioxide laser in otology and neurotology has not yet been fully defined. Some surgeons advocate its use in stapedotomy and intracranial tumor removal; others await research findings concerning the transmission of heat to surrounding structures during its use. The use of the argon laser in otologic surgery is still controversial but is being explored.

Evaluation

Intraoperative nursing care should be evaluated at the completion of the surgical procedure before the patient is transported to PACU or the nursing unit (if a local anesthetic has been given). If the patient has had a local anesthetic, the nurse will have had the opportunity to evaluate the patient throughout the procedure. The patient can communicate any discomfort during the procedure and indicate any instructions not heard, such as when the surgeon asks, "Can you hear my voice clearly?" or "Are you comfortable?"

During evaluation, the perioperative nurse determines whether the patient met the goals established in the nursing care plan. Some goals can be reached during the preoperative and intraoperative phases of care; they are evaluated prior to the patient's discharge from the operating room. Others require ongoing monitoring and measurement in the postoperative phase. Part of the nursing report to the PACU or nursing unit should include the outcomes of care provided:

- The patient expressed himself or herself effectively and with minimal frustration.
- The patient's anxiety was reduced.
- The patient demonstrated effective coping mechanisms.
- The patient was free from injury.

SURGICAL INTERVENTIONS
Incisional approaches

The endaural (vertical) incision frequently is used for temporal operations, except for simple mastoidectomy. The first incision extends from the superior meatal wall, and the second extends directly upward to a point between the meatus and the upper edge of the auricle, where the two incisions join.

The high posterior incision may be used in operations on infants or young children. The incision is placed at a higher posterior level than the endaural incision and thereby prevents possible damage to the facial nerve.

The postaural incision may be used to expose the mastoid process. It follows the curve of the postaural fold, beginning at the upper attachment of the auricle and continuing behind the postaural fold downward to the tip of the mastoid process.

For stapes surgery, a circumferential incision is made in the posterior half of the canal, starting at the inferior aspect of the anulus and ending posterior to the short process of the malleus.

For myringotomy, a circumferential (posteroinferior) incision is made. It provides for wide drainage and removal of pus or fluid under pressure from the middle ear.

Myringotomy

Myringotomy is the incision of the tympanic membrane. It is performed to treat acute otitis media in the presence of an exudate. Otitis media can be very difficult to diagnose because it is asymptomatic in many patients. The only symptom may be some conductive hearing loss.

Serous otitis media is very common in children between the ages of 6 months and 2 years. About 50% to 60% of children in this age group have effusion in the middle ear at the time tested. The incidence may again peak between the ages of 4 and 6 years; 30% of this age group have fluid in the middle ear with hearing loss.

Ninety-five percent of children with serous otitis media have spontaneous resolution. Hearing loss is the main concern when fluid is present in the middle ear. This hearing loss could affect language development and IQ level if fluid persists for a long period of time. The accepted practice is removal of the fluid and placement of ventilating tubes in the eardrum if the fluid persists more than 6 weeks and is accompanied by hearing loss.

Otitis media is primarily a pediatric problem, but adult cases are seen. It may respond to one treatment only to return and require another type of therapy. Tympanic fibrosis is common in adults and is a result of repeated infections that have occurred in childhood.

Acute otitis media requires prompt surgical drainage known as myringotomy. The patient may have severe pain and bulging of the tympanic membrane (Fig. 19-14). By release of the pus or fluid, hearing is restored and the infection can be controlled. The procedure may be performed for chronic serous otitis media in which the presence of fluid in the middle ear produces a hearing loss. Frequently, tubes are inserted into the tympanic membrane (Fig. 19-15) to allow ventilation of the middle ear. Care must be taken to avoid getting water in the ears while the tubes are in place. Myringotomy is usually performed on an ambulatory surgery basis.

Procedural considerations. Myringotomy is considered a clean procedure. The patient is usually not prepped or draped. The surgeon may wear gown and gloves or gloves only, depending upon the policy related to universal precautions at the institution in which the procedure is performed. The instrument setup includes the following:

1 Myringotomy knife
2 Aural applicators, metal
1 Hartmann aural forceps, delicate type
  Aural specula, assorted sizes
3 Buck ear curettes
1 Suction tip and tubing
1 Culture tube
  Cotton, absorbent

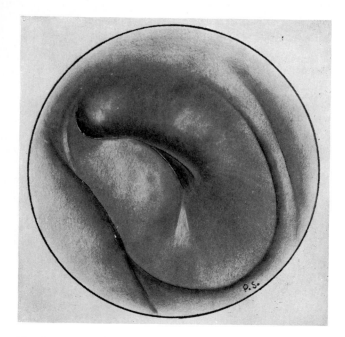

Fig. 19-14. In purulent otitis media, pus under pressure pushes eardrum outward, resulting in bulging tympanic membrane. (From DeWeese, D.D., and Saunders, W.H.: Textbook of otolaryngology, ed. 6, St. Louis, 1982, The C.V. Mosby Co.)

Several disposable myringotomy sets are available commercially. They are relatively inexpensive and afford an expedient procedure.

Operative procedure

1. With microscopic visualization, the aural speculum is inserted in the ear canal. The excess cerumen is removed with a wire loop curette or Toby forceps. With a sharp myringotomy knife, a small, curved incision is made in the anterior inferior quadrant of the pars tensa, and the membrane is cut (Fig. 19-16).
2. A culture may be taken to determine the type of organism present.
3. Pus and fluid are suctioned from the middle ear.
4. A tube may be inserted into the incision with alligator forceps or a tube inserter.
5. Antibiotic drops may be instilled following the positioning of the tube.

Several types of disposable myringotomy tubes are available for implantation, depending on the length of time the surgeon wishes the tube to remain in place (Fig. 19-15, *C*). Once the tube falls out, the tympanic membrane incision usually heals.

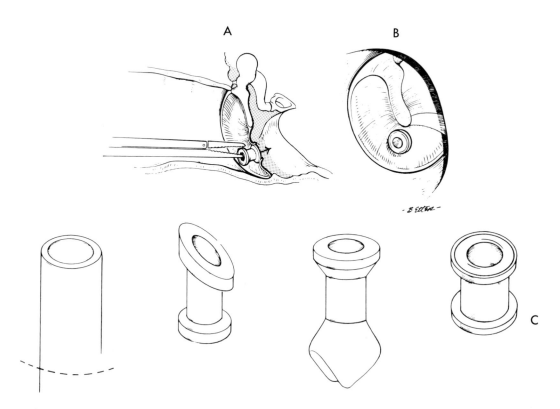

Fig. 19-15. A, Tube (placed on end of alligator forceps) being inserted into tympanic membrane. **B,** Tube in place. **C,** Several types of plastic tubes that may be inserted into tympanic membrane. Purpose of tubes is to aerate middle ear and reduce middle ear infections. (From Saunders, W.H., and others: Nursing care in eye, ear, nose, and throat disorders, ed. 4, St. Louis, 1979, The C.V. Mosby Co.)

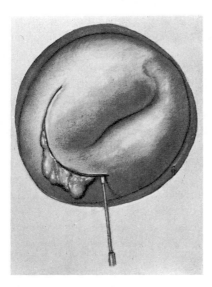

Fig. 19-16. Circumferential incision provides for visibility of eardrum without damage to ossicles and for removal of pus or fluid from middle ear. (From DeWeese, D.D., and Saunders, W.H.: Textbook of otolaryngology, ed. 6, St. Louis, 1982, The C.V. Mosby Co.)

Tympanoplasty

Tympanoplasty was first performed in the eary 1950s. The success rate of the procedure at that time was about 30%. With progress in surgical technique and use of the operating microscope, antibiotic therapy, and better grafting tissue, the success rate soon grew to 90% to 95%.

Tympanoplasty is a surgical procedure performed on the middle ear structures, including the eardrum and ossicles, which usually leads to improved hearing and prevention of recurrent infection.

Perforation of the "eardrum" (tympanic membrane) is the most common serious ear injury necessitating surgical intervention. Perforations may result from:

1. Direct injury (for example, cotton applicators, pencil)
2. Blow to the ear
3. Tears from temporal bone fracture
4. Lightning injury

Early diagnosis is the key to proper management.

Conductive hearing loss is caused by an obstruction in the external canal or middle ear, which impedes the passage of sound waves to the inner ear. It may be due to disease of the middle ear or tympanic membrane. Occasionally the tympanic membrane does not heal following myringotomy.

Ossicular discontinuity may result from chronic otitis media, trauma, or cholesteatoma. Various methods and materials are being used in constructing a closed, air-contained middle ear cavity and restoring a sound-pressure transforming action. Among these materials are homo-

grafts and Teflon, Plastic-Pore, silicone, and metal prostheses.

Procedural considerations. The ear is prepped and draped as previously described. An endaural or postauricular approach may be used. Both these approaches provide similar functional results. The procedure is most often performed under local anesthesia.

Operative procedure

1A. When an *endaural approach* is used, the ear speculum is introduced into the external meatus of the ear canal, and the microscope is brought into place. The surgeon injects local anesthetic into the external meatus and external auditory canal and postauricularly, using a 1-ml or 3-ml syringe. Lidocaine (Xylocaine) with epinephrine is generally used unless the patient's general medical condition necessitates a substitute. The purpose of the injection of local anesthetic is twofold: to make the operation painless (if the patient is having a local anesthetic) and to reduce the amount of bleeding. An endaural incision is then made, using a no. 15 knife blade.

1B. When a *postauricular approach* is used, the surgeon injects local anesthetic (lidocaine with epinephrine) postauricularly using a 3-ml or 5-ml syringe. An ear speculum is introduced, and the microscope is brought into place. The surgeon injects local anesthetic into the external auditory canal using a 1-ml syringe. The microscope head is moved from directly over the patient's ear. The skin incision is made behind the fold of the ear with a no. 10 or no. 15 knife blade. The bleeding vessels are coagulated or clamped and tied. An incision is made in the periosteum down to the bone, and the periosteum is elevated from behind the incision with a Lempert elevator.

2. At this point the temporalis fascia is usually harvested to provide the graft material for the repair of the tympanic membrane. Lidocaine with epinephrine may be injected under the fascia to separate it from the temporalis muscle. A narrow Shambaugh elevator or duckbill elevator is used to separate the fascia. Small, sharp scissors or a knife blade serves to remove the amount of fascia needed. The fascia is trimmed of excess tissue with small, sharp scissors and either laid flat or molded onto an ear speculum. Some surgeons prefer to thin the fascia by using a House Gelfoam press. The fascia is then set aside to dry while the tympanic membrane is prepared.

3. The canal skin may be elevated from the canal with a duckbill elevator, Rosen needle, gimmick, or similar microinstrument, or it may be removed, depending on the size and location of the tympanic membrane perforation.

4. The edges of the tympanic membrane are prepared for the graft by removing all epithelium from the drum surrounding the perforation, usually with a sickle

knife, Rosen needle, 45- or 90-degree pick, or cup forceps.

5. If an edge of the perforation or tympanic membrane cannot be visualized because of the bony canal, the surgeon uses a microcurette or drill to remove the overhang of bone.

6. The middle ear is explored with a pick or similar instrument, and any epithelium present is removed with an alligator or cup forceps. The ossicular chain is tested for mobility. Each ossicle is inspected to ensure that it is intact.

7. If the malleus or incus is diseased or eroded, it may be removed and replaced with a partial ossicular replacement prosthesis (PORP). If the incus is eroded, it may be removed, reshaped with the aid of a drill and small burr, and replaced. If all ossicles are diseased or eroded, they may be removed and replaced with a total ossicular replacement prosthesis (TORP). This step is accomplished with microinstrumentation such as Bellucci scissors, cup forceps, malleus nipper, incudostapedial joint knife, sickle knife, picks, and Rosen needle.

8. Once confident that the middle ear has been explored and corrected, the surgeon prepares the graft for insertion. The edges are trimmed with a no. 15 knife blade or sharp scissors. The surgical site is suctioned with a microsuction. Hemostasis may be achieved by applying very small, epinephrine-soaked dental cotton balls with an alligator forceps and suctioning on the cotton ball. These cotton balls are not radiopaque, and the scrub nurse must ensure the removal of all of them before the graft insertion. Radiopaque microcottonoids are available for this use.

9. Placement of the graft is performed by two main techniques: lateral grafting and medial grafting. Medial grafting provides better functional results than lateral grafting and allows less chance for the development of cholesteatoma, but it is more surgically demanding.

   Different tissues, such as temporal area fascia, tragus perichondrium, and vein grafts, have been used for a tympanoplasty procedure. The most common tissue used is temporalis fascia. Most surgeons prefer to use autograft tissue, although homograft tympanic membranes have also been used.

   For easier manipulation, the graft may be dipped in water, saline, or a Tis-U-Sol solution before its insertion with an alligator forceps. A gimmick, Bileau loop, pick, Rosen needle, or similar microinstrument is used to position the graft into place. Small pledgets of absorbable gelatin sponge may be packed around the graft to ensure support and position. Some surgeons prefer to pack the middle ear before the graft insertion to provide support.

10. The external ear canal is packed with moistened absorbable gelatin sponge pledgets, ½- × 8-inch gauze packing, or a rosebud pack consisting of rayon strips and cotton balls soaked in an antibiotic solution or ointment.

11. The incision is closed with suture of the surgeon's preference.

12. A pressure dressing may be applied for the first 24 hours to prevent dislodgment of the new graft. This dressing usually consists of fluffed gauze placed around the ear and an elastic gauze wrapped around the affected ear and the head.

Mastoidectomy

Mastoidectomy is the removal of the diseased bone of the mastoid, along with the cholesteatoma present in the middle ear and mastoid (Fig. 19-17).

Cholesteatoma is the result of accumulation of squamous epithelium and its products in the middle ear and mastoid. It occasionally forms an encysted, puttylike mass. As it expands, it is destructive to the middle ear and mastoid. As a result, the diseased bone (ossicles and mastoid bone) must be removed to prevent recurrence of the cholesteatoma.

There are three types of mastoidectomy. A *simple mastoidectomy* is removal of the diseased bone of the mastoid while the ossicles, eardrum, and canal wall are left intact. The simple mastoid procedure performed to evacuate a coalescent abscess is rarely performed today. Most procedures of the mastoid are performed for cases of acute suppurative otitis media that have failed to respond to antibiotic therapy. These cases proceed to a coalescent mastoiditis.

The most common serious surgical accident during a simple mastoid procedure is injury to the facial nerve. Other complications are injury to the sigmoid sinus, mastoid vein, or dura. Injury to the dura, however, is the least common.

A *modified radical mastoidectomy* is removal of the diseased bone of the mastoid along with some of the ossicles and the canal wall. The eardrum and some of the ossicles remain, thus leaving a mechanism for the patient to hear. A *radical mastoidectomy* is the removal of the canal wall along with the ossicles. The patient has a large cavity created to allow ease in cleaning the ear.

Procedural considerations. General anesthesia is usually selected but local anesthesia can be used. The patient is prepped and draped as for a tympanoplasty. An endaural or postauricular incision may be used (Fig. 19-18), but most surgeons believe that the postauricular incision offers better exposure to all areas of the mastoid and middle ear. A drill is used to remove diseased bone and tissue while the surgeon continually observes for anatomical structures, such as the facial nerve, within the mastoid.

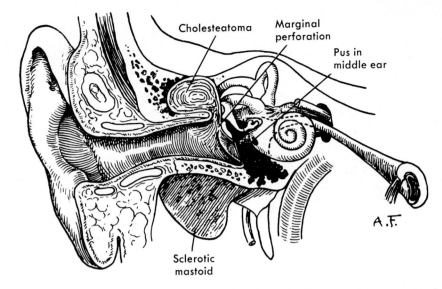

Fig. 19-17. Cholesteatoma of middle ear is mass of epidermoid cells arranged in concentric layers, intermingled with cholesterin crystals. Squamous epithelium grows through tympanic perforation to form pouch, which finally lines middle ear cavity and adjacent mastoid cells. Center of pouch tends to become necrotic and houses infectious bacteria. These lesions increase in size slowly at margins of tympanic membrane. (From Davis, H., and Fowler, E.P. In Davis, H., and Silverman, S.R., editors: Hearing and deafness, rev. ed., New York, 1960, Holt, Rinehart & Winston, Inc.)

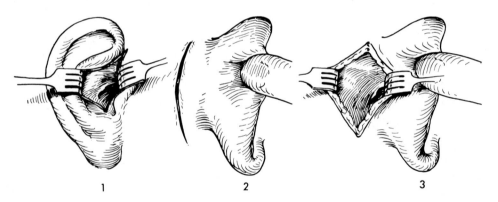

Fig. 19-18. Mastoidectomy incision. *1,* Endaural. *2,* Postauricular. *3,* Postauricular incision retracted. (From DeWeese, D.D., and Saunders, W.H.: Textbook of otolaryngology, ed. 6, St. Louis, 1982, The C.V. Mosby Co.)

Operative procedure

1-6. These steps are as for tympanoplasty.

7. The mastoid bone is drilled initially with a large cutting burr, usually under direct vision. As the mastoid cavity is created, the scrub nurse should be able to anticipate changes needed in burr size. Once the vital structures have been identified, diseased bone is usually removed from them by use of diamond burrs of the appropriate size. The surgeon may interrupt drilling to explore areas of the mastoid with a pick, Rosen needle, mastoid searcher, gimmick, or other microinstrument to identify surrounding structures.

8. On completion of the mastoidectomy, the surgeon focuses on the middle ear. Diseased ossicles are removed, middle ear mucosa is inspected and removed if necessary, and all evidence of cholesteatoma is removed. Depending on the extent of the disease and the reliability that the patient will be available for follow-up, the surgeon then reconstructs the ossicular chain or prepares the cavity created by a radical mas-

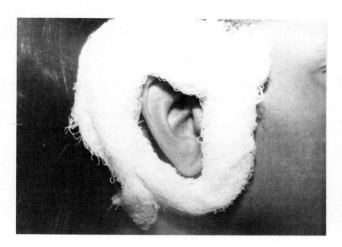

Fig. 19-19. Initial dressing after mastoidectomy. Space behind ear is well padded to prevent pain if ear is pressed against skull.

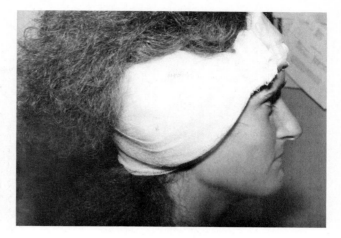

Fig. 19-20. Completed dressing following mastoidectomy. Fluffs and gauze bandage comprise the dressing. Dressing is placed high enough that it does not fall over eyes.

toidectomy. Some surgeons do not reconstruct at the time of mastoidectomy but follow the patient for a specified time. If cholesteatoma does not recur during that period, the patient receives a reconstructive procedure to restore hearing.

9. The mastoid cavity and middle ear may be packed with absorbable gelatin sponge. The external auditory canal may be packed with absorbable gelatin sponge, a strip of ½-inch gauze, or a rosebud pack consisting of rayon strips and cotton balls soaked in an antibiotic solution or ointment.

10. The incision is closed with suture of the surgeon's preference.

11. A pressure dressing is applied and kept in place for the first 24 hours. This dressing usually consists of fluffed gauze around the ear and plain or elastic gauze wrapped around the head and affected ear (Figs. 19-19 and 19-20).

Stapedectomy

Stapedectomy is removal of the stapes for treatment of otosclerosis and replacement with a prosthesis to restore ossicular continuity and improve hearing.

Otosclerosis is the overgrowth of bone around the stapes footplate, resulting in immobility of the footplate. Sound waves cannot be transmitted adequately through the oval window and round window to be changed into electrochemical impulses in the cochlea.

There are two types of procedures for replacing the immobile stapes. In *stapedotomy* the footplate of the stapes is not removed; only the superstructure is removed. A hole is made in the stapes footplate, and the prosthesis is secured laterally to the long process of the incus and positioned medially over the hole created in the footplate. In *stapedectomy* the entire stapes (superstructure and foot-

plate) is removed, a graft is placed over the oval window, and a prosthesis is attached laterally to the long process of the incus and positioned medially on the graft over the oval window.

Procedural considerations. Various materials are used as the prosthesis for the stapes; the most common are stainless steel and Teflon (Fig. 19-21). The prosthesis of choice is determined by the surgeon.

The scrub nurse must be aware of each step in the procedure and hand the instruments to the surgeon expediently. Because the oval window is left uncovered, some perilymph may leak from the inner ear into the middle ear. This leak subjects the patient to the possible complication of a sensorineural hearing loss postoperatively or, more seriously, a "dead ear."

Microsuctions (18- to 25-gauge) are used in this procedure because other suction tips are too large and may suction perilymph from the oval window as well as promote bleeding in the middle ear.

Following the incision and reflection of the flap, footplate hooks are used because the tips on picks are so large and long that they may cause damage rather than assist in the procedure.

Operative procedure
Stapedectomy

1. A temporalis fascia, fat, perichondrium, or vein graft may be harvested before the procedure. This graft is used to cover the oval window. Depending on the surgeon's preference, the ear, hand, or a portion of the abdomen may be prepped for the graft.

2. The ear speculum is introduced, and the microscope is brought into position. The ear canal is cleansed of wax and debris and may be gently washed with Tis-U-Sol and suctioned with a Baron or microsuction tip.

3. The surgeon injects lidocaine with epinephrine into the ear canal.

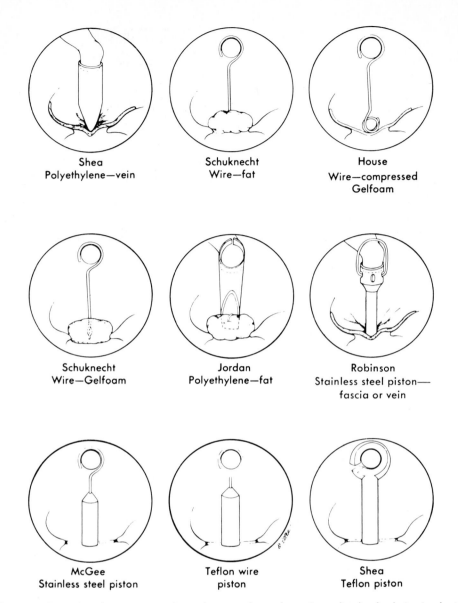

Shea
Polyethylene—vein

Schuknecht
Wire—fat

House
Wire—compressed
Gelfoam

Schuknecht
Wire—Gelfoam

Jordan
Polyethylene—fat

Robinson
Stainless steel piston—
fascia or vein

McGee
Stainless steel piston

Teflon wire
piston

Shea
Teflon piston

Fig. 19-21. Examples of more commonly used ear prostheses shown immediately after being implanted. Grafts gradually thin out and become continuous with mucoperiosteum in ear. (From Saunders, W.H., and others: Nursing care in eye, ear, nose, and throat disorders, ed. 4, St. Louis, 1979, The C.V. Mosby Co.)

4. An ear speculum is inserted, the tympanomeatal flap is created (using a flap knife, roller knife, or sickle knife), and the tympanic membrane is reflected forward (using duckbill elevators or a drum elevator), exposing the middle ear (Fig. 19-22).
5. If visualization of the ossicles is inadequate owing to the overhang of bone, the surgeon may use micro-curettes or a drill to remove enough bone to allow proper visualization. If the chorda tympani nerve obstructs the view of the stapes, the surgeon may transect this nerve. However, attempts to save the chorda tympani nerve are usually made because it controls taste from the anterior two thirds of the tongue.

6. The surgeon may measure the distance from the incus to the stapes footplate at this time or after the removal of the stapes. It is accomplished with a measuring stick and done to ensure the proper fit of the prosthesis.
7. The incudostapedial joint is disarticulated to allow fracture and subsequent removal of the stapes, usually accomplished through the use of a House or Guilford-Wright joint knife.
8. Both crura of the stapes are fractured laterally, usually with a footplate pick or Rosen needle, and the superstructure is removed with an alligator forceps. The surgeon may take this opportunity to ensure hemo-

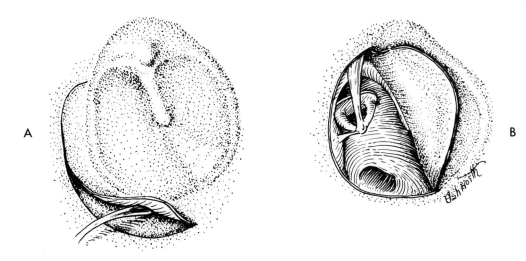

Fig. 19-22. Stapedectomy. **A,** Incision in posterior ear canal wall. **B,** Operative field seen through aural speculum. (From DeWeese, D.D., and Saunders, W.H.: Textbook of otolaryngology, ed. 6, St. Louis, 1982, The C.V. Mosby Co.)

stasis using tiny dental cotton balls or a sponge soaked in epinephrine along with a microsuction tip.

9. To prevent a suction effect on the underlying perilymph, the footplate is fractured in the middle portion, usually with a footplate pick or similar sharp microinstrument. If the footplate is extremely thick, a microdrill may be used. Each half of the footplate is then removed, using a Hough hoe, footplate pick, or footplate hook.

10. The oval window is then inspected, and the graft is placed over the oval window with alligator forceps or a pick. The edges of the graft are smoothed and positioned with a Hough hoe, pick, or gimmick.

11. The prosthesis is passed on an alligator forceps to the surgeon, who introduces it into the middle ear with the shaft of the prosthesis resting against the oval window graft.

12. The wire is positioned over the long process of the incus by using picks, Hough hoes, or footplate hooks. Once it is in proper position, the surgeon uses a crimper to crimp the wire onto the long process of the incus and thus ensure its attachment to the incus.

13. The surgeon may test the patient's hearing by softly whispering to the patient (if the procedure is performed under local anesthesia) or by touching the malleus with a pick and observing for mobility of the malleus, incus, and stapes prosthesis (if performed under general anesthesia).

14. Tiny squares of moistened, compressed, gelatin sponge may then be placed around the base of the prosthesis to enure its stability. Alligator forceps, picks, gimmick, and similar instruments may be used for this step in the procedure.

15. The tympanomeatal flap is returned to its original lo-

cation, using a drum elevator, duckbill elevator, or Rosen needle, and the external ear canal may be packed with a cotton ball, a moistened compressed gelatin sponge, or a rosebud pack.

16. The external dressing may consist of a gauze bandage wrapped around the head and affected ear, or a Band-Aid may be used as covering for the external ear canal. A Band-Aid or small dressing is usually applied to the graft site.

Stapedotomy. The stapedotomy procedure is similar to stapedectomy but has these differences:

1. No graft is taken before the procedure.
2. The footplate is not removed. A hole is made in the footplate, using perforators or hand drills of increasing size, and the prosthesis is inserted when the perforation in the footplate is the appropriate size.
3. Following the positioning and the crimping of the prosthesis, either a moistened, compressed, gelatin sponge or a few drops of the patient's blood may be placed around the junction of the prosthesis and the footplate to ensure stability of the prosthesis.

Stapedotomy has been performed with the argon laser utilized to perforate the footplate. Some surgeons believe that this method is more efficient, whereas others think that the procedure is prolonged through the positioning and preparation of the laser. The scrub and circulating nurses must be knowledgeable in the operation, safety, and procedure for use of the laser if the surgeon elects to perform stapedotomy with a laser (Chapter 10).

Ossicular reconstruction

Ossicular reconstruction is commonly performed for the replacement of the incus portion of the ossicular chain.

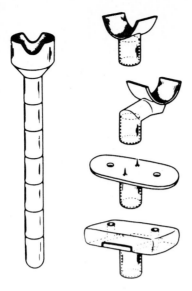

Fig. 19-23. Middle ear reconstruction kit is composed of a Teflon piston cup prosthesis measuring approximately 7 to 8 mm in length and 0.5 mm in width, and various types of caps to accommodate different anatomic circumstances. (Courtesy Dr. Moshe Ziv, designer, Columbus, Ohio.)

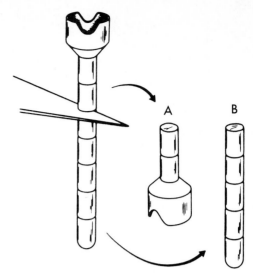

Fig. 19-24. Teflon piston cup prosthesis. The shaft of the prosthesis has fine lines 1 mm apart that provide a measuring rod incorporated in each prosthesis. The shaft is cut according to the length necessary to obtain the appropriate height from the capitulum of the stapes or from the footplate of the stapes. Each of these two pieces can be used with any of the four caps (Fig. 19-23) to fit the prosthesis in the most desirable position up to the handle of the malleus or to the tympanic membrane when the malleus is absent. **A** is a piston cup segment; **B** is a piston shaft segment. (Courtesy Dr. Moshe Ziv, designer, Columbus, Ohio.)

There are many surgical techniques for ossicular reconstruction. Autografts of ossicles taken from the patient's ear may be used, but they must be reshaped to reestablish the ossicular chain. Preserved homografts have been used in the past; however, patients are refusing to even consider these grafts since HIV has become so prevalent.

About 50% to 60% of ossicular problems are related to the incus, and 10% affect the stapes as a result of otosclerosis. Malleus dysfunction accounts for 10% of ossicular problems and is mainly due to the formation of cholesteatoma.

Alloplastic materials have been produced and improved upon for use in ossicular reconstruction. This material is used in the manufacturing of partial and total ossicular reconstruction prostheses.

An interesting concept in ossicular reconstruction using an assembly system (Ziv Middle Ear Reconstruction System) has been introduced (Figs. 19-23, 19-24, and 19-25). It is assembled in the operating room by the surgeon, based on the ossicle or ossicles that require replacement. The exact measurements are taken during the operation, and the size is tailored according to the patient's needs. The different combinations cover all possible ossicular problems that may occur in the middle ear. The reconstruction system can be placed between the most favorable points and brought to the handle of the malleus and not to the tympanic membrane. The advantage of this is that improved functional results occur as well as decreased possibility of extrusion of the prosthesis.

Procedural considerations. The patient is prepped and draped as for stapedectomy.

Operative procedure. The procedural steps for stapedectomy are followed.

Endolymphatic shunt

An endolymphatic shunt procedure is the creation of an opening into the endolymphatic sac and the insertion of a shunt to allow drainage of excess endolymph into the cerebrospinal fluid or into the mastoid cavity.

The endolymphatic shunt is a nondestructive procedure designed to drain excess endolymph from the endolymphatic sac in Ménière's disease. The theory is that the inability of the endolymphatic sac to resorb endolymph results in an overaccumulation of endolymph. This surplus leads to vertigo, in which patients feel that they are stationary and the environment is spinning around them. Movement usually increases the vertigo, which may be accompanied by severe nausea and vomiting. The vertigo attacks appear to be periodic and may last from several minutes to several hours. Most patients with Ménière's disease complain of tinnitus, usually low pitched. They often describe the sound as a roar or buzz and can predict an attack of vertigo by an increase in the loudness or pitch of the tinnitus. Patients with Ménière's disease usually complain of pressure or fullness in the ear, as well as hearing loss in lower frequencies. Diagnostic audiometry

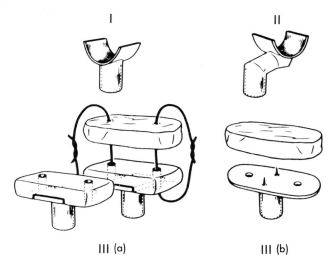

Fig. 19-25. Types of caps that fit snugly to the piston cup prosthesis. Cap I is designed to fit the manubrium of the malleus once it is incorporated into the Teflon cup with the shortened piston (Fig. 19-24, *A*) to replace the incus or into the Teflon piston (Fig. 19-24, *B*) to replace the incus and the stapes. Cap II is a variation of Cap I that fits an anatomic situation in which the manubrium of the malleus is in a more anterior position. Cap III(a) has a Plastipore plate to be used with cartilage underneath the tympanic membrane if the malleus is absent or if the manubrium is too close to the promontory and does not allow enough room for the prothesis to be inserted in the middle ear. Cap III(b) is a variation of Cap III(a) that may require suturing of the cartilage to the top plate before its placement underneath the tympanic membrane. (Courtesy Dr. Moshe Ziv, designer, Columbus, Ohio.)

reveals the hearing loss to be sensorineural. These patients require emotional support because the vertigo is often so severe that it disrupts their lives. Frequently they continue to experience the vertigo and progressive hearing loss despite a medical regimen of tranquilizers, diuretics, vasodilators, and a low-sodium or sodium-free diet.

Procedural considerations. Preoperative assessment by the perioperative nurse confirms that the patient's electrolyte levels (especially potassium) are adequate and provides a basis for the support system to be carried out intraoperatively and postoperatively. Because Ménière's disease may develop bilaterally, conservative therapy is often employed.

The patient is prepped and draped as for tympanoplasty.

Operative procedure
1-7. These steps are as for mastoidectomy.
8. Drilling with a diamond burr over the posterior fossa dura is continued until the endolymphatic sac is identified.
9. An incision is made into the lateral wall of the sac with a microknife such as a sickle, Beaver blade, or Ziegler. An incision is then made through the medial wall, exposing the subarachnoid space.

10. A shunt (commercially prepared tube, Silastic tubing, or Silastic sheeting) is inserted with microforceps and is manipulated into place, usually with microinstruments such as a Rosen needle, fine pick, or gimmick. When the shunt is designed to drain into the mastoid, only the lateral wall of the sac is incised.
11. The dural incision may be covered with temporalis fascia, and the mastoid cavity may be packed with moistened absorbable gelatin sponge.
12. The incision is closed with suture of the surgeon's preference.
13. A pressure dressing of elastic gauze is applied around the head and affected ear.

Labyrinthectomy

Labyrinthectomy is a procedure that destroys membranous labyrinth to relieve the patient of severe vertigo. The procedure is usually performed when the disease is unilateral, a shunt has been ineffective, and the patient's hearing is poor. Because the inner ear is destroyed, the patient may be very dizzy for several days until the brainstem begins to compensate for the destroyed labyrinth. The operation also leaves the ear deaf.

Procedural considerations. This procedure may be performed on the patient via the transmastoid or transtympanic approach. The patient is prepped and draped as described for tympanoplasty.

Operative procedure
Transmastoid approach
1-7. These steps are as for mastoidectomy.
8. A hole is drilled into the horizontal semicircular canal with a small diamond burr.
9. The membranous labyrinth is removed with a fine pick or hook and microsuctions. Streptomycin-soaked absorbable gelatin sponge may be placed in the inner ear to ensure destruction of all nerve elements.
10. The hole may be covered with bone or temporalis muscle or fascia. Absorbable gelatin sponge may be used to pack the mastoid cavity.
11. The incision is closed with suture of the surgeon's choice.
12. A pressure dressing of elastic gauze is applied.
Transtympanic approach
1-9. These steps are as for stapedectomy.
10. The incus is separated from the malleus, usually with a pick, and removed with an alligator or cup forceps.
11. The membranous labyrinth is removed by means of picks and microsuctions. Streptomycin-soaked absorbable gelatin sponge is introduced into the inner ear.
12. Moistened absorbable gelatin sponge may be placed in the oval window and middle ear space.
13. The tympanomeatal flap is returned via a gimmick, drum elevator, picks, or Rosen needle.
14. The external auditory canal may be packed with ab-

sorbable gelatin sponge or a rosebud pack as described for the tympanoplasty procedure.

15. An external pressure dressing of elastic gauze is applied.

Vestibular neurectomy

In vestibular neurectomy, the vestibular portion of the eighth cranial nerve (acoustic nerve) is transected, but the cochlear portion is left intact to relieve the patient of severe vertigo. Vestibular neurectomy is performed when a patient has adequate hearing and a labyrinthectomy is not indicated.

Procedural considerations. The patient's abdomen or lateral thigh is prepped and draped for the purpose of obtaining fat or a segment of muscle and fascia to be used for obliteration of the mastoid cavity at the end of the procedure. If the abdomen is used, most surgeons prefer to take fat from the left side to avoid future confusion with an appendectomy scar. Setups for the graft and neurectomy procedure are separate to avoid cross-contamination. The graft may be taken before the procedure or after the vestibular nerve has been transected, depending on the surgeon's preference. The patient is prepped and draped as for tympanoplasty.

Operative procedure

1. Lidocaine with or without epinephrine is injected subcutaneously using a 3- or 5-ml syringe.
2. A retrolabyrinthine U-shaped incision is made slightly posterior to the area of the postauricular incision used in other otologic surgery.
3. An incision is made in the mastoid muscles with a no. 10 or no. 15 blade. These muscles are elevated with a Lempert, Joseph, or similar elevator.
4. A self-retaining retractor is inserted after the muscles and periosteum are elevated.
5. The surgeon begins drilling, usually with a large cutting burr, and continues until a complete mastoidectomy is performed. The sigmoid sinus and posterior and inferior semicircular canals are skeletonized with a diamond burr. The posterior fossa bone is removed, exposing the posterior fossa dura. During the drilling process, burr sizes and types (cutting and diamond) may be changed as vital structures are identified. The scrub nurse must ensure that irrigation and suction are adequate. The surgeon may pause during the drilling to verify vital structures with a microinstrument such as a Rosen needle, gimmick, pick, or searcher.
6. The posterior fossa dura is incised with a sickle or Ziegler microknife. Hemostasis may be achieved by the use of bipolar forceps, a moistened absorbable gelatin sponge covered by a cottonoid, or Surgicel. Cottonoids, Surgicel, and gelatin sponge may be loaded onto bayonet forceps before the forceps is placed in the surgeon's hand or may be introduced into the field by the scrub nurse with the use of bayonet

forceps while the surgeon controls another bayonet forceps.

7. As exploration and dissection of the cochleovestibular nerve are carried out, cottonoids may be used to cover vital structures and thus maintain orientation. The vestibular portion of the eighth cranial nerve (acoustic) nerve is identified by the surgeon and transected with Bellucci scissors, other microscissors, or a microknife.
8. Hemostasis is achieved by the methods mentioned in Step 6.
9. The dural incision is closed with suture of the surgeon's preference, usually no. 4-0 silk or nylon on a very small needle.
10. Fat from the abdomen or fascia and muscle from the lateral aspect of the thigh are packed over the closed dural incision, and the skin incision is closed.
11. A pressure dressing of elastic gauze is applied.

Facial nerve decompression

Facial nerve decompression is a procedure designed to identify and relieve an area of compression of the facial nerve. The most common form of facial paralysis is Bell's palsy. It provokes more controversy regarding proper management than any other disorder of the facial nerve. The cause is unknown, although clinical and laboratory evidence suggests a virus of the herpes simplex group. The patient experiences multiple problems such as decreased tearing, inability to close the affected eye, and drooping of the affected corner of the mouth with pooling of oral secretions. Preoperatively, the eye is protected by ointments and the eyelid is taped closed, or an adhesive bubble is placed over the eye to trap moisture. This protection is continued into the postoperative period unless a tarsorrhaphy (suturing the eyelid closed) is performed intraoperatively. The patient is taught to place food at the back of the tongue on the unaffected side to assist in mastication. Tilting the head to the unaffected side while eating decreases the pooling of oral secretions and drooling. The patient must be taught proper mouth care because the pooling of oral secretions may lead to dental caries or gingivitis. This regimen is continued until the nerve manifests its regeneration by the return of facial movement. Controversy exists regarding whether the facial nerve should be decompressed in the middle cranial fossa as well as in the transmastoid, translabyrinthine area. Both approaches are discussed here because current theory suggests that transmastoid decompression alone is not effective.

Transmastoid, translabyrinthine approach

Procedural considerations. The patient is prepped and draped as described for tympanoplasty.

Operative procedure

1–7. These steps are as for mastoidectomy.
8. Following complete mastoidectomy, the dissection is

carried out by the use of cutting and diamond burrs until the internal auditory canal and the posterior fossa bone are removed.

9. The bone immediately over the facial nerve is removed by the use of nerve excavators and picks.

10. The facial nerve sheath is incised with a facial nerve knife, neurectomy knife, sickle knife, neurectomy scissors, or micropicks. The incision and decompression are carried out from the stylomastoid foramen to the brainstem.

11. Hemostasis is achieved by the use of moistened absorbable gelatin sponge, cottonoids, Surgicel, bipolar forceps, or a combination.

12. The incision is closed with suture of the surgeon's preference.

13. A pressure dressing of elastic gauze is applied.

Middle cranial fossa approach

Procedural considerations. The patient's hair is shaved almost to the midline on the affected side. Povidone-iodine is usually used for the prep, which includes the portion of the head that has been shaved, the affected side of the face, and the neck.

Lidocaine with or without epinephrine is usually injected subcutaneously above the ear to assist in hemostasis.

Operative procedure

1. The temporalis muscle is incised and elevated with a Lempert, Shambaugh, or similar elevator.

2. Hemostasis is achieved by clamping and tying vessels or with electrocoagulation.

3. A square of bone is drilled from the temporal bone to expose the middle cranial fossa dura. (The bone is saved for replacement at the end of the procedure.)

4. A self-retaining retractor with a blade for retraction of the middle fossa (for example, a Fisch middle fossa retractor or House-Urban retractor) is inserted.

5. The microscope is brought into place, and the dura is elevated from the floor of the middle fossa with the use of Fisch excavators, nerve excavators, a gimmick, or similar instruments.

6. Once hemostasis is achieved and the blade is inserted over the dura to expose the middle fossa, drilling may proceed.

7. When the bone becomes quite thin, the surgeon may remove the remaining bone with excavators to avoid damaging the nerve sheath.

8. The facial nerve sheath is incised with a facial nerve knife, neurectomy knife, neurectomy scissors, or microknife.

9. The retractor is removed when hemostasis is achieved, and the bone flap is replaced.

10. The temporalis muscle is approximated and sutured. The incision is closed with suture of the surgeon's preference.

11. A pressure dressing of elastic gauze is applied.

Damage to the facial nerve from trauma, infection, or tumors may be treated surgically by these approaches. Facial nerve grafting requires the use of a separate setup for obtaining a nerve for grafting and microinstrumentation for handling the nerves as well as suturing them. Microsutures such as no. 8-0 to 11-0 are used.

Removal of acoustic neuroma

An acoustic neuroma arises from the Schwann cells of the vestibular portion of the eighth cranial (acoustic) nerve. These tumors are benign but may grow to a size that produces symptoms of cerebellar and brainstem origin.

Acoustic neuroma was a rare clinical finding in the past. With the extension of life expectancy and improved diagnostic technology, the diagnosis of acoustic neuroma has become more frequent. Brainstem auditory evoked responses is a highly sensitive noninvasive test for this tumor. If this test yields suspicious findings, an MRI of the brain and internal auditory canals is performed.

Depending on the rate and direction of tumor growth, symptoms may include hearing loss, tinnitus, vertigo, headaches, double vision, diplopia, decreased corneal reflex, decreased blink reflex, impaired taste, reduced lacrimation, diminished gag reflex, vocal cord paralysis, atrophy or fasciculation of the tongue, weakness of the sternocleidomastoid and trapezius muscles, disturbance in balance and gait, hydrocephalus, lethargy, confusion, drowsiness, and coma. Most patients complain of only a unilateral hearing loss, the main symptom of a possible acoustic neuroma.

Several centers have developed great expertise in acoustic neuroma surgery, which requires a combined team of an otologist and a neurosurgeon.

Procedural considerations. The translabyrinthine approach for the removal of an acoustic tumor has increased in popularity over the past decade. It reduces mortality and morbidity and offers a good chance of saving the facial nerve, if the tumor has not directly invaded the nerve. It also relieves tinnitus by destroying the vestibular apparatus.

The patient should be informed preoperatively about the presence of a Foley catheter, arterial line, temperature probe, shaved head, and graft site incision during the postoperative period. Postoperative complications may include a cerebrospinal fluid leak, vertigo, facial nerve weakness or paralysis, and wound infection.

These patients require considerable postoperative teaching in preparation for discharge. Areas addressed in discharge instructions include activity, oral care, diet, medication, return office visit, eye care, and graft site and suture line care. Emotional support is vital because of the severity of the disease, the operative procedure, and the altered body image patients experience as a result of removal of their hair and facial weakness or paralysis. Members of the national support group, the Acoustic Neuroma

Association, will visit the patient before and after surgery if requested by the surgeon or nurse.

The patient's hair is shaved to the midline of the affected side. Some patients prefer to have the entire head shaved to facilitate wearing a wig. The options should be presented preoperatively to enable the patient to make a decision before surgery.

The patient is prepped and draped as described for labyrinthectomy. Lidocaine with or without epinephrine may be injected subcutaneously behind the ear.

Operative procedure

1. A postauricular incision is made slightly longer and wider than the incision in mastoidectomy. The periosteum is elevated from the mastoid bone with a Lempert, Shambaugh, or similar elevator.
2. Self-retaining retractors are inserted, and the cortical mastoidectomy is begun with a large cutting burr.
3. The microscope is brought into position, and the attic is opened to visualize the ossicles. The sigmoid sinus, middle fossa dura, and superior petrosal sinus are left with a thin covering of bone. The semicircular canals are exposed. The incus is removed with an alligator or cup forceps and suction.
4. The semicircular canals are excised with the drill. The utricle and saccule are removed, and the aqueduct of the vestibule is drilled out.
5. On completion of the drilling, the remainder of bone is removed with nerve excavators, Fisch dissectors, or picks from the dura of the internal meatus, posterior fossa, middle fossa, and petrosal angle. The wedge of bone between the facial and superior vestibular nerves (Bill's bar) is removed.
6. The dura is opened with a no. 11 blade or microknife. Dissection of the tumor ensues with a gimmick, micro Freer elevator, microinstrument, and bipolar forceps (with or without suction, depending on the surgeon's preference). Hemostasis is frequently achieved through the use of a moistened absorbable gelatin sponge, cottonoids, Surgicel, and a bipolar coagulator.
7. When the tumor has been removed by the use of pituitary cup forceps, long alligator forceps, and similar instruments, hemostasis is achieved.
8. Graft material is obtained to pack the mastoid cavity created from the drilling. It may be fat, fascia, or muscle. The packing is performed meticulously to avoid a cerebrospinal fluid leak postoperatively.
9. On completion of the packing, the wound is closed with suture of the surgeon's choice.
10. A thick pressure dressing, consisting of gauze for absorbency and elastic gauze for pressure, is applied.

The patient is placed in an intensive care setting for close observation for 48 to 72 hours. Initial postoperative nursing care includes monitoring of neurologic and routine vital signs, monitoring of facial nerve function on the affected side, observation of the dressing for drainage, close monitoring of temperature, monitoring of intake and output, observation and testing of nasal drainage to determine cerebrospinal fluid leak, positioning, deep breathing by the patient (coughing is discouraged because of the possibility of dislodging the graft), administering medications for pain and nausea, antibiotics, and stool softeners (to prevent straining, which might dislodge the graft), and providing emotional support to the patient. Early ambulation is advised to maintain proper circulation and avoid pulmonary complications, which could lead to coughing and subsequent dislodgment of the graft. While the patient's opposite vestibular system is compensating for the removed system, the patient needs assistance in moving and ambulating. The family is advised to help as needed, while allowing the patient to move at his or her pace to avoid sudden vertigo and nausea.

If facial function is altered on the affected side because of manipulation, edema, or surgical excision, the patient must use supportive measures until adequate function returns. These include lubrication, covering, and inspection of the eye to avoid corneal injury, frequent brushing and rinsing of the oral cavity to prevent dental caries from the pooling of secretions on the affected side, a semisoft to soft diet to allow the patient more ease in directing the food toward the back of the unaffected side of the mouth, and tilting the head toward the unaffected side. The soft diet and head tilting are designed to decrease the collection of food and the spillage of food from the affected side yet allow the patient to maintain dignity while eating.

As mentioned previously, the Acoustic Neuroma Association is available to visit the patient, share experiences, give helpful suggestions, or listen to the patient. On notification by the surgeon or nurse, members visit the patient in the hospital setting and follow up with home visits.

Cochlear implantation

Cochlear implantation is the placement of an electrode device in the winding, cone-shaped tube called the *cochlea.*

Approximately half a million people in the United States have complete deafness. Cochlear implantation seems to be beneficial for a certain segment of that group. The most important prerequisite for candidacy for cochlear implantation is a previous history of lingual skill prior to becoming deaf. This criterion basically excludes all patients who were born deaf. Appropriate auditory training and psychologic counseling is also needed following appropriate selection of candidates.

Technologic advancements have given the deaf patient new hope in the area of cochlear implantation. The device is implanted in the cochlea, with the receiver resting in the mastoid. As the device receives sound through the receiver, it emits electrical impulses through the transmitter into the cochlea and along the acoustic nerve. These impulses are interpreted as sound in the temporal cortex of the cerebrum. The patient must be taught to interpret these sounds through extensive training sessions with an audiology department.

There is a risk of meningitis in some of these patients. Therefore, all patients who have had cochlear implantation should be followed closely postoperatively.

Operative procedure

1. A U-shaped incision is made, creating a skin flap well behind the mastoid. The flap including the temporalis muscle is elevated, exposing the underlying bone. The site of the internal coil is identified, and with a special drill a circular depression in the squamous portion of the temporal bone is made to house the internal coil.
2. A mastoidectomy is accomplished with preservation of the bony ear canal and opening of the facial recess.
3. The coil is secured in the depressed area in the temporal bone, and the active electrode is introduced through the facial recess and through the round window 6 mm into the cochlea. It is secured in place with a piece of temporalis fascia. The other wire attached to the internal coil (ground wire) is introduced into the temporalis muscle.
4. The wound is closed. The patient is observed for several months until complete wound healing has occurred. Then the external device is applied over the internal coil.

Computerized facial nerve monitoring

Technology enables the surgeon to monitor movement and function of the facial nerve intraoperatively. This monitoring decreases trauma to the facial nerve during tumor dissection and assists the surgeon in determining the point of surgical intervention in idiopathic facial nerve palsy.

The mechanism of hearing can also be tested during surgical intervention to determine the effectiveness of a procedure and thus predict the patient's postoperative result.

Implantable hearing aids

A good deal of research in the development of implantable hearing aids is going on in different parts of the world. At the present time, conductive hearing aids are available for a small percentage of the hard-of-hearing who have conductive hearing loss due to chronic ear disease and cannot benefit from a hearing aid.

Implantable hearing aids for sensorineural hearing loss are the challenge of the future.

BIBLIOGRAPHY

Bray, C.A.: Benign but fatal: acoustic neuroma, Todays OR Nurse 6(1):8, 1984.

DeWeese, D.D., and Saunders, W.H.: Textbook of otolaryngology, ed. 6, St. Louis, 1982, The C.V. Mosby Co.

Goodhill, V.: Ear diseases, deafness and dizziness, Hagerstown, Md., Harper & Row.

Guyton, A.C.: Textbook of medical physiology, ed. 7, Philadelphia, 1986, W.B. Saunders Co.

Hanson, C., and others: Comprehensive care of patient undergoing stapedectomy for otosclerosis, Periop. Nurs. Q. 1(2):21, 1985.

Hood, G.H., and Dincher, J.R.: Total patient care: foundations and practice, ed. 6, St. Louis, 1984, The C.V. Mosby Co.

Iadarola, G., and Kerrigan, M.B.: Do you hear what I hear? Cochlear implants aid the deaf, AORN J. 43:478, 1986.

Kneedler, J., and Dodge, G.: Perioperative patient care, ed. 2, Boston, 1987, Blackwell Scientific Publications.

Long, B.C., and Phipps, W.J.: Essentials of medical-surgical nursing, St. Louis, 1985, The C.V. Mosby Co.

Sabiston, D.C., Jr., editor: Davis-Christopher textbook of surgery: the biological basis of modern surgical practice, ed. 13, Philadelphia, 1986, W.B. Saunders Co.

Saunders, W.H., Paparella, M., and Miglets, A.W., Jr.: Atlas of ear surgery, ed. 4, St. Louis, 1986, The C.V. Mosby Co.

Saunders, W.H., and others: Nursing care in eye, ear, nose, and throat disorders, ed. 4, St. Louis, 1979, The C.V. Mosby Co.

Shambaugh, G.E.: Surgery of the ear, ed. 3, Philadelphia, 1980, W.B. Saunders Co.

20 Rhinologic and sinus surgery

KAREN S. McNEELY

The nose is covered with skin and is supported internally by bone and cartilage. The two external nares provide openings through which air can enter and leave the nasal cavity. These openings contain internal hairs that help prevent coarse particles sometimes carried by air from entering the nose.

Surgery of the nose is performed to treat internal and external injuries and malformations and to provide for effective functioning of the respiratory system.

SURGICAL ANATOMY

The nose is divided into the prominent external portion and the internal portion known as the nasal cavity (Fig. 20-1). The chief purpose of the nose is the preparation of air for use in the lungs.

The *external* nose projects from the face. The upper portion of the external nose is formed by the nasal bones and the frontal process of the maxillae, and the lower portion is formed by a group of nasal cartilages and connective tissue covered with skin (Fig. 20-2). The nostrils and the tip of the nose are shaped by the major alar cartilages. The nares are separated by the columella, which is formed by the lower margin of the septal cartilage, the medial parts of the major alar cartilages, and the anterior nasal spine, all of which are covered by skin. The nasal cavity is a hollow space behind the nose that is divided

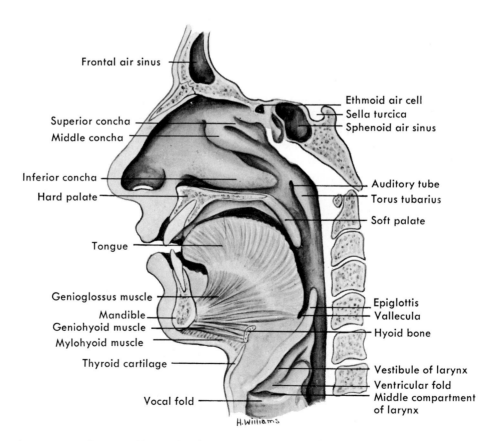

Fig. 20-1. Sagittal section of face and neck. (From Francis, C.C., and Martin, A.H.: Introduction to human anatomy, ed. 7, St. Louis, 1975, The C.V. Mosby Co.)

528

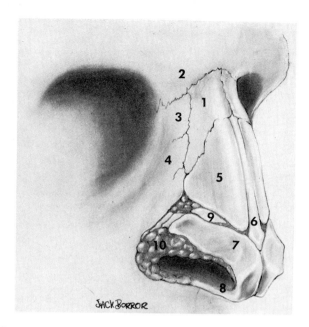

Fig. 20-2. Nasal bony framework. *1,* Nasal bone; *2,* frontal bone; *3,* lacrimal bone; *4,* maxillary bone; *5,* upper lateral cartilage; *6,* nasal septum; *7,* lower lateral cartilage, lateral crus; *8,* lower lateral cartilage, medial crus; *9,* sesamoid cartilage; *10,* fibrofatty tissue. (From Saunders, W.H., and others: Nursing care in eye, ear, nose, and throat disorders, ed. 4, St. Louis, 1979, The C.V. Mosby Co.)

medially into right and left portions by the nasal septum.

The nasal septum is composed of three structures: the nasal cartilage, the vomer bone, and the perpendicular plate of the ethmoid bone. The septum is covered by mucous membrane on either side. The deviated or fractured septum may be repaired surgically by mobilization of the fracture or removal of the deformed cartilage or bone.

The *internal* portion, or nasal cavity, is divided by the nasal septum into two parts at its midline. The nasal cavity communicates with the outside by its external openings, called the *nares.* The nares open into the nasopharynx through the choanae. The nasal cavity is also associated with each ear by means of the eustachian tube and with the paranasal sinuses (frontal, maxillary, ethmoidal, and sphenoidal) through their respective orifices (meatuses). The nasal cavity also communicates with the conjunctiva through the nasal duct. The nasal cavity is separated from the lingual cavity by the hard and soft palates (Fig. 20-1) and from the cranial cavity by the ethmoid bone. The nasal cavity is held together by periosteal covering and by perichondrium, which extends over the cartilages.

The *turbinate bones* of the nasal structure are arranged one above the other, separated by grooves and meatuses. These act as drainage passages of the accessory sinuses and are known as the sphenoethmoidal recesses and the superior, middle, and inferior meatuses, respectively (Fig. 20-3).

The nasal sinuses serve as air spaces and communicate with the nasal cavity through the meatuses. Anteriorly, on each side of the skull, the frontal sinus, the anterior ethmoidal sinus, and the maxillary sinus (antrum of Highmore) drain into the middle meatus; posteriorly, the ethmoidal and the sphenoidal sinuses drain into the superior meatus and the sphenoethmoidal recess. A passageway for the flow of air is provided by the irregular air spaces between these structures. Because of their shape, the air is forced to flow in thin air waves.

The sensory nerve supply of the nasal cavity is derived from the trigeminal nerve.

The nose and sinuses receive their blood supply (Fig. 20-4) from the branches of the internal maxillary, anterior ethmoid, sphenopalatine, nasopalatine, pharyngeal, and

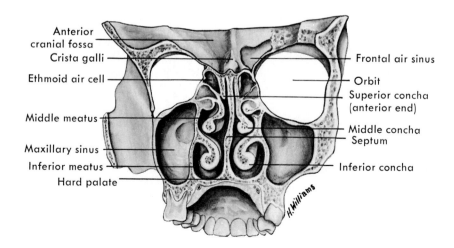

Fig. 20-3. Vertical section through nose. Plane of section passes slightly obliquely through left first molar tooth and behind second right premolar tooth. Posterior wall of right frontal sinus removed. (From Francis, C.C., and Martin, A.H.: Introduction to human anatomy, ed. 7, St. Louis, 1975, The C.V. Mosby Co.)

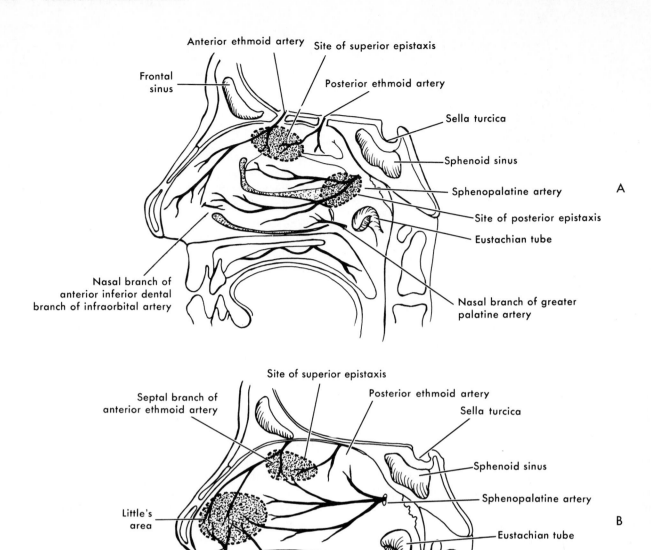

Fig. 20-4. A, Blood supply of lateral nasal wall. **B,** Arteries of nasal septum. (Modified from Ryan, R.E., and others: Synopsis of ear, nose, and throat diseases, ed. 3, St. Louis, 1970, The C.V. Mosby Co.)

posterior ethmoid arteries. Masses of communicating veins lie below the epithelial layer of the turbinate bones, and the veins just beneath the skin anastomose freely. Dilation of the superficial veins may cause the turbinate bones to swell, whereas contraction of these vessels may cause the bones to shrink.

PERIOPERATIVE NURSING CONSIDERATIONS
Assessment/nursing diagnosis

Because nasal surgery is sometimes performed with the patient under a local anesthetic, the perioperative nurse must collect comprehensive baseline data during preop-

erative assessment of the patient to facilitate accurate monitoring during the surgical procedure. That assessment should include vital signs, allergies, skin condition, sensory deficits, central nervous system problems, and mental status of the patient. Close attention should be paid to any past drug reactions experienced by the patient, especially if related to the administration of local anesthetics. Questions about previous dental experiences involving this type of anesthesia and the patient's tolerance to it can provide a clue to how the patient will react to the anesthetic agents.

Cardiac status should be noted because many surgeons use epinephrine as an additive to the local anesthetic. The epinephrine acts as a vasoconstrictor and reduces the blood loss during surgery but may also contribute to cardiac dysrhythmias. In addition, cocaine is often preoperatively administered intranasally to afford the patient more comfort during injection of local anesthetic and to achieve local vasoconstriction.

Respiratory patterns and any respiratory conditions, such as asthma, should be noted. Physical limitations of the patient can determine additional aspects that should be included in the intraoperative care of the patient.

Nursing diagnoses appropriate to patients undergoing rhinological or sinus surgery are as follows:

- Sensory/perceptual alterations (olfactory and gustatory) related to nasal packing postoperatively
- Potential for pain related to local anesthesia
- Anxiety related to fear of the unknown
- Potential for infection related to surgical site

Planning

Planning of the patient's care is based on the preoperative assessment and the nurse's knowledge of the scheduled surgical procedure and associated events, such as the administration of local anesthesia. Development of a meaningful care plan enables the perioperative nurse to meet the patient's needs effectively during surgical intervention.

Supplies necessary to assure comfort of the patient should be obtained. They may include a foam headrest, a pillow for under the knees, and warm blankets.

Preparation of the operating room includes checking the availability and functional capability of suction, the surgeon's headlight, the pulse oximeter to measure oxygen saturation, oxygen administration equipment, a cardiac monitor, and a blood pressure cuff.

Because local anesthesia is frequently utilized for nasal surgical procedures, the nurse must be prepared to react quickly to signs of allergic reactions or toxic responses. Symptoms of adverse drug reactions include changes in skin such as rash or itching, restlessness, unexplained anxiety or fearfulness, diaphoresis, complaints of blurred vision, tinnitus, dizziness, nausea, palpitation, disturbed respiration, pallor or flushing, and syncope. Emergency drugs, suction apparatus, and resuscitation equipment should be readily available.

The Sample Care Plan on p. 532 shows a generic care plan addressing the needs of patients undergoing rhinologic or sinus surgery.

Implementation

For most procedures the patient is placed on the operating room bed in a dorsal recumbent (supine) position. The hair in the nostrils may be clipped with fine, curved scissors. An antibiotic ophthalmic ointment may be put into the eyes of the patient to protect them from the prep solutions. The face may be scrubbed with povidone-io-dine. Prepping and draping of the patient are usually done before injection of the local anesthetic. However, the surgeon may request that the topical anesthetic be placed on the prep table so the nose may be topically anesthetized for a period before the anesthetic injections are started. This allows the topical anesthetic to take effect earlier and affords more comfort for the patient. Some surgeons also request that the local anesthetic be placed on the prep table so it can be injected before the skin is prepared. The circulating or monitor nurse should observe any changes in the vital signs of the patient. The amount of both topical and local anesthetic agents used and any additions to the local anesthetics, such as epinephrine, should be recorded on the appropriate records.

Several principles of nursing care are basic to all types of nasal surgery. The following information should be given to the patient.

1. Some discomfort may occur during the initial administration of a local anesthetic. If the surgeon uses a topical anesthetic (usually cocaine) as the first phase of anesthesia, it is applied to the nose with applicators. The patient may find the applicators or packing uncomfortable or may have the urge to sneeze. These sensations disappear as the anesthetic takes effect. The needle may cause momentary discomfort, and a burning sensation may occur as an anesthetic is injected. If the surgeon uses epinephrine with the local agent, the resulting weak, quivery feeling and the increased heart rate are effects of the epinephrine and disappear after a few minutes. The patient's cardiac status should be noted at this time.

2. Certain procedures may be performed on entry to the operating room or holding area in accordance with operating room policies, for example, insertion of intravenous lines, application of monitoring devices, and oxygen administration.

3. During the surgical procedure the patient feels the surgeon working and may feel pressure at some point, but should *not* feel pain. The patient should let the surgeon know if any discomfort is felt during the procedure, and more anesthetic can be given.

4. After surgery the head of the bed is elevated to facilitate breathing and drainage.

5. A nasal pack will probably be inserted, and there may be some difficulty in swallowing. When the patient attempts to swallow, a sucking action occurs in the throat because the packing does not allow air passage through the nose, thereby creating a partial vacuum.

6. Measures to maintain oral hygiene are frequently offered and encouraged because of the postoperative mouth breathing.

7. Some bruising and swelling can be expected after surgery but gradually subside.

Sample Care Plan

NURSING DIAGNOSIS:
Sensory/perceptual alterations (olfactory and gustatory) related to nasal packing postoperatively
GOAL:
The patient will verbalize understanding of the anticipated alteration in the senses of smell and taste.
INTERVENTIONS:
Explain to the patient that a "moustache" dressing will be in place postoperatively and that it will greatly interfere with the sense of smell.
Inform the patient that the sense of taste will also be altered, as with having a head cold.
Assure the patient that these alterations are usually temporary.
Encourage the patient to maintain proper dietary intake even if the food does not smell or taste as it should.

NURSING DIAGNOSIS:
Potential for pain related to local anesthesia
GOAL:
The patient will verbalize knowledge of the physical and psychologic responses to surgical pain.
INTERVENTIONS:
Explain to the patient that some initial discomfort (for example, pin prick, followed by slight burning, then numbness) may be felt during the administration of the local anesthetic.
Inform the patient prior to the injection of the local anesthetic; provide support and reassurance as needed.
Describe the sequence of events to the patient to prevent unrealistic expectations.
Monitor nurse should observe for, document, and report any changes in the patient's vital signs (blood pressure, heart rate and rhythm, respiratory rate, and oxygen saturation), skin condition, or mental status.

Monitor nurse should be aware of the maximum recommended doses of local anesthetics (Chapter 4) and alert for signs of allergic reactions or toxic responses.
Ask the patient whether he or she is experiencing any pain; communicate the presence of pain sensation to the surgeon.

NURSING DIAGNOSIS:
Anxiety related to fear of the unknown
GOAL:
The patient will verbalize knowledge of the steps of the perioperative process.
INTERVENTIONS:
Using a teaching guide such as a photo album, inform the patient and family of what the preop holding area, OR, and PACU look like. Explain the function of each.
Explain all activities performed by the nursing staff and provide the rationale for each.
Assure the patient that he or she will be informed before any procedure is done.
Provide time for the patient to express fears and concerns.
Include family if appropriate.

NURSING DIAGNOSIS:
Potential for infection related to surgical site
GOAL:
The patient will be free from signs and symptoms of infection.
INTERVENTIONS:
Review chart for recent lab results and vital signs.
Obtain baseline data (skin integrity, color).
Maintain aseptic technique and handwashing practices.
Explain the importance of the "moustache" dressing.
Demonstrate correct procedure for "moustache" dressing change.

8. Forceful nose blowing must be avoided for a time to prevent movement of the rearranged nasal structures.
9. The sense of smell is diminished for a time after surgery but gradually returns.
10. Some numbness may be noticed postoperatively, but this gradually disappears.
11. A moderate amount of discomfort should be expected after surgery; medication is ordered for this.
12. There is a procedure for changing the "moustache" dressing that is in place postoperatively to absorb any drainage. This procedure should be reviewed with the patient.

Draping

The patient is draped as follows.

1. A small sheet with two towels on top of it is placed over the head of the bed and under the patient's head ("head drape").
2. The uppermost towel is brought around the head, including the hairline.
3. The ends of the uppermost towel are secured with a towel clamp, and the free ends are tucked under the patient's head.
4. A split sheet is applied.
5. Moist gauze pads, tape, Band-Aids, or a towel is placed over the patient's eyes to protect them from injury by instruments and from nasal drainage.

Instrumentation

Sterile instruments, supplies, and other items required for rhinologic surgery include the following:

Local anesthesia setup

Cocaine crystals, 4 grains
Cocaine topical solution, 4% or 10%
Lidocaine 1% or 2% (usually with epinephrine 1:100,000)
Luer-Lok syringes, 3 and 5 ml
Needles, 27-gauge (1½ inches) and 30-gauge (1 inch)
Bayonet tissue forceps
Metal applicators
Cotton balls
Gauze packing in ½ × 12 inch strips

Supplies

1 ENT drape pack
1 Split sheet (if not included in the pack)
1 Gauze packing (plain or petrolatum) ½ inch by 48 inches
3 Medication cups
1 Marking pen
1 Package of labels
1 Basin set
  Gloves
2 Gowns
1 Skin prep tray
1 Tube of antibiotic ointment or cream
1 Headlight

Cutting instruments (Figs. 20-5 and 20-6)

2 Knife handles no. 3 or no. 7 for intranasal procedures with no. 15 blades
1 Myles septum-cutting forceps
1 Ballenger swivel knife
1 Freer septum knife
1 Septal forceps
1 Kerrison rongeur
1 Freer septum chisel
1 Freer dissecting elevator
1 Ballenger nasal gouge
1 Knight scissors
1 Fomon scissors
1 Joseph knife (sharp)
1 Joseph knife (blunt)
1 McKenty knife
1 Button knife
1 Maltz rasp
1 Glabella rasp
1 Fomon rasp
2 Freer nasal saws (right and left)
2 Neivert osteotomes (right and left)
2 Narrow osteotomes
1 Bone cutter
2 Jansen-Middleton forceps (open and closed)
6 Coakley curettes (assorted shapes and angles)
1 Suture scissors

Holding and clamping instruments

5 Towel clamps
2 Kelly hemostats, straight
1 Mayo forceps, curved
2 Bayonet tissue forceps
1 Adson tissue forceps

Exposing instruments (Fig. 20-7, p. 536)

2 Killian nasal specula
1 Cottle nasal speculum
4 Skin hooks (two single and two double)
  Retractors, assorted sizes

Suturing items

1 Needle holder, small
1 Jacobson bayonet needle holder (for intranasal procedures)
  Suture of the surgeon's preference

Accessory items (Fig. 20-8, p. 536)

1 Ruler
3 Frazier suction tips (various sizes)
1 Suction tubing
  Obturators for suction tips
1 Mallet
1 Yankauer suction tube
1 Caliper
1 Antrum suction tip

Postoperative care of instruments

Care of the instruments used in nasal surgery follows the general care regimen of any other surgical instruments. Chisels, gouges, and other cutting instruments should be inspected carefully for any nicks and for dullness and sent for repair as needed. Using damaged instruments may cause tissue damage in succeeding procedures. Rasps and files should be thoroughly cleaned and all bone debris removed. Special attention should also be given to suction tips. Lenses on headlights used during the procedure should be checked for cleanliness. Spatter on lenses should be removed according to the manufacturer's instructions.

Evaluation

The patient should be assessed postoperatively for any difficulties in breathing. Nasal packing inhibits breathing; however, the patient should be able to breathe normally through the mouth. Reddened or bruised areas related to positioning should be noted and treatment begun. The amount of drainage present on the moustache dressing should be noted. The head of the PACU bed should be elevated before transport to the unit. A thorough report is called to PACU and any variances reported. Goals of the nursing care plan are reviewed and may be communicated and documented as outcome statements:

- The patient verbalized understanding of anticipated postoperative alteration in the senses of smell and taste.

- The patient demonstrated effective coping with the physical and psychological effects of pain.
- The patient's anxiety was reduced.
- The patient will experience no signs and symptoms of infection postoperatively

SURGICAL INTERVENTIONS
Rhinologic surgery
Submucous resection of the septum, or septoplasty

A septoplasty is removal of either the cartilaginous or osseous portions of the septum that lie between the flaps of the mucous membrane and the perichondrium.

When the nasal septum is deformed, fractured, or injured, normal respiratory function and nasal drainage may be impaired. Deviations of the septum involving cartilage, bony parts (spurs), or both may block the meatus and compress the middle turbinate on that side, thereby resulting in an obstruction of the sinus opening. Septal deviations tend to produce sinus disease and nasal polyps.

The objective of a submucous resection is to establish an adequate partition between the left and right nasal cav-

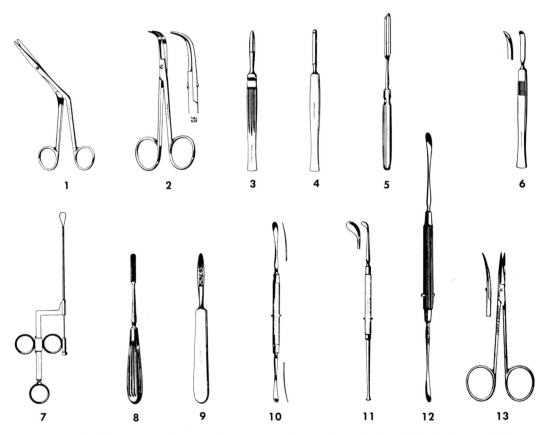

Fig. 20-5. Cutting instruments for operations on external nose and nasal cavity. *1,* Nasal scissors, angled; *2,* Fomon upper lateral scissors; *3,* cartilage knife, beveled blade; *4,* cartilage knife, straight; *5,* cartilage knife, swivel blade; *6,* cartilage nasal knife, curved; *7,* nasal snare; *8,* nasal rasp, narrow; *9,* nasal rasp; *10,* double-ended elevator; *11,* golf stick elevator-dissector; *12,* Freer dissecting elevator; *13,* iris scissors, straight and curved. (Courtesy Codman & Shurtleff, Inc., Randolph, Mass.)

ities, thereby providing a clear airway through both the internal and external cavities of the nose.

Procedural considerations. The setup is as described in the general preparation for nasal surgery.

Operative procedure

1. The nostril is opened with a speculum. An incision is made through the mucoperichondrium and mucoperiosteum of the septum with a knife having a no. 15 blade. The tissues are separated and elevated with a Freer knife (Fig. 20-9).

2. The cartilage is incised with a knife, and the mucous membrane is elevated with a Ballenger knife and a septal elevator; deviated cartilage and bony, thickened structures are removed with a septum punch and a nasal cutting forceps.

3. The mucous membrane is freed from the bony septal base by means of a chisel, gouge and mallet, or punch forceps. Bleeding is controlled by gauze sponges; suctioning is used to expose the field.

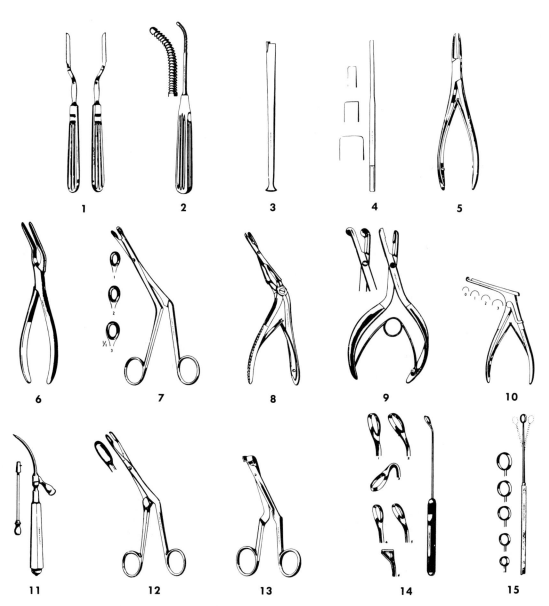

Fig. 20-6. Cutting instruments for operations on external nose and nasal cavity, continued. *1*, Freer nasal saws, right and left; *2*, reamer; *3*, nasal chisel with guard; *4*, osteotome, narrow widths; *5*, nasal bone cutter; *6*, Asch septum forceps; *7*, Bruening septum forceps; *8*, double-action nasal rongeur; *9*, McCoy septum forceps; *10*, Kerrison rongeur; *11*, antrum trocar and stylet; *12*, septum-cutting forceps; *13*, septal ridge—cutting forceps; *14*, Coakley ethmoidal sinus curettes; *15*, Myles antrum ring curettes. (Courtesy Codman & Shurtleff, Inc. Randolph Mass.)

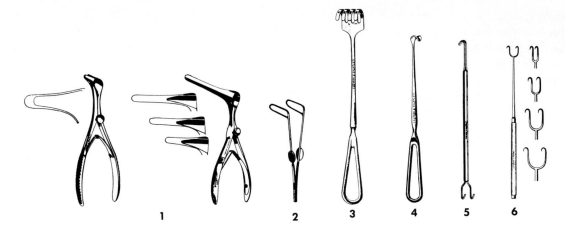

Fig. 20-7. Exposing instruments for operations on external nose, nasal cavity, and sinuses. *1*, Vienna and Killian nasal specula; *2*, Bosworth nasal wire speculum; *3*, Volkmann rake retractor; *4*, Cushing vein retractor; *5*, one- and two-pronged retractor, double-ended; *6*, two-pronged retractors, sharp, various sizes. (Courtesy Codman & Shurtleff, Randolph, Mass.)

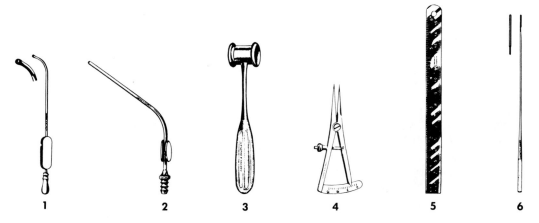

Fig. 20-8. Accessory instruments for operations on external nose and nasal cavity. *1*, Antrum suction tip; *2*, Frazier suction tip; *3*, metal mallet; *4*, caliper; *5*, ruler; *6*, nasal applicator. (Courtesy Codman & Shurtleff, Inc., Randolph, Mass.)

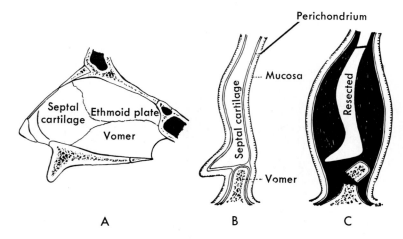

Fig. 20-9. A, Primary components of septum. Incision line is for Killian type of submucous resection. **B,** Septum with deviated cartilage and spur at junction of vomer and septal cartilage. **C,** Resection of obstructive parts after careful elevation of mucoperichondrium and mucoperiosteum. (From DeWeese, D.D., and Saunders, W.H.: Textbook of otolaryngology, ed. 6, St. Louis, 1982, The C.V. Mosby Co.)

4. The perpendicular plate of the ethmoidal sinus, as well as the vomer, may be removed by means of the retractor, chisel and mallet, and suitable septum-cutting forceps (Fig. 20-6).
5. The incision may be sutured with plain no. 4-0 atraumatic suture on a small straight needle.
6. Nostrils are packed with gauze impregnated with antibiotic ointment or cream to keep the septal flaps in a midline position. Some surgeons use nasal tampons that provide a patent airway while maintaining support for the septum. They are used instead of packing. The face is cleansed with moist and dry compresses. A moustache dressing may be applied. External dressings or splints depend on the surgeon's preference, as does application of a small ice bag to the nose. A surgical glove filled with ice is an excellent ice bag because it is small and lightweight.

Corrective rhinoplasty

A corrective rhinoplasty is removal of the hump, narrowing and shortening of the nose, and reconstruction of the tip of the nose.

Rhinoplasty may help solve the patient's physiologic or psychologic problems.

Procedural considerations. The patient's face is prepped as described in the general preparation for nasal surgery. The patient is usually placed in a dorsal recumbent position. The rhinoplasty and nasal instruments are shown in Figs. 20-10 and 20-11.

Operative procedure
1. An incision is made through the skin of one nostril with a knife and no. 15 blade. A second incision is made in the other nostril and carried around the columella to join the first incision. A nasal speculum, sponges, and skin hooks are used.
2. The skin of the nose is undermined by elevators, knives, and scissors. The periosteum and periochondrium are freed with elevators, saws, and a periosteal dissector.
3. The nasal bone or upper lateral cartilage is fractured. The hump and possibly the septal cartilage are removed by means of cutting forceps, such as the Jansen-Middleton; osteotomes, such as the Kazanjian action type; mallet; plastic scissors; and Adson forceps. The field is cleared by suctioning and by sponging with bayonet forceps.

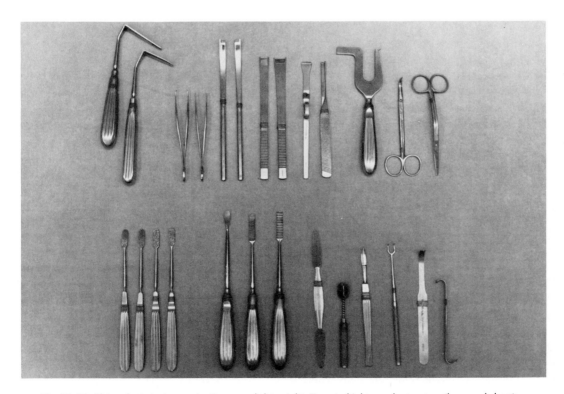

Fig. 20-10. Rhinoplasty instruments. *Top row, left to right:* Two Aufricht nasal retractors (long and short); Beasley Babcock tissue forceps; Adson Brown tissue forceps; Converse curved, guarded chisel, left; Converse curved, guarded chisel, right; Cinelli osteotome, 10 mm; Cinelli osteotome, 14 mm; Rubin osteotome, 14 mm; Parkes lateral osteotomy chisel; Rubin nasofrontal osteotome; Fomon upper lateral scissors; Fomon dorsal scissors. *Bottom row, left to right:* Four diamond rasps (two curved, two straight); Aufricht glabellar rasp; two Parkes rasps (fine and medium); Converse rasp; wire brush; Cottle knife; double-pronged skin hook; Parkes nasal retractor; S-shaped blade retractor.

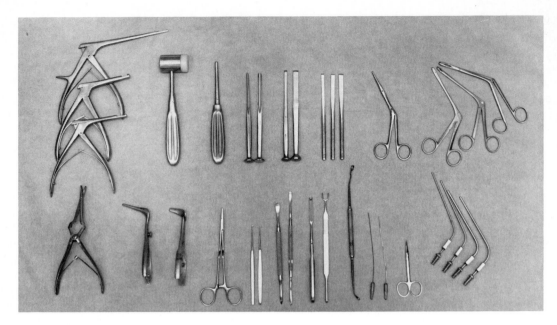

Fig. 20-11. Nasal instruments. *Top row, left to right:* Kerrison rongeurs, 2, 4, and 6 mm; mallet; septal displacer; gouges; small chisels; small osteotomes; Knight nasal scissors; Knight polyp forceps, small medium, and large. *Bottom row, left to right:* Jansen-Middleton forceps; medium and short nasal specula; Jacobson-Bayonet needle holder; single skin hooks; Alberg periosteal elevator; Freer elevator; Ballenger swivel knife; Cottle knife guard/retractor; Faulkner antrum curette (double ended); University of Iowa cotton applicators; Knapp scissors, light curve; Frazier suction tips, sizes 1, 2, 3, and 4.

4. The edges of the cartilages are trimmed by means of septum forceps and scissors.
5. To prevent or control infection and the formation of a hematoma, the blood is suctioned from the nose, and the wound is cleansed.
6. The cartilage and bones are molded into proper postion. The columella is sutured back onto the septum with fine silk sutures. The membranous septal edges are closed; dressings with a pressure splint are applied and held in place with tape. A moustache dressing may be secured below the nares to absorb any bleeding. The head is elevated, and ice packs may be applied to the eyelids.

Sinus surgery

Intranasal antrostomy (antral window)

An intranasal antrostomy is an opening made in the lateral wall of the nose under the middle turbinate and the removal of the anterior end of the inferior turbinate (Figs. 20-3 and 20-4). The objective of this procedure is to relieve edema or infection of the membrane lining the sinuses and resultant headaches.

Procedural considerations. The setup is as described in the general preparation for nasal surgery. The instrument setup includes the following:

5 Towel clamps
2 Nasal specula

4 Dean applicators
1 Metal tongue depressor
1 Yankauer suction tube
2 Antrum suction tips
1 Universal handle with punches
1 Dean antrum rasp, concave
2 Dean antrum rasps, left and right
2 Wiener rasps, dull and sharp
6 Coakley curettes
1 Freer elevator
1 Dean elevator
2 Bayonet forceps
1 Suture scissors
2 Knife handles, no. 7, with no. 15 blades
1 Polyp forceps
1 Nasal snare with wires
2 Syringes

Operative procedure

1. When the patient has been anesthetized, prepped, and draped, the inferior turbinate is explored with bone-cutting forceps, elevators, and dissectors (Fig. 20-5).
2. An opening is made into the maxillary sinus (Fig. 20-3) beneath the inferior turbinate by means of a gouge, perforator, or rasp (Fig. 20-6). The opening is enlarged with cutting forceps and antrum punches. Accessory polyps and degenerate mucosa are removed with a snare, polyp forceps, and suction.
3. The sinus can be irrigated with saline solution and suctioned. The sinus is packed with gauze impregnated

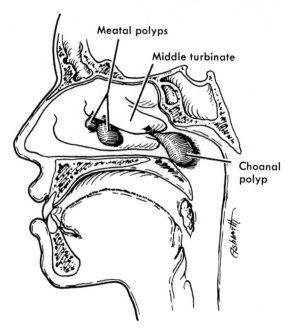

Fig. 20-12. Nasal polyps. Choanal polyp is usually single and originates in maxillary sinus; however, most polyps are found in middle meatus. (From DeWeese, D.D., and Saunders, W.H.: Textbook of otolaryngology, ed. 6, St. Louis, 1982, The C.V. Mosby Co.)

with antibiotic ointment or cream. The face is cleansed, and a drip pad (moustache dresssing) is applied under the nostrils.

Nasal polypectomy

A nasal polypectomy is the removal of polyps from the nasal cavity (Fig. 20-12).

The tissues become edematous, resulting in the formation of polyps that obstruct the free passage of air and make breathing difficult.

Procedural considerations. For polyps arising from the border of the middle turbinate, the instruments are as described for submucous resection. An intranasal setup is used if the polyps arise above or from the semilunar hiatus. In some cases polyps are removed in conjunction with a Caldwell-Luc operation, ethmoidectomy, enlargement of the frontal sinus, or opening of the sphenoidal sinus.

Operative procedure. The operation is as described for the intranasal antrostomy or other types of operations on the sinuses with removal of the polyps and degenerated tissue.

If the intranasal approach is used, the surgeon applies local and topical anesthetics to shrink the mucosa and ensure vasoconstriction and then removes the polyps with a nasal snare, obtains hemostasis, and packs the nose with an antibiotic-impregnated gauze. A drip pad or moustache dressing is then applied under the nostrils.

Radical antrostomy (Caldwell-Luc operation)

A radical antrostomy entails an incision into the canine fossa of the upper jaw and exposure of the antrum for removal of bony diseased portions of the antral wall and contents of the sinus (Fig. 20-13), or establishment of drainage by means of a counteropening into the nose through the inferior meatus.

In the presence of pus in acute sinus disease, the mucous membrane may become thickened and polyps may form, resulting in an obstruction of the nasal cavity and external passageway. In such cases the patient suffers from nasal catarrh, headaches, and cough. Chronic sinusitis may be associated with asthma.

The purpose of a radical antrostomy is to establish a large opening in the nasoantral wall of the inferior meatus, which ensures adequate gravity drainage and aeration and permits removal, under direct vision, of all diseased tissues in the sinus.

Procedural considerations. The setup is as described for intranasal antrostomy, plus the following:

2 Jansen-Middleton septum-cutting forceps
2 Kerrison rongeurs (upbiting and straight)
1 Ferris-Smith forceps
1 Killian dressing forceps
1 Weil nasal forceps
1 Ethmoid curette
2 Caldwell-Luc retractors
1 Mallet
2 Kelly hemostats
2 Allis forceps
8 Towel clamps
1 Adson tissue forceps with teeth
1 Adson-Brown tissue forceps
2 Single skin hooks
2 Double skin hooks
2 Freer elevators (sharp and dull)
1 Pennington elevator
1 Ball-ended elevator
1 Ballenger V-shaped chisel
1 Knight nasal scissors
1 Takahashi forceps
2 Ethmoid forceps (straight and upbiting)
1 Metzenbaum scissors
2 Mayo scissors (curved and straight)
2 Scissors, curved, small, blunt and sharp
1 Suture scissors
2 Knife handles, no. 3 and no. 7, with no. 15 blades
2 Straight chisels, 2 mm and 4 mm

The patient is usually given a general anesthetic.

Operative procedure (Fig. 20-13)
1. The upper lip is elevated with a Caldwell-Luc retracor, and a transverse incision is made in the gingivolabial sulcus just above the teeth; the incision is carried down to the underlying bone. Periosteum and soft tissue are elevated with dissectors and periosteal elevators.
2. The thin bony plate is perforated with a chisel, the antrum is entered, and its opening is enlarged with nasal rongeurs. The anterior angle of the sinus may be opened

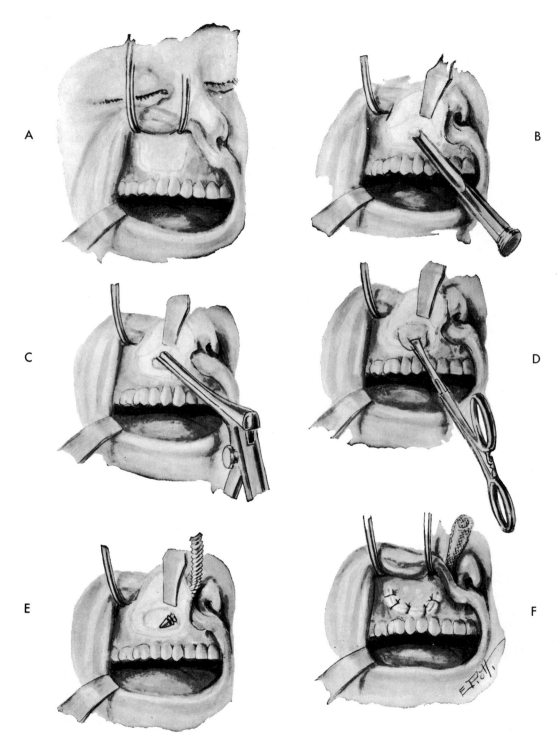

Fig. 20-13. Caldwell-Luc operation. **A,** Incision. **B,** Flap retracted and perforation made in canine fossa. **C,** Perforation enlarged with Kerrison rongeur. **D,** Removal of diseased antral membrane. **E,** Rasp used to make nasoantral window. **F,** Incision closed. (From Thoma, K.H.: Oral surgery, ed. 5, St. Louis, 1969, The C.V. Mosby Co.)

by enlarging the window with Jansen-Middleton septum-cutting forceps, double-action rongeurs, and Kerrison rongeurs.

3. The mucous membrane of the antrum is removed with Coakley curettes and Takahashi forceps.
4. Nasoantral drainage may be established by removal of a portion of the nasoantral wall below the inferior turbinate by means of cutting forceps and rasps.
5. The nose and sinus are packed with antibiotic or petrolatum-impregnated gauze.
6. The labial incision may be sutured with chromic no. 3-0 atraumatic suture on a small curved needle. The patient's face is cleansed and dried. If iodoform packing is used, the patient should be warned that there may be a foul taste in the mouth postoperatively.

Endoscopic sinus surgery

Endoscopic sinus surgery involves the endoscopic resection of inflammatory and anatomic defects of the sinuses. The amount of disease resected is much less than that removed by the more traditional methods.

The purpose of endoscopic sinus surgery is to ensure adequate ventilation and to restore mucociliary clearance in the sinuses. If there is contact between the mucosa and the sinuses, mucociliary clearance is inhibited and secretions are retained in the sinus, which predisposes the patient to sinus infections.

Endoscopic sinus surgery can bring relief to patients with chronic sinus problems. This procedure is preferred to the Caldwell-Luc procedure because there is decreased morbidity.

Candidates for endoscopic sinus surgery are patients who have had recurrent acute or chronic sinusitis that is not treatable with antibiotics. Chronic sinusitis can be caused by anatomic deformities or an allergy history. Immunologic abnormalities, fluctuations in hormone levels, and environmental factors may also contribute to chronic sinusitis. Patients who are considered candidates for endoscopic sinus surgery undergo an office endoscopic exam preoperatively. During this procedure none of the sinus cavities is opened. These patients must also have CT scans done to determine the areas affected by the sinusitis.

Procedural considerations. Endoscopic sinus surgery instruments include (Fig. 20-14):

    0-degree, 30-degree, 70-degree, 120-degree endoscopes
4 Straight forceps
4 Angled forceps
3 Nasal specula
6 Ethmoid curettes
2 Curved suction tips

This procedure may be done under local anesthesia with IV sedation. The patient is placed in a supine position.

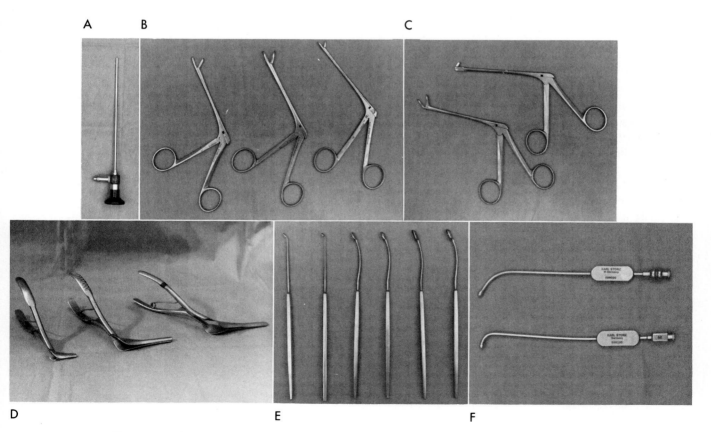

Fig. 20-14. Endoscopic sinus surgery instruments. **A,** Endoscope. **B,** Straight forceps. **C,** Angled forceps. **D,** Nasal specula. **E,** Ethmoid curettes. **F,** Curved suction tips.

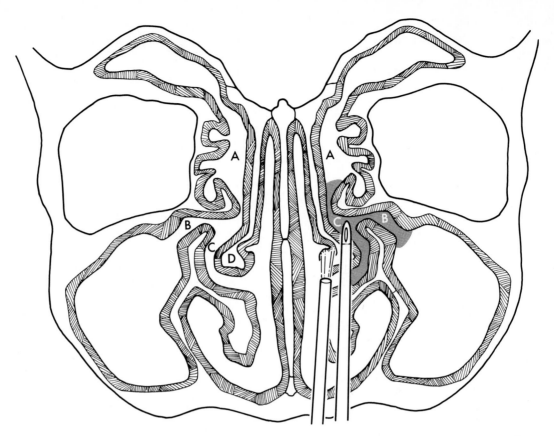

Fig. 20-15. Surgery is performed using an endoscope and forceps via an intranasal approach. Diseased tissue is being removed from the shaded areas depicting **(A)** the ethmoid sinus area, **(B)** the maxillary sinus ostia, and **(C)** the middle meatus. The **(D)** middle turbinate is unaffected. (From Thawley, S.E., and Garrett, H.: Endoscopic sinus surgery: an outpatient procedure that minimizes tissue removal, AORN J. 47:902, 1988. Copyright © AORN, Inc., 10170 East Mississippi Avenue, Denver, Colo. 80231)

The face and throat are prepped, and the patient is draped as for other nasal procedures.

Operative procedure

1. The surgeon may apply topical anesthesia, followed by the local anesthesia.
2. The anterior wall of the maxillary sinus (Fig. 20-3) is entered through a 5-mm incision.
3. The diseased tissue is visualized through a 0-, 30-, 70-, or 120-degree endoscope. Straight or angled forceps may be used to remove only the diseased tissue (Fig. 20-15).
4. If an anterior ethmoidectomy is indicated, the endoscope is inserted through the middle meatus (Fig. 20-3) into the frontal recess, and the ethmoidectomy is performed.
5. Due to the small incisions made, no sutures are required.
6. Antibiotic ointment is applied intranasally using a 10-cc syringe with a small catheter on the end to ensure proper placement.
7. Nasal packing is not required. A moustache dressing is applied.

Frontal sinus operation (external approach)

A frontal sinus operation involves making an incision through the anterior wall of the floor of the frontal sinus for removal of diseased tissue, cleansing of the sinus cavity, and drainage.

In acute frontal sinusitis, in which the patient suffers from persistent headaches and edema of the upper eyelid, and in cases in which medical therapy has failed, surgical treatment may be indicated. Drainage of the frontal sinus may be performed by a simple trephine opening through the floor of the sinus. In the presence of chronic suppuration with repeated acute attacks of frontal sinusitis, surgery may be done to remove the diseased lining of the sinus and to reconstruct the nasofrontal duct, thereby ensuring adequate drainage.

Procedural considerations. The setup is as described for intranasal antrostomy, plus the following items:

1 Power saw with oscillating blade
2 Brawley or Spratt frontal rasps
1 Potts or Cushing nerve hook, blunt
2 Cushing forceps, straight, fine
2 Adson tissue forceps

Dural hooks
Raney clip appliers and clips

The patient is given a general anesthetic.

The surgical approach used depends on the preference of the surgeon and the patient. If a coronal incision is to be made, the hair should be shaved from the hairline to slightly past the crown of the head. If a brow incision is to be made, no shaving is necessary. Fat may be taken from the abdomen for subsequent use in obliterating the sinus space.

The patient's eyes are usually protected during the procedure with tarsorrhaphies (suturing the eyelids closed), sterile ocular occluders, or tape. The patient's head and face are prepped with a povidone-iodine scrub and solution.

Operative procedure

1A. When a *coronal* approach is used, the incision is made in the scalp skin from ear to ear, well behind the hairline. The edges of the skin are compressed by the application of Raney clips. The flap is reflected to expose the upper portion of the nose, thus exposing the anterior of the sinus.

1B. When a *brow* approach is used, the incision is made in the superior margin of the eyebrow(s), hemostasis is obtained, and the flap is elevated, exposing the anterior sinus wall.

2. A template (steam-sterilized radiological outline of the frontal sinus) is placed over the sinus and marked on the pericranium with a marking pen.

3. The pericranium is elevated.

4. An oscillating saw is used to cut through the bone overlying the frontal sinus. An elevator may be used to free the bone from the sinus.

5. The mucosa of the sinus is removed in its entirety through the use of elevators and a drill.

6. Absorbable gelatin sponge or a fat graft taken from the abdomen is placed in the sinus to obliterate the space.

7. The bone flap is replaced, and the pericranium is repositioned and sutured.

8. The skin incision is closed with suture of the surgeon's preference.

9. A pressure dressing of elastic gauze is applied for 48 to 72 hours.

Potential postoperative complications include osteomyelitis, meningitis, cerebrospinal fluid leak, abscess, and stenosis of the nasofrontal duct.

Frontal sinus trephination

Frontal sinus trephination is the creation of a hole in the frontal sinus to drain pus or fluid accumulation. This procedure is performed for early signs of frontal sinusitis. After the procedure the patient should be observed for signs of intracranial involvement.

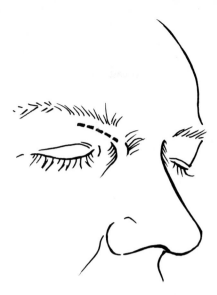

Fig. 20-16. Incision to expose ethmoidal and frontal sinuses. Resulting scar is almost invisible.

Procedural considerations. The patient's face is prepped with a povidone-iodine scrub and solution. The face is draped as previously described. The skin under the eyebrow is injected with lidocaine with or without epinephrine.

Operative procedure

1. The incision is made medially below the eyebrow, along the same contour of the brow (Fig. 20-16).

2. The periosteum is elevated from the bone, and a small diamond or cutting burr is used to create a hole into the sinus.

3. Cultures are generally taken before the aspiration of the pus present in the sinus.

4. A large Silastic or Teflon tube or a large catheter is placed through the incision into the sinus to facilitate postoperative irrigation.

5. The incision is closed with suture of the surgeon's preference.

6. A small dressing is usually applied to absorb drainage from the incision and catheter.

Ethmoidectomy

An ethmoidectomy is the removal of the diseased portion of the middle turbinate, removal of ethmoidal cells, and removal of diseased tissue in the nasal fossa through a nasal or an external approach.

The purpose of an ethmoidectomy is to reduce the many-celled ethmoidal labyrinth into one large cavity to ensure adequate drainage and aeration.

Procedural considerations. The setup for the *nasal approach* is as described for intranasal antrostomy; for the *external approach* the setup is as described for the frontal sinus operation.

Operative procedure. For the nasal route, the procedure is similar to intranasal antrostomy described previously. For the external route, the procedure is similar to the frontal sinus operation described previously.

Sphenoidectomy

A sphenoidectomy is the making of an opening into one or both of the sphenoidal sinuses by the intranasal or external ethmoidectomy approach. In surgical treatment of sinusitis of the sphenoidal sinus, visualizing the cavity is difficult because of its depth. Surgery of the sphenoidal sinus is usually performed intranasally or through an external ethmoidectomy approach.

Procedural considerations. The setup is as described for intranasal antrostomy, with the addition of long sphenoid curettes, antrum rasps, and antrum punches.

Operative procedure. The operation is as described for intranasal antrostomy.

Turbinectomy

Anterior inferior turbinectomy is removal of the anterior end of the inferior turbinate. *Inferior turbinectomy* is removal of the greater part of the lower border of the hypertrophied inferior turbinate. *Anterior middle turbinectomy* is removal of the anterior end of the middle turbinate body. In all cases, turbinectomy may include removal of polyps (Fig. 20-12). A turbinectomy is preferred to provide adequate ventilation and drainage and relieve pressure against the floor of the nose.

Procedural considerations. The setup is as described for intranasal antrostomy.

Operative procedure. The nose is packed with petrolatum-impregnated gauze on all sides of the turbinate. An incision is made. The affected turbinate is amputated and removed, the polyps are removed, and the cavity is packed, as described for intranasal antrostomy.

Crushing of turbinates

Turbinate crushing is similar to turbinectomy, except that the turbinate is compressed with heavy forceps, such as a morselizer.

Repair of nasal fracture

Repair of a nasal fracture involves manipulation and mobilization of nasal bones. When the nose is struck by a direct frontal blow, usually both nasal bones are fractured, displaced outward, and depressed into the ethmoidal sinus (Fig. 20-3). The septal cartilages are displaced. Prompt reduction should be done.

Procedural considerations. The patient is placed on the operating room bed in a dorsal recumbent position, and a topical anesthetic may be applied.

The setup includes a topical anesthesia set, plus a rubber-covered Salinger elevator or Asch septum-straightening forceps, a straight hemostat, petrolatum-impregnated gauze packing, a plastic mold or aluminum splint, and adhesive tape.

Operative procedure. A rubber-shod narrow forceps is inserted into the nostril; the nasal bones are elevated and molded into place by external manipulation.

BIBLIOGRAPHY

Aminio, P.A.: Perioperative nursing documentation, AORN J, 46:1, 1987.

Association of Operating Room Nurses: Recommended practices for monitoring the patient receiving local anesthesia. In AORN standards and recommended practices for perioperative nursing, Denver, 1990, The Association.

DeWeese, D.D., and Saunders, W.H.: Textbook of otolaryngology, ed. 6, St. Louis, 1982, The C.V. Mosby Co.

Guyton, A.C.: Textbook of medical physiology, ed. 7, Philadelphia, 1986, W.B. Saunders Co.

Hood, G.H., and Dincher, J.R.: Total patient care: foundations and practices, ed. 6, St. Louis, 1984, The C.V. Mosby Co.

Ivey, D.F.: Local anesthesia: implications for the perioperative nurse, AORN J. 45:3, 1987.

Karmody, C.S.: Textbook of otolaryngology, Philadephia, 1983, Lea & Febiger.

Kleinbeck, S.V. M.: Developing nursing diagnoses for a perioperative care plan, AORN J, 49:6, 1989.

Long, B.C., and Phipps, W.J.: Essentials of medical-surgical nursing, St. Louis, 1985, The C.V. Mosby Co.

Sabiston, D.C., Jr., editor: Davis-Christopher textbook of surgery: the biological basis of modern surgical practice, ed. 13, Philadelphia, 1986, W.B. Saunders Co.

Saunders, W.H., and others: Nursing care in eye, ear, nose, and throat disorders, ed. 4, St. Louis, 1979, The C.V. Mosby Co.

Thawley, S.E., and Garrett, H.: Endoscopic sinus surgery, AORN J, 47:4, 1988.

21 Laryngologic and head and neck surgery

SUE SILCOX

SURGICAL ANATOMY

The *throat* includes the structures of the neck in front of the vertebral column; these are the mouth, tongue, pharynx, tonsils, larynx, and trachea.

The *mouth* extends from the lips to the anterior pillars of the fauces. The portion of the mouth outside the teeth is the buccal cavity, and that on the inner side of the teeth is the lingual cavity. The tongue occupies a large portion of the floor of the mouth. The hard and soft palates form the upper and posterior boundaries of the oral cavity, separating it from the nasal cavity and the nasopharynx. The soft palate emerges from the posterior border of the hard palate to form the uvula, a fingerlike movable projection. On either side the uvula joins the base of the tongue anteriorly and the pharynx posteriorly.

The *pharynx* serves as a channel for both the digestive and respiratory systems. It is situated behind the nasal cavities, mouth, and larynx. The food and air passages cross each other in the pharynx. The pharynx is a funnel-shaped structure, wider above and narrower below, about 12 cm in length. It is composed of muscular and fibrous layers and lined with mucous membrane. It is associated above with the sphenoidal sinus and the basilar part of the occipital bone, and it joins the esophagus below. Seven cavities communicate with the pharynx: the two nasal cavities, the two tympanic cavities, the mouth, the larynx, and the esophagus. The cavity of the pharynx may be subdivided from above downward into three parts: nasal, oral, and laryngeal. Infection may spread from the pharynx to the middle ear through the eustachian tube.

The nasopharynx communicates with the oropharynx through the pharyngeal isthmus, which is closed by muscular action during swallowing. The oropharynx and the laryngopharynx cannot be closed off from each other; both serve respiratory and digestive functions.

The pharynx comprises three groups of constrictor muscles (Fig. 21-1). Each muscle fits within the one below, and each inserts posteriorly in the median line with its mate from the opposite side. The constrictor muscles provide constriction of the pharynx for swallowing. Between the origins of the constrictor muscle groups are so-called intervals through which ligaments, nerves, and arteries

pass. The recurrent laryngeal nerve is closely associated with the lower portion of the pharynx.

The *tonsils* are situated one on each side of the oropharynx, lodged in a tonsillar fossa that is attached to folds of membrane containing muscle. One pair, the palatine tonsils, are the only lymphatic organs covered with stratified squamous epithelium. The lateral surface of each tonsil is usually covered with a fibrous capsule. The anterior and posterior tonsillar pillars join to form a triangular fossa, with the posterior lateral aspects of the tongue at its base. The lingual tonsils are lodged in each fossa. The adenoids or pharyngeal tonsils are suspended from the roof of the nasopharynx and consist of an accumulation of lymphoid tissue.

The arteries of the tonsils enter the upper and lower poles. The tonsils are supplied with blood by tonsillar branches of the ascending palatine branch of the facial artery (branch of the external carotid artery). The external carotid artery on each side lies behind and lateral to each tonsil. The nerves supplying the tonsils are derived from the middle and posterior palatine branches of the maxillary and glossopharyngeal nerves.

Larynx and associated cartilages and muscles
Larynx

The larynx is located at the upper end of the respiratory tract. It is situated between the trachea and the root of the tongue, at the upper front part of the neck. The larynx has three main functions: as a passageway for air, as a valve for closing off air passages from the digestive system and the pharynx, and as a voice box on which sound and speech depend to a degree.

The larynx is a cartilaginous box situated in front of the fourth, fifth, and sixth cervical vertebrae. The upper portion of the larynx is continuous with the pharynx above, and its lower portion joins the trachea. The skeletal structure provides for patency of the enclosed airway. The complex muscle action and arrangement of tissues within the structure provide for closure of the lumen for protection against trauma and entrance of foreign bodies and for speech.

545

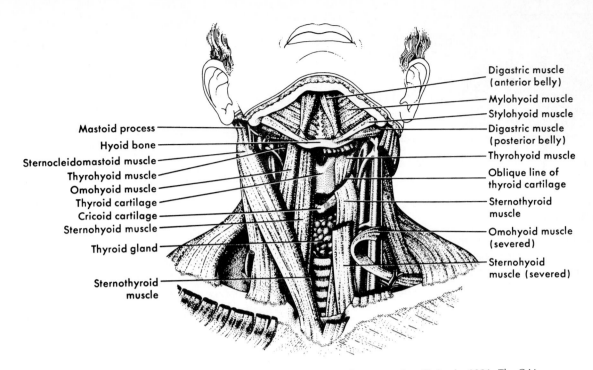

Mastoid process
Hyoid bone
Sternocleidomastoid muscle
Thyrohyoid muscle
Omohyoid muscle
Thyroid cartilage
Cricoid cartilage
Sternohyoid muscle
Thyroid gland
Sternothyroid muscle

Digastric muscle (anterior belly)
Mylohyoid muscle
Stylohyoid muscle
Digastric muscle (posterior belly)
Thyrohyoid muscle
Oblique line of thyroid cartilage
Sternothyroid muscle
Omohyoid muscle (severed)
Sternohyoid muscle (severed)

Fig. 21-1. Extrinsic muscles of the larynx. (From Marino, L.B.: Cancer nursing, St. Louis, 1981, The C.V. Mosby Co.)

Cartilages

The skeletal framework of the larynx consists of cartilages and membranes. Of the nine separate cartilages, three are single and six are arranged in pairs. The main cartilages of the larynx include the thyroid, cricoid, epiglottis, two arytenoid, two corniculate, and two cuneiform. The thyroid cartilage, or Adam's apple, forms the anterior portion of the voice box. The cricoid cartilage, which resembles a signet ring, rests beneath the thyroid cartilage (Fig. 21-2). The epiglottis is a slightly curled, leaf-shaped, elastic fibrous membrane. It is prolonged be-

low into a slender process, attached in the midline to the upper border of the thyroid cartilage. When the cricothyroid muscle contracts, it pulls the thyroid cartilage and the cricoid cartilage, thereby tightening the vocal cords and, if unopposed, closing the glottis. The arytenoid cartilages, which rest above the signet ring portion of the cricoid cartilage, support the posterior portion of the true vocal cords.

Laryngeal ligaments

The extrinsic ligaments of the larynx are those connecting the thyroid cartilage and epiglottis with the hyoid bone and the cricoid cartilage with the trachea (Fig. 21-3). The intrinsic ligaments of the larynx are those connecting several cartilages of the organ to each other. They are considered the elastic membrane of the larynx.

The mucous lining of the larynx blends with the fibrous tissue to form two folds on each side of the larynx. The upper set is known as the false cords. The lower set is called the true vocal cords because they are primarily concerned with the speaking voice and protection of the lower respiratory channels against the invasion of food and foreign bodies.

Laryngeal muscles

The laryngeal muscles perform two distinct functions: the extrinsic muscles open and close the glottis, and the intrinsic muscles regulate the degree of tension on the vocal cords.

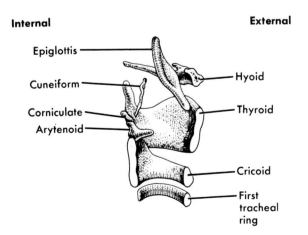

Internal

Epiglottis
Cuneiform
Corniculate
Arytenoid

External

Hyoid
Thyroid
Cricoid
First tracheal ring

Fig. 21-2. Skeletal framework. (From Marino, L.B.: Cancer nursing, St. Louis, 1981, The C.V. Mosby Co.)

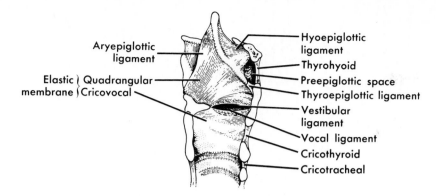

Fig. 21-3. Ligaments of larynx. (From Marino, L.B.: Cancer nursing, St. Louis, 1981, The C.V. Mosby Co.)

The spoken voice also depends on the sphincter action of the soft palate, tongue, and lips. The muscle action of the larynx permits the glottis to close either voluntarily or involuntarily by reflex action. The closure of the inlet by this mechanism protects the respiratory passages. The closure of the glottis and the action of the vocal cords are precisely coordinated to produce the spoken voice.

Two branches of the vagus nerve supply the intrinsic muscles. The recurrent laryngeal nerve branch of the vagus nerve is the important motor nerve of the intrinsic muscles of the larynx. The sensory nerve, which is derived from the branches of the superior laryngeal nerve, supplies the mucous membrane of the larynx.

When both the recurrent laryngeal nerves become divided or paralyzed, the glottis remains closed so tightly that air cannot be drawn into the lungs. As a lifesaving measure an endotracheal or tracheostomy tube is inserted immediately.

The larynx derives its blood supply from the branches of the external carotid and subclavian arteries.

Trachea

The trachea, a cylindrical tube about 15 cm in length and 2 to 2.5 cm in diameter, begins in the neck and extends from the lower part of the larynx, on a level with the sixth cervical vertebra, to the upper border of the fifth thoracic vertebra. The tube descends in front of the esophagus, enters the superior mediastinum, and divides into right and left main bronchi. The trachea is composed of a series of incomplete rings of hyaline cartilage. The carina is a ridge on the inside of the bifurcation of the trachea. It is a landmark during bronchoscopy and separates the upper end of the right main branches from the upper end of the left main branches of the bronchi. Branches given off from the arch of the aorta—the brachiocephalic (innominate) and left common carotid arteries—are in close relation to the trachea. The cervical portion of the trachea is related anteriorly to the sternohyoid and sternothyroid muscles and to the isthmus of the thyroid gland.

Salivary glands

The salivary glands consist of three paired glands: the sublingual, submaxillary, and parotid. They communicate with the mouth and pour their secretions into its cavities. Saliva is the combined secretion of all these glands. The salivary glands consist of tissues found in the mucosa of the cheeks, tongue, palates, floor of the mouth, pharynx, lips, and paranasal sinuses. A tumor of a salivary gland may occur in any of these structures.

The external carotid artery supplies the salivary glands and divides into its terminal branches: the internal maxillary and superficial temporal. The superficial temporal and internal maxillary veins unite to form the posterior facial vein.

The *sublingual gland* lies on the undersurface of the tongue beneath the mucous membrane of the floor of the mouth at the side of the tongue, on the inner surface of the mandible.

The sublingual gland is supplied with blood from the submental arteries. Its nerves are derived from the sympathetic nerves. The many tiny ducts of each gland separately enter the oral cavity on the sublingual fold.

The *submandibular gland* lies partly above and partly below the posterior half of the base of the mandible and on the mylohyoid and hyoglossus muscles. This gland is closely associated with the lingual veins and the lingual and hypoglossal nerves. The external maxillary artery lies on the posterior border of the gland. Its duct (Wharton's duct) enters the mouth at the frenulum of the tongue.

The *parotid gland,* the largest of the salivary glands, lies below the zygomatic arch in front of the mastoid process and behind the ramus of the mandible. This gland is enclosed in fascia, attached to surrounding muscles, and divided into two parts—a superficial and a deep portion—by means of the facial nerve. The parotid duct (Stensen's duct) pierces the buccal pad of fat and the buccinator muscle, finally opening into the oral cavity opposite the crown of the upper second molar tooth. The superficial temporal artery and small branches of the external carotid artery arise in the parotid gland behind the neck of the mandible.

General structures of the neck

The general topography of the organs lying in front of the prevertebral fascia has been described. A layer of deep cervical fascia surrounds the neck like a collar and is attached to the trapezius and sternocleidomastoid muscles. In front of the neck the deep fascial layer is attached to the lower border of the mandible.

The *pretracheal fascia* of the neck lies deep in the strap muscles (sternothyroid, sternohyoid, and omohyoid) and partially encloses the thyroid gland, trachea, and larynx. The pretracheal fascia is pierced by the thyroid vessels. It fuses with the front of the carotid sheath on the deep surface of the sternocleidomastoid muscle. The carotid sheath consists of a network of areolar tissue surrounding the carotid arteries and vagus nerve.

Laterally, the carotid sheath is fused with the fascia on the deep surface of the sternocleidomastoid muscle; anteriorly, it is fused with the middle cervical fascia along the lateral border of the sternothyroid muscle. Lying between the floor and roof of this triangular formation of muscles are the lymph glands and the accessory nerve. Arteries and nerves traverse and pierce this triangle.

Lymphatic system of the neck

The lymph glands of the neck are closely associated with the salivary glands and the lymph plexus. The submaxillary nodes, located in the submaxillary triangle, drain the cheek, side of the nose, upper lip, side of the lower lip, gums, side of the tongue, and medial palpebral commissure. Lymph from the facial and submental nodes also drains to these glands (Fig. 21-4). The superficial cervical nodes, following the external jugular vein, drain the ear and parotid area to the superior deep cervical nodes. The cervical nodes are in close contact with the larynx, thyroid gland, nasal cavities, ears, nasopharynx, palate, esophagus, and skin and muscles of the neck.

PERIOPERATIVE NURSING CONSIDERATIONS
Assessment/nursing diagnosis

The nursing history must be thorough, including definite and questionable risk factors such as: sun exposure, tobacco use, ethanol use, radiation, family history of carcinoma, and the patient's dental history. Specific factors that should be assessed include:

The patient's respiratory status. Note the quality and character of respirations; note the quality and character of the voice, hoarseness, "hot potato" voice, or hyponasal speech; inspiratory stridor, expiratory stridor, hemoptysis, or dyspnea; a lesion in the oral cavity, nasopharynx, or larynx; bleeding from the oral cavity or nasopharynx.

The patient's nutritional status. Note weight loss and length of time; dysphagia.

The patient's metabolic status. Note lab values.

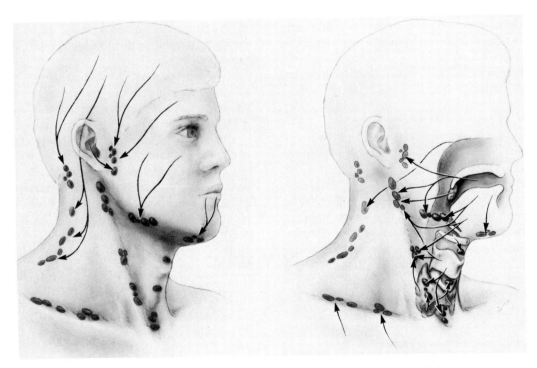

Fig. 21-4. Location of common lymphatic and glandular masses of head and neck. *Stippled areas* represent congenital masses. *Arrows* indicate lymphatic drainage pathways. (From Cummings, C.W., and Schuller, D.E.: *Otolaryngology—head and neck surgery,* Vol. 2, St. Louis, 1986, The C.V. Mosby Co.)

The patient's circulatory status. Note pedal pulses and color of the nailbeds, especially in children, elderly patients, and patients in respiratory distress. Note preoperative vital signs compared with vital signs on admission to the patient care unit; note the presence of antiembolism stockings (the perioperative nurse should ensure proper fit of these stockings when checking pedal pulses).

Infection. Note the temperature, color, and turgor of the skin over the affected site; note lesions and their characteristics.

The patient's dentition. Note dentures and their fit, lesions, loose teeth, persistent bad breath, and poor oral hygiene.

The patient's anxiety level. Note restlessness, poor eye contact, facial tension, increased perspiration; note the area around the patient's eyes for signs of crying (edema, redness).

Pain. Note location and character, odynophagia, sore throat, facial pain, otalgia; note preoperative medications and the time they were administered.

The patient's musculoskeletal system. Note problems in range of motion in all four extremities; note joint replacements, back or neck stiffness or pain, trismus.

The patient's allergies.

The patient's understanding of the surgical procedure. Note questions and give answers or ask surgeon to clarify information for the patient.

The presence of a mass. Note the length of time involved with the mass; note if decrease in size of the mass followed antibiotic therapy; note a fixed versus mobile mass; note cranial nerve palsies involving VII, IX, X, XI, XII.

The availability of replacement blood. Note if the patient has designated donor units (the patient usually will have been typed and the blood samples held, or typed and cross-matched for two units, minimally, depending on the anticipated extent of the procedure).

The patient's support personnel. Note family members' names and their location during the surgical procedure, introduce them to the nurse who will be in contact with them during the procedure, and establish initial communication and the intervals between which the nurse will be in contact with them regarding the patient.

Laboratory/diagnostic studies

Chest x-ray (to rule out mediastinal/pulmonary involvement and tracheal compression and to assess the patient's pulmonary status)

CT or MRI of neck (to delineate normal and abnormal soft tissue structures)

Ultrasound of mass (to determine solid versus cystic mass)

ECG

Complete blood count

Urinalysis

Prothrombin time (PT), partial thromboplastin time (PTT)

Blood chemistries

If the thyroid gland is suspect, the following tests may be indicated:

Serum calcium levels (to determine parathyroid functioning)

Serum calcitonin (to assess potential for medullary carcinoma)

Thyroid scan (to assess presence of "cold" nodule, which is often indicative of carcinoma)

Thyroid antibody tests (may show decreased levels in carcinoma)

Serum thyrotoxin (T_4)

TSH

T_3 resin uptake

The patient should be given explanations about the operating room environment and perioperative routines to decrease apprehension. Warm blankets, thermadrapes, reassurance, and a quiet environment should be provided to ensure that the patient is comfortable, calm, and warm prior to the surgical experience.

Nursing diagnoses that pertain to many patients undergoing laryngologic or head and neck surgery include:

- Impaired gas exchange due to airway obstruction
- Anxiety related to impending surgery
- Potential for infection
- Body image disturbance

Planning

Development of a meaningful perioperative nursing care plan assists nursing personnel in meeting the needs of patients undergoing laryngologic or head and neck surgery. A Sample Care Plan for this type of patient is shown on p. 550.

Implementation

The patient with a neck mass seldom undergoes surgical excision of the neck mass as a primary procedure. Endoscopic evaluation may be the initial surgical procedure, unless the primary lesion is clearly delineated.

Positioning

Routine positioning of the laryngologic or head and neck surgical patient involves placement of the patient in a supine position on the operating room bed. A shoulder roll may be utilized for hyperextension of the neck, depending on the surgeon's preference. The headrest should allow easy movement of the head from side to side yet maintain support. The extremities are well padded at pressure points and at major nerves. A pillow should be placed under the thighs and the legs slightly "frogged" to decrease pressure on the patient's back; this positioning should be carried out before the patient is anesthetized to ensure comfort.

Prepping

The male patient should be instructed to shave his face on the morning of surgery. Further removal of hair intra-

Sample Care Plan

NURSING DIAGNOSIS:
Impaired gas exchange due to airway obstruction
GOAL:
Patient will experience adequate gas exchange.
INTERVENTIONS:
Check BP, rate and quality of respirations, rate and quality of pulse, and apical pulse preoperatively.
Auscultate chest for breath sounds preoperatively.
Elevate head of bed 45 to 60 degrees as tolerated, preoperatively and intraoperatively.
Check arterial blood gases as ordered.
Monitor oxygen saturation perioperatively.
Administer steroids as ordered.
Monitor preoperatively for and report signs of impaired gas exchange, such as stridor, confusion, hypoxia, restlessness, and irritability.
Provide equipment, instruments, and supplies for a tracheotomy.

NURSING DIAGNOSIS:
Anxiety related to impending surgery
GOAL:
The patient will demonstrate effective coping skills and a decreased level of anxiety.
INTERVENTIONS:
Assess patient's level of anxiety (alertness, ability to comprehend, ability to perform ADL).
Maintain calm and safe environment.
Assist patient in identifying possible sources of stress.
Allow patient to ventilate and ask questions.

NURSING DIAGNOSIS:
Potential for infection
GOAL:
Patient will not exhibit signs of infection.
INTERVENTIONS:
Note temperature and WBC preoperatively.
Note temperature, color, and turgor of skin at operative site.
Note and report lesions in close proximity to the surgical site.
Note patient's nutritional status.
Ensure sterile environment during surgical procedure.
Monitor traffic patterns during surgical procedure.
Monitor blood loss and fluid replacement during surgical procedure.
Note patient's temperature during surgical procedure.
Ensure that initial dressing is dry and clean.

NURSING DIAGNOSIS:
Body image disturbance
GOAL:
The patient will experience a sense of self-worth and self-respect.
INTERVENTIONS:
Encourage the patient to verbalize feelings and changes related to health status and surgical procedure.
Involve family and/or significant others in initial communication with patient.
Encourage patient to ask questions.

---

operatively depends on the site of surgery and the anticipated extensiveness of the surgical intervention. Parotid surgery may require shaving the patient's hair from just below the temple to a line even with or slightly behind the pinna of the ear. Head and neck surgery often requires removal of hair on the chest to the nipple area on both sides.

Laryngeal procedures for benign lesions do not usually involve preparation of the skin, due to the intraoral approach. Head and neck procedures involve extensive preparation and usually include the entire area from the chin to the nipples. Some surgeons prefer the patient's face to be included in the prep, depending on the type of surgery anticipated and the site of the lesion. Povidone-iodine scrub and solution are generally preferred for preparation of the skin. If a flap may be raised to reconstruct a defect, saline should be available to remove the discoloration from the skin and allow the surgeon to check for flap viability.

Draping

As with prepping, draping of the patient for a laryngeal procedure for a benign lesion is minimal, with the primary focus being protection of the patient's eyes and face. This may be accomplished by: (1) placing ointment in the patient's eyes, (2) taping the eyelids closed with a nonabrasive, nonirritating tape, (3) applying moist cotton balls over the tape (especially if use of the carbon dioxide laser is anticipated), and (4) placing self-adhering eyepads over the cotton balls. A huck towel may be placed over the patient's face to expose only the lips and chin.

Draping for head and neck procedures often varies according to surgeon preference. If the preference is to have the patient's face exposed, a commercially prepared head drape may be used. When they are not available, a head drape may be made by utilizing a sterile sheet folded in half with a sterile huck towel on the innermost side to wrap the patient's hair. A towel clamp or sterile tape may be used to secure the head drape in place. Towels may be opened fully, "crushed," and placed in the space at both sides of the patient's neck and shoulder area to prevent contact with the unsterile operating room bed linen during the procedure. The area of the endotracheal tube may be isolated by a self-adherent, clear drape. Sterile towels are utilized to drape the neck, shoulder, and chest areas. An impervious drape is used to cover the patient from the chest to the foot of the operating room bed. A split sheet may then be used to drape over the huck towels and body drape. Commercially prepared split sheets have adhesive backing along the split that facilitates adherence to the area to be draped out and decreases slippage with subsequent contamination resulting from manipulation of the head during the surgical procedure.

Instrumentation

The instrumentation used in laryngologic surgery is quite specific and is discussed with each surgical intervention. *Head and neck instrumentation* consists of general surgical instruments such as:

Mosquito hemostats	Long tenotomy scissors
Kelly hemostats	Adson forceps with teeth
Crile hemostats	Vascular forceps
Mayo-Pean forceps	Towel clamps
Allis forceps	Needle holders
Babcock forceps	Yankauer suction tubes
Thyroid tenacula	Frazier suction tips
Right-angle clamps	Rake retractors
Skin hooks	Army-Navy retractors
Mayo scissors	Vein retractors
Metzenbaum scissors	Green retractors

Intraoral, laryngeal, and mandibular procedures require the addition of periosteal elevators (such as Joseph, Freer, Cleoid), cartilage scissors, bone cutter, rongeurs (such as Lempert, Adson), tracheal hooks, tracheal spreader, and saws. Although a Gigli saw and handles may be used on rare occasions, technology has made the sagittal saw standard in operating room armamentarium. Saws are either nitrogen powered or electric. The choice of power source should be a collaborative effort among the perioperative nursing staff, supervisor, and surgeon. A dermatome may be used if skin grafting of surgical defects or flap recon-

struction is anticipated. In the case of large reconstructive surfaces, a skin mesher may be used to extend the skin graft.

Equipment

Equipment that may be utilized in head and neck surgery includes an electrosurgical unit (both monopolar and bipolar), a hypothermia-hyperthermia unit, headlights (both fiberoptic and nonfiberoptic), pulse oximeter, blood warmer, temperature recorder, and humidifier. Although the last four items of equipment are primarily the responsibility of anesthesia personnel, the circulating nurse collaborates in providing access to electrical outlets to power the equipment and participates in interventions based on the results of patient monitoring.

Safety in head and neck surgery is primarily patient related with the exception of lasers, which warrant both patient and staff safety. All equipment should be checked prior to use to ensure that it is in proper working condition. Visual inspection should ensure that all equipment is clean. Headlights, in particular, should be inspected for blood prior to and following each use. Personnel should be reminded to wear safety glasses for eye protection in accordance with OSHA regulations. The circulating nurse should inspect the masks of the scrub team during the procedure for contamination by blood and body fluids and assist them in changing masks as needed.

Medications

Medications used in laryngeal surgery are targeted at decreasing bleeding and edema in the airway. Typical medications include:

Steroids are often given intraoperatively and postoperatively yet may be given preoperatively in the presence of edema or airway obstruction.

Epinephrine may be placed topically when vocal cord lesions are excised manually or biopsies are taken to identify a primary tumor site.

Xylocaine is instilled into the trachea to decrease coughing immediately prior to insertion of a tracheotomy tube.

Medications used in head and neck surgery include antibiotics and steroids. They are primarily given intravenously; however, an antibiotic may also be added to irrigating solution. Chemotherapeutic agents are often an important aspect of adjuvant therapy for the head and neck cancer patient. The perioperative nurse should be familiar with the chemotherapeutic agents prescribed for the patient. Suggested reading about these agents has been provided in the Bibliography.

Monitoring

Intraoperative monitoring of the patient includes assessment of the patient's circulatory, metabolic, urinary, respiratory, and musculoskeletal systems at regular intervals. Assessment of fluid volume is a collaborative effort. Blood loss and urinary output are communicated to anesthesia personnel. The perioperative nurse participates in the administration of fluid replacement therapy, assists in maintaining patency of lines, and notes the patient's response. Pedal pulses and pressure points should be checked without disturbing the surgical field or team. The scrub and circulating nurses must be aware of significant findings during the surgical procedure to anticipate changes or additional supplies and equipment needed. Communication with the patient's family or support persons is vital during the surgical procedure to decrease their anxiety.

Additional methods of monitoring the laryngologic or head and neck surgical patient include:

Pulse oximeter: usually monitored via the great toe due to the BP cuff on one arm of the patient and the arterial line and intravenous infusion line in the other arm

Blood pressure cuff: preferably automatic because of the necessity of frequent monitoring when dissecting around vital structures in the neck

Arterial line: detects sudden changes in BP and serves as a vehicle to obtain PO_2 and PCO_2 levels

Foley catheter: monitors the patient's urinary function, especially important for the elderly or debilitated patient

Temperature monitoring: usually via rectal probe or endotracheal tube probe

Esophageal stethoscope: usually contraindicated in head and neck procedures because of the interruption of the esophagus or structures adjacent to the esophagus

Computerized anesthesia monitoring system: standardized method of ensuring the safety of the patient while the anesthetic is being administered

Accurate and thorough monitoring is critical to safe and effective patient outcomes. Perioperative nurses should be familiar with monitoring equipment, able to interpret results, and remain responsive to implementing collaborative interventions based on those results.

Evaluation

Postoperative evaluation includes reassessing potential patient problems identified in the preoperative assessment as well as assessing the electrosurgical pad site, surgical incision, dressing, drains, respiratory status, skin turgor, and color of the head and extremities. Preoperative assessment findings, intraoperative changes in the patient's condition, and the postoperative evaluation must be documented and communicated to ensure continuity of care and patient safety. The report should also include relevant nursing diagnoses, goals, and outcomes of care. Some nursing diagnoses may have already been resolved; others

are ongoing and require continued planning and intervention during the patient's recovery from anesthesia and postoperative rehabilitation. A complete nursing report allows the PACU or ICU nurse to detect significant changes in the patient's condition in an early stage. Special considerations should also be reported, such as the necessity of flexion of the neck to avoid disruption of the suture line of the trachea in a patient who has undergone tracheal resection. Documentation should include the postoperative report given and the name of the RN to whom that report is given, prior to the patient's discharge from the operating room. Based on the nursing diagnoses selected for the patient undergoing laryngologic or head and neck surgery, the nursing report might include the following outcome statements:

· The patient's gas exchange remained normal.
· Anxiety was decreased.
· Infection will be prevented (ongoing).
· The patient verbalized feelings regarding disturbances in body image.

SURGICAL INTERVENTIONS
Laryngoscopy

Laryngoscopy is direct visual examination of the interior of the larynx by means of a lighted speculum known as a laryngoscope (Fig. 21-5) to obtain a specimen of tissue or secretions for pathologic examination.

Procedural considerations. To facilitate this examination, the patient should be sufficiently relaxed by psychologic reassurance and drug preparation. Sedatives are usually ordered before surgery.

Immediate preoperative assessment should include the presence of any dental appliances and condition of dental work and loose teeth. Any stiffness or immobility of the neck or shoulders should be evaluated. Respiratory problems such as asthma must receive careful attention.

The patient should be cautioned about not eating or drinking after surgery until the gag reflex has returned and swallowing occurs without difficulty.

Infants usually do not require an anesthetic; children and adults who cannot relax are given a general anesthetic; adults who are well prepared preoperatively do very well with the application of a local anesthetic of lidocaine (Xylocaine), tetracaine (Pontocaine), or cocaine.

The setup includes the following:

Local anesthesia setup

Gauze sponges, 4 × 4 inches
Laryngeal mirror
Cotton balls
Small cup of hot water (to warm the laryngeal mirror so it does not fog when inserted into the mouth to view the vocal cords)
Emesis basin
Syringe, 5 ml, and Abraham cannula

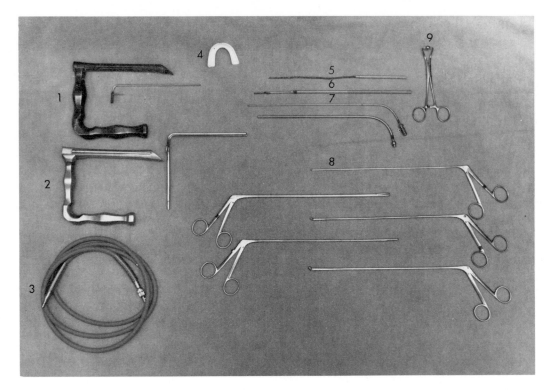

Fig. 21-5. Laryngoscopy instruments. *1*, Anterior commissure laryngoscope and light carrier; *2*, Dedo Pilling laryngoscope and light carrier; *3*, fiberoptic light cord; *4*, tooth guard; *5*, laryngeal pigtail applicator; *6*, long knife handle; *7*, laryngeal suction tubes, small and medium; *8*, assorted laryngeal cup forceps and laryngeal alligator forceps; *9*, nonperforating towel clamp.

Medication cup
Jackson laryngeal applicating forceps
Cetacaine spray, with angulated tip, or other topical anesthetic
  for the oral mucosa

Instrument setup

1 Laryngoscope (surgeon's choice), size suitable to the patient (adult, child, or infant)
2 Laryngeal suction tubes
1 Light carrier, fiberoptic
2 Laryngeal biopsy forceps, 1 straight and 1 upbiting
2 Sponge-carrier forceps with extra sponges
1 Tooth guard
1 Fiberoptic light cord

Accessory items

Suction tubing
Specimen jar
Basin of sterile saline
Gauze sponges
Sterile towels
Gloves

If the surgeon wishes to perform a suspension laryngoscopy, a self-retaining laryngoscope holder is added to
the instrument table. A special platform may be mounted
onto the operating room bed, or a Mayo stand may be
placed above the patient's chest and over the operating
room bed to provide a place for the laryngoscope holder

to rest. The surgeon usually requests the operating microscope for use during suspension laryngoscopy.

The patient is placed in a supine position to facilitate
visualization of the vocal cords.

Operative procedure

1. Moist gauze pads should be put over the patient's eyes
   to protect them from the light of the instrument and to
   prevent injury and irritation from secretions during the
   procedure. The head may also be wrapped in a sterile
   towel. Some surgeons may request a sterile drape to
   cover the patient.
2. The spatula end of the laryngoscope is introduced into
   the right side of the patient's mouth and directed toward
   the midline; then the dorsum of the tongue is elevated,
   exposing the epiglottis.
3. The patient's head is first tipped backward and then
   lifted upward as the laryngoscope is advanced into the
   larynx.
4. The larynx is examined, a biopsy is taken, secretions
   are aspirated, and bleeding is controlled.
5. The patient's face is cleansed. The patient is reassured
   and then taken to own room or to PACU.

Microlaryngoscopy

Microlaryngoscopy facilitates improved diagnoses and
allows the laryngologist to view with relative ease areas

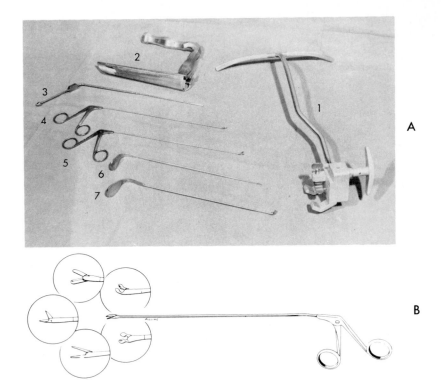

Fig. 21-6. Jako microlaryngeal instrumentation. **A,** Basic setup for microlaryngoscopy. *1,* Lewy self-retaining laryngoscope holder; *2,* Jako laryngoscope; *3,* suction tube; *4,* grasping forceps; *5,* cup forceps; *6,* probe; *7,* mirror. **B,** Closeup of working ends of instruments. (**A** from DeWeese, D.D., and Saunders, W.H.: Textbook of otolaryngology, ed. 6, St. Louis, 1982, The C.V. Mosby Co.; **B** courtesy Pilling Co., Philadelphia.)

that were previously inaccessible or difficult to visualize. It may also be used for minor surgery of the larynx, especially for the removal of polyps or nodes on the vocal cords.

Procedural considerations. If the procedure is done to remove polyps or nodes from the vocal cords, the patient must be cautioned about not speaking for a period of time postoperatively. The patient should be provided with a pencil and paper or a Magic Slate to aid in communication. The patient's restriction on speaking should be noted on the nursing care plan and on the front of the chart.

The basic instrument setup for laryngoscopy is used; however, the patient may receive a general anesthetic instead of a local. Microlaryngeal instruments are added to the setup and include the following (Fig. 21-6):

Self-retaining laryngoscope holder
Jako microlaryngeal grasping forceps
Jako microlaryngeal cup forceps, straight and upbiting cups
Jako microlaryngeal scissors, straight, angled, and upbiting
Jako microlaryngeal knives, straight and curved
Laryngeal probe
Microlaryngeal mirror
Open-ended microlaryngeal suction tube
Laryngoscope (dual light channel)

The aforementioned instruments have a length of 22 cm to allow use with the microscope, being long enough to keep the surgeon's hands out of the visual field.

The microscope is used. The head is adjusted to allow visualization of the larynx. The surgeon usually adjusts the microscope.

The microscope lens should have a 400-mm focal length. Focal length is the distance from the lens to the operative area and is the point at which the field can be clearly viewed through the microscope. Beyond this point the field becomes fuzzy. The 400-mm lens gives the surgeon a 40-cm focal length, or working distance. A general rule for determining focal length of a lens is to divide the millimeter power, for example, 400 mm, by 10. In this instance it is 40 cm.

Care of endoscopic equipment

Endoscopic equipment is fragile and should be handled carefully. Rigid endoscopes should be thoroughly cleaned and lumina checked for cleanliness. Long, narrow brushes and long pipe cleaners are available for cleaning the lumen and suction and light channels. The scopes should be dried carefully before sterilization. The light carriers are stored in the endoscopes. The endoscope should be checked for any dents, roughened edges, or deep scratches on the surface. Any of these can cause tissue damage or lead to corrosion of the instrument. Endoscopes should be handled individually.

Fiberoptic equipment is also fragile. The light cables should be handled with care and not allowed to drop or swing free while being carried. This can break the filaments inside the cords, rendering them unusable. Most cables can be autoclaved, but according to manufacturer's instructions only. They should be coiled loosely when not in use, and care should be taken not to put anything heavy on top of the cables. Kinking and sharp bending of the cables must be avoided.

The main advantage of fiberoptic light is that the light, although very bright, remains cool when used for a relatively long time. A simple test for the integrity of the cable is to hold one end of the cable to a bright light and inspect the opposite end. Dark spots are an indication that some of the fibers are broken. If more than 25% of the fibers are broken, the cable should be sent for repair, or replacement should be considered.

Telescopes for rigid equipment, as used for bronchoscopy, should also be handled carefully to prevent damage. The telescope should be cleaned carefully, thoroughly dried, and returned to its case for protection during storage. Telescopes may be sterilized, but strict adherence to manufacturer's instructions must be followed. Gas sterilization is the method of choice. If a telescope is dropped or hit against another object, it should be sent to the manufacturer for examination and repaired if required.

Suction tubes should be flushed thoroughly with running water. An instrument-cleaning solution may also be used for this purpose. The lumen should be cleaned with a long pipe cleaner to remove remaining debris. The tube is then rinsed again, and the lumen dried with a clean, dry pipe cleaner. The suction tube should be inspected for dents or nicks, especially on the end, to prevent damage to delicate tissues.

Biopsy forceps should be thoroughly cleaned, and the edges of the cups inspected for chips or nicks. They should also be checked periodically for sharpness. If the forceps are dull, nicked, or chipped, tissue will be torn or ripped instead of cut cleanly when a biopsy is taken, resulting in more bleeding than usual. It is a good practice to rotate the use of biopsy forceps on a regular basis depending on the frequency of use. All forceps should be thoroughly cleaned, dried, and inspected for damage after use and should be sent for repair if necessary.

Proper care of endoscopic equipment can extend the service life of these instruments indefinitely.

Carbon dioxide laser surgery of the larynx

The advent of the carbon dioxide laser has added a new dimension to the laryngologist's treatment of lesions of the larynx and vocal cords. The carbon dioxide laser is efficient and has a high power output. It uses a combination of carbon dioxide, nitrogen, and helium gases that becomes energized to a high degree by an electric current. As the energy level subsides, light beams are produced and are reflected off the mirror-lined walls of the laser tube. These beams eventually form a single beam of light that has a high intensity in the ultraviolet range and is therefore invisible to the eye. For this reason a red beam from a helium-neon laser is added to the carbon dioxide beam so it can be properly aimed at the affected tissue. The beam destroys tissue at a precise point with minimal destruction of the surrounding tissue. It is especially useful in surgeries such as removal of webs in the larynx, vocal cord papillomas, and carcinoma in situ of the larynx, as well as benign endobronchial lesions.

Procedural considerations. The basic setup for laryngoscopy and microlaryngoscopy is used. All instrumentation used for laser laryngoscopy should be ebonized. General anesthesia is usually given. Suggested equipment placement is shown in Fig. 21-7.

The operating microscope with a 400-mm lens is used. The laser micromanipulator is attached to the microscope head (Fig. 21-8). The manufacturer's instructions for attaching it must be followed. The beam should also be tested for proper working order. Signal lights on the console illuminate if any malfunction occurs in the equipment or if the gas supply is low. Extreme care should be used when handling this delicate equipment.

Precautions. Because of the pinpoint tissue destruction, specific precautions are necessary.

1. Laser light is reflected by shiny surfaces or absorbed by moisture. Because silicone, latex, and red rubber endotracheal tubes are combustible, they must be protected by being carefully wrapped with adhesive sensing tape. In addition, saline-soaked gauze or

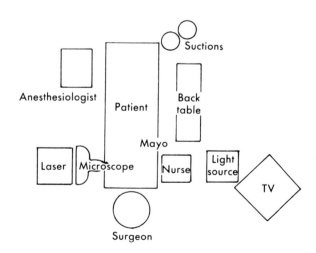

Fig. 21-7. Operating room arrangement of equipment for laser surgery. (From Pilcher, L: AORN J. 33:1402, 1981.)

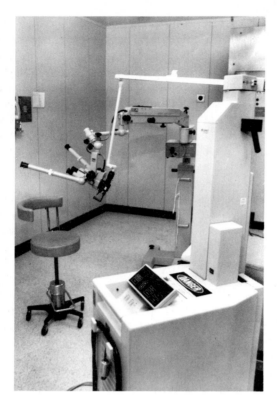

Fig. 21-8. Operating microscope with laser micromanipulator attached.

cottonoid patties with strings are placed just above the tube cuff. These precautions eliminate the possibility of the tube or cuff being punctured or set afire by a stray laser beam. A safer alternative is the use of copper (Carden), stainless steel (Porch), or commercially prepared laser-retardant endotracheal tubes and a jet ventilation system.

2. Because the laser beam can destroy tissue, the patient's healthy tissue must be protected. This is best done by covering the areas such as the eyes, the oral cavity, and the peritracheal area with wet gauze pads or cottonoid patties. Cottonoid patties covering the balloon on the endotracheal tube are effective in preventing rupture of the cuff. *It is imperative that all gauze pads or patties be kept wet during the surgery to prevent damage to healthy tissue from stray or reflected beams of light.* Moisture is the most effective barrier to stop the laser energy from penetrating healthy tissue or igniting materials in the area. Should the endotracheal tube be ignited for some reason (not a common occurrence but the most dangerous of complications) during the procedure, a ventilating bronchoscope, grasping forceps of some type, and a tracheostomy tray should be available.

3. Operating room personnel must wear eyeglasses or special plastic protective goggles when the CO_2 laser

is in use. Contact lenses do not protect the eyes from stray laser beams. The corneas are especially vulnerable to stray laser radiation and must be protected. If the corneas are left unprotected and energy is absorbed, corneal opacification can result.

4. Signs indicating that a laser is in use should be placed on the operating room door during the procedure to keep extra people out of the room while the laser is used.

5. If the laser equipment does not test properly before the procedure, it should be checked by biomedical engineering personnel or the manufacturer before being used.

The use of this equipment requires thorough education of perioperative nursing personnel, anesthesia staff, and surgeons. The teaching should include the assembly and disassembly of the equipment, proper techniques for the immediate preoperative testing of the equipment, precautions that must be taken while in use, and a basic explanation of the principles of laser use (see Chapter 10). These points should be clearly understood by all involved to prevent any undue tissue damage to the patient or injury to personnel.

Bronchoscopy

The trachea, bronchi, and lungs are visualized directly with a rigid or flexible bronchoscope that has a fiberoptic lighting system. A rigid scope gives a larger viewing area, whereas a flexible scope is easily inserted into the patient and manipulated. Bronchoscopy is fully described in Chapter 25.

Esophagoscopy

Esophagoscopy is the direct visualization of the esophagus and the cardia of the stomach. This procedure is utilized to observe the area for extension of tumor, remove tissue and secretions for study, or observe for primary tumor site.

Procedural considerations. Esophagoscopy facilitates the diagnosis of esophageal carcinoma, diverticula, hiatal hernia, stricture, benign stenosis, or varices. Patients with suspected obstruction, symptoms of bleeding, or regurgitation may require endoscopy. Esophagoscopy may also be used for therapeutic manipulations, such as removal of a foreign body or insertion of an esophageal bougie.

Prior to esophagoscopy, a member of the surgical team must be designated to be responsible for holding and moving the patient's head throughout the procedure. The movement of the patient's head during the procedure ensures the examination of all areas of the esophagus, as it is not a rigid structure like the bronchus.

The setup includes the following:

Esophagoscopes, desired type, size and length (Figs. 21-9 and 21-10)
Suction tubing

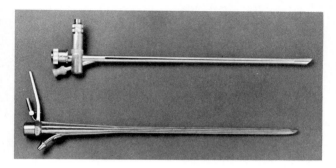

Fig. 21-9. Pediatric and adult esophagoscopes.

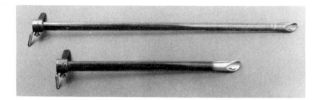

Fig. 21-10. Jesberg adult esophagoscopes.

Fiberoptic light source and light cords
Bougies, if desired
Forceps, desired type and length
Specimen containers
Water-soluble lubricating jelly
Gauze sponges
Basin with sterile saline
Suction tubes (velvet-eye tips to avoid suctioning the mucosa
of the esophagus into the tip)

Operative procedure

1. The fiberoptic light carrier is inserted into the esophagoscope, and a fiberoptic light cord is attached. A thin layer of lubricant is applied to the scope. The scope is passed into the mouth. The tongue, epiglottis, laryngeal inlet, and cricopharyngeal lumen are identified. The person holding the patient's head may tip the patient's head backward while extending the neck anteriorly. Usually the esophagoscope is passed to the right side of the tongue and the patient's head is turned slightly to the left.
2. When the scope has passed the inferior constrictors, the patient's head is moved in various directions so that all areas of the esophageal wall may be examined.
3. Specimens of secretions from the esophageal lumen may be obtained with an aspirating tube and suctioning apparatus. In some cases, saline may be injected through the esophagoscope's aspirating channel and the fluid withdrawn immediately for histologic study. A biopsy of tissue may be taken using forceps of the surgeon's preference. Following biopsy, the area is assessed for bleeding, and the esophagoscope is then removed.

Triple endoscopy

When laryngoscopy, bronchoscopy, and esophagoscopy are performed on a patient, the procedure is termed *triple endoscopy*. The order in which the procedures are performed depends on the surgeon's preference. The purpose of triple endoscopy is usually diagnostic. While inspecting for a malignancy, the surgeon views the structures, takes biopsies, and possibly makes smears or washings of the suspect areas.

Tonsillectomy and adenoidectomy

The tonsils and adenoids are removed by sharp or blunt dissection. Enlarged tonsils and adenoids are usually associated with difficulty in breathing and hearing, chronic colds, enlarged glands of the neck, otitis media, and pressure on the eustachian tubes caused by adenoiditis. Rheumatism, bronchitis, and hearing loss may be associated with diseased tonsils.

Special preoperative teaching and orientation sessions for pediatric patients have decreased the stress of the perioperative period for children undergoing this surgery. During these sessions, parents are instructed in the essentials of postoperative care.

Procedural considerations. The patient is anesthetized and then placed in slight Trendelenburg's position. The neck is hyperextended by placing a roll under the shoulders. A small headrest may be necessary if the patient's head is unstable. The patient's face may be cleaned with an antimicrobial solution. Typical draping includes application of a head drape and an impervious sheet over the patient.

The instruments and supplies required include the following (Fig. 21-11):

1 Knife handle, no. 7 with no. 12 blade
1 Tonsil knife
1 Tonsil snare with additional wires
1 LaForce or Sluder tonsil guillotines, if desired
1 Metzenbaum scissors, curved, 7½ inches
1 Mayo scissors
  Adenoid curettes, assorted sizes
1 Adenoid punch
  LaForce Adenotomes, assorted sizes
1 Hurd dissector and pillar retractor
2 Sponge-holding forceps
1 Towel clamp
2 Tonsil-grasping forceps, straight and curved
2 Dean hemostatic forceps
  Jennings mouth gag, suitable size
  Self-retaining mouth gag with tongue blades, if desired
1 Uvula or palate retractor
1 Tongue depressor
1 Needle holder, 7 inches
  Plain no. 2-0 atraumatic sutures on half-circle tonsil needle
1 Yankauer suction tube with suction tubing
  Tonsil sponges of assorted sizes
  Gauze sponges
  Basin set

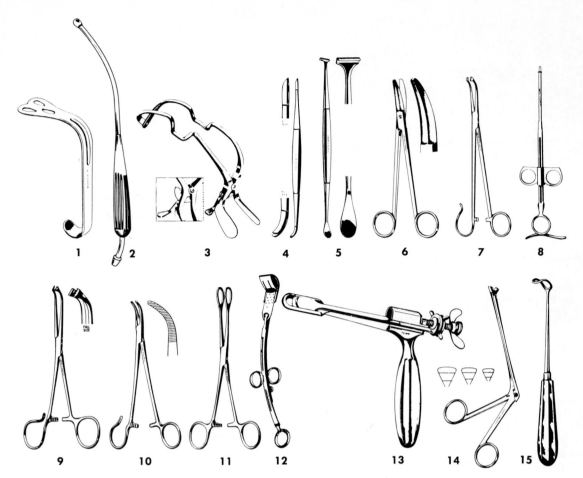

Fig. 21-11. Instruments for tonsillectomy and adenoidectomy. *1,* Tongue depressor; *2,* Yankauer suction tube; *3,* Jennings mouth gag; *4,* tonsil knife; *5,* Hurd dissector and pillar retractor; *6,* Boettcher tonsil scissors; *7,* White tonsil-grasping forceps; *8,* Eves tonsil snare; *9,* Allis-Coakley forceps, curved; *10,* Dean hemostatic forceps; *11,* Ballenger sponge-holding forceps, serrated jaw; *12,* LaForce adenotome; *13,* Daniel tonsillectome; *14,* adenoid punch; *15,* Barnhill adenoid curette. (Courtesy Codman & Shurtleff, Inc., Randolph, Mass.)

Cold sterile saline solution
Electrosurgical handpiece, with suction attached
Electrosurgical unit
Headlight of surgeon's preference

Operative procedure

1. When a general anesthetic is used, an endotracheal tube is inserted, the mouth is retracted open with a self-retaining retractor, and the tongue is depressed with a blade retractor. Efficient suction is most important. The metal suction tube is introduced gently and passed along the floor of the mouth, over the base of the tongue, and into the pharynx. During the procedure the suctioning ensures adequate exposure of the operative site and prevents blood from reaching the lungs.

2. The tonsil is grasped with a pair of tonsil-grasping forceps, and the mucous membrane of the anterior pillar is incised with a knife; the tonsil lobe is freed from its attachments to the pillars with a tonsil dissector, curved

scissors, and gauze sponges on a holder. The tonsil is withdrawn with forceps.

3. The posterior pillar is cut with scissors, and the tonsil is removed with a snare (Fig. 21-12). In some cases a tonsil guillotine clamp may be used.

4. A tonsil sponge is placed in the fossa with a sponge-holding forceps.

5. Bleeding vessels are clamped with tonsil forceps and tied with slipknot ligatures of plain no. 0 and the free ligature ends are cut, or the vessels are electrocoagulated.

6. The adenoids are removed with an adenotome or curette. Bleeding is controlled by pressure with tonsil sponges, sometimes soaked in a tannic acid solution.

7. The fossa is carefully inspected, and any bleeding vessels are clamped and tied. Retractors and endotracheal tube are removed, the patient's face is cleaned, and the head is turned to one side. The patient is placed in the

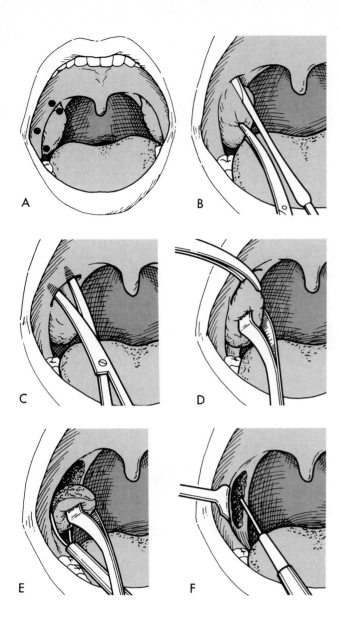

Fig. 21-12. The surgical method of tonsillectomy. **A,** Local anesthesia infiltration points. **B,** A tonsil knife is used to make an incision at the tonsil anterior pillar superiorly. **C** and **D,** Scissors are used to dissect the superior pole of the tonsil. **E,** A snare is used to separate the tonsil from the lower pole. **F,** Hemostasis is achieved by electrocoagulation or tying of bleeding vessels. (From Luckmann, J., and Sorenson, K.C.: Medical-surgical nursing, ed. 3, Philadelphia, 1987, W.B. Saunders Co.)

semirecumbent (Fowler's) position or on one side, horizontally, to prevent aspiration of blood and venous engorgement postoperatively.

Surgery of the oral cavity

Benign or malignant lesions of the tongue, floor of the mouth, alveolar ridge, buccal mucosa, or tonsillar area are excised. Benign or small malignant tumors of the oral

cavity may be excised without neck dissection. In the presence of tongue cancer without evidence of metastasis, a "prophylactic" neck dissection may be performed in an effort to control a cancerous growth in the upper jugular chain of the neck.

In the treatment of typical carcinoma of the floor of the mouth with involvement of the mandible, a portion of the tongue is removed in the combined operation—a radical neck dissection and resection of both the mandible and the tongue. When the primary intraoral lesion is confined to the tongue, a neck dissection and a hemiglossectomy are performed without resection of the mandible.

In the presence of a lesion of the tonsil or an extensive lesion at the base of the tongue with pharyngeal wall involvement, a resection of the ascending ramus of the mandible is necessary, and portions of the base of the tongue, pharyngeal wall, and soft palate are removed to secure an adequate margin of normal tissue around the lesion.

Psychologic preparation of the patient is extremely important, as these procedures may be done for a minor lesion in the oral cavity or they may be the first part of much more extensive surgery in the head and neck area. A supportive and accepting family is most important to the patient at this time because of the possibility of disfigurement after surgery.

Procedural considerations. The patient is placed in a supine position with shoulders elevated. Generally, endotracheal anesthesia is used, and a pharyngeal pack of moist gauze is inserted in the mouth. Instruments and supplies include the following items:

2 Knives, nos. 3 and 7, with nos. 10 and 15 blades
1 Metzenbaum scissors, curved, 7¼ inches
1 Mayo scissors, straight
1 Mayo scissors, curved
1 Suture scissors
4 Foerster or Ballenger sponge-holding forceps
6 Towel clamps
2 Tissue forceps without teeth, 5½ inches
2 Tissue forceps with teeth, 5½ inches
2 Adson forceps
2 Brown-Adson forceps
2 Nasal dressing forceps
4 Allis forceps, 3 and 4 teeth
6 Mayo-Pean forceps, curved, 6½ inches
3 Mayo-Pean forceps, curved, 9¼ inches
6 Crile hemostats, straight
2 Rochester-Carmalt forceps, 8 inches
3 Tonsil artery forceps
1 Metal anesthesia tube
1 Mouth gag
2 McBurney retractors
3 Bosworth tongue depressors
1 Cheek retractor
2 Parker retractors
1 Cushing loop retractor
1 Nerve hook
1 Crile-Wood needle holder, 8 inches
1 Crile-Wood needle holder, 5½ inches

Chromic, nos. 2-0 and 3-0, for ligatures
Silk, no. 3-0, taper point needles
Silk, no. 4-0 atraumatic on cutting-edge needles
1 Catheter, whistle-tipped, with open end, 14 Fr
1 Petrolatum-gauze packing
2 Yankauer suction tubes and tubing
1 Tracheostomy instrument set
1 Local anesthesia set for nerve block, if desired
1 Minor throat pack, including gauze compresses and tonsil
    sponges

1 Minor neck drape pack
    Tracheostomy tubes, assorted sizes
1 Syringe, 10 ml
    Electrosurgical unit

Operative procedure. Although the procedure may be scheduled as a local excision, frequently lesions of the oral cavity require more extensive excisions than planned preoperatively. The setup should be designed to include the

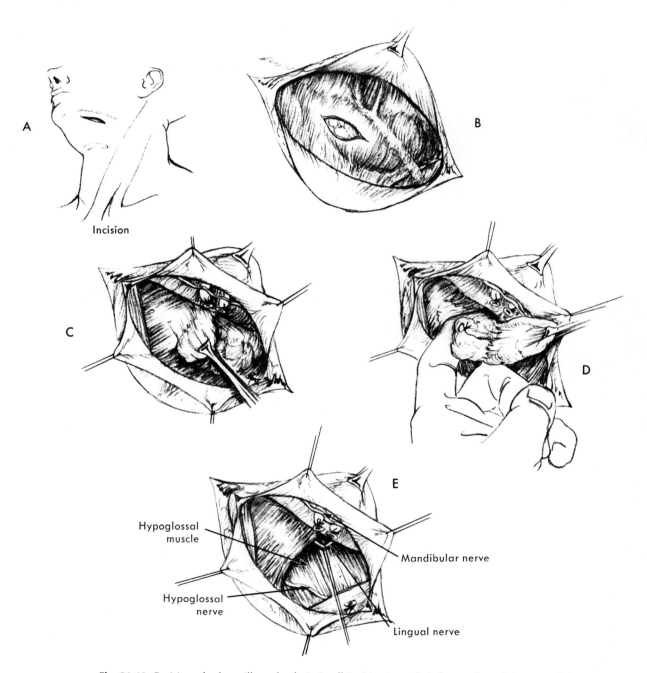

Fig. 21-13. Excision of submaxillary gland. **A,** Small incision is made below and parallel to mandible and extending forward beneath chin. **B,** Skin flaps and platysma are dissected, and cervical fascia is incised to expose gland. **C,** Gland is grasped and freed by blunt dissection. **D,** Posterior lobe delivered. **E,** Dissection completed. (From Wilder, J.R.: Atlas of general surgery, ed. 2, St. Louis, 1964, The C.V. Mosby Co.)

instruments for a neck dissection, or they should be readily available. For most tumors of the oral cavity a tracheostomy is performed to ensure an airway after surgery.

Excision of the submaxillary gland

This operation is performed to remove mixed tumors and multiple calculi associated with extensive chronic inflammation. An incision is made in the neck beneath the chin to remove the gland and tumor.

Procedural considerations. The patient is placed on the operating room bed in a supine position, with the affected side uppermost, and prepped as for neck surgery.

The instruments include a minor neck dissection setup. A tracheostomy tube should be available. A set of lacrimal probes should also be added to the instrument setup if exploration of the submaxillary (Wharton's) duct is necessary during surgery.

Operative procedure

1. A small skin incision is made below and parallel to the mandible, extending forward to beneath the chin (Fig. 21-13, A). The platysma is incised with scissors; the skin flaps and undersurface of the platysma and cervical fascia covering the gland are undermined with fine hooks, tissue forceps, and Metzenbaum scissors (Fig. 21-13, B).
2. The mandibular branch of the facial nerve is retracted away with a small loop retractor.
3. The submaxillary gland is elevated from the mylohyoid muscle (Fig. 21-13, C). The edge of the muscle is retracted to expose the lingual veins and nerve and the hypoglossal nerve.
4. The gland is freed by blunt dissection, and the submaxillary duct is clamped, ligated, and divided.
5. The external maxillary artery is clamped, ligated, and divided. The submaxillary gland is removed (Fig. 21-13, D and E).
6. The wound is closed with interrupted fine silk or chromic sutures. The skin edges are approximated with nylon sutures. A drain is inserted in the submaxillary bed and secured to the skin. Dressings are applied.

Parotidectomy

The tumor and a portion of or the entire parotid gland are removed through a curved incision in the upper neck and behind the lobe of the ear (Fig. 21-14) or through a Y type of incision on both sides of the ear and below the angle of the mandible.

The majority of benign tumors of the salivary glands occur in the parotid gland. These benign tumors are of the same types as are those found in soft tissues in other parts of the body. In the parotid gland the closeness of the facial nerve makes removing the entire tumor difficult. Parotidectomy is indicated for removal of all benign and some malignant tumors, for inflammatory lesions, for vascular anomalies, and for metastatic cancer involving lymph nodes overlying the gland.

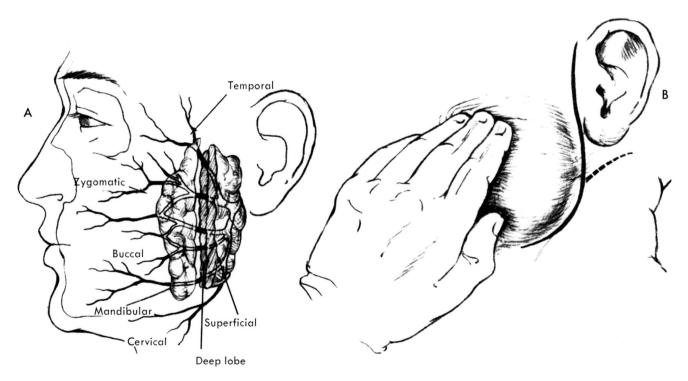

Fig. 21-14. A, Anatomy of facial nerve. **B,** Site of incision for parotidectomy. (From Wilder, J.R.: Atlas of general surgery, ed. 2, St. Louis, 1964, The C.V. Mosby Co.)

If the removal of malignant tumors involves adjacent structures, such as the mandible or cheek, the operation may become a radical removal of the involved structures. The patient must be aware of the possible complication of facial nerve weakness or paralysis.

Procedural considerations. The patient is placed on the operating room bed in a supine position with the entire affected side of the face uppermost. The entire side of the face, the mouth, the outer canthus of the eye, and the forehead are prepped and left exposed.

The instrument setup is a neck dissection set. A nerve stimulator should be available for use. A set of lacrimal probes should be included in the setup if exploration of the ductal system of the parotid is necessary during the course of surgery.

Operative procedure (Fig. 21-15)
1. The incision may extend from the posterior angle of the zygoma downward in front of the tragus of the ear and behind the lobule of the ear backward over the mastoid process, then downward and forward on the

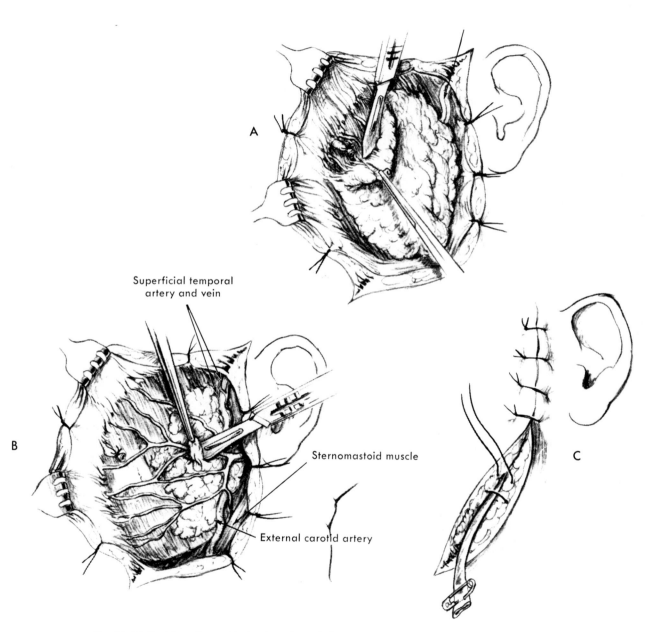

Fig. 21-15. Excision of parotid gland. **A,** Parotid duct is exposed and identified. By sharp and blunt dissection, duct is mobilized, ligated with fine chromic suture, and divided. **B,** Following anterior lobe mobilization and identification of facial nerve and vessels, posterior lobe is removed. **C,** Wound is cleansed, and bleeding is controlled. A drain is inserted and wound is closed. (From Wilder, J.R.: Atlas of general surgery, ed. 2, St. Louis, 1964, The C.V. Mosby Co.)

neck parallel to and below the body of the mandible. (A chin incision may also be used.) Bleeding vessels are controlled by hemostats and fine ligatures.

2. With fine-toothed tissue forceps and scissors, the skin flaps are elevated as described for thyroidectomy (Chapter 16). The skin wound edges are retracted by means of silk sutures fastened to clamps.

3. The upper portion of the sternocleidomastoid muscle is exposed and retracted, the auricular nerve is identified, and the lower part of the parotid gland is elevated with curved hemostats.

4. The superficial temporal artery and vein and external jugular vein are identified by means of blunt dissection.

5. The parotid tissue is dissected from the cartilage of the ear and the tympanic plate of the temporal bone. The temporal, zygomatic, and mandibular and cervical branches of the facial nerve are identified and preserved.

6A. The superficial portion of the parotid gland containing the tumor is removed. In some cases the entire superficial portion is removed, followed by ligation and division of the parotid duct.

6B. When the deep portion of the parotid gland must be removed, the facial nerve is retracted upward and outward by nerve hooks, and then the parotid tissue is removed from beneath the nerve. Kocher retractors are used to retract the mandible. The external carotid artery is identified. In many cases the internal maxillary and superficial temporal arteries are clamped, ligated, and divided.

7. The wound is closed in layers with fine silk sutures. A small drain is inserted, and a pressure dressing is applied.

Tracheostomy

Tracheostomy is opening of the trachea and insertion of a cannula through a midline incision in the neck, below the cricoid cartilage. It is used as an emergency procedure to treat upper respiratory tract obstruction and as a prophylactic measure in the presence of chronic lung disease or sleep apnea in which an obstruction could occur. A prophylactic tracheostomy is performed at the time of surgery to permit easy and frequent aspiration of the tracheobronchial tree and diminish the dead space that exists from the opening of the mouth down to the supraclavicular region. The creation of a new clearance (tracheostomy) nearer to the functional areas in the lung provides for a greater volume of air for the patient with a partly destroyed lung. Anesthesia may be maintained through a prophylactic tracheostomy.

The patient's psychologic status should be carefully evaluated because of the altered body image and physical status, which may be either temporary or permanent, depending on the disease entity involved. Tracheostomy care should be explained carefully and thoroughly so the patient will understand why it must be done so frequently, especially the suctioning of the tube.

Reinforcement should be given about the ability to communicate with others by means of a pencil and paper. As recovery progresses, the patient can be shown how to occlude the opening of the tube for brief periods to be able to speak a few words.

Procedural considerations. The patient is placed in a supine position, with the shoulders raised by a folded sheet to hyperextend the neck and head. The neck is prepped, and sterile drapes are applied. Along with a basic minor drape pack, the following instruments and supplies should be included:

2 Knife handles, no. 3 with nos. 10 and 15 blades
1 Metzenbaum scissors, curved
1 Mayo scissors, straight
1 Suture scissors
2 Allis forceps, straight
1 Needle holder
2 Tissue forceps with fine teeth
2 Tissue forceps without teeth
2 Adson forceps
4 Towel clamps
2 Sponge-holding forceps
4 Mosquito hemostats, straight
4 Kelly hemostats, curved
1 Mayo-Pean forceps, curved
2 Crile hemostats, curved
2 Volkmann rake retractors
2 Army-Navy retractors
2 Frazier skin hooks
1 Jackson tracheal hook
1 Tracheal dilator
1 Cushing nerve hook
2 Brophy tenaculum hooks
  Plain no. 3-0 sutures
  Chromic no. 3-0 atraumatic sutures on fine, ½-circle, taper point needles
  Silk no. 2-0 atraumatic sutures on ⅜-circle, cutting-edge needles
2 Catheters, whistle-tipped, open-ended, 14 Fr
1 Yankauer suction tube
1 Frazier suction tip
2 Suction tubings
  Tracheostomy tubes (Fig. 21-16), appropriate for age and size of patient
  Cardiac arrest setup, oxygen, and thiopental (Pentothal) sodium setup
  Local anesthesia set

Operative procedure

1. A vertical or transverse incision may be used. A vertical incision is made in the midline from approximately the cricoid cartilage to the suprasternal notch. When a transverse incision is made, it extends approximately one fingerbreadth above the suprasternal notch parallel to it and from the anterior border of one sternocleidomastoid muscle to the opposite side. Soft tissues and muscle are divided, and the isthmus of the thyroid gland that joins both lobes of the gland in the midline over

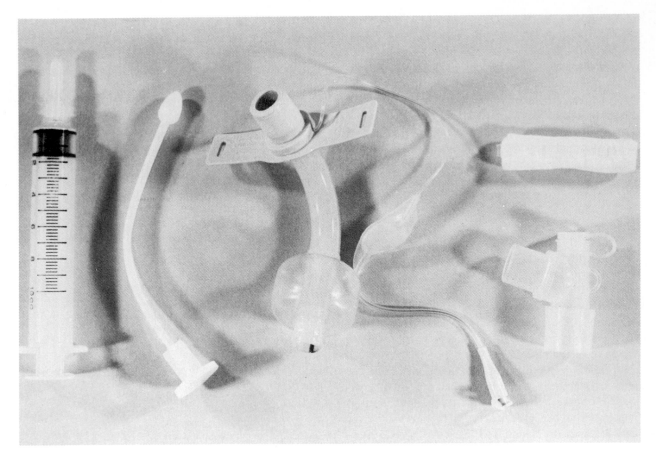

Fig. 21-16. Portex tracheostomy tube with cuff inflated, obturator, syringe, adapter, and neck ties.

the trachea is retracted in an upward direction with retractors, resulting in exposure of the underlying tracheal rings, usually the third and fourth (Fig. 21-17, *A*). In some cases two curved clamps may be inserted through this incision across the isthmus and the isthmus transected (Fig. 21-17, *B*). The transected ends of the isthmus are secured with chromic sutures.

2. Lidocaine, 1% (1 or 2 ml), may be instilled into the trachea to reduce the coughing reflex when the tube is inserted. Air is first drawn into the syringe to ensure that the needle point is located in the lumen. With a knife and no. 15 blade, an incision is made in the trachea directly across the two tracheal rings. The cut ends of the cricoid cartilage are elevated with a hook (Fig. 21-17, *C*).

3. A tracheostomy tube is inserted into the trachea (Fig. 21-17, *D*), the obturator is quickly removed, and the trachea is suctioned with a catheter.

4. The wound edges are lightly approximated with silk sutures no. 2-0, or the wound edges are allowed to fall together around the tube. One or two skin sutures are inserted above the tube. The lower angle of the wound may be left open for drainage.

5. The tracheostomy tube is held in place with tapes tied

with a square knot to the side of the neck. The inner tube is then inserted. A gauze dressing split around the tube is applied to the wound.

6. An additional tracheostomy tube of the same size should be kept adjacent to the patient at all times, in the event the tube becomes dislodged or plugged with secretions. This practice expedites changing the tracheostomy tube with minimal potential for complications to the patient.

Uvulopalatopharyngoplasty (UPPP)

UPPP is primarily performed to relieve obstructive sleep apnea and snoring. Indications for the procedure include:

1. An O_2 saturation that drops below 80
2. Apnea index worse than 20
3. Significant daytime sleepiness
4. Heroic snoring, producing social or marital problems
5. Cardiac arrhythmias, other than tachycardia, or bradycardia during sleep

Any two or more of these indications are reason to perform the operation (Cummings and Schuller, 1986).

Procedural considerations. A tracheostomy may be

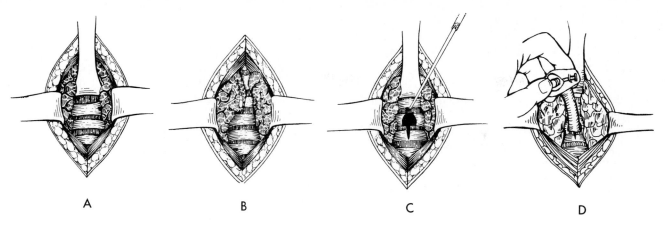

Fig. 21-17. Operative technique for elective tracheostomy. **A,** Retractor exposing trachea by drawing isthmus of thyroid upward. **B,** Alternative method to that shown in **A.** Isthmus of thyroid is divided to expose trachea. **C,** Two tracheal rings are cut, and upper ring is partially resected. Tracheal hook pulls trachea from depth of wound nearer surface. **D,** Insertion of tube. (Modified from DeWeese, D.D., and Saunders, W.H.: Textbook of otolaryngology, ed. 6, St. Louis, 1982, The C.V. Mosby Co.)

performed in conjunction with UPPP because of postoperative edema with subsequent airway obstruction. The tracheostomy tube is removed and the incision closed when the danger of postoperative edema and bleeding has passed (if the surgical procedure is successful). Because some of these patients are obese (causing the tissue of the pharynx to sag during sleep), preoperative planning should include obtaining an assortment of tracheostomy tubes, including extralong tubes, prior to the start of the procedure. Care must be taken in positioning the obese patient to ensure proper body alignment. Emergency tracheostomy or bronchoscopy should be planned, in the event of airway obstruction following anesthetic induction. The surgeon may choose to perform the tracheostomy under local anesthesia with anesthesia personnel monitoring the patient, and then induce general anesthesia after an adequate airway is established.

Instrumentation and positioning are similar to those discussed under tracheostomy and tonsillectomy, with the

exception noted previously of the need to properly position the obese patient.

Operative procedure
1. The mouth gag (usually self-retaining) is inserted.
2. The tissue to be resected may be outlined by an electrosurgical blade. A no. 3 knife handle with no. 15 blade or a no. 7 knife handle with a no. 12 blade may be used to make the incision in the soft palate and anterior to the tonsillar pillar (if the patient has not previously had a tonsillectomy), or posterior to the tonsillar pillars if the patient has had a tonsillectomy (Cummings and Schuller, 1986) (Fig. 21-18).
3. The tissue is resected via Metzenbaum scissors and long forceps with teeth or by hand-controlled electrosurgical pencil.
4. Larger blood vessels may be clamped until the tissue is removed, or a suction coagulator or hand-controlled electrosurgical pencil may be used to obtain hemostasis as the tissue is excised.

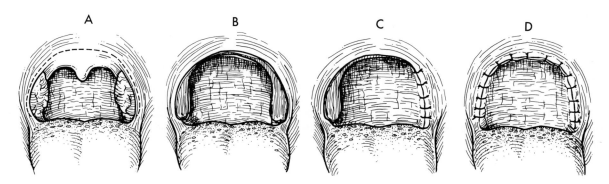

Fig. 21-18. Technique of palatopharyngoplasty as advocated by Simmons et al. (From Luckmann, J., and Sorenson, K.C.: Medical-surgical nursing, ed. 3, Philadelphia, 1987, W.B. Saunders Co.)

5. Once the tissue is removed and hemostasis is obtained, absorbable sutures are used to approximate the edges of the mucosa. Depending on the surgeon's preference, no. 2-0 and 3-0 chromic suture should be available. Needle holders should be long enough to allow the surgeon ease in delivering the atraumatic needle to the edges of the mucosa.

6. The oral cavity should be rinsed of blood and debris, and the incision inspected prior to patient discharge from the operating room.

Care should be taken when inspecting the incision in the postoperative period not to disturb the incision with a tongue blade, if one is used to provide access for inspection. The patient must not be provided with a straw for fluid intake, as it may disturb the suture line. Gentle oral cavity rinsing is recommended several times daily to decrease the chance of postoperative infection and to increase patient comfort.

Laryngofissure

Laryngofissure is opening the larynx for exploratory, excisional, or reconstructive procedures.

Procedural considerations. A laryngofissure is performed whenever access to the intrinsic larynx is necessary. The thyroid cartilages are split in the midline, and the true vocal cords and false vocal cords are incised at the midline anteriorly.

A neck dissection instrument set is required, plus an oscillating power saw.

Operative procedure

1. A tracheostomy is performed, and an endotracheal tube inserted. A general anesthetic is administered. (This procedure may also be done with the patient under local anesthesia.)

2. A transverse incision is made through the skin and first layer of the cervical fascia and platysma muscles, approximately 2 cm above the sternoclavicular junction or in the normal skin crease. The upper skin flap is undermined to the level of the cricoid cartilage, and the lower flap is undermined to the sternoclavicular joint.

3. Bleeding vessels are clamped with mosquito hemostats and ligated. The strap muscles are elevated and incised in the midline.

4. The thyroid cartilages are cut with an oscillating saw, and the true vocal cords are visualized through an incision into the cricothyroid membrane. The true vocal cords are divided in the midline (anterior commissure), and the interior of the larynx is exposed.

5. The tracheostomy tube must be left in place after surgery to ensure an airway.

Partial laryngectomy

Partial laryngectomy is removal of a portion of the larynx. It is done to remove superficial neoplasms that are confined to one vocal cord or to remove a tumor extending up into the ventricle on the anterior commissure or a short distance below the cord. Cancers confined to the intrinsic larynx (Fig. 21-19, *A*) are generally a low-grade malignancy and tend to remain localized for long periods.

Procedural considerations. The patient is placed in the supine position. The operative site is prepped and draped as described for thyroidectomy (Chapter 16).

The setup for partial laryngectomy includes a neck dissection setup, oscillating saw, tracheostomy tubes, and an electrosurgical unit.

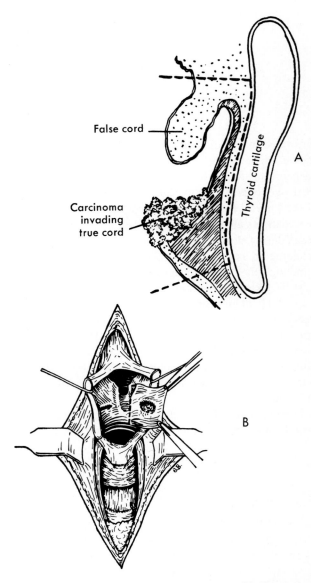

Fig. 21-19. Partial laryngectomy. **A,** Lesion suitable for removal. *Dotted line* indicates wide margin of normal tissue removed along with tumor. When limits of tumor are known, false cord may not be excised. **B,** Incision into larynx is from thyroid notch above to cricoid below. Drawing shows excision of lesion on true cord along with wide margin of normal tissue. (Modified from DeWeese, D.D., and Saunders, W.H.: Textbook of otolaryngology, ed. 6, St. Louis, 1982, The C.V. Mosby Co.)

Operative procedure

1. A tracheostomy is performed as previously described, and an endotracheal tube is inserted.
2. A vertical incision or a thyroid incision with elevation of a flap may be employed (Fig. 21-19, *B*).
3. The sternothyroid muscles are separated in the midline and retracted by means of Green retractors.
4. The fascial covering over the thyroid cartilage is incised with a knife, and with a Freer periosteal elevator the perichondrium is elevated from the cartilage on the side of the tumor.
5. The thyroid cartilage is divided longitudinally in the midline by means of an oscillating saw.
6. The cartilages are retracted, and the cricothyroid membrane is incised with a knife. A blunt-nosed laryngeal scissors is introduced between the vocal cords to divide the mucosa of the anterior wall of the glottis.
7. The divided cartilages are retracted with Kocher retractors to expose the interior of the larynx. A small, moist gauze pack may be placed in the trachea to prevent aspiration of blood or mucus. A small amount of a topical anesthetic may be applied to the larynx to prevent laryngeal muscular spasm. The extent of the intrinsic laryngeal tumor is determined.
8. With a small periosteal elevator, the mucosa on the involved side of the larynx is freed; the false cord and mucosal layer of the region are lifted by means of a periosteal elevator and hooks. The involved cord is excised with straight scissors (Fig. 21-19, *B*).
9. In some cases the thyroid cartilage may be removed with a knife and straight scissors. Bleeding is controlled with hemostats, fine chromic ligatures and sutures, and electrocoagulation.
10. The gauze pack is removed from the trachea. The perichondrium is approximated with chromic no. 2-0 sutures. The strap muscles are approximated in the midline with chromic no. 2-0 sutures. The platysma and the skin edges are approximated separately with fine silk sutures.
11. A tracheolaryngeal tube is left in place and removed at a later date when the airway is adequate. Dressings are applied to the wound and around the tube.

Supraglottic laryngectomy

Supraglottic laryngectomy is excision of the laryngeal structures above the true vocal cords.

Procedural considerations. Supraglottic laryngectomy is indicated in cancer of the epiglottis and false vocal cords. It is designed to remove the cancer, yet preserve the phonatory, respiratory, and sphincteric functions of the larynx. A neck dissection is almost always performed.

The instrument setup is as described for neck dissection.

Operative procedure. The procedure is similar to that described for partial laryngectomy.

Total laryngectomy

Total laryngectomy is complete removal of the cartilaginous larynx, the hyoid bone, and the strap muscles connected to the larynx and possible removal of the preepiglottic space with the lesion. A wide-field laryngectomy is done when there is a loss of mobility of the cords and to treat cancer of the extrinsic larynx and hypopharynx. Malignant tumors of the extrinsic larynx are more anaplastic and tend to metastasize. When laryngeal carcinoma involves more than the true cords, a prophylactic (preventive) radical neck dissection is done to remove the lymphatics. In the presence of malignant tumors, the patient usually has no previous hoarseness, and the first symptom is often the appearance of a lump in the neck.

Laryngectomy presents many psychologic problems. The loss of voice that follows total laryngectomy is psychologically traumatic for the patient and family. The patient may be taught to talk either by using esophageal voice or with an artificial larynx. Esophageal voice is produced by the air contained in the esophagus rather than by that in the trachea. Speech requires a sounding air column. With instruction and practice, the patient is able to control the swallowing of air into the esophagus and reintroduction of this air into the mouth with phonation. The sounding air column is then transformed into speech by means of the lips, tongue, and teeth. A Blom-Singer procedure for tracheoesophageal fistula facilitates insertion of a duckbill prosthesis for purpose of speech.

Because the stump of the trachea is brought out to the skin of the neck, all the patient's breathing is done directly into the trachea. This air is no longer moistened by the nose. Drying and crusting of the tracheal secretions occur. Humidification may be provided by covering the opening with a moist gauze compress.

The patient will be anxious to know about postoperative voice quality, which depends on the specific procedure performed. Table 21-1 lists surgical procedures and associated predictions of postoperative voice qualities.

Procedural considerations. The patient is placed on the operating room bed in a supine position with neck extended and shoulders elevated by a shoulder roll or folded sheet.

An endotracheal anesthetic is administered. An effective suction apparatus is essential. The proposed operative site, including the anterior neck region, the lateral surfaces of the neck down to the outer aspects of the shoulders, and the upper anterior chest region, is prepped and draped in the usual manner.

The instrument setup is a neck dissection set.

Operative procedure

1. A tracheostomy may be performed to control the airway.
2. A midline incision is made from the suprasternal notch to just above the hyoid bone. Skin flaps are undermined on each side. The sternothyroid, sternohyoid,

Table 21-1. Surgical procedures for laryngeal carcinomas and predictions of vocal quality after surgery

Structures removed	Structures left	Postoperative condition
TOTAL LARYNGECTOMY		
Hyoid bone	Tongue	Loses voice
Entire larynx (epiglottis, false cords, true cords)	Pharyngeal walls	Breathes through tracheostomy stoma
	Lower trachea	No problem swallowing
Cricoid cartilage		
Two or three rings of trachea		
SUPRAGLOTTIC OR HORIZONTAL LARYNGECTOMY		
Hyoid bone	True vocal cords	Normal voice
Epiglottis	Cricoid cartilage	May aspirate occasionally, especially liquids
False vocal cords	Trachea	Normal airway
VERTICAL (OR HEMI) LARYNGECTOMY		
One true vocal cord	Epiglottis	Hoarse but serviceable voice
One false cord	One false cord	Normal airway
Arytenoid	One true vocal cord	No problem swallowing
One-half thyroid cartilage	Cricoid	
LARYNGOFISSURE AND PARTIAL LARYNGECTOMY		
One vocal cord	All other structures	Hoarse but serviceable voice; occasionally almost normal voice
		No airway problem
		No swallowing problem
ENDOSCOPIC REMOVAL OF EARLY CARCINOMA		
Part of one vocal cord	All other structures	May have a normal voice
		No other problems

From Saunders, W.H., and others: Nursing care in eye, ear, nose, and throat disorders, ed. 4, St. Louis, 1979, The C.V. Mosby Co.

and omohyoid muscles (strap muscles) on each side are divided by means of curved hemostats and a knife.

3. The suprahyoid muscles are severed from the portion of the hyoid to be divided. The hyoid bone is divided at the junction of its middle and lateral thirds with bone-cutting forceps. Bleeding vessels are clamped and ligated.

4. The superior laryngeal nerve and vessels are exposed and ligated on each side with long curved fine hemostats and fine chromic or silk ligatures.

5. The isthmus of the thyroid gland is divided between hemostats. Each portion of the thyroid gland is dissected from the trachea with Metzenbaum scissors and fine tissue forceps. The superior pole of the thyroid is retracted. The superior thyroid vessels are freed from the larynx by sharp dissection.

6. The larynx is rotated. The inferior pharyngeal constrictor muscle is severed from its attachment to the thyroid cartilage on each side.

7. The endotracheal tube is removed. The trachea is transected just below the cricoid cartilage over a Kelly or Crile hemostat previously inserted between the trachea

and esophagus. The upper resected portion of the trachea and the cricoid cartilage are held upward with Lahey forceps (Fig. 21-20, A). A balloon-cuffed wire-reinforced endotracheal tube with a Murphy eye is inserted in the distal trachea.

8. The larynx is freed from the cervical esophagus and attachments by sharp and blunt dissection. A moist pack is placed around the endotracheal tube to help prevent leakage of blood into the trachea.

9. The pharynx is entered. In most cancers of the intrinsic larynx, the pharynx is entered above the epiglottis. The mucous membrane incision is extended along either side of the epiglottis; the remaining portion of the pharynx and cervical esophagus is dissected well away from the tumor by means of fine-toothed tissue forceps, Metzenbaum scissors, knife, and fine hemostats. The specimen is removed en masse.

10. A nasal feeding tube is inserted through one naris into the esophagus; closure of the hypopharyngeal and esophageal defect is begun with continuous, inverting fine sutures of chromic no. 3-0. The nasal tube is guided down past the pharyngeal suture line.

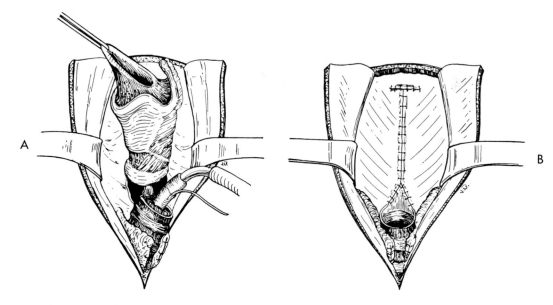

Fig. 21-20. Total laryngectomy. **A,** Usually one or two tracheal rings and hyoid bone are included with specimen. **B,** Mucous membrane and muscles of pharynx are closed in layers. (From DeWeese, D.D., and Saunders, W.H.: Textbook of otolaryngology, ed. 6, St. Louis, 1982, The C.V. Mosby Co.)

11. The pharyngeal suture line is reinforced with interrupted sutures; the suprahyoid muscles are approximated to the cut edges of the inferior constrictor muscles (Fig. 21-20, *B*).

12. The diameter of the tracheal stoma is increased by means of a knife and heavy scissors. The two portions of the thyroid behind the tracheal opening are approximated with interrupted silk sutures, thereby obliterating dead space posterior to the upper portion of the trachea.

13. A closed wound drainage system is used, and the suction drains are appropriately placed (Fig. 21-21).

14. The edges of the deep cervical fascia and the platysma are closed separately with interrupted fine silk sutures. When a great amount of the fascia and platysma has been removed, the wound edges are approximated with silk sutures.

15. A laryngectomy tube of desired size is inserted into the tracheal stoma; a pressure dressing is applied to the wound and neck. (A cuffed tracheostomy tube may be inserted for 24 to 48 hours postoperatively until edema subsides; then it is replaced with a laryngectomy tube.)

Radical neck dissection

In a radical neck dissection, the tumor, surrounding structures, and lymph nodes are removed en masse through a Y-shaped or trifurcate incision in the affected side of the neck. This procedure is done to remove the tumor and metastatic cervical nodes present in malignant lesions, as well as all nonvital structures of the neck. Metastasis occurs through the lymphatic channels by way of the bloodstream. Diseases of the oral cavity, lips, and thyroid gland may spread slowly to the neck. Radical neck surgery is done in the presence of cervical node metastasis from a cancer of the head and neck that has a reasonable chance of being controlled.

A prophylactic neck dissection implies elective radical neck surgery when there is no clinical evidence of metastatic cervical cancer.

Procedural considerations. The patient is placed on the operating room bed in a supine position. General endotracheal anesthesia is administered before the patient is positioned for surgery. During the operation the anesthesiologist works behind a sterile barrier, away from the surgical team. The patient's head is moderately extended with the entire affected side of the face and neck facing uppermost. During surgery the face of the patient is turned away from the surgeon.

The preoperative skin prep is extensive. The patient's neck is draped, leaving a wide operative field. The thigh area is also prepped and draped with sterile towels in readiness for obtaining a dermal graft before closure of the neck wound; it is usually more convenient to use the thigh on the same side as the neck dissection.

The instrument setup includes the following:

50 Mosquito hemostats, curved
 8 Allis forceps
 8 Kelly hemostats
 8 Pean forceps
 4 Thyroid tenacula
 4 Babcock forceps

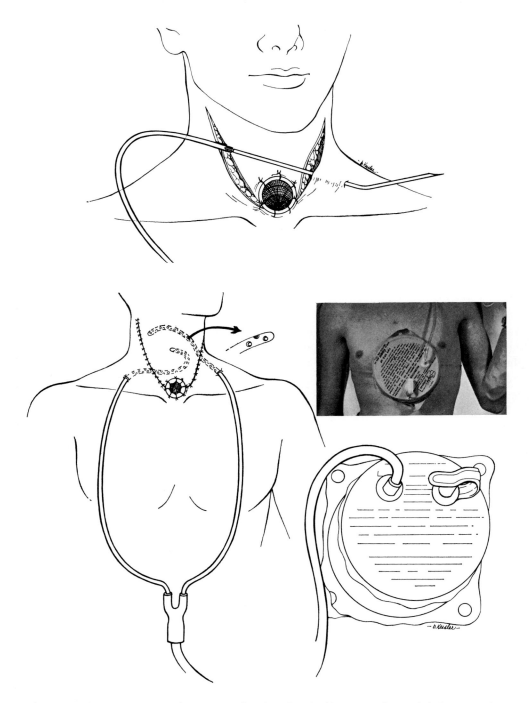

Fig. 21-21. Hemovac apparatus for constant closed suction. In this system of wound drainage, suction is maintained by plastic container with spring inside that forces apart lids and thereby produces suction, which is transmitted through plastic tubing. Neck skin is pulled down tight, and no external dressing is required. Container serves as both suction source and receptacle for blood. It is emptied as required, and drainage tubes are usually left in neck for 3 days. (From DeWeese, D.D., and Saunders, W.H.: Textbook of otolaryngology, ed. 6, St. Louis, 1982, The C.V. Mosby Co.)

2 Right-angle clamps
Needle holders, assorted
12 Towel clamps
2 Tonsil suction tubes
1 Trousseau tracheal dilator
2 Rake retractors
2 Army-Navy retractors
2 Richardson retractors
2 Vein retractors
4 Skin hooks, 2 single and 2 double
1 Gelpi retractor
4 Knife handles no. 3, with nos. 10 and 15 blades
1 Tracheal hook
1 Upper-lateral scissors
1 Cartilage scissors
2 Mayo scissors, straight and curved
2 Metzenbaum scissors
2 Scissors, small, curved, sharp and blunt
4 Tissue forceps, 2 with and 2 without teeth
2 Adson tissue forceps
2 Brown-Adson tissue forceps
1 Periosteal elevator
2 Freer elevators
1 Bayonet forceps
Brown or Stryker dermatome

Operative procedure

1. One of several types of incisions may be used, including the Y-shaped, H-shaped, or trifurcate incision (Fig. 21-22, *A*).
2. The upper curved incision is made through the skin and platysma with a knife, tissue forceps, and fine hemostats; ligatures are used for bleeding vessels. The upper flap is retracted; then the vertical portion of the incision is made, and the skin flaps are retracted anteriorly and posteriorly with retractors. The anterior margin of the trapezius muscle is exposed by means of curved scissors. The flaps are retracted to expose the entire lateral aspect of the neck (Fig. 21-22, *B*). Branches of the jugular veins are clamped, ligated, and divided.
3. The sternal and clavicular attachments of the sternocleidomastoid muscle are clamped with curved Pean forceps and then divided with a knife (Fig. 21-22, *C*). The superficial layer of deep fascia is incised. The omohyoid muscle is severed between clamps just above its scapular attachment.
4. The internal jugular vein is isolated by blunt dissection and then doubly clamped, ligated with medium silk, and divided with Metzenbaum scissors. A transfixion suture is placed on the lower end of the vein.
5. The common carotid artery and vagus nerve are identified. The fatty areolar tissue and fascia are dissected away, using Metzenbaum scissors and fine tissue forceps. Branches of the thyrocervical artery are clamped, divided, and ligated.
6. The tissues and fascia of the posterior triangle are dissected, beginning at the anterior margin of the trapezius muscle and continuing near the brachial plexus and the levator scapulae and the scalene muscles. During the dissection, branches of the cervical and suprascapular arteries are clamped, ligated, and divided.
7. The anterior portion of the block dissection is completed. The omohyoid muscle is severed at its attachment to the hyoid bone. Bleeding is controlled. All hemostats are removed, and the operative site is covered with warm, moist laparotomy packs.
8. The sternocleidomastoid muscle is severed and retracted. The submental space is dissected free of fatty areolar tissue and lymph nodes from above downward.
9. The deep fascia on the lower edge of the mandible is incised; the facial vessels are divided and ligated.
10. The submaxillary triangle is entered. The submaxillary duct is divided and ligated. The submaxillary glands with surrounding fatty areolar tissue and lymph nodes are dissected toward the digastric muscle. The facial branch of the external carotid artery is divided. Portions of the digastric and stylohyoid muscles are severed from their attachments to the hyoid bone and on the mastoid. The upper end of the internal jugular vein is elevated and divided. The surgical specimen is removed (Fig. 21-22, *D*).
11. The entire field is examined for bleeding and then irrigated with warm saline solution. A skin graft is placed, covering the bifurcation of the carotid artery extending down approximately 4 inches, and sutured with no. 4-0 chromic on a very small cutting needle. Closed wound suction drains are placed in the wound (Fig. 21-21).
12. The flaps are approximated with interrupted, fine silk or nylon sutures (Fig. 21-22, *E*) or with skin staples. Mastisol liquid is applied to the wound edges, or a bulky pressure dressing may be applied to the neck.

Modified neck dissection

Modified neck dissection is removal of neck contents with the exception of the sternocleidomastoid muscle, internal jugular vein, and eleventh cranial nerve.

Procedural considerations. When performed by an experienced surgeon, this type of neck dissection can facilitate removal of a tumor and lymph nodes suspected of metastases and allow the patient a minimal defect and unimpaired shoulder function.

With radical and modified neck dissection, the surgeon and radiologist may decide on a course of postoperative radiation therapy or chemotherapy. The decision depends on the type and location of tumor, stage of disease, and condition of the patient.

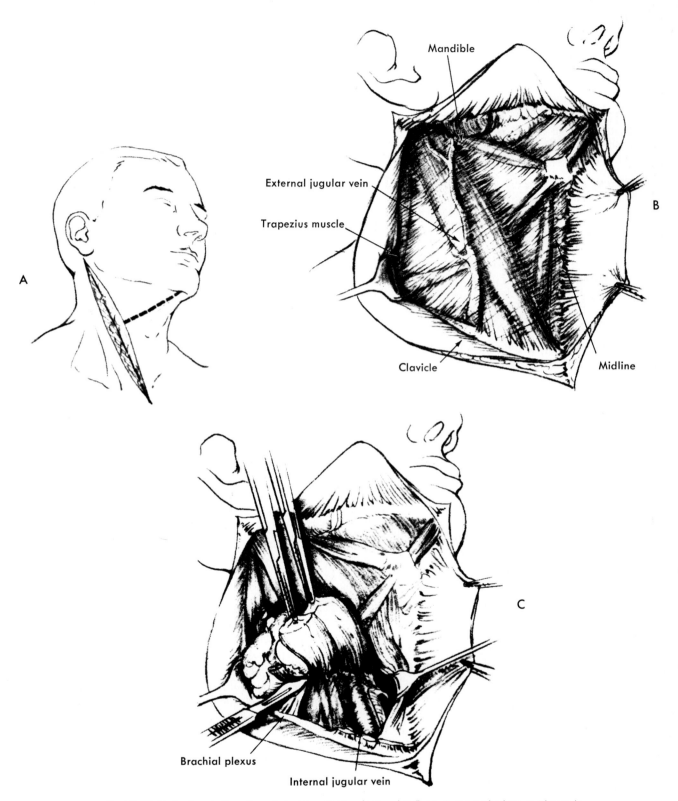

Fig. 21-22. Radical neck dissection. **A,** Incision. **B,** Developing skin flaps. **C,** Sternocleidomastoid muscle divided.

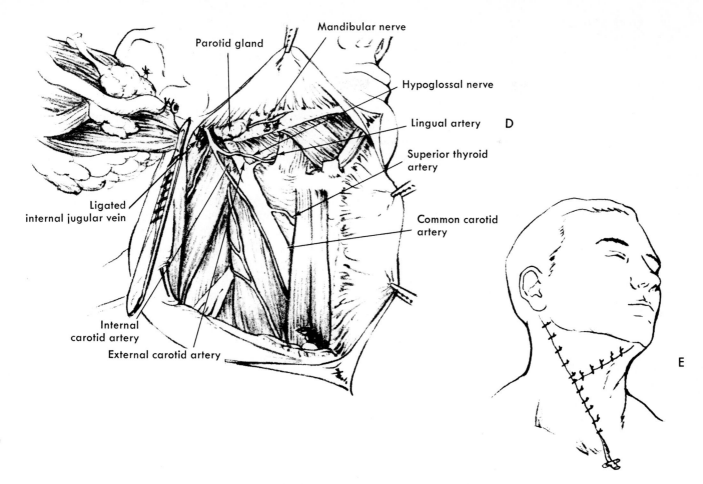

Fig. 21-22, cont'd. D, Dissection completed, and surgical specimen removed. **E,** Closure. (Modified from Wilder, J.R.: Atlas of general surgery, ed. 2, St. Louis, 1964, The C.V. Mosby Co.)

REFERENCE

Cummings, C.W., and Schuller, D.E.: Otolaryngology—head and neck surgery, 3 vols., St. Louis, 1986, The C.V. Mosby Co.

BIBLIOGRAPHY

American Academy of Facial Plastic and Reconstructive Surgery: Plastic and reconstructive surgery of the face and neck, St. Louis, 1984, The C.V. Mosby Co.

American Academy of Otolaryngology—Head and Neck Surgery Foundation: Common problems of the head and neck region, Philadelphia, 1986, W.B. Saunders Co.

Carrell, B.L.: Laser treatment of laryngeal polyps, AORN J 38:232, 1983.

Cummings, C.W., and others: Atlas of laryngeal surgery, St. Louis, 1984, The C.V. Mosby Co.

DeWeese, D.D., and Saunders, W.H.: Textbook of otolaryngology, ed. 6, St. Louis, 1982, The C.V. Mosby Co.

Freund, H.R.: Principles of head and neck surgery, ed. 2, New York, 1979, Appleton-Century Crofts.

Gates, G.A.: Current therapy in otolaryngology—head and neck surgery, St. Louis, 1984, The C.V. Mosby Co.

Guyton, A.C.: Textbook of medical physiology, ed. 7, Philadelphia, 1986, W.B. Saunders Co.

Hood, G.H., and Dincher, J.R.: Total patient care: foundations and practice, ed. 7, St. Louis, 1989, The C.V. Mosby Co.

Karmody, C.S.: Textbook of otolaryngology, Philadelphia, 1983, Lea & Febiger.

Long, B.C., and Phipps, W.J.: Essentials of medical-surgical nursing, St. Louis, 1985, The C.V. Mosby Co.

Luckmann, J., and Sorenson, K.C.: Medical-surgical nursing, ed. 3, Philadelphia, 1987, W.B. Saunders Co.

Lyons, R.J.: Surgical implants: voice prostheses, AORN J 37:1369, 1983.

Lyons, R.J., and Coren, D.A.: The head and neck patient: a team approach to rehabilitation, AORN J 40:751, 1984.

Marino, L.B.: Cancer nursing, St. Louis, 1981, The C.V. Mosby Co.

Minx, S.M., and Stellwagon, G.: Pediatric airway obstruction: nursing care of the patient undergoing endoscopy, AORN J 40:338, 1984.

Paparella, M., and Shumrick, D.: Otolaryngology, vol. 3, Head and neck, ed. 2, Philadelphia, 1980, W.B. Saunders Co.

Potter, P., and Perry, A.G.: Fundamentals of nursing, ed. 2, St. Louis, 1989, The C.V. Mosby Co.

Protocol for laser surgery described, Anesth. News 8(7):1, 1982.

Sabiston, D.C., Jr., editor: Davis-Christopher textbook of surgery: the biological basis of modern surgical practice, ed. 13, Philadelphia, 1986, W.B. Saunders Co.

Saunders, W.H., and others: Nursing care in eye, ear, nose, and throat disorders, ed. 4, St. Louis, 1979, The C.V. Mosby Co.

Ward, S.: Rigid endoscopy of respiratory tract, AORN J 34:1058, 1981.

22 Orthopedic surgery

JANE SCOTT WITCHEY

Nicholas André first used the word "orthopaedia" in 1741 as the title for a book dealing with the prevention and correction of skeletal deformities in children. The word is derived from the Greek *orthos,* meaning straight, and *paidios,* meaning child. Orthopedic surgery has been defined by the American Academy of Orthopaedic Surgeons as "the medical specialty that includes the investigation, preservation, restoration and development of the form and function of the extremity, spine and associated structures by medical, surgical and physical methods."

SURGICAL ANATOMY

To be an efficient member of the operating team, the perioperative nurse must be aware of the anatomic structures involved in orthopedic surgery. Following is a brief summary of the anatomy of the musculoskeletal system.

The bones of the body form a stable framework that supports the weight of the soft tissues. Diarthrodial joints consist of (1) the ends of the articulating bones that are covered with hyaline cartilage, (2) the supporting ligaments and capsule, and (3) a filmy synovium that forms the inner lining of the joint. Hyaline cartilage provides a smooth gliding surface for joint movement and cushions the joint to help soften impact. Musculotendinous units originate and insert on adjacent bones and pass across the joints. Contraction of muscles produces motion at the joints and brings about body movements.

Bones are divided into four types, according to their shapes: long, short, flat, and irregular (Fig. 22-1). *Long* bones are present in the limbs and consist of a shaft and two ends; the ends are covered with articular cartilage and provide a surface for articulation and muscle attachment. *Short* bones, such as the carpals and tarsals, are present where strength but limited movement is required. *Flat* bones are found in the shoulder and pelvis. *Irregular* bones are found in the skull and vertebral column. Sesamoid bones (resembling a sesame seed) are a type of irregularly shaped bones that are found specifically within tendons. For the most part they are small bones located between the metacarpal and proximal phalanx in the thumb but include the triangular patella, the largest of the sesamoid bones.

Long bones are divided into three sections: the diaphysis and two epiphyses. The *diaphysis,* or shaft, is the midportion, and each articulating end is an *epiphysis*. Until skeletal maturity a line of cartilage called the *epiphyseal plate* separates the epiphyses from the diaphysis.

There are two types of bone tissue: cortical and cancellous bone. *Cortical* bone is the main supporting tissue, the hard bone that forms the shell of all bones. *Cancellous* bone is the soft, spongy bone contained inside cortical bone at the ends of long bones and permeating the bodies of short and flat bones. *Trabeculae* are located within cancellous bone and consist of an interconnecting network of bone oriented along the lines of stress. These structures are important for weight bearing, providing the strength to withstand the stresses placed upon the specific bone. *Bone marrow* is a soft substance located in the center of bones. A thin layer of connective tissue called *periosteum* covers all bone.

Shoulder and upper extremity

The *clavicle,* which is a long, doubly curved bone, serves as a prop for the shoulder and holds it away from the chest wall. The clavicle rests almost horizontally at the upper and anterior part of the thorax, above the first rib. It articulates medially with the manubrium of the sternum and laterally with the acromion of the scapula and is tethered to the underlying coracoid process of the scapula by the coracoclavicular ligaments.

The *scapula* (shoulder blade) is a flat, triangular bone that forms the posterior part of the shoulder girdle, lying superior and posterior to the upper chest. The glenoid cavity provides a socket for the humerus, and the acromion process articulates with the clavicle. The scapula is attached to the trunk by muscles.

The *acromioclavicular joint* is the articulating structure (joint) between the outer end of the clavicle and a flattened articular facet situated on the inner border of the acromion.

The *shoulder joint,* a ball-and-socket joint, is formed by the head of the humerus and the shallow glenoid cavity. This joint is surrounded by a loose capsule that allows considerable motion (Fig. 22-2).

The muscles immediately surrounding the shoulder joint are the supraspinous, infraspinous, teres minor, and subscapular muscles; together, they are referred to as the *rotator cuff*. These muscles stabilize the shoulder joint while the entire arm is moved by the powerful deltoid,

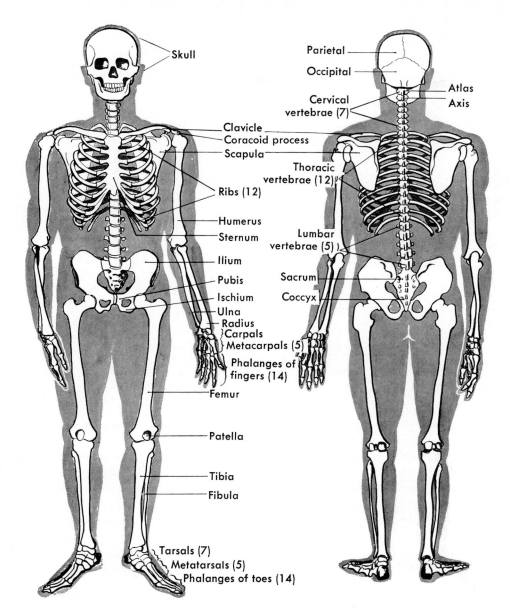

Fig. 22-1. Human skeleton, ventral and dorsal views. Numbers in parentheses indicate number of bones in that unit. In comparison with skeletons of other mammals, the human skeleton is a patchwork of primitive and specialized parts. Erect posture brought about by specialized changes in legs and pelvis enabled primitive arrangement of arms and hands (arboreal adaptation of human's ancestors) to be used for manipulation of tools. Development of skull and brain followed as consequence of premium natural selection based on dexterity, better senses, and ability to appraise environment. (Modified from Hickman, C.P., Jr., Roberts, L.S., and Hickman F.M.: Integrated principles of zoology, ed. 7, St. Louis, 1984, The C.V. Mosby Co.)

pectoralis major, teres major, and latissimus dorsi muscles.

The *humerus*, the longest and largest bone of the upper extremity, is composed of a shaft and two ends. The proximal end, or head, has two projections, the greater and lesser tuberosities (Figs. 22-1 and 22-3).

The head articulates with the glenoid cavity of the scapula. The circumference of the articular surface of the humerus is constricted and is termed the *anatomic neck*. The constriction below the tuberosities is called the *surgical neck* and is the site of most fractures. The anatomic neck marks the attatchment to the capsule of the shoulder joint.

The greater tuberosity is situated at the lateral side of the head. Its upper surface has three impressions where the supraspinous, infraspinous, and teres minor tendons insert. This tendinous insertion is known as the rotator cuff. The lesser tuberosity is situated in front of the neck and has an impression for the insertion of the tendon of the subscapular muscle. The tuberosities are separated

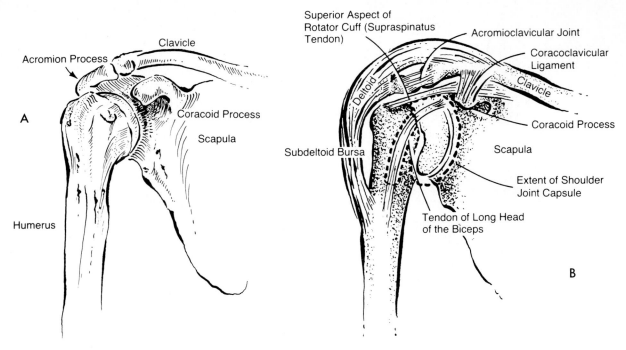

Fig. 22-2. Shoulder joint and related parts: anterior view. **A,** Without soft tissue; **B,** Soft tissue added. (Redrawn from Lewis, R.C.: Primary care orthopedics, New York, 1988, Churchill Livingstone.)

from each other by a deep groove (bicipital groove) in which lies the tendon of the biceps muscle of the arm. The tendon of the pectoralis major inserts on the lateral margin of the bicipital groove, and the latissimus dorsi and teres major insert on the medial margin.

The lower portion of the humerus is flattened and ends below in a broad articular surface, which is divided into two parts by a slight ridge. On either side of the ridge are projections, the lateral and medial condyles. On the lateral condyle the rounded articular surface is called the *capitellum;* it articulates with the head of the radius. On the medial condyle the articular surface is termed the trochlea; the articular surface articulates with the ulna (Fig. 22-4, *A*).

The *ulna* is located medial to the radius. The proximal portion of the ulna, the olecranon, articulates with the trochlea of the humerus at the elbow (Fig. 22-4, *B*).

The *radius* rotates around the ulna. At the proximal end is the head, which articulates with the capitellum of the humerus and also the radial notch of the ulna. The tendon of the biceps muscle is attached to the tuberosity just below the radial head (Fig. 22-4, *C*). The distal end of the radius is divided into two articular surfaces. The distal surface articulates with the carpal bones of the wrist, and the surface on the medial side articulates with the distal end of the ulna.

Wrist and hand

The skeletal bones of the wrist and hand consist of three distinct parts: (1) the carpals, or wrist bones; (2) the meta-

carpals, or bones of the palm; and (3) the phalanges, or bones of the digits.

There are eight carpal bones arranged in two rows. The distal row, proceeding from the radial to the ulnar side, includes the trapezium, trapezoid, capitate, and hamate; the proximal row consists of the scaphoid, lunate, triquetrum, and pisiform. Functionally, the scaphoid links the rows as it stabilizes and coordinates the movement of the proximal and distal rows (Fig. 22-5).

Each carpal bone consists of several smooth articular surfaces for contact with the adjacent bones, as well as rough surfaces for the attachment of ligaments. No tendons or muscles are attached to the wrist bones. Consequently, the movement of the carpal bones is dependent on the tendons, which pass across the dorsal and volar surfaces to insert into the metacarpals and phalanges distally.

The five metacarpal bones are situated in the palm. Proximally they articulate with the distal row of carpal bones, and distally the head of each metacarpal articulates with its proper phalanx. The heads of the metacarpals form the knuckles (Fig. 22-6).

The phalanges, or *finger bones,* consist of 14 bones in each hand, two in the thumb and three in each finger. Each phalanx consists of a shaft and two ends.

Hip and femur

The *hip joint,* a ball-and-socket joint, is formed by the acetabular portion of the innominate (pelvic) bone and the proximal end of the femur. The hip joint is surrounded by a capsule, ligaments, and muscles (Fig. 22-7).

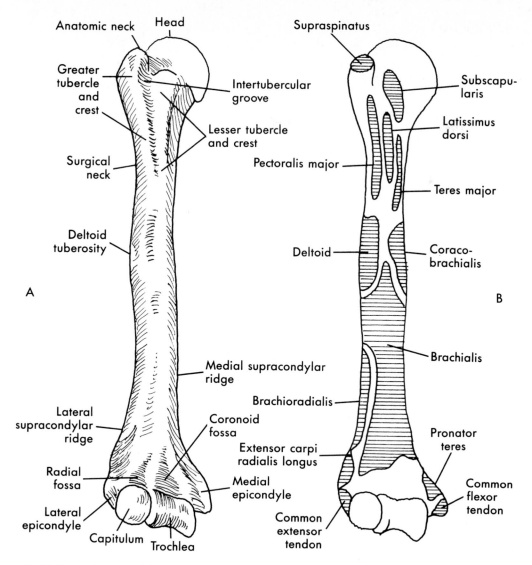

Fig. 22-3. Anterior views of the humerus. In **B** muscle attachments are shown. (Redrawn from Hollinshead, W.H.: Anatomy for surgeons, vol. 3, ed. 3, Philadelphia, 1982, Harper & Row Publishers.)

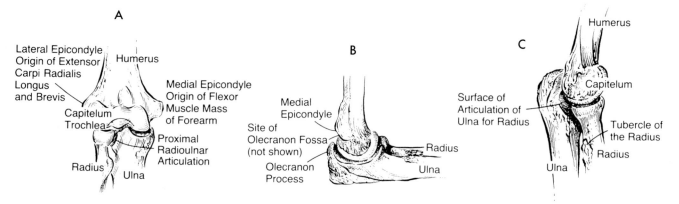

Fig. 22-4. Anatomy of the elbow. **A,** Anterior view: Note the lateral and medial epicondyles, the capitellum and trochlear portions of the articular surface, and the articulation between the radial head and capitellum superiorly and the radial head and ulna medially. **B,** Lateral view. **C,** Oblique view: Note the relationship between the radial head and capitellum of the humerus, the articulation with the ulna, and the tuberosity below the radial head where the biceps attaches. (Redrawn from Lewis, R.C.: Primary care orthopedics, New York, 1988, Churchill Livingstone.)

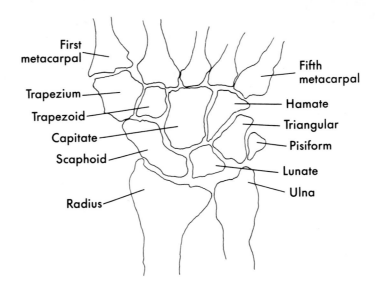

Fig. 22-5. Anatomy of the wrist and carpus. (Redrawn with permission from AORN J., Vol. 49, p. 760, March 1989. Copyright AORN Inc, 10170 East Mississippi Avenue, Denver, Colo. 80231.)

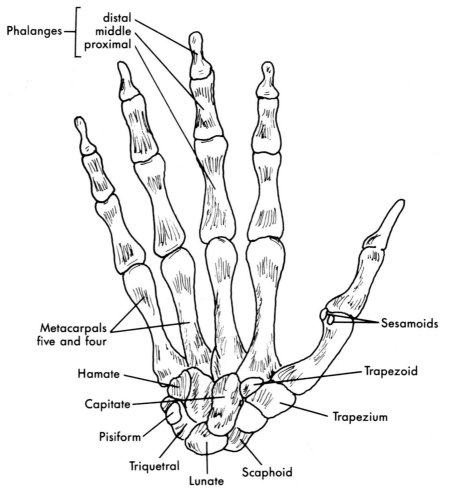

Fig. 22-6. Anatomy of the hand, palmar view. (Redrawn from Hollinshead, W.H.: Anatomy for surgeons, vol. 3, ed. 3, Philadelphia, 1982, Harper & Row Publishers.)

Fig. 22-7. Right hip joint: **A,** anterior view; **B,** frontal section. (From Seeley, R.R., Stephens, T.D., and Tate, P.: Anatomy and physiology, St. Louis, 1989, Times Mirror/Mosby College Publishing.)

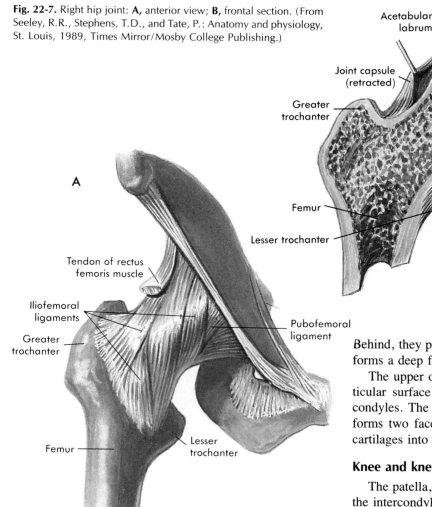

The acetabulum is a deep, round cavity that holds the head of the femur. The proximal end of the femur consists of the femoral head and neck, the upper portion of the shaft, and the greater and lesser trochanters.

The greater trochanter is a broad process of cancellous bone that protrudes from the outer upper portion of the shaft and projects upward from the junction of the superior border of the neck with the outer surface of the shaft (Fig. 22-7). It serves as a point of insertion for the abductor and short rotator muscles of the hip.

The lesser trochanter is a conical process projecting from the posterior and inferior portion of the base of the neck of the femur at its junction with the shaft (Fig. 22-7). It serves as a point of insertion for the iliopsoas muscle. The lower end of the femur terminates in the two condyles. In front, the condyles are separated from one another by a smooth depression, called the *intercondylar* or *patellar groove,* forming an articulating surface for the patella.

Behind, they project slightly, and the space between them forms a deep fossa, the *intercondylar fossa* (Fig. 22-8).

The upper or condylar end of the tibia presents an articular surface corresponding with those of the femoral condyles. The articular surface of the two tibial condyles forms two facets, which are deepened by the semilunar cartilages into fossae for the femoral condyles.

Knee and knee joint

The patella, or *kneecap,* is anterior to the knee joint in the intercondylar groove of the distal femur. It is a sesamoid bone within the quadriceps tendon. The anterior surface of the patella is united with the patellar tendon. The posterior surface of the patella articulates with the femur (Fig. 22-9).

The knee joint consists of three articular surfaces: two condyle articulations, one between each condyle of the femur and the corresponding meniscus and condyle of the tibia, and a third articulation between the patella and femur. The bones of the knee joint are connected by extraarticular and intraarticular structures. The extaarticular attachments are the capsule, the quadriceps muscle, and two collateral ligaments. The intraarticular ligaments are the two cruciate ligaments and the attachments of the menisci (semilunar cartilages) (Fig. 22-10).

The capsule of the knee joint is attached proximally to the femoral condyles, and it is attached distally to the condyles of the tibia and to the upper end of the fibula. The capsule is reinforced—in front by the patellar and quadriceps tendon, on the sides by the medial and lateral collateral ligaments, and posteriorly by the popliteus and gastrocnemius muscles.

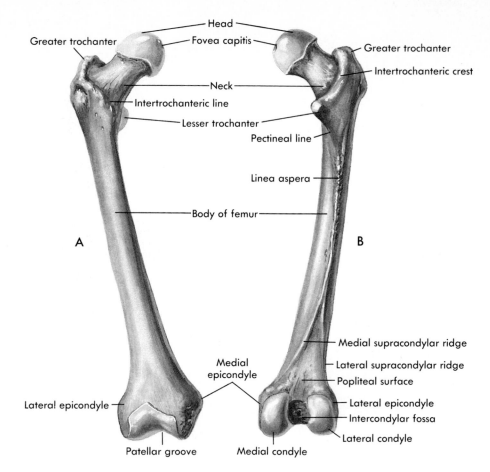

Fig. 22-8. A, Anterior and B, posterior views of the right femur. (From Seeley, R.R., Stephens, T.D., and Tate, P.: Anatomy and physiology, St. Louis, 1989, Times Mirror/Mosby College Publishing.)

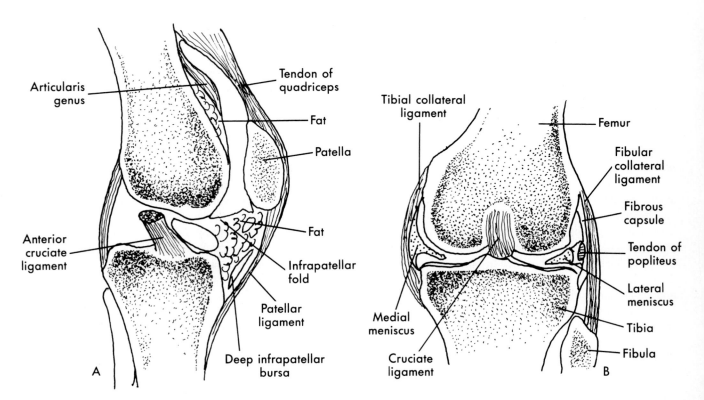

Fig. 22-9. A, Sagittal and B, frontal sections of the knee joint. (Redrawn from Hollinshead, W.H.: Anatomy for surgeons, vol. 3, ed. 3, Philadelphia, 1982, Harper & Row, Publishers.)

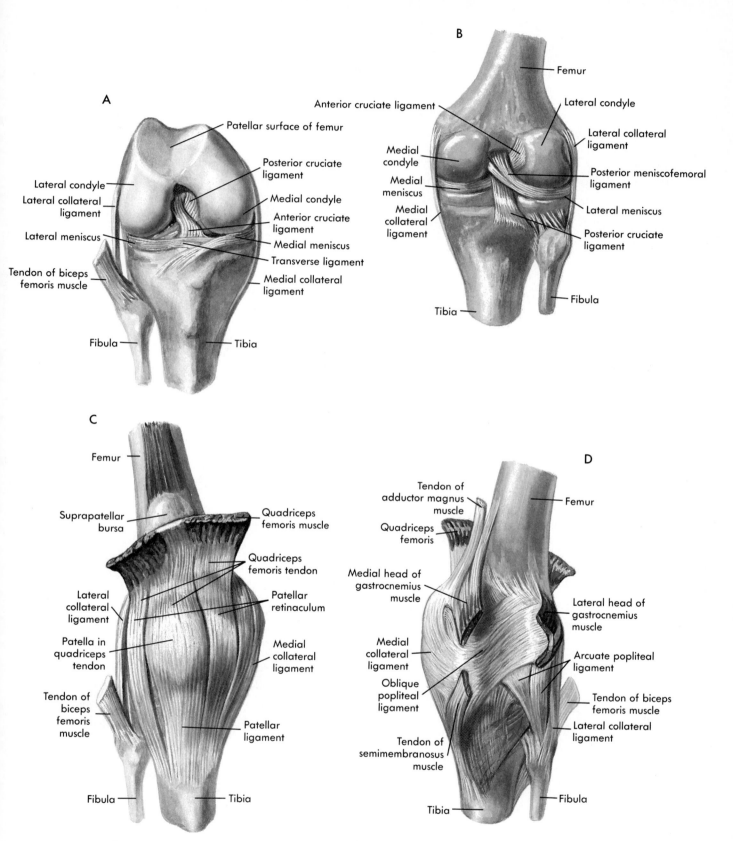

Fig. 22-10. Anatomy of the right knee joint. **A,** anterior view with knee flexed; **B,** posterior view; **C,** anterior superficial aspect; and **D,** posterior superficial aspect. (From Seeley, R.R., Stephens, T.D. and Tate, P.: Anatomy and physiology, St. Louis, 1989, Times Mirror/Mosby College Publishing.)

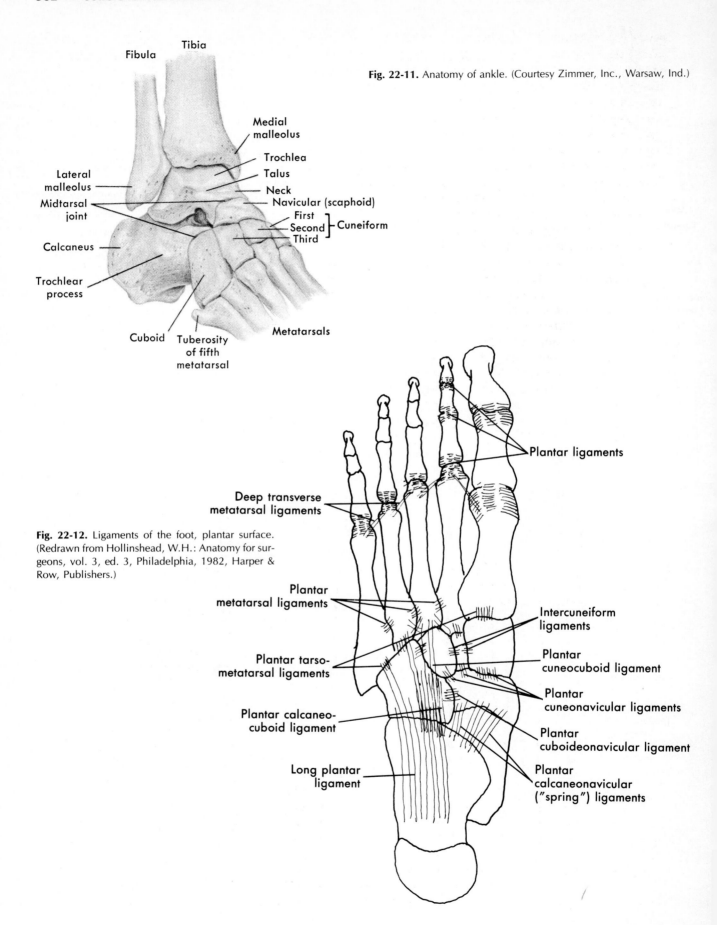

Fibula

Tibia

Medial
malleolus

Trochlea

Talus

Neck

Navicular (scaphoid)

First ⎫
Second ⎬ Cuneiform
Third ⎭

Lateral
malleolus

Midtarsal
joint

Calcaneus

Trochlear
process

Cuboid

Tuberosity
of fifth
metatarsal

Metatarsals

Fig. 22-11. Anatomy of ankle. (Courtesy Zimmer, Inc., Warsaw, Ind.)

Plantar ligaments

Deep transverse
metatarsal ligaments

Fig. 22-12. Ligaments of the foot, plantar surface.
(Redrawn from Hollinshead, W.H.: Anatomy for sur-
geons, vol. 3, ed. 3, Philadelphia, 1982, Harper &
Row, Publishers.)

Plantar
metatarsal ligaments

Plantar tarso-
metatarsal ligaments

Plantar calcaneo-
cuboid ligament

Long plantar
ligament

Intercuneiform
ligaments

Plantar
cuneocuboid ligament

Plantar
cuneonavicular ligaments

Plantar
cuboideonavicular ligament

Plantar
calcaneonavicular
("spring") ligaments

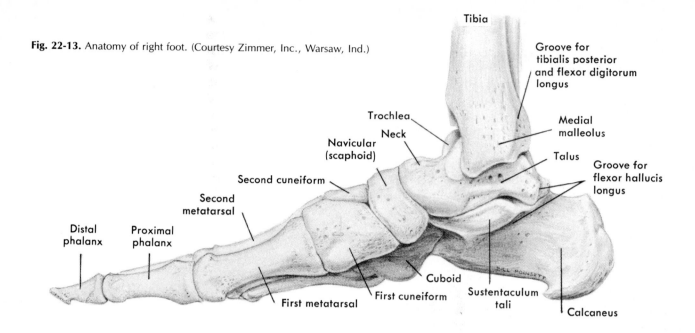

Fig. 22-13. Anatomy of right foot. (Courtesy Zimmer, Inc., Warsaw, Ind.)

The cruciate ligaments, consisting of two fibrous bands, extend from the intercondylar fossa of the femur to attachments in front of and behind the intercondylar surface of the tibia (Fig. 22-10, *A, B*).

The semilunar cartilages, known as the *menisci*, are interposed between the condyles of the femur and those of the tibia (Fig. 22-10 *A, B*). Each meniscus is attached to the joint capsule. The ends of the cartilages are attached to the tibia in the middle of its upper articular surface.

Synovial membrane lines the capsule of the joint and covers the infrapatellar fat pad, parts of the cruciate ligaments, and portions of the bone.

The portion of the knee joint cavity that extends upward in front of the femur is called the *suprapatellar pouch* or *bursa* (Fig. 22-10, *C*).

Ankle and foot

The *ankle joint,* a hinge joint, is formed by the lower end of the tibia and its malleolus, as well as the malleolus of the fibula. These structures form a mortise for the reception of the upper surface of the talus and its facets (Fig. 22-11).

The bones are connected by ligaments, which spread out from the malleoli to be attached to the calcaneus and navicular bones (Fig. 22-12). The joint is surrounded by a thin capsule.

The *talus* consists of a body, neck, and head. It is an irregular bone that fits into a mortise formed by the malleoli. It articulates with the calcaneus and navicular bones (Fig. 22-13).

The bony framework of the foot comprises seven tarsal bones, five metatarsal bones, and 14 phalanges.

The calcaneus forms the heel and gives support to the talus. The cuboid bone articulates proximally and posteriorly with the calcaneus and distally with the fourth and fifth metatarsals and the third cuneiform bones.

The navicular bone articulates with the cuneiform bones, which lie side by side in front of the scaphoid. The metatarsal bones articulate proximally with the tarsal bones and distally with the bases of the first phalanges of the corresponding toes. There are two phalanges for the great toe and three for each of the other toes (Fig. 22-13).

PERIOPERATIVE NURSING CONSIDERATIONS
Assessment/nursing diagnosis

In the perioperative care of the orthopedic patient, a nursing assessment is done in each phase of care and treatment.

Included in the preoperative assessment is a nursing history and physical examination. In obtaining the history, interview techniques are employed for collecting data. Information specific to orthopedics includes onset of the problem (that is, congenital or developmental), specifics of onset (for example, accident or injury), and functional limitations. Observation skills are needed to perform the physical examination. Appearance of the extremity, range of motion, gait abnormalities, and neurovascular status are noted. The results of the preoperative assessment are documented. This information will be used throughout the patient's hospital or ambulatory surgery course.

Communication between nursing and surgical personnel is essential for intelligent planning for the orthopedic surgical patient. Information concerning the patient's diagnosis, radiologic studies, physical disabilities, surgical approach, position, special equipment, and instruments or supplies needed enables the nurse to plan for the surgical procedure. This preparation can significantly reduce both anesthesia and operating time.

In the operating room the nurse conducts an assessment while admitting the patient to the surgical suite. In addition to the standard assessment, the orthopedic nurse is concerned with range of motion, mobility, level of pain on mobility, and x-ray findings. Immobilization materials, bandages, and traction equipment are observed. Ascertaining the extremity to be treated with both the patient and the chart is imperative. Once the perioperative nurse has assessed the orthopedic patient, nursing diagnoses can be formulated. Nursing diagnoses related to the patient having orthopedic surgery might include:

- Potential for infection related to the surgical procedure
- Potential for injury related to the surgical position
- Knowledge deficit related to the surgical procedure
- Pain related to the orthopedic injury
- Potential for impaired skin integrity

Planning

Planning the care of the orthopedic patient in the operating room requires specialized skills that come from experience. Infection is a main concern in orthopedic surgery. Incisions are usually deep, increasing the potential for infection locally or in the joint, if the joint is entered. Another concern is positioning the patient on the standard

Sample Care Plan

NURSING DIAGNOSIS:
Potential for infection related to the surgical procedure
GOAL:
Patient will not have postoperative signs of infection caused by the surgical procedure.
INTERVENTIONS:
Review chart for recent lab results and vital signs.
Determine wound classification.
Isolate genitals and buttocks from operative site with adhesive drape.
Apply surgical skin prep according to policy and procedure.
Provide iodine-impregnated (Ioban) incisional drape for surgical draping per surgeon's request.
Utilize laminar air flow, exhaust system, or ultraviolet lighting system for total joint replacement surgery.
Deliver antibiotic wound irrigation to the field per surgeon's order.
Enforce and implement aseptic technique.
Keep traffic in and out of the room to a minimum.
Keep movement within operating room to a minimum.

NURSING DIAGNOSIS:
Potential for injury related to the surgical position
GOAL:
Patient will be free of injury related to positioning.

INTERVENTIONS:
Ensure that adequate equipment and provisions are available for positioning of the patient.
Obtain assessment of pain-related areas, and transfer and position patient accordingly to minimize pain and prevent further injury.
Maintain body alignment and obtain assistance with transfer and positioning.
Utilize padding and positioning and safety devices as needed to support patient in desired position and protect bony prominences and dependent pressure areas.
Note changes in mobility and function of musculoskeletal system preoperatively to postoperatively, if able.
Report to postanesthesia care unit nurse special positioning needs required postoperatively.

NURSING DIAGNOSIS:
Knowledge deficit related to the surgical procedure
GOAL:
Patient will understand the surgical procedure and sequence of perioperative events.

or orthopedic operating room bed. Various positions are used for orthopedic surgery including supine, sitting, prone, lateral, and modifications of each. The nurse must know the hazards and precautions, special equipment, and accessory items needed to support patients in these positions.

A Sample Care Plan for a patient having orthopedic surgery is shown below.

Implementation
Positioning

The orthopedic patient requires special handling. The patient with a fractured hip should not be moved from the bed onto a stretcher to be taken to the operating room but should be transported in the bed to avoid unnecessary pain.

Proper positioning of the patient on the operating room bed provides for good body alignment without undue strain or pressure on nerves and muscles, adequate exposure of the operative area, optimum respiratory and circulatory functions, and adequate stabilization of the body.

The surgeon is responsible for supervising the surgical team as they position the patient on the operating room bed. The operating room staff should know the meaning of terms such as flexion, extension, abduction, and adduction, which are used in positioning a patient. All nursing personnel should know how to manipulate the orthopedic surgical table and apply the attachments (Fig. 22-14).

Sample Care Plan—cont'd

INTERVENTIONS:

Determine patient's understanding of the impending surgery during the preoperative visit.

Explain the sequence of perioperative events; utilize teaching resources.

Answer questions and listen to patient's concerns regarding the surgery.

Orient patient to the operating room environment upon arrival to the operating room.

Explain procedures such as transfers, ESU dispersive pad placement, safety belt, and anesthesia monitors before they are carried out.

NURSING DIAGNOSIS:

Pain related to the orthopedic injury

GOAL:

Patient will maintain an adequate level of comfort throughout perioperative phase.

INTERVENTIONS:

Determine specific areas of patient's discomforts before transfers are made.

Assure patient that postoperative pain relief will be available.

Assist patient in transfers to and from the surgical bed, supporting a limb fracture from above and below injury.

Provide positioning aids that support injured and painful areas.

Dispense medications to field for postoperative pain relief per surgeon's order.

Report to postanesthesia care unit nurse the patient's specific needs for comfort, such as elevate the leg.

NURSING DIAGNOSIS:

Potential for impaired skin integrity

GOAL:

Patient will maintain skin integrity during perioperative experience

INTERVENTIONS:

Assess preoperative skin integrity.

Use eggcrate mattress for surgical procedures over 4 hours and for elderly and thin patients.

Pad all bony prominences.

Avoid pooling of prep solutions to prevent chemical burns and skin breakdown; use gel prep when available.

Assess skin for erythema or induration after surgical drapes have been removed and compare to preoperative skin assessment; document changes.

Inform surgeon of changes in skin integrity.

Move patient to postanesthesia care unit stretcher with a pull sheet or a patient transfer roller.

Report to postanesthesia care unit nurse any changes in skin integrity.

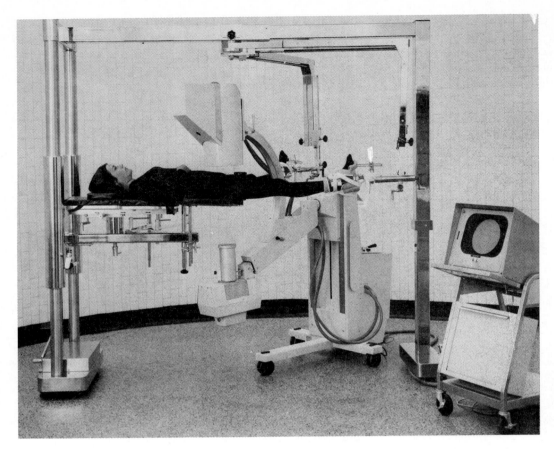

Fig. 22-14. Orthopedic surgical table with image intensifier in position. (Courtesy Chick Orthopedic, Oakland, Calif.)

The principles of positioning and the different types of positions used in orthopedic surgery are described and illustrated in Chapter 6.

The selection of the position depends on several factors: (1) the type of operation to be performed, (2) the location of the injury or lesion, (3) the age and physical condition of the patient, and (4) the preference of the surgeon.

Most orthopedic operations are performed with the patient in the supine position. However, to operate on a patient in the prone position, it is necessary to use special devices that permit proper respiratory exchange. Operations on the spine not only require provisions for proper air exchange but also must allow for flexion at the operative site. Most surgeons have a preference as to what positioning devices they use when performing spinal operations. Following are some available choices:

1. *Doughnut*—foam rubber pad about 4 inches thick made in the shape of a slightly oblong doughnut that supports the skeleton but does not compress the viscera

2. *Wilson convex frame*—provides adjustable flexion of the lumbosacral spine without flexing the operating room bed (Fig. 22-15, *A*)

3. *Chest rolls*—custom-made or made by rolling and taping two sheets, bath blankets, or large foam pads together; used when flexion is not necessary

4. *Andrews spinal surgery frame*—used for exposure of a large number of vertebrae for spinal fusion (Fig. 22-15, *B*)

Prepping

A primary concern in orthopedic surgery is the prevention of infection. The orthopedic surgical prep must be meticulously carried out with proper technique. A general principle in the orthopedic prep is to extend the prep one joint above and one joint below the operative site.

If hair removal from the incisional site is necessary, surgical clippers should be utilized. If it is essential to shave the patient for the surgical procedure, shaving should be done immediately preceding surgery. The skin is often defatted with a skin degreaser before the operative prep is performed. The operative scrub is then carried out under sterile conditions. The most common skin preparation solutions used in orthopedic surgery are halogen agents containing organic iodides such as povidone-iodine soap and solution, or gel. Gel preps are recommended due to their

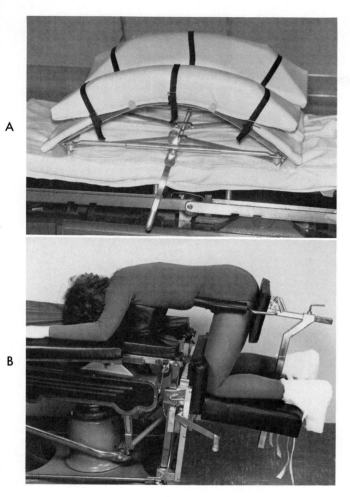

Fig. 22-15. A, Wilson convex frame. **B,** Andrews spinal surgery frame. (Courtesy Orthopedic Systems, Inc., Hayward, Calif., and E. Trent Andrews, M.D., F.A.C.S.)

better surface contact and absence of pooling. The prep is applied, beginning in the central area of the incision and proceeding peripherally. If solutions are used instead of gel, pooling of solutions should be avoided to prevent chemical burns to the patient's skin.

Draping

Application of sterile drapes is the final step in preparing the patient for the operation. The sterile packs containing sheets, towels, and other drapes should be standardized (Chapter 5). The sterile drapes, towels, and stockinette for operations on the ankle and foot, the knee and midthigh, the hip, the spine, and the upper extremity are described in Chapter 5. Iodophor-impregnated adhesive drapes have been found to contribute to low infection rates; they are often used in orthopedic surgery.

Equipment/supplies

Orthopedic operating rooms require a variety of special accessories in addition to routine operating room equip-

ment. Although these vary from hospital to hospital, they serve the same basic purposes.

Orthopedic surgical tables, commonly referred to as fracture tables, are designed to enable the surgeon to apply traction to a lower extremity while maintaining good alignment and control of the patient. These tables are equipped with radiotranslucent components, trays, and cassette holders to allow x-ray examination of any part of the body. Use of these tables makes it possible to apply a cast to a large body area while properly supporting the patient. The orthopedic surgical table with equipment is shown in Fig. 22-14. Tables most widely used are made by Chick, Stryker, and Amsco.

At times, Wedge frames and Circo-Electric beds are used in orthopedics. Wedge frames enable the surgeon to maintain the patient in cervical or halo traction during the procedure, eliminating the need for postoperative transfer. The Circo-Electric bed is often employed for postoperative care following spinal procedures. Manufacturer's pamphlets with illustrations on each table are available. A working knowledge of the table before use is very important.

Tourniquets are used during most operations on the extremities (Fig. 22-16 and 22-17). They prevent venous oozing but do not totally obstruct the arterial blood supply, thereby leaving the operative field as clear of blood as possible. While elevated, the extremity is wrapped distally to proximally with a 4- or 6-inch Ace wrap or Esmarch rubber bandage to exsanguinate the limb. The tourniquet is then inflated.

Most surgeons now prefer to inflate the tourniquet to 50 mm to 75 mm Hg above the patient's systolic pressure for an upper extremity and 100 mm to 150 mm Hg above the patient's systolic pressure for a lower extremity. Tourniquet pressures usually range between 135 mm to 255 mm Hg for an upper limb and 175 mm to 305 mm Hg for a lower limb.

Tourniquets can be very dangerous if not used properly. The following checks are essential:

1. *Application.* To be most effective, tourniquets should be placed on single long bones, such as a femur or humerus. Placing a tourniquet at the elbow or knee interferes with the superficial neurovascular structures. Webril, stockinette, or a tourniquet cover is wrapped smoothly around the limb as high on the extremity as possible, being careful not to pinch the skin folds, where the tourniquet will be applied. An encircling role of adhesive tape may be placed around the outside of the secured tourniquet as an extra precaution against loosening. A tourniquet of sufficient length and width for the extremity is essential. The ends must overlap at least 2 to 3 inches.
2. *Setting.* The original setting is determined by the

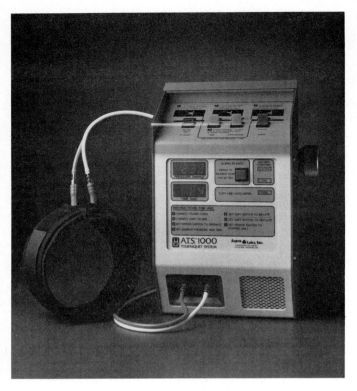

Fig. 22-16. ATS 1000 tourniquet system. (Courtesy Aspen Labs, Inc., Englewood, Colo.)

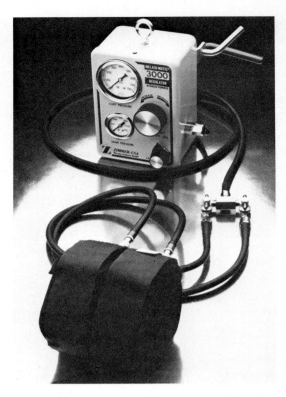

Fig. 22-17. Double-cuffed tourniquet and gauge used for regional anesthesia. (Courtesy Zimmer, Inc., Warsaw, Ind.)

surgeon and should be checked at intervals by operating room personnel and reported to the surgeon. The tubing should also be checked for leaks or kinks.

3. *Skin preparation.* The cleansing solution must not be allowed to pool under the cuff because tourniquet burns may result.

4. *Tourniquet time.* Accurate tourniquet time must be recorded and maintained as part of the anesthesia and nursing records. The surgeon should be informed of the tourniquet time at hourly intervals. Tourniquets are usually released every 2 hours for several minutes. Freon and nitrogen are used most frequently for inflation of tourniquets.

5. *Accurate gauge.* Tourniquet paralysis can occur and is usually caused by an inaccurate tourniquet gauge. The accuracy of the gauge must be checked on a regular basis to prevent this complication. Commercial testers are available.

Radiographic apparatus is essential for an orthopedic operating room. For some procedures the standard fixed or portable x-ray machine is required to take still films. Anterior-posterior (A-P) and lateral views are commonly requested to assess the reduction of a bone fracture, to determine the position of an implant, or to determine the anatomic site. The mobile image intensifier, also referred to as fluroscopy or x-ray image (Fig. 22-14), allows the surgeon to view the progression of a procedure on a television screen. Fluoroscopy is used during the operative treatment of long bone fractures, specifically for intramedullary pinning or nailing procedures. Sterile plastic drapes to cover the arm of the image intensifier are available from manufacturers. Lead aprons and thyroid shields are worn by all personnel in the operating room while x-rays are being taken or fluroscopy utilized. The patient is also protected by placing a lead apron under the drapes over the torso, if the area is not within the surgical field.

Instrumentation and accessory items

The successful management of an active orthopedic operating room suite depends on the maintenance of adequate inventory levels of standard implants. Types, styles, and sizes of necessary implants are usually determined by the operating surgeon, and the number of each depends on the usage. Appropriate companion instruments, such as drivers and extractors, must also be available.

Lot and implant serial numbers must be recorded on the patient's chart. An appropriate space should be provided on the operating room record. If one has not been provided or the record is not a permanent part of the patient's chart, the serial numbers should be recorded in the progress notes. Operating rooms should maintain a logbook for all implants that have lot and serial numbers. Then the patient can be contacted if for some reason the manufacturer recalls a specific lot number.

Many different alloys are used in manufacturing orthopedic implants. However, the insertion of implants with different metallic composition must be avoided to prevent galvanic corrosion; internal fixation implants used during an orthopedic procedure should be of the same metal. Screws, for example, should be of the same composition as the metal plate they fix to the bone. Alloys most frequently used include stainless steel, cobalt-chromium, and titanium-vanadium-aluminum.

Internal fixation devices should never be reused. Laboratory testing has demonstrated that scratches, abrasions, and the like critically affect the strength of an orthopedic implant. These imperfections are inevitable with use. Bending implants to conform to the contour of the bone should be avoided whenever possible to prevent loss of strength. When bending is necessary, the proper bending press should be used. Once an implant is bent, any attempt to rebend or straighten it should not be allowed. An internal fixation device that has become damaged as a result of improper storage or handling is not usable for similar reasons.

Orthopedic instruments, equipment, and implants require special care, storage, and handling. All precautions must be taken to prevent the most minute scratches on orthopedic implants. During sterilization, implants should not be placed in a position in which knocking or bumping might occur. Appropriate sterilizing cases and trays should be used. Implants should be sterilized according to the manufacturer's instructions. Cleaning of instruments frequently presents a problem because of areas that are inaccessible to the cleaning brushes. The most effective cleaning method available is an ultrasonic cleaner.

Instruments and equipment that do not function properly (as a result of dullness, poor adjustment, lack of lubrication, damage, improper fit, or incomplete cleaning) are primary sources of complaints and problems in the operating room. The same instruments and equipment, properly maintained and in good repair, make the operation much easier. The proper maintenance of delicate instruments, such as those used in hand surgery, is particularly important. The perioperative nurse is responsible for ensuring such maintenance.

Following are basic instrument sets that should be available in the orthopedic operating room. Additional instruments and appliances are added as needed for specific procedures.

Minor soft tissue set (Fig. 22-18)

2 Knife handles, no. 3
1 Knife handle, no. 7
2 Towel clamps, non-perforating, 5¼ inches
8 Towel clamps, 3 inches
  Clamps: mosquito, Crile artery, Oschner, Pean, tonsil, Mixter, Allis, Babcock
1 Sponge-holding forceps
2 Needle holders: Mayo Hegar, Webster
  Scissors: 1 each, Mayo dissecting, bandage, Metzenbaum, iris sharp (curved, straight), iris blunt (curved, straight)
  Forceps: 2 each, tissue, Brophy, Adson tissue, De Bakey
1 Dressing forceps
2 Skin hooks: double, single-pronged
  Retractors: 2 each, USA, Volkman rake (sharp, blunt), Senn, Weitlaner, Cushing vein
  Richardson retractors: 1 each, ¾ × 1 inch, 1⅛ × 1⅛ inch, 1½ × 1½ inches, ¾ × 2 inches
1 Freer elevator
1 Probe and groove director
1 Ruler
  Suction: 1 each, Yankauer, Frazier (8 fr, 12 fr)

Small bone set (Fig. 22-19)

1 Beaver blade handle
2 Mixters, baby
1 Litler scissors
1 Tendon passer
1 Volkman hook, small
2 Alar retractors
2 Ragnell retractors
2 Mini Hohmann retractors
2 Miltex self-retaining retractors
1 Carroll elevator
  Hoke osteotomes: 1 each, ⅛, 3/16, ¼, 5/16, ⅜
  Curettes: 1 each, 000, 0
1 Home double-ended curette
1 Bone rasp
  Rongeurs: 2 each, Lempert (straight), Carroll (curved)
1 Mallet, small
1 Liston bone cutter
1 Pin cutter

Ortho soft tissue set (Fig. 22-20)

  Knife handles, 1 each, no. 4 and no. 7
2 Knife handles, no. 3
2 Towel clamps, nonperforating, 5¼ inches
8 Towel clamps, 5¼ inches
  Clamps: mosquito, Crile artery, Pean, Allis, Oschner, tonsil, Mixter
1 Sponge-holding forceps
  Scissors: 1 each, Metzenbaum dissecting curved (5½, 7 inches), Mayo dissecting straight and curved (6¾ inches), wire cutting, bandage
4 Mayo Hegar needle holders
  Forceps: 2 each, tissue, Russian, Brophy, Adson, Curtis, De Bakey
  Retractors: 2 each, Israel, Volkman rake (sharp, blunt), Senn, Gelpi, Weitlaner, USA, Richardson (¾ × 2 inches)
  Kelly retractors: 1 each, 1½ × 2 inches, 2 × 2½ inches, 2½ × 3 inches
  Richardson retractors: 1 each, ¾ × 1 inch, 1 × 1¼ inches, 1½ × 1½ inches

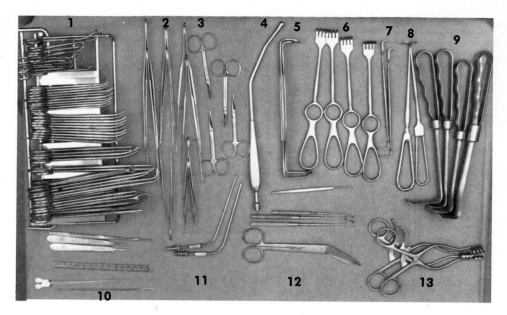

Fig. 22-18. Minor soft tissue set. *1,* On stringer *(top to bottom):* nonperforating towel clamps; 5¼-inch towel clamps; 3-inch towel clamps; Crile, Allis, Pean, Oschner, Babcock, tonsil, and Mixter forceps; needle holders; sponge-holding forceps; Metzenbaum dissecting scissors; Mayo scissors (curved, straight); *2,* DeBakey, tissue, dressing, Russian, and Adson forceps; *3,* iris scissors (straight, curved, sharp, blunt); *4,* Yankauer suction; *5,* USA (Army-Navy) retractors; *6,* Volkman rakes (sharp, blunt); *7,* Senn retractors; *8,* vein retractors; *9,* Richardson retractors; *10,* knife handles (no. 7, no. 3), ruler, probe, and groove director; *11,* Frazier suctions; *12,* skin hooks (single and double), bandage scissors; *13,* Weitlaner self-retaining retractors.

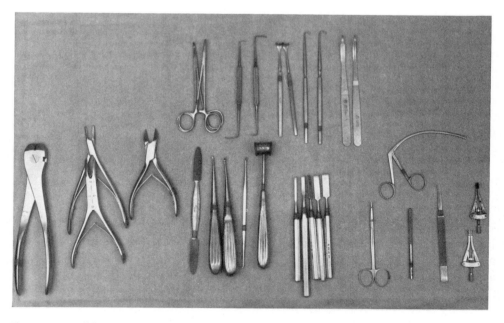

Fig. 22-19. Small bone set. *Top (left to right):* baby Mixters, Ragnell retractors, Alar retractors, Volkman hooks, mini Hohmann retractors. *Bottom (left to right):* pin cutter, Lempert and Carroll rongeurs, Liston bone cutter, bone rasp, small curettes, fine double-ended curette, small mallet, Hoke osteotomes, Litler scissors, tendon passer, Beaver blade handle, Carroll elevator, Miltex self-retaining retractors.

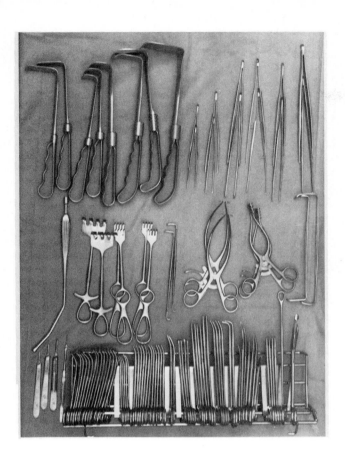

Major bone set (Fig. 22-21)

Brun bone curettes: 1 each, 3/0, no. 2, no. 5 (straight, curved)

Hibbs osteotomes: 1 each, ¼, ½, 1 (straight, curved)

Langenbeck periosteal elevators: 1 each, wide, narrow

1 Cushing periosteal elevator

Hohmann retractors: 2 each, wide, narrow-sharp, narrow-blunt

2 Bennett retractors

1 Bone hook, large

1 Metal ruler

Rongeurs: 1 each, Stille-Luer, Zaufal-Jansen, Adson-cranial

Pliers: 1 each, heavy, needle-nose

1 Buttie double-ended rasp

1 Mallet, 2 pound

1 Stille-Liston bone-cutting forceps, straight

1 Bone tamp

1 Pin cutter

Fig. 22-20. Ortho soft tissue set. *Bottom (left to right):* knife handles; towel clamps; mosquito, Crile, Pean, Allis, Oschner, tonsil, and Mixter forceps; Metzenbaum, Mayo, and wire cutting scissors; needle holders; sponge-holding forceps; bandage scissors. *Middle (left to right):* Yankauer suction; Israel, Volkman, and Senn retractors; Gelpi and Weitlaner self-retaining retractors; USA (Army-Navy) retractors. *Top (left to right):* Richardson and Kelly retractors; Adson, tissue, Russian, Brophy, De Bakey, and Curtis forceps.

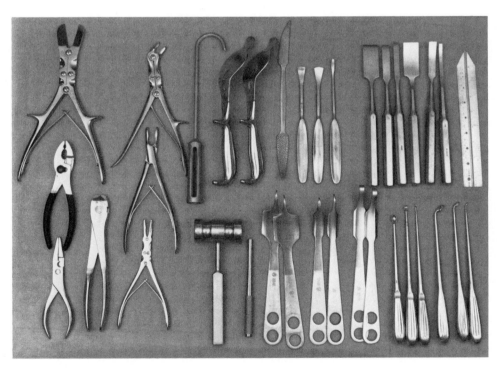

Fig. 22-21. Major bone set. *Top (left to right):* Stille-Liston bone-cutting forceps, Stille-Luer rongeur, bone hook, Bennett retractors, rasp, Langenbeck periosteal elevators (wide and narrow), Cushing periosteal elevator, osteotomes (straight, curved), ruler. *Middle (left to right):* pliers, Adson-cranial rongeur. *Bottom (left to right):* needle-nosed pliers, pin cutter, Zaufal-Jansen rongeur, mallet, bone tamp, Hohmann retractors (wide sharp, narrow sharp, and blunt), curettes (straight, curved).

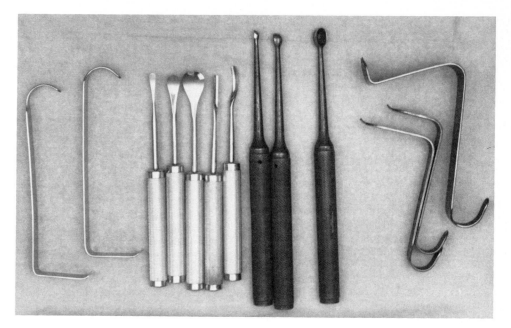

Fig. 22-22. Bone graft instrument set. *Left to right:* Hibbs retractors, Cobb periosteal elevators, Cobb gouges, McElroy curettes, spinal retractors, iliac graft retractor.

Bone graft instrument set (Fig. 22-22)

    Taylor Spinal retractors: 1 each, small, large
1 Iliac graft retractor
2 Hibbs retractors
    Cobb periosteal elevators: 1 each, ⅜, ¾, 1¼ inches
    Cobb gouges: 1 each, ³⁄₃₂, ⁵⁄₃₂ inches; curved, straight
    McElroy curettes: 1 set

Air-powered instruments

The use of air-powered surgical instruments in the operating room has eliminated the need for many hand-operated tools, thereby reducing operating time and improving technical results. Fingertip control allows the surgeon to control speed and power instantly. This is especially important in total joint replacement procedures. While using air-powered instruments, it is important to be aware of the manufacturer's recommended cleaning and lubricating instructions. With proper care, air-powered tools have an indefinite life span and many uses (Figs. 22-23 and 22-24).

Medications/suture material

Many orthopedic procedures involve contaminated wounds or tissues that are highly susceptible to infection. An infected bone may cause lifelong problems or even lead to amputation. Orthopedic surgeons usually request an antibiotic to be dispensed to the field for wound irrigation. An intravenous antibiotic is also used when the operative procedure is expected to last more than 2 hours, or when orthopedic implants are used. The antibiotic of choice is a cephalosporin such as cefazolin sodium. One

to 2 grams are administered intravenously preoperatively, and 1 gram is administered every 6 hours thereafter for 24 hours.

Orthopedic tissues include tendons, ligaments, periosteum, and bone. Most of these tissues are very fibrous, contain few cells, and lack a rich blood supply. Due to their lack of vascularity, these tissues heal slowly. Nonabsorbable suture material is commonly preferred for tendons and ligaments. Tendons require close apposition of their ends; therefore, durable suture with little elasticity is desired. Surgical steel and polyester are often used. Bone is not usually sutured; however, when attachment of tendons to bone is necessary, wire suture is used. Periosteum heals more rapidly than other orthopedic tissues; therefore, absorbable material such as surgical gut or polyglactin is preferred.

Evaluation

Immediately after the surgery the perioperative nurse assesses the condition of the patient. Evaluation of all nursing diagnoses is imperative in order to determine whether the goals of the nursing care plan were met. The desired outcome is that the patient will have no signs or symptoms of postoperative wound infection and only normal postoperative inflammation. The patient's ability to move all extremities, except those that have been purposely immobilized, and to maintain proper body alignment without complaining of more than the expected postoperative discomfort assures the nurse that the patient has remained free from injuries related to improper position-

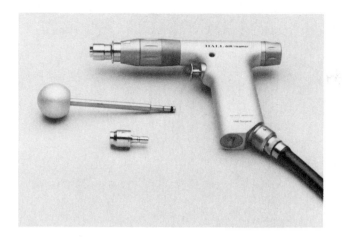

Fig. 22-23. Power drill/reamer with trinkle adaptor and handle attachment. (Courtesy Zimmer, Inc., Warsaw, Ind.)

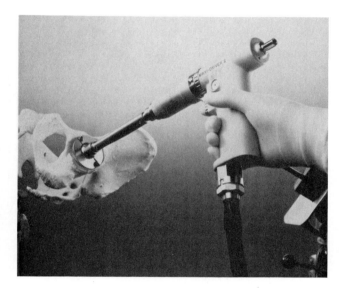

Fig. 22-24. Example of an air-powered tool and its use. Power acetabular reamer cuts through cartilage and sclerotic bone. (Courtesy Orthopedic Products Division/3M, St. Paul, Minn.)

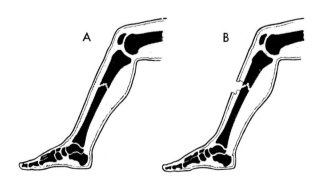

Fig. 22-25. A, Closed, or simple, fracture. No communication between fractured bone and body surface. **B,** Open, or compound, fracture. Wound leading down to site of fracture. Organisms may gain access through wound and infect bone. (From Adams, J.C.: Outline of fractures, ed. 4, Edinburgh, 1964, E. & S. Livingston.)

ing. Special consideration must be given to the neurovascular status of any operative extremity. The affected extremity is usually elevated and checked for warmth, color, sensation, and the presence or absence of pulses. Immobilization techniques are also checked, and stabilization is ensured.

As part of the report to PACU nursing personnel, the perioperative nurse should review outcomes of the care plan, based on reassessment and evaluation. For the nursing diagnoses selected for the orthopedic patient, the following outcomes would be desired:

- The patient will evidence no signs and symptoms of postoperative wound infection.
- The patient was free of injury related to the surgical position.
- The patient understood the surgery and the sequence of perioperative events.
- The patient's pain was controlled and/or minimized.
- The patient's skin integrity was maintained.

SURGICAL INTERVENTIONS
Fractures and dislocations

A fracture is a break in the continuity of a bone. The care of fractured bones or dislocation of a joint is always complicated because of trauma to the soft tissues, including the muscles, nerves, and blood vessels.

Types

Fractures are classified into two main groups: closed fractures and compound or open fractures (Fig. 22-25).

Closed (Fig. 22-25, *A*) fractures are those in which there is no communication between the bone fracture and the skin surface. *Incomplete* fractures are those in which the whole thickness of the bone is not broken but is bent or buckled, as in greenstick fractures that occur in children before puberty.

Open (Fig. 22-25, *B*) fractures exist when the break in the bone communicates with a wound in the skin. Because these fractures are usually considered contaminated, measures must be carried out to control potential infection.

There are many varieties of fracture architecture (Fig. 22-26), including (1) *transverse* fracture, in which the fracture line runs at a right angle to the longitudinal axis of the bone; (2) *longitudinal* fracture, which runs along the length of the bone; (3) *oblique* fracture and *spiral* fracture, in which bone has been twisted apart (are similar except that oblique is shorter than spiral); (4) *comminuted* fracture, in which the bone fragments splinter into more than two pieces; (5) *impacted* fracture (Fig. 22-27), in which one fragment is driven into the other end and is relatively fixed in that position; and (6) *pathologic* fracture in which a bone is weakened by disease, thereby causing the bone to break, even with minor trauma.

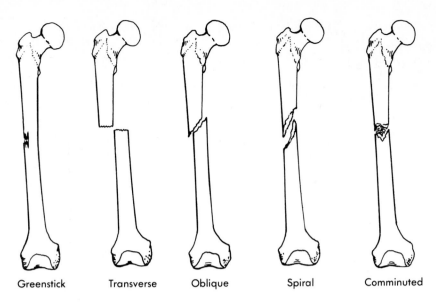

Greenstick   Transverse   Oblique   Spiral   Comminuted

Fig. 22-26. Types of fractures. Greenstick fracture is closed and incomplete. Other fractures shown are open. (From Phipps, W.J., Long, B.C., and Woods, N.F.: Medical-surgical nursing, St. Louis, 1987, The C.V. Mosby Co.)

An *epiphyseal separation* occurs when a fracture passes through or lies within the growth plate of a bone.

An *avulsion fracture* may result from a joint displacement where the ligament or tendon avulses its bony attachment instead of rupturing its fibers. A *dislocation* is a complete displacement of one articular surface of a joint from the other. A *subluxation* is a partial dislocation.

A fracture in the shaft of a long bone is usually described as being in the proximal, middle, or lower third or at the junction of two of these divisions.

A fracture of one of the bony prominences of the end of a long bone is described as a fracture of that prominence by name, for example, a fracture of the olecranon, a fracture of the medial malleolus, or a fracture of the lateral condyle of the femur.

Principles of treatment

The purpose of fracture treatment is to reestablish the length, shape, and alignment of the fractured bones or joints and restore their anatomic function to normal or as near normal as possible.

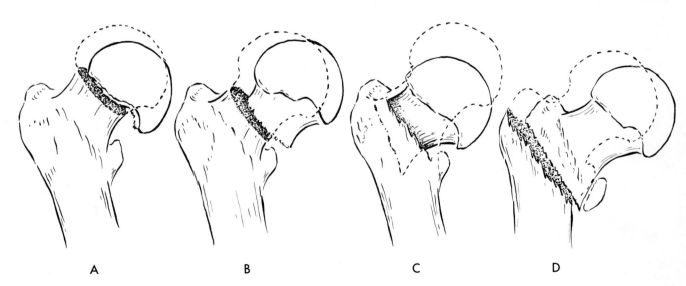

A   B   C   D

Fig. 22-27. Fractures of the hip. **A,** Subcapital fracture. **B,** Transcervical fracture. **C,** Impacted fracture of base of neck. **D,** Intertrochanteric fracture. (From Phipps, W.J., Long, B.C., and Woods, N.F.: Medical-surgical nursing, St. Louis, 1987, The C.V. Mosby Co.)

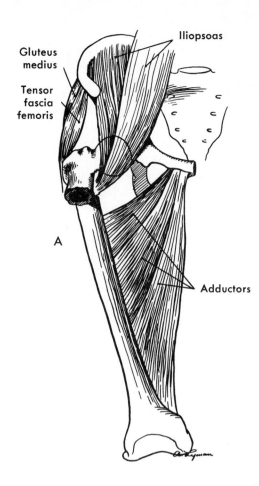

Gluteus medius

Tensor fascia femoris

Iliopsoas

A

Adductors

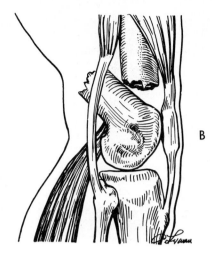

B

Fig. 22-28. A, Muscle action in subtrochanteric fracture of femur. B, Supracondylar fracture of femur (transverse). Note pull exerted by gastrocnemius muscle. (Modified from Larson, C.B., and Gould, M.: Orthopedic nursing, ed. 9, St. Louis, 1978, The C.V. Mosby Co.)

Fractures of a bone involve two parts: the proximal and the distal fragments. The position of the proximal fragment is controlled by the pull of the attached muscles (Fig. 22-28). For this reason the distal fragment must be manipulated into the position that is assumed by the proximal fragment. The surgeon selects the method whereby this can be accomplished.

In fractures involving an upper extremity, the surgeon endeavors to preserve mobility because the individual needs a wide range of motion to perform skilled and delicate work. In fractures of a lower extremity, the objectives of surgery are to restore alignment and length and provide stability of the extremity for weight bearing.

In the presence of open fractures involving soft tissues, several associated conditions may arise, including (1) secondary hemorrhage, (2) infection, (3) severe damage to soft tissues, (4) damage to blood vessels and nerves, and (5) Volkmann's contracture.

To meet the demands of orthopedic surgery, the surgical team should keep in mind the following principles: (1) the extremity must be handled gently, (2) the patient must receive initial general medical treatment, (3) proper equipment and personnel must be readily available to treat impending or existing shock and to control hemorrhage, (4) aseptic surgical techniques and care must be maintained

to prevent infection, (5) the patient must be positioned properly to provide for adequate circulatory and respiratory functioning, and (6) the comfort of the patient must be considered.

Bone-healing processes

The healing process involves several stages (Fig. 22-29). When a bone is fractured, bleeding occurs. The amount of extravasated blood depends on the vascularity of the fracture site. The blood exudate infiltrates the surrounding area, where it forms a clot. Fibroblasts invade the hematoma and form a fibrin meshwork.

As osteoblasts invade the fibrin meshwork, blood vessels develop to build collagen. After several days, calcium deposits may form in the granulation tissue. These deposits eventually form new bone, known as *callus*. Within the callus, cartilage cells develop a temporary semirigid tissue that helps stabilize the bone fragments. The callus is immature bone that is remodeled by new connective tissue cells (osteoblasts of the periosteum and the inner membrane of the bone cavity). Through this process, mature bone is formed, excess callus is reabsorbed, and trabecular bone is laid down (Fig. 22-29).

After several months, depending on the age and physical condition of the individual, the fractured bone becomes firmly united, although the ossification process is not yet completed. Complete union of the fractured bone or joint is determined by means of clinical and radiologic examination.

Nonunion of a fracture signifies that the process of healing has ended without producing bony union.

Delayed union signifies that a specific fracture has not

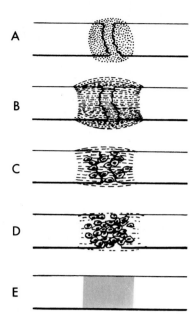

Fig. 22-29. Schematic drawing of the five stages of bone healing: **A,** hematoma formation, **B,** fibrin network formation, **C,** invasion of osteoblasts, **D,** callus formation, and **E,** remodeling. (From Phipps, W.J., Long, B.C., and Woods, N.F.: Medical-surgical nursing, St. Louis, 1987, The C.V. Mosby Co.)

healed in the time considered average for that fracture. The average time for healing of a fracture depends on many factors, and delayed unions must not be considered nonunions until the healing process has ceased without bony union.

Malunion signifies that the fracture has united with deformity sufficient to cause impairment of the function or a significant cosmetic defect.

Basic treatment techniques
Closed reduction by manipulation

Whenever possible, fractures are treated by manipulating the fragments into position without incising the skin. If fractures can be treated by this closed method, there is less chance of infection and greater chance for union (healing) of the fracture, as long as soft tissue is not caught in the fracture site.

Procedural considerations. The closed reduction can be performed with (1) infiltration of local anesthetic agent into the fracture site, (2) intravenous regional anesthesia, (3) regional or spinal nerve block, or (4) general anesthesia. The choice of anesthesia depends on the site of the fracture and the condition of the patient.

Operative procedure
1. The fragments are manipulated into alignment by the surgeon with the aid of fluoroscopy.
2. After the fracture has been reduced, it is immobilized.

Immobilization by cast. Cast immobilization is a form of external mold that places the fractured extremity or joint

at rest by immobilizing the joint and both ends of the fractured bone in a rigid casing.

Types of casts. A *short leg cast* applied from below the knee to the toes may be used for fractures of the foot and the ankle. A *long leg cast* applied from the groin to the toes may be used to treat fractures of the tibia, fibula, and ankle (Fig. 22-30). A rubber heel or cast shoe may be used with the long leg or short leg cast to allow walking. A *cylinder cast* from the groin to the ankle is used to treat fractures of the patella and to immobilize the knee.

Spica casts are desinged to immobilize different parts of the body; for example, a *single hip spica cast* involving the trunk, the affected leg, and foot may be applied to treat a fracture of the femur (Fig. 22-30). A *body jacket cast* encircling the body but not the extremities may be used to treat spinal conditions.

A *short arm cast* is applied from below the elbow to the knuckles and is used for wrist fractures. A *long arm cast* is applied from above the elbow to the knuckles and is used to treat fractures of the elbow or the forearm (Fig. 22-30).

The *femoral cast brace* is designed to immobilize a fracture of the femoral shaft without immobilizing the hip joint. It consists of (1) a snug-fitting thigh cast with a specially molded quadrilateral socket at the proximal opening, which controls rotation of the cast brace on the extremity; (2) a short leg walking cast distal to the knee; and (3) hinges at the knee that join the other two components. The hinges allow active knee motion. The cast brace (Fig. 22-31) is usually applied after 4 to 6 weeks of skeletal traction, when callus formation has been initiated at the fracture site.

Splints are frequently employed in the immediate postoperative period. They do not completely encircle the limb, and therefore the degree of swelling and staining can be directly observed.

Casting materials. Plaster of Paris is the least expensive casting material available, is easily molded, and is used for acute fractures when maintenance of bone alignment is critical (Fig. 22-32). Proper handling of plaster is illustrated in Fig. 22-33.

Synthetic casting materials frequently have a role in the treatment of fractures. They are lightweight, waterproof, and relatively easy to apply. In using synthetic casting materials, the manufacturer's instructions must be followed explicitly. Figs. 22-34 and 22-35 show synthetic casting materials.

Traction

Fractures that are difficult to reduce and immobilize in a cast can be treated by applying distal traction to the extremity. Traction provides a steady pull on the distal part of the body. Balanced suspension, in which the body part is suspended, not pulled, is often used in conjunction with traction.

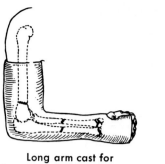

Long arm cast for
fractures of elbow, forearm,
and comminuted
fractures of wrist

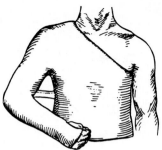

Shoulder spica cast for
injuries about shoulder
or humerus requiring com-
plete immobilization of arm

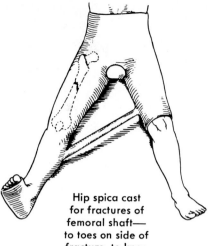

Hip spica cast
for fractures of
femoral shaft—
to toes on side of
fracture, to knee
on uninjured side

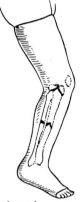

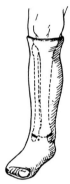

Long leg cast
for fractures of tibia—
30-degree flexion of knee

Short leg cast
for ankle fractures—
molded to tibial
condyles

Fig. 22-30. Several types of plaster casts and some fractures for which they may be indicated. (From Compere, E.L., Banks, S.W., and Compere, C.L.: Pictorial handbook of fracture treatment, ed. 5, Chicago, 1963, Year Book Medical Publishers, Inc.)

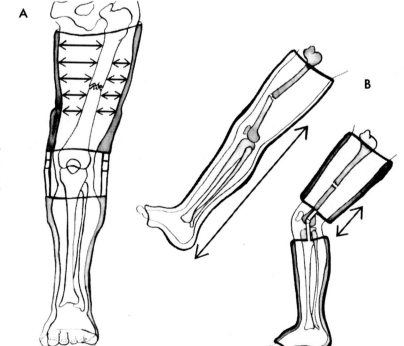

Fig. 22-31. A, Cast brace. **B,** Comparative length of lever arm distal to fracture site, with long-leg cast and with cast brace. (From Larson, C.B., and Gould, M.: Orthopedic nursing, ed. 9, St. Louis, 1978, The C.V. Mosby Co.)

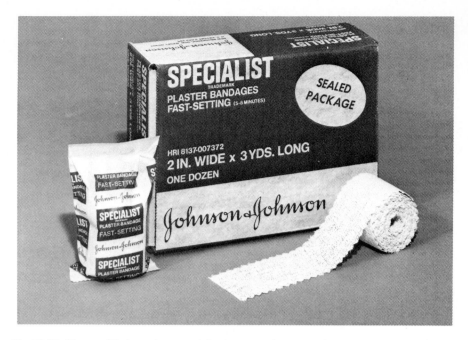

Fig. 22-32. Plaster of Paris casting material. (Courtesy Johnson & Johnson, New Brunswick, N.J.)

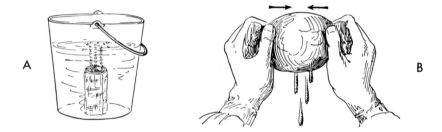

Fig. 22-33. Correct handling of plaster roll. **A,** Roll of plaster placed on end in pail of water. Roll is saturated when bubbles cease to appear. **B,** Excess water squeezed (*not* twisted) from plaster roll by pushing both ends toward middle. (From Compere, E.L., Banks, S.W., and Compere, C.L.: Pictorial handbook of fracture treatment, ed. 5, Chicago, 1963, Year Book Medical Publishers, Inc.)

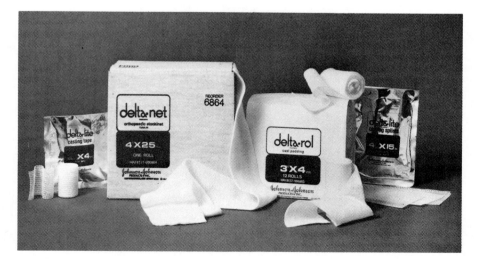

Fig. 22-34. Synthetic casting materials. (Courtesy Johnson & Johnson, New Brunswick, N.J.)

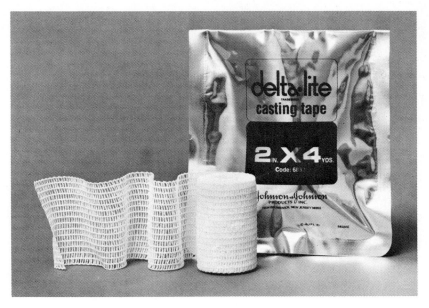

Fig. 22-35. Synthetic casting tape. (Courtesy Johnson & Johnson, New Brunswick, N.J.)

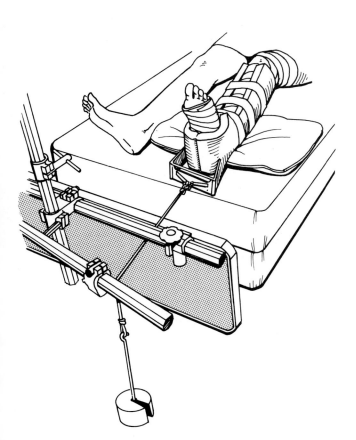

Fig. 22-36. Buck's skin traction. Heel is supported off bed to prevent pressure on heel. Weight hangs free of the bed. (From Phipps, W.J., Long, B.C., and Woods, N.F.: Medical-surgical nursing, St. Louis, 1987, The C.V. Mosby Co.)

There are two types of traction: *skin traction* and *skeletal traction*. Common forms of skin traction are Buck's extension and Russell traction (Figs. 22-36 and 22-37). Skeletal traction is applied directly to the bone distal to the fracture. Balanced suspension with a Thomas or Hodgen splint and Pearson attachment is a frequently seen skeletal traction on the lower extremity (Fig. 22-38). The problem for the patient with traction is the long period of confinement in bed, but the incidence of infection and nonunion of the fracture is less with this treatment than with open reduction.

Procedural considerations. For skeletal traction application, a local or general anesthetic may be administered. This procedure may be performed in the cast room, emergency department, patient's room, or operating room, depending on the patient's condition. Aseptic technique is followed to prevent wound infection. The area is prepped with prep solution or gel. The following items are sterilized and placed on a sterile table (Fig. 22-39):

Scalpel
Hand drill with chuck key
Kirschner wires or Steinman pins, desired type and size
Bolt cutter
Ruler
Gauze dressing

Nonsterile items

Traction equipment, desired type

Operative procedure

1. Under sterile conditions, a pin is passed through the bone distal to the fracture site.
2. A traction bow is attached to the pin and is connected

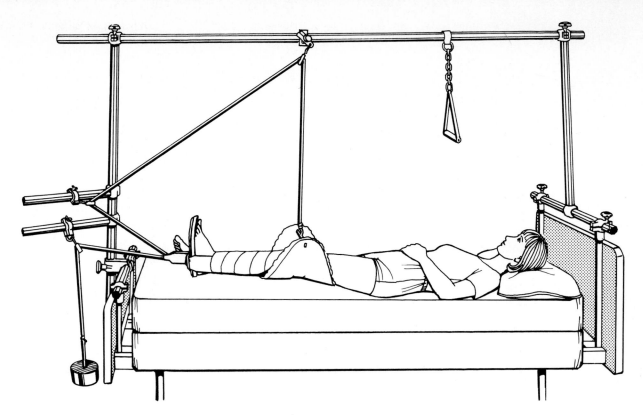

Fig. 22-37. Russell skin traction. Hip is slightly flexed. Pillows may be utilized under lower leg to provide support and keep the heel free of the bed. (From Phipps, W.J., Long, B.C., and Woods, N.F.: Medical-surgical nursing, St. Louis, 1987, The C.V. Mosby Co.)

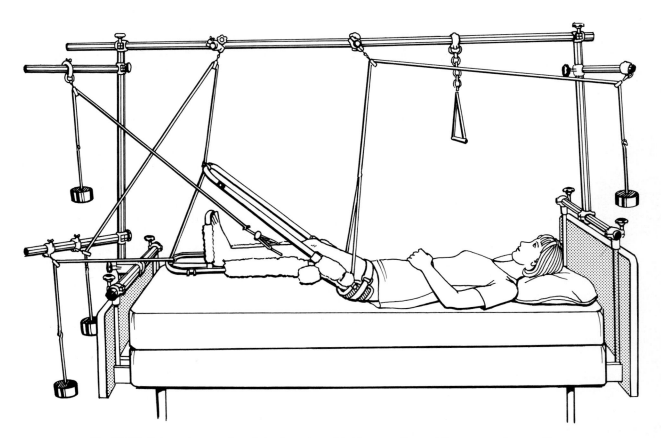

Fig. 22-38. Balanced suspension skeletal traction with Thomas splint and Pearson attachment. (From Phipps, W.J., Long, B.C., and Woods, N.F.: Medical-surgical nursing, St. Louis, 1987, The C.V. Mosby Co.)

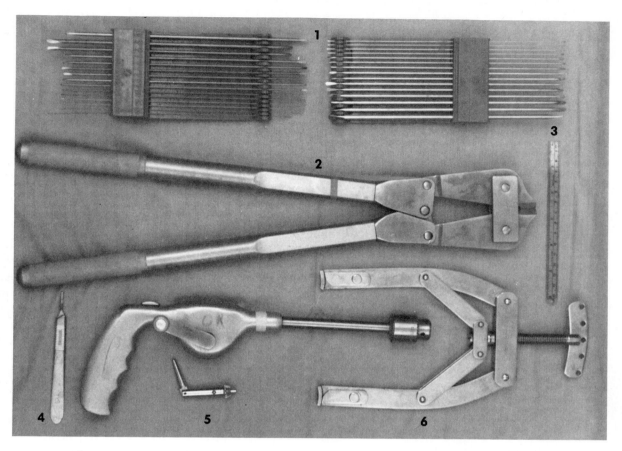

Fig. 22-39. Instruments for insertion of skeletal traction: *1,* Kirschner wires and Steinman pins; *2,* bolt cutter; *3,* ruler; *4,* knife handle (use no. 15 blade); *5,* hand drill with chuck key; *6,* traction bow.

by ropes to weights that pull on the fracture fragments and override the deforming muscle forces, thereby reducing the fracture.

External fixation

Because of the increased chance of infection in patients with an open fracture, external fixation is often the preferred treatment. External fixation offers great versatility in the treatment of bone and soft tissue injuries and defects. In fractures with a substantial amount of soft tissue damage, rigid immobilization is mandatory. Advantages of external fixation include the absence of plaster, fracture stabilization at a distance from the injury site, ability to perform subsequent procedures such as skin grafts, minimal joint interference, early mobilization, and the ability to use internal fixation or other skeletal fixation devices at the same time or sequentially.

Indications for external fixation include (1) severe open fractures, (2) highly comminuted closed fractures, (3) arthrodesis, (4) infected joints, (5) infected nonunion, (6) fracture stabilization to protect arterial or nerve anastomosis, (7) major alignment and length deficits, (8) congenital deformities, and (9) static contractures.

Many improvements have been made in the design and articulations of external fixators in the past years. The many external fixators that are available vary greatly in design; however, they all contain three main components: (1) bone anchoring devices (threaded pins or Kirschner wires), (2) longitudinal supporting devices (threaded or smooth rods), and (3) connecting elements (clamps and partial or full rings).

Procedural considerations. External fixators are applied under general or regional anesthesia using sterile technique. X-ray intensification aids in proper pin placement and fracture reduction.

Major bone and soft tissue sets are required, plus the following:

Irrigation basin
Suction irrigator
Power drill
Pin cutter, large
Bone-holding forceps
Fixation device of choice with instrumentation: Hoffman (Fig. 22-40), Vidal-Sudrey, Ace-Fischer, AO/ASIF (Fig. 22-41), Ilizarov (Fig. 22-42)
Gauze wrap

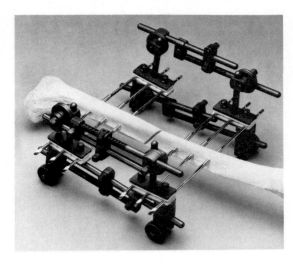

Fig. 22-40. Hoffman external fixation device. (Courtesy Zimmer, Inc., Warsaw, Ind.)

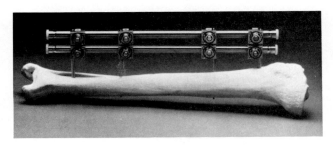

Fig. 22-41. AO/ASIF tubular external fixation device. (Courtesy Synthes, U.S.A., Paoli, Pa.)

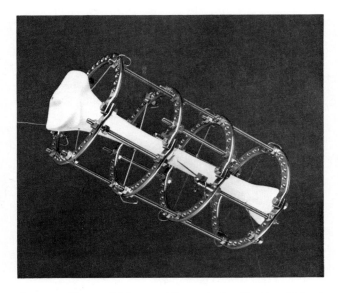

Fig. 22-42. Ilizarov tibial external fixator device. (Courtesy Richards Medical Co., Memphis, Tenn.)

Operative procedure—simple frame Hoffman

1. Three transfixing pins are inserted proximally and distally with the drill and pin guide.
2. The fracture is reduced using manipulation or bone clamps if the wound is open.
3. A 10-hole ball joint is positioned on each set of pins.
4. A longitudinal connecting rod is passed through the ball joints.
5. The entire apparatus is then tightened using the provided wrenches.
6. The pin sites are wrapped with sterile gauze.

Internal fixation

Closed method. The fracture is reduced using closed reduction methods and then fixed with percutaneous insertion of pins, or a small incision is made to place screws or an intramedullary nail (Fig. 22-43, *E*). Improved instrumentation and image intensification control have made closed reduction with internal fixation a safe and common practice in the treatment of some fractures. The advantages of closed reduction, internal fixation over open reduction, internal fixation are (1) a lower incidence of infection, (2) absence of additional soft tissue or vascular damage, and (3) good bone stability.

Open method. Through an open wound, the fracture site is exposed, the bone is manually realigned, and the fragments are fixed by pins, wire, nails, screws, or plates and screws (Figs. 22-43 through 22-46). The procedure is frequently called open reduction, internal fixation (ORIF). Open reduction, internal fixation is used when satisfactory reduction of a fracture cannot be obtained or maintained by closed methods and when skeletal traction is not indicated. The advantage is that anatomic alignment of the fracture can usually be obtained, and the patient does not have to be confined to bed. However, the incidence of infection and nonunion is increased.

Bone grafting may be used to promote union of fractures at the time of open reduction or to fill cavities and defects in the bone. The type of graft to be used depends on the location of the fracture or defect, the condition of the ends of the fragments, and the preference of the surgeon.

Bone graft may be the patient's own bone (autogenous) or cadaver bone (homogenous). Homogenous allografts are used when bone is not available from the patient due to lack of sufficient quantity or because a secondary procedure is undesirable for the patient.

Procedural considerations. Cancellous grafts may be taken from the ilium, olecranon, or distal radius; cortical grafts may be taken from the tibia, fibula, or ribs. When taking an autogenous graft and the recipient site is contaminated by a disease process, instruments used for the recipient site must not cross over to the donor site. Either the bone graft must be harvested before the recipient site is touched, or clean, unused instruments from a separate small table are used to harvest the graft. The operating

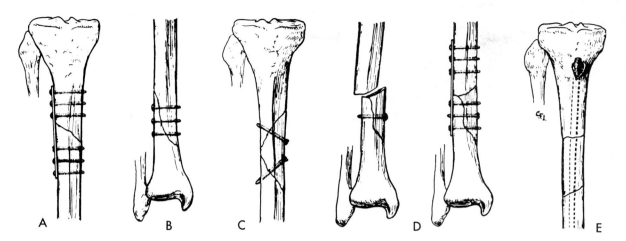

Fig. 22-43. Techniques of internal fixation. **A,** Plate and six screws for transverse or short oblique fracture. **B,** Transfixion screws for long oblique or spiral fractures. **C,** Transfixion screws for long butterfly fragment. **D,** Fixation of fracture with short butterfly fragment. **E,** Medullary fixation. (From Edmonson, A.S., and Crenshaw, A.H., editors: Campbell's operative orthopaedics, ed. 7, St. Louis, 1987, The C.V. Mosby Co.)

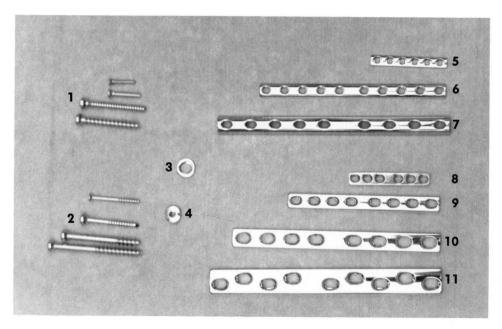

Fig. 22-44. Screws and plates used for internal fixation: *1,* cortical screws; *2,* cancellous screws; *3,* washer; *4,* nut; *5,* ¼ tubular plate; *6,* ⅓ tubular plate; *7,* semitubular plate; *8,* 2.7 dynamic compression plate (DCP); *9,* 3.5 DCP plate; *10,* narrow DCP plate; *11,* broad DCP plate.

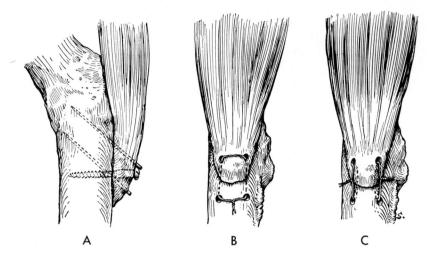

Fig. 22-45. Fixation of osseous attachment of tendon to bone. **A,** Fixation by Vitallium screw or nail. **B,** Fixation by mattress suture of stainless steel wire through holes drilled in bone. **C,** Fixation by wire loops. (From Crenshaw, A.H., editor: Campbell's operative orthopaedics, ed. 7, St. Louis, 1987, The C.V. Mosby Co.)

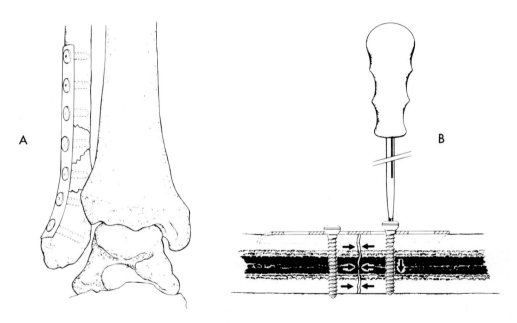

Fig. 22-46. A, Internal fixation of fracture with compression plate and screws. **B,** Forces applied during compression plating. (Courtesy Zimmer, Inc., Warsaw, Ind.)

team must change their gowns and gloves to take the bone graft to prevent cross-contamination.

The instrumentation for taking a bone graft includes soft tissue and major bone sets, plus the following:

Bone graft instruments
Power saw and drill
Saw blades and drill bits of surgeon's choice

Operative procedure—cancellous bone graft. A *cancellous bone graft* consists of spongy bone usually taken from the anterior or posterior crest of the ilium.

Exposure of the ilium is relatively easy because the crest is located subcutaneously.

1. An incision is made along the border of the iliac crest, and the muscles on the outer table of the ilium are elevated and retracted.
2. Strips of the iliac crest can be removed with an osteotome parallel to the crest.
3. A cortical window can be made in the outer table instead, and the cancellous bone chips can be obtained with curettes or gouges.

Operative procedure—cortical bone graft. A *cortical bone graft* consists of hard, dense bone that can be taken from the tibia.

1. A curved anteromedial incision is made along the tibia.
2. The periosteum is incised and reflected, and the size and shape of the graft are outlined with drill holes.
3. The graft is removed with an osteotome or an oscillating bone saw.
4. Once harvested, the cortical graft is placed across the fracture site and secured.

Bone banking

Many institutions have developed programs for storing bone allograft. The American Association of Tissue Banks (AATB) accredits and periodically inspects bone banking programs to assure that specific guidelines are followed in the retrieval, processing, storage, and distribution of bone allograft. Accredited programs comprise a national tissue network that provides hospitals and surgeons with various types of high-quality allografts.

Patients who consent to donate, usually first-time total-hip or total-knee replacement patients, are thoroughly screened. Screening procedures include HIV and hepatitis testing, among others. A detailed medical and social history are also taken. The harvesting process must be done under strict sterile technique. Cultures and a specimen are taken and sent to the respective labs for testing. The allograft is placed in a sterile container, labeled, frozen, and then sent to an institution that performs further testing. Once the tissue has been determined acceptable, it is returned to the bone bank for storage. Frozen allografts are stored in plastic and/or cloth wraps to ensure sterility and prevent the grafts from drying out. Vacuum-sealed freezers are monitored with an alarm that sounds if the temperature rises above $-70°$ C. Allografts are kept frozen until use. Tissue maintained at $-70°$ C or colder may be stored for up to 5 years before expiration (Buckham, 1989).

When requested for a procedure, the bone allograft is delivered to the field, slightly thawed, cultured, and then washed with an antibiotic solution.

Records are kept on both donors and recipients. Donor records provide the donor's identification, medical history (with circumstances of death if applicable), lab results, and graft description. Recipient records include recipient's identification, surgeon and organization implanting the graft, surgical procedure, culture results, and any adverse reactions. Like any other implant, the recipient's operative record should include the name of the bone bank from which the allograft was received, type of allograft, tissue number, and expiration date, if applicable.

Electrical stimulation to induce osteogenesis

Electrical stimulation is artificially applied electrical current that induces or influences osteogenesis. Types include noninvasive, implantable, and percutaneous. The choice of bone stimulator varies according to the patient and pathologic condition (Fig. 22-47). Electrical bone

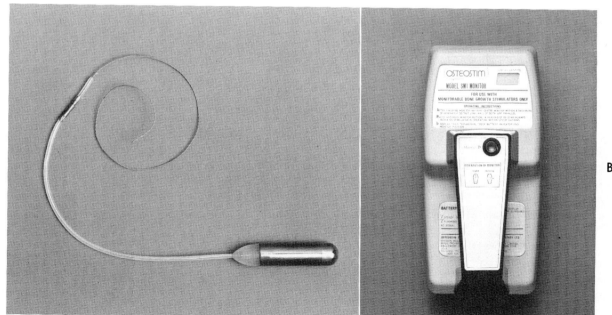

Fig. 22-47. A, Bone growth stimulator cathode and lead. **B,** Monitor for bone growth stimulator. (Courtesy Orthopaedic Division of Telectronics Proprietary, Ltd., Englewood, Colo.)

stimulation works on the principle that bone, when stressed, produces an electrical charge. The area under compression is electronegative, and the area under tension is electropositive.

The bone growth stimulator is used in patients in whom the risk of nonunion is high. It can be used to provide electrical stimulation for the treatment of nonunion, delayed union, congenital pseudarthrosis, and bone defects. It may be used with or without internal fixation devices, external fixation devices, or bone grafting. Patients who have undergone previous surgery, who have sustained significant tissue loss, or in whom bone grafting is contraindicated are candidates. Along with their use in accelerating fracture healing, bone growth stimulators have been successfully used in infected nonunions because the electrical stimulation retards bacterial growth. The normal range of use is 18 to 22 microamperes.

Procedural considerations. The position of the patient depends on the fracture site. A soft tissue set is used, along with straight osteotomes, curettes, rasp, power drill and drill bits, implant instrumentation, orthopedic instrument set appropriate to the surgical area, implant monitor, and bone growth implant according to the surgeon's preference. The stimulator is supplied gas sterilized. Instructions and components vary according to the type. The entire surgical team should familiarize themselves with the appropriate technique.

Operative procedure
1. The fracture site is exposed, creating a mortise or slot spanning the nonunion. Dimensions of the slot are proportional to the size of the bone in question.
2. To ensure medullary canal continuity, the canal on either side of the nonunion should be cleared by curetting, drilling, or rasping.
3. A second incision is made about 8 to 10 cm from the first one, in the appropriate intermuscular tissue. Before implantation of the generator, it is imperative that hemostasis via electrosurgical equipment be accomplished. The nurse should be aware that electrosurgical equipment may interfere with functioning of the bone growth stimulator.
4. A subcutaneous channel for the cathode is created, using digital dissection or a hemostat.
5. The long cathode lead is guided through the channel created in step 4.
6. The generator is carefully implanted near the skin surface. The generator should be in soft tissue and not against bone or metal fixation devices, nor should it create a bulge beneath the skin.
7. The inside diameter of the medullary canal is measured with the gauge so the helix can be formed by wrapping the noninsulated portion of the cathode around the correspondingly sized section of the mandrel. The helix expands approximately 25% once the mandrel is removed.

8. The helix is placed into the prepared bone slot with equal lengths above and below the fracture site. The coils should not be stretched more than 1 cm (⅜ inch) apart. The connection between the stainless steel lead and the titanium cathode is checked to ensure that it has not been loosened during implantation.
9. Cancellous bone grafts are placed between the coils of the helix if large bony defects are being treated.
10. Routine closure of the subcutaneous and skin tissue is carried out.

Once the union has occurred (in 5 to 6 months), the generator can be removed. Explantation can be done with local anesthesia and requires no special instrumentation.

Operations on the shoulder
Correction of acromioclavicular joint separation

Acromioclavicular joint separation is frequently seen in athletes. Not only is the ligamentous support of the acromioclavicular joint disrupted, but also the coracoclavicular ligaments that tether the clavicle to the underlying coracoid process of the scapula. The result is either a posterior or superior displacement of the lateral end of the clavicle.

The purpose of surgery in an acutely injured patient is to reestablish the proper relationship between the clavicle and the coracoid process. This is done by replacing the coracoclavicular ligament with heavy suture or Mersilene tape or by inserting a screw through the clavicle and into the coracoid process. It may also be necessary to stabilize the acromioclavicular joint with a smooth Steinman pin placed across the acromium and into the clavicle. Sometimes the outer one third of the clavicle is resected as well.

Procedural considerations. The patient is placed in the supine or semisitting position with a sandbag or folded sheet under the affected shoulder. The head is tilted as far as possible to the opposite side. The extremity is draped with a stockinette to the midhumeral level, so it is free to be manipulated.

The soft tissue and major bone sets and shoulder instruments (Fig. 22-48) are required, plus the following:

Screw set with instrumentation
Power drill
Micro power drill and saw (Fig. 22-49)
Bone clamps (Fig. 22-50)
Roux retractors
Aneurysm needles (ligature carriers)

Operative procedure—Weaver and Dunn procedure
1. A short anterior curvilinear incision is made over the distal clavicle, and dissection is carried down to expose the acromioclavicular joint.
2. The coracoacromial ligament is detached from the acromium end to the coracoid process, retaining the attachment at the coracoid end.

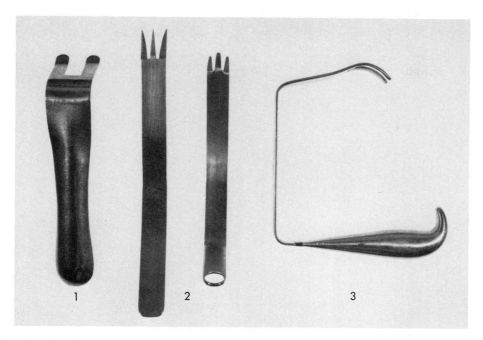

Fig. 22-48. Shoulder instruments. *1*, Rowe modified humeral head retractor; *2*, two Rowe capsule retractors (pitch-forks); *3*, humeral head retractor.

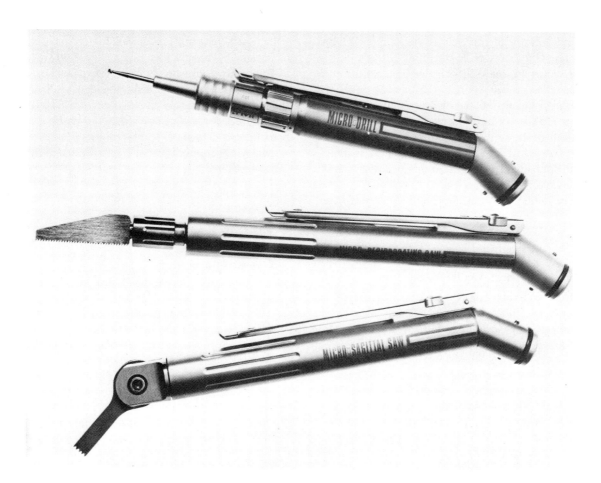

Fig. 22-49. Air-powered microdrill and microsaws. (Courtesy Zimmer, Inc., Warsaw, Ind.)

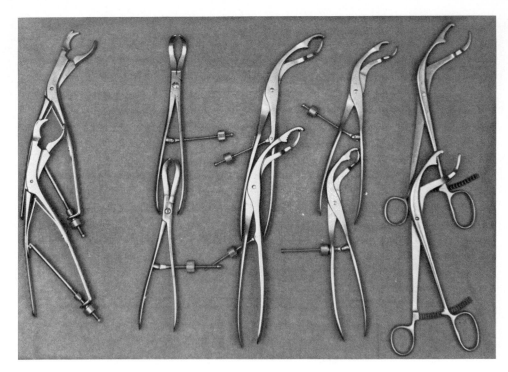

Fig. 22-50. Large bone clamps, reduction.

3. The lateral 2 cm of the clavicle is then removed with a microsaw, Gigli saw, or bone-cutting forceps.
4. Two drill holes are made into the superior cortex end of the clavicle.
5. A heavy no. 1 nonabsorbable mattress suture is placed at the dissected end of the coracoacromial ligament and passed through the drill holes in the clavicle.
6. With the clavicle held in reduction, the suture is tightened. This pulls the ligament into the medullary canal of the clavicle.
7. The suture is tied, and muscle layers are closed over the joint.
8. The wound is closed in the usual fashion, and a sling is applied postoperatively.

Correction of sternoclavicular dislocation

Dislocation and subluxation of the sternoclavicular joint are uncommon. Sternoclavicular dislocation usually is treated nonoperatively with immobilizing bandages. In certain severe cases, open reduction may be necessary.

Clavicular fracture

Fractures of the clavicle are common. The most common site of clavicular fractures is the middle third portion of the bone, mainly at the middle and outer third junction. Clavicular fractures are usually treated by immobilization in a figure-of-eight splint (Fig. 22-51). Surgery is necessary when the fracture is displaced enough to cause underlying damage to the vessels and brachial plexus. Open reduction is accomplished with a tubular plate and screws or intramedullary pin fixation.

Procedural considerations. The patient is placed in the supine or semisitting position with a sandbag or folded sheet under the affected shoulder and the head tilted as far as possible to the opposite side. The entire extremity is prepped and draped.

Major bone and soft tissue sets are required, plus the following:

Power drill
Kirschner wires
Plate and screw set or fixation appliance of choice
Bone graft instruments

Operative procedure

1. An 8-cm incision is made just above or below the clavicle.
2. Dissection is carried down to the fracture site, avoiding injury to vessels and nerves.
3. The fracture site is exposed and reduced, using bone-holding clamps.
4. A one-third tubular plate is fitted across the fracture site; if necessary, the plate is contoured with bending irons.
5. Bone screws are used to secure the plate. The plate hole sites are drilled, measured for depth, and tapped, cutting the threads from the appropriate screw.
6. Bone graft is added superiorly and posteriorly if the fracture is a nonunion.

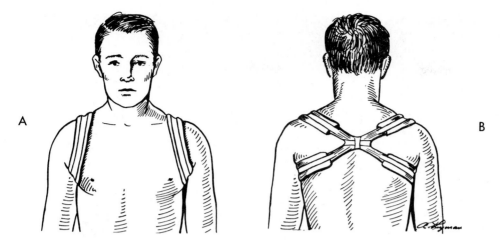

Fig. 22-51. Figure-of-eight splint. **A,** Front view. **B,** Back view. Felt, bias flannel bandage, and adhesive tape are used. Splint should be changed every week to 10 days for cleanliness. (From Larson, C.B., and Gould, M.: Orthopedic nursing, ed. 9, St. Louis, 1978, The C.V. Mosby Co.)

7. The wound is closed, and a sling is applied postoperatively.

Correction of rotator cuff tear

A rotator cuff tear is one occurring through the inserting tendinous fibers of the infraspinous, supraspinous, teres minor, and subscapular muscles on the humerus.

Rotator cuff tears frequently follow trauma in patients with weakened tendinous fibers who have degenerative changes within the joint. Patients with this problem are unable to initiate abduction of the shoulder because the stabilizing forces of the ruptured tendons on the humeral head are lost. Many rotator cuff tears can be treated conservatively with special splints or braces.

Procedural considerations. If surgery is necessary, the patient is placed in the supine or semisitting position with a sandbag or folded towel under the affected shoulder. The head is tilted to the opposite side as far as possible.

Soft tissue and major bone sets are required, plus the following:

Power drill and drill bits
Shoulder instruments

Operative procedure

1. A superior incision that extends both anteriorly and posteriorly is made.
2. The muscles are then detached from the scapula and clavicle.
3. Small, simple tears can be repaired by suturing the torn edges with heavy, nonabsorbable sutures.
4. Massive tears may require attaching the torn edges to the greater tuberosity through drill holes or into a wedge-shaped osteotomy using cotton or synthetic sutures.

5. Once the repair is complete, the wound is closed and dressed with a sterile dressing.
6. The shoulder is placed in a sling or shoulder immobilizer postoperatively.

Correction of recurrent anterior dislocation of the shoulder

The anterior fibers of the shoulder capsule are stretched and weakened as a result of frequent dislocations of the shoulder joint. There are several different methods of repair, but all of the procedures are designed to strengthen the anterior joint capsule. The surgical incision and instruments used for all of the procedures are similar.

Procedural considerations. The patient is placed in the supine or semisitting position with a sandbag or folded sheet under the shoulder. The arm is draped free so the extremity can be manipulated. An anterior curved incision or a longitudinal incision in the anterior axillary fold is made over the shoulder joint.

A regular soft tissue instrument set and a major bone set are required, plus the following:

Shoulder instruments
Power drill and drill bits
Bankart instruments (Fig. 22-52)
Mayo needles, no. 5

Operative procedures

Bankart procedure (Fig. 22-53). The attenuated anterior capsule is reattached to the rim of the glenoid fossa with heavy sutures. The glenoid fossa rim is roughened with a chisel to provide a raw surface to which the capsule is attached. Special instruments designed for the Bankart procedure are desirable (Fig. 22-52). Instruments such as an angled drill, a curved awl, or drill bits are necessary for making the suture holes in the rim of the glenoid fossa.

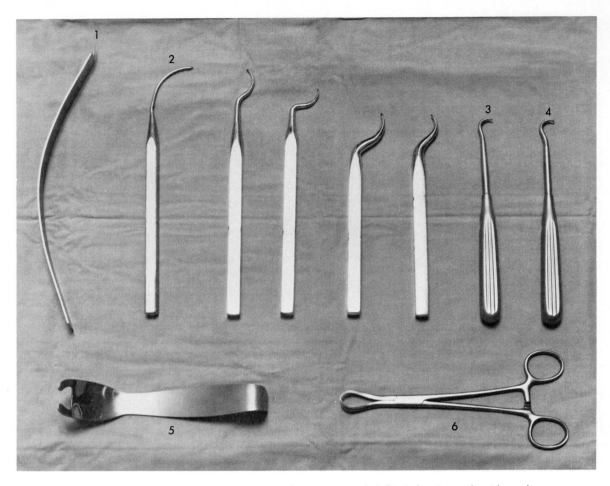

Fig. 22-52. Bankart instruments. *1,* Rowe capsule retractor (pitch-fork); *2,* five Rowe glenoid punches; *3,* curved awl; *4,* ligature retriever; *5,* humeral head retractor; *6,* glenoid reaming forceps.

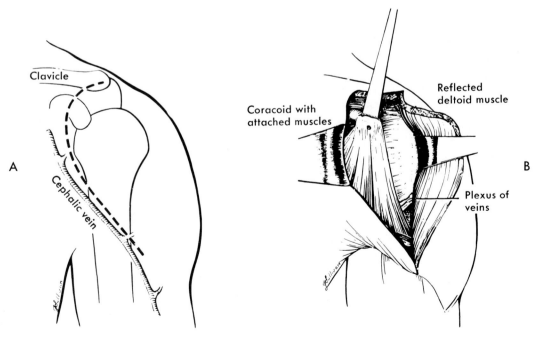

Fig. 22-53. Bankart operation (technique of Cave and Rowe). **A,** Skin incision. **B,** Coracoid divided.

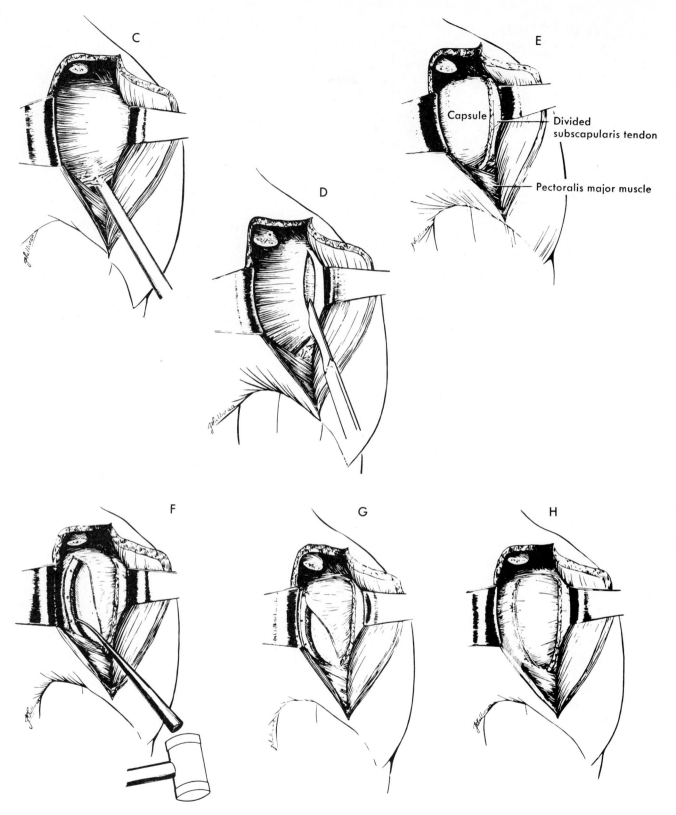

Fig. 22-53, cont'd. C, Inferior margin of subscapular tendon identified. **D,** Subscapular tendon divided near lesser tuberosity. **E,** Subscapular tendon retracted medially. **F,** Holes made through rim of glenoid. **G,** Free lateral margin of capsule sutured to rim of glenoid. **H,** Medial margin of capsule lapped over lateral part and sutured in place. (From Edmonson, A.S., and Crenshaw, A.H., editors: Campbell's operative orthopaedics, ed. 7, St. Louis, 1987, The C.V. Mosby Co.)

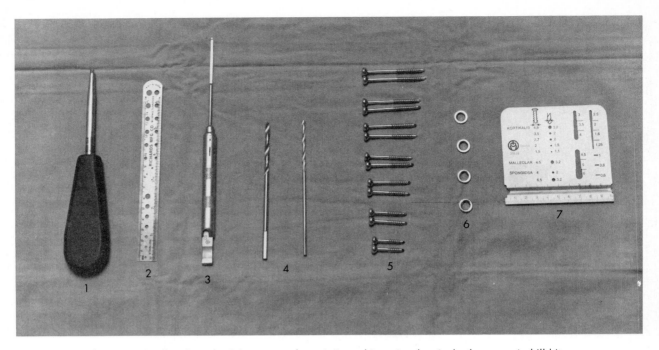

Fig. 22-54. Small A-O set for Bristow procedure. *1*, Screwdriver; *2*, ruler; *3*, depth gauge; *4*, drill bits (4.5 and 3.2 mm); *5*, screws; *6*, washers; *7*, measuring gauge for screws and ruler.

If the coracoid process is to be removed to obtain better operative exposure, a drill and drill bits should be available. Postoperatively, the extremity is immobilized in a sling or shoulder immobilizer. See Fig. 22-53 for the operative procedure.

Putti-Platt procedure

1. The subscapularis tendon is divided approximately 1 inch medial to its insertion on the lesser tuberosity.
2. The free edge of the lateral part of the subscapularis is taken across the joint and sutured to the soft structures along the anterior rim of the glenoid cavity.
3. The free edge of the medial part of the subscapularis is taken across laterally to the area of the greater tuberosity and sutured to the rotator cuff. This overlapping and shortening of the subscapularis limits external rotation and thus prevents dislocation.

Bristow procedure. The coracoid process, along with the attached muscles, is detached and inserted onto the neck of the glenoid cavity, where it is held with a screw. This stabilizes the anterior joint capsule and prevents recurrent dislocation. Bristow instrumentation is shown in Fig. 22-54.

Correction of fracture of the humeral head

Comminuted fractures of the humeral head with displacement may require open reduction and internal fixation with screws or pins or closed reduction with a humeral fixation device. However, if the fracture is badly comminuted, a prosthetic replacement is indicated. Traumatic or degenerative arthritic shoulder joints may be so painful that a total shoulder joint replacement is necessary. Several total shoulder joint prostheses (Dana, Bechtol, Neer [Fig. 22-55], Fenlin) are available.

The need for good shoulder function, extensive rehabilitation for the shoulder, and an intact or repairable rotator cuff are essential for a good result from this procedure. In no other joint surgery are these factors so important.

The shoulder is the most difficult joint in the body to rehabilitate because it has (1) the greatest range of motion, (2) a second space beneath the acromion that must be mobilized, and (3) many muscles, weakened by trauma, that enter into complex movements. The prosthesis alone does not give the desired results but offers the patient the means by which necessary exercises can be performed to restore function.

Procedural considerations. The patient is placed in a 30-degree, "beach-chair" position with the arm on a padded armboard and draped free so it can be moved at the side of the table. The head is supported to avoid neck extension. A pad is placed under the scapula to hold it forward. An adherent plastic skin drape is applied. Antibiotics are given.

Soft tissue and major bone sets are used, plus the following:

Curette set, long
Power drill and drill bits, 3 × 6 inches long, ¼, ⅜, and ½ inch in diameter
Shoulder instruments

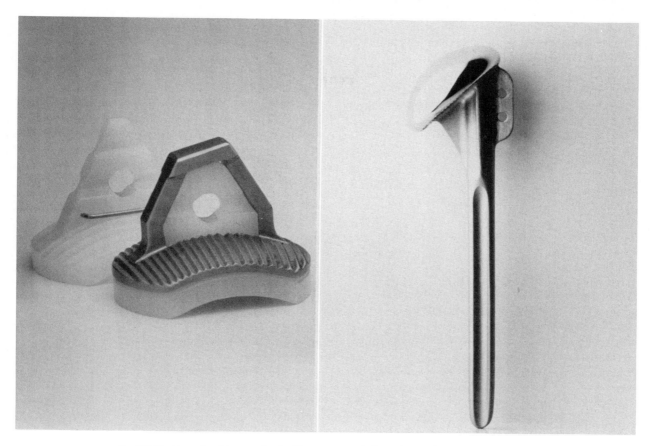

Fig. 22-55. Neer shoulder prosthesis. (Courtesy 3M Orthopedic Products, St. Paul, Minn.)

Intramedullary rasp
Intramedullary tapered reamers, ⅜ and ½ inch in diameter
Methyl methacrylate and cement instrumentation (see Fig. 22-83)
Shoulder trials and prosthesis of choice
Prosthesis impactor
Simpulse suction/irrigator and 3000-ml bag of normal saline, or Pulse Lavage (see Figs. 22-87 and 22-88)

Operative procedure

1. A 16-cm incision is made from the clavicle passing over the coracoid and downward to the level of the deltoid insertion.
2. The cephalic vein may or may not be ligated, and the deltopectoral interval is opened. The deltoid origin is not detached from the clavicle.
3. The coracoacromial ligament and clavipectoral fascia are divided, and the clot is irrigated. Blunt retraction is used on the coracoid muscles and deltoid.
4. With the arm in maximum external rotation, the subscapularis is elevated from the underlying capsule. A stay suture is placed, and the subscapularis is divided 2 cm medial to the bicipital groove. The biceps muscle is left intact.
5. The anteroinferior two thirds of the capsule is exposed by elevation. The elevator is placed beneath the cap-

sule to protect the axillary nerve, and the capsule is divided.
6. The head is presented by further external rotation. The long head of the biceps is left undisturbed and free in its groove so it will continue to function as a depressor of the head after surgery.
7. Marginal osteophytes are trimmed, and the head is removed in line with sulcus of the normal head.
8. With the glenoid exposed, measurements are taken for prosthesis fit.
9. A central hole for prosthesis fit is made into the glenoid with a high-speed burr and curette.
10. With the shaft held forward and upward, the intramedullary canal is located with a long curette. A ¼-, ⅜-, or ½-inch drill is selected to correspond to the diameter of the canal; depending on stem length of the prosthesis, 5 or 6 inches down the medullary canal is drilled. Final preparation of the shaft for the 9.5-mm (⅜-inch) or 12.7-mm (½-inch) diameter prosthesis is accomplished with the appropriately sized tapered reamer.
11. A check for 35- to 40-degree retroversion is done by palpating the epicondyles at the elbow. The implant is seated on the calcar with a driver and mallet, with

its articular surface protected with a moist sponge. Just before final seating, further trimming of high spots with a chisel or power drill may be required. Acrylic cement is used except in a young patient in whom a firm press fit can be achieved.

12. The shoulder joint is reduced and irrigated. The capsule is not closed, but the subscapularis is reattached anatomically with nylon sutures.

13. A closed drainage system is inserted between cuff and deltoid, avoiding contact of the drainage tubes with the axillary artery. Routine closure is accomplished.

14. Pads are placed between arm and body; a sling, sling and swathe, or shoulder immobilizer is applied postoperatively.

Operations on the humerus, radius, and ulna
Correction of fractures of the shaft of the humerus

Reduction of the fractured humerus is usually accomplished by closed manipulation and immobilization. When closed reduction is impossible or when nonunion of the fracture has occurred, surgery is indicated. The fracture is reduced and held with medullary nails, a heavy compression plate, or lag screw. Bone graft may be used, de-

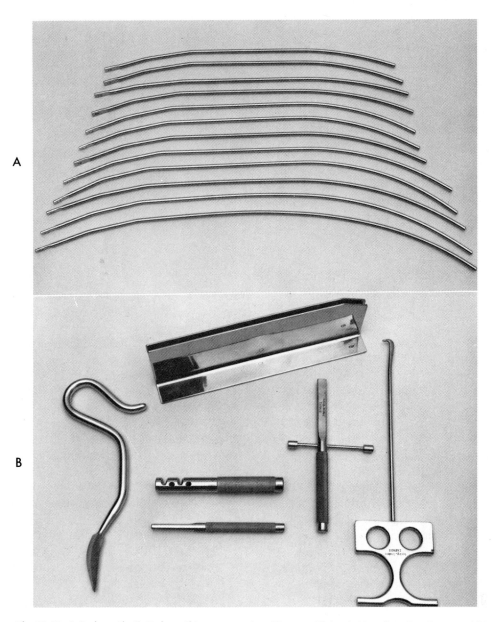

Fig. 22-56. A, Ender nails. **B,** Ender nail instrumentation. (Courtesy Richards Manufacturing Co., Memphis, Tenn.)

pending on both the extent of the fracture and the time since injury.

Procedural considerations. The patient is supine with the extremity prepped and draped from the middle of the chest to below the elbow.

Soft tissue and major bone sets are required, plus the following:

Power drill
Plates and screws with instrumentation
Steinman pins
Nails and instrumentation (Ender [Fig. 22-56] or Kuntschner nails; Rush Rods)
Bone graft instruments
Methyl methacrylate (for pathologic fractures)

Operative procedure—Ender nailing

1. A skin incision is made over the proximal humerus metaphysis, medial to the bicipital groove.
2. Entry into the medullary canal is initiated with a drill, and then an awl is used to pass through the deltopectoral groove.
3. Nail length is determined by external placement of the nail along the humerus in conjunction with image intensification. The nail should lie from the canal entrance point to just above the distal end of the medullary canal.
4. Two to three flexible Ender nails of appropriate size are driven down the humeral shaft, across the fracture line, and into the distal fragment. Fluoroscopy is used to aid in nail placement.
5. The proximal wound is irrigated and closed. A sterile dressing is applied.

Correction of distal humerus fractures (supracondylar, epicondylar, intercondylar)

Distal humerus fractures are particularly difficult to treat by closed methods. Screws, pins, and a variety of different plates can be used for internal fixation. There are circumstances in which it is necessary to transfer the ulnar nerve anteriorly to prevent compression of the nerve.

Procedural considerations. General or regional anesthesia is administered. The patient may be prone with the elbow flexed over a small table, supine with the arm over the chest, supine with the arm on a hand table, or lateral. A tourniquet is useful during this procedure.

Soft tissue and major bone sets are required, plus the following:

Power drill
Bone-holding clamps
Kirschner wires
Screw and plate set with instrumentation

Operative procedure

1. An incision is made over the distal humerus fracture site.
2. The fracture is exposed and reduced.

3. Any intraarticular fractures are treated with Kirschner wires and a screw.
4. If a one-third tubular, DCP (dynamic compression plate), or semitubular plate (Fig. 22-44) is used, it is contoured to the fracture site and secured with screws.
5. The wound is irrigated and closed.
6. An arm cast is applied for postoperative immobilization.

Correction of olecranon fracture

If the olecranon fracture fragment is small, it may be excised and the triceps tendon reattached to the ulna shaft. This does not result in loss of stability of the elbow joint. However, larger fragments must be reduced and held with internal fixation.

Procedural considerations. Compression (small fragment) screws (Fig. 22-57), Kirschner wires, Steinman pins, and figure-of-eight wire may be used (Fig. 22-58). Small bone and soft tissue sets are required, plus the following:

Small bone clamps
Fragment compression screws, small, with instrumentation
Power drill and bits
Wire and wire tightener
Steinman pins
Kirschner wires

Operative procedure

1. An incision is made over the olecranon, and the fracture is exposed.
2. A drill hole is made in the distal fragment from side to side.
3. An 18-gauge stainless steel wire is passed around the tip of the olecranon.
4. One end of the wire is then passed obliquely across the fracture to the other side of the triceps.
5. The fracture is reduced with distal traction, and the wire is twisted tightly.
6. A Kirschner wire or bone screw may be required through the olecranon and into the medullary canal of the ulna if more stability is required.
7. The wound is closed, and a posterior splint is applied.

Transposition of the ulnar nerve

Transposition of the ulnar nerve involves freeing the ulnar nerve from its groove at the back of the medial epicondyle of the humerus and bringing it to the front of the condyle.

The ulnar nerve is frequently divided or damaged in fractures or wounds of the elbow. Dislocation of the elbow may also cause ulnar nerve damage. Late traumatic neuritis results from stretching of the ulnar nerve caused by an old injury. The hand appears atrophied, and sensory loss is high. In severe cases a clawhand deformity occurs.

Procedural considerations. The patient is placed in the supine position with the extremity slightly flexed on a

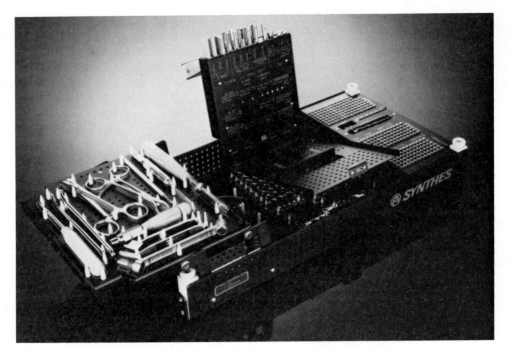

Fig. 22-57. Small fragment compression set. (Courtesy Synthes, U.S.A., Paoli, Pa.)

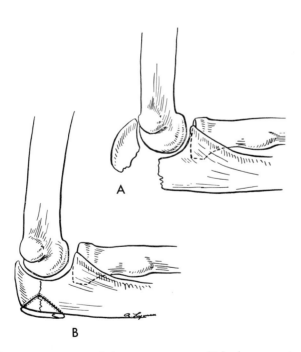

Fig. 22-58. Fracture of olecranon process, which always requires open reduction if fragments are separated. **A,** Fracture. **B,** Wire suture that should be fairly superficial for best results. (From Larson, C.B., and Gould, M.: Orthopedic nursing, ed. 9, St. Louis, 1978, The C.V. Mosby Co.)

hand table or flexed over the chest. A tourniquet is applied to the upper arm, and the entire arm (fingers to tourniquet) is prepped and draped.

Minor and small bone sets are required.

Operative procedure

1. An incision is made on the lateral aspect of the elbow near the epicondyle.
2. The fascia and the flexor carpi ulnaris muscle are divided.
3. The ulnar nerve is freed, and the medial intermuscular septum is cut away.
4. The nerve is then drawn anteriorly and placed deep in the brachialis flexor muscle origin.
5. A right-angled plaster cast is applied to the elbow postoperatively.

Excision of the head of the radius

A congruous radial head is essential for proper rotation of the forearm at the elbow. Consequently, in an adult it is necessary to excise the radial head if a severely comminuted fracture of the radial head with angulation interferes with rotation (Fig. 22-59). The radial head should never be excised in children.

Procedural considerations. The patient is supine with the arm over the chest or on a hand table. A tourniquet is used.

A minor set, small bone set, and micro oscillating saw with blades are required.

Operative procedure

1. An oblique incision is made over the posterior surface

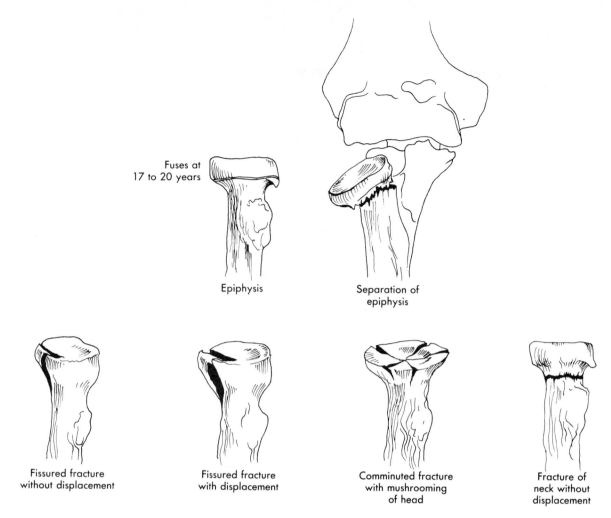

Fig. 22-59. Types of fractures of head and neck of radius. (From Moseley, H.F., editor: Textbook of surgery, ed. 3, St. Louis, 1959, The C.V. Mosby Co.)

of the lateral humeral condyle and continued over the posterior border of the ulna just distal to the tip of the olecranon.

2. Dissection is continued between the anconeus and extensor carpi ulnaris muscle to the joint capsule.
3. With the head and neck of the radius exposed through the joint capsule, the joint is irrigated of bone debris and blood clots.
4. The radial head is then excised just proximally to the radial tuberosity. The remaining annular ligament is excised as well.
5. The wound is closed, and a posterior plaster splint is applied.

Total elbow replacement

Total elbow replacement (Fig. 22-60) is indicated in patients with posttraumatic lesions or excessive bone loss from rheumatic or degenerative arthritis, resulting in elbow instability and pain. The Tri-Axial, Schlein, and Pritchard are among the prostheses available. This procedure is not done frequently because of the many potential problems. Postoperative stability of the elbow implant depends largely on the soft tissues surrounding the joint. The prosthesis may be used with or without methyl methacrylate (cement), depending on the quality of the diseased bone and the design of the implant. If no cement is employed, grafting with the bone resected off the distal humerus may be required to seat the ulnar component snugly and achieve adequate bony contact with the porous coating of the metal ulnar component.

After implantation of the prosthetic parts, closure of the joint is achieved with heavy, nonabsorbable suture material. A suction drain is inserted. Routine skin closure is performed, and a bulky dressing and plaster splint are applied.

Postoperative instability and dislocation are the major complications associated with total elbow replacement.

Procedural considerations. In the operative proce-

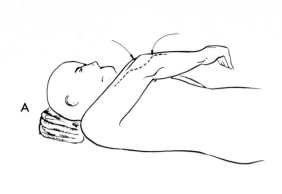

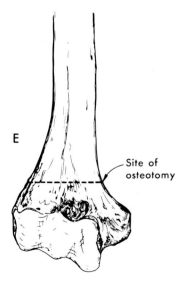

Fig. 22-60. Total elbow replacement procedure. **A,** Patient positioning. **B,** Triceps tendon and periosteum stripped together intact. **C,** Bone removal from proximal ulna gives excellent exposure and can include almost entire olecranon and notch. **D,** Alternative resection removes articular surfaces while preserving major portion of olecranon. **E,** Bone removal from distal humerus can include both epicondyles so as to correctly seat humeral stem. **F,** Total elbow prosthesis and trial. (Courtesy Zimmer, Inc., Warsaw, Ind.)

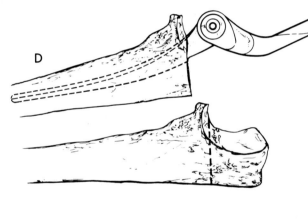

Site of osteotomy

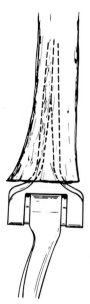

dure, the patient is positioned supine with the arm over the chest. A tourniquet is used. The elbow joint is exposed through a lateral incision.

Small and major bone and ortho soft tissue sets are required, plus the following:

Power drill, drill bits, and burrs
Power saw
Total elbow trials and implants
Replacement instrumentation
Methyl methacrylate, with instrumentation
Awl
Simpulse or Pulse Lavage (see Figs. 22-87 and 22-88), and 3000-ml bag of normal saline

See Fig. 22-60 for the operative procedure.

Correction of fractures of the radius and ulna

Fractures of the radius and ulna frequently occur in children. As long as there is apposition of the fracture fragments, any angular deformity will be corrected as the child grows, so an operation is not indicated. However, an adult does not correct angular deformities, so anatomic reduction is necessary to permit proper rotation of the forearm. Consequently, open reduction and internal fixation (ORIF), using intramedullary pins or compression plates, is frequently necessary for displaced fractures of one or both of these bones. Bone graft may also be used.

Procedural considerations. The patient is supine with the arm extended on the hand table. Minor soft tissue and small bone sets are used, plus the following:

Small bone clamps (Fig. 22-61)
Nail set with instrumentation (Rush rods)

Kirschner wires
Power drill
Small compression plate and screw set with instrumentation
Bone graft instruments

Operative procedure

1. A longitudinal incision is made directly over the fractures, and the fractures are exposed.
2. Once the fracture sites are debrided, they are reduced with small bone clamps.
3. The ulnar fracture is plated first, preferably with the plate fitted on the posterior side.
4. The previously reduced radius is then fitted with a 5- to 6-hole DCP plate, contoured as needed and placed on the dorsal surface over the fracture.
5. The plate is held over the fracture with two bone-holding forceps, and the plate holes on one side of the fracture are drilled, measured for depth, tapped, and filled with a bone screw of appropriate length and diameter. The same steps are then followed to secure the opposite end of the plate.
6. Sometimes a compression device is used to apply compression to the fragments while the opposite end of the plate is secured (Fig. 22-62).
7. Autogenous iliac bone graft may be necessary for additional stabilization.
8. The subcutaneous tissue and skin are closed and a pressure dressing or cast is applied.

Correction of Colles' fracture

Colles' fracture is a dorsally angulated fracture of the distal radius. It usually is treated with closed reduction

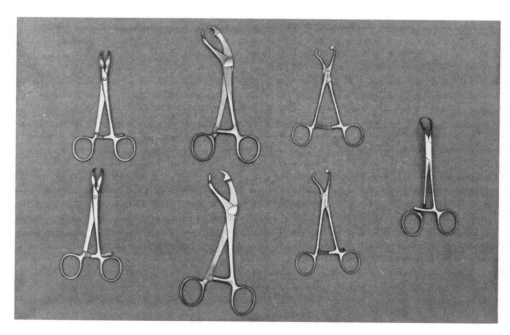

Fig. 22-61. Small bone clamps. *Left to right:* reduction, Verbrugge bone holding, plate holding, reduction with points.

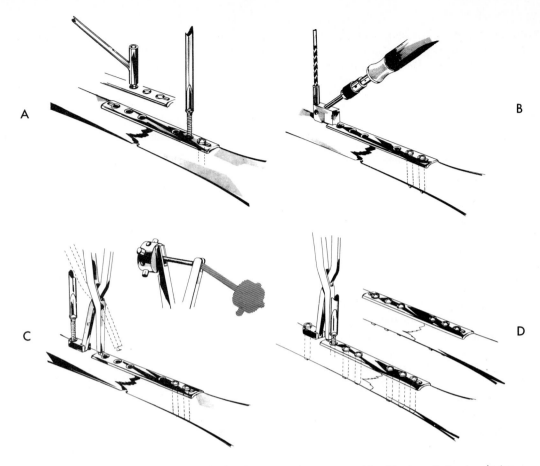

Fig. 22-62. A, Compression plate attached with screws to bone on one side of fracture. **B,** Tension device fixed into bone. **C,** Fracture reduced, using tension and compression devices. **D,** Internal fixation completed. Screws are used to fix other end of compression plate into place. Tension device is removed before incision is closed. (Courtesy Zimmer, Inc., Warsaw, Ind.)

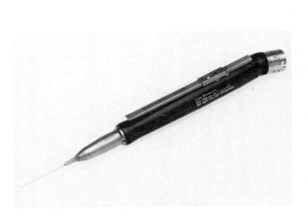

Fig. 22-63. Micro wire driver. (Courtesy Micro-aire Surgical Instruments, Inc., Valencia, Calif.)

and immobilization with a cast or external fixator. Internal fixation is indicated when the distal radius is severely comminuted. In these cases Kirschner wires are used for internal fixation.

Procedural considerations. The patient is in the supine position with the arm extended on a hand table. Minor soft tissue and small bone sets are used, plus a micro wire driver (Fig. 22-63) and Kirschner wires.

Operative procedure

1. Percutaneous pins are placed through the styloid, across the fracture, and into the opposite cortex.
2. Another method of Kirschner wire insertion is to drive one wire transversely through the proximal ulna and another transversely through the bases of the second and third metacarpal.
3. Casting is applied for postoperative immobilization.

Operations on the hand

Certain aspects of hand surgery are covered in Chapter 24. Air-powered microdrills are frequently used (Fig. 22-49).

Carpal tunnel release

Carpal tunnel syndrome is an entrapment process in which the median nerve becomes compressed at the volar surface of the wrist because of thickened synovium, trauma, or aberrant muscles. Carpal tunnel syndrome is frequently seen in patients with rheumatoid synovitis or malaligned Colles' fracture and is associated with obesity, Raynaud's disease, and pregnancy. The symptoms are pain, numbness, and tingling of the fingers and weakness of the intrinsic thumb muscles. These symptoms are usually reversible after the flexor retinaculum is incised, which relieves the compressed median nerve.

Procedural considerations. The patient is placed in the supine position with the arm extended on a hand table. A tourniquet is applied to the upper arm. Minor soft tissue and small bone sets are required.

Operative procedure

1. A curvilinear, longitudinal volar incision is made from the proximal palm across the wrist joint.
2. The deep transverse carpal ligament is divided, and a synovectomy is done if necessary.
3. A pressure dressing is applied with or without a volar splint.

Correction of fractures of the carpal bones

Most fractures of the carpal bones are treated by closed reduction and immobilization. However, it is occasionally necessary to operate on a fracture because of acute instability, delayed union, or nonunion. The scaphoid is the most commonly fractured carpal bone. Internal fixation is accomplished with Kirschner wires, small compression screws, or small plates and screws. Bone graft from the distal radius or olecranon is frequently added.

Procedural considerations. The patient is supine with the arm extended on a hand table. A tourniquet is applied. Minor soft tissue and small bone sets are required, plus the following:

Kirschner wires
Micro wire driver
Power drill
Mini screw or plate and screw set, such as Mini fragment compression (Fig. 22-64), Wurzburg or Herbert bone screw set (Fig. 22-65).

Operative procedure

1. An anterior incision is made over the scaphoid bone.
2. The superficial palmar branch of the radial artery is ligated and divided.
3. The flexor carpi radialis tendon sheath is incised and retracted to expose the capsule of the wrist.
4. The capsule is entered, and the scaphoid fracture is identified.
5. The fracture is reduced by manipulation and temporarily held with small Kirschner wires.
6. Bone graft is frequently added.
7. The fixation screw of choice is then inserted across the fracture after drilling, depth measuring, and tapping is completed.
8. The wound is closed and dressed with a firm bandage or splint.

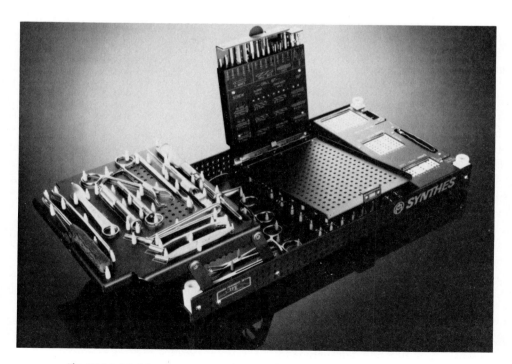

Fig. 22-64. Mini fragment compression set. (Courtesy Synthes, U.S.A., Paoli, Pa.)

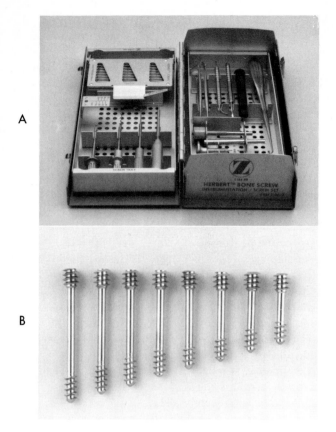

Fig. 22-65. Herbert bone screw set. **A,** system. **B,** bone screws. (Courtesy Zimmer, Inc., Warsaw, Ind.)

Excision of ganglia

Ganglia are benign outpouchings of the synovium from the intercarpal joints or tendon sheaths that become filled with synovial fluid, causing pain and weakness. Ganglia are usually found on the dorsal surface of the wrist or on the tendon sheath over the metacarpophalangeal joint but can also be found on the volar surface. Ganglia appear as firm masses that vary in size. Frequently ganglia resolve spontaneously, but occasionally they are excised because of discomfort or for cosmetic reasons.

Procedural considerations. The patient is supine with the arm extended on a hand table. Minor soft tissue and small bone sets are required.

Operative procedure
1. A transverse incision is made over each ganglion.
2. Generous margins are removed around the base to prevent recurrence.
3. The wound is irrigated and closed, and a pressure dressing is applied.

Metacarpal arthroplasty

Metacarpal joint replacement is most often performed in patients who have pain or a disabling deformity asso-

ciated with rheumatoid or degenerative arthritis of the metacarpophalangeal or interphalangeal joints. The results of rheumatoid reconstructive surgery are generally good, and pain can be eliminated and joint alignment and joint stability restored in the majority of patients. The greatest problems following an operation are weakness of grasp and pinch and progression of the disease in adjacent joints.

Procedural considerations. The patient is placed in the supine position with the arm extended on a hand table. A tourniquet is applied, and the entire extremity is prepped and draped.

Swanson small bone instruments (Fig. 22-66) and a minor set are required, plus small reamers and trials and permanent implants (Fig. 22-67).

Operative procedure
1. Incisions are made on the dorsum of the appropriate fingers.
2. The proximal and distal portions of the joints are excised, and intramedullary canals are reamed.
3. Trial implants are inserted to facilitate correct fit of the prosthesis.
4. Once the appropriate sized implant is determined, it is positioned into the canal, and appropriate tendon and ligament repairs are made to improve stability.
5. The joint is irrigated and closed, and a bulky dressing is applied.
6. A 3-inch posterior splint is applied for immobilization.

Operations on the hip and femur
Correction of fractures of the acetabulum

Fractures of the acetabulum usually result from high-energy injuries such as motor vehicle accidents. The fracture is directly related to the force transmitted to the femoral head via the greater trochanter or lower extremity. Indications for internal fixation of acetabular fractures include (1) more than 2 mm of displacement, (2) presence of intraarticular loose bodies, (3) inability to reduce under closed methods, and (4) unstable fractures of the posterior acetabular wall. Internal fixation is usually delayed 3 to 10 days to allow time for the patient to be systematically evaluated and clinically stabilized. Meanwhile, the fracture is reduced under closed methods and maintained in skeletal traction. General anesthesia may be required for closed reduction and skeletal traction when the acetabular fracture is severely displaced or dislocated. The most common fractures are posterior wall or column fractures, high transverse fractures, fractures of the weight-bearing dome, and fractures with interposition with bone or soft tissue. Internal fixation is accomplished with reconstruction plates and screws, total hip replacement, or fusion if the fracture can not be reduced.

Procedural considerations. The surgical approach depends on the type and area of the fracture and the surgeon's preference. The patient is placed on a fracture table or

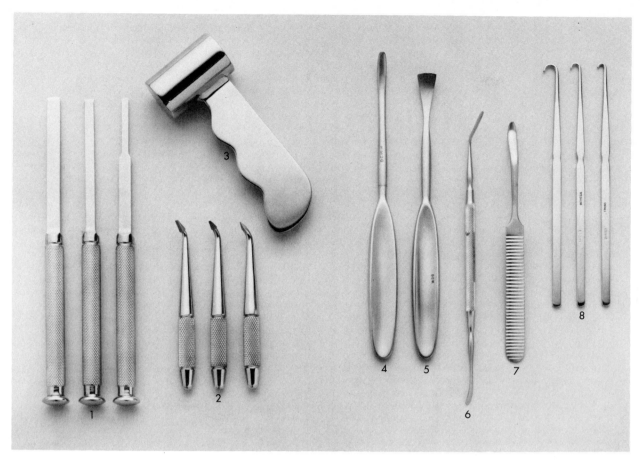

Fig. 22-66. Swanson small bone instruments. *1,* Swanson osteotomes: size A (8.5 mm blade width), size B (6.5 mm blade width), size C (4.5 mm blade width); *2,* Swanson awls (scaphoid/lunate): large, small, pointed end; *3,* Swanson mallet; *4,* Langenbeck (narrow) subperiosteal elevator; *5,* Langenbeck (wide) subperiosteal elevator; *6,* Freer-Swanson (narrow) ganglion knife; *7,* Swanson elevator; *8,* tendon hooks, large, medium, small. (Courtesy Dow Corning Wright, Arlington, Tenn., and Alfred B. Swanson, M.D.)

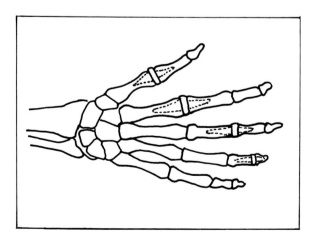

Fig. 22-67. Metacarpal implants, Swanson design. (Courtesy Dow Corning Wright, Arlington, Tenn.)

standard operating room bed in the lateral or supine position. General anesthesia along with a continuous epidural is given.

Soft tissue and major bone sets are required, plus the following:

    Acetabular fracture instruments (Fig. 22-68)
        Pelvic reduction clamp
        Femoral distractor with 5-mm Schanz screw
        Faraboef forceps
        Initial incision retractor with deep blades
        Reconstruction plates, 3.5 mm and 4.5 mm
        Long cancellous and cortical bone screws
        Long depth gauge
        Long drill bits, 2.5, 3.2, and 3.5
        Long taps, 3.5 and 4.5
        Plate-bending irons for reconstruction plates
        Ball spike
        Screwdriver, small and large
    Kirschner wires
    Power drill

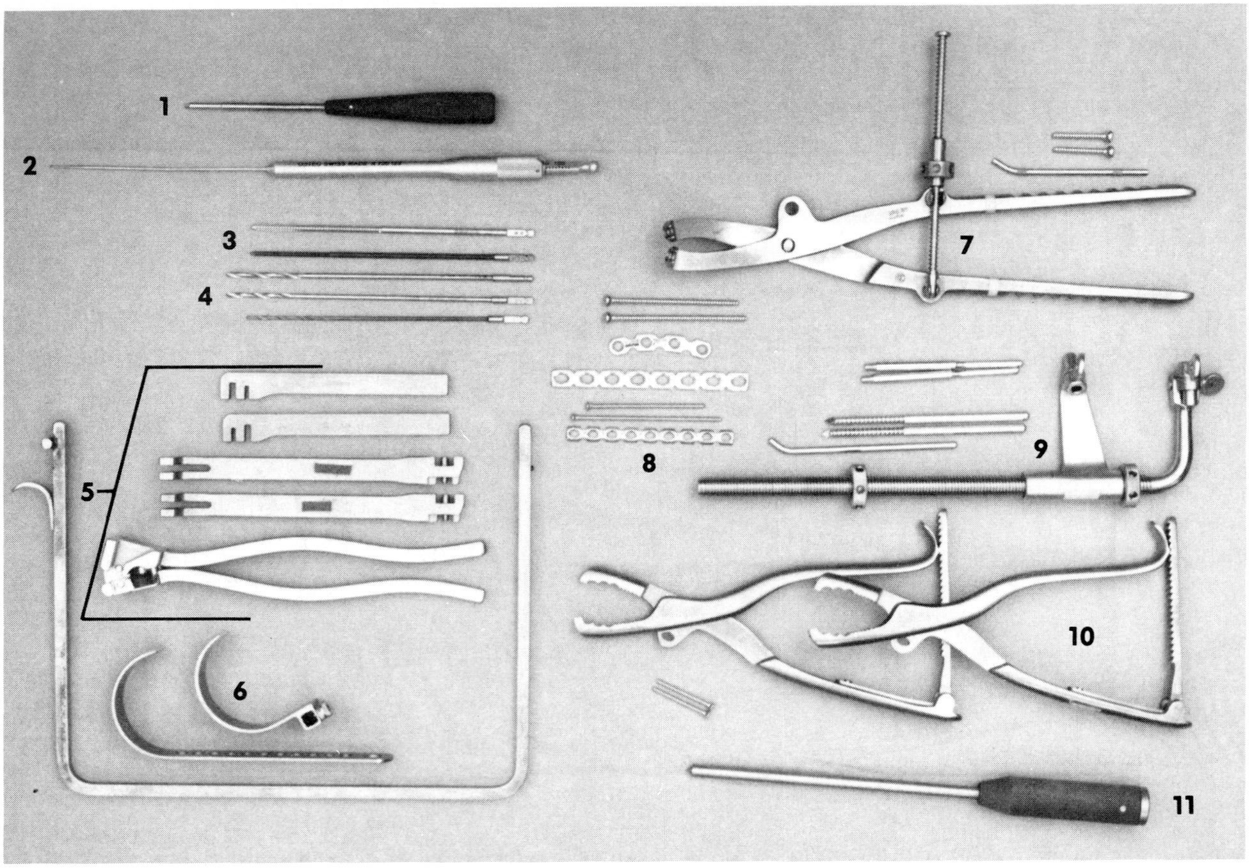

Fig. 22-68. Acetabular fracture instruments with implants: *1*, screwdriver, small and large (not shown); *2*, depth gauge; *3*, taps; *4*, drill bits; *5*, plate bending irons; *6*, initial incision retractor with blades; *7*, pelvic reduction clamp with accessories; *8*, reconstruction plates and screws; *9*, femoral distractor and accessories; *10*, Faraboef forceps with screws; *11*, ball spike.

Large bone clamps

Small and large compression plate and screw set with instrumentation

Bone graft instruments (have available)

Operative procedure—posterolateral approach

1. A lateral incision is made over the acetabular fracture site.
2. A femoral distractor may be applied to provide exposure of the articular surface of the acetabulum.
3. The fracture is reduced using bone clamps, Faraboef forceps, and a ball spike.
4. Reduction is accomplished in gradual steps using Kirschner wires to hold the fragments temporarily in place.
5. Reconstruction plates are fitted and contoured to the fracture site and secured with screws. Long cancellous lag screws are also used to provide interfragmentary compression.
6. Bone graft may be needed for additional fixation.
7. The wound is irrigated and closed over drains.
8. A compression dressing is applied.

Correction of hip fractures

Hip fractures include extracapsular intertrochanteric fractures and intracapsular femoral neck fractures (Fig. 22-27). Manipulation, reduction, and internal fixation of these fractures are greatly facilitated by use of a fracture table, which also permits adequate x-ray examination to determine whether the internal fixation devices are properly placed.

Intertrochanteric fractures

Intertrochanteric fractures most frequently occur in older people. The fractures usually unite without difficulty. However, because the lower extremity is externally rotated at the fracture site, internal fixation is necessary to prevent malunion. Internal fixation allows patients to get out of bed and helps prevent complications such as thrombophlebitis, pulmonary emboli, pneumonia, and decubitus ulcers.

Procedural considerations. The patient is placed in the supine position on the fracture table, and the fracture is reduced by manipulation of the extremity.

Various internal fixation devices, including Ambi, Free-lock (Figs. 22-69 through 22-71), DHS hip screws, De-yerle plate, Ender nails, and compression hip plates and screws may be used. Blood loss is minimal because the hip joint is not opened. Soft tissue and major bone sets are needed, plus the following:

Large bone clamps
Power drill
Fixation device of choice with instrumentation
Bone screw set with instrumentation

Operative procedure (Fig. 22-72)

1. A lateral incision is made from the tip of the greater trochanter distally about 15 cm.
2. The incision is carried down through the soft tissue and muscle layers to expose the lesser trochanteric region.
3. Using an angled guide, a guide pin is placed into the center of the neck and head of the femur.
4. Placement of the pin is checked with anteroposterior and lateral views under fluoroscopy.
5. A measuring gauge is used to determine the length of the pin inside the femur.
6. The reamer is set to the appropriate length and placed over the guide pin to ream the lag screw channel.
7. Tube plate trials are used to check the angle of fixation and fit.
8. The channel is then tapped for the lag screw threads.

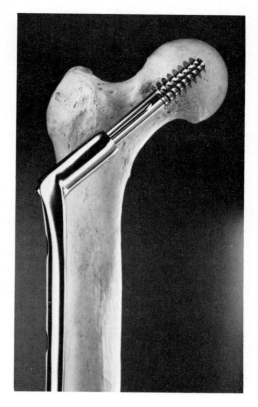

Fig. 22-69. Free-Lock® compression hip screw fixation system. (Courtesy Zimmer, Inc., Warsaw, Ind.)

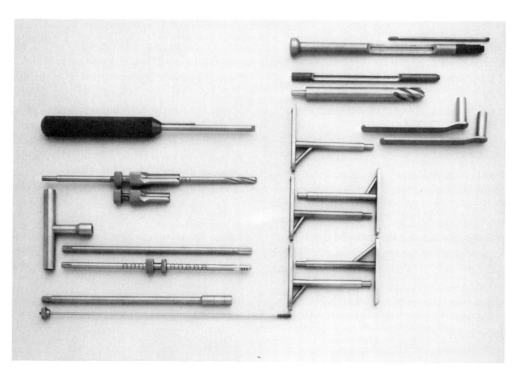

Fig. 22-70. Free-Lock® compression hip screw fixation system instruments. (Courtesy Zimmer, Inc., Warsaw, Ind.)

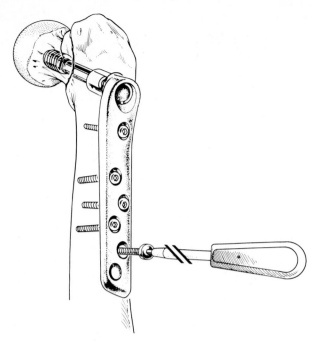

Fig. 22-71. Free-Lock℗ compression hip screw fixation system (line drawing). (Courtesy Zimmer, Inc., Warsaw, Ind.)

9. The appropriate length lag screw and tube plate are assembled together and introduced through the lag screw channel.
10. If desired, the implant is keyed (locked) for additional rotational stability.
11. Using bone screws, the side plate is secured to the femoral shaft.
12. A compression screw is inserted through the lag screw to achieve further impaction and to ensure overlap of the lag screw.
13. The wound is closed, and a pressure dressing is applied.

Femoral neck fractures

Internal fixation. Anatomic reduction is necessary before internal fixation of femoral neck fractures because of the high incidence of associated complications, such as nonunion and aseptic necrosis of the femoral head. Growing children may sustain fractures through the epiphyseal growth plate (slipped capital femoral epiphysis). These injuries are treated by reduction and internal fixation of the femoral head, similar to the procedures used in the adult. Pins of various designs, such as Deyerle, Knowles, and Universal cannulated screws, are used for fixation (Figs. 22-73 through 22-75).

Procedural considerations. The patient is placed on a fracture table under general anesthesia. Soft tissue and major bone sets are used, plus the following:

Fixation device of choice with instrumentation
Kirschner wires
Power drill
Large bone-holding forceps

Operative procedure—cannulated screw fixation

1. The fracture is exposed through a lateral incision over the greater trochanter.
2. A guide wire is placed through the neck and head of the femur with the aid of fluoroscopy.
3. The wire is measured to determine the length of screw needed.
4. Reaming and tapping are carried out over the guide wire with the cannulated instruments.
5. The cannulated screw is then inserted across the fracture site. The process is repeated for the number of screws necessary for adequate fixation.
6. X-rays are taken to check the position of the screws, and the wound is closed. A pressure dressing is applied.

Femoral head prosthetic replacement. A femoral endoprosthesis is indicated in (1) a displaced femoral neck fracture that cannot be reduced by manipulation, (2) a nonunion of a femoral neck fracture where the acetabulum is uninvolved and bone grafting and electrical stimulation are not feasible, (3) severe aseptic necrosis of the femoral head, and (4) degenerative arthritis involving the femoral head with a healthy acetabulum. Austin-Moore, Thompson, Mueller, and bipolar designs are among the many prostheses available (Figs. 22-76 to 22-78).

With conventional unipolar designs, the regular stem Austin-Moore prosthesis approximates the anatomic configuration of the femur; the straight stem Austin-Moore prosthesis may be indicated if there is also a fracture of the femoral shaft. Austin-Moore prostheses have openings in the stem for bone to grow into, forming a bridge for additional stability. The Thompson prosthesis has a large collar for weight distribution on the calcar femorale.

The development of modular systems (see discussion of total hip replacement arthroplasty) has allowed the orthopedic surgeon the ability to design a unipolar or bipolar endoprosthesis that fits on various stem designs. Bipolar endoprostheses were introduced to reduce the shear stresses affecting the acetabular surface. Bipolar design prostheses eliminate some of the motion and friction between the prosthetic head and the acetabulum that is seen with conventional endoprostheses. A femoral head prosthesis is snapped into a rotating polyethylene-lined cup that, when inserted, moves as one unit. Friction occurs between the ball and plastic instead of between the head and the acetabulum. Bipolar cups available include the self-centering cup, Universal Head Replacement (UHR), Bateman Universal Proximal Femur (UPF), Giliberty II, and Centrax. The femoral stem may or may not be cemented; the femoral cup is never cemented.

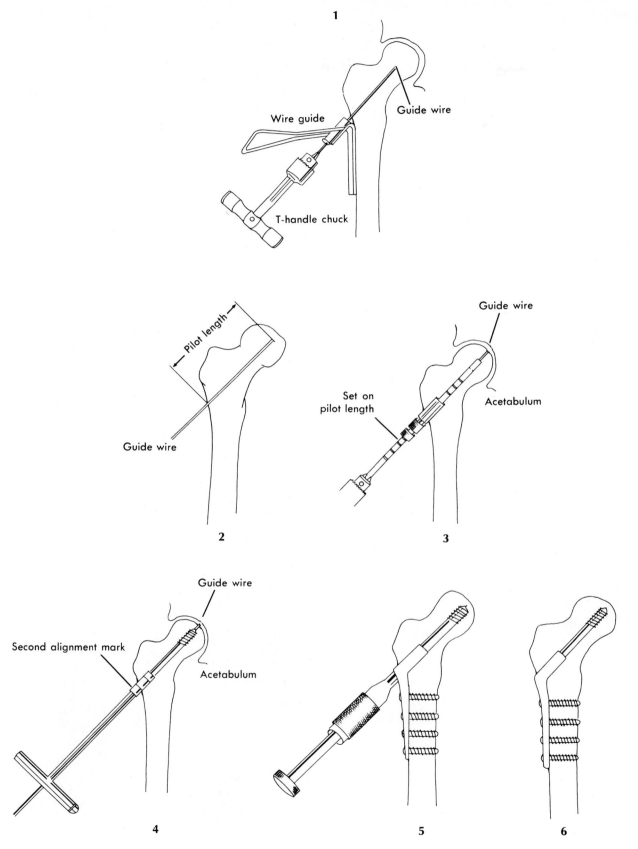

Fig. 22-72. Summary of basic hip fixation technique. (Courtesy Zimmer, Inc., Warsaw, Ind.)

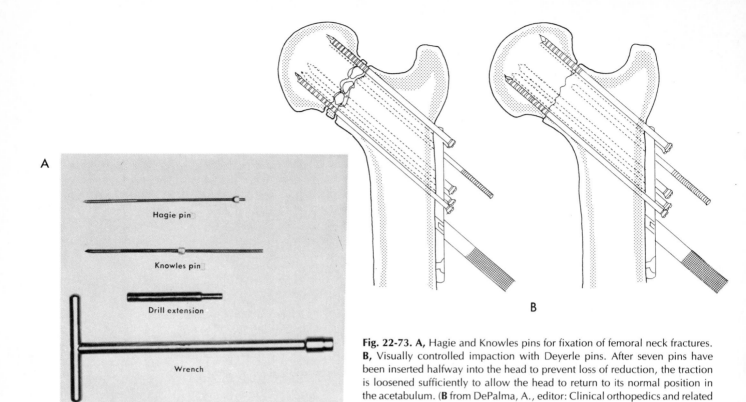

Fig. 22-73. **A,** Hagie and Knowles pins for fixation of femoral neck fractures. **B,** Visually controlled impaction with Deyerle pins. After seven pins have been inserted halfway into the head to prevent loss of reduction, the traction is loosened sufficiently to allow the head to return to its normal position in the acetabulum. (**B** from DePalma, A., editor: Clinical orthopedics and related research, vol. 39, Philadelphia, 1965, J.B. Lippincott Co.)

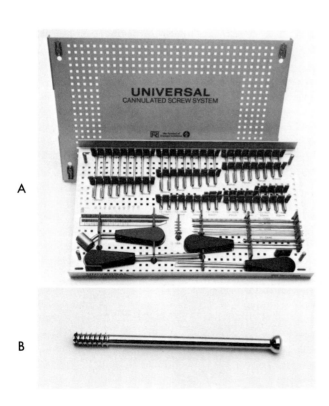

Fig. 22-74. **A,** Universal cannulated screw system: **B,** Universal cannulated screw. (Courtesy Richards Medical Co., Memphis, Tenn.)

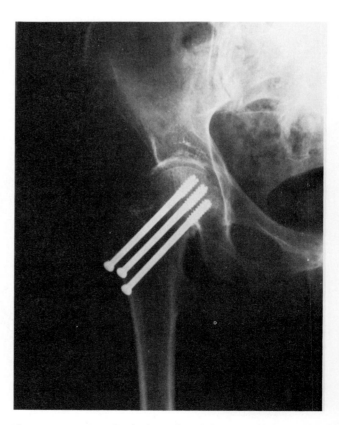

Fig. 22-75. Fixation of right femoral neck fracture with cannulated screws. (Courtesy Richards Medical Co., Memphis, Tenn.)

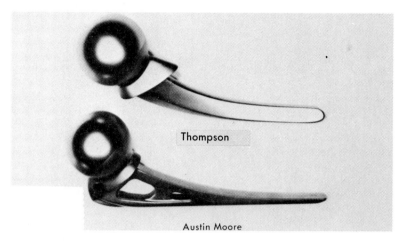

Fig. 22-76. Femoral head prostheses. (Courtesy Zimmer, Inc., Warsaw, Ind.)

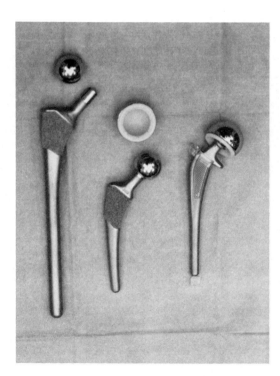

Fig. 22-77. Bipolar endoprostheses. (Courtesy Howmedica, Inc., Rutherford, N.J.)

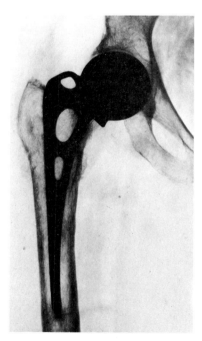

Fig. 22-78. Roentgenogram of hip after replacement arthroplasty with Austin-Moore metal prosthesis in 75-year-old woman who had nonunion of femoral neck fracture and vascular necrosis of femoral head. (From Brashear, H.R., and Raney, R.B.: Handbook of orthopaedic surgery, ed. 10, St. Louis, 1986, The C.V. Mosby Co.)

Procedural considerations. The patient is placed in the supine position if an anterior approach is used (Fig. 22-79) and in the lateral position if a lateral or posterolateral incision is used. The prep extends from the nipple line to below the knee for the supine position and from the toes to umbilical level for the lateral position.

Total hip no. 1 and no. 2 instrument sets (Figs. 22-80 and 22-81) are required, plus the following:

Trial prostheses, with instrumentation and implants of choice
Air-powered saw (Fig. 22-82)
Cement instrumentation (if methyl methacrylate is used) (Fig. 22-83)
Osteotomes (have available)
Gigli saw blade and handles (have available)
Intramedullary reamers with guide rods

Total hip set no. 1

2 Knife handles, no. 3
1 Knife handle, no. 3, long
2 Knife handles, no. 4
1 Knife handle, no. 7
1 Metal ruler
2 Nonperforating towel clamps

8 Perforating towel clamps
8 Moynihan towel clamps
   Clamps: Crile artery, wire-pulling, Allis, Pean, Mixter, Oschner, and tonsil forceps
2 Sponge-holding forceps
2 Needle holders: Mayo Hegar, short and long
2 Mayo dissecting scissors: 1 each straight and curved
1 Metzenbaum scissors, curved
1 Bandage scissors
   Forceps: 2 each Brophy tissue, regular tissue, Curtis tissue, Adson tissue, Russian
   Retractors: 1 each Richardson (¾ × 2, 1½ × 1½, 1⅛ × 1⅛, 1⅝ × 2⅜), St. Mary's (1½ × 4, ¾ × 4), USA, Hohmann (narrow blunt and sharp; broad and extrawide sharp), Volkman rake (sharp and blunt), Weitlaners (sharp), initial incision with blades, ball-and-chain, Aufranc femoral neck (superior, inferior) Adson-Beckman, horizontal

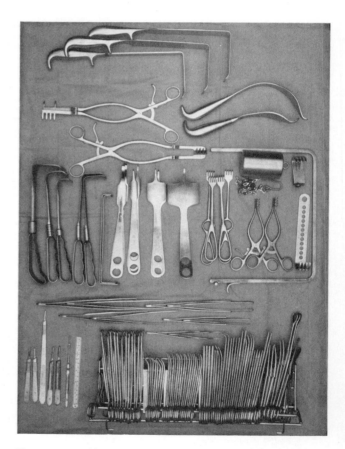

Fig. 22-80. Total hip set no. 1. *First row, bottom (left to right):* Knife handles, ruler, nonperforating towel clamps, Moynihan towel clamps, perforating towel clamps; Crile artery, wire-pulling, Allis, Pean, Mixter, Oschner, and tonsil forceps; needle holders (short, long), Mayo scissors (straight, curved), Metzenbaum scissors, sponge-holding forceps, bandage scissors. *Second row (left to right):* Adson tissue, Brophy, tissue, Curtis, and Russian forceps. *Third row (left to right):* Richardson, Army-Navy, Hohmanns (narrow blunt and sharp, broad and extrabroad sharp), Volkman (sharp, blunt) Weitlaners, initial incision with blades, and ball-and-chain retractors. *Fourth row:* horizontal retractor *(top)*; Adson-Beckman retractor *(bottom)*; *Fifth row:* Aufranc femoral neck retractors (superior and inferior); St. Mary's retractors.

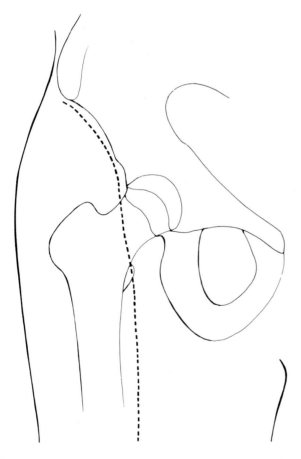

Fig. 22-79. Anterior approach to hip. (Modified from Nicola, T.: Atlas of orthopaedic exposures, Baltimore, 1966, The Williams & Wilkins Co.)

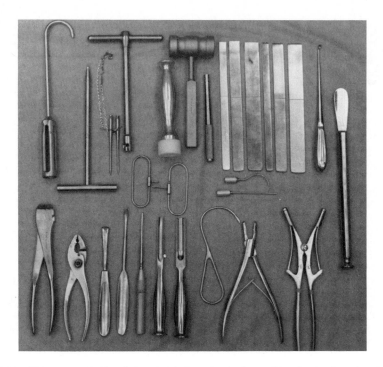

Fig. 22-81. Total hip set no. 2. *Top (left to right):* Bone hook, femoral head extractor, pin retractors with T-handle extractor, femoral prosthesis driver, mallet, bone tamp, osteotomes (curved, straight) no. 2 angled Brun curette. *Middle:* Gigli saw handles, small wire passers (curved, straight), Watson-Jones gouge (hip skid). *Bottom:* Pin cutter, pliers, Langenbeck periosteal elevators (wide, narrow), navicular gouge, Smith Peterson gouge (⅜, ⅝), Charnley trochanteric wire passer, Adson-cranial rongeur, Harris wire tightener.

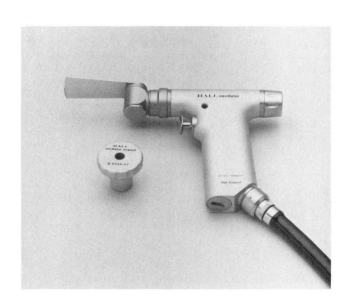

Fig. 22-82. Air-powered saw. (Courtesy Zimmer, Inc., Warsaw, Ind.)

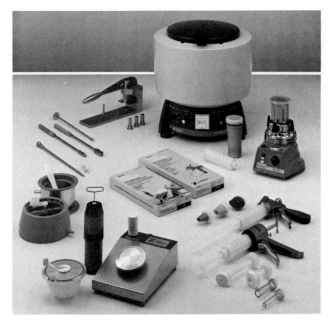

Fig. 22-83. Bone cement instruments and supplies. (Courtesy Zimmer, Inc., Warsaw, Ind.)

Total hip set no. 2

1 Bone hook, large
1 Femoral head extractor (corkscrew)
1 Pin retractor with T-handle extractor
2 Gigli saw handles
1 Femoral prosthesis driver
1 Mallet
1 Bone tamp
    Osteotomes: 1 each 1½, ½, ⅜ (straight and curved)
1 Brun bone curette, no. 2 angled
    Wire passers: 1 each small (curved, straight), Charnley
        trochanteric
    Elevators: 1 each Langenbeck periosteal, wide and narrow
    Gouges: 1 each Smith Peterson (⅜, ⅝), navicular,
        Watson-Jones
1 Wire cutter, heavy
1 Pliers, regular
1 Adson cranial rongeur
1 Harris wire tightener

Operative procedure—posterolateral approach

1. A linear incision is made from 5 cm below the posteroinferior iliac spine toward the posterior aspect of the greater trochanter and distally along the posterior aspect of the proximal femur for 7 cm.
2. The capsule is entered, and the femoral head is removed and sized.
3. The femoral neck is fashioned to achieve an accurate prosthetic fit.
4. A punch is then used to open the medullary canal from the femoral neck.
5. The intramedullary canal is reamed, rasped, and broached to accommodate the prosthesis.
6. Once the canal is prepared, the prosthesis of choice is inserted with or without bone cement.
7. The hip is reduced, and closure is accomplished in layers over suction drains.

Total hip replacement arthroplasty

Total hip replacement arthroplasty is a common orthopedic procedure. It is indicated for patients with hip pain due to degenerative joint disease or rheumatoid arthritis.

In the past, reconstructive surgery of the hip consisted of subtrochanteric osteotomy, cup arthroplasty, and prosthetic femoral head replacement. Since the development of the total hip arthroplasty, these procedures are rarely performed.

Total hip arthroplasties are cemented, noncemented, or hybrid. Hybrid arthroplasties involve cementing one component, usually the femoral stem, and not cementing the other component, the acetabular cup. Hybrid arthroplasties are becoming increasingly popular. Excellent short-term results have been achieved with cemented total hip replacement; however, long-term studies have reported loosening or migration in 20% to 50% of femoral and acetabular components, 10 to 15 years after surgery. The concern of component loosening has led to the development of porous ingrowth and anatomic press-fit designs. Porous-coated components contain surface pores that allow bone ingrowth that results in attachment of the component to the bone. Press-fit femoral components involve using a larger stem than the reamed canal, providing a firm fit. Press-fit femoral components that are partially porous with the remainder of the stem designed for press-fit are also available. This design depends on bone ingrowth as well as on press-fit for prosthesis maintenance. Although porous-coated devices are not yet officially approved by the FDA for cementless application, many orthopedic surgeons elect to insert these components without methyl methacrylate. When porous-coated and press-fit prostheses are cemented, the rough surfaces help to enhance cement fixation.

Noncemented acetabular cups have threaded outer surfaces for immediate press-fit. Other designs require fixation to the acetabulum with bone screws. Porous-coated acetabular cups are available for cemented or noncemented application. Cups with irregular outer surfaces are usually designed for cement fixation.

No one prosthesis is suitable for every patient's needs. For this reason modular hip systems (Fig. 22-84) that allow the orthopedic surgeon to choose from an array of interchangeable components have been developed. Various femoral head sizes (22 mm, 26 mm, 28 mm, 32 mm, 38 mm) are available with standard, plus 5 mm, and plus 10 mm femoral neck lengths. Femoral stems may be collared or without collars and with distal stem diameters ranging

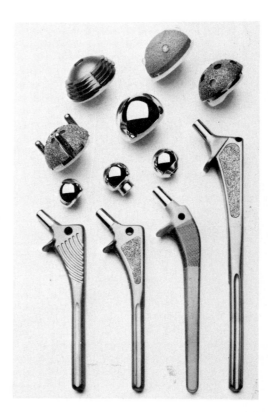

Fig. 22-84. Modular hip system prostheses. (Courtesy Zimmer, Inc., Warsaw, Ind.)

from 10 to 18 mm; primary, intermediate, and long stems range from 115 to 300 mm in length. Acetabular components are metal backed and range from size 40 to 73 mm. Cups contain polyethylene liners that may be snap-fit, low profile, or deep profile, which adds additional thickness to the medial wall.

In revision cases, if a new neck length is required for

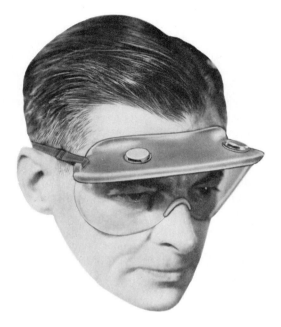

Fig. 22-85. Visorgogs, designed to protect eyes from flying particles or liquids, as well as from glaring overhead ultraviolet lights. (Courtesy Johns & Co., East Providence, R.I.)

leg length considerations, the modular system allows the surgeon to change the head and/or replace the acetabular component without disturbing the femoral stem.

With modular systems, unipolar or bipolar cups are also an option when the acetabulum is relatively normal. The unipolar and bipolar cups with appropriate head sizes are designed to fit on various modular system stems.

The newest development in hip designs is a custom-fit femoral stem. Custom prostheses are not new; traditional customized hip prostheses take up to 6 to 8 weeks for delivery. The newest custom hip is designed to fit the patient's measurements exactly and be available for implant in 45 minutes. A laser-driven computer located within the hospital mills the prosthesis from a mold taken while the patient is in the operating room.

Young, active individuals with strong healthy bones are ideal candidates for noncemented total hip replacement arthroplasties. Elderly patients with osteoporosis and poor-quality bone are usually candidates for cemented components because their bones may lack the compressive strength to support weight-bearing forces. The thin cortices may also lack the strength to resist the impaction forces of initial implant insertion.

Because of the possible disastrous effects of wound infection, special precautions are usually observed during total joint replacement and may include the following:

1. Laminar airflow rooms
2. Ultraviolet lights, eye protectors (Fig. 22-85)
3. Exhaust system (space suits) (Fig. 22-86)
4. Antibiotic irrigation solution administered by hand or by mechanical means

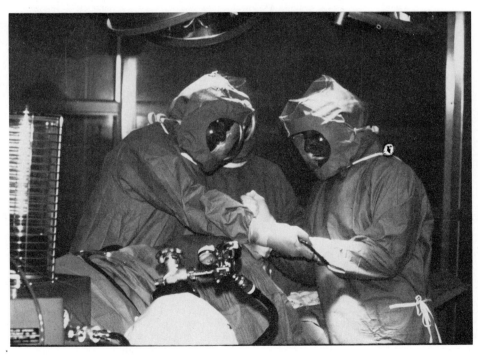

Fig. 22-86. Exhaust system. (Courtesy Stackhouse Associates, Manhattan Beach, Calif.)

5. Limited movement of personnel in and out of the operating room

6. Impervious nonwoven gowns and drapes

The patient is usually placed in the lateral decubitus position with the dependent leg flexed at the hip and the knee. All bony prominences are padded.

Hip reconstruction (cemented)

In cemented total hip arthroplasty an acetabular cup and femoral component are held in place with methyl methacrylate. The numerous total hip implants include Charnley, Aufranc-Turner, Harris, PCA, Precision, Omnifit, and Harris/Galante.

Methyl methacrylate (sometimes labeled by the misnomer "cement") adheres to the polyethylene and metal but not to the bone. It fills the cavity and interstices of the bone and forms a mechanical bond. Methyl methacrylate usually takes 10 to 12 minutes to harden. Methyl methacrylate is manufactured as liquid monomer and a powder and is mixed under sterile conditions by the scrub nurse in the operating room at the time of implantation. Because of the potential harmful effects of methyl methacrylate fumes to the nasal epithelium, some type of exhaust system should be used during the mixing process.

In total hip arthroplasty, cement integrity is essential to implant durability. The main problem with total hip replacement is femoral and acetabular loosening. Methods have been employed to increase the density of polymethyl methacrylate (PMMA) by the use of cement guns, ace-tabular and femoral compactors, and the introduction of bone and cement plugs distal to the femoral prosthesis. These methods have improved the cementing technique but have not greatly reduced the high degree of cement porosity generated during mixing. Trapped air pockets significantly weaken the density of acrylic bone cement, thereby threatening the longevity of the implant. The centrifugation process reduces the size of the air pockets in the cement, which results in a denser bone cement with improved strength and strain, increased fatigue life, and overall improved implant longevity.

When methyl methacrylate is being used, the patient may experience adverse reactions. Studies have reported that cardiovascular and pulmonary changes occur, especially after the impaction of bone cement down the femoral canal (Orsini and others, 1987). The rise in intramedullary canal pressure, not the nature of the inserted substances, causes these effects. Various reactions including bradycardia, hypotension, hypoxemia, microembolisms, and even cardiac arrest and death have been reported. Venting the cement in the femoral canal, using canal cement plugs, and lavaging of the intramedullary canal before insertion of cement seem to prevent severe cardiopulmonary changes. Because of the potential adverse reactions to methyl methacrylate, extremely careful monitoring of the patient's blood pressure and pulse is essential while cement is being forced into the canal.

Procedural considerations. In addition to total hip no. 1 and no. 2 instrument sets, the following instrumentation

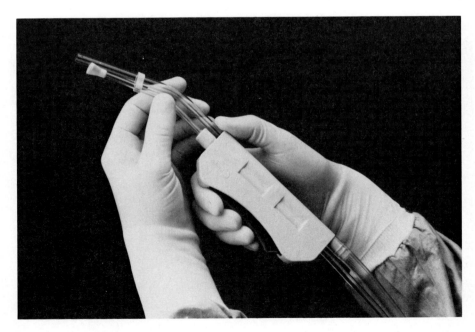

Fig. 22-87. Simpulse suction irrigator. Applications in orthopedics include debridement of bone in joint replacement and revision procedures, debridement of open fractures, cleansing, irrigation, and debridement of traumatic wounds, irrigation of soft tissue injuries, irrigation of contaminated wounds, and irrigation and debridement of surgical wounds. (Courtesy Davol, Inc., Cranston, R.I.)

is required for cemented total hip replacement arthroplasties:

Power drill/reamer

Power saw with blades

Methyl methacrylate insertion and mixing devices

Simpulse or Pulse Lavage and 3000-ml bag of normal saline solution (Figs. 22-87 and 22-88)

Hip system instrumentation with trials and implants of choice (Fig. 22-89)

Intramedullary reamers with guide rods (Fig. 22-90)

Acetabular reamers (Fig. 22-91)

Femoral canal suction tampons

Buck cement plugs and inserter (Fig. 22-92)

Femoral canal and acetabular brush

Cement compression instruments with disposable attachments

Osteotomes, extra (have available)

Revision of total hip arthroplasties requires the same instrumentation as cemented total hip, plus the following:

Midas Rex instrumentation (Figs. 22-93 and 22-94)

Cement removal instruments

Image intensifier (have available)

Long (sigmoidoscopy) suction tube

Headlight

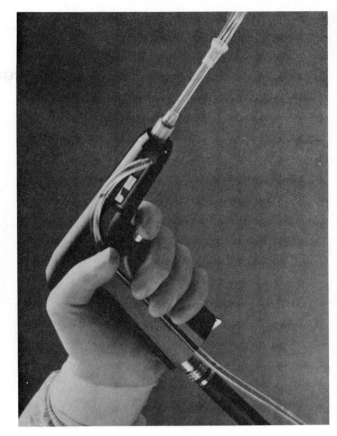

Fig. 22-88. Pulse Lavage. (Courtesy Micro-Aire Surgical Instruments, Inc., San Fernando, Calif.)

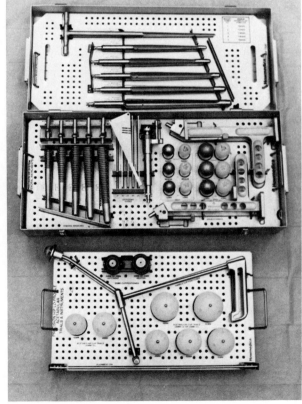

A

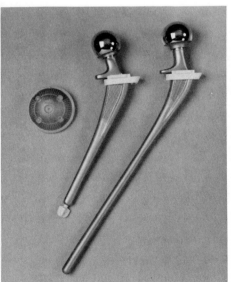

B

Fig. 22-89. Precision Total Hip System. **A,** Instrumentation; **B,** implants. (Courtesy Howmedica, Inc., Rutherford, N.J.)

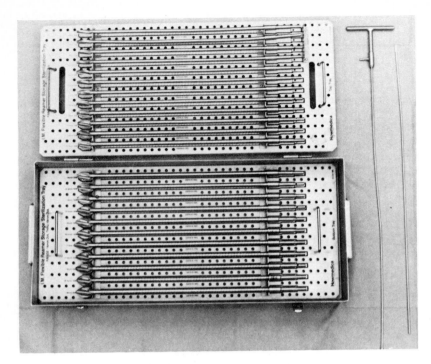

Fig. 22-90. Intramedullary reamers with guide rods. (Courtesy Howmedica, Inc., Rutherford, N.J.)

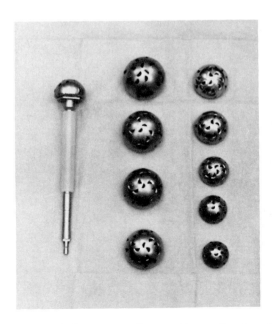

Fig. 22-91. Acetabular reamers. (Courtesy Howmedica, Inc., Rutherford, N.J.)

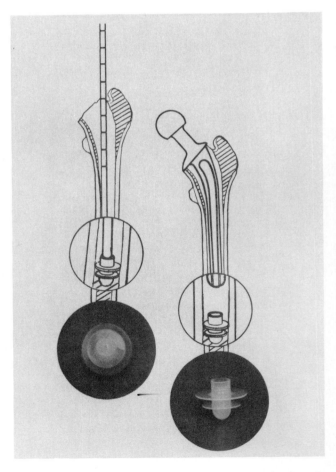

Fig. 22-92. Buck femoral plug and insertor. (Courtesy Richards Medical Co., Memphis, Tenn.)

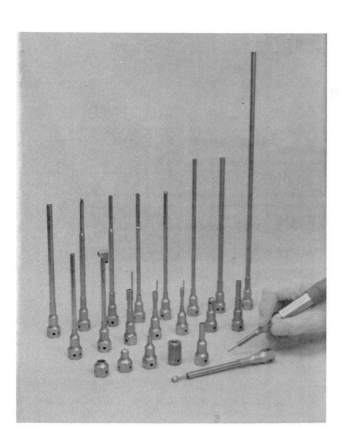

Fig. 22-93. Midas Rex bone scalpel instrumentation with a variety of attachments for many bone-working applications in hip revision procedures. (Courtesy Midas Rex Psychomotor Institute, Fort Worth, Tex.)

Operative procedure—cemented total hip replacement arthroplasty using the Precision Total Hip System

1. A lateral skin incision is made in the axis of the femoral shaft, extending down 3 to 4 inches from the tip of the trochanter and curving posteriorly proximal to the greater trochanter (Fig. 22-95, *A*).
2. Femoral neck exposure is accomplished by identifying and releasing the external rotators (Fig. 22-95, *B*).
3. Once a capsulotomy is performed (Fig. 22-95, *C*), the hip can be dislocated (Fig. 22-95, *D*).
4. The femoral osteotomy guide is used for transection of the femoral head and neck (Fig. 22-95, *E* and *F*).
5. The acetabulum is then exposed and reamed (Fig. 22-95, *G*). The retained acetabular bone in the reamers may be set aside for bone grafting if needed.
6. After reaming, acetabular trials are placed in the acetabulum to test for proper fit (Fig. 22-95, *H*).
7. At least three holes are drilled in the ilium, ischium, and pubis for anchoring the implant (Fig. 22-95, *I*).
8. The acetabulum is then lavaged, dried, and prepared with bone cement before the acetabular cup is implanted (Fig. 22-95, *J*).
9. A tapered awl is placed into the posterolateral region of the femoral neck to open the proximal canal (Fig. 22-95, *K*).
10. Flexible reamers are passed over a guide wire into the canal in progressive sizes until resistance to distal passage is felt (Fig. 22-95, *L*).
11. Midshaft area preparation is carried out with a conical

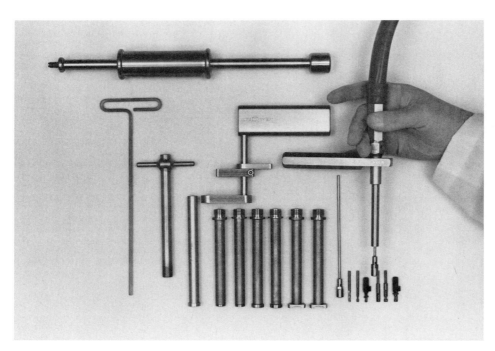

Fig. 22-94. Midas Rex stem extraction equipment that enables surgeon to preserve cortex without fenestration. (Courtesy Midas Rex Psychomotor Institute, Fort Worth, Tex.)

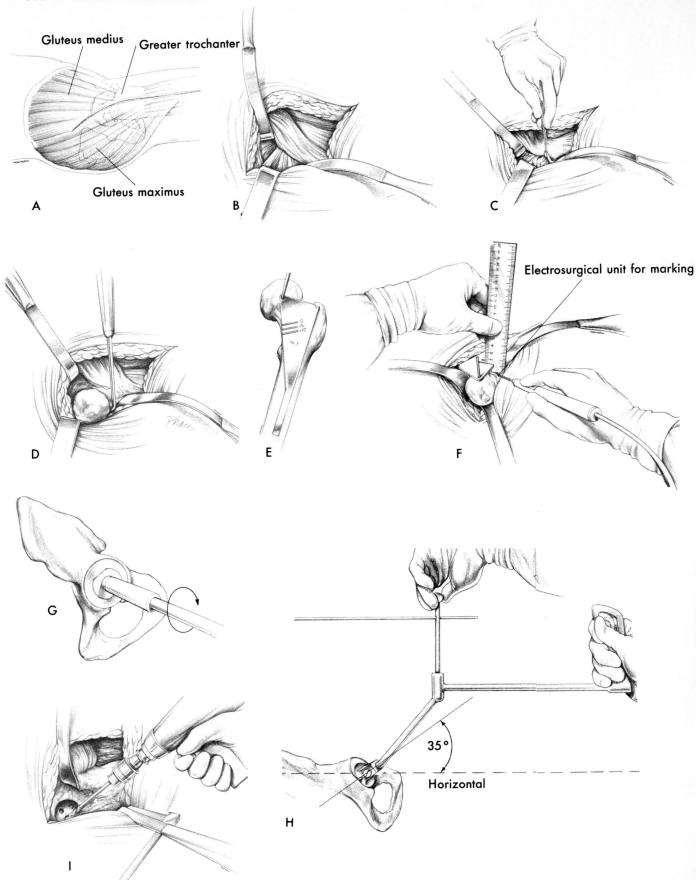

Fig. 22-95. Surgical techniques for cemented total hip arthroplasty using Precision Total Hip System. (Courtesy Howmedica, Inc., Rutherford, N.J.)

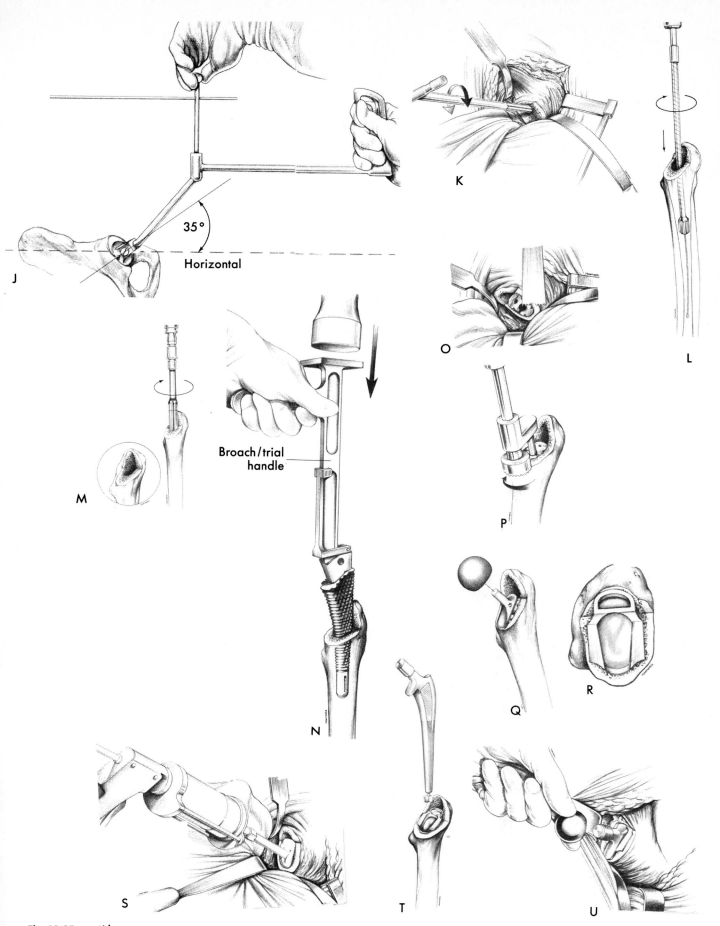

Fig. 22-95, cont'd.

reamer one size smaller than the preoperative femoral template size (Fig. 22-95, *M*).

12. Femoral broaches are then inserted into the femoral canal to prepare the proximal metaphyseal (Fig. 22-95, *N*).

13. Final preparation is accomplished by cutting off excess bone above the level of the broach and using a calcar planing device for collar-calcar contact (Fig. 22-95, *O* and *P*).

14. A collar neck trial and head trial are positioned (Fig. 22-95, *Q*), and a trial reduction is carried out. The appropriate size of trial proximal spacer is also fitted if desired (Fig. 22-95, *R*).

15. The trial is removed, and the canal is lavaged and brushed to accommodate the methyl methacrylate.

16. A bone plug is inserted, followed by cementing of the canal (Fig. 22-95, *S*).

17. Insertion of the proximal spacer, if used, and femoral component with preselected PMMA distal centralizer is performed under manual pressure (Fig. 22-95, *T*).

18. The appropriate size of femoral head is positioned onto the stem, and reduction is carried out (Fig. 22-95, *U*).

19. Depending on the surgeon and the surgical approach, the greater trochanter may or may not have been removed for better exposure of the hip joint. If removed, it is reattached with 18-gauge wire or a trochanteric fixation device.

20. The wound is closed in layers over suction drains.

The skin is closed with staples, and a sterile dressing is applied to provide compression to the wound.

21. An abduction pillow is placed between the patient's legs postoperatively (Fig. 22-96).

Hip reconstruction (noncemented)

Fixation with a noncemeted prosthesis is initially accomplished by a tight fit of the implants within bone of substantial strength. As with all prosthetic designs, it is essential to fill the medullary canal and wedge the prosthesis in as tightly as possible to provide temporary press-fit fixation. Sufficient time is then allowed for the fractured cancellous bone of the marrow to heal by growing into the porous portions of the prosthesis.

The healing process is identical to and requires the same amount of time as a long bone cortical fracture (approximately 3 months). Extreme caution is taken postoperatively to protect the operative hip from excessive compression, rotation, and shear stresses.

There are numerous noncemented implants, such as the Anatomical Medullary Locking (AML) (Fig. 22-97), Harris/Galante, Osteolock, Omnifit, and bias long revision stems.

Procedural considerations. The position and incision are the same as for the total hip replacement (cemented).

Operative procedure—noncemented total hip replacement arthroplasty using the AML hip system

1. After the incision is made and the capsule is entered, the femoral head is dislocated.

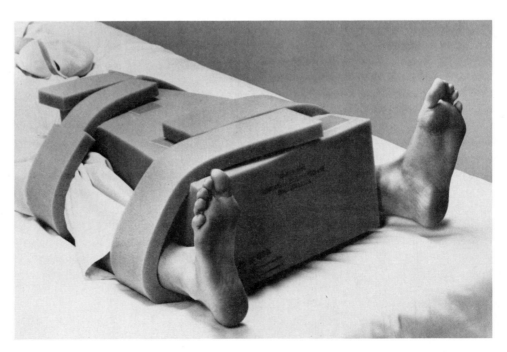

Fig. 22-96. Abduction pillow aids in immobilizing hip joints after surgery. (Courtesy Span & Aids, McGaw Park, Ill.)

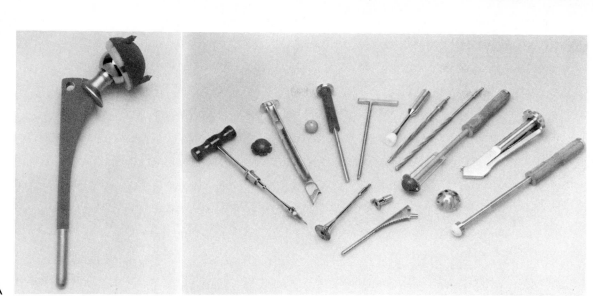

Fig. 22-97. Anatomical Medullary Locking (AML) Total Hip System. **A,** Implant; **B,** instrumentation. (Courtesy DePuy, Warsaw, Ind.)

2. A pilot hole is established in the trochanteric fossa as an intramedullary reference point (Fig. 22-98, A).

3. Reaming of the intramedullary canal is then performed in a progressive manner with fully fluted rigid reamers (Fig. 22-98, B).

4. A femoral neck osteotomy is achieved by positioning an osteotomy template along the axis of the femur and cutting at the level of the collar (Fig. 22-98, C).

5. Attention is directed to the acetabulum, which is cleared of all soft tissue and reamed with hemispherical reamers (Fig. 22-98, D).

6. Trial acetabular sizers are positioned in the acetabulum to determine correct position and size of the prosthetic component.

7. Returning to the femoral canal, a hollow osteotome is used to connect the pilot hole to the osteotomy site (Fig. 22-98, E).

8. Femoral broaches are then inserted to enlarge the intramedullary space for trial insertion (Fig. 22-98, F).

9. A power calcar planer may be placed over the trunion of the broach and used to contour the femoral neck (Fig. 22-98, G).

10. A trial head neck component is positioned onto the fitted broach, and a trial reduction is carried out (Fig. 22-98, H).

11. If trial reduction is satisfactory, all trial components are removed.

12. The appropriate-sized AML acetabular component is inserted into the acetabulum, and a polyethylene insert is locked into place (Fig. 22-98, I).

13. The femoral component is placed into the canal, and the modular head is seated on the trunion (Fig. 22-98, J and K).

14. Reduction of the hip is followed by standard closure with drains.

15. Abduction of the hip is maintained postoperatively with a foam abduction pillow.

Correction of congenital dislocation of the hip

A congenital dislocation of the hip is an abnormal development of the hip present at birth. It is considered a lateral or upward dislocation of the femoral head from the acetabulum. When alignment is disrupted, soft tissue and bony changes result in contractures of the hip muscles, a shallow acetabulum, and possibly a deformed femoral head. Treatment of congenital dislocation of the hip varies depending on the age of the patient and the stability of the hip. Treatment modalities include application of a Pavlik harness, closed reduction, and spica cast application; or surgical correction. Surgery involves soft tissue release and/or acetabular and femoral procedures.

Procedural considerations. The patient is usually in the lateral position for these procedures. An anterior incision is usually made for open reduction, whereas a lateral incision is made for the subtrochanteric osteotomy. The surgeon's preference dictates the incision for an innominate osteotomy.

Soft tissue and major bone sets are required, plus the following:

Steinman pins
Angled blade plate, screws, and instrumentation (Fig. 22-99)
Power drill
Power saw with assorted blade sizes

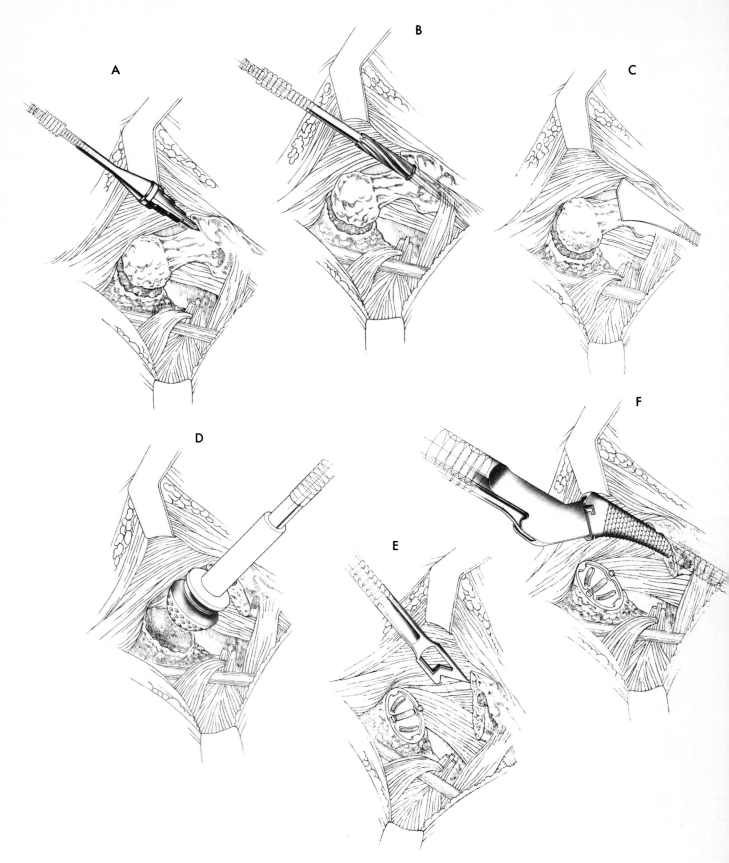

Fig. 22-98. Surgical technique for noncemented total hip arthroplasty using Anatomical Medullary Locking (AML) Total Hip System. (Courtesy DePuy, Warsaw, Ind.)

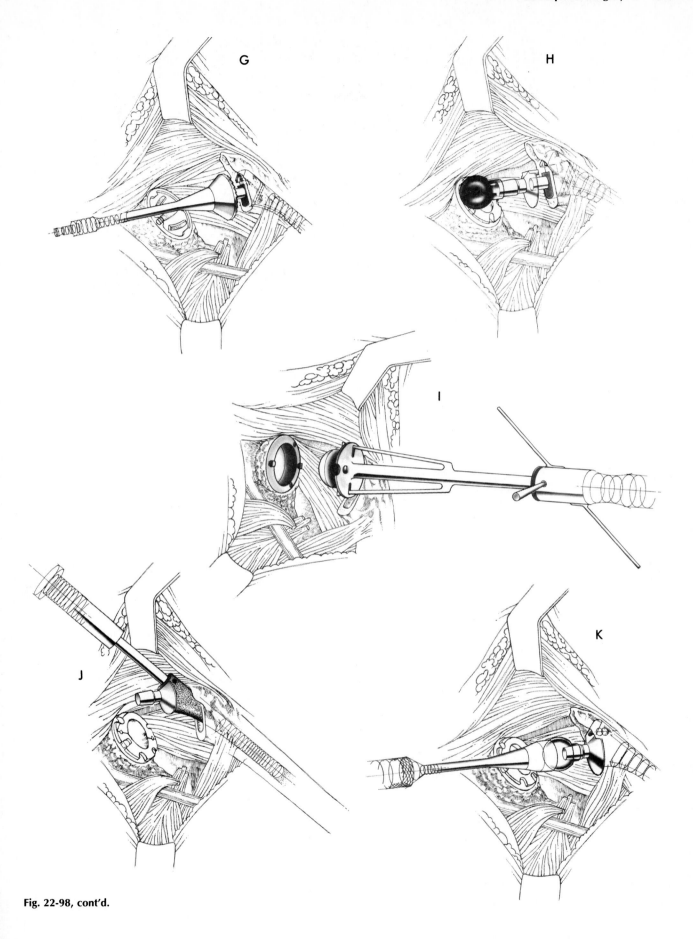

Fig. 22-98, cont'd.

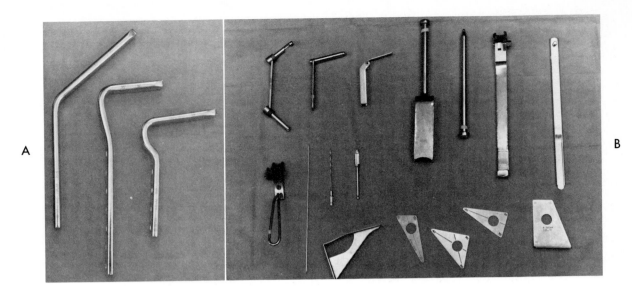

Fig. 22-99. A, Angled blade plates and **B,** instrumentation.

Operative procedures. Following are standard operative procedures.

Open reduction

1. The hip joint is opened, and the soft tissue in the acetabulum is excised.
2. The femoral head can then be reduced into the acetabulum and held by suturing the capsule.

Derotational osteotomy.
A derotational osteotomy is performed when the head is improperly seated in the acetabulum.

1. The femur is placed in internal rotation and divided.
2. The distal fragment is rotated externally to place the knee and foot straight ahead.
3. If the patient is a young child, the osteotomy is frequently performed in the supracondylar region, and the patient is immobilized in a plaster spica cast.
4. For an older child, the osteotomy is frequently done in the subtrochanteric region, and the osteotomized fragments are held with an osteotomy blade plate or an intermediate compression screw. Immobilization may not be necessary.

Innominate osteotomy

1. A complete division of the wing of the ilium is made by an osteotomy from the sciatic notch to the anterior margin of the ilium, superior to the acetabulum.
2. The ilium is then wedged down to increase the depth of the acetabulum by opening the osteotomy site and inserting a bone graft.
3. The bone graft is held in place with two heavy wires.
4. Heavy suture is used to close the capsule, and a spica cast is applied for postoperative immobilization.

Correction of femoral shaft fracture

Fractures of the femoral shaft occur at any age, usually due to high-impact injuries. The femoral shaft is also a common site for pathologic fractures due to carcinoma. Conservative treatment involves skeletal traction until sufficient callus formation is present at 4 to 6 weeks. At this time the extremity is immobilized in a spica cast or femoral cast brace. When surgical treament is indicated, the femoral fracture is fixed with an intramedullary nail, seldom with compression plates. Intramedullary nailing is the most rigid form of fixation.

There are two methods of nail insertion: open and closed. If the fracture can be reduced by manipulation with or without the use of traction, nailing should be performed without exposing the fracture site. This closed method involves driving a nail over a guide wire inserted into the canal from the proximal end of the bone. If the fracture cannot be reduced by the closed method, the fracture must be exposed through an incision. Reduction is accomplished under direct visualization.

Closed intramedullary nailing of the femur is preferred when possible because (1) it prevents disruption of periosteal blood supply, (2) less soft tissue trauma occurs, (3) healing is accelerated, (4) infection and nonunion are less likely, (5) early knee motion and quadricep function is possible, and (6) no scars are left over the femoral shaft.

The latest development in intramedullary nailing of shaft fractures is the locking nail. Locking nails have greatly expanded the indications for intramedullary nailing because of their ability to prevent rotation and control shortening. Locking nails can be either static or dynamic. Static locking is achieved by inserting screws proximally and distally through the nail and bone. Static locking neutralizes rotational stresses and prevents telescoping from the fracture site. Screws farthest from the fracture site are removed to convert a static nail to a dynamic nail. Dynamic locking nails neutralize rotation but allow compression at the fracture site. Dynamic locking is achieved by inserting

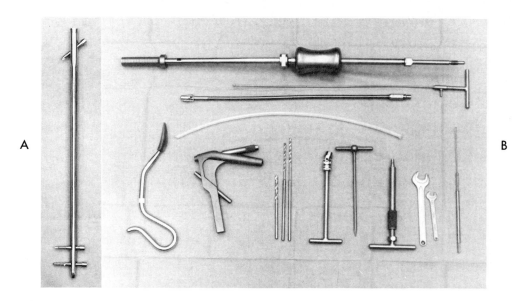

Fig. 22-100. Grosse-Kempf femoral intramedullary nailing system. **A,** Femoral interlocking nail; **B,** instrumentation. (Courtesy Howmedica, Inc., Rutherford, N.J.)

screws closest to the fracture site, either proximally or distally.

Procedural considerations. The patient is positioned in the lateral or supine position on the fracture table with traction applied to the affected leg by a traction pin or fracture table boot. If a traction pin is desired and not already in place, it is inserted through the proximal tibia before transferring the patient to the fracture table. The extremity is prepped and draped from above the iliac crest to mid-calf. Fluoroscopy is used intermittently throughout the nailing procedure to check progress.

Soft tissue and major bone sets are used, plus the following:

Large bone-holding clamps (open method)
Power intramedullary reamer driver
Power drill
Nail of choice with instrumentation

For insertion or removal of traction pin:

Hand drill
Kirschner wire
Bolt cutter
Traction pin

Numerous intramedullary nails are available for femoral shaft fixation. Noninterlocking nails include Kuntschner, AO, and Ender; interlocking nails include Precise, AO, Grosse-Kempf (Fig. 22-100), and Russell-Taylor.

Operative procedures
Closed nailing method

1. Reduction is accomplished by manipulation and mechanical traction under image intensification.
2. A small incision is then made over the top of the greater trochanter and carried down to expose the proximal femur (Fig. 22-101, *A*).
3. Once an awl has been used to enter the intramedullary canal (Fig. l22-101, *B*), an olive-tipped guide wire is passed down the shaft, across the fracture site, and into the distal femur (Fig. 22-101, *C*).
4. The guide wire is overreamed with flexible reamers to the desired size. Fluoroscopy is used.
5. The size of the nail is determined by the last size reamer used and the length of the guide wire within the bone.
6. The olive-tipped guide wire is replaced with a plain-tipped guide wire for nail insertion.
7. The nail is attached to the driver or proximal target device and driven over the wire, down the canal, and across the fracture (Fig. 22-101, *D*). Progress is checked with fluoroscopy. To avoid incarceration proximally, the guide wire is removed once the nail has been introduced.
8. If a locking nail has been used and locking is desired, the guide sleeve is positioned in the oblique hole of the proximal target device.
9. The cortices are then drilled after an awl is used to engage the lateral cortex (Fig. 22-101, *E* and *F*).
10. The depth is measured, and the appropriate proximal screw is inserted (Fig. 22-101, *G* and *H*).
11. The distal holes are locked with the same technique, using a targeting jig or freehand. The distal holes are drilled, and then the lateral cortex is redrilled with a larger drill bit to accept the distal screws.

Open nailing method

1. Two incisions are required, one to expose the greater

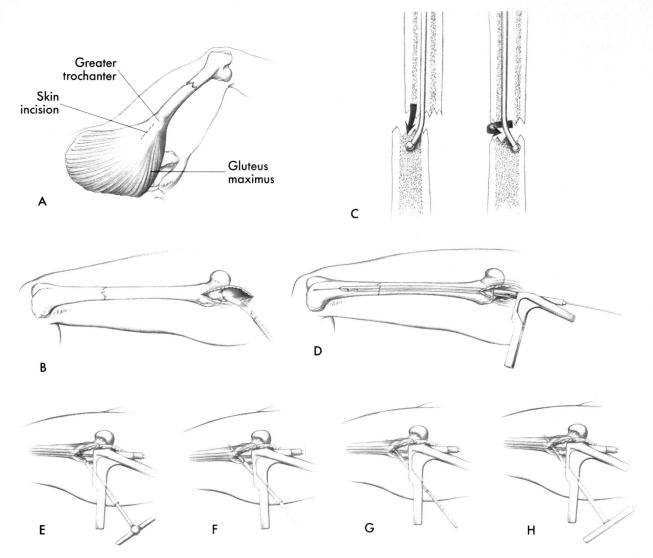

Fig. 22-101. Grosse-Kempf femoral intramedullary nailing technique. (Courtesy Howmedica, Inc., Rutherford, N.J.)

trochanter for nail insertion and another to expose the fracture.

2. The skin and muscle are retracted over the fracture site, and the area is cleared of blood clot and soft tissue.
3. The fracture is reduced with large bone clamps, manipulation, and traction.
4. An olive-tipped guide wire is passed down the femoral canal and across the fracture site.
5. Flexible intramedullary reamers are used to overdrill the guide wire.
6. The olive-tipped guide wire is removed and replaced with a plain-tipped guide wire for nail insertion.
7. Once the nail is inserted, the proximal and/or distal end of the nail is locked by predrilling and inserting the appropriate-length locking screws through the nail and femur.

8. The wounds are closed, and the traction pin is removed. No external support should be necessary.

Arthroscopy

Learning the art of arthroscopy is an enormous task; it requires superb technical skills. With advancements in arthroscopic video cameras and specialized instrumentation, many procedures that previously required an arthrotomy can now be performed through an arthroscope. The advantages of an arthroscopic procedure over an open procedure are (1) lower risk of infection, (2) small incision, (3) no disruption of extensor mechanisms, (4) decreased postoperative pain, (5) decreased hospital stay, and (6) earlier rehabilitation.

Modern arthroscopy equipment includes antifog arthroscopes that provide excellent visualization with clarity and a wide field of vision. New light sources automatically control light levels, depending on the reflectivity of the background. More than adequate light is delivered to the field for direct or television-aided visualization. Small handheld cameras are easier for the surgeon to manipulate and are less likely to compromise the sterility of the field because they are completely soakable. Adequate inflow and outflow and safe pressures in the joint can be regulated with the arthroscopy pump. Acufex, Concept, Dyonics, Storz, 3M, and Wolf are among the companies that manufacture arthroscopic equipment.

Arthroscopic equipment has certain requirements for care and handling. Ethylene oxide sterilization is recommended because steam sterilization is known to cause deterioration of arthroscopes and lens cement. Proper ethylene oxide sterilization usually takes 3 to 7 hours, plus aeration time. Most equipment used with the scopes can be steam sterilized.

Although sterilization is optimum and should be encouraged, liquid disinfection according to the manufacturer's instructions is often performed. "Cold sterilization" (disinfection) with an activated glutaraldehyde solution, followed by thorough rinsing with sterile water, is the standard of practice among some established arthroscopists.

The fiberoptic cords used in the surgery should never be kinked or twisted. When they are mishandled, gradual deterioration occurs in the cables, fibers in the cable break, and light cannot be transmitted. When stored, the cords should be loosely coiled or hung.

Two types of arthroscopy may be performed:

1. *Diagnostic arthroscopy* for patients whose diagnosis cannot be determined by history, physical examination, or arthrogram—findings insufficient to warrant surgical exploration
2. *Operative arthroscopy* for patients who show an intraarticular abnormality or ligamentous injury

Diagnostic arthroscopy may be performed before an anticipated arthrotomy. Frequently, surgical treament is modified on the basis of the findings of the arthroscopic examination.

Arthroscopy of the knee

Visualization of the intraarticular structures is facilitated through a small-diameter arthroscope. Arthroscopic surgery of the knee is indicated for diagnostic viewing, synovial biopsies, removal of loose bodies, resection of plicae, shaving of the patella, synovectomy, meniscus repair, and anterior and posterior cruciate ligament repairs.

Procedural considerations. The patient is placed in the supine position on a standard operating room bed. The foot end of the bed may be flexed 90 degrees. A tourniquet is almost always applied but may not be inflated, depending on the amount of bleeding that occurs within the joint. The bed should have the appropriate attachment in place to connect the "surgical assistant" or other leg holders approximately 4 inches above the patella (Figs. 22-102 through 22-104). These devices provide a fixed fulcrum for manipulation of the knee and also reduce the fatigue

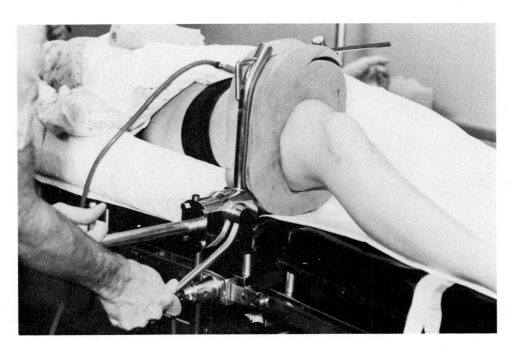

Fig. 22-102. Surgical assistant device is secured to patient manually and with pumping of cam action lever. (From Johnson, L.L.: Diagnostic and surgical arthroscopy: the knee and other joints, ed. 2, St. Louis, 1981, The C.V. Mosby Co.)

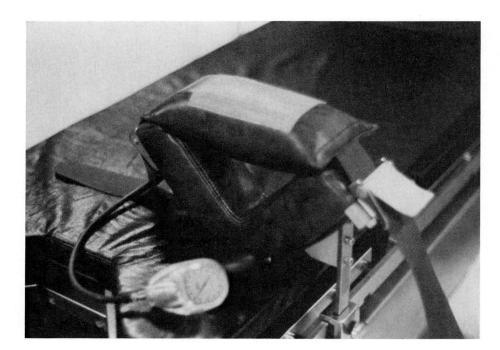

Fig. 22-103. Surg-Assist. (Courtesy Medmetric Corporation, San Diego, Calif.)

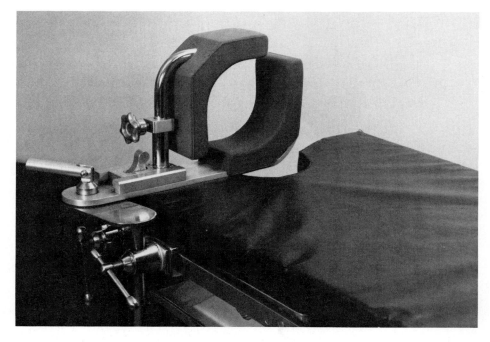

Fig. 22-104. Arthroscopic leg holder. (Courtesy Orthopedic Systems, Inc., Hayward, Calif.)

of the person holding the extremity. General anesthesia is usually preferred, whether the procedure is inpatient or outpatient. Sometimes a local block is chosen, and in these cases the surgeon will inject the local anesthetic. The leg is prepped (foot-holding devices [Fig. 22-105] may be used) and draped in the routine manner.

With the completely soakable miniature arthroscopy cameras, reprepping and redraping are no longer required if subsequent arthrotomy is to be performed after initial arthroscopy.

Instruments and equipment needed for an arthroscopy include the following:

Diagnostic arthroscopy

Arthroscopy instruments (Fig. 22-106)
Arthroscopes (surgeon's preference), usually 4 mm, 30 and 70 degrees (Fig. 22-107)
2 Plastic 60-cc Toomey syringes
1 Plastic 10-cc control syringe
1 Needle for injection of Marcaine, 21 gauge, 1½ inches
2 to 6 3-liter bags of lactated Ringer's or normal saline solution
T irrigation tubing or arthroscopy pump tubing
Light cord
Cannulae for scope, irrigation, and suction (Fig. 22-107)
Camera (Fig. 22-108)
Video (television) equipment (Fig. 22-109)
Light source
Arthroscopy pump, surgeon's preference (Fig. 22-110)

Operative arthroscopy

All instruments and supplies for a diagnostic arthroscopy, plus any of the following:

Suction container with trap to catch specimen
Operative arthroscopy instruments (Fig. 22-111)

Manipulation instruments (Fig. 22-112)
Acufex arthroplasty instruments (Fig. 22-113)
Fat pad retractor (Fig. 22-114)
Oretorp meniscus instruments (Fig. 22-115)
Meniscus stitching needles (Fig. 22-116)
Arthroscopic anterior cruciate ligament (ACL) reconstruction instrumentation (Fig. 22-117)
Arthroscopic power system, power unit, and foot pedal (Fig. 22-118)

Diagnostic arthroscopy

Operative procedure

1. The anteromedial and anterolateral joint lines are marked with a skin marker.
2. A Verres or other irrigation cannula and trocar are inserted into the lateral suprapatellar pouch near the superior pole of the patella.
3. Lactated Ringer's or normal saline solution is connected to the cannula, and the joint is distended. An arthroscopy pump with pressure-sensitive tubing may be used instead.
4. A stab incision is then made anterolaterally or anteromedially 2 to 3 mm above the tibial plateau or patellar tendon at the joint line. Diluted epinephrine solution may be injected in the skin at the site of the scope insertion.
5. A sharp trocar and sheath are inserted through the stab wound and just through the capsule.
6. A blunt trocar is then used to pass the sheath into the knee joint.
7. The trocar is removed and a 4-mm, 30-degree scope is inserted into the sheath. The light source and video camera are connected to the scope.

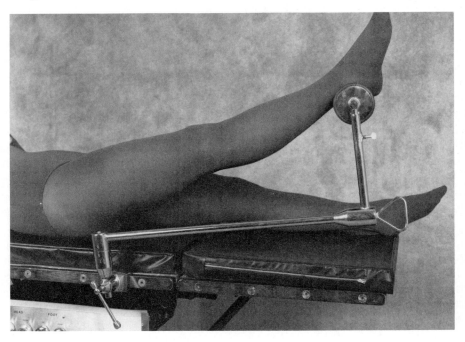

Fig. 22-105. Prep-Assist. (Courtesy Orthopedic Systems, Inc., Hayward, Calif.).

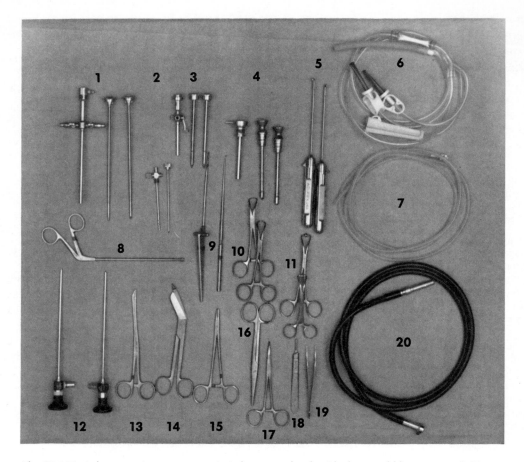

Fig. 22-106. Arthroscopy instrument set. *1,* Arthroscope sheath with sharp and blunt trocars; *2,* Verres needle cannula with trocar; *3,* and *4,* cannulae with their sharp and blunt trocars; *5,* rotary basket punch and scissors; *6,* TURP inflow tubing; *7,* outflow tubing; *8,* cup forceps; *9,* probes; *10,* perforating towel clamps; *11,* nonperforating towel clamps; *12,* arthroscopes, 30 degrees and 70 degrees; *13,* meniscus clamp; *14,* bandage scissors; *15,* needle holder; *16,* suture scissors; *17,* hemostat; *18,* no. 3 knife handle; *19,* Adson tissue forceps; *20,* light source cable.

8. The inflow may remain in the suprapatellar area and the drain-off tubing connected to the arthroscope, or the position may be reversed.

9. Another stab wound incision is made to establish the opposite portal, and by inserting a probe the cruciate ligaments and meniscus can be examined.

10. Moving the scope to the opposite portal and changing the position of the knee allow a complete examination to be performed.

11. The joint is always thoroughly irrigated at the end of the procedure until it is clear of blood and any particles.

12. The portals are closed with nylon or undyed Vicryl suture and ½-inch Steri-Strips.

13. Bupivacaine 0.25% (Marcaine), 30 ml, with epinephrine 1:200,000 may be injected intraarticularly to minimize bleeding and postoperative pain.

14. Gauze dressing, Webril, and 4-inch and 6-inch Ace bandages are applied.

15. Procedures may be recorded on videocassette tapes for instruction and research.

Operative arthroscopy

Arthroscopic meniscus repair. Menisci are important structures in the knee joint that distribute load across the knee joint and provide capsular stability. A tear in the meniscus is the most common knee injury requiring arthroscopic surgery (Fig. 22-119). Although both menisci can sustain tears, the medial meniscus is injured much more frequently than the lateral.

Treatment of meniscus tears is aimed at preserving the structures. Some minor tears heal with cast immobilization, but some persist and cause symptoms. In these more severe cases, surgical intervention is necessary. Arthroscopic meniscal repair is widely accepted as the standard of care. Arthroscopy provides much greater exposure than an arthrotomy and enables the surgeon to approach the meniscus from the inner margin where most tears begin.

Text continued on p. 656.

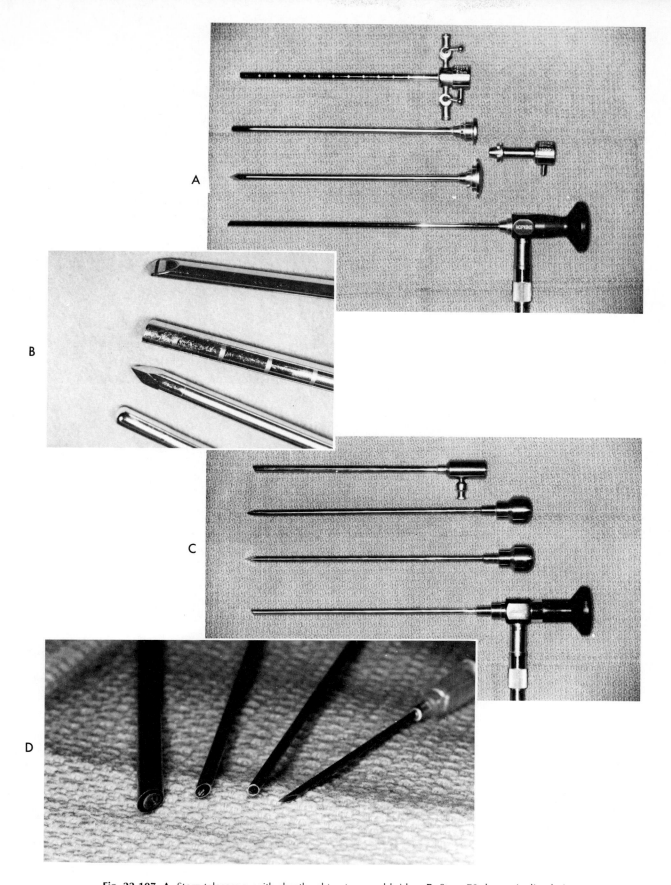

Fig. 22-107. A, Storz telescope, with sheath, obturators, and bridge. **B,** Storz 70-degree inclined view rod-lens telescope, with cannula and sharp and blunt obturators. This telescope is used in viewing posterior compartment. **C,** Dyonics rod-lens system, with insertion instrumentation. **D,** *Left to right,* 4-mm-diameter Dyonics rod-lens endoscope; 2.2-mm Needlescope seen in end view; 1.7-mm Needlescope; 18-gauge needle, shown for relative size comparison.

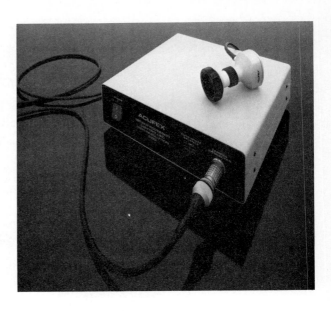

Fig. 22-108. Arthroscopy camera. (Courtesy Acufex Microsurgical, Inc., Norwood, Mass.)

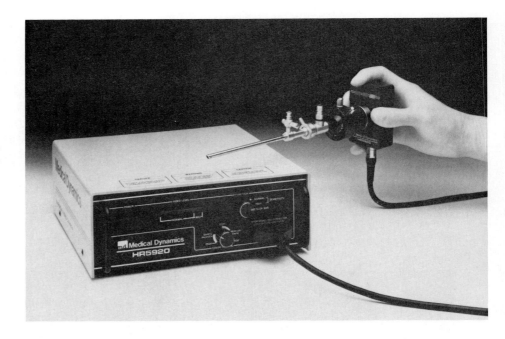

Fig. 22-109. High-resolution, solid-state, surgical video camera. (Courtesy Medical Dynamics, Inc., Englewood, Colo.)

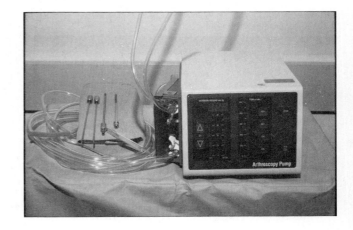

Fig. 22-110. Arthroscopy pump with cannulae and tubing. (Reprinted with permission from AORN Journal, vol. 48, p. 1091, December 1988, copyright AORN Inc., 10170 East Mississippi Avenue, Denver, Colo. 80231).

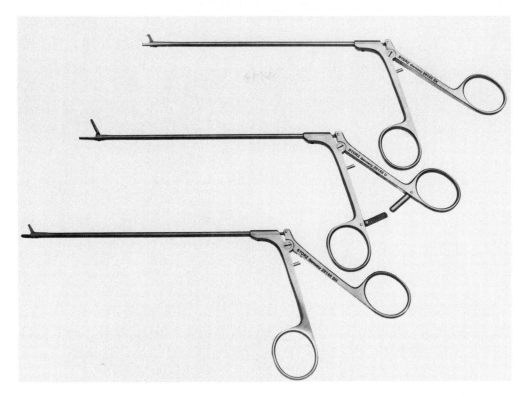

Fig. 22-111. Operative arthroscopy instruments can be introduced through accessory trocar and cannula or stab incision. These have 3.5-mm diameters and lengths of 13 cm. *From top,* hook scissors, alligator grasping forceps with ratchet handle, and cutting forceps. (Courtesy Karl Storz Endoscopy—America, Inc.)

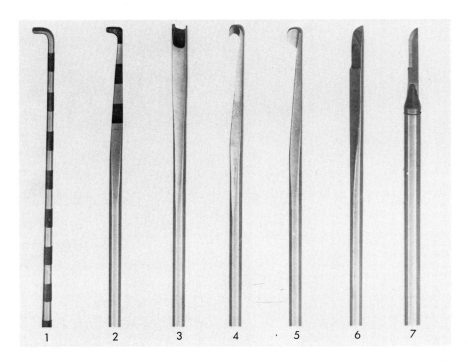

Fig. 22-112. Manipulation instruments to be introduced through second trocar and cannula or through skin incision. These have diameters of 3.5 mm and are available in 13-cm lengths. *1,* Hook and retractor; *2,* graduated right-angle hook; *3,* Smillie-type knife; *4,* hook knife; *5,* retrograde knife; *6* and *7,* pointed knives. (Courtesy Karl Storz Endoscopy—America, Inc.)

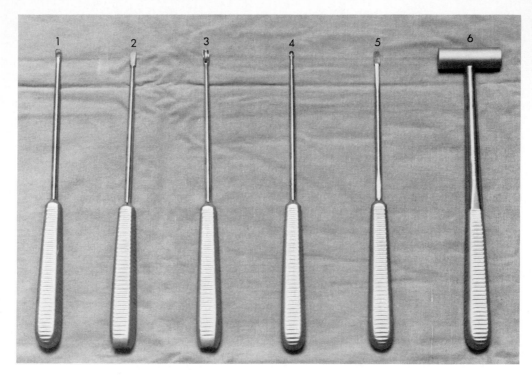

Fig. 22-113. Acufex arthroplasty instruments. *1,* Open 4-mm curette; *2,* straight osteotome; *3,* curved gouge; *4,* 3-mm closed curette; *5,* convex rasp; *6,* mallet.

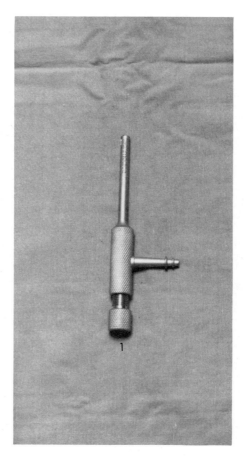

Fig. 22-114. Fat pad retractor.

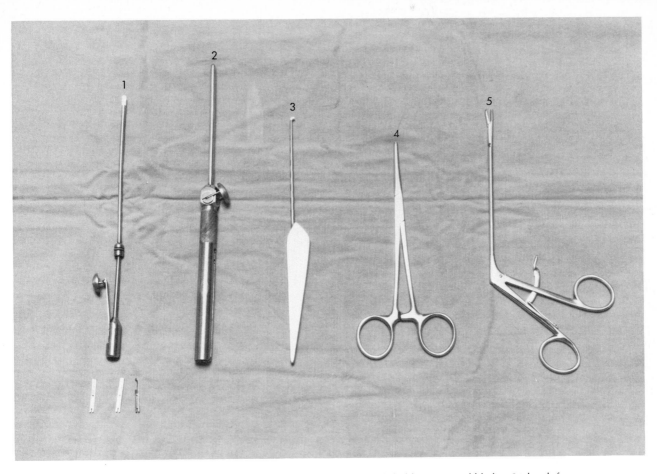

Fig. 22-115. Oretorp arthroscopic meniscus instruments. *1,* Knife holder insert and blades; *2,* sheath for knife holder; *3,* Stille probe; *4,* 6-inch fine tip Kocher forceps; *5,* tissue grasper. (Courtesy Depuy Co., Warsaw, Ind.)

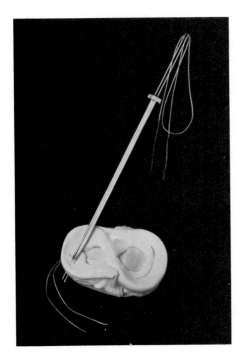

Fig. 22-116. Meniscus stitching needles. (Courtesy Acufex Micro-surgical Inc., Norwood, Mass.)

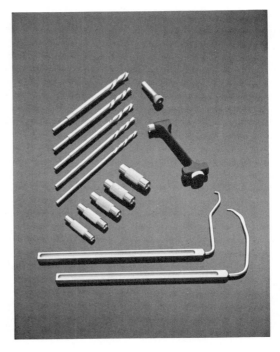

Fig. 22-117. Arthroscopic ACL reconstruction instrumentation. (Courtesy Acufex Microsurgical Inc., Norwood, Mass.)

A

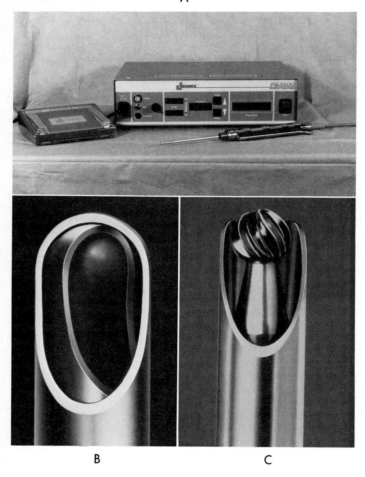

B   C

Fig. 22-118. A, Arthroscopic power system, power unit, and foot pedal; **B,** and **C,** disposable blades for power system. (Courtesy Dyonics, Inc., Andover, Mass.)

There are two methods of arthroscopic treatment of meniscus tears. The first method involves resection of the meniscus. Complete meniscectomy can lead to severe degenerative changes; therefore, a partial meniscectomy is preferred. The second method of treatment is suture repair of the torn meniscus. Suture repair is most suitable for meniscal tears occurring in the vascular peripheral portion of the meniscus in a stable knee without degenerative changes.

Operative procedure

1. The anteromedial and anterolateral portal sites are marked with a surgical skin marker.
2. A Verres needle or other irrigation cannula and trocar are inserted into the suprapatellar pouch.
3. The joint is distended with lactated Ringer's or normal saline solution.
4. Once the joint has been distended, a stab wound incision is made at the anterolateral portal site.
5. A sharp trocar with scope sheath is used to penetrate the capsule, and then a blunt trocar is used to enter the joint.
6. The arthroscope is inserted through the sheath and attached to the drain-off tubing, light source cord, and video camera. The inflow remains at the suprapatellar site or may be switched with the outflow.
7. Another stab wound incision is made over the anteromedial portal site, where instruments are usually directly inserted.
8. Basket forceps and a knife or a power meniscus cutter are placed into the anteromedial portal and used to resect part of the medial meniscus.
9. When the medial meniscus is to be sutured, a cannula is placed next to the inner edge of the tear. Two long meniscus stitching needles with absorbable Vicryl or PDS suture are inserted into the cannula, through the meniscus, across the tear, and through the capsule.
10. The needle tips are felt under the skin and a small incision is made to pull the suture out of the joint.

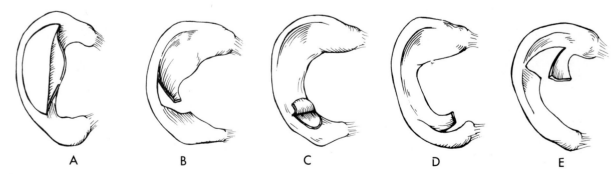

A   B   C   D   E

Fig. 22-119. Meniscal cartilage injury. **A,** Longitudinal splitting (bucket-handle type). **B,** Tear of middle third. **C,** Tear of anterior tip. **D,** Longitudinal splitting of anterior third. **E,** Tear of posterior third. (Modified from Brashear, H.R., and Raney, B.R.: Handbook of orthopaedic surgery, ed. 10, St. Louis, 1986, The C.V. Mosby Co.)

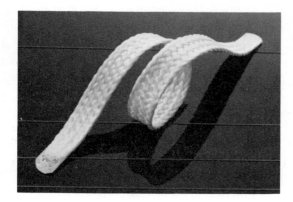

Fig. 22-120. Kennedy ligament augmentation device. (Courtesy 3M Health Care, St. Paul, Minn.)

11. The sutures are tied over the capsule. Positioning the cannula enables either horizontal or vertical sutures to be placed. As many sutures as necessary are used.
12. After completing partial meniscectomy or suture repair, the joint is thoroughly irrigated.
13. The incisions are closed, and the knee is lightly dressed and wrapped with Webril and Ace bandages.

Arthroscopic anterior cruciate ligament repair. The anterior cruciate ligament is an important stabilizing structure of the knee and the most frequently torn ligament. Injury is usually a result of simultaneous anterior and rotational stresses. Candidates for anterior cruciate ligament reconstruction are active individuals with instability that is sufficient to interfere with their activities and that has failed to respond to bracing, rehabilitation, exercises, and other nonoperative treatment methods. The selected treat-

ment method depends on the classification and severity of the tear, the experience and preference of the surgeon, and whether a previous repair has failed.

Reconstruction of the anterior cruciate ligament may be intraarticular, extraarticular, or a combination of both. Arthroscopic repair causes less patellar pain and less disturbance of extensor mechanisms and therefore is becoming the treatment of choice if there is no other significant capsular instability or gross disruption of the knee joint.

Anterior cruciate ligament repair most often involves replacement of the ligament with a substitute. Substitutes include autografts, allografts, and synthetic ligaments. Autografts are currently the method of choice, with a free central-third patellar tendon graft attached to patellar and tibial bone blocks used most often. The semitendinosus tendon and iliotibial band are sometimes used instead. Autografts may be used alone or augmented. A ligament augmentation device (Fig. 22-120) strengthens the graft and protects it from rupture during early postoperative healing.

Procedural considerations. Instrumentation for an anterior cruciate ligament repair includes all instruments required for an operative arthroscopy, plus the following:

Ortho soft tissue and major bone sets
Microsaw with blades
Power drill
Fixation device of choice (staple set, bone screws with spiked washers, interference screws, ligament button (Fig. 22-121)
Tendon leader
Tension isometer (Fig. 22-122)
Bone tunnel plugs (Fig. 22-123)

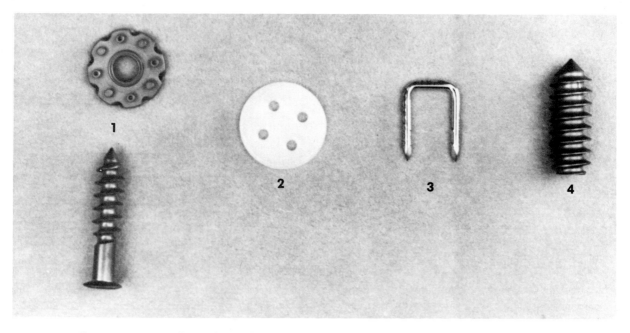

Fig. 22-121. Fixation devices for attachment of knee ligament substitutes. *1,* bone-anchoring screw with spiked washer; *2,* ligament button; *3,* barbed knee staple; *4,* interference screw.

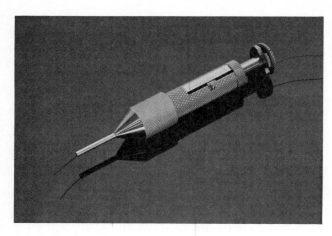

Fig. 22-122. Tension isometer used to determine isometric placement of ligament substitute. (Courtesy Acufex Microsurgical Inc., Norwood, Mass.)

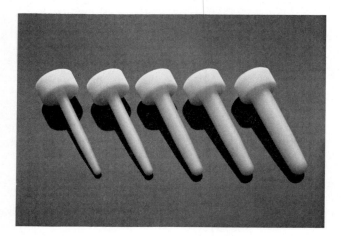

Fig. 22-123. Bone tunnel plugs. (Courtesy Acufex Microsurgical Inc., Norwood, Mass.)

Operative procedure—using patellar tendon graft

1. An exam under anesthesia is performed immediately after induction to further evaluate the instability of the knee.
2. A diagnositc arthroscopy is then carried out through the standard anteromedial and anterolateral portals.
3. Any meniscal tears or other intraarticular injuries are treated before attending to the ligament.
4. The remaining anterior cruciate ligament tissue is debrided with a full-radius resector.
5. A notchplasty is then performed, widening the intracondylar notch with a 4.5-mm arthroplasty burr, rasp, osteotome, and curettes. Notchplasty aids in arthroscopic visualization and protects the graft from abrasion.
6. After preparation of the intracondylar area, a small incision is made on the distal lateral aspect of the

femur and carried down to the flare of the lateral femoral condyle.

7. A femoral aiming device is positioned, and a guide pin is inserted from the femoral site into the posterior-superior region of the intercondylar notch at an isometric point (Fig. 22-124).
8. Another small incision is made anteriorly, below the knee and medial to the tibial tubercle.
9. The tibial aiming device is positioned and a guide pin is inserted from the anterior tibial incision into the intercondylar notch, anterior and medial to the center of the tibial anatomic attachment site of the anterior cruciate ligament (Fig. 22-125).
10. The pins are then replaced with a heavy suture passing through the femoral and tibial pin sites.
11. Isometric placement of the guide pins is checked with a tensioning device that is attached to the heavy suture. The knee is put through a range of motion to determine correct isometric measurement.
12. Once isometric positioning is determined, a longitudinal skin incision is made medial to the midline near the patellar tendon.
13. The central-third portion of the patellar tendon with tibial and patellar bone plugs is harvested with a minisaw and osteotome.
14. The graft is sized to the appropriate width, usually 10 mm to 12 mm, using sizing tubes (Fig. 22-117).
15. Heavy (Ethibond, Mersilene, or Ti·Cron) suture is placed through drill holes made at each end of the graft in the bone plugs.
16. The guide pins are then reinserted and overdrilled with cannulae that are close in width to the prepared graft. Overdrilling establishes the tunnels so they are in the center of the previous insertion sites of the anterior cruciate ligament.
17. The femoral and tibial osseous tunnels are smoothed with curettes, a rasp, or an abrader. If the tunnels are made before the graft is harvested, they are temporarily occluded with bone tunnel plugs (Fig. 22-123) to minimize fluid extravasation.
18. Both ends of the graft are fixed with a barbed staple, bone screw with washer, interference screw, or ligament button.
19. The incisions and joint are irrigated and closed.
20. A hinged knee brace is applied over the dressing. The brace allows 10 to 90 degrees of motion.

Arthroscopic posterior cruciate ligament repair. Tears of the posterior cruciate ligament are not commonly reconstructed because of poor results. Patients usually return to adequate function without operative treatment. Surgery should be considered only if significant disabling instability occurs. The arthroscopic procedure for repair of the posterior cruciate ligament is similar to the technique used to repair the anterior cruciate ligament, except that iso-

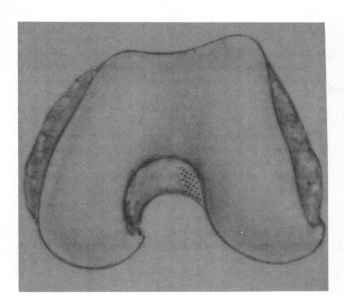

Fig. 22-124. Femoral isometric point. (Courtesy Acufex Microsurgical Inc., Norwood, Mass.)

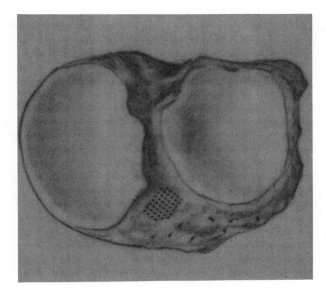

Fig. 22-125. Tibial isometric point. (Courtesy Acufex Microsurgical Inc., Norwood, Mass.)

metric placement is posterior within the joint and the femoral attachment is proximal to the medial epicondyle.

Arthroscopy of the shoulder

Shoulder arthroscopy is a useful diagnostic and therapeutic tool in the management of shoulder disorders. It is particularly beneficial in the evaluation and management of patients with chronic shoulder problems. Arthroscopy provides extensive visualization of the intraarticular aspect of the shoulder joint. Indications for shoulder arthroscopy include removal of loose bodies; lysis of adhesions; sy-

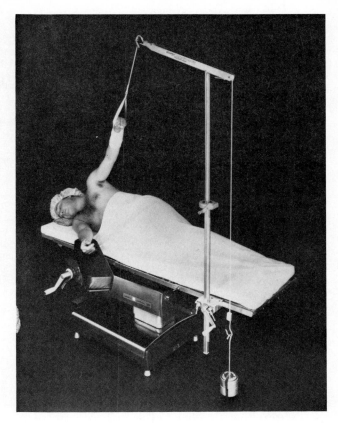

Fig. 22-126. Shoulder arthroscopy holder. (Courtesy Acufex Microsurgical Inc., Norwood, Mass.)

novial biopsy; synovectomy; bursectomies; stabilization of dislocations; correction of glenoid labrum, biceps tendon, and rotator cuff tears; and relief of impingement syndrome. General endotracheal anesthesia is administered.

Procedural considerations. The patient is placed in the lateral position. The position is maintained by using a vacuum beanbag positioning device or lateral rolls with a kidney rest. Three-inch adhesive tape is secured across the patient's hips. Proper padding of the uninvolved axilla and lower extremity is important to prevent soft tissue or neurovascular problems. The affected extremity is placed in an overhead traction device (Fig. 22-126) and Buck's traction or a Velcro immobilizer is applied to the forearm to achieve adequate distraction to the glenohumeral joint. The extremity is abducted 40 to 60 degrees and forward flexed 10 to 20 degrees, with 5- to 15-pound weights placed on the pulley system.

The shoulder is prepped and draped free, permitting full range of motion during the procedure. The surgeon stands posterior to the patient.

The operative instruments and arthroscope commonly used for the knee may also be used in the shoulder, plus an 18-gauge needle, switching sticks, and a Wissinger rod (Fig. 22-127).

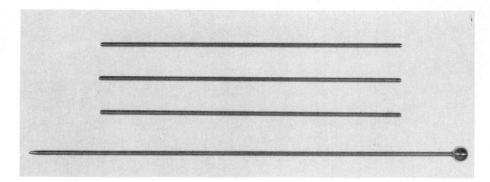

Fig. 22-127. Switching sticks *(top)* and Wissinger rod *(bottom)*. Switching sticks are used during shoulder arthroscopy to switch cannula without losing place in tissue. Switching stick is placed in already inserted cannula. Cannula is removed over stick, and new cannula can be replaced over stick in exactly same spot. Wissinger rod is used to determine opposite-side portal during shoulder arthroscopy. Rod is placed in anterior incision and worked through tissue until it is just under skin in posterior shoulder. Surgeon can then palpate rod and make incision posteriorly at exact spot needed.

Operative procedure

1. An 18-gauge spinal needle is inserted through the posterior soft spot and directed anteriorly toward the coracoid process, where the surgeon's index finger has been positioned (Fig. 22-128, *A*).
2. The glenohumeral joint is distended with saline or lactated Ringer's solution. This facilitates entry of the arthroscope.
3. Bupivacaine 0.25% (Marcaine), 2 to 3 ml, with epinephrine 1:200,000 is injected along the needle track to minimize bleeding.

4. With the needle removed, a stab incision is made with a no. 11 blade over the needle site (Fig. 22-128, *B*).
5. The arthroscope sleeve and sharp trocar are then introduced through the posterior joint capsule.
6. Once the capsule has been penetrated, a blunt obturator replaces the sharp trocar to enter the joint (Fig. 22-128, *C*).
7. The arthroscope is inserted and attached to inflow and outflow tubings, the video camera, and light source (Fig. 22-128, *D*).
8. Operative instruments are placed through an anterior

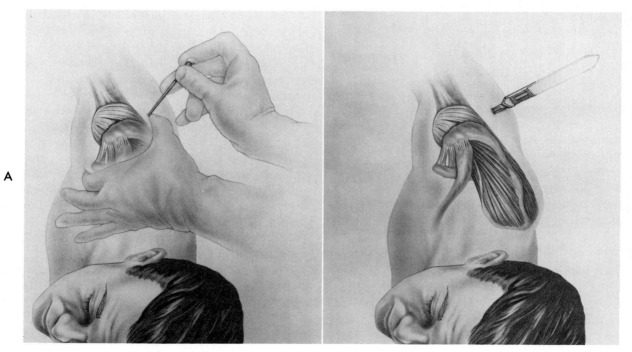

Fig. 22-128. Shoulder arthroscopy. (Courtesy Dyonics, Inc., Andover, Mass.)

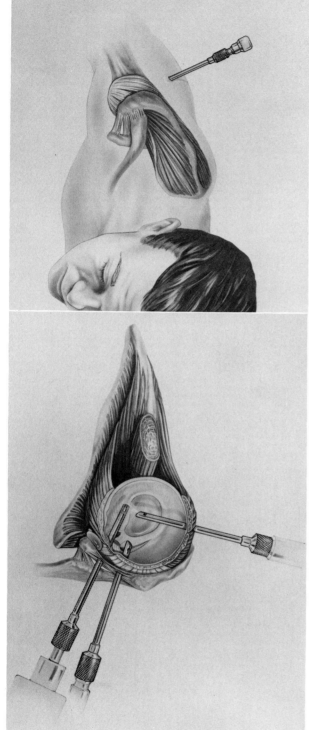

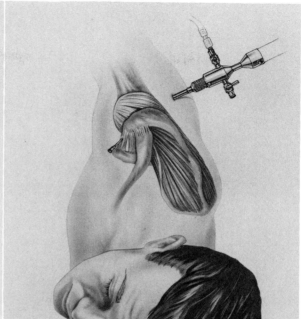

Fig. 22-128, cont'd.

portal that is established lateral to the coracoid process (Fig. 22-128, *E*) by using a Wissinger rod (Fig. 22-127).

9. A third portal can be established near the anterior portal or supraspinous fossa portal. Switching sticks (Fig. 22-127) are used to change portals.

10. The arm is moved and rotated as needed to visualize various structures in and around the joint.

11. At the conclusion of the procedure, the joint is irrigated. The surgeon may inject a long-acting local anesthetic drug into the joint and subacromial space through the portal to minimize postoperative discomfort.

12. The puncture wounds are closed and dressed with a sterile 4 × 4 gauze pad. The patient's arm is placed into a sling for recovery.

Arthroscopy of the elbow

The elbow joint is accessible to arthroscopic examination, although it requires more attention to detail than the knee because instruments must be placed through deeper muscle layers and close to important neurovascular structures.

Arthroscopy of the elbow, both diagnostic and operative, has become fairly routine. Indications for its use include extraction of loose bodies, evaluation or debridement of osteochondritis dissecans of the capitellum and radial head, partial synovectomy in rheumatoid disease, debridement and lysis of adhesions of posttraumatic or degenerative processes at or near the elbow, diagnosis of a chronically painful elbow when the diagnosis is obscure,

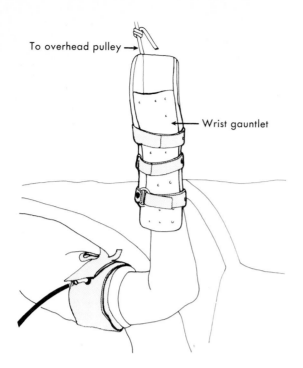

To overhead pulley →

Wrist gauntlet

Fig. 22-130. Portals commonly used for arthroscopy of elbow. **A,** Anterolateral. **B,** Anteromedial. **C,** Posterolateral. (From Andrews, J.R., and Carson, W.G.: J. Arthroscopic Rel. Surg. 1[2]:97, 1985.)

Fig. 22-129. Arm positioned for arthroscopy of elbow. (From Andrews, J.R., and Carson, W.G.: J. Arthroscopic Rel. Surg. 1[2]:97, 1985.)

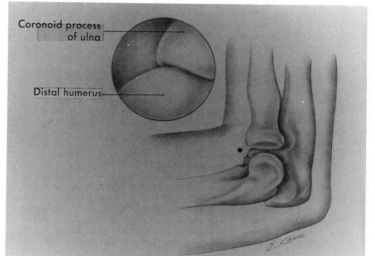

Coronoid process of ulna

Distal humerus

A

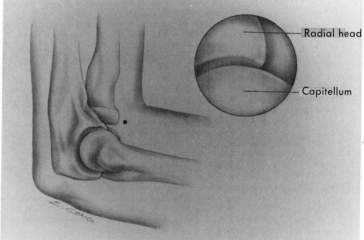

Radial head

Capitellum

B

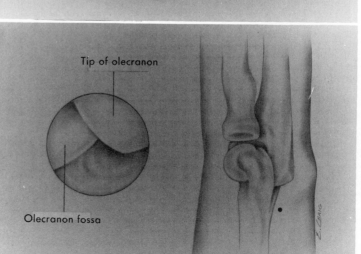

Tip of olecranon

Olecranon fossa

C

and evaluation of fractures of the capitellum, radial head, or olecranon.

Procedural considerations. General anesthesia is preferred to local anesthesia because it affords complete comfort to the patient and provides total muscle relaxation.

The patient is placed in the supine position on an operating room bed. The forearm is flexed on an armboard or placed in a prefabricated wrist gauntlet connected to an overhead pulley device and tied off at the end of the operating room bed (Fig. 22-129). If lifted overhead, the entire arm is allowed to hang free over the side of the operating room bed with the elbow flexed approximately 90 degrees. This provides excellent access to both the medial and lateral aspects of the elbow, allows the forearm to be freely pronated and supinated, and places the important neurovascular structures in the antecubital fossa at maximum relaxation. A tourniquet is routinely used for hemostasis. The entire arm, including the hand, is prepped and draped.

The three portals most commonly used for diagnostic and operative arthroscopy of the elbow are the anterolateral, the anteromedial, and the posterolateral (Fig. 22-130).

Operative arthroscopy instruments commonly used for the knee may also be used in the elbow. However, smaller-diameter scopes and instruments may be desired instead.

Operative procedure

1. The bony anatomic landmarks are outlined with a marking pen before initiation of the procedure. Lateral structures to be marked and identified are the radial head and the lateral epicondyle. The medial structure to be marked is the medial epicondyle.
2. An 18-gauge needle is inserted anterior to the radial head from the lateral side, and the joint is distended.
3. Once joint distention has been achieved with approximately 15 to 30 cc of lactated Ringer's or normal saline solution, a stab wound incision is made and the sharp trocar with cannula is inserted just through the joint capsule.
4. The sharp trocar is replaced with the blunt obturator to provide safe entry of the cannula into the joint.
5. The scope replaces the blunt obturator and is attached to the video and light source.
6. A second and third portal are established anteromedially and posterolaterally for triangulation. With the patient's elbow flexed to 90 degrees and adequate distention maintained at the time of insertion of the instruments, the neurovascular structures are displaced anteriorly, and this provides more area above the medial and lateral humeral epicondyles in which to insert the various instruments.
7. Outflow and inflow are controlled by alternating the valve on the scope or using a separate 18-gauge needle with drainage tubing.
8. After diagnostic and/or operative procedures have been

completed, the joint is irrigated, the puncture sites are sutured, and a compression dressing is applied with Webril and Ace bandages.

Arthroscopy of the ankle

The talocalcaneal articulations are complex and play an important role in the movements of inversion and eversion of the foot. The subtalar joints function as a single unit, but anatomically they are divided into anterior and posterior joints. The surgeon and nurse must be familiar with the extraarticular anatomy of the ankle to prevent neural or vascular damage.

Indications for ankle arthroscopy include osteochondral fragments or loose bodies, persistent ankle pain following trauma and despite adequate conservative treatment, biopsy, posttraumatic arthritis of the ankle joint, an unstable ankle before lateral ligamentous reconstruction, and osteochondritis dissecans of the talus.

Procedural considerations. General anesthesia is preferable because manipulation and distraction of the joint to obtain adequate arthroscopic viewing require muscle relaxation. The position of the patient depends on the surgeon's preference. The patient may be supine with the knee flexed approximately 70 degrees or supine with a sandbag under the buttock of the operative side. Ankle and thigh holders may be used; when better posterior visualization is necessary, a distractor may be used to increase the space between the tibia and talus. A tourniquet is placed around the upper thigh but not used unless excessive bleeding, uncontrolled by irrigation, is encountered. Routine skin prepping and draping are done.

Operative instruments and the arthroscope commonly used for the knee may also be used for the ankle; however, miniaturized instruments and needle scopes for the ankle are becoming more available.

Operative procedure

1. The important extraarticular anatomic structures are outlined on the skin using a sterile marking pen.
2. Examination of the ankle joint using the anterolateral portal (Fig. 22-131) is then performed. The anteromedial joint line is palpated, and an 18-gauge, 1½-inch needle is inserted into the joint.
3. Sterile plastic extension tubing is attached to the needle, and a 50-ml plastic Luer-Lok syringe filled with normal saline is connected to the tubing to distend the joint. Approximately 15 to 20 cc are needed.
4. After intraarticular injection is confirmed by the ease with which the saline can be injected and by palpation of the joint as it is distended, a small incision is made with a no. 11 blade on a no. 3 knife handle over the site of the anterolateral portal.
5. A hemostat is then inserted and used to spread the incision down to the capsule.
6. The sheath of the arthroscope and sharp trocar are placed into the incision, angled approximately 30 to

Fig. 22-131. Ankle arthroscopy. Posterior needle and anterior arthroscope positions.

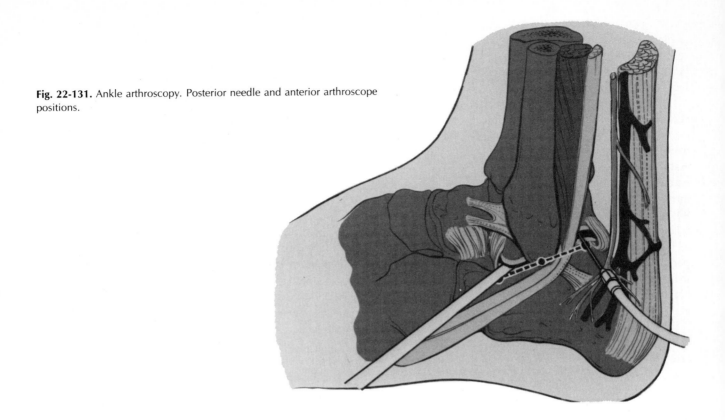

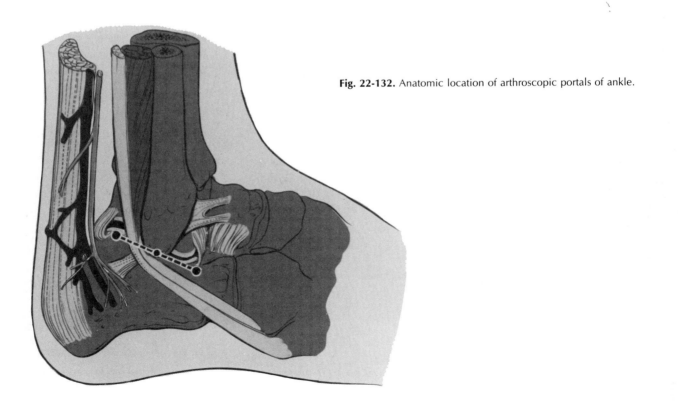

Fig. 22-132. Anatomic location of arthroscopic portals of ankle.

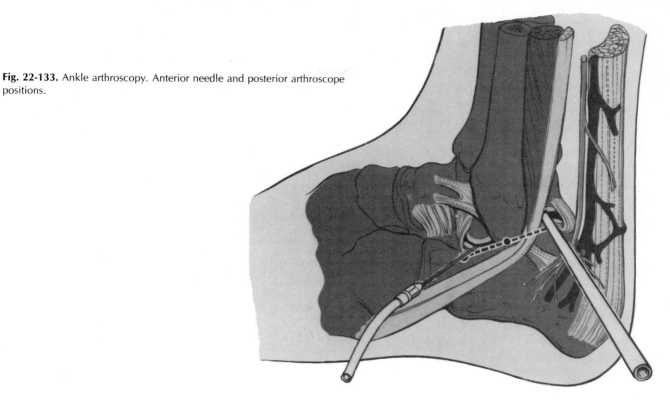

Fig. 22-133. Ankle arthroscopy. Anterior needle and posterior arthroscope positions.

45 degrees laterally, and inserted with a sharp plunge as joint distention is maintained. Entrance into the joint is felt as the sleeve and trocar "pop" through the capsule and is confirmed by the rush of saline on removal of the trocar from the sheath.

7. The arthroscope is inserted into the sheath, the needle is removed, and the plastic tubing and syringe are attached to the stopcock on the arthroscope sleeve. The video camera and light source are connected to the scope. Joint distention must be maintained.

8. Triangulation through other portals (Fig. 22-132) is easily done by first inserting the 18-gauge needle for localization while viewing with the arthroscope. Posterior viewing is done in the same fashion (Fig. 22-133), except that the patient is usually placed in the prone position and instruments are inserted through the posterior portals.

9. After the procedure is completed, the joint is irrigated and wounds are closed with Steri-Strips or a single suture and covered with a dressing and short leg compression Ace wrap.

Operations on the knee and tibia

Most operations on the knee are performed with the patient in the supine position and the leg prepped and draped from the groin to the middle of the calf or including the entire foot. It is occasionally necessary for the surgeon to operate with the foot of the operating room bed dropped and the patient's knee flexed to 90 degrees. Consequently, it is important to position the patient so the knee is at a "break" in the bed; then if necessary the lower leg can be flexed at the knee during the operation. One of many possible incisions is used for surgery of the knee joint (Fig. 22-134).

A basic set of specifically designed instruments must be available for all open operations involving the knee joint (Fig. 22-135).

Correction of femoral condyle and tibial plateau fractures

Anatomic alignment of the articular surfaces of the distal femur and proximal tibia is necessary to provide joint stability and decrease the chance of posttraumatic arthritis. Fractures of the femoral condyle are uncommon; however, when they do occur, they are most often the result of direct trauma to the knee. Condylar fractures can be single condylar fractures or multicondylar fractures that separate both condyles. They are referred to as T or Y fractures. Undisplaced fractures can usually be treated by plaster and immobilization. Displaced fractures are treated with open reduction if distal tibial traction and manipulation attempts fail. Fixation is accomplished with long cancellous screws and/or a right-angled condylar blade plate.

Tibial plateau fractures most often involve the lateral condyle. The most common type of tibial plateau fracture is a comminuted compression fracture in which the lateral

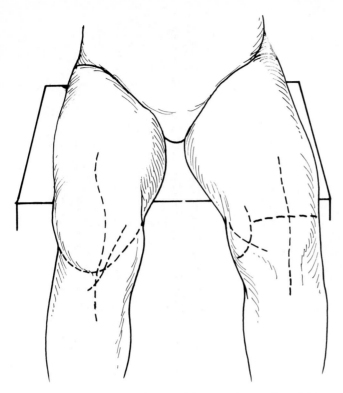

Fig. 22-134. Various incisions used for operations on knee joint.

condyle and articular surface are crushed and fragmented (Fig. 22-136). Injury is a result of the tibia abducting upon the femur while the foot is planted on the ground. The lateral femoral condyle is driven into the tibia. Central depression fractures like this require elevation of the articular surface and fixation of the fragments. Long cancellous screws and/or buttress plates and cancellous bone graft are used.

Procedural considerations. The patient is placed in the supine position under general anesthesia. The leg is prepped and draped free with a stockinette.

Ortho soft tissue and major bone sets are required plus the following:

Knee retractors
Power drill
Kirschner wires
Large bone clamps
Compression screw set with instrumentation
Assortment of plates (angled blade plates, condylar plates, T and L buttress plates (Fig. 22-137)
Bone graft instruments

Operative procedures
T or Y femoral condyle fracture
1. A curvilinear incision is made anterior to the lateral collateral ligament and extended distally to the level of the knee joint, curving just lateral to the tibial tuberosity.

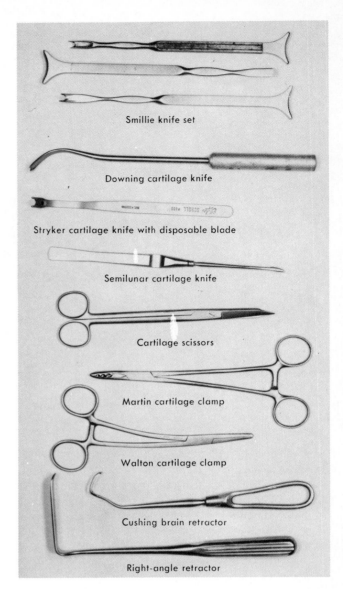

Fig. 22-135. Specifically designed instruments necessary for all open knee operations.

2. The knee joint is entered anterior to the collateral ligament, providing exposure and reduction of articular surfaces.
3. The condyles are reduced with the knee flexed, and the fragments are temporarily held with Kirschner wires.
4. Two 6.5 cancellous screws with washers are then inserted across the condyles. Washers prevent the heads of the screws from sinking into the cortex. The wires are removed.
5. The supracondylar component is reduced with bone clamps and held in place with Kirschner wires.
6. The fracture is fixed with condylar lag screws and an angled blade plate or condylar plate. The wires are removed.
7. Iliac bone graft may be required for medial defects.

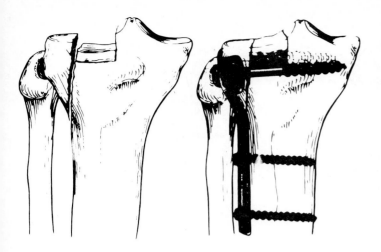

Fig. 22-136. Type II tibial plateau fracture. Reduction requires elevation of fragments with bone grafting of resultant hole in metaphysis. Lateral wedge is lagged on lateral cortex protected with buttress plate. (From Schatzker, J., McBroom, R., and Bruce, D.: Clinical Orthopaedics 138:94, 1979.)

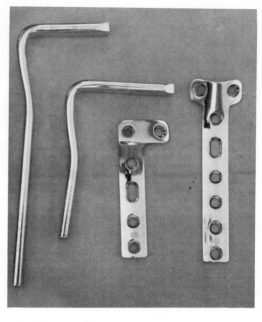

Fig. 22-137. Plates used for fixation of femoral condylar and tibial plateau fractures. *Left to right:* 95-degree angled condylar plates, L and T buttress plates.

Tibial plateau fracture

1. An incision is made lateral to the superior pole of the patella and carried distally to a point lateral to the tibial tuberosity, curving distally and posteriorly to the joint line.
2. The head of the fibula and lateral aspect of the joint are exposed.
3. After incising the capsule, the joint is inspected for injury.
4. Further exposure of the lateral condyle and articular surface allows visualization of the tibial plateau fracture.
5. A periosteal elevator is inserted into the anterolateral cortex of the tibia beneath the depressed fragments in order to elevate the fragments and compressed cancellous bone.
6. The cavity resulting from elevation of the depressed fragments and cancellous bone is filled with cancellous bone graft to hold the articular surface in place.
7. Small Kirschner wires are inserted to fix the fragments until an L or T buttress plate is placed across the anterolateral tibial condyle and proximal metaphysis.
8. The plate holes are secured with cancellous screws.
9. The meniscus is repaired if needed, and the wound is closed.
10. A posterior plaster splint is applied for postoperative immobilization.

Patellectomy and reduction of fractured patella

It is possible to excise a portion of the patella (for comminuted fracture) or the entire patella (for painful degenerative arthritis) without significantly affecting the function of the knee joint. Removal of the entire patella

may result in relative lengthening of the knee extensor mechanism, which necessitates imbrication of the quadriceps tendon at the time of operation to prevent a lag in knee extension. If the fracture consists of two large fragments that can be anatomically reduced, fixation is accomplished with suture and tension band wiring or a screw. Tension band wiring produces compression forces across the fracture site and results in earlier union and immediate motion and exercise of the knee (Fig. 22-138).

In a patient with mild chondromalacia of the patella, the softened and frayed articular cartilage can be shaved or excised, and range-of-motion exercises are begun early in the postoperative period.

Procedural considerations. Ortho soft tissue and major bone sets as well as knee instruments are required, plus the following:

Power drill and bits
Compression screw set with instrumentation
Ortho wire, wire tightener, and wire passers
Large bone clamps

Operative procedure

1. A transverse curved incision is made over the patella.
2. Dissection is carried down to expose the surface of the patella, the quadriceps, and patellar tendons.
3. The joint is irrigated, and the fracture is reduced with bone-holding forceps.
4. A heavy orthopedic wire is passed transversely through the insertion of the quadriceps tendon and

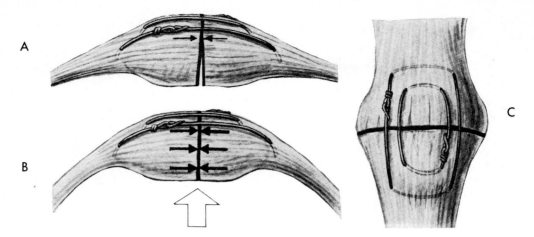

Fig. 22-138. Tension band wiring of patella fracture. **A,** Wire that has been passed around the insertion of the patellar tendon and quadriceps tendon is tightened until fracture is slightly overcorrected or opened on articular surface. Second wire is then passed more superficially but through bone fragments. **B,** On flexing knee or contracting quadriceps muscle, pressure of condyles against patella compresses bony fragments together. **C,** Anterior view of both wires. (From Müller, M.E., Allgöwer, M., and Willenegger, H.: Manual of internal fixation, New York, 1970, Springer-Verlag, Inc.)

then passed anteriorly over the superficial surface of the patella.

5. The wire is passed through the patellar tendon insertion and tightened until the fracture is overcorrected.
6. A drill is used to make holes through the superior and inferior poles of the anterior patellar surface.
7. A second wire is then passed through the distal transverse holes and tightened.
8. Repair of capsular tears is acccomplished with interrupted sutures.
9. The quadriceps and synovial membrane are repaired from the outer ends toward the midline of the joint.
10. The wound is completely closed and 4 × 4 sterile gauze, Webril, and an Ace wrap are applied.
11. The knee is placed in a long leg splint or knee immobilizer to allow full weight bearing.

Correction of recurrent dislocation of the patella

Teenagers with a shallow femoral condylar groove and a patella proximal to the normal anatomic position may have recurrent lateral dislocation of the patella. If the condition persists, chondromalacia may occur. Numerous operations have been designed to realign the knee extensor mechanism. All the operations include incising the lateral quadriceps tendon and shifting the insertion of the patellar tendon medially or distally to the original insertion of the tibia.

Procedural considerations. Ortho soft tissue and major bone sets, knee instruments, a drill and drill bits, and a screw set are required.

Operative procedure

1. An anteromedial incision is made parallel to the quadriceps tendon, patella, and patellar tendon.

2. Tight and contracted soft tissue, including the vastus lateralis insertion lateral to the patella, are released.
3. Structures medial to the patella are reinforced, plicated, or transferred to strengthen medial support.
4. The patellar tendon insertion is transferred medially to properly align the extensor mechanism or distally to align the inferior pole of the patella at the level of the joint line.
5. The wound is closed, and a posterior plaster or metal splint is applied.

Repair of collateral or cruciate ligament tears

The stability of the knee depends on the integrity of the cruciate and collateral ligaments. If any of these supporting structures is damaged, an unstable knee is likely unless properly repaired. Injuries to these supporting structures are usually not isolated. More frequently, several of the ligaments are injured at the same time. For example, common injuries referred to as the "terrible triad" include a torn anterior cruciate ligament, torn medial meniscus, and torn medial collateral ligament.

The knee demonstrates grave disability with major ligamentous disruption. The collateral ligaments reinforce the knee capsule medially and laterally. They resist varus and valgus stresses on the knee. The cruciate ligaments control anteroposterior stability. Along with the ligaments, the muscle groups stabilize the joint and control movement. Because muscle strength is the first line of defense for the knee, damage is repaired to protect the ligaments. For optimum function of the joint, damaged structures should be reconstructed as close as possible to the original anatomy. If the knee is left untreated, osteoarthritis will develop.

Various types of ligament grafts may be utilized to stabilize the patient's knee. Autografts, allografts, and artificial substitutes are available. Artificial ligament substitutes function as scaffolds, stents, augmentation devices, or a combination of the three. Scaffolds support the soft tissue initially to allow ingrowth of the host tissue. Stents protect the joint from excessive stress while the permanent ligament substitute is healing. Augmentation devices protect the graft initially and can be temporary or permanent. Synthetic ligaments include carbon fiber grafts, polyglycolic acid material, Dacron, polyester, and Gortex. All synthetic grafts are subject to mechanical failure from weakening with fragmentation and synovitis; therefore, they are recommended for salvage procedures only when conventional reconstruction has failed and when all other autogenous tissue is unavailable for substitution. Biologic materials from animals, such as bovine xenografts, are also available for ligament substitution, although they are subject to increased risk of infection, synovitis, and rejection. Homogenous allografts are the substitute of choice for knee reconstruction when no autogenous graft is available from the patient. Disadvantages of homogenous allografts include long-term weakening, possible rejection, and the possibility of HIV transfer in tissue. Autogenous tissues are currently the substitute of choice, with the mid-third patellar tendon being the most reliable. To minimize necrosis and maintain graft strength, the fat pad with its blood supply may be preserved along with the patellar tendon. With the combination of a torn anterior cruciate ligament, medial meniscus, and medial collateral ligament, an open procedure (arthrotomy) is properly indicated.

Procedural considerations. The patient is placed in the supine position with a tourniquet applied to the upper thigh. The extremity is prepped and draped for a routine knee procedure.

Ortho soft tissue and major bone sets, knee instruments, and a power drill are required, plus the following:

Nerve hook
Microsaw and drill with assorted blades and burrs
Wire passer
Kirschner wires
Fixation device of choice—polyethylene buttons, knee staples, bone screws with spiked washers, interference screws (Fig. 22-121)
Arthroplasty instruments (Fig. 22-113)
Tension isometer (Fig. 22-122)
Meniscal repair instruments (Fig. 22-116)
Ligament guide set
Anterior cruciate ligament reconstruction instruments (Fig. 22-117)
Suture retriever

Operative procedure

1. An examination under anesthesia is performed immediately after induction to evaluate completely the severity of the ligamentous injury.

2. A straight midline or slightly medial incision is made across the knee.
3. Meniscus tears are repaired with arthroscopic meniscal repair instruments or cutting needles with a size 0 nonabsorbable suture to repair the meniscofemoral and meniscotibial ligaments. If the meniscus is not repairable, partial meniscectomy is performed.
4. The mid-third patellar tendon with patellar and tibial bone plugs is harvested, using a power saw and osteotome.
5. A notchplasty is then performed, debriding and smoothing the lateral intercondylar wall with a burr and curette.
6. The femoral and tibial osseous tunnels are developed by using the ligament guide to pass guide wires from the lateral femoral condyle and tibial tubercle into the intercondylar notch at isometric points near the anatomic attachment site of the anterior cruciate ligament.
7. The pins are temporarily removed to measure isometric positioning with a tension isometer.
8. The pins are then replaced and overdrilled with cannulated drills as close to the size of the patellar tendon graft as possible. The tunnels are smoothed with a curette.
9. Sutures are placed through drill holes at both ends of the graft in order to pass the graft through the tunnels.
10. Once the graft is passed through the femoral and tibial osseous tunnels, it is fixed at both ends with staples, screws, or polyethylene buttons.
11. The medial collateral ligament and posterior oblique ligament are then individually repaired at their insertion sites with bone screws and spiked washers.
12. Additional extraarticular repair is done if necessary.
13. The wound is closed over intraarticular and subcutaneous drains, and a cast is applied.

Popliteal (Baker's) cyst excision

Baker's cyst excision is removal of a cyst from the popliteal fossa. Baker's cysts are frequently painful and can become very large, especially when associated with rheumatoid arthritis. Whereas cysts in the popliteal fossa occur without a precipitating cause in children, in adults they often indicate an intraarticular disease process, such as rheumatoid arthritis, or a torn medial meniscus.

Procedural considerations. In contrast to other operative procedures on the knee, the patient is placed in the prone position with chest rolls under the thorax during surgery.

Ortho soft tissue and major bone sets are required.

Operative procedure
1. An oblique incision is made in the popliteal area over the mass.
2. The deep fascia is divided to expose the mass.
3. The cyst is then freed by blunt dissection and clamped at its attachment to the joint capsule.

4. The cyst is divided, and the pedicle is inverted and closed.

5. After the mass has been removed, the wound is irrigated and closed.

6. The knee is immobilized in extension with a posterior splint.

Total knee joint replacement arthroplasty

Total knee joint arthroplasty is a surgical procedure designed to replace the worn surfaces of the knee joint. Patients with severe destruction of the knee joint resulting from degenerative rheumatoid or traumatic arthritis or destruction of only the medial or lateral compartments of the knee joint as a result of extreme varus or valgus deformity complain of pain and instability. Total knee joint replacement arthroplasty has been successful in relieving pain and providing a stable knee.

Many models of knee prostheses are available, but basically only two types of knee joint replacement designs exist. The nonhinge type is similar to the total hip replacement in that a stainless steel distal femoral component articulates with a high-density polyethylene tibial component. The Porous Coated Anatomic (PCA), Insall/Burstein, Microloc, Modular, and Miller/Galante are among the many models of this type available (Figs. 22-139 through 22-142).

The second design is the hinge type of total knee prosthesis. For increased stability a metallic implant is placed in the distal femoral shaft and is fixed to another metallic implant in the proximal tibial shaft by a bolt, forming a hinge. The Kinematic II Rotating Hinge and Offset Hinges are among the available hinge models (Fig. 22-143).

Both the nonhinge and hinge implants usually have a stem extending into the femoral and tibial medullary canals. The components are held in the bone with methyl methacrylate. The hinge type of prosthesis is used when there is marked instability of the knee with destroyed supporting ligament, fixed flexion contractures greater than 25%, or failed total knee arthroplasty of other types. More bone is cut away with this type of implant. Due to rapid improvements in the field of total joint arthroplasties, hospitals are recommended to stock total knee, as well as total hip, prostheses on a consignment basis.

Procedural considerations. The patient is placed in the supine position. A tourniquet is applied to the upper thigh. A knee holder (Fig. 22-144) may be used.

Major bone and soft tissue sets are required, plus the following:

Knee instruments (Fig. 22-135)
Power drill
Power saw and appropriate blades
Nerve hooks
Total knee system with trials and instrumentation
Methyl methacrylate instruments and supplies if cement is to be used (Fig. 22-83)
Simpulse (Fig. 22-87) or Pulse Lavage (Fig. 22-88) with 3000-ml bag of normal saline

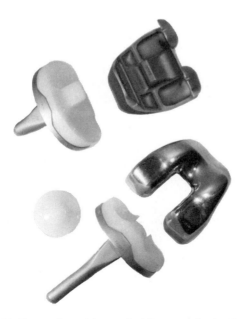

Fig. 22-139. Porous-Coated Anatomical Knee prosthesis. (Courtesy Howmedica, Inc., Rutherford, N.J.)

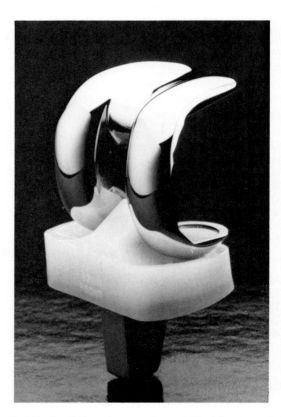

Fig. 22-140. Insall/Burstein posterior stabilized knee prosthesis. (Courtesy Zimmer Inc., Warsaw, Ind.)

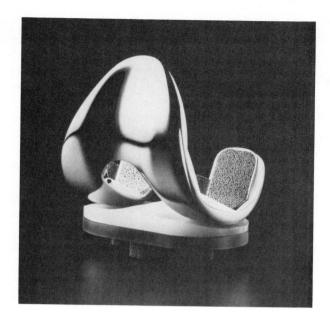

Fig. 22-141. Microloc porous-coated knee prosthesis. (Courtesy Johnson & Johnson Co., New Brunswick, N.J.)

Fig. 22-142. A, Miller/Galante knee prostheses; **B,** Miller/Galante knee system components; **C,** intramedullary knee instruments. (Courtesy Zimmer Inc., Warsaw, Ind.)

Operative procedure

1. An anterior longitudinal incision is made over the knee.
2. The capsule is entered anteromedially, and the patellar ligament is elevated.
3. With exposure established, osteophytes are removed, and the patella is everted.
4. Medial and lateral tibial plateaus are now presented; with a portion of the infrapatellar fat pad excised and the tibia subluxed, the plateau surfaces can be seen.
5. Fixed varus, fixed valgus, and fixed flexion are corrected with soft tissue and tendon releases.
6. Bony cuts are made to remove diseased bone and provide correct prosthesis fit. Cutting blocks from the knee system instruments are used to make the distal femoral resection, proximal tibial resection, and anterior femoral resection. Certain components may require additional cuts.

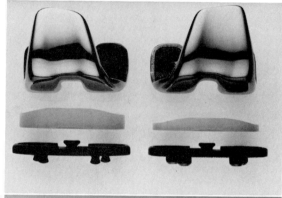

A

B

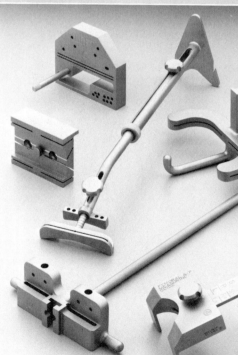

C

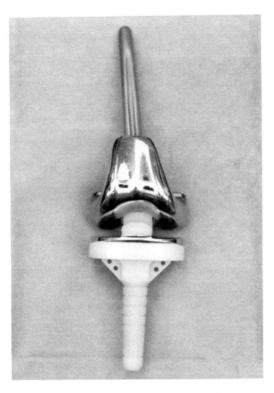

Fig. 22-143. Kinematic rotating hinge knee prosthesis. (Courtesy Howmedica, Inc., Rutherford, N.J.)

7. Patellar resection may be done freehand; it involves excising the worn surface on the back of the patella with a power saw and rongeur.

8. The tibial and femoral component trials are positioned for trial reduction before the permanent implants are dispensed to the field.

9. If cement is to be used, it is prepared and placed onto the ends of the femur and tibia, and the implants are inserted.

10. A polyethylene patella button is cemented to the prepared patella.

11. Once the knee components have been implanted and excess cement removed, the wound is irrigated and closed over a suction drain.

12. A knee immobilizer is applied before the patient is extubated.

Passive motion devices therapy

Postoperative care of the patient with total knee joint replacement and other procedures frequently includes use of a passive motion device. Application may be done immediately when the patient is still in the postanesthesia care unit. Two types of devices are shown in Figs. 22-145 and 22-146.

Indications for passive motion devices include these conditions and procedures related to the *knee:* total knee replacement, supracondylar fractures, tibial plateau fractures, infections, and ligament repairs. Indications related

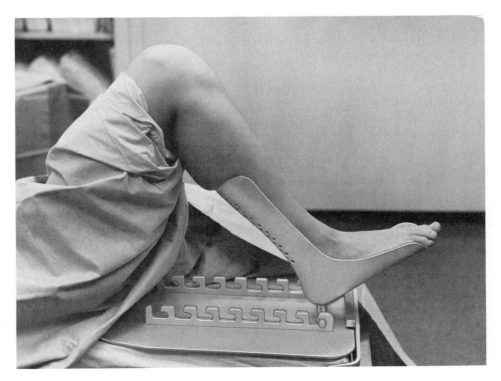

Fig. 22-144. Alvarado knee holder. (Courtesy Zimmer, Inc., Warsaw, Ind.)

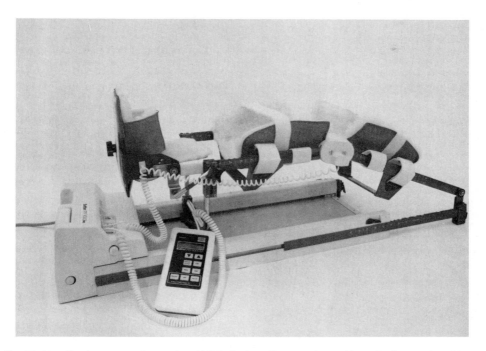

Fig. 22-145. Continuous passive motion (CPM) device. (Courtesy Sutter Biomedical, Inc., San Diego, Calif.)

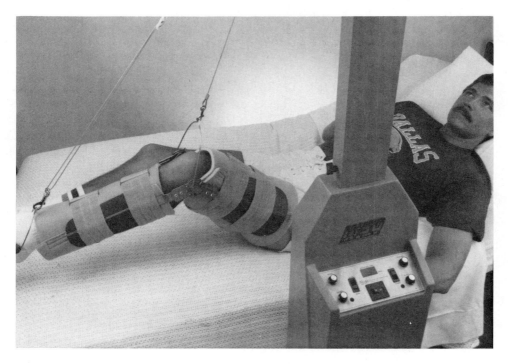

Fig. 22-146. Articular motion device (AMD). (Courtesy Medsurg Design (MSD), Inc., Chardon, Ohio.)

to the *hip* are total hip replacement, cup arthroplasty, hip fractures, and post–femoral shaft fracture fixation. Indications related to the *elbow* and *shoulder* include total elbow and shoulder replacements, rotator cuff repairs, and removal of loose bodies.

Beneficial effects of this mode of treatment are inhibition of formation of adhesions, improvement in articular cartilage nutrition because of better fluid mechanics, improvement in clearance of enzymes and exudate from the joint, improvement in matrix formation by stimulation of the chondrocytes, early functional range of motion postoperatively, decrease in postoperative pain, decrease in joint stiffness and swelling, and decrease in the length of hospital stay.

Correction of fractures of the tibial shaft

Tibial shaft fractures are difficult to treat. Open fractures are more common in the tibia than other major bones because one third of its surface is subcutaneous. Rotational deformities are seen often; delayed union, nonunion, and infection are fairly common complications. Closed reduction and plaster casting provide excellent healing without significant nonunion or infection. Surgical reduction and internal fixation are indicated when soft tissue is caught between fragments, initial treatment has been delayed, and severe rotational defect is present in the segmental fracture.

Internal fixation is accomplished with compression plates and screws (Fig. 22-147) or intramedullary nails (Fig. 22-148). Closed intramedullary nailing is the treatment of choice in tibial shaft fractures because infection is less likely to occur and periosteal blood supply is preserved. Interlocking nails are preferred in most cases. They can control rotation of fragments by proximal and/or distal locking. Static locking nails (locking both proximal and distal ends of the nail) are indicated for fractures with comminution, bone loss, and lengthening osteotomies. Dynamic locking nails (locking the end closest to the fracture site) are indicated for proximal or distal tibia fractures, nonunions, and malunions. Locking tibial nails include Universal and Grosse-Kempf (Fig. 22-148).

Procedural considerations. The patient is usually induced with general anesthesia while still on the hospital bed and then transferred to the fracture table. The patient is positioned supine on the fracture table with the affected hip flexed approximately 45 degrees and the knee at 90 degrees. A calcaneal traction pin is inserted under sterile conditions and attached to the traction mechanism on the fracture table. After rotational alignment is obtained, the leg is prepped and draped. The image intensifier is also draped into the sterile field.

Ortho soft tissue and major bone sets are used, plus the following:

Large bone clamps (open nailing procedure only)
Power drill
Power intramedullary reamer
Nail of choice with instrumentation
Compression plate and screw set (open plating procedure only)

Operative procedure

1. A 5- to 6-cm incision is made from the joint line along the medial margin of the patellar tendon to expose the tibial tuberosity (Fig. 22-149, *A*).

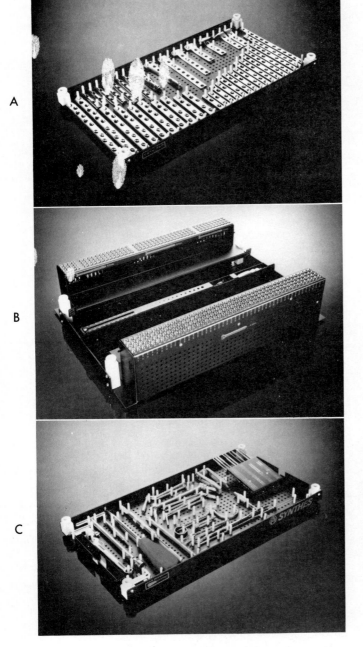

Fig. 22-147. Large fragment compression plating system. **A,** Plate set; **B,** screw set; **C,** basic instrumentation. (Courtesy Synthes, U.S.A., Paoli, Pa.)

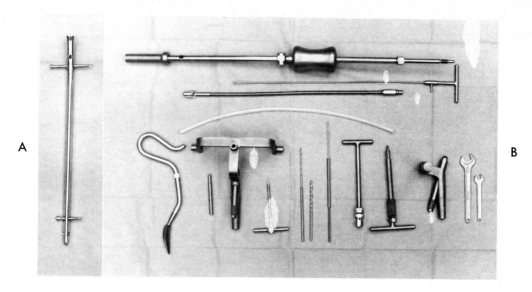

Fig. 22-148. Grosse-Kempf tibial intramedullary nailing system: **A,** Tibial interlocking nail; **B,** instrumentation. (Courtesy Howmedica Inc., Rutherford, N.J.)

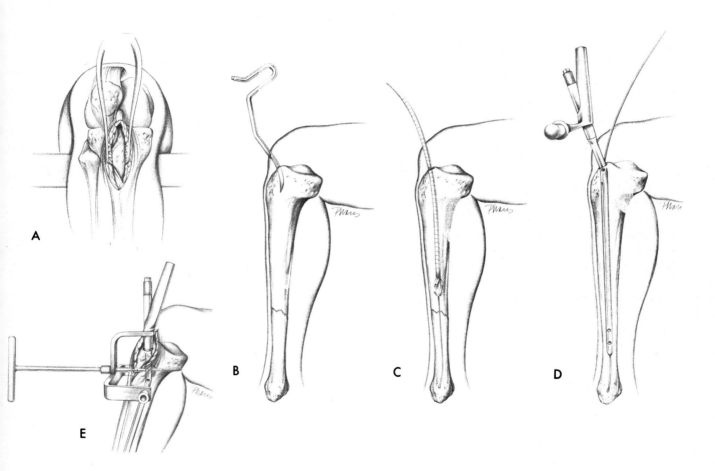

Fig. 22-149. Grosse-Kempf tibial nailing technique. (Reprinted with permission from Howmedica, Inc., Rutherford, N.J.)

2. The medullary canal is entered with a pointed awl (Fig. 22-149, *B*).

3. An olive-tipped guide pin is then passed down the canal across the fracture site and into the distal epiphysis under x-ray image.

4. Flexible intramedullary reamers are used to overdrill the guide pin to the appropriate diameter (Fig. 22-149, *C*).

5. A straight guide rod is then inserted in place of the olive-tipped guide pin to drive the appropriate-sized tibial nail across the fracture site (Fig. 22-149, *D*).

6. The nail can then be locked proximally with screws placed in the anterior-posterior plane and/or the medial-lateral plane (Fig. 22-149, *E*). Distal locking can be accomplished by placing transverse screws in the distal nail holes.

7. Once the nail has been inserted and locked if desired, the wound is irrigated and closed.

8. Sterile 4 × 4 gauze, Webril, and Ace wraps are applied.

Operations on the ankle and foot
Correction of ankle fractures

Ankle fractures include fractures of the medial malleolus (tibia), lateral malleolus (fibula), and posterior malleolus (posterior aspect of the articular surface of the distal tibia). The terms *malleolar*, *bimalleolar*, and *trimalleolar* are used depending on the number of fractures involved. Because medial malleolar and posterior malleolar fractures involve the distal weight-bearing articular surface of the tibia, open reduction and anatomic alignment are necessary.

Anatomic reduction prevents the occurrence of degenerative joint disease. Displaced fractures are treated with pins, malleolar or bone screws, or plates and screws (Fig. 22-150). Sometimes wire is needed for reinforcement. The lateral malleolus is important for lateral and rotational stability of the joint, and open reduction with internal fixation, using Steinman pins, Rush rods, or long bone screws, is frequently necessary. In trimalleolar fractures, the posterior, lateral, and then medial malleolus are fixed in order.

Procedural considerations. Incisions are made directly over the fracture (Figs. 22-151 and 22-152). The patient is in the supine position for most malleolar fracture procedures.

Small bone and minor soft tissue sets are required, plus the following:

Kirschner wires
Steinman pins
Rush rods, with instrumentation
Ortho wire and wire tightener
Bone clamps
Power drill
Compression set, small or large fragment or universal screw set

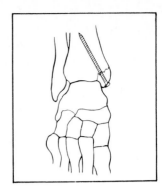

Fig. 22-150. Reduction of medial malleolar fracture with insertion of screw. (Courtesy Zimmer, Inc., Warsaw, Ind.)

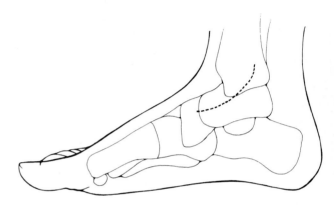

Fig. 22-151. Medial approach to ankle. (Modified from Nicola, T.: Atlas of orthopaedic exposures, Baltimore, 1966, The Williams & Wilkins Co.)

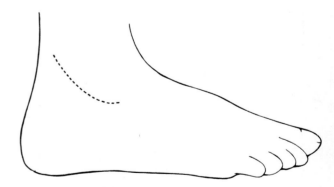

Fig. 22-152. Lateral approach to ankle. (Modified from Nicola, T.: Atlas of orthopaedic exposures, Baltimore, 1966, The Williams & Wilkins Co.)

Operative procedure—trimalleolar fracture

1. Incisions are made both medially and laterally across the ankle.

2. The posterior malleolar fracture is exposed and reduced with bone-holding clamps and manipulation.

3. The fracture is temporarily held in reduction with two

Kirschner wires inserted above the anterior tibial lip and directed anterior to posterior, engaging both fragments.

4. A drill hole is made anterior to posterior through both fragments. After measuring with a depth gauge, a malleolar, small cancellous, or other preferred screw is inserted through the fracture. The wires are removed.
5. The lateral malleolar fracture is then manipulated into reduction.
6. If the fracture is oblique and not comminuted, it is reduced with one or two lag screws placed anterior to posterior. If the fracture is transverse, a long screw or medullary pin is inserted across the fracture line into the canal of the proximal fragment. A small semitubular or one-third tubular plate is applied if the fracture occurs above the syndesmosis.
7. Once the posterior and lateral malleolar fractures have been fixed, the medial malleolar fracture is finally reduced with bone clamps.
8. The reduction is held with two Kirschner wires while a hole is drilled through the medial malleolus into the metaphysis of the tibia.
9. Once the appropriate length of screw is determined by a depth gauge, a malleolar screw is inserted across the fracture site. The Kirschner wires are removed.
10. If rotational stability is needed, an additional smaller screw or compression wiring is added.
11. The wounds are irrigated and closed, and a short or long leg cast is applied.

Triple arthrodesis

The talocalcaneal (subtalar), talonavicular, and calcaneocuboid joints must be fused in patients with marked inversion or eversion deformities of the foot. Such deformities occur in clubfoot, poliomyelitis, and rheumatoid arthritis. Occasionally, this operation is necessary for patients who have pain resulting from degenerative or traumatic arthritis. This triple fusion does not interfere with flexion and extension of the foot at the ankle joint (Fig. 22-153).

Procedural considerations. The patient is placed in the supine position. Instrumentation includes the ortho soft tissue and major bone sets, a small bone set, plus the following:

Bone graft instruments
Small vertebral spreader
Kirschner wires
Compression plate and screw set
Bone staple set
Micro power saw with blades

Operative procedure

1. An oblique incision is made laterally over the sinus tarsi.
2. To correct either eversion or inversion deformities, articular surfaces and bone wedges of the subtalar, calcaneocuboid, and talonavicular bones are resected.
3. Bone graft, compression plates, or bone staples are used to secure the bone surfaces together.
4. The wounds are closed, and cast immobilization is applied.

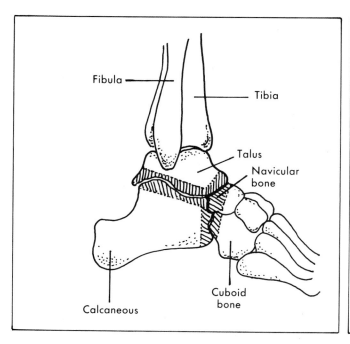
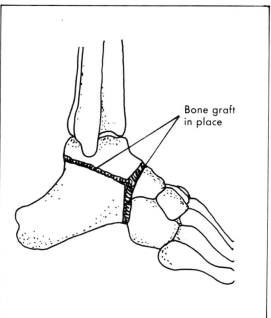

Fig. 22-153. Lateral views of joint fusion—triple arthrodesis. *Shading,* Area of bone to be resected. (From Brantley, P., and Analla, M.: The nurse and orthopedic surgery, Rutherford, N.J., 1980, Howmedica, Inc.)

Total ankle joint replacement

Because flexion and extension of the ankle joint are of great importance to weight bearing and ambulation, all efforts should be made to maintain this motion (Fig. 22-154). Ankle arthrodesis should be considered first in joint reconstructions; in certain situations, however, an ankle prosthesis is indicated. Indications include (1) failed arthrodesis, (2) bilateral ankle arthritis when arthrodesis has already been performed on one ankle, (3) after talectomy owing to avascular necrosis, and (4) revision of a previous arthroplasty. Total ankle replacement prostheses with high-density polyethylene and metal components have been developed. The Oregon, Imperial College London Hospital (ICLH), Waugh, University of California–Irvine (UCI), Newton (Fig 22-155), and Schultz are among the models available.

Procedural considerations. Ideally, total ankle joint replacement arthroplasty is performed in a laminar air flow room. A broad-spectrum antibiotic is given immediately prior to surgery and continued for 24 to 48 hours postoperatively.

Soft tissue, major bone, and small bone sets are required, plus the following:

Air-powered saw, small
Air-powered drill, small
Total ankle joint replacement system with implants
Methyl methacrylate, with instrumentation
Simpulse or Pulse Lavage (Figs. 22-87 and 22-88) and 3000-ml bag of normal saline solution

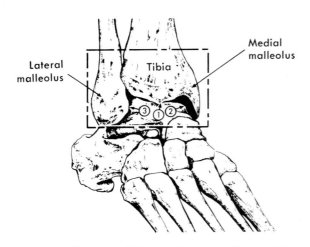

Fig. 22-154. Ankle joint with three motion points. (Courtesy Zimmer, Inc., Warsaw, Ind.)

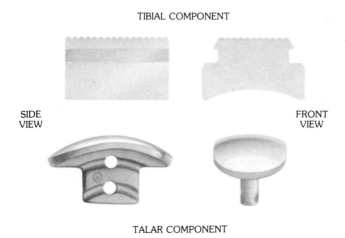

TIBIAL COMPONENT

SIDE VIEW   FRONT VIEW

TALAR COMPONENT

Fig. 22-155. Newton total ankle prosthesis. (Courtesy Howmedica Inc., Rutherford, N.J.)

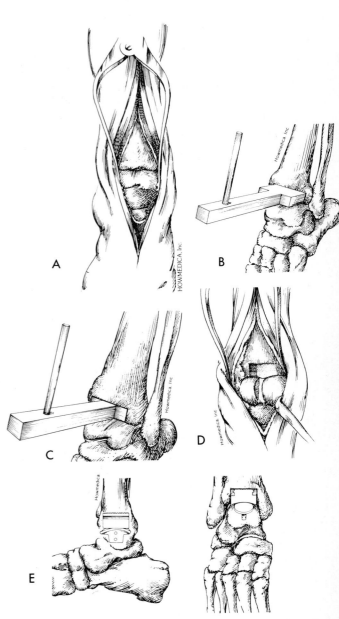

Fig. 22-156. Newton total ankle replacement technique. (Reprinted with permission from Howmedica, Inc., Rutherford, N.J.)

Operative procedure

1. An anterior incision is made over the ankle joint (Fig. 22-156, *A*).
2. Exposure of the tibiotalar joint and talus dome is achieved with dissection.
3. Once the center of the talus is identified and marked, a sizing template is used to mark the tibia (Fig. 22-156, *B*).
4. A 1-inch-wide by ⅜-inch-deep defect is made using the air drill, and then anchoring holes can be made in the tibia.
5. The template is positioned in the defect while the foot is distracted (Fig. 22-156, *C*).
6. The talus is marked and a ½-inch-deep by ³⁄₁₆-inch groove is made with a reciprocating saw to accommodate the talar component (Fig. 22-156, *D*).
7. A trial fit is carried out to assure that the talar unit is in the center of the talus and that the tibial unit is parallel to the plane of the floor, both centered over the dome of the talus.
8. Once trial reduction is complete, the talar and tibial components are cemented into place (Fig. 22-156, *E*).
9. A medium-sized suction drain is placed in the operative site, and the wound is closed.
10. A large, bulky pressure dressing (Robert-Jones) and a posterior splint are applied.

Bunionectomy

A bunion (hallux valgus) is a soft tissue or bony mass at the medial side of the first metarsal head. It is associated with a valgus deformity of the great toe (Fig. 22-157). A bunion is caused by a basic structural defect of the foot, which predisposes to the development of this deformity. Ill-fitting shoes accentuate the situation and speed the development of bunions. Bunions are 40 times more common in women because of their shoes (high heels and pointed toes). Other factors that may contribute to this deformity are heredity, flatfeet, foot pronation, longer first toe, muscle imbalance, and inflammatory disturbances of the feet.

Symptoms include pain on the dorsomedial aspect of the first metatarsal head or directly over the medial exostosis, swelling of the big toe, painful plantar callus, plantar keratosis, and discomfort to the entire foot as the forefoot in general becomes more fatigued and symptomatic, with pain radiating to the leg and knee.

Hallux valgus is treated with a variety of surgical procedures (Keller, McBride, Silver, Lapidus, Akin, and Mayo). All these procedures remove the exostosis and attempt to realign the great toe by removal of bone, transfer of tendons, osteotomy of the first metatarsal shaft, or appropriate imbrication of soft tissue.

The goals of surgery are correction of the deformity (cosmesis), resection of the abnormal bony components (reconstruction), and normal or near-normal range of motion (function).

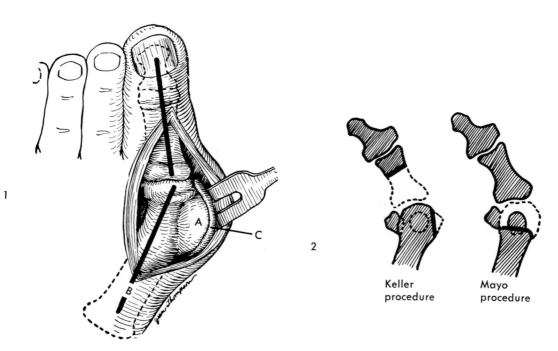

Fig. 22-157. 1, Bunion: *A,* exostosis of metatarsal head; *B,* hallux valgus deformity; *C,* overlying bursa. **2,** Operations for hallux valgus. (From Richards, V.: Surgery for general practice, St. Louis, 1956, The C.V. Mosby Co.)

Keller procedure

Mayo procedure

Procedural considerations. The patient is given general anesthesia, and a tourniquet is applied to the proximal thigh. The foot and leg are prepped and then draped free using a sterile stockinette. Small bone and minor soft tissue sets are required, plus the following:

Minidriver and microsaw
Kirschner wires
Microsaw blades

Operative procedure

1. A dorsal medial, curvilinear incision extending from the distal portion of the proximal phalanx of the great toe to the metatarsal cuneiform joint is commonly used.
2. Dissection is carried down through the joint capsule.
3. A flap incision is made to expose the underlying bone in order to resect the hypertrophic bone found at the dorsomedial aspect of the first metatarsal head.
4. One third of the proximal phalanx is also resected with a power oscillating saw.
5. The wound is then irrigated and closed, and a bandage is applied to maintain the toe in the rectus position. Postoperative convalescence requires a minimum of 6 weeks.

Correction of hammer-toe deformity

A hammer-toe flexion deformity develops at the proximal interphalangeal joint of four lateral toes. This deformity causes painful calluses on the dorsal joints of the four lateral toes, as the cocked-up digits rub against the shoes. The deformity is treated by incising the long extensor tendon to the toes and fusing the middle joint. A smooth Kirschner wire is frequently used to stabilize the fusion and position the toe properly during the postoperative period.

Procedural considerations. Small bone and minor soft tissue sets, Kirschner wires, pliers, and a microsaw and minidriver are needed.

Operative procedure

1. A straight, longitudinal incision is made over the dorsal medial or dorsal lateral area of the affected digits.
2. The capsular tissue of the distal third of the proximal phalanx and proximal interphalangeal joint is entered to expose the defect completely.
3. A small rongeur or microsaw is used to resect the distal third portion of the proximal phalanx.
4. Once the capital fragment is excised, the remaining portion of the distal proximal phalanx is debrided with a rongeur or rasp.
5. Digital alignment can be maintained with small Kirschner wires.
6. The wounds are irrigated and closed, and a sterile dressing and orthopedic wooden shoe are applied for postoperative recovery.

Correction of metatarsal fractures

Metatarsal fractures occur in various sites. These fractures have a reduced healing potential because metatarsals mainly consist of cortical bone, which lacks much vascularity. Treatment is determined by the extent of the fracture; the greater the displacement, the greater the need for reduction. In general, transverse and short, oblique midshaft fractures of the metatarsals are internally fixed because of their instability and displacement. Pins, wires, screws, and plates are used for internal fixation of metatarsal fractures. The simplest method is Kirschner wire fixation.

Procedural considerations. The patient is placed in the supine position. Minor soft tissue and small bone sets, a miniwire driver, and small Kirschner wires are needed.

Operative procedure

1. A small incision is made over the fracture.
2. The distal fragment is identified and retracted.
3. A smooth Kirschner wire is driven down distally, exiting the skin.
4. The miniwire driver is then switched and attached to the end protruding from the skin.
5. The pin is then driven back proximally into the canal of the proximal fragment.
6. If the fracture is more complex or comminuted, the fracture site is transfixed by crossing two Kirschner wires through the fracture.
7. The small incision is closed, and a short leg cast is applied.

Metatarsal head resection

Patients with rheumatoid arthritis frequently have dorsally dislocated toes and prominent and painful metatarsal heads on the plantar surfaces of the feet. Excision of all the metatarsal heads commonly relieves the pain and corrects an associated bunion deformity.

Procedural considerations. The patient is placed in a supine position, and a tourniquet is applied. The heads of the metatarsals are excised through a transverse plantar incision.

Small bone and minor soft tissue sets are required, plus the following:

Kirschner wires	Wire cutter
Microdrill	Pliers
Minidriver	

Metatarsal arthroplasty

Silastic implantation is indicated in the treatment of deformities associated with rheumatoid arthritis, hallux valgus, hallux rigidus, and a painful or unstable joint.

Procedural considerations. The patient is placed in the supine position. A tourniquet is applied, and the entire extremity is prepped and draped.

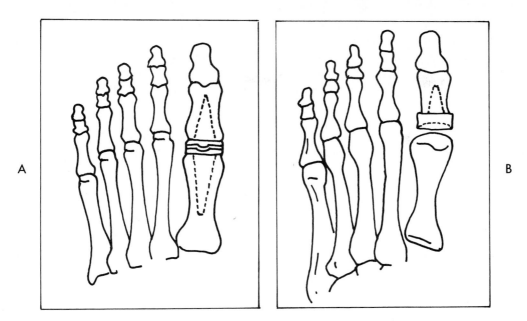

Fig. 22-158. A, Metatarsal implant, Swanson design. **B,** Great toe implant, Swanson design. (Courtesy Dow Corning Wright, Arlington, Tenn.)

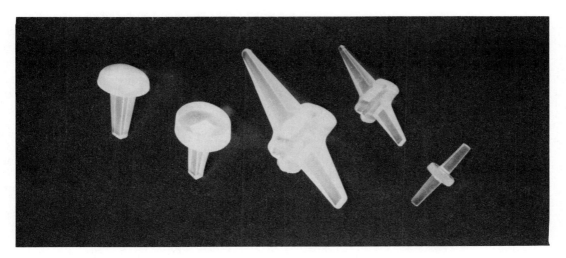

Fig. 22-159. Silastic orthopedic implants for the foot. (Courtesy Dow Corning Wright, Arlington, Tenn., and Alfred B. Swanson, M.D.)

Small bone and minor soft tissue sets are required, plus the following:

Microreamers
Minidriver
Trial and permanent implants (Figs. 22-158 and 22-159)
Microsaw with small blades

Operative procedure
1. The incision is made over the appropriate joints.
2. Resection of the proximal phalanx with removal of exostosis of the metatarsal head is carried out.

3. The medullary canal is reamed, and trial implants are fitted.
4. Once the appropriate-sized metatarsal implant is determined, it is seated.
5. The wound is irrigated and closed.
6. A bulky compression dressing and wooden shoe are applied for early ambulation.

Operations on the spinal column

Surgery of the spine, other than procedures for the treatment of scoliosis, is covered in Chapter 23.

Treatment of scoliosis

Scoliosis is a lateral deviation of the spinal column from the midline; it may include rotation or deformity of the vertebrae (Fig. 22-160). School screening programs provide quick and simple detection. For effective treatment of scoliosis, early detection is critical.

Some form of scoliosis occurs in one in ten people (Dell and Regan, 1987), affecting a million people in the United States. Two in 100 require medical treatment. Of all treated patients, 8% are female. Scoliosis can be idiopathic (80% of the time) or congenital and may result from muscular or neurologic diseases or unequal leg lengths (Dell and Regan, 1987).

Posterior spinal fusion with Harrington rods

Posterior spinal fusion is most frequently performed in adolescence, when the laterally deviated curve is still flexible.

Harrington rods are internal splints that help maintain the spine as straight as possible until the vertebral body fusion has become solid. The distraction rods are placed

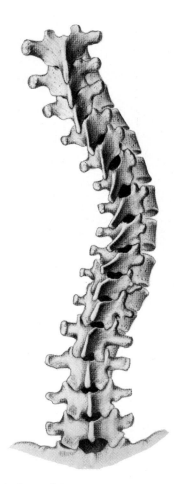

Fig. 22-160. Scoliosis deformity. (Courtesy Zimmer, Inc., Warsaw, Ind.)

on the concave side of the curve, and compression rods are placed on the convex side. On the convex side of the curve, three to eight hooks are inserted in the transverse processes of the vertebrae and pulled together with a threaded rod. In this way the scoliotic deformity can be corrected as much as the flexibility of the spine allows.

The posterior elements of the vertebrae are denuded of soft tissue, and the bone graft is added. Considerable blood is lost in this extensive operative procedure, and an accurate record of the loss must be maintained. After surgery the patient is placed in an immobilizing jacket.

Some disadvantages of the Harrington rod system over other systems are that there is only end-point fixation, rod breakage is increased, fixation is less, sagittal plane curves are difficult to manage, distraction for correction is not always desired, and the patient will have to wear a postoperative cast or brace.

Procedural considerations. The patient is placed in the prone position on the Wilson (Fig. 22-15, *A*) or Andrews frame (Fig. 22-15, *B*) or with rolls under the chest and abdomen to facilitate respiration. Before the procedure begins, an x-ray cassette is placed under the patient so an x-ray film for accurate identification of the vertebrae to be fused can be taken during the operation. A single straight longitudinal incision is made down the midline of the back. Because of the amount of bleeding, the skin and subcutaneous tissues are often infiltrated with a vasoconstricting solution, such as epinephrine.

Basic back instrumentation and Harrington rod instrumentation include the following (Fig. 22-161):

Distraction rods (relatively heavy rods, ratcheted on one end)
Compression rods (somewhat flexible threaded rods with nuts designed to maintain force against each of separate hooks used with compression rods)
Distraction and compression hooks (anchor distraction and compression rods to vertebrae)
Hook clamps (hold hooks during insertion and manipulation)
Rod clamps (hold and stabilize rod as corrective forces are applied with spreader)
Spreader (advances the ratchets through hooks)
Drivers (drive various hooks into prepared area of vertebrae)
Wrench (turns nuts on compression rod)
Outrigger (designed to apply distracting forces temporarily during operation but is out of operative field; replaced by distraction rod after vertebrae have been prepared to receive bone graft)
Heavy wire or washer (placed between distraction hook in last ratchet on rod to prevent slippage)
Large pin cutter (designed to cut large pins but provided with small end so it will fit in wound)

A separate instrument table is used for the Harrington rod equipment.

Operative procedure

1. The appropriate hooks are selected and inserted. A Harrington distraction rod of appropriate length is inserted through the two proximal self-adjusting hooks, which have been placed under the laminae.

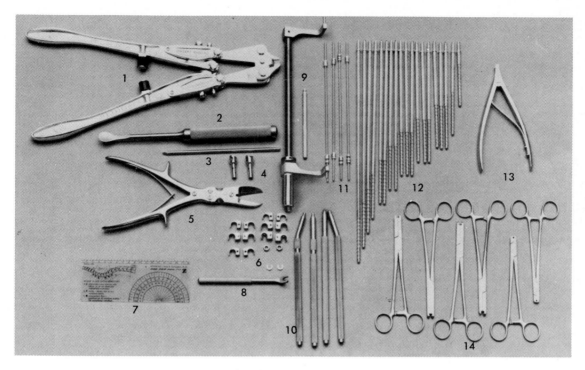

Fig. 22-161. Harrington rod instruments. *1,* Pin cutter; *2,* Harrington special elevator; *3,* Steinman pin; *4,* sacral rod, nut, and eyelet; *5,* large bone cutter; *6,* hooks for distraction rod; *7,* protractor; *8,* flat wrench; *9,* outrigger distraction unit; *10,* drivers; *11,* compression rod assembly; *12,* distraction rods; *13,* spreader; *14,* hook clamps.

2. A rod clamp is clamped onto the Harrington rod just below the hook, and a single regular spreader is used to obtain the first inch of distraction.
3. The Bobechko spreader is used to span over the first hook, closest to the smooth part of the rod, to apply distraction force on the most proximal hook.
4. Two C locking rings are inserted around the first ratchet immediately below the hook to prevent dislodgment of the hooks. The excessive length of protruding rod above the most proximal hook is cut off with a rod cutter. The compression is tightened.

Luque segmental spinal rod procedure

The Luque segmental method employs smooth, L-shaped, stainless steel rods, usually ³⁄₁₆ or ¼ inch in diameter, with sublaminar wires placed at every level possible. It is more secure and longer than the Harrington rod system, does not require distraction, and needs no postoperative cast. However, patients lose approximately 1 unit of blood for each hour of surgery, the rods are difficult to remove, and there is increased risk of neurologic trauma.

Luque instrumentation applies corrective forces to the spinal segments at each level, thereby spreading the corrective forces throughout the length of the deformity. Two Luque rods are wired to both sides of the spine. The rods are contoured to achieve no more than 10 degrees of in-creased correction beyond that exhibited on preoperative x-ray study.

Procedural considerations. The patient is placed in the prone position on the Wilson (Fig. 22-14, *A*) or Andrews frame (Fig. 22-14, *B*) or with rolls under the chest and abdomen to facilitate respiration. A straight midline incision is made in the back. Because of the amount of bleeding, the skin and subcutaneous tissues are often infiltrated with a vasoconstricting solution such as epinephrine.

Basic back instrumentation, Luque rods and instrumentation (Figs. 22-162 through 22-164), a wire tightener, and a wire cutter are needed.

Operative procedure
1. The ligamentum flavum is detached, exposing the neural canal.
2. Doubled stainless steel suture wire is passed under the lamina. The wire loop will be cut later to form two wires at each level.
3. Total bilateral facetectomies are made, forming posterolateral troughs for subsequent bone grafts.
4. Wedge osteotomies may be necessary in severe immobile curves to avoid stretching the spinal cord during correction.
5. The wire loop is cut, resulting in two separate wires at each level.

6. Rod migration is prevented by securing the L bend to the base of the spinous process.
7. Initial placement of the convex rod is made.
8. Initial placement of the concave rod is made.
9. Transverse wiring is done to add increased stability to the system.
10. Stabilization of the lumbosacral joint is corrected by bending the rods distally to form sacral bars.

Wisconsin compression system procedure

The Wisconsin compression system is a refinement of the Harrington compression instrumentation designed for correcting and stabilizing deformities and fractures. It was developed to overcome technical difficulties observed during surgery with compression instrumentation.

The Wisconsin compression system (Fig. 22-165) considerably reduces operating time and provides a valuable addition for treatment of kyphotic deformities, the convex side of thoracic scoliosis, unstable spine fractures and dislocations, and neuromuscular scoliosis.

Procedural considerations. The patient is placed in the prone position, as with Harrington rod insertion. Basic back instrumentation and the Wisconsin compression unit are needed.

Operative procedure
1. A midline incision is made, and the spine is exposed by a subperiosteal dissection.
2. A sharp Keene hook is used to create the purchase sites on the transverse processes or laminae.

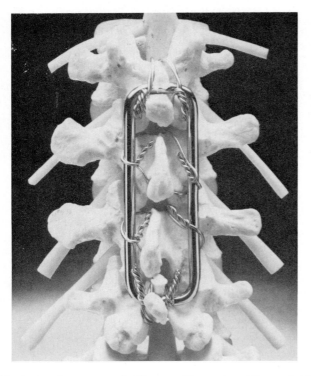

Fig. 22-162. Luque rectangle. (Courtesy Zimmer, Inc., Warsaw, Ind.)

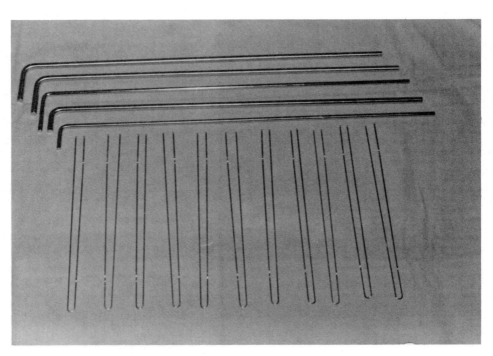

Fig. 22-163. Luque rods and wires. (Courtesy Zimmer, Inc., Warsaw, Ind.)

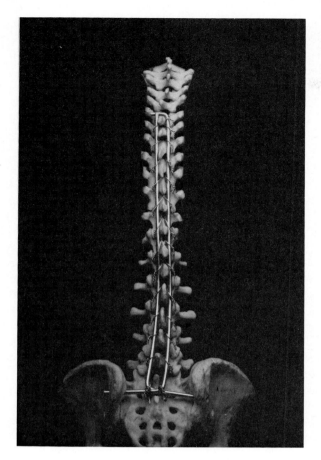

Fig. 22-164. Luque segmental spinal rod technique. (Courtesy Zimmer, Inc., Warsaw, Ind.)

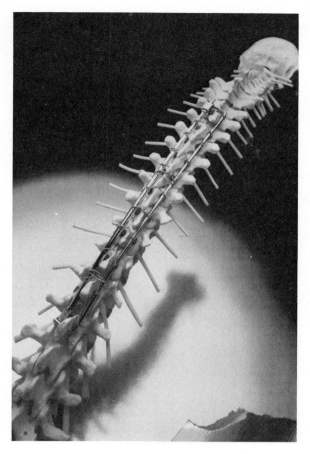

Fig. 22-165. Wisconsin segmental spinal unit. (Courtesy Zimmer, Inc., Warsaw, Ind.)

3. Blunt Keene hooks are placed at each level as desired. Each hook is controlled by a Drummond hook holder.
4. The compression rod with mounted bushings and nuts is passed through windows in all the holders.
5. The rod is pressed down into the hook, and the bushing is advanced into the slot of the hook, sequentially securing each hook to the rod.
6. The nut is advanced to adjust the compression, and the threads behind each nut are crimped to secure the assembly permanently.

Cotrel Dubousset system procedure

The Cotrel Dubousset system provides three-dimensional correction of spinal deformities without sublaminar wiring and its neurologic risks. This instrumentation permits distraction, compression, or derotation. Correction of scoliosis is brought about by derotation and, at the same time, restoration of the normal sagittal contours. In addition to correction of scoliosis, the Cotrel Dubousset system can be applied to correct kyphosis or lordosis and to stabilize and rebuild the spine after tumor resection or after traumatic injury. No external support is necessary. The Cotrel Dubousset system (Fig. 22-166) has no ratchets or notches. It consists of metallic rods with diamond crosscut patterns on which hooks and screws can be positioned in any position, level, or degree of rotation. The rod is held in the open hooks with blockers. The rods are then interlocked by means of devices for transverse traction (DTT).

Procedural considerations. The patient is placed in the prone position under general anesthesia. Basic back instrumentation, bone graft instruments, and the Cotrel Dubousset system and instrumentation are required (Fig. 22-167).

Operative procedure
1. Closed hooks are inserted at both ends of the surgical site, and open hooks are inserted at various levels in between.
2. Decortication and facet excision are done at the remaining interposed vertebrae levels for rod placement.
3. Bone graft is placed in the areas that will be under the rod.
4. The appropriate concave rod is bent to shape for sagittal plane correction and manipulated into the end hooks.
5. Stabilization along the length is achieved with blockers that anchor the rod into the open hooks.

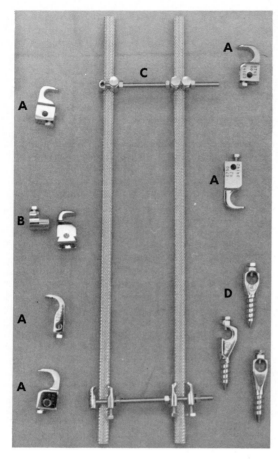

Fig. 22-166. Cotrel-Dubousset spinal system. **A,** Closed hooks. **B,** Open hook with blocker. **C,** Spinal rods with attached devices for transverse traction (DTT). **D,** Sacral screws. (With permission from Stuart, Greensburg, Pa.)

6. The spine is then derotated using the rod holders. The frontal plane scoliosis curve becomes the sagittal plane kyphosis.
7. Hooks are reseated for secure fixation.
8. To correct kyphosis, the convex rod is then bent to shape and seated.
9. Once the rods have been placed, final stabilization is completed by applying the DTT, usually near the ends of the rods.
10. Remaining bone graft is applied to the fusion area.

Texas Scottish Rite Hospital (TSRH) crosslink system

The TSRH crosslink system (Fig. 22-168) is a multi-component stainless steel implant used to rigidly lock spinal rods together. Locking the rods increases construct stiffness and prevents rod migration. The system was originally designed for the Luque segmental system to prevent migration between the rods and wires before complete fusion occurred. By rigidly crosslinking the rods, loss of scoliotic correction was reduced. This system can also be utilized with the Harrington and Cotrel Dubousset systems. Crosslinks are indicated when the rigidity of a spinal system alone is not sufficient to generate fusion in a reasonable amount of time.

Operative procedure
1. Eyebolts are placed on the spinal rods before the rods are implanted.
2. The rods are secured with hooks or wires, depending on the system used.
3. Once the rods are positioned, cross plates of varying widths accommodating different rod-to-rod distances are bolted in placed between the rods and nuts.

Anterior spinal fusion with Dwyer instrumentation

Anterior spinal fusion is most frequently performed in patients with idiopathic thoracolumbar scoliosis and lordosis, especially when associated with posterior spinal deficiencies or congenital anomalies of the spine. This system is sometimes combined with Harrington instrumentation for the correction of paralytic scoliosis or pelvic obliquity.

Procedural considerations. The patient is placed in the lateral decubitus position with the convex side of the curve superior. The upper arm is brought forward so the scapula rotates away from the vertebral column. The kidney rest is elevated at the apex of the curve. An anterolateral incision is made over the curvature area to provide exposure. A rib is exposed, resected, and saved for the bone graft.

Routine thoracotomy and spinal instrumentation is required, plus Dwyer instrumentation (Fig. 22-169), which consists of the following:

Cables	Cable tensioner
Staples	Staple starter
Screws	Staple introducer (functions as
Buttons	staple holder and impactor)
Collar	Screwdriver
Crimper	Ratchet spanner

Operative procedure
1. The lateral portion of the spinal column is exposed, and the intervertebral discs along the curve are removed using a rongeur.
2. The vertebral end plates are excised, using a chisel or curette.
3. Using the staple starter, a purchase site for the first staple leg is prepared in the disc above the first vertebra to receive instruments. The proper size staple is selected according to the calibrations on the staple starter.
4. The selected staple is placed on the staple introducer, and the handle is tightened. With a mallet the staple is placed snugly over the vertebral body. During impaction of the staple, the staple introducer also makes a starter hole for the screw.
5. A cancellous screw of proper length is selected and, with the screwdriver, is inserted into the first vertebral body. The staple and screw insertions are repeated for

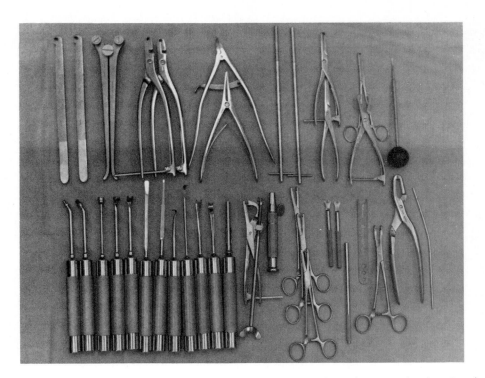

Fig. 22-167. Cotrel-Dubousset spinal system instrumentation. *Top (left to right):* In-situ benders, French bender, rod grippers, curved spreader, DTT spreader, hex screwdrivers, rod holder, DTT shaft holder, set screw holder, pedicle locator. *Bottom:* Inserter for closed hook, inserter for open hook, bone pusher, blocker pushers, 10-mm osteotome, 3-mm osteotome, laminar elevator, transverse process elevator, rod driver, pedicle elevator, screwdriver for sacral screws, bulb hook holder, staple inserter, hook holders, wrenches, DTT hook holder, open wrench, curved hook holder, hook compressor, malleable guide. (With permission from Stuart, Greensburg, Pa.)

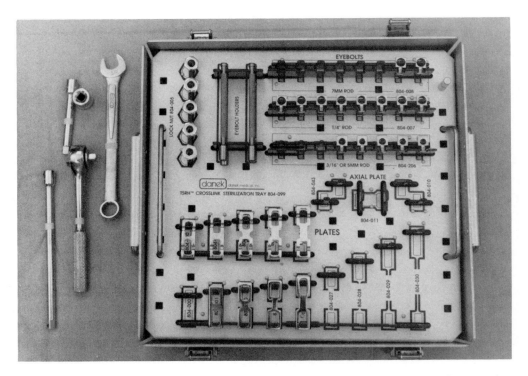

Fig. 22-168. Texas Scottish Rite Hospital (TSRH) crosslink spinal system. (With permission from Danek, Memphis, Tenn.)

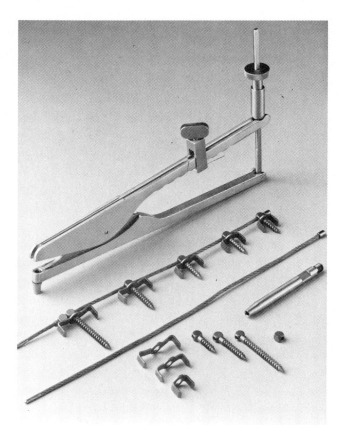

Fig. 22-169. Dwyer instrumentation. (Courtesy Zimmer, Inc., Warsaw, Ind.)

the second vertebral body, except that the second screw is not completely tightened down until after the cable has been passed through.

6. A cable is passed through the cancellous screw head, and the second screw is tightened down so the cable is straight.

7. A bone graft is prepared from the resected rib. The rib is cut into small pieces, some of which are placed between the vertebral bodies.

8. The cable tensioner is applied to shorten the distance between the screws. As the cable is tightened, the curve is straightened.

9. To keep the cable from slipping, the cannulated screw heads are crimped to the cable with a crimper before the cable tightener is removed.

10. Following crimping of the last screw head, the cable is passed through an end button. The end button is positioned adjacent to the last screw head and is crimped onto the cable as a safety lock. A collar is slipped onto the cable and clamped adjacent to the end button to prevent the cable from unraveling. Finally, the cable is cut off flush with the collar.

Anterior spinal fusion with Zielke instrumentation

Zielke instrumentation involves screw fixation into each vertebral body, complete disc excision and grafting, and segmental connection of the vertebral bodies. A semirigid rod connects the segments. The Zielke technique is the preferred method of anterior spinal instrumentation for thoracolumbar and lumbar scoliosis. The average blood

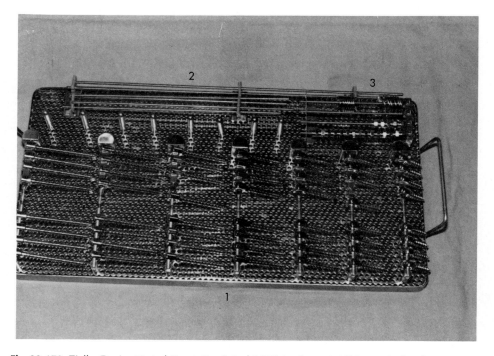

Fig. 22-170. Zielke Device Ventral Derotating Spinal (VDS) implants. *1,* VDS superior head open screws, 25, 30, 35, 40, 45, 50, and 55 mm, and VDS lateral head open screws, 25, 30, 35, 40, 45, 50, and 55 mm (four each); *2,* VDS compression rods, 200 mm (four) and 300 mm (two); *3,* VDS hex nuts (20).

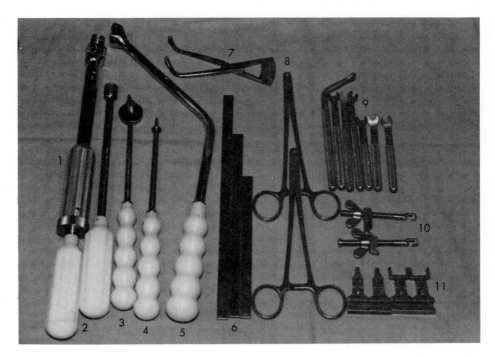

Fig. 22-171. Zielke Device Ventral Derotating Spinal (VDS) fusion instrumentation. *1*, Cardan screwdriver (angle adjustable); *2*, VDS screwdriver with plastic handle; *3*, rectangular awl; *4*, straight awl; *5*, Zielke derotation level; *6*, derotator splints, long, 150, 200, and 250 mm; *7*, goniometer; *8*, two Harrington rod clamps; *9*, seven VDS wrenches; *10*, two tension screws for derotator; *11*, two single and two double slides.

loss for the patient is 1300 ml. The advantages of anterior spinal fusion and instrumentation are correction of pelvic obliquity, increase in fusion rate when combined with posterior fusion, and shorter fusion.

Procedural considerations. The patient is positioned 20 degrees back from the lateral position on a vacuum beanbag positioning device, with the convex side of the scoliosis upward. The top leg is extended, and the bottom leg is flexed to obtain stability. The rib to be resected is one or two levels above the top vertebra to receive implants in the curve.

The skin incision is started at the edge of the paraspinous muscles and extended to the costochondral junction over the chosen rib.

Basic back instrumentation, Zielke implants and instrumentation (Figs. 22-170 and 22-171), and a rib tray are required.

REFERENCES

Buckham, K.R.: Surgical bone banking: recommendations for setting up a program, AORN J. 50:764, 1989.

Dell, D.D., and Regan, R.: Juvenile idiopathic scoliosis, Orthopaedic Nursing 6(6):23, 1987.

Orsini, E.C., and others: Cardiopulmonary function and pulmonary microemboli during arthroplasty using cemented or non-cemented components, J. Bone Joint Surg. 69A:822, 1987.

BIBLIOGRAPHY

Aiello, D.H.: Congenital dysplasia of the hip, AORN J. 49:1566, 1989.

Alexander, J.P., and Barron, D.W.: Biomechanical disturbances associated with total hip replacement, J. Bone Joint Surg. 61B:101, 1979.

Allen, B.L., and Ferguson, R.L.: The Galveston technique for L-rod instrumentation of the scoliotic spine, Spine 7:276, 1982.

Andrews, J.R., and Carson, W.B.: Shoulder joint arthroscopy, Orthopaedics 6:1157, 1983.

Andrews, J.R., and Carson, W.B.: Arthroscopy of the elbow, Arthroscopy 1(2):97, 1985.

Andrews, J.R., Farrell, J., and Carson, W.G.: Arthroscopy of the elbow, videotape no. 119, American Academy of Orthopaedic Surgeons, 1983.

Beaudet, F., and Dixon, J.: Posterior subtalar joint synoviography and corticoid injection on rheumatoid arthritis, Ann. Rheum. Dis. 40:132, 1981.

Blauvelt, C.T., and Nelson, F.R.T.: A manual of orthopaedic terminology, ed. 2, St. Louis, 1981, The C.V. Mosby Co.

Brown, C.: Continuity of care for the orthopedic patient, AORN J. 31:1128, 1980.

Brown, C.: The child undergoing anterior spinal surgery, Orthop. Nurs. 1:33, 1982.

Caspari, R.B.: Shoulder arthroscopy: a review of the present state of the art, Contemp. Orthop. 4:523, 1982.

Chandler, H.P., and others: Total hip replacement in patients younger than 30 years old: a five year follow-up, J. Bone Joint Surg. 63A(9):1426, 1981.

Chao, E.Y., and others: Symposium: external fixators—scientific research and clinical applications, Contemporary Orthopedics 18:65, 1989.

Chapman, M.W.: Operative orthopedics, Philadelphia, 1988, J.B. Lippincott Co.

Clancy, W.G., and Graf, B.K.: Arthroscopic meniscal repair, Orthopaedics 6(9):1125, 1983.

Connolly, J.F.: DePalma's the management of fractures and dislocations: an atlas, Philadelphia, 1981, W.B. Saunders Co.

Crenshaw, A.H., editor: Campbell's operative orthopaedics, ed. 7, St. Louis, 1987, The C.V. Mosby Co.

Donahoo, C.A., and Spickler, L., editors: Core curriculum of orthopedic nursing, Atlanta, 1980, Orthopedic Nurses Assocation.

Dorr, L.D., Carn, R.M., and Bloebaum, R.: Proximal femoral metaphyseal porous-coated implants for hip replacement arthroplasty, Contemp. Orthop. 9(5):15, 1984.

Dorr, L.D., Takei, G.K., and Conaty, J.P.: Total hip arthroplasty in patients under 45 years, J. Bone Joint Surg. 65A:450, 1983.

Drummond, D., and Keene, J.: A technique of segmental spinal instrumentation without the passing of sublaminar wires, Mediguide Orthop. 6(2):1, 1985.

Dwyer, A.P., and Schafer, M.F.: Anterior approach to scoliosis, J. Bone Joint Surg. 56B:218, 1974.

Electrical stimulation: an alternative to bone grafting, Englewood, Colo., 1980, Teletronics Orthopedic Division of Teletronic Proprietary, Ltd.

Engh, C.A.: Hip arthroplasty with a Moore prosthesis with porous coating, Clin. Orthop. 176:52, 1983.

Feagin, J.A.: Arthroscopy—assisted patellar tendon substitution for anterior cruciate ligament insufficiency: surgical technique, Am. J. Knee Surg. 2:3, 1989.

Ferris, B.D., and Kinsella, M.: Fatal complications of the distal fractures of the femur, Injury 16:207, 1984.

Freeman, M.A.R., McLeod, H.C., and Levai, J.P.: Total arthroplasty of the knee and hip, Clin. Orthop. 176:88, 1983.

Gallagher, L.L.: Shoulder arthroplasty, Nursing '80 10(7):46, 1980.

Gibson, T.P., and Turick-Gibson, T.: The Insall procedure: a method of anterior cruciate ligament reconstruction, AORN J. 48:466, 1988.

Glousman, R., and others: Treatment of femoral neck fractures with total hip replacements vs. cemented and uncemented hemiarthroplasty. Submitted to Western Orthopaedic Association Meeting for presentation, October 1984.

Goldstein, T.B.: Chemonucleolysis: another look, Contemp. Orthop. 10(4), 1985.

Green, S.A.: Ilizarov methods: innovations from a Siberian surgeon, AORN J. 49:215, 1989.

Hales, A.L.: Arthroscopically assisted anterior cruciate ligament reconstruction, AORN J. 49:234, 1989.

Hampel, G.: Closed interlocking nailing in the lower extremity, AORN J. 47:1203, 1988.

Harris, W.H., and others: Bony ingrowth fixation of the acetabular component in canine hip joint arthroplasty, Clin. Orthop. 176:7, 1983.

Hendler, R.C.: Arthroscopic meniscal repair: surgical technique, Clin. Orthop. 190:163, 1984.

Hilt, N.E., and Cogburn, S.B.: Manual of orthopedics, St. Louis, 1980, The C.V. Mosby Co.

Hoek, K.J., Bowen, W.W., and Schulz, W.P.: Cement removal techniques in revision hip arthroplasty, Contemp. Orthop. 10(1):83, 1985.

Hollinshead, W.J.: Anatomy for surgeons, Philadelphia, 1982, Harper & Row.

Jackson D.W., and Drez, D., Jr.: The anterior cruciate deficient knee, St. Louis, 1987, The C.V. Mosby Co.

Jackson, R.W.: Arthroscopic surgery, J. Bone Joint Surg. 65(3):416, 1983.

Jahss, M.H.: Disorders of the foot, Philadelphia, 1982, W.B. Saunders Co.

Jay, R.M.: Current therapy in podiatric surgery, Toronto, 1989, B.C. Decker.

Johnson, L.L.: Diagnostic and surgical arthroscopy: the knee and other joints, ed. 2, St. Louis, 1981, The C.V. Mosby Co.

Kane, W.J.: A technique for insertion of the totally implantable bone growth stimulator, Englewood, Colo., 1979, Telectronics Orthopedic Division of Teletronic Proprietary, Ltd.

Kleinbeck, S.V.M.: Developing nursing diagnoses for a perioperative care plan: a classroom research project, AORN J. 49:1613, 1989.

Larson, R.L.: Combined instabilities of the knee, Clin. Orthop. 147:68, 1980.

Lewis, R.C.: Primary care orthopedics, New York, 1988, Churchill Livingstone.

Lombardo, S.J.: Arthroscopy of the shoulder, Clin. Sports Med. 2:309, 1983.

Lopez, J.O., and Silva, I.: Shoulder arthroscopy: a diagnostic and therapeutic tool, AORN J. 48:1078, 1988.

Luque, E.R.: The anatomic basis and development of segmental spinal instrumentation, Spine 7:256, 1982.

Lynch, M., Henning, C.E., and Glick, K.R.: Knee joint surface changes, Clin. Orthop. 172:148, 1983.

Mann, R.A., editor: Surgery of the foot, ed. 5, St. Louis, 1986, The C.V. Mosby Co.

Matthews, L.S.: Shoulder anatomy for the arthroscopist, Arthroscopy 1(2):83, 1985.

Metcalf, R.W.: Arthroscopic knee surgery, Adv. Surg. 17:197, 1984.

Morscher, E.W.: Cementless total hip arthroplasty, Clin. Orthop. 181:76, 1983.

Neer, C.S., Watson, K.C., and Stanton, F.J.: Recent experience in total shoulder replacement, J. Bone Joint Surg. 64A(3):319, 1982.

Nichols, C.D.: Wrist arthroscopy: an ambulatory surgery procedure, AORN J. 49:759, 1989.

Parisien, J.S., and Vangsness, T.: Arthroscopy of the subtalar joint, Arthrosc. Relat. Surg. 1(1):53, 1985.

Patel, D., and Denoncourt, P.: Arthroscopic surgery: coordinating portals for operative arthroscopy, Contemp. Orthop. 10(1):43, 1985.

Paterson, D.C., Lewis, G.N., and Cass, C.A.: Treatment of delayed union and nonunion with an implanted direct current stimulator, Clin. Orthop. 148:117, 1980.

Quattro, L.S.: Spinal stabilization: an introduction to Cotrel-DuBousset instrumentation, AORN J. 46:54, 1987.

Richardson, W.J., and Garrett, W.E., Jr.: Clinical uses of continuous passive motion, Contemp. Orthop. 10(1):75, 1985.

Roaf, R., and Hopkinson, L.J.: Textbook of orthopedic nursing, ed. 3, Oxford, 1980, Blackwell Scientific Publications.

Rowe, C.R.: The shoulder, New York, 1988, Churchill Livingstone.

St. Anthony Medical Center Tissue Bank: Bone donation: answers to commonly asked questions, Columbus, 1988, Franciscan Health Systems of Central Ohio.

Schonholtz, G.J., and Ling, B.: Arthroscopic chondroplasty of the patella, Arthroscopy 1(2):92, 1985.

Silo, H.M.: Perioperative nursing research, AORN J. 49:1627, 1989.

Skinner, H., and Cook, S.: Fatigue failure stress of femoral neck, Am. J. Sports Med. 10(4):245, 1982.

Spiegel, P.G.: Topics in orthopaedic trauma, Baltimore, 1984, University Park Press.

Sprague, N.F.: Arthroscopic surgery: degenerative and traumatic flap tears of the meniscus, Contemp. Orthop. 9(4):23, 1984.

Stone, R.G., Nolan, S.E., and Ryan, J.P.: Meniscus preservation. Presented at AANA Annual Meeting, 1984.

Taillard, W., Meyer, J., Garcia, J., and Blanc, Y.: The sinus tarsi syndrome, Int. Orthop. 5:117, 1981.

Tobiason, S.J.: The arthritis patient comes to surgery, AORN J. 32:608, 1980.

Tomford, W.W., and others: Methods of banking bone and cartilage for allograft transplanting, Orth. Clin. North Am. 18(2):241, 1987.

Wilde, A.H., and Borden, L.S.: Experience with the Neer total shoulder replacement, Orthop. Transact. 5:397, 1981.

23 Neurosurgery

RUTH E. VAIDEN

Perioperative nurses must understand the structure and function of the nervous system to provide intelligent, safe, humanistic care for neurosurgical patients. From a range of variables of normal development, they must identify those critical for each patient and recognize and respond to a variety of dependency needs, such as the normal response to preoperative sedation, as well as pathologic conditions such as paralysis, aphasia, or coma. Based on an understanding of the many pathologic conditions that result in surgical intervention, they must plan and manage complex patient care. They must be familiar with the use, care, working order, and safety factors of sophisticated instrumentation. They need to appreciate the limitations and stresses facing neurosurgeons. Anticipating and responding to potential complications inherent in specific patients, procedures, and neurosurgical emergencies require great speed but the same care and precision as elective situations. Basic general information to assist perioperative nurses to function effectively in their own clinical settings is presented here.

SURGICAL ANATOMY

The nervous system, the most complex and least understood of body systems, has been divided in various ways to simplify study. Structural divisions are the central nervous system (brain and spinal cord) and the peripheral nervous system (cranial and spinal nerves)

Nervous system tissue is composed of neurons and neuroglial cells that support the neurons. The brain and spinal cord are protected by bony structures. The cranial nerves originate within the brain and emerge through openings in the skull to run peripherally. The spinal nerves that emerge from the spinal cord through the vertebral foramina also run peripherally. In this chapter, therefore, peripheral nerves are those outside the cranial cavity and vertebral canal.

The nervous system is divided functionally into voluntary and autonomic (involuntary) systems. The nervous system functions as the communication system for the rest of the body. The functions of all body systems are dependent, in part, on nervous system function. In turn, the nervous system is directly dependent on circulatory system function for life-sustaining glucose and oxygen. Nervous system functions include orientation, coordination, conceptual thought, emotion, memory, and reflex response.

Within the framework of neurosurgical techniques, logical divisions of the nervous system are the head, or cranium; the back, or spine; and the peripheral nerves. These subdivisions lend themselves to meaningful discussion of supporting structures, body positions, instrumentation, and other considerations useful to the nurse providing care for neurosurgical patients during the intraoperative phase of care.

Head

Scalp layers of the head (Fig. 23-1) include skin, subcutaneous tissue, galea, and occipitofrontal musculature. Scalp skin is thick. The subcutaneous tissue, which is exceptionally dense, tough, and vascular, is firmly attached to the galea. Most of the blood vessels lie superficial to the galea. The subgaleal space contains loose areolar tissue that permits mobility of the scalp. The pericranium, or outer periosteum of the skull, separates the galea from the cranium.

The arterial supply of the scalp comes from the external carotid artery through the superficial temporal, posterior auricular, occipital, frontal, and supraorbital branches. Most veins roughly follow the course of the arteries, except emissary veins that drain directly through the skull into the intracranial venous sinuses. Unlike the arteries, the surface veins of the brain have many large anastomoses. The scalp, the extracranial arteries, and portions of the dura mater are the only pain-sensitive structures that cover the brain, which itself is insensitive.

The skull is formed by 24 bones, joined by serrated bony seams called *sutures*. Eight bones form the walls of the cranial cavity, which houses the brain. There are four single bones—frontal, occipital, ethmoid, and sphenoid—and four paired bones—temporal and parietal (Fig. 23-2). The coronal suture joins the frontal and parietal bones. The squamous sutures border the squamous part of the temporal bones. The lambdoid suture joins the occipital and parietal bones. The sagittal suture lies in the medial plane and joins the two parietal bones (Fig. 23-3).

At the top of the skull in front of and behind the parietal bones are the anterior and posterior fontanelles, which are open at birth. The posterior fontanelle is closed by 2 months and the anterior by about 18 months after birth.

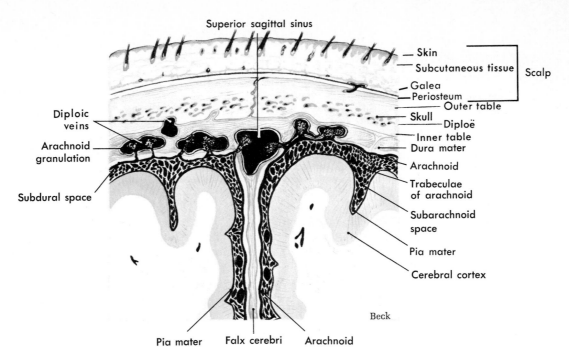

Fig. 23-1. Scalp is composed of following layers: skin, subcutaneous tissue, galea, and periosteum of skull. Skull bone has three tables: outer, diploë or spongy layer, and inner. Dura mater lies beneath skull and completely encapsulates brain. Other structures are identified for reference and are described in text. (Modified from Anthony, C.P., and Kolthoff, N.J.: Textbook of anatomy and physiology, ed. 9, St. Louis, 1975, The C.V. Mosby Co.)

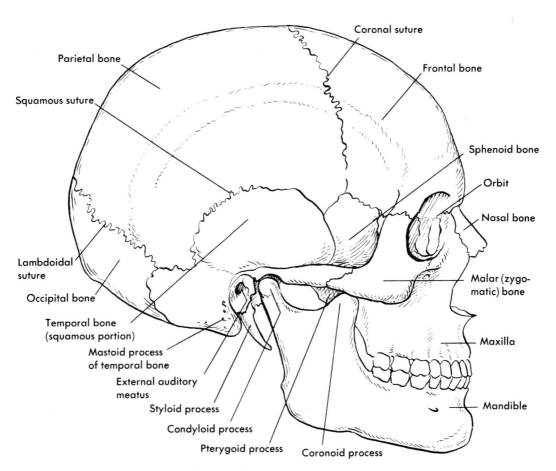

Fig. 23-2. Skull viewed from right side. (From Anthony, C.P., and Kolthoff, N.J.: Textbook of anatomy and physiology, ed. 9, St. Louis, 1975, The C.V. Mosby Co.)

If the suture lines close prematurely, the skull cannot expand as the brain grows. This condition, *craniosynostosis,* demands early surgical intervention.

The skull is ovoid and is wider in back than in front. The flattened, irregular bones consist of two tables of compact bone that enclose a layer of spongy bone, or *diploë* (Fig. 23-1).

The interior of the skull is anatomically divided into three cranial fossae: anterior, middle, and posterior (Fig. 23-4). The anterior fossa is limited posteriorly by the sphenoid ridge, along which pituitary tumors and aneurysms of the circle of Willis are generally approached. The frontal lobes and olfactory bulbs and tracts lie in the anterior fossa. The temporal lobes lie in the middle fossa, which is shaped like a butterfly. The sella turcica, formed by the sphenoid bone, is the most central part of the middle fossa and houses the pituitary gland. The floor and lateral walls of the middle fossa are shaped from the greater wings of the sphenoid bone and parts of the temporal bone, which house the internal and middle ear structures (Fig. 23-4). The posterior fossa, the largest and deepest fossa, is formed by the occipital, sphenoid, and petrous portions of the temporal bones; the cerebellum, pons, and medulla lie

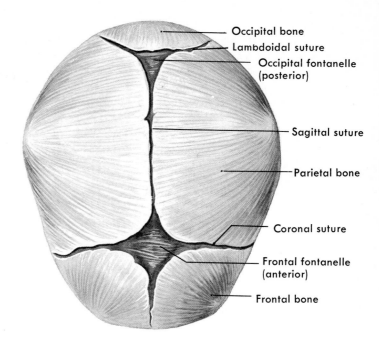

Fig. 23-3. Skull at birth viewed from above. (Modified from Anthony, C.P., and Kolthoff, N.J.: Textbook of anatomy and physiology, ed. 9, St. Louis, 1975, The C.V. Mosby Co.)

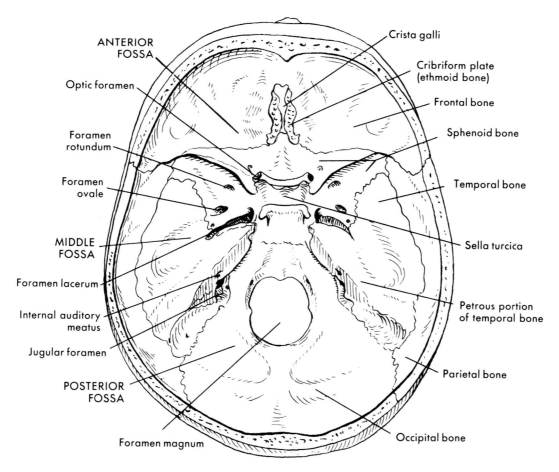

Fig. 23-4. Floor of cranial cavity. (Modified from Anthony, C.P., and Kolthoff, N.J.: Textbook of anatomy and physiology, ed. 9, St. Louis, 1975, The C.V. Mosby Co.)

here, as do many cranial nerves. The foramen magnum, the largest opening in the skull, permits the spinal cord to join the brainstem in the posterior fossa. There are numerous other openings in the base of the skull for passage of arteries, veins, and cranial nerves (Fig. 23-4).

Between the skull and brain are the meninges, three covering membranes: the dura mater, arachnoid, and pia mater (Fig. 23-1).

The *dura mater* is a tough, shiny, fibrous membrane that is close to the inner surface of the skull and folds to separate the cranial cavity into compartments. The largest fold is the falx cerebri (Fig. 23-1), an arch-shaped, vertically placed, midline structure separating the right and left cerebral hemispheres. A smaller fold of dura mater, the falx cerebelli, separates the cerebellar hemispheres vertically. A transverse fold, the tentorium cerebelli, forms the roof of the posterior fossa. The tentorium supports the temporal lobe and occipital lobes of the cerebral hemispheres. Below the tentorium lie the cerebellum and brainstem. Structures above the tentorium are referred to as supratentorial, and those below as infratentorial (Fig. 23-5).

At margins of these dural folds lie large venous sinuses that drain blood from the intracranial structures into the jugular veins. Several arteries also lie within the layers of the dura. The largest is the middle meningeal, a source of serious hemorrhage if torn by an overlying fracture of the skull. The rigid skull makes hemorrhage and swelling in the brain critical. Pressure on brain tissue may cause irreparable damage.

Beneath the dura mater is a fine membrane, the *arachnoid*. The outer layer of arachnoid closely approximates the dura mater. The inner layer forms innumerable weblike filaments that bridge to the surface of the brain (Fig. 23-1). The outer surface of the arachnoid membrane adheres closely to the dura mater with no space normally between the two membranes. The inner surface is separated from the pia mater beneath it by the subarachnoid space, which is filled with cerebrospinal fluid that bathes the brain. Around the base of the brain particularly, this space becomes enlarged to form cisterns. The major intracranial nerves and blood vessels pass through these compartments. Intracranial approaches can be charted in terms of the basal cisterns.

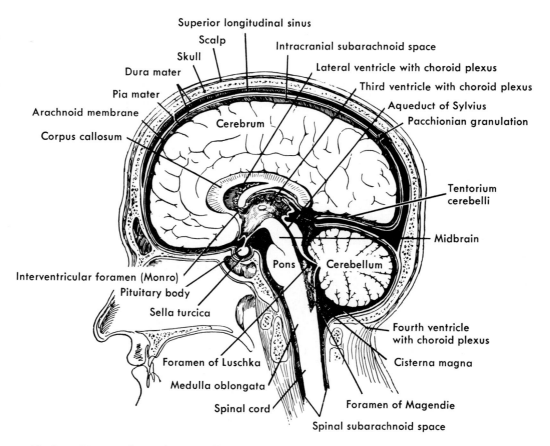

Fig. 23-5. Diagram of sagittal section of head showing cerebrospinal fluid spaces and their relationship to venous circulation and principal subdivision of the brain and its coverings. (From Conway-Rutkowski, B.L.: Carini and Owens' neurological and neurosurgical nursing, ed. 8, St. Louis, 1982, The C.V. Mosby Co.)

The *pia mater,* the innermost membrane, is like gossamer and attaches to the gray matter, dipping into the sulci and gyri. The pia mater has a rich vascular network that helps form the choroid plexus of the ventricles.

The brain is divided into the cerebral cortex, basal ganglia, hypothalamus, midbrain, brainstem, and cerebellum (Figs. 23-5 and 23-6).

The right and left cerebral hemispheres are the largest parts of the brain. Each hemisphere is composed of cerebral cortex and is divided into frontal, parietal, occipital, and temporal lobes; insula; rhinencephalon; basal ganglia; and hypothalamus. The two hemispheres are divided by a longitudinal fissure and joined underneath the falx by a large transverse bundle of nerve fibers, the corpus callosum (Fig. 23-6). Each of the cerebral hemispheres controls sensation and motor activity to and receives sensory stimuli from the opposite half of the body.

The surfaces of the hemispheres form convolutions called *gyri* and intervening furrows called *sulci.* Two sulci of anatomic importance to the surgeon are the central sulcus, or fissure of Rolando, which separates the motor from the sensory cortex, and the lateral sulcus, or fissure of Sylvius, which marks off the temporal lobe (Fig. 23-7). The insula (island of Reil) lies deep within the fissure of Sylvius and can be exposed by separating the upper and lower lips of the fissure. The frontal lobe is anterior to the fissure of Rolando and controls the higher functions of intellect and abstract reasoning. The motor cortex lies anterior to the fissure of Rolando. Destruction leads to loss of voluntary motor function on the opposite side of the body (Fig. 23-8).

Posterior to the fissure of Rolando is the parietal lobe, extending back to the parieto-occipital fissure. This area contains the final receiving and integrating station for sensory impulses from the contralateral side of the body. The occipital lobe lies posterior to the parieto-occipital fissure. It receives and integrates visual impulses and registers them as meaningful images (Figs. 23-7 and 23-8).

Inferior to the fissure of Sylvius, in the middle fossa, is the temporal lobe. Lesions of the left temporal lobe in right-handed individuals and in many left-handed persons may affect the comprehension and verbalization of words, resulting in aphasia. Rhinencephalic structures, such as the anterior limbic area, may exert an inhibitory effect on brain mechanisms in the expression of emotions, such as anger. Restlessness and hyperactivity may result from lesions of this area. The rhinencephalon has many connections with the hypothalamus. Malfunctions may affect sexual behavior, emotions, and motivation. Loss of recent memory may indicate a lesion of this area.

The convoluted surface of the cerebrum consists of gray matter, the *cerebral cortex,* which contains the cell bodies

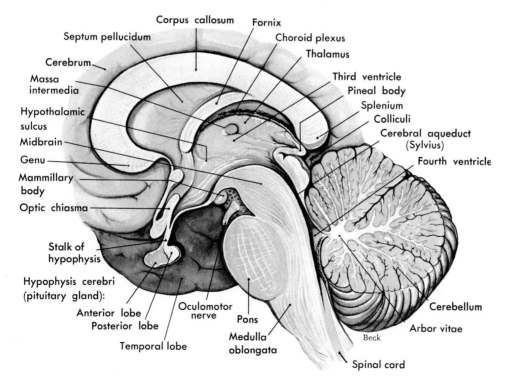

Fig. 23-6. Sagittal section through midline of brain showing structures around third ventricle including corpus callosum, thalamus, and hypothalamus. (From Anthony, C.P., and Kolthoff, N.J.: Textbook of anatomy and physiology, ed. 9, St. Louis, 1975, The C.V. Mosby Co.)

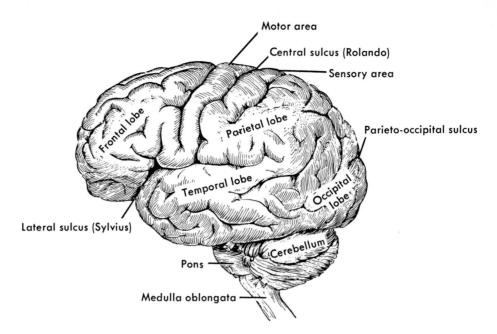

Fig. 23-7. Lateral view of cerebral hemisphere (showing lobes and principal fissures), cerebellum, pons, and medulla oblongata. (From Conway-Rutkowski, B.L.: Carini and Owens' neurological and neurosurgical nursing, ed. 8, St. Louis, 1982, The C.V. Mosby Co.)

of the many nerve pathways of the brain. The underlying white matter contains millions of myelinated nerve axons and is relatively avascular compared with the cortex. The nerve pathways, or fiber tracts, are of three types: (1) commissural fibers, which pass from one cerebral hemisphere to the other; (2) association fibers, which connect gyri regions and lobes longitudinally within a cerebral hemisphere; and (3) projection fibers, including the great motor and sensory systems, which run vertically to connect the cortical regions with other portions of the central nervous system.

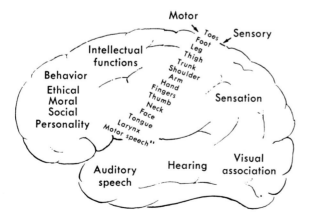

Fig. 23-8. Principal functional subdivisions of cerebral hemispheres. (Modified from Conway, B.L.: Carini and Owens' neurological and neurosurgical nursing, ed. 7, St. Louis, 1978, The C.V. Mosby Co.)

In prefrontal lobotomy, association fibers in the frontal lobe were divided to effect changes in personality that may be beneficial in certain psychiatric disorders. *Cingulotomy,* in which the cingulum is interrupted, also may be performed for treatment of these disorders.

Deep in the brain are five *basal ganglia,* or collections of nuclei, of the extrapyramidal system. Three of them, the caudate nucleus, putamen, and globus pallidus, collectively referred to as the corpus striatum, associate with the thalamus for motor control (Fig. 23-6). Lesions here cause rigidity of the skeletal muscles and various types of spontaneous tremors. The basal ganglia and thalamus can be selectively destroyed surgically in an effort to relieve the tremors and rigidity associated with multiple sclerosis, Parkinson's disease, various forms of cerebellar degeneration, and late effects of severe brain trauma. In addition to rhythmic processing of brain activity and its influence on affect and higher brain activity, the thalamus is the major relay station for incoming sensory stimuli. Many of these stimuli are subsequently relayed to a final destination in the parietal cortex. Because of its central role in perception of body sensations, surgical lesions can be made in the thalamus in an attempt to alleviate pain.

Along the floor of the third ventricle is the *hypothalamus* (Fig. 23-6), which is principally concerned with the autonomic regulation of the body's internal environment and is intimately connected with the pituitary gland.

The short, stocky portion of the brain, between the cerebral hemispheres and pons, is the *midbrain* (Fig. 23-5), also referred to as the mesencephalon. It is made up of the cerebral peduncles, numerous nerve tracts and nuclei, and association centers that control the majority of eye movements. The hindbrain, or *brainstem*, immediately below the midbrain, consists of the pons and medulla oblongata (Fig. 23-7). The midbrain and brainstem form the floor of the fourth ventricle in the posterior fossa of the skull and contain many large efferent and afferent tracts and nuclei of most cranial nerves. The brainstem contains the cardiovascular and respiratory regulatory centers. Surgery directly on the brainstem is extremely dangerous.

The *cerebellum*, which occupies most of the posterior fossa, forms the roof of the fourth ventricle (Figs. 23-6 and 23-7). It has two lateral lobes and a medial portion, the *vermis*. The fissures of the cerebellum are small and run transversely. The cerebellum is principally concerned with balance and coordination of movement. It has many complex connections with higher and lower centers and exerts its influence homolaterally, in contrast to the cerebral hemispheres, which act contralaterally. At least half the brain tumors in children originate in the cerebellum. In adults and children the most common surgical lesions in this area are tumors and abscesses. By splitting the vermis in the exact midline, a satisfactory exposure of tumors that lie in the fourth ventricle is obtained without sacrificing the important cerebellar functions.

Cerebrospinal fluid system

Within the brain are four communicating cavities, or *ventricles,* filled with cerebrospinal fluid (CSF). In the lower medial portion of each cerebral hemisphere lies a large lateral ventricle, which resembles a wishbone and is separated anteriorly from its counterpart by a thin pellucid septum (Fig. 23-9). Each lateral ventricle has a body and three horns: frontal, occipital, and temporal. Below the bodies of the lateral ventricles is a central cleft, or third ventricle. It communicates anteriorly with the lateral ventricles through the foramen of Monro and posteriorly with the fourth ventricle through the aqueduct of Sylvius, a long narrow channel passing through the midbrain. The fourth ventricle is a rhomboid cavity in the posterior fossa, between the cerebellum and the brainstem. In the roof of the fourth ventricle is the foramen of Magendie, an opening into the cisterna magna; at the lateral margins are the two foramina of Luschka, which open into the cisterna pontis.

Much of the CSF originates in the *choroid plexuses* of the ventricles. These are tufted, vascular structures that allow certain fluid elements of the blood to pass through their ependymal linings. A choroid plexus is found along the floor in each lateral ventricle, on the roof of the third ventricle, and in the posterior portion of the fourth ventricle. Most of the fluid is formed in the lateral ventricles and flows through the interventricular foramen of Monro to the third ventricle and through the aqueduct of Sylvius to the fourth ventricle, where it escapes into the subarachnoid space of the basal cisterns through the foramina of Magendie and Luschka. From the basal cisterns the fluid flows around the spinal cord, over the cerebellar lobes, around the medulla and the base of the brain, and over the cerebral hemispheres in the subarachnoid space. The fluid is absorbed into the venous circulation through villi of the arachnoid (pacchionian granulations) into the great dural venous sinuses, particularly the superior sagittal sinus, and by diffusion through perivascular, perineural, and periradicular channels (Fig. 23-1).

The total amount of circulating CSF averages 125 to 150 ml in the adult. Each lateral ventricle contains 10 to

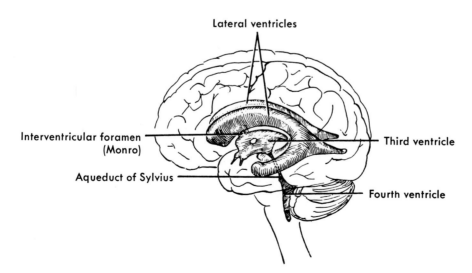

Fig. 23-9. Diagram of ventricular system showing its relationship to various parts of the brain. (From Conway-Rutkowski, B.L.: Carini and Owens' neurological and neurosurgical nursing, ed. 8, St. Louis, 1982, The C.V. Mosby Co.)

15 ml, the rest of the ventricular system contains 5 ml, the cranial subarachnoid space averages about 25 to 35 ml, and the spinal subarachnoid space contains about 75 to 90 ml. The ventricular fluid normally has 5 to 15 mg/100 ml protein content, whereas the spinal fluid has 25 to 45 mg/100 ml. These values may be considerably elevated in pathologic conditions of the central nervous system.

The characteristics of normal spinal fluid are as follows:

- Appearance: clear and colorless
- Pressure: 70 to 200 mm H_2O
- pH: 7.35 to 7.4
- Specific gravity: 1.005 to 1.009
- Glucose: 50 to 75 mg/100 cc (⅔ of blood sugar)
- Chlorides: 120 to 130 mEq/liter
- Cells: 0 to 10 (lymphocytes only)
- Protein: lumbar 15 to 45 mg/100 ml
  cisternal 10 to 25 mg/100 ml
  ventricular 5 to 15 mg/100 ml
- Culture: negative
- Gamma globulin: 6% to 13% of total protein

Spinal fluid bathes the brain and spinal cord, helps support the weight of the brain, and acts as a cushion for the brain and spinal cord by absorbing some of the force of external trauma. By variation in its volume, it aids in keeping intracranial pressure relatively constant. If the brain atrophies, the CSF increases in amount to fill the dead space; if the brain swells, the CSF decreases in amount to compensate for the increase in brain mass. The fluid can carry certain drugs to diseased parts of the brain. It does not, however, play a significant role in supplying nutrition to the structures that it bathes.

The rate of formation and absorption of CSF is related to the osmotic and hydrostatic pressure of the blood. When intracranial pressure rises, an intravenous injection of hypertonic mannitol or a nonosmotic diuretic is employed to dehydrate the blood and decrease the volume of cerebrospinal fluid.

Elevations in CSF pressure can be caused by an expanding mass within the skull, such as a tumor, hemorrhage, or cerebral edema; an increase in formation of fluid, as in meningitis, encephalitis, and other febrile conditions; an increase in venous pressure within the skull from an obstruction to normal venous drainage; a blockage of absorption by inflammatory conditions of the arachnoid and perivascular spaces; any mechanical obstruction of the ventricular or subarachnoidal fluid pathways; or problems with the absorption of CSF. Some of these conditions are amenable to surgical intervention.

Blood supply

The *arterial* supply to the brain, which requires 20% more oxygen than any other organ, enters the cranium through the two internal carotid arteries anteriorly and the two vertebral arteries posteriorly. These communicate at the base of the brain through the basilar artery and the circle of Willis (Fig. 23-10), which ensures continuity of the circulation if any one of the four main channels is

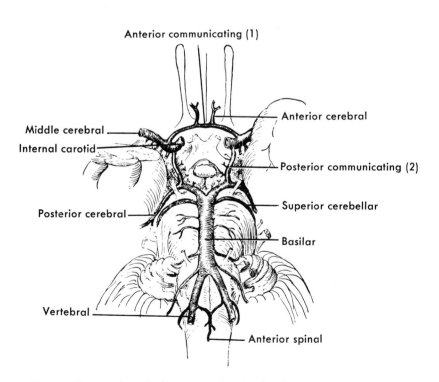

Fig. 23-10. Diagram of principal cerebral arteries and circle of Willis. (From Conway-Rutkowski, B.L.: Carini and Owens' neurological and neurosurgical nursing, ed. 8, St. Louis, 1982, The C.V. Mosby Co.)

interrupted. The main branches for distribution of blood to each hemisphere of the brain from the internal carotid arteries are the anterior, middle, and posterior cerebral arteries. Each artery nourishes a specific area of the brain (Fig. 23-11). The anterior cerebral artery supplies the anterior two thirds of the medial surface and adjacent region over the convexity of the hemisphere, thus including about half of the frontal and parietal lobes. The middle cerebral artery supplies most of the lateral surface of the hemisphere, including half of the frontal, parietal, and temporal lobes. The posterior cerebral artery supplies the occipital lobe and the remaining half of the temporal lobe, principally on the inferior and medial surfaces. The brainstem and cerebellum are supplied by branches of the basilar and vertebral arteries.

The circle of Willis is of particular interest surgically because of the development of aneurysms in this area. An aneurysm is a weakness in the wall of a large artery. Aneurysms usually develop in or near the crotch of a bifurcation of the circle of Willis. It is thought that the weakness develops because of the superimposition of two lesions: a congenital absence of the media and a degen-

eration of the internal elastic lamina that normally strengthens the arterial wall. Erosion of the lamina results from the wear and tear of pulsatile pressure.

The most common sites of intracranial aneurysms are (1) adjacent to the anterior communicating artery, (2) at the junction of the posterior communicating artery and the internal carotid artery, (3) at the origin of the anterior cerebral arteries, (4) at the first bifurcation of the middle cerebral artery, and (5) on the basilar arteries.

The cerebral *veins* do not parallel the arteries as do the veins in most other parts of the body. The external cortical veins anastomose freely in the pia mater, forming larger cerebral veins, and as such they pierce the arachnoid membrane, cross the subdural space, and empty into the great dural venous sinuses. A subdural hemorrhage following head trauma may arise from disruption of these bridging vessels; an epidural hemorrhage often results from lacerations of the middle meningeal artery, a branch of the external carotid artery that supplies the dura mater. The deep cerebral veins, which drain the interior of the hemispheres, empty principally into the great vein of Galen and the inferior sagittal sinus (Figs. 23-12 and 23-13).

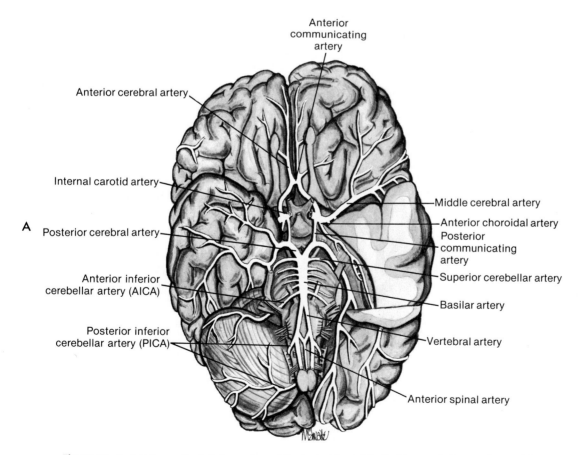

Fig. 23-11. A, Arteries on the inferior surface of the brain. The left half of the cerebellum and part of the left temporal lobe have been removed.

Continued.

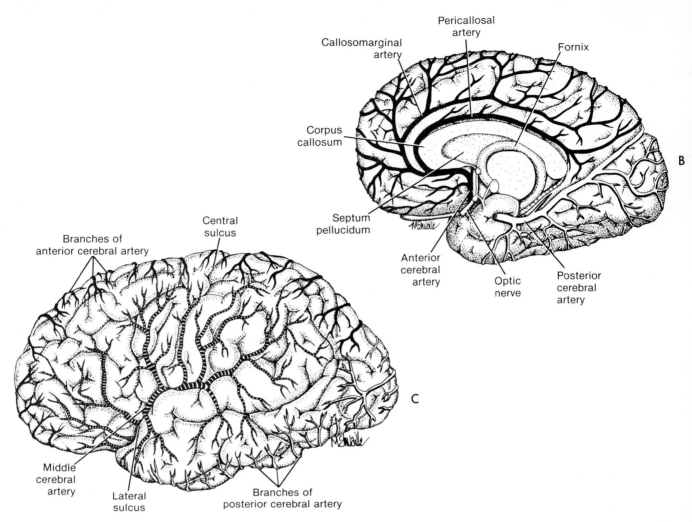

Fig. 23-11, cont'd. B, Arteries of the medial surface of the brain. The anterior cerebral artery and its branches are shown in black, the posterior cerebral artery and its branches are shown in white. **C,** Arteries of the lateral surface of the brain. The middle cerebral artery and its branches are shown striped. The small branches of the anterior cerebral artery reaching around from the medial surface are shown in black, and those of the posterior cerebral artery are shown in white. (From Nolte, J.: The human brain: an introduction to its fundamental anatomy, ed. 2, St. Louis, 1988, The C.V. Mosby Co.)

The blood transports oxygen, nutrients, and other substances necessary for the proper functioning of living tissue. The needs of the brain for oxygen and glucose are critical. The brain can store only small amounts of oxygen and energy-producing nutrients. Constant flow of blood to the brain must be maintained.

The brain uses oxygen in the metabolism of glucose, the chief source of energy. Protein and fat metabolism play little part in energy production. In the face of an oxygen deficit, the survival time of central nervous system tissue is very short. In the face of low blood sugar, central nervous system function is compromised and unconsciousness results.

Generally, all factors affecting the systemic blood pressure indirectly affect the cerebral circulation. The brain normally receives 20% of the cardiac output. The cerebral blood flow is kept constant by an autoregulation phenomenon. When the mean arterial pressure falls below 60 mm Hg, the autoregulation mechanism usually fails. Thus controlled hypotension may be safely used in intracranial surgery.

Cranial nerves

Twelve pairs of cranial nerves arise within the cranial cavity (Fig. 23-14). From a surgical standpoint, they are considered with the head.

First cranial nerve

The olfactory nerve, a fiber tract of the brain, is located under the frontal lobe on the cribriform plate of the ethmoid

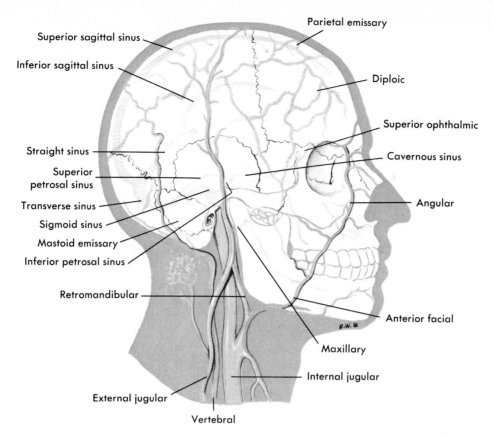

Fig. 23-12. Semischematic projection of large veins of head. Deep veins and dural sinuses are projected on skull. Note connection (emissary veins) between superficial and deep veins. (From Anthony, C.P., and Thibodeau, G.A.: Textbook of anatomy and physiology, ed. 11, St. Louis, 1983, The C.V. Mosby Co.)

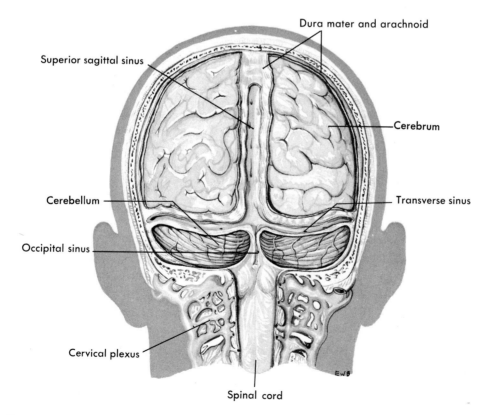

Fig. 23-13. Venous sinuses shown in relation to brain and skull. (From Anthony, C.P., and Thibodeau, G.A.: Textbook of anatomy and physiology, ed. 11, St. Louis, 1983, The C.V. Mosby Co.)

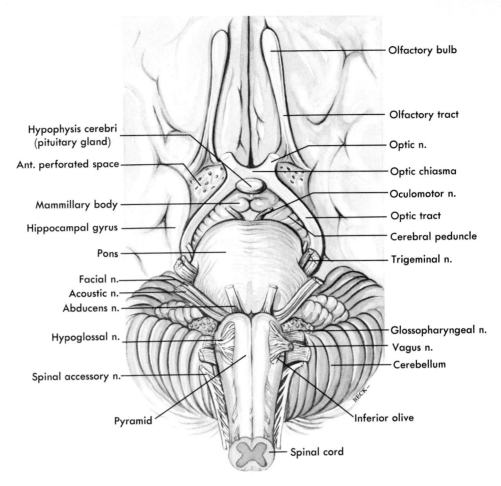

Fig. 23-14. Ventral surface of brain showing attachment of cranial nerves. (From Anthony, C.P., and Kolthoff, N.J.: Textbook of anatomy and physiology, ed. 9, St. Louis, 1975, The C.V. Mosby Co.)

bone. It transmits the sense of smell. Frontal lobe tumors, fractures of the anterior fossa of the skull, and lesions of the nasal cavity may affect the olfactory nerve.

Second cranial nerve

The optic nerve is a fiber tract of the brain. Originating in the ganglion cells of the retina, it passes through the optic foramen in the apex of the orbit to reach the optic chiasma, where a partial crossing of the fibers occurs, so the fibers from the nasal half of each retina pass to the opposite side. Posterior to the chiasma, the visual pathway is called the *optic tract;* still farther back, it becomes the optic radiation. Lesions in various parts of this pathway produce characteristic defects in the visual fields. For example, a lesion of the chiasma usually destroys the temporal vision of each eye (bitemporal hemianopia), whereas a lesion of the occipital lobe produces impairment of vision (homonymous hemianopia) affecting the right or left halves of the visual fields of both eyes.

Lesions that affect the optic nerve and are treated by neurosurgery include primary gliomas of the nerve, pituitary tumors that press on the optic chiasma, and, oc-

casionally, meningiomas in the region of the sella turcica and olfactory groove. The optic nerves and chiasma are best exposed through a frontal craniotomy, along the floor of the anterior fossa, or through a frontotemporal approach along the sphenoid ridge.

Third, fourth, and sixth cranial nerves

These three pairs of nerves—the oculomotor, the trochlear, and the abducens, respectively—are conveniently considered together because they are the motor nerves to the muscles of the eyes. They are affected by many toxic, inflammatory, vascular, and neoplastic lesions. The third nerve may be affected by aneurysms of the internal carotid artery, and pressure against this nerve accounts for pupillary dilation when temporal lobe herniation resulting from increased intracranial pressure is present.

Fifth cranial nerve

The trigeminal nerve has two functions: (1) sensory supply to the forehead, eyes, meninges, face, jaw, teeth, hard palate, buccal mucosa, tongue, nose, nasal mucosa,

Divisions of trigeminal nerve:

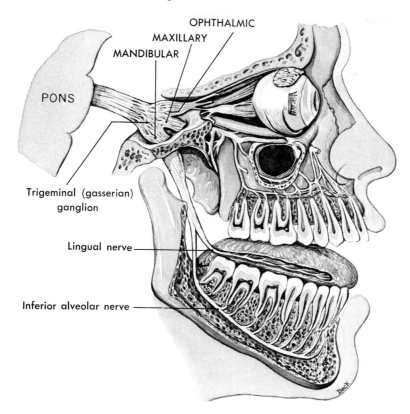

OPHTHALMIC
MAXILLARY
MANDIBULAR
PONS
Trigeminal (gasserian) ganglion
Lingual nerve
Inferior alveolar nerve

Fig. 23-15. Trigeminal (fifth cranial) nerve and its three main divisions. (From Anthony, C.P., and Kolthoff, N.J.: Textbook of anatomy and physiology, ed. 9, St. Louis, 1975, The C.V. Mosby Co.)

and maxillary sinus, and (2) motor innervation of the muscles of mastication. The sensory fibers that arise from cells in the gasserian ganglion travel along the medial wall of the middle cranial fossa and then extend peripherally in three divisions: ophthalmic, maxillary, and mandibular. Behind the ganglion the fibers enter the brainstem by way of the sensory root. The motor root, which originates from cells in the brainstem, follows the course of the larger sensory component (Fig. 23-15).

Trigeminal neuralgia (tic douloureux) is characterized by excruciating, piercing paroxysms of pain, affecting one or more of the major peripheral divisions. The recurrent attacks are usually brought on by stimulation of trigger zones present about the face, nares, lips, or teeth. This affliction, of unknown cause, tends to occur unilaterally and in older persons. Medical treatment is frequently unsuccessful. A great variety of neurosurgical procedures have been proposed for its control. Peripheral neurectomies of the supraorbital or infraorbital nerves may easily be performed with the patient under local anesthesia, but the effect is temporary because the nerves regenerate. Trigeminal neuralgia can also be treated by a posterior fossa approach using the operating microscope. The microscope allows decompression of the trigeminal nerve

from normal surrounding blood vessels and selection of its various fibers. Sensations of pain and temperature are eliminated, and the sensation of touch and corneal reflex are preserved.

Trigeminal neuralgia can be treated by retrogasserian rhizotomy with radiofrequency current and chemical rhizolysis.

Seventh cranial nerve

The facial nerve supplies the musculature of the face and the anterior two thirds of the tongue (for taste). It originates in the brainstem, passes through the skull with the eighth nerve by way of the internal acoustic meatus, continues along the facial canal, and exits just posterior to the parotid gland. The nerve may be damaged by acoustic neurinomas, fractures at the base of the skull, mastoid infections, or surgical procedures in the vicinity of the parotid gland.

Bell's palsy, a facial lower motor neuron paralysis, can affect the seventh nerve. It may last for a few weeks to a few months, but recovery usually takes place. When permanent interruption of the nerve occurs, useful operations for restoration of function include spinal accessory–facial or hypoglossal-facial anastomosis. These operations are performed high in the neck behind the parotid gland, using the operating microscope.

Eighth cranial nerve

The acoustic nerve has two parts, both sensory—the cochlear for hearing and the vestibular for balance. The former receives stimuli from the organ of Corti, the latter from the semicircular canals. The major surgical lesion of the eighth nerve is acoustic neurinoma, a histologically benign tumor growing from the nerve sheath at its entrance into the internal auditory meatus. This tumor arises deep in the angle between the cerebellum and pons. Symptoms may include unilateral deafness, tinnitus, unilateral impairment of cerebellar function, numbness of the face from involvement of the fifth cranial nerve, and, late in the course, papilledema caused by pressure on the pons. The operative approach is usually through a unilateral suboccipital craniectomy; in some instances a translabyrinth approach may be used. Great care must be taken to prevent injury to the pons, and an attempt is made to preserve the facial nerve.

Ménière's disease is an affliction of the eighth nerve characterized by a recurrent and usually progressive group of symptoms including dizziness and a sensation of fullness or pressure in the ears. When medical measures fail to alleviate the problem, section of the eighth nerve may be performed; this procedure has given consistently excellent results.

Ninth cranial nerve

The glossopharyngeal nerve supplies the sense of taste to the posterior third of the tongue and sensation to the tonsils and pharyngeal region and partially innervates the pharyngeal muscles. Rarely, it is involved in a painful tic similar to trigeminal tic. Its sensory component can be sectioned for this reason, to treat a hypersensitive carotid sinus, or, along with the fifth nerve, to treat painful malignancies of the face, mouth, and pharynx. The ninth nerve lies near the eighth nerve in the posterior fossa and is exposed in a similar way.

Tenth cranial nerve

The vagus nerve has many motor and sensory functions, chief among which are innervation of pharyngeal and laryngeal musculature, control of heart rate, and regulation of acid secretion of the stomach. In neck surgery the surgeon carefully avoids the recurrent laryngeal branch; in gastric surgery the surgeon may sever the vagus nerve at the lower end of the esophagus to treat a peptic ulcer. The neurosurgeon is concerned mainly with preventing damage to the vagus nerve during posterior fossa surgery.

Eleventh cranial nerve

The spinal accessory nerve is a motor nerve to the sternocleidomastoid and trapezius muscles. To restore mo-

bility to the face, it may be anastomosed to the peripheral end of a damaged facial nerve.

Twelfth cranial nerve

The hypoglossal nerve innervates the musculature of the tongue. Its neurosurgical interest is similar to that of the spinal accessory nerve.

Pathologic lesions of the brain

Brain tumors are not as rare, nor is their prognosis as poor, as is often believed. Early diagnosis simplifies surgical treatment because increased intracranial pressure and severe neurologic changes are not usually present. Brain tumors are either malignant or benign, depending on the cell type. Primary tumors generally do not resemble the carcinomas and sarcomas found elsewhere in the body and rarely metastasize outside the central nervous system. If both primary and metastatic tumors of the brain and its covering membranes are included in the term *intracranial tumors,* such tumors may be classified pathologically as germ cell, mesodermal, neuroepithelial, metastatic, and miscellaneous as follows:

A. Germ cell tumors
   1. Teratoma
   2. Germinoma
   3. Embryonal carcinoma
   4. Choriocarcinoma
   5. Craniopharyngioma (occurs in children and adults and arises from the region of the pituitary stalk; usually cystic; calcification above the sella turcica is often seen on x-ray films. In addition to headache, vertigo, vomiting, and papilledema, diabetes insipidus and visual field changes are common.)
B. Meningeal lesions
   1. Meningioma (slow-growing tumors, originating in the arachnoidal tissue; very vascular and may adhere to the dural venous sinuses or major arteries, making their complete removal difficult)
C. Neural sheath tumor
   1. Neurinoma (usually arise from the neurolemma sheath cells of the vestibular portion of the eighth cranial nerve within the auditory meatus, grow to fill the cerebellopontine angle, and may indent the brainstem)
D. Vascular tumors
   1. Angioma (often congenital arteriovenous malformation)
   2. Hemangioblastoma (may be solid or cystic; likely to occur in cerebellar hemispheres; sometimes present in association with angiomas of the retina and other organs)
E. Neuroepithelial tumors
   1. Gliomas
      a. Glioblastoma multiforme is an infiltrative, fast-

growing, rapidly recurring cerebral tumor that occurs most frequently in middle age. It may invade both cerebral hemispheres by crossing in the corpus callosum. Areas of necrosis are characteristic. Astrocytomas (astroblastomas) and oligodendrogliomas may transform into this malignant tumor with time.

b. Medulloblastoma is a fast-growing, rapidly recurring tumor of the vermis of the cerebellum and fourth ventricle that usually occurs in young children. It characteristically metastasizes in the subarachnoid spaces, usually spreading to the base of the brain by this route.

c. Ependymoma occurs most frequently in children and is likely to arise in or near the ventricular walls. It commonly occurs in the fourth ventricle, where it abuts or involves vital medullary centers. It also frequently metastasizes in the subarachnoid spaces.

d. Astrocytoma usually occurs in the cerebellum of children and the cerebrum of adults. It is often cystic and discrete in children, infiltrating and ill defined in adults.

e. Oligodendroglioma is usually found in the cerebral hemispheres and is infiltrating but occasionally moderately well defined.

f. Astroblastoma is a rare glioma occurring in the cerebral hemisphere of middle-aged adults. It may share the growth characteristics of astrocytoma and glioblastoma multiforme.

g. Spongioblastoma occurs predominantly in the optic chiasma and nerves of children and in the pons. This lesion grows in vital structures and is rarely amenable to even partial removal.

h. Others not mentioned include choroid plexus papillomas, pinealomas, and microgliomas.

2. Pituitary tumors

a. Chromophobe tumor is relatively common in the anterior pituitary glands of adults. It causes compression of the pituitary, adjacent optic chiasma, and hypothalamus. The latter may lead to diabetes insipidus.

b. Eosinophilic adenomas are secretory, causing an excessive amount of growth hormone in the serum.

c. Basophilic adenomas are responsible for the excessive secretion of corticotropic, gonadotropic, and thyrotropic hormones. Acromegaly or, less commonly, Cushing's syndrome may occur and cause the patient to seek help long before the tumor has expanded sufficiently to compromise the optic chiasma.

d. Prolactinoma or prolactin cell adenoma exhibits considerable differences in clinical presentation depending on the sex of the patient. In women of reproductive age, the onset of amenorrhea and galactorrhea with associated infertility are obvious signs. The diagnosis of a prolactinoma is established early in the course. In men the clinical endocrinal symptoms, which include decreased libido and impotence, are not as conspicuous and initially may be disregarded by the patient. As a result, male patients frequently do not seek medical attention until the tumors are large and have spread beyond the confines of the sella.

F. Metastatic tumors usually arise from carcinoma, more rarely from sarcoma, and occasionally from melanomas and retinal tumors. The most common sources are bronchogenic carcinoma and carcinoma of the breast. Tumors not discussed here are eosinophilic granulomas, tuberculomas, and other granulomas; brain abscesses; colloid cysts; fibrous dysplasia; and lymphomas.

A brain lesion is diagnosed by history, neurological examination, and diagnostic studies. The manifestations of an intracranial tumor fall into two classes: those resulting from irritation or impairment of function in specific areas of the brain directly affected by the tumor and those resulting from diffuse increased intracranial pressure.

Lesions in the left frontotemporal region, where motor speech originates, lead to aphasia; occipital tumors produce hemianoptic visual defects; large frontal lobe tumors may cause striking personality changes. Cortical tumors frequently produce focal seizures of diagnostic value. The onset of epileptiform seizures in an adult is often associated with an intracranial neoplasm. Pituitary tumors characteristically press on the optic chiasma and impair the temporal vision of each eye. They disturb pituitary glandular function, resulting in hypopituitary states, pituitary dwarfism, or acromegaly. Posterior fossa tumors often manifest their presence by blocking the cerebrospinal fluid circulation, but they may also destroy cerebellar function, resulting in incoordination, ataxia, scanning speech, and deafness.

Back

The spinal column consists of 33 vertebrae: seven cervical, twelve thoracic, five lumbar, five sacral (fused as one), and one coccygeal (fused from four small vertebrae) (Fig. 23-16).

The first cervical vertebra, or atlas, supports the skull. The second cervical vertebra, or axis, can be identified by its odontoid process, a vertical projection extending into the foramen of the atlas like a stick in a hoop, and rests against the anterior tubercle. Ligaments hold the two together but allow considerable rotational movement.

The other cervical, thoracic, and lumbar vertebrae are more alike in structure. Each has a body, an oval block of spongy bone situated anteriorly. An intervertebral disc, a fibrocartilaginous elastic cushion, separates one body from another (Figs. 23-17 and 23-18). The spinal cord

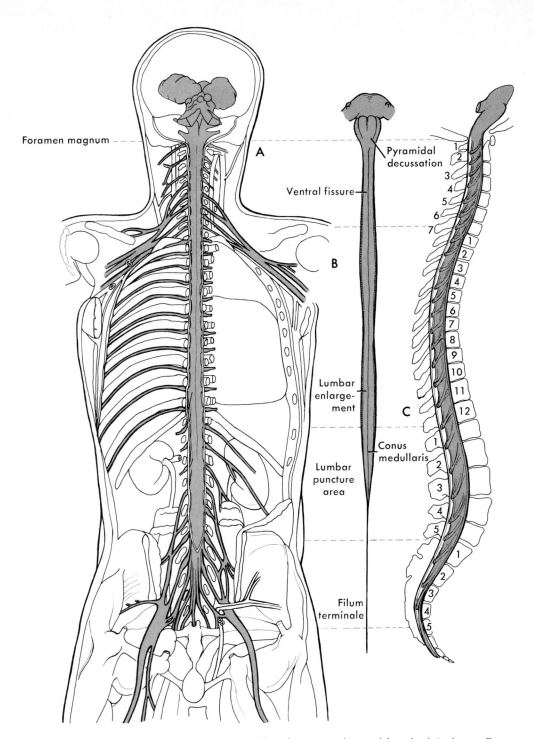

Fig. 23-16. Posterior view of brainstem and spinal cord. **A,** Torso dissected from back is shown. Dura mater has been opened and cord exposed. Levels concerned can be easily determined by referring to ribs on left side of thorax. Cord proper terminates opposite body of second lumbar vertebra (**B**) as conus medullaris. **B,** Ventral surface of cord stripped of dura mater and arachnoid. It is symmetrical in structure, two halves of which are separated by ventral fissure. This fissure stops at foramen magnum. Caudally, pia mater leaves conus medullaris as glistening thread or filum terminale. **C,** Cord is exposed from lateral side. Dura mater has been opened. Since cord is shorter than canal and spinal nerves leave through intervertebral foramina, one at a time, lowest portion of canal is occupied only by a bundlelike accumulation of nerve roots, the cauda equina. Caudal end of dural sac, enclosing spinal cord and cauda equina, lies somewhere between bodies of first and third sacral vertebrae. Size and position of the three views correspond, and delimitation of major vertebral levels is indicated by transverse lines for all three figures. (Modified from Mettler, F.A.: Neuroanatomy, ed. 2, St. Louis, 1948, The C.V. Mosby Co.; from Conway-Rutkowski, B.L.: Carini and Owens' neurological and neurosurgical nursing, ed. 8, St. Louis, 1982, The C.V. Mosby Co.)

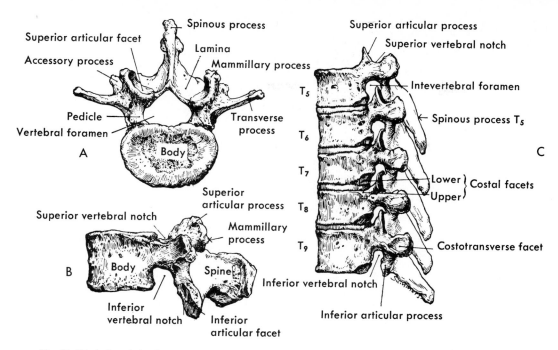

Fig. 23-17. A, Fourth lumbar vertebra from above. **B,** Fourth lumbar vertebra from side. **C,** Fifth to ninth thoracic vertebrae, showing relationships of various parts. (From Mettler, F.A.: Neuroanatomy, ed. 2, St. Louis, 1948, The C.V. Mosby Co.)

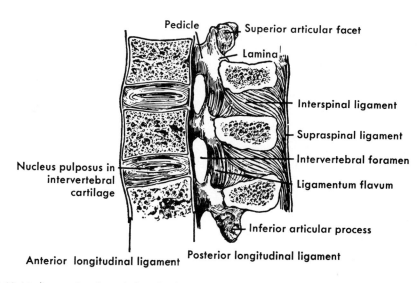

Fig. 23-18. Median section through three lumbar vertebrae, showing intervertebral discs (nuclei pulposi). (From Mettler, F.A.: Neuroanatomy, ed. 2, St. Louis, 1948, The C.V. Mosby Co.)

lies in a canal formed by the vertebral bodies, pedicles, and laminae. Articular surfaces or facets project from the pedicles and form joints with the facets of the vertebrae above and below. Transverse processes extend laterally and serve as hitching posts for muscles and ligaments. Spinous processes extend posteriorly (Fig. 23-17) and can be palpated in all except obese persons. The vertebrae are held together by multiple ligaments and muscles. Motion

of the spine occurs at the articular facets and through the elastic intervertebral discs (Fig. 23-18).

The spinal cord is protected by this bony framework. The dura mater is separated from its bony surroundings by a layer of epidural fat. Beneath the dura mater is the arachnoid, a continuation of the same structure in the head. The subarachnoid space contains spinal fluid. A thin layer of pia mater adheres to the cord, and cerebrospinal fluid

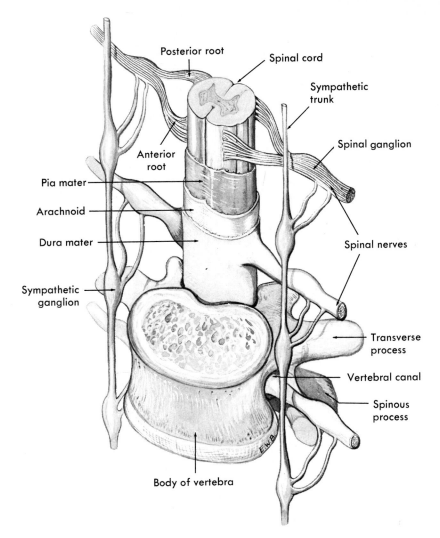

Fig. 23-19. Spinal cord, showing meninges, formation of spinal nerves, and relations to vertebra and to sympathetic trunk and ganglia. (From Anthony, C.P., and Kolthoff, N.J.: Textbook of anatomy and physiology, ed. 9, St. Louis, 1975, The C.V. Mosby Co.)

also circulates from the fourth ventricle into the central canal of the cord.

The spinal cord is a downward prolongation of the brainstem, starting at the upper border of the atlas and ending at the upper border of the second lumbar vertebra. The cord is oval in cross-section. It is slightly flattened in the anteroposterior diameter. A cross-section looks like a gray H surrounded by a white mantle split in the midline, anteriorly and posteriorly, by sulci (Fig. 23-19).

The peripheral white matter carries long myelinated motor and sensory tracts; the central gray matter consists of nerve cell bodies and short unmyelinated fibers (Figs. 23-16 and 23-19). The principal long pathways are the laterally placed pyramidal tracts, carrying impulses down from the cerebral cortex to the motor neurons of the cord; the dorsal ascending columns, mediating sensations of

touch and proprioception; and the anterolaterally placed spinothalamic tracts, carrying pain and temperature sensations to the thalamus, the sensory receiving station of the brain (Fig. 23-20).

At each vertebral level are two pairs of spinal nerves (Fig. 23-19): an anterior or motor root, the cell bodies of which lie in the anterior horn of the spinal gray matter, and a posterior root, the cell bodies of which lie in the spinal ganglia in the intervertebral foramina, through which the nerves exit from the spinal canal and emerge from the cord. Each pair of roots forms one spinal nerve. The cervical nerves pass out horizontally, but at each lower level they take on an increasingly oblique and downward direction. In the lumbar region, the course of the nerves is nearly vertical, forming the cauda equina (Fig. 23-16). This phenomenon is explained by the fact that the spinal

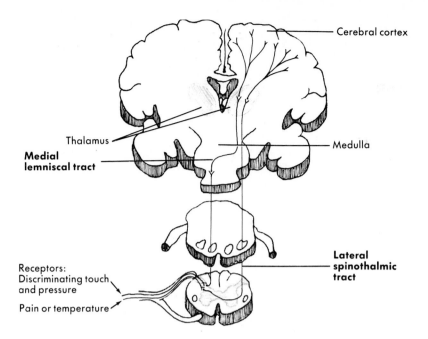

Fig. 23-20. Lateral spinothalamic and medial lemniscal neural tracts.

cord, which fills the entire spinal canal in the fetus, grows at a slower rate than the bony spine, thus leaving the lower nerves a progressively longer course to their exit.

The vasculature of the spinal cord and vertebral column is a rich, delicate network. The arterial blood supply to the spinal cord arises from the vertebral arteries as the anterior spinal artery and the posterior spinal arteries. These vessels branch and anastomose on both sides of the cord and within the substance of the cord. They also branch into anterior and posterior radicular arteries that form spinal rami as they accompany the spinal nerve roots through the intervertebral foramina.

A series of venous plexuses surround and innervate the spinal cord at each level in the vertebral canal. They anastomose with each other and form the intervertebral veins as they exit through the intervertebral foramina with the spinal nerves to join the intercostal, lumbar, and sacral veins. The lateral longitudinal veins near the foramen magnum empty into the inferior petrosal sinus and cerebellar veins. The venous network innervates the bony structures and musculature as well as the spinal cord and nerve roots. Venous bleeding during spinal surgery is a potential problem for which the nurse must be prepared.

Pathologic lesions of the spinal cord and adjacent structures

Operations are performed to correct congenital malformations, injuries, tumors, herniated and degenerative intervertebral discs, abscesses, and intractable pain.

The most common congenital lesion encountered is a lumbar *meningocele*, or *meningomyelocele*, a failure of the union of the vertebral arches during fetal development. The fluid-filled, thin-walled sac often contains neural elements. Surgical correction is necessary when the sac lining is so thin that there is a potential or actual CSF leak. The operation consists of excising the sac wall to preserve adhering nerves, closing the dura mater, and reinforcing the closure with fascial flaps swung from the paraspinal muscles. Skin closure without tension is essential for primary healing. Large skin and subcutaneous flaps must occasionally be fashioned to ensure healing.

Injuries to the spinal cord are serious. No regeneration of destroyed or divided nerve tracts occurs. Recovery may take place with lesser degrees of injury, such as contusion or compression. Surgery can be of value in preventing further damage by debridement of penetrating wounds, removal of foreign bodies, relief of pressure on the cord or roots, open reduction of certain dislocations and fractures, and measures aimed at stabilizing the spine. In cervical injuries, skeletal traction by means of tongs applied to the skull is often the preferred treatment.

Spinal cord tumors are classified according to location as extradural (outside the dura mater) or intradural (inside the dura mater). Intradural tumors may be either extramedullary (outside the cord) or intramedullary (within the cord). Extradural tumors include sarcomas and carcinomas, which may be metastatic from adjacent structures in or about the vertebrae. Other extradural lesions include Hodgkin's disease, lipomas, neurofibromas, chondromas, angiomas, abscesses, and granulomas.

Intradural tumors can be extramedullary, in which case they are usually benign and originate from the dura mater and arachnoid surrounding the cord and from the root sheaths of spinal nerves. Neurinomas are especially common in the thoracocervical area and may be part of generalized neurofibromatosis. Meningiomas also commonly occur in intradural extramedullary locations. Less frequently, lipomas or other types of tumors are found. Gliomas are the most common intramedullary tumors and have a less favorable prognosis. These tumors infiltrate the cord tissue and are much more difficult to remove than extramedullary tumors.

The majority of intradural tumors are extramedullary and benign and, if diagnosed early before severe neurological deficits occur, offer an excellent prognosis. They manifest their presence by pain of a radicular nature and various motor and sensory disabilities below their segmental locations.

Cord tumors frequently produce spinal fluid blockage and can be pinpointed accurately with MRI, which is now the procedure of choice with or without enhancement. Intraspinal injection of contrast material (myelography) is another option. A standard laminectomy is used for exposure and removal.

The rare surgical infections of the spinal cord take the form of extradural abscesses and granulomas. Treatment consists of a combination of excision, drainage, chemotherapy, and occasionally spinal fusion.

The most frequently encountered neurosurgical problem is the herniated intervertebral disc. Because of weakness or rupture of the circular ligament (anulus fibrosus), which confines the soft center of the disc (nucleus pulposus), herniation of the latter may occur and give rise to pain from nerve root compression. When pain is severe or nerve damage excessive, surgical excision of the disc offers the most satisfactory relief. The procedure entails interlaminar exposure and piecemeal removal of the displaced nucleus. If the spine is unstable or there are other incontrovertible reasons for operative stabilization of the bony spine, a fusion of one type or another may be combined with the disc surgery (Chapter 22).

Another method of treating disc disease is chemonucleolysis, a technique whereby primary lumbar intervertebral disc disease is treated by an intradiscal injection of the enzyme chymopapain. Chymopapain is a proteolytic enzyme in the form of a sterile lyophilized powder. However, the injection of chymopapain into the lumbar nucleus pulposus is not an innocuous procedure. Hypersensitivity to the drug and anaphylactic reactions have been reported. Reports of transverse myelitis and subsequent paraplegia associated with chymopapain injection have raised serious questions about its use in young and otherwise healthy patients.

A newer concept is that of percutaneous lumbar discectomy, through a posterolateral approach. The method entails gaining access to the disc space through the use of an introduction system and cannulae. A 2-mm aspiration probe (called a Nucleotome) is then placed through the cannula into the disc space, and the nucleus pulposus is aspirated.

Certain painful spinal lesions, usually of a malignant nature, can be controlled by epidural opiates or by dividing the pain fibers supplying the affected area. It may be accomplished by sectioning the sensory roots intraspinally (posterior rhizotomy) or by incising the spinothalamic tracts (anterolateral cordotomy) that carry pain and temperature impulses. A laminectomy is necessary for exposure.

Peripheral nerves

Within the context of this discussion, the peripheral nervous system includes the cranial nerves outside the cranial cavity, the spinal nerves, the autonomic nerves, and the ganglia. This division is artificial and only for the purpose of delineating surgical approaches. The cranial nerves have been described under the section on the head because all arise within the cranial cavity, and most are approached neurosurgically through the head.

There are 31 pairs of spinal nerves, each pair numbered for the level of the spinal column at which it emerges: cervical one (C1) through eight (C8), thoracic one (T1) through twelve (T12), lumbar one (L1) through five (L5), sacral one (S1) through five (S5), and coccygeal one. The thoracic region is sometimes referred to as the dorsal region with D1 being synonymous with T1 and so on. The first pair of cervical spine nerves emerges between C1 and the occipital bone. The eighth cervical nerves emerge from the intervertebral foramina between C7 and T1. The first thoracic nerves emerge between T1 and T2.

In the cervical and lumbosacral regions, the spinal nerves regroup in a plexiform manner before they form the peripheral nerves of the upper and lower extremities; those in the thoracic region form cutaneous and intercostal nerves. The principal nerves of the upper plexus include the musculocutaneous, median, ulnar, and radial; those of the lumbosacral plexus include the obturator, femoral, and sciatic.

Each spinal nerve divides into anterior, posterior, and white rami. Anterior and posterior rami contain voluntary fibers; white rami contain autonomic fibers. Posterior rami further branch into nerves going to the muscles, skin, and posterior surfaces of the head, neck, and trunk. Most anterior rami branch to the skeletal muscles and the skin of extremities and anterior and lateral surfaces. In the process they form plexuses, such as the brachial and sacral plexuses. Spinal nerves contain sensory dendrites and motor axons; some have somatic axons, and some have axons of preganglionic autonomic motor neurons.

The autonomic (involuntary) nervous system consists of all the efferent nerves, through which the cardiovascular apparatus, viscera, glands of internal secretion, and peripheral involuntary muscles are innervated (Fig. 23-21). A major anatomic difference between the somatic and autonomic nervous systems is that in the former an impulse from the brainstem or spinal cord reaches the end organ through a single neuron, whereas in the latter an impulse passes through two neurons—the first ending in an autonomic ganglion and the second running from the ganglion to the end organ. Some of the ganglia lie adjacent to the vertebral column to form the sympathetic trunks or

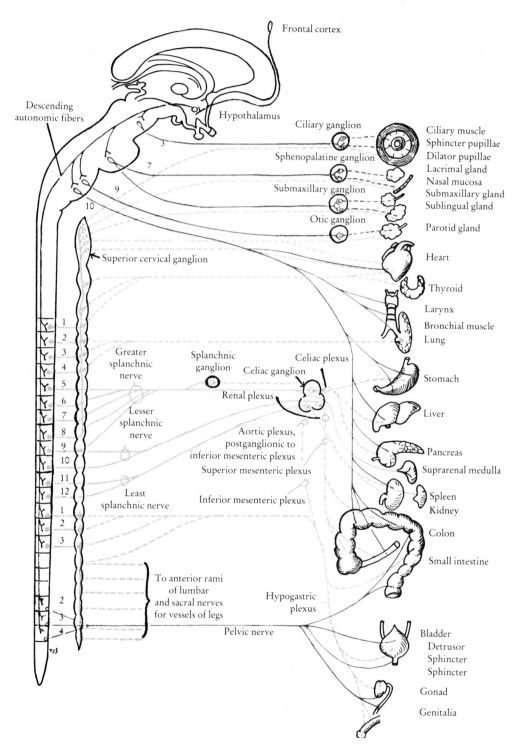

Fig. 23-21. Sympathetic division of the autonomic nervous system. (From Conway-Rutkowski, B.L.: Carini and Owens' neurological and neurosurgical nursing, ed. 8, St. Louis, 1982, The C.V. Mosby Co.)

chains; others are closely associated with the end organs.

The preganglionic neurons from the brainstem, which go out along the cranial nerves, and those from the second, third, and fourth sacral segments to the pelvic viscera end in ganglia in proximity to their end organs; thus their postganglionic fibers are very short. This is known as the *parasympathetic* or craniosacral division of the autonomic nervous system. The preganglionic fibers from the thoracic and lumbar spinal cord end in the paravertebral ganglia, making up the sympathetic chain, and their postganglionic fibers are relatively long. This is termed the *sympathetic* or thoracolumbar division of the autonomic nervous system.

The two divisions are distinct anatomically and physiologically. The chemical substance mediating transmission of impulses at most postganglionic sympathetic nerve endings is norepinephrine, and at all parasympathetic and preganglionic sympathetic neurons, acetylcholine.

The majority of organs have dual innervation, part from the craniosacral and part from the thoracolumbar divisions. The functions of these two systems are antagonistic. Together they work to maintain homeostasis. In general the thoracolumbar division functions as an emergency protection mechanism, always ready to combat physical or psychologic stress. The craniosacral division functions to conserve energy when the body is in a state of relaxation.

Stimuli arising from internal organs or from outside the body traverse visceral and somatic afferent nerve fibers to make reflex connections with preganglionic autonomic neurons in the brainstem and spinal cord. Such stimuli trigger activity of these involuntary systems automatically. When these automatic mechanisms break down or overact, surgery may be indicated. Thoracolumbar sympathectomy was once performed in hypertension to try to decrease blood vessel tone and lower the blood pressure. Vagotomy is done to decrease acid secretion to the stomach in peptic ulcer patients. Lumbar sympathectomy is used to relieve vasospastic disorders of the legs.

PERIOPERATIVE NURSING CONSIDERATIONS
Assessment/nursing diagnosis

Communication between the perioperative nurse and surgeon, either directly or through a knowledgeable person, such as a clinical nurse specialist, operating room supervisor, privately employed nurse, or resident who has direct communication with the surgeon, is essential for intelligently planning care for the neurosurgical patient in the operating room. Information the nurse needs before the arrival of the patient in the operating room includes the diagnosis; the diagnostic studies done and reports needed at the time of operation; the age, size, level of consciousness, physical disabilities resulting from neuropathologic conditions (as well as those from other causes), and communication problems of the patient; the specific surgical approach and body position to be used; the need

for any special equipment, instruments, or supplies not ordinarily used; the amount of blood ordered and available; the method or methods planned to reduce intracranial pressure in the case of cranial surgery; the need for radiologic support during the procedure; and the planned preliminary procedures, such as carotid ligation, lumbar puncture, placement of monitoring lines, and Foley catheter insertion. This information permits the nurse to plan for needed equipment, instruments, and supplies.

Most diagnostic procedures are performed before the patient arrives in the operating room. Studies of greatest significance to the perioperative nurse are radiologic studies that produce either positive or negative images the surgeon can use during the operation to locate the pathologic condition. The nurse is responsible for having these images in the operating room before the procedure begins. The studies include the following:

1. *Myelography*—injection of contrast medium into the spinal subarachnoid space to demonstrate a defect by radiography.
2. *Pneumonencephalography (PEG)*—injection of air into the subarachnoid space, usually through a lumbar or cisternal puncture, to outline the ventricular system and the cranial subarachnoid space to identify deviations from normal. Because of advances in radiologic techniques, this procedure has become somewhat dated.
3. *Ventriculography*—injection of air directly into the lateral ventricles when a block exists between the spinal canal and the lateral ventricles.
4. *Angiography (arteriography)*—injection of contrast medium into the brachial, carotid, vertebral, or femoral arteries to study the intracranial blood vessels for size, location, and configuration and to diagnose space-occupying lesions and vascular abnormalities.

   Digital subtraction angiography (DSA)—a computerized radiologic procedure. An intravenous rather than arterial injection is required; a contrast medium injection to allow examination of selected arterial circulation is used. DSA provides an alternative to cerebral angiography for high-risk patients by using computer technology.
5. *Venography*—dural sinus studies for narrowing sinuses and interference with cranial drainage, which often occur in lesions of the posterior fossa. This study is necessary for glomus jugular tumors.
6. *Computed tomography (CT scan)*—use of x-ray studies with or without instilled contrast medium and computer technology to produce a sequential series of positive images of transverse sections of the brain and spinal cord in which differences in tissue density can be detected and deviations from normal identified.
7. *Isotope brain scan*—injection of radioactive substance intravenously to demonstrate brain lesions.

8. *Echoencephalography*—method of recording referred ultrasound from reflecting surfaces; especially helpful in the identification of subdural hematomas.

   Echo doppler—noninvasive technique used to assess the blood flow in the carotid artery. The procedure can be done in or out of the surgical suite.

9. *Magnetic resonance imaging (MRI)*—use of powerful magnetic and radiofrequency waves to reproduce details of the human body with no known risk to patients; uses no radiation. Advances in MRI scanning provide enhancement of the scan with the use of gadolinium. Many patients experience extreme feelings of claustrophobia during MRI.

Five nursing diagnoses to be considered in caring for the neurosurgical patient are as follows:

- Anxiety related to surgery/surgical outcome
- Knowledge deficit related to diagnostic tests and surgical procedures
- Potential for ineffective breathing patterns related to location of tumor, surgical position, or effects of general anesthesia
- Potential for pain related to pathophysiologic alterations
- Potential for infection related to surgical intervention

Planning

Preparation can significantly reduce both anesthesia and intraoperative time for the patient as well as physical and psychologic stress for both the surgeon and the perioperative nurse. Planning for the patient's care in the operating room is based on the results of nursing assessment and the identification of relevant nursing diagnoses. The plan of care then includes goals derived from the nursing diagnoses; priorities are set and nursing interventions designed to assist the patient to reach the desired goals. Nursing interventions identified for the patient's plan of care may include reassessment, teaching, counseling, referrals, and specific interventions to assist the patient in achieving expected goals. The Sample Care Plan shown on pp. 714-715 could be utilized by the perioperative nurse for the patient who is undergoing a neurosurgical procedure.

Implementation

Neuropathologic conditions requiring surgical intervention can be found in any age group.

The most common problems requiring neurosurgical procedures in infants and children include meningocele, myelomeningocele, encephalocele, craniosynostosis, hydrocephalus, brain tumors, and trauma. The nurse plays a vital role in maintaining blood volume, body temperature, and fluid balance in pediatric patients. The nurse's role in maintaining blood volume includes planning for minimizing and monitoring blood loss, as well as for blood replacement. The surgeon may minimize blood loss by infiltrating the tissues at the site of incision with normal saline solution; minimizing or eliminating periosteal stripping and carefully attending to intracranial emissary veins and sinuses; and using electrosurgery and bipolar coagulation, bone wax, Gelfoam, thrombin, or Surgicel. The surgeon's preferences for instruments and supplies must be prepared and ready for use before needed. Sponges from the operative field must be continuously placed within view of the anesthesiologist or weighed as they are discarded from the field. Blood or blood products must be available in the surgical suite. A blood warmer must be ready to use as careful, accurate fluid replacement therapy is carried out. When the anesthesiologist is unable to see the operative field (which is usually the situation during *any* cranial surgery), the nurse must inform the anesthesiologist immediately of active bleeding at the operative site.

The nurse must place a warming blanket on the operating room bed before the pediatric patient arrives. If the room temperature can be individually regulated, the nurse should regulate the thermostat to a temperature about 22.2° C (72° F) after consultation with the anesthesiologist. The child's body and extremities can be wrapped in plastic materials. Body temperature is monitored with a rectal, intraaural, or esophageal thermistor probe. The thermistor unit must be calibrated and placed within the view of the anesthesiologist before surgery.

Some means to control and monitor fluid intake and output must be planned with the anesthesiologist and neurosurgeon: microdrip intravenous tubing or an electronic drip regulator such as an I-Vac unit may be used for regulating intravenous intake; a Foley catheter may be inserted into the bladder and attached to a urinometer and closed drainage system if the child is to undergo a prolonged procedure; output should be recorded at time intervals decided on by the nurse and anesthesiologist and based on the child's general condition. Irrigation fluid and suction bottle contents are measured and recorded.

Parents of infants and children are usually extremely anxious, as are the families of most surgical patients. Arrangements by which families can have contact with the patient through a nurse who has direct access to the operating room during the operation and the postanesthesia recovery relieve anxiety and diminish perceived waiting time for them.

Older children, adolescents, and adults come to the operating room fearful and apprehensive about the outcome of the surgical procedure and its effect on them and their life-style. Both male and female patients are devastated by having their hair removed. This procedure is best done by a nurse who can provide psychologic support and give realistic reassurance and information to both conscious, responsive patients and patients who may be incoherent or unconscious but still hear what is going on around them and feel what is being done to them. Hair removal from the head, like all other forms of preoperative

Sample Care Plan

NURSING DIAGNOSIS:
Anxiety related to surgery/surgical outcome
GOAL:
The patient's anxiety will be reduced or controlled.
INTERVENTIONS:
Broadly classify the patient's anxiety (low, moderate, high).
Provide reassurance and explanations; repeat as necessary.
Provide ongoing opportunity for patient (and/or family) to ask questions and express fears.
Involve other support persons (social worker, case manager, chaplain) as appropriate.
Determine the patient's coping skills.
Assist the patient to utilize personally effective coping skills.
Use touch to communicate caring (as appropriate).

NURSING DIAGNOSIS:
Knowledge deficit related to diagnostic and/or surgical procedures
GOAL:
Patient and/or family will verbalize knowledge of diagnostic and/or surgical procedures.

INTERVENTIONS:
Determine patient or family knowledge level (and desire for knowledge).
Correct misinformation; refer to other health care team members as appropriate.
Identify patient or family readiness and motivation to learn.
Provide information about procedures; use understandable terms.
Explain perioperative routine; include both factual information and expected sensations associated with tests, surgical procedure, perioperative environment, and postoperative care.
Base psychoeducational interventions on individual needs.

NURSING DIAGNOSIS:
Potential for ineffective breathing patterns related to location of tumor, surgical position, or effects of anesthesia
GOAL:
The patient will maintain effective breathing patterns.
INTERVENTIONS:
Provide appropriate positioning accessories; assist in their placement.

---

preparation, should be done as close to the time of skin incision as possible to decrease the possibility of postoperative wound infection. Some surgeons prefer complete hair removal because dressings are easier to apply, hair regrowth is more even, a better wig fit can be obtained, and it is far easier to prepare a sterile field around such an operative site. However, because of the severe disturbances in body image caused by total hair removal, an effort should be made to facilitate a compromise between patient and surgeon. Whenever possible, minimal hair removal is recommended. There may be a relationship between hair removal and postoperative recovery, especially in the areas of orientation, social interaction, and compliance. Also, when the patient's wishes are considered, the patient has a degree of control over what is happening.

An aged person undergoing neurosurgical intervention brings a potential range of problems such as hearing, sight, or mobility deficiencies unrelated to the neuropathologic condition. Responses to stimuli generally are slower in the elderly. The skin is more prone to pressure sores. The ability to heal may be impaired. More time and greater care must be taken with older patients. Communication can be established and reassurance given by touching and by being nearby while the patient is conscious. Vigilant monitoring of blood loss, temperature, and urine output is also required in caring for the older patient in the operating room. Surgery may be performed under local anesthesia, and the nurse may be responsible for monitoring vital signs, as well as for providing a human communication link for the patient. Sitting with the patient and explaining the procedure and the sensations that will be experienced makes the patient more comfortable and cooperative and diminishes fears.

Among neurosurgical patients are those who have little or no apparent loss of function, those who are coping with chronic pain and are looking forward to the operation for

Sample Care Plan—cont'd

Monitor ABGs; interpret and report variations from expected values.

Review results of pulse oximetry for blood oxygen saturation.

Collaborate with anesthesiologist in monitoring end-tidal volume carbon dioxide.

Maintain open suction line.

Note respiratory rate, depth, and characteristics of breath sounds.

Encourage patient to cough and breathe deeply on emergence from anesthesia.

Communicate with PACU regarding postoperative requirements for ventilatory assistance.

Check airway patency frequently during transport to PACU.

NURSING DIAGNOSIS:

Potential for pain related to pathophysiologic alterations

GOAL:

The patient will report a reduction in pain.

INTERVENTIONS:

Determine effectiveness of preoperative medications; communicate ineffectiveness.

Administer additionally prescribed medications to control pain and/or anxiety; monitor patient response.

Assist patient to utilize personally effective pain control measures.

Provide physical comfort measures (such as warm blankets) and emotional support.

Explain postoperative regimens for control of pain.

NURSING DIAGNOSIS:

Potential for infection related to surgical intervention

GOAL:

Patient will be free of signs and symptoms of infection.

INTERVENTIONS:

Adhere to strict aseptic technique.

Implement environmental precautions.

Control traffic patterns.

Document wound classification.

Identify and correct breaks in technique.

Dress wound, intravenous line sites, and drain exit sites aseptically.

Monitor for postoperative indications of infection (elevated temperature; redness, swelling, warmth, or drainage at incision site; persistent incisional pain).

Provide patient or family with specific information regarding wound care and the signs and symptoms that should be reported.

---

the relief it will bring, and those who are totally or partially dependent for everything because they are unconscious, quadriplegic, or aphasic. If pain is present, the nurse should know the type and site of the pain and aim to make the patient as comfortable as possible while conscious. If the patient is acutely and severely traumatized, the nurse must be aware of injuries other than those for which the patient is being treated neurosurgically so these injuries can be taken into consideration. A nurse with prior knowledge of a given situation is better prepared to cope with that situation and can plan individualized care based on that knowledge.

Basic neurosurgical maneuvers

Scientific advances that enable surgeons to control pain, hemorrhage, infection, and other physiologic responses have contributed largely to the neurosurgeon's ability to operate successfully on the nervous system. The extent of a modern neurosurgical operation may be determined not so much by the physiologic hazards involved as by the degree of neurologic disability that may be expected after surgery. Knowing the hazards and having everything ready in advance will enhance the ability of the surgeon to achieve a favorable outcome.

Preliminary procedures

A number of procedures or therapeutic measures may be performed by the neurosurgeon or other member of the team in a holding or induction room before positioning, prepping, and draping take place. It is important that the nurse know why these procedures are done in order to anticipate them and be prepared to facilitate them.

A Foley catheter is often inserted into the bladder to monitor urinary output during the procedure. It is essential for prolonged procedures and when mannitol is to be given intravenously, so the bladder does not become distended.

A Foley catheter is also required when hypothermia or hypotension will be induced, when excessive bleeding is anticipated, and in trauma patients for continuous assessment of kidney function.

A right atrial or central venous pressure line is required for management of air embolism. An air embolus can occur in operations on the head and neck when the patient is in an upright position. A left atrial pressure line may also be inserted in the operating room immediately before the surgical procedure is begun.

When excessive intracranial bleeding is a possibility, the neurosurgeon may choose carotid cutdown and temporary ligation or tourniquet placement for occlusion of the carotid arteries during bleeding. Carotid cutdown is a separate surgical procedure and requires a special sterile setup, including drapes and instruments. Procedures that may require such management include intracranial vascular surgery and removal of meningiomas.

In some situations, CSF drainage may be required. This can be done by placement of a ventricular cannula, such as the Scott or Seletz, or by placement of a spinal needle in the lower lumbar spinal canal. The stylet of either needle is left in place until drainage is required. The surgeon can remove the ventricular sylet, but the nurse must be able to remove the spinal needle stylet. When the lumbar puncture method is used, the patient is placed in a semilateral position and stabilized, so the patient does not roll onto the needle and the nurse can remove the stylet without contaminating it during the procedure. An extension tubing and stopcock can be attached to the needle at the time of lumbar puncture. When this is done, the tubing and stopcock are supported so traction is not put on the needle and are placed where they are accessible to the nurse or anesthesiologist. The stopcock can be opened for drainage.

Induced hypotension may be required to manage bleeding. Intracranial vascular surgery and removal of some tumors also may require induced hypotension. Sodium nitroprusside (Nipride) is an effective agent. Very little of the drug is required to produce an immediate and dramatic hypotensive state. Recovery from the effects of the drug is immediate. When mixed in solution for intravenous administration, sodium nitroprusside is unstable in light. The nurse must have a roll of aluminum foil available to cover the intravenous bottle and tubing completely when the drug is hanging and in use or ready for immediate use; an electronic device to measure and control the amount administered must also be set up.

Some surgeons prefer to use antibiotics in the immediate preoperative period. The regimen includes streptomycin, 50 mg in 1000 ml of saline irrigation. Before the surgical procedure begins, vancomycin, 1 g, is given intravenously and tobramycin, 80 mg, is given intramuscularly. If this regimen is used, postoperative antibiotics may not be needed.

Skin preparation

Head hair is best removed after the patient has arrived in the surgery department but before arrival in an operating room. The hair is first clipped with an electric clippers, which is cleaned and disinfected after each use. The hair is placed in a container, labeled with the patient's name, and kept with the patient after surgery. The scalp is then shaved, using warm, soapy water and either a straight razor or several disposable safety razors. As soon as the patient experiences any pulling, the razor blade should be changed. The nurse should explain to the patient exactly what is being done and what sensations to expect during the procedure.

For surgery on the cervical spine, it is possible to secure long hair on top of the head and remove neck hair with a clippers to a level even with the top of the ears or just below the occipital protuberance. Postoperatively, patients with long hair can comb it down over the shaved area until the hair regrows.

Patients undergoing thoracic or lumbar spine surgery may not need to be shaved. If hair is present, it can be removed by depilatory or clipping just before surgery.

After hair removal, the skin should be inspected carefully for any signs of inflammation or infection. If any such signs are noted, they should be reported to the surgeon immediately.

An antiseptic skin prep is done after the patient is positioned and before draping. Skin prepping may be done by the perioperative nurse, surgeon, or resident. General principles and precautions cited in Chapter 5 apply to neurosurgical preparations, regardless of who performs them.

Many neurosurgeons mark the incision line with a marking pencil, a marking solution and wooden stick, or a scalpel. If a marking solution is used, indigo carmine, gentian violet, or brilliant green is recommended. Methylene blue should *never* be found in a neurosurgical operating room because it produces an inflammatory reaction in central nervous system tissue and could be disastrous if accidentally injected into the subarachnoid space, for example.

After marking, the surgeon may inject the incision site and the sites for application of towel clamps with a local anesthetic agent or with normal saline solution. Any solution will apply pressure within the tissues and decrease bleeding at the time of incision. The local anesthetic agent has the additional effect of decreasing the effect of the stimulus of the skin incision.

Positioning

The basic body positions and their modifications are used in neurosurgery. The nurse must know the position for each procedure; the hazards and precautions of each position; and the equipment, supportive positioning devices, and time necessary to place a patient in a given position (Chapter 6). General considerations of special importance in positioning for neurosurgery include protecting the eyes from pressure, chemical burns, and corneal scratches; maintaining joints in functional alignment with no pressure or tension on superficial nerves and vessels; and checking the Foley catheter for tension and kinks to ensure drainage.

The dorsal recumbent, or supine, position or some modification of it is used for supratentorial craniotomy, subtemporal decompression, and anterior cervical fusion. The lateral position is used for thoracic and lumbar laminectomy by some surgeons and for lumbar sympathectomy. Modifications of the prone position can be used for lumbar, thoracic, and cervical laminectomy and for posterior fossa craniectomy. The sitting, or upright, position can be used for cervical laminectomy, posterior fossa craniectomy, temporal craniectomy, and ventriculography. Only specific aspects of the sitting position for neurosurgical procedures and the knee-chest position, a modification of the prone position, are covered in this chapter.

The extreme sitting, or upright, position may be the neurosurgeon's choice for infratentorial cranial surgery and posterior cervical laminectomy when acute trauma is not the cause of cervical cord disease. Advantages of this position include optimum visibility of the operative field and decreased blood loss because of the lowered arterial and venous pressures. However, hypotensive changes also pose potential problems: some patients cannot tolerate the upright position under general anesthesia; thus the patient is slowly placed in this position as the anesthesiologist monitors the blood pressure. Most patients have a drop in arterial pressure but rapidly adapt to the position; those who do not are placed in the prone position. In the sitting position, the venous pressure in the head and neck may be negative, predisposing to air embolism. Other potential problems with this position include neck flexion with airway compromise and difficulty in achieving and maintaining functional alignment.

Preoperatively, elastic bandages, wrapped from the patient's toes to groin, special tensor stockings, such as TED hose, or sequential compression stockings may be applied. All these help prevent venous stasis in the lower extremities and help maintain the blood pressure. Other precautions during positioning and throughout the procedure include checking the heels, soles of feet, and popliteal areas to prevent pressure; checking male genitals to ensure that pressure will not compromise circulation and cause necrosis and female breasts to prevent any unnecessary pressure; preventing thighs from contacting the metal crossbar table attachment; stabilizing the head in the headrest; and stabilizing the shoulders and torso to prevent neck flexion.

Preparations should be made in collaboration with the anesthesiologist to manage air embolism if this complication should occur. The patient may be placed in a G-suit before positioning to prevent this complication. The G-suit also assists in maintaining the blood pressure. A right atrial line can be placed under direct vision fluoroscopy either in the cardiac catheterization laboratory or radiology department, before arrival of the patient in the operating room, or in the operating room, using the image intensifier. After anesthesia induction, the anesthesiologist may place an esophageal stethoscope or attach the patient to a Doppler unit to hear air entering the right atrium. The air can be withdrawn through the atrial line with a 50-ml syringe and three-way stopcock connection. If the management of air embolism includes repositioning the patient with the surgical wound open, the repositioning must be accomplished quickly, without endangering the patient in other ways, such as contamination of the surgical wound, displacement of a joint, or dislodgement of the endotracheal tube.

The most common position for lumbar and thoracic laminectomy is prone. Both legs are wrapped with elastic bandages, or tensor hose are used to prevent venous stasis in the extremities. Anesthesia induction and intubation take place on the transport vehicle. The patient is then placed on the operating room bed in the prone position. Special bed attachment supports or a chest roll must be placed under the chest on each side from the shoulder to the iliac crest to permit lung expansion during the procedure. The bottom of the bed is dropped to about a 25-degree angle. The patient's knees are flexed, and the lower legs elevated and supported on two large pillows and the bed mattress, under which the footboard is placed at right angles to the bed. The knees are padded with foam. The arms are flexed at the elbows and supported by pillows on wide armboards. Care is taken to prevent pressure or tension on the brachial plexus. The Wilson back frame can be used. The patient is placed prone on the frame with pillows under the legs and pillows or sheets supporting each arm. For surgery on the neck and posterior skull, the foot of the bed is not dropped; the ankles and feet are supported on a large pillow; and the arms are secured at the patient's sides, protecting the ulnar, median, and radial nerves. A horseshoe or Mayfield point headrest may be used.

The major problems encountered with the prone position include increase in venous pressure and bleeding at the operative site, peripheral venous stasis, and decrease in vital capacity. Precautions include checking female breasts, male genitals, and knees to prevent pressure on these areas; avoiding hyperextension of shoulders and pressure on the brachial plexus when turning the patient to begin positioning and during the procedure; preventing abduction of the arms and occlusion of the subclavian and axillary arteries; and protecting the eyes from pressure, corneal scratches, and chemical burns.

The knee-chest, or "tuck," position is also used for lumbar laminectomy. This is a modification of the prone position, in which the patient's hips and knees are flexed so the body is supported on the thighs and lower legs, with the abdomen and chest hanging free or supported on chest rolls. The Hicks spinal surgery frame (Butt Board®) may be used for the knee-chest position. Advantages of this position include decreased bleeding because of the collapse of epidural veins, better exposure resulting from hyperflexion of the spine, absence of pressure on the vena cava, and increased ease of ventilation. Operating time is usually reduced when this position is used.

Disadvantages of the knee-chest position include the difficulty of maintaining physical stability on the operating room bed, hypotension, and pooling of blood in the lower extremities.

Draping

Most neurosurgeons do their own draping. Draping for some procedures is complex and requires the cooperation of surgeon, assistant and nurse. Four or more towels are placed around the operative site. They may be secured by disposable skin staples, small towel clamps, or silk sutures on a heavy cutting needle. When sutures are used, the surgeon also needs a heavy, 6-inch toothed tissue forceps and a suture scissors. Forceps, scissors, needle holders, and needles are discarded after towels have been secured in place.

A plastic adhesive drape may be placed either before or after the towels. The skin must be completely dry for the drape to adhere tightly to the skin.

Fluid-impervious barrier drape sheets and towels are essential. If an overhead instrument table is used, it should be covered with a sheet large enough that the front edge can be fanfolded at the front edge of the table until the table is brought forward over the patient toward the operative site. The fanfolded sheet can then be secured at the lower border of the operative site to bridge the gap between the unsterile undersurface of the table and the sterile field. Mayo stands should also be covered with effective barriers. The particulars of draping for neurosurgical procedures vary and are influenced by the patient's position, the surgeon's preferences, and what is available in each hospital. Therefore, a detailed description of the draping for each procedure is not provided here. The particulars of draping for each procedure should be clearly described on the neurosurgeon's preference card. Doubts can be clarified by communication with the neurosurgeon before the operation.

As a general rule, neurosurgeons prefer to have all equipment ready before making the incision. Therefore, they can be helpful to the nurse in attaching and hooking up suction tubings, electrosurgical cords, and other equipment that will be needed for the operation.

Hemostasis

Meticulous hemostasis is of particular importance in neurosurgery. The first consideration is control of hemorrhage from the highly vascular scalp. Compression of the edges of the wound with gauze sponges and fingers during the initial incision is followed by application of hemostatic clips and clamps. When clips are used, they are applied so that they include the galea and skin edge, whereas clamps are attached directly to the galea and then everted. Before the incision is made, normal saline solution or a local anesthetic agent may be injected to minimize scalp bleeding.

Bone wax, a hemostatic material described in Chapter 7, is prepared for all cranial and spinal cord operations. The surgeon firmly rubs the wax into the bleeding surface of the bone after all periosteum has been scraped off. When the skull flap has been elevated, bone wax is also rubbed into the diploë to control bleeding from the bone edge. During spinal surgery, bone wax is used on the cut edges of the laminae.

Electrosurgery is routine for neurosurgical procedures. Nursing personnel must understand the uses and hazards of the electrosurgical unit and be familiar with the safety measures. Electrocoagulation may be used to stop bleeding in the galea, in the periosteum, on the surface of the dura, on the spinal cord, and in the brain. The coagulation current seals the blood vessels. The electrical current is applied to the forceps, a metal suction tip, or other instrument, which acts as a conducting tool. To be effective, the coagulating current must contact the vessel in a dry field. For this reason, suctioning is necessary to remove the blood as the contact is made between the instrument carrying the current and the bleeding point.

Bipolar electrosurgical units are frequently used (Fig. 23-22). Bipolar units provide a completely isolated output with negligible leakage of current between the tips of the forceps, permitting use of coagulating current in proximity to structures where ordinary unipolar coagulation would be hazardous. Ringer's lactate or normal saline irrigation is used during bipolar coagulation to minimize tissue heating, shrinkage, drying, and adherence to the forceps. Some bipolar units have built-in irrigating systems. Need for a dispersive pad is eliminated. The use of the bipolar coagulation technique allows hemostasis of almost any size vessel encountered. Vessels as large as the superficial temporal artery, as well as those too small for suture or clip ligation, may be coagulated with bipolar units.

Electrosurgery is also used for cutting with a lower power setting. When the surgeon is using a cutting electrode to remove a tumor, the circulating nurse should stand by the machine to adjust the settings as needed. As the surgeon uses the cutting electrode, an assistant holds a suction tip to one side of the area of dissection to remove smoke.

Gauze sponges are used to control bleeding before the skull or spinal canal is entered. Coarse gauze sponges injure fragile tissues such as the brain or spinal cord, so wet compressed rayon cotton (cottonoid) pledgets or strips

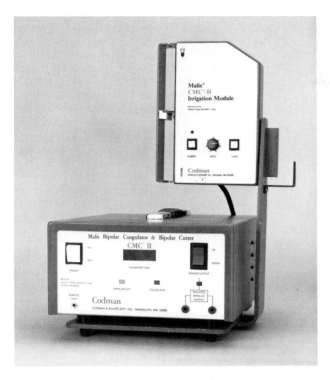

Fig. 23-22. Malis bipolar coagulator and bipolar cutter, with irrigation module. (Courtesy Codman & Shurtleff, Inc., Randolph, Mass.)

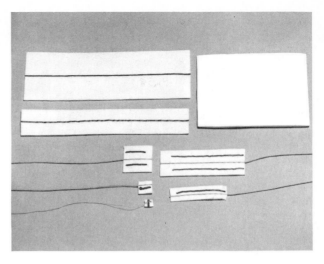

Fig. 23-23. Cottonoid strips and neuro patties. (Courtesy Codman & Shurtleff, Inc., Randolph, Mass.)

are used in place of gauze sponges to control bleeding beneath the skull and around the spinal cord. Sterile cottonoid strips and pledgets, or "patties," must be available in a variety of sizes (Fig. 23-23). Strips are usually 6 inches long, although some surgeons prefer them 3 inches in length. The standard widths are ¼, ½, ¾, and 1 inch. Strips have x-ray-detectable markers or strings attached. Pledgets should have both x-ray-detectable markers and strings attached.

Standard sizes for pledgets are ¼ × ¼ inch, ½ × ½ inch, ¾ × ¾ inch, and 1 × 1 inch. All strips and pledgets must be counted. Some surgeons prefer to use Biocal or Telfa strips, which the nurse cuts to size before use. During the procedure the nurse maintains a supply of these special neurosurgical sponges, thoroughly soaked with normal saline or Ringer's lactate solution, within reach of the surgeon's forceps. They may be displayed on a waterproof surface, such as a towel; a sterile inverted metal basin (emesis basin, small bowl); a plastic drape, such as 3M or Vi-Drape; a piece of rubber clipped to a folded towel; or a "patty plate," a flat piece of metal that attaches to the Mayo tray with two small towel clamps. The surgeon may prefer that the nurse keep a supply of these moist sponges on the palm or back of one hand and extend them toward the surgeon as needed. The sponges are aligned on the display surface in order of size. As soon as one is used, the nurse replaces it.

Loose wet cotton balls may be used as a temporary pack or tamponade in a bleeding tumor bed after a tumor has been removed. The gentle pressure of the cotton balls along with time and patience on the part of the surgeon may stop bleeding not controllable by other means. The scrub nurse is responsible for counting the number of cotton balls placed in the tumor bed and ensuring that none is left behind at closure.

A variety of hemostatic clips are available and used by neurosurgeons to occlude both superficial and deep vessels. The original clip used by Cushing and later modified by McKenzie is made of silver. Newer clips such as the Samuels hemoclip and the Ligaclip are of tantalum or an alloy that is compatible with the MRI scanner. The nurse removes the clips from a special cartridge with the appropriate applicator and passes them to the surgeon for application to a vessel. Such clips enable the surgeon to occlude vessels in areas difficult to reach by other means and to ligate superficial vessels of the brain before cutting them and without destroying any surrounding tissues. Clips can be obtained in a variety of sizes.

Hemostatic scalp clips include Raney, Adson, and LeRoy clips. Autoclips and Michel clips are still used occasionally (Fig. 23-24). There are also plastic disposable scalp clips of the Raney and Leroy Raney types. Each type of clip has a specific clip applier by which the clips are placed on the scalp edges. At time of closure, clips are removed by a hemostat, a special clip remover, or the applier, which simultaneously serves as a remover. A minimum of two clip appliers is essential; the nurse loads one clip applier while the surgeon is using the other to place the clip on the scalp. The Adson clips are loaded on the appliers from a special rack. After use they must be reshaped before replacement on the clip rack; there is a

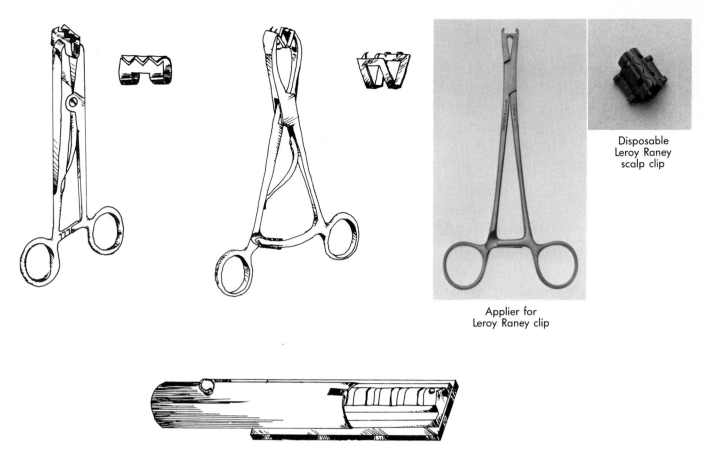

Fig. 23-24. Scalp clip appliers and clips, disposable Leroy Raney scalp clip, and applier for Leroy Raney scalp clip. (Courtesy Codman & Shurtleff, Inc., Randolph, Mass.)

special instrument for this purpose. The Raney and Michel clips are loaded by hand. If the Raney clips are non-disposable, they are difficult to clean by hand and should be placed in a sonic cleaner or soaked in hydrogen peroxide.

Numerous special clips are used for permanent or temporary occlusion of vessels or an aneurysm neck in the surgical treatment of intracranial aneurysm. These are discussed under "Microneurosurgery."

Neurosurgeons almost routinely use certain hemostatic agents in addition to mechanical hemostasis. Gelfoam is one of these agents. It comes in two forms: a powder and a compressed sponge. The sponge is produced in three sizes: nos. 12, 50, and 100. The sponge form can be applied to an oozing surface dry or saturated with saline solution or topical thrombin. The larger pieces of Gelfoam are cut into a variety of sizes of strips and pledgets. The surgeon's preference dictates the exact method of preparation and use. Gelfoam is absorbable and can be left in the body.

Surgicel, a rayonlike cellulose gauze, and Oxycel, an absorbable hemostatic agent that comes in both cotton and gauze forms, are used to control bleeding from oozing

surfaces, vessels, and sinuses in the brain and spinal canal. These hemostatic substances are also cut into suitable sizes and shapes and are handed to the surgeon dry, followed by a moist cottonoid strip or patty. The hemostatic material adheres to the bleeding area as gentle pressure is applied to the cottonoid material for several minutes.

Pieces of fresh muscle tissue can be used to tamponade and control bleeding where the usual forms of hemostasis are not possible.

Most surgeons use Polyglactin synthetic absorbable; black, braided nylon; or silk suture material for traction sutures and wound closure.

Irrigating the wound with Ringer's lactate or normal saline solution may facilitate hemostasis. This procedure definitely helps the surgeon identify active bleeding points. Two completely filled bulb or Asepto syringes should always be within reach of the surgeon. Suction is the best means of keeping the wound dry and permitting control of bleeding. Therefore, suction and irrigation are used together.

Metal suction tips, such as the Cone, Sachs, Frazier, Bucy, or Adson (Fig. 23-25), are used because they not only keep the wound dry but also can be used to conduct

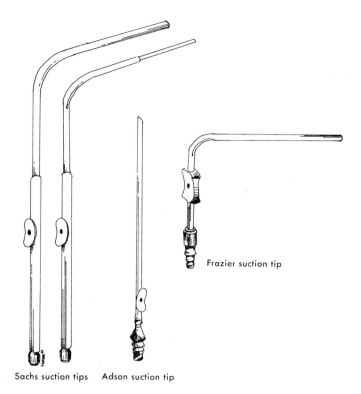

Frazier suction tip

Sachs suction tips   Adson suction tip

Fig. 23-25. Suction tips.

coagulation current from a monopolar unit to the bleeding point. The Bucy-Frazier tip is insulated and attached to both suction and electrosurgical units to become the active coagulating electrode. Use of the suction-coagulation unit is limited to areas in which gross coagulation can be done safely, for example, during the opening phase of a surgical procedure.

Suction can be used to remove necrotic or traumatized brain tissue or soft brain tumors rapidly after a sample has been obtained for pathologic examination. It is also useful in evaluating abscess cavities, removing fluid from a ventricle or the subarachnoid space, holding a solid tumor during its removal, and applying compression to a bleeding vessel.

Many neurosurgeons irrigate surgical wounds with an antibiotic solution before wound closure. The antibiotic must be mixed with irrigation solution according to the surgeon's preference so it is ready for use when needed. Gelfoam may be soaked in antibiotic solution before use.

Equipment

An operating room used for neurosurgical procedures should be large enough to accommodate the equipment needed for procedures done by the neurosurgeons on the hospital staff. The emphasis of this discussion is equipment that is *necessary* for neurosurgery in any setting.

Essential built-in equipment includes a minimum of four electrical outlets per wall, four overhead spotlights with autoclavable handles to permit persons at the operative field to adjust the lights as needed, six single or three double x-ray view boxes, and four wall or ceiling vacuum suction outlets capable of high negative pressure. Other equipment that can be built in if the situation demands includes a two-way telephone communication line, a ceiling-mounted operating microscope with camera, a closed-circuit television unit with monitor, an electrocardiogram-electroencephalogram monitor with readouts, and a wall or ceiling source of nitrogen or compressed air to operate air-powered equipment.

Some basic mobile equipment is needed for any setting in which neurosurgery is done. An operating room bed and complete set of bed attachments and neurosurgical headrests are essential. The best headrest is one that can be adapted for use in any body position, such as the Amsco multipoise, the Gardner, and the Mayfield skull clamp (Fig. 23-26, *B*). Each of these headrests has a three-pin suspension and skull clamp that attaches to a headrest bed attachment for secure fixation of the skull during the operation. This is especially useful when the patient is placed in a sitting position. Two or three sterile pins are placed in the head after the insertion sites are prepared with an antiseptic, such as an iodophor. The headrest skull clamp is first attached to the pins and then to the bed attachment. Precautions during insertion of the pins include avoiding the frontal sinuses and superficial temporal arteries. Other headrests, such as the Light-Veley or Multipoise (Fig. 23-26, *A* and *B*), that are of more limited use may be preferred by the individual neurosurgeon. In many instances, especially for supratentorial craniotomy, the head can be stabilized by a rubber doughnut. A mobile cart should be used for storage of the neurosurgical headrests and bed parts, as well as any other positioning devices and aids used by the neurosurgeon.

One special neurosurgical overhead instrument table, such as the Mayfield table (Fig. 23-27), is preferable, but two large Mayo trays can be used for any neurosurgical procedure. One large instrument back table is a must. It should be at least 6 to 8 inches higher than the standard table because the scrub nurse must frequently work on a high lift to see the operative field and perform effectively. The extra height of the back table enables the nurse to maintain a sterile field and to work more comfortably.

Eight to 10 footstools are needed. They can be arranged side by side or on top of each other for the safety, efficiency, and comfort of the personnel. Kickbuckets are needed for trash and sponges. Also useful are two small utility tables for preparation and special equipment and supplies.

A cooling-heating unit with two blankets, such as the K-thermia unit, should be available for use. An electronic temperature monitoring device with esophageal, intraaural, and rectal probes is essential.

Other essential equipment includes a monopolar elec-

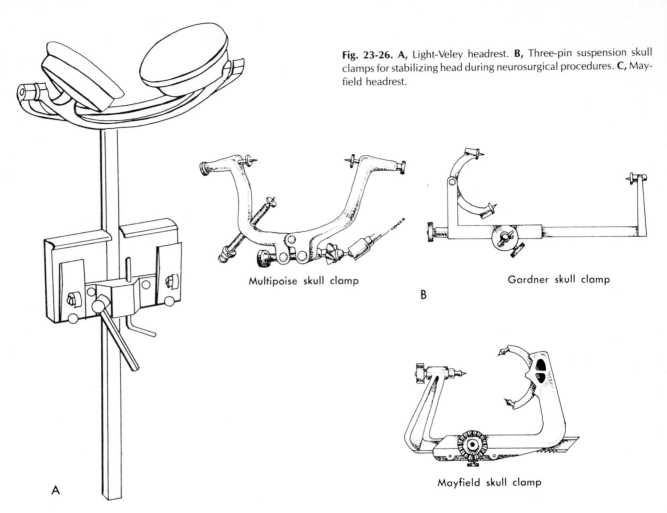

Fig. 23-26. A, Light-Veley headrest. **B,** Three-pin suspension skull clamps for stabilizing head during neurosurgical procedures. **C,** Mayfield headrest.

Multipoise skull clamp

Gardner skull clamp

Mayfield skull clamp

A

B

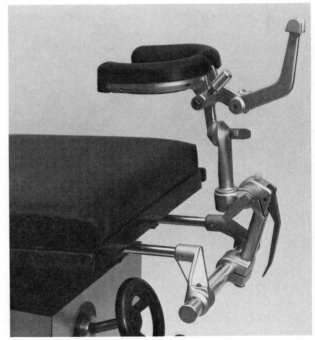

C

trosurgical unit, a bipolar electrosurgical unit, at least one fiberoptic headlight, and one fiberoptic light source for lighted retractors and telescopes, if they are used. Also needed is an operating microscope such as the Zeiss or Storz, a portable tank of nitrogen with a special pressure gauge for operating air-powered instruments, four pressure bags and bulb pumps for infusion of blood, two blood-warming units, one or two electronic intravenous rate control units such as I-Vac units, a solution warmer, and a nerve stimulator. A cryosurgical unit, an image intensifier, and a stereotaxic apparatus may be needed if the surgical procedure requires them. A laser, ultrasonic surgical aspirator, and intraoperative ultrasound should be available (Fig. 23-28).

Instrumentation

Scientific developments in other fields have been applied to the health care delivery system in general. Some of the developments with application to neurosurgery in the forms of specialized instrumentation and equipment have been discussed previously. A few items require further discussion.

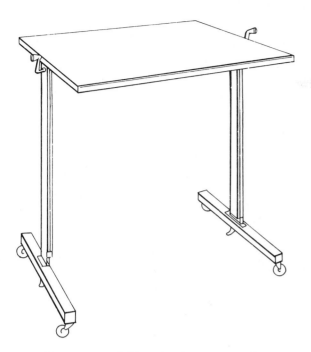

Fig. 23-27. Mayfield overhead instrument table.

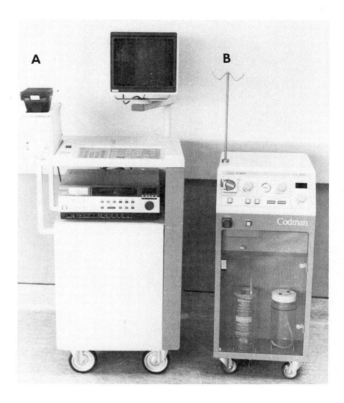

Fig. 23-28. A, Intraoperative ultrasound. **B,** Ultrasonic aspirator. (Courtesy Codman & Shurtleff, Inc., Randolph, Mass.)

Air-powered instrumentation has become popular with neurosurgeons over the years since the first Hall air drill was developed. Modifications of the original instrument continue today. These instruments decrease open wound time and anesthesia time for the patient and conserve energy for the surgeon.

The basic air driver has been adapted by means of special attachments for neurosurgery. Because improvements and new developments in air-powered instruments are on-going, specific instructions for use and care of such equipment should be obtained from the manufacturer at the time of purchase. Basic general information is included here.

The Air Drill 100 (Fig. 23-29) has replaced the Surgairtome or Hall II air drill for precision cutting, shaping, and repair of bone. Its use increases the ease of bone work and reduces operating time. Compressed nitrogen is the power source, as with other air-powered equipment. The Air Drill 100 can be used to widen the graft area in anterior fusions and to unroof the auditory canal in eighth cranial nerve surgery. For use in less accessible areas, such as the sphenoidal sinus, pituitary fossa, and vertebral bodies, 20-degree and 90-degree angle attachments are available. A range of burrs and guards is available.

The Craniotome C-100 (Fig. 23-30) is the newest adaptation of the original Hall Neurairtome. A perforator driver attachment reduces the speed to 1000 rpm for drilling burr holes. Both 12-mm and 7-mm perforators are available, disposable or reusable. The perforator driver attachment can be removed, and a saw blade and dura guard attached to adapt the instrument for cutting a cra-

niotomy bone flap. The saw blade is interchangeable with a wire-pass drill bit for drilling holes and placing wires, when a bone flap is to be wired in place. A cranioplasty burr and skull contour burr, as well as guards for each type of burr, are available.

Electrically powered instruments were popular and widely used before the introduction of the air-powered models. Some surgeons prefer power drills such as the Light-Veley or the Codman-Shurtleff drills with a Smith perforator.

Another versatile pneumatic tool is the Midas Rex Whirlwind instrument (Chapter 22). The variety of disposable cutting tools of this foot-controlled instrument and its attachments provides the neurosurgeon with a wide capability in bone cutting, including small rectangular holes in place of burr holes; bone flaps of any size and shaping; and unroofing areas such as the sphenoid wing. Manufacturer's precautions and instructions must be followed.

The operating microscope (Chapter 18) has revolutionized neurosurgery, making possible procedures never done before and making other neurosurgical procedures on vessels, such as aneurysm surgery and surgery on nerves, more precise and therefore more successful.

The lens system for neurosurgery and the angle of the microscope are different from those used in otologic surgery. If a microscope is shared by neurologic and otologic

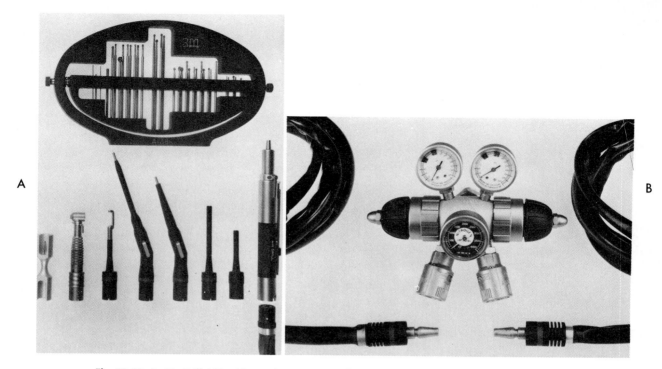

Fig. 23-29. A, Air Drill 100 with attachments. **B,** Dual nitrogen regulator. (Courtesy 3M Co., St. Paul, Minn.)

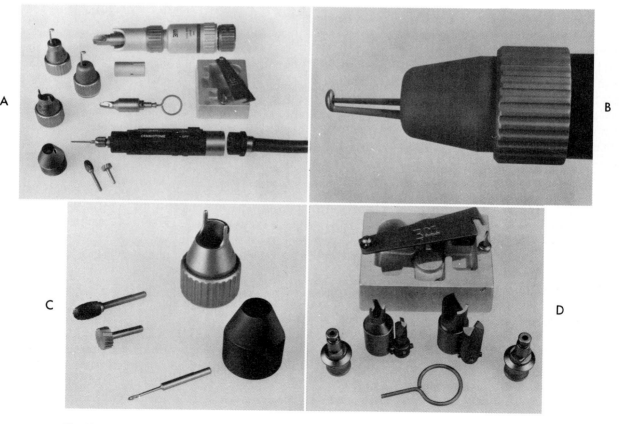

Fig. 23-30. A, Craniotome C-100 with attachments. **B,** Craniotome with neuroblade. **C,** Cranioplasty and wire-pass attachments. **D,** Skull perforators. (Courtesy 3M Co., St. Paul, Minn.)

services, the nurse must be able to adapt the microscope for use in neurosurgery by attachment of the appropriate pieces, and the surgeon must check it for focal length and focus before scrubbing. Disposable drapes are available for the microscope, as are assistant and observer lenses. Cameras and closed-circuit television monitors are also available for use with the operating microscope, if the situation warrants such sophisticated equipment.

The routine use of video cameras, recorders, and television monitors, if available, is invaluable to teach staff and enhance interest and understanding of the surgical procedure by nurses who are otherwise unable to visualize the surgeon's actions directly.

Many surgeons routinely use the carbon dioxide laser for precise dissection and hemostasis. The laser produces a concentrated infrared energy beam, generated by carbon dioxide, that can be precisely focused on any point at which it is aimed. The beam, which is made visible by a superimposed red aiming light, causes flash vaporization of cellular water at 100° C. Advantages of the laser include improved hemostasis and healing with decreased tissue trauma, swelling, and risk of metastasis. Postoperative morbidity is minimal. The laser is especially advantageous in microvascular surgery and is used to occlude vessels less than 0.5 mm in diameter in operations for aneurysms and arteriovenous malformations, as well as to remove tumors with minimal or no damage to surrounding structures. Tissue damage depends on amounts of energy generated and exposure duration.

Precautions include the need to wear protective glasses or plastic goggles to prevent accidental damage to eyes of personnel in the room and the need to keep all cottonoid, sponge, and towel materials thoroughly damp to prevent fire that could result from contact between a dry combustible material and the beam. The carbon dioxide and other gas sources must be checked before use to ensure adequate supply for the procedure. Nonflammable anesthetic agents must be used.

Direct image intensification is essential for an increasing number of neurosurgical procedures, such as placement of nerve stimulator electrodes in brain or spinal areas and stereotaxic procedures. If possible, a C-arm and monitor should be available in the operating room. Otherwise these procedures can be done in the radiology department. Procedures requiring use of the CT scan can also be done in the radiology department.

Choice of instrumentation for a given neurosurgical procedure is largely controlled by the surgeon or, in some operating rooms, by the chief of the department. Exactly what the neurosurgeon needs for a specific procedure is highly individual. Factors that influence the choices include training, experience, type of setting in which the surgery is performed, pathologic condition of the patient, surgical approach planned, and equipment available.

Some hospitals provide a full range of highly specialized neurosurgical instrumentation; some supply only instruments that can be used in orthopedic, otologic, or nasal surgery as well as in neurosurgery. Many neurosurgeons in private practice carry some or all of their own special instruments from hospital to hospital.

Usually several instruments can be used to perform one function. The choice depends on what is available and the surgeon's preference. Therefore, only instrument types and examples of each type are listed here. The exact instrument list for any neurosurgeon for each procedure must be written by the nurse in collaboration with that surgeon.

Basic instruments include the following list (specific names in parentheses are examples):

    1 Hudson brace (or craniotome) with burrs and perforators
    1 Drill guide
    1 Hand drill with drill bits and key
    2 Cranial saw handles
    2 Cranial saw guides (Cushing, Bailey, Poppen)
    6 Cranial saws (Gigli, Tyler)
    2 Double-action rongeurs, 9¾ inches (Stille gooseneck, Leksell)
    2 Double-action rongeurs, 6¾ inches (Zaufel-Jansen, Beyer, Fulton)
    2 Single-action rongeurs (Adson, Stookey, Lempert)
    2 Cloward punches, 40-degree, 5 mm and 3 mm
    1 Raney punch
    1 Kerrison rongeur, 5 mm
    5 Penfield dissectors, nos. 1, 2, 3, 4, and 5
    5 Bone curettes, nos. 0, 00, 1, 3, and 4
    2 Four-prong rake retractors, dull
    2 Cushing subtemporal decompression retractors
    4 Self-retaining retractors, dull, 8 inches (Cone, Weitlaner, Anderson-Adson)
    1 Jansen mastoid retractor
   36 Scalp clips (Adson, Raney, Michel)
    2 Scalp clip appliers for the specific clip used
    1 Scalp clip remover (Adson, Michel)
    4 Bayonet forceps, smooth, 7¼ inches
    2 Tissue forceps with teeth, 6 inches
    2 Cushing forceps, smooth, 7 inches
    2 Cushing forceps with teeth, 7 inches
    2 Adson tissue forceps, 5 inches
   18 Towel clamps, Backhaus type, 3½ inches
   18 Halsted mosquito hemostats, 12 curved and 6 straight
   36 Hemostatic scalp forceps (Dandy, Crile, Kolodney, Kelly)
   10 Rochester-Pean forceps
    4 Kocher forceps, straight, 6 inches
   12 Towel clamps, Peers type
    6 Fishhook retractors
    4 Periosteal elevators (Cushing, Adson, Langenbeck)
    1 Dura separator (Sachs, Frazier, Hoen)
    1 Adson elevator, no. 3
    1 Cushing periosteal elevator (joker)
    2 Freer dissectors (Olivecrona, Woodson)
    4 Ventricular needles with obturators, 3½ inches (Cone, Seletz, Scott)
    1 Brain-aspirating needle with cannula
    1 Aneurysm needle
    2 Brain spoons, 1 small and 1 large (Cushing)
    6 Suction tips, 2 each large, medium, and small (Frazier, Bucy, Sachs, Cone, Adson)
    2 Suction tubings

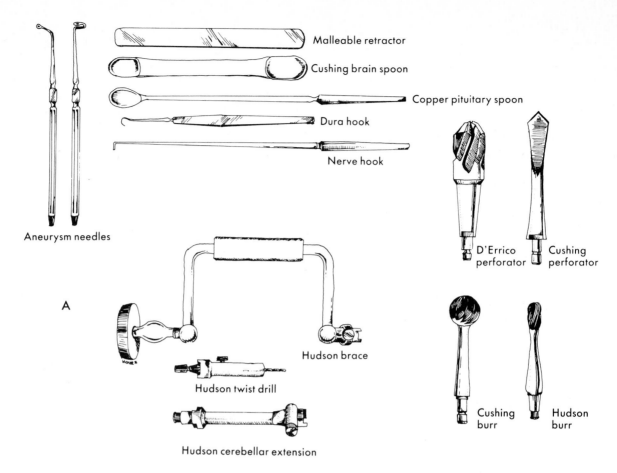

Malleable retractor

Cushing brain spoon

Copper pituitary spoon

Dura hook

Nerve hook

Aneurysm needles

A

Hudson brace

Hudson twist drill

Hudson cerebellar extension

D'Errico perforator

Cushing perforator

Cushing burr

Hudson burr

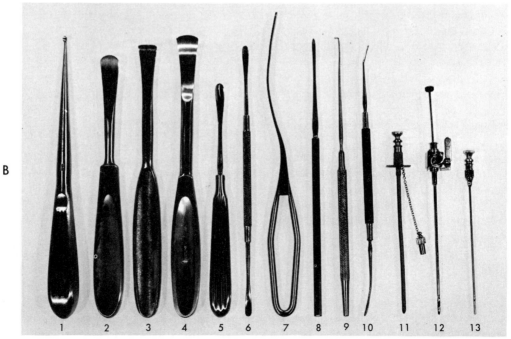

B

1 2 3 4 5 6 7 8 9 10 11 12 13

Fig. 23-31. A, Some basic instruments for craniotomy. **B,** *1,* Spinal curette, straight; *2,* Cushing periosteal elevator, blunt; *3,* Cushing periosteal elevator, sharp; *4,* Adson periosteal elevator, wide; *5,* Adson elevator no. 3 (joker); *6,* Freer elevator; *7,* Sachs dura separator; *8,* Sunday staphylorrhaphy elevator; *9,* nerve hook: *10,* Olivecrona double-ended dissector; *11,* Scott ventricular cannula; *12,* Seletz ventricular cannula; *13,* Cone ventricular needle.

1 Electrosurgical pencil with spatula and needlepoint tip
6 Gerald bayonet forceps: 2 each fine with teeth; fine, smooth; and heavy with teeth
6 Davis brain retractors, 2 each narrow, medium, and wide
4 Clip appliers, 2 each medium and small (Hemoclips, Ligaclips, McKenzie)
4 Clip cartridges, 2 each medium and small
1 Clip rack
2 Alligator clip appliers (Penfield, Samuels-Weck)
1 Stainless steel metric ruler
2 Dura hooks, 6 inches
6 Needle holders: 2 each fine, 7½ inches; fine, 6 inches; and heavy, 7¼ inches
3 Adson (tonsil) hemostatic forceps, straight, 7¼ inches
3 Nerve hooks, 7¾ inches, 1 each small, medium, and large
3 Copper pituitary spoons, 1 each small, medium, and large (Cushing)
1 Self-retaining brain retractor with assorted blades (Leyla-Yasargil, Edinborough, DeMartel, Hamby, Greenberg)
6 Knife handles, 2 each nos. 3, 4, and 7
1 Mayo scissors, curved, 7 inches
2 Metzenbaum scissors, 5 and 7 inches
5 Alligator pituitary/disc rongeurs with assorted cup sizes
1 Bipolar electrosurgical forceps and cord
3 Irrigating syringes (Asepto, ear bulb)
6 Syringes, 10 ml, 2 each plain tip, Luer-Lok, and control grip
1 DeVilbiss bone-cutting instrument with 2 blades

The foregoing instrument list is very basic and compiled to help a nurse in a general hospital rather than a nurse in a large neurosurgical center. A hospital with an active neurosurgical service has its own basic craniotomy instrument list. The nurse should use that list and add the special preferences of a given neurosurgeon.

In addition to the basic types of instruments essential for supratentorial craniotomy (Figs. 23-31 through 23-34), suture scissors, a wire scissors, and a 6-inch Russian forceps should be included. A bone punch (Cone or Ingram), a drill guide and dura protector (Adson or Hamlin), a twist

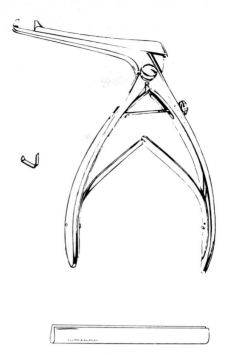

Fig. 23-32. Setup for craniosynostosis may include Ingraham-Fowler tantalum clips, Ingraham-Fowler guillotine applicators, and preformed silicone strip. (Courtesy Codman & Shurtleff, Inc., Randolph, Mass.)

drill that fits the Hudson brace or a Raney brace and perforator, hemostatic clips and applicators, trephines, burr hole covers (Silastic, such as the Todd-Crue buttons, or tantalum), Ray pituitary curettes, a Rayport dura knife, pituitary forceps (Adson or D'Errico), Bonney forceps, Penfield watchmaker's forceps, Hartmann forceps, monopolar electrosurgical bayonet forceps (Davis, Raney, Hoen, Jansen), bulldog clamps, angled dura scissors (Tay-

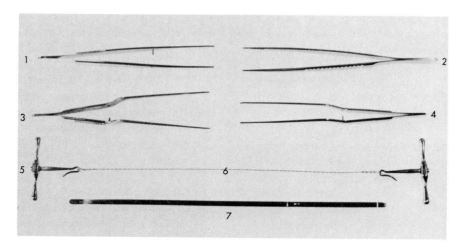

Fig. 23-33. *1,* Cushing tissue forceps; *2,* Cushing dressing forceps; *3,* Cushing bayonet dressing forceps; *4,* Cushing bayonet tissue forceps; *5,* Gigli saw handle; *6,* Gigli saw wire; *7,* Bailey saw guide.

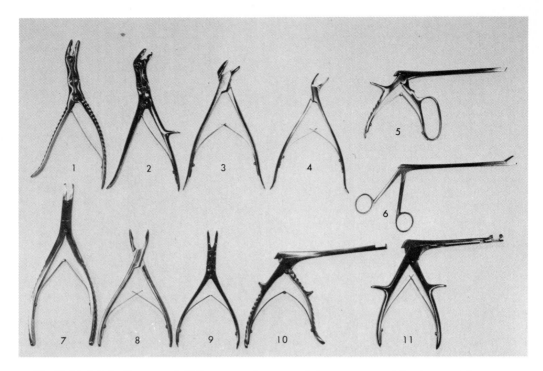

Fig. 23-34. *1,* Leksell rongeur; *2,* Stille gooseneck rongeur; *3,* Bacon rongeur; *4,* Stookey cranial rongeur; *5,* Cloward 40-degree-angle punch rongeur; *6,* pituitary disc rongeur; *7,* Fulton rongeur; *8,* Lempert rongeur; *9,* Zaufal-Jansen rongeur; *10,* Kerrison rongeur; *11,* Raney punch.

lor, Frazier, DeBakey, Potts-Smith), or a myriad of other instruments that a given neurosurgeon may desire can be included.

Many neurosurgeons prefer Allis forceps, rather than towel clamps or Peers clamps, to attach suction, electrosurgical pencils, and other devices to the drapes. Allis forceps used for this purpose should not be used for any other surgical procedures. They can be marked for neurosurgery and kept with the special neurosurgical instruments. They will not effectively hold tissue, such as the edge of the small bowel, after continued use on drape materials.

Two 10-ml Luer-Lok and two 10-ml plain-tip syringes should be included in every craniotomy setup. Also included should be six to 12 rubber bands, one or two Penrose drains, two medicine cups, suture material and needles of the surgeon's choice, and dressing headrolls (Kling or Kerlix).

Many neurosurgeons use magnifying loupes. They should be available.

Posterior fossa or infratentorial craniectomy requires the same instrumentation as supratentorial craniotomy, minus saws, saw handles, and saw guides. A cerebellar extension for the Hudson brace must be included, as well as a larger assortment of double-action and Kerrison rongeurs.

Additional instruments required for laminectomy, an-terior fusion, surgery of peripheral nerves, microsurgery and aneurysm surgery are included in the descriptions of the surgical procedures.

An example of a back table setup for craniotomy is shown in Fig. 23-35.

Evaluation

After the surgical procedure is completed, the patient is transported to the PACU. The patient is evaluated for the outcomes of the established goals. Bony prominences and pressure points are checked for skin integrity. A report along with documentation is given to the PACU nurse. Included are the outcomes from the identified goals. These may be evaluated as follows:

- The patient demonstrated a reduction in anxiety, verbalized feeling less anxious, coped with perioperative routines adequately, and verbalized an understanding of the planned procedure(s).
- The patient and/or family verbalized knowledge of diagnostic and surgical procedures and had realistic expectations of tests, routines, and postoperative care.
- The patient maintained effective breathing patterns; ventilation was maintained, ABGs were within normal limits, and breath sounds were bilateral.
- The patient will continue to report a reduction in pain, ask for pain medication, and verbalize relief or absence of pain.

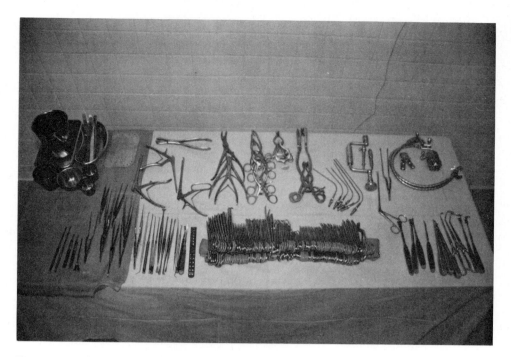

Fig. 23-35. Back table instrument setup for craniotomy. (Courtesy Humana Hospital, St. Luke's, Richmond, Va.)

• The patient will exhibit no signs and symptoms of infection; the wound will be clean and well-healed.

SURGICAL INTERVENTIONS

It is not possible in this chapter to provide a detailed approach to each neurosurgical procedure. Specific neurosurgical procedures are numerous, and each has a number of modifications or variations. The operating surgeon decides exactly which procedure and what variation will be performed. Basic general approaches, however, are limited and can be described in detail. Therefore, only a few step-by-step descriptions of basic approaches are presented. The nurse who is familiar with neurosurgical anatomy and pathologic conditions can learn these basic approaches and adapt them to the specific procedure.

Operations on the head
Burr holes

Burr holes are placed to remove a localized fluid collection beneath the dura mater. Fluid not composed of clot can be easily evacuated through a burr hole. Burr holes are also made to tap a lateral ventricle to relieve pressure. Burr holes are used by many surgeons when treating a brain abscess. The abscess may be aspirated, and antibiotics instilled. Other surgeons prefer to treat abscess by craniotomy. Occasionally burr holes are used to locate or drain subdural hematomas. However, a craniectomy is usually necessary to gain adequate exposure in these cases (Fig. 23-36). A burr hole is one of the steps in procedures

to shunt ventricular fluid to another body system for absorption or elimination.

Burr holes are placed to introduce air into the lateral ventricles for ventriculography (Fig. 23-37). The air makes the ventricles visible in x-ray studies.

Trephination

Trephination is the formation of an opening into the skull. This term usually applies when the opening is larger than the average burr hole. A piece of bone is cut with a circular saw that attaches to a Hudson brace. Procedures performed by trephination include prefrontal lobotomy, topectomy, cingulotomy, leukotomy, and thalamotomy. Today some of these procedures may be a part of stereotaxic neurosurgery.

Craniotomy

Craniotomy is an incision into the skull to expose and surgically treat intracranial disease.

Procedural considerations. Depending on the location of the pathologic condition, a craniotomy may be frontal, parietal, occipital, temporal, or a combination of two or more of these. When turning a scalp flap for a craniotomy, the surgeon may peel the scalp back off the periosteum (osteoplastic), or the periosteum may be stripped off the skull as the scalp is being lifted off the bone (osteoclastic).

The bone plate may be separated from the soft tissues, removed from the skull, and set aside for replacement at the end of the procedure. It may be placed in an antibiotic solution or an iodophor solution or wrapped in a saline-

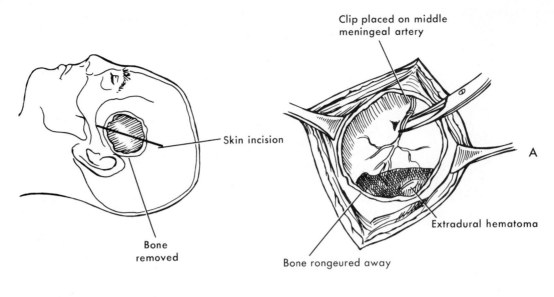

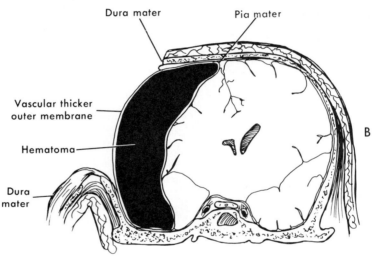

Fig. 23-36. **A,** Extradural hematoma. **B,** Subdural hematoma. (From Richards, V.: Surgery for general practice, St. Louis, 1956, The C.V. Mosby Co.)

moistened sponge or one that has been saturated with an antibiotic solution or an iodophor solution. The bone plate is not removed from the sterile field. If it is not replaced, it may be frozen in a sterile container or saved and stored in a marked, unsterile container to use as a template for forming a cranioplastic plate at a later date. The defect can be repaired without use of this template, however. If the bone is not separated from the soft tissues, it is turned back with the temporal muscle and soft tissues.

Operative procedure. After draping and attachment of suctions and electrosurgical cords, the procedure is begun:

1. The surgeon and the assistant apply digital pressure over folded 4 × 4 inch radiopaque sponges on both sides of the incision line. The skin and galea are incised in segments, the length of each segment being

equal to that over which the finger pressure is applied. The tissue edges are held with a 6-inch toothed forceps as scalp clips are placed on the flap edges. Hemostatic clamps are placed on the outside edge of the incision in adults and are grouped in segments and secured together by rubber bands placed around the handles or by a Penrose drain or open 4 × 4 inch sponge threaded through the handles and tied or clamped together with heavy forceps, such as a Pean (Fig. 23-38). Any remaining active arterial bleeding is controlled by electrocoagulation. If the incision extends into the temporal area, bleeding in the temporal muscle is managed by electrocoagulation, hemostats, tamponade, or suture ligature. A Mayo scissors may be used to incise temporal muscle and fascia.

2. The soft tissue is peeled off the periosteum by sharp

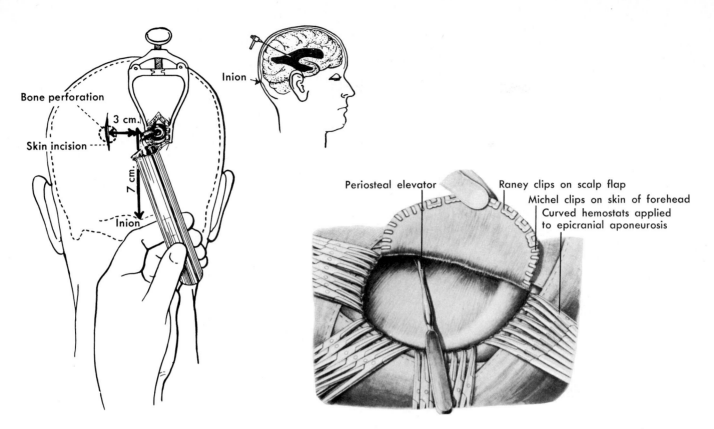

Fig. 23-37. Occipital burr holes for ventriculography. (From Richards, V.: Surgery for general practice, St. Louis, 1956, The C.V. Mosby Co.)

Fig. 23-38. Elevation of scalp flap. Hemostats on outer rim of incision and Raney clips and Michel clips on scalp flap. (From Kempe, L.G.: Operative neurosurgery, vols. 1 and 2, New York, 1968, Springer-Verlag New York, Inc.)

or blunt dissection or by electrodissection (see Fig. 23-38). The scalp flap is turned back over folded sponges and retracted by use of small towel clamps and rubber bands or muscle hooks on rubber bands. In either case the traction is maintained by securing the rubber band to the drapes with heavy forceps. The flap may be covered with a moist sponge or Telfa strips and a sterile towel. Bleeding is controlled by electrocoagulation.

3. When a free bone flap is planned, the muscle and periosteum are incised. Muscle and periosteum are elevated with the skin-galea flap, turned back, and retracted as a unit, as described previously.

4. The periosteum and muscle are incised with a scalpel or electrosurgical knife except at the inferior margins, which are left intact to preserve blood supply to the bone flap. The periosteum is stripped from the bone at the incision line with a periosteal elevator. Bone wax is used to control bleeding.

5. The scalp edges and muscle are retracted from the bone incision line by a Sachs or Cushing retractor. Two or more burr holes are made with either a hand or power cranial drill (Fig. 23-39). As each hole is drilled, the assistant must hold the patient's head to

diminish the agitation and prevent displacement from the headrest. A great deal of heat is generated by the friction of the perforator or burr against the bone. The nurse or assistant must irrigate the drilling site to counteract the heat and remove bone dust, which collects as the holes are made. Some surgeons prefer that the nurse collect the bone dust for replacement in the burr holes at closure. The dust is placed in a medicine glass and kept moist with a small amount of normal saline solution. A large-gauge suction tip is used to remove both irrigating solution and debris from the field. As the inner table is perforated and the dura exposed, the burr hole may be temporarily tamponaded with bone wax or a cottonoid strip or patty. Each hole is eventually debrided by a no. 0 or 00 bone curette or small periosteal elevator (joker). The dura mater is freed at the margins with a no. 3 Adson elevator, no. 3 Penfield dissector, or right-angle Frazier elevator or similar instrument. The hole is irrigated and suction applied simultaneously. Active bleeding points in the bone are identified, and bone wax is applied.

6. When all burr holes have been made, the bone flap is cut by sawing between holes after the dura mater

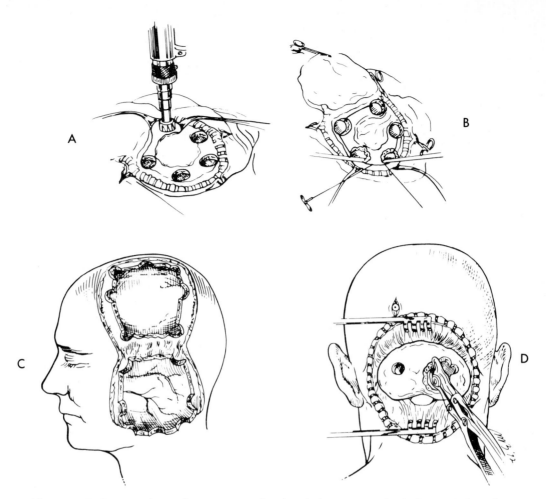

Fig. 23-39. Techniques of cranial surgery. **A,** Drilling burr holes. **B,** Using the Gigli saw. **C,** Bone flap turned down. **D,** Modification for cerebellar craniotomy. (From Barber, J., Stokes, L., and Billings, D.: Adult and child care, ed. 2, St. Louis, 1977, The C.V. Mosby Co.)

has been separated from the bone by a dural separator, such as the Sachs, or by a no. 3 Penfield dissector. Dural separation is done to prevent tearing of the dura mater, especially over venous sinuses. Using a rongeur, the surgeon may cut channels in the two burr holes at the inferior edge of the planned bone flap under the muscle. When the rest of the bone flap has been sawed, this segment can be easily cracked as the bone is elevated and turned back. If the sawing is done by hand, a dural separator is passed from one hole to the next under the bone. A saw guide-passer with a saw attached is passed from one hole to the next in the same manner (Fig. 23-40). The saw is detached from the guide, saw handles are attached to both ends of the saw, and the bone is incised by sawing in a back-and-forth motion. Friction generates heat, so irrigation and suction must be used during the process. The procedure is repeated until all segments but the one under the muscle have been cut. Usually a new saw is used each time. An air craniotome or

Midas Rex drill can also be used for the opening. Irrigation and suction are required as the bone flap is cut. Soft tissue edges are retracted with Sachs or Cushing retractors.

7. The bone flap with muscle attached is lifted off the dura mater by two periosteal elevators. As it is forced up the back, the bridge of bone under the muscle cracks. Bleeding from the bone is controlled with bone wax. A double-action rongeur is used to remove sharp, irregular edges where the bone cracked (Fig. 23-41). The bone flap is covered with a moist sponge, cottonoid material, or Telfa pads and then a clean sterile towel and is retracted in the same manner as the scalp flap.

8. The dura mater is irrigated. Moist cottonoid strips or patties or Telfa pads may be inserted between the dura mater and bone and folded back to cover the exposed bone edges. Clean sterile towels may be placed around the operative site.

9. The dura mater is opened (Fig. 23-42). A dura hook

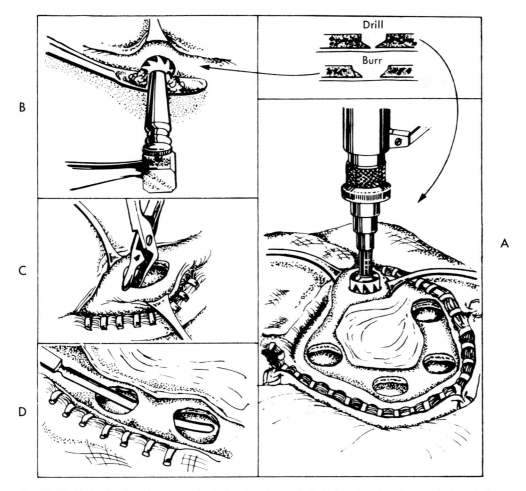

Fig. 23-40. Methods of making osteoplastic flap (craniotomy). **A,** Using electric drill to make burr hole. **B,** Using hand perforator to make burr hole. **C,** Using rongeur to enlarge burr hole. **D,** Separating dura mater from skull. (From Carini, E., and Owens, G.: Neurological and neurosurgical nursing, ed. 6, St. Louis, 1974, The C.V. Mosby Co.)

may be used to elevate the dura mater from the brain, and a small nick is made in the dura mater with a no. 15 blade on a no. 3 or no. 7 knife handle; or a small opening may be made in the dura mater without elevating it, after which the dural edges are grasped with straight mosquito hemostats or two Adson or Cushing forceps with teeth and are elevated. A narrow, moist cottonoid strip is inserted with a smooth forceps (bayonet or Cushing) into the opening to protect the brain as the dura mater is incised and elevated. The dural incision can be made with a Metzenbaum scissors, special dura scissors, or a Rayport dura knife. Usually traction sutures are placed at the outer edge of the dura mater and are tagged with small bulldog clamps or mosquito hemostats. Sometimes the tag instruments are attached to the drapes to increase traction and keep tension on them. As the dural veins are approached during dural opening, they are ligated or coagulated before cutting. Ligation is done with

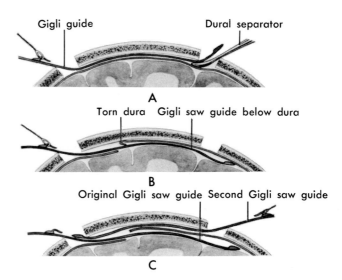

Fig. 23-41. Gigli saw insertion. **A** to **C,** Steps to be taken if Gigli saw tears dura mater. (From Kempe, L.G.: Operative neurosurgery, vols. 1 and 2, New York, 1968, Springer-Verlag New York, Inc.)

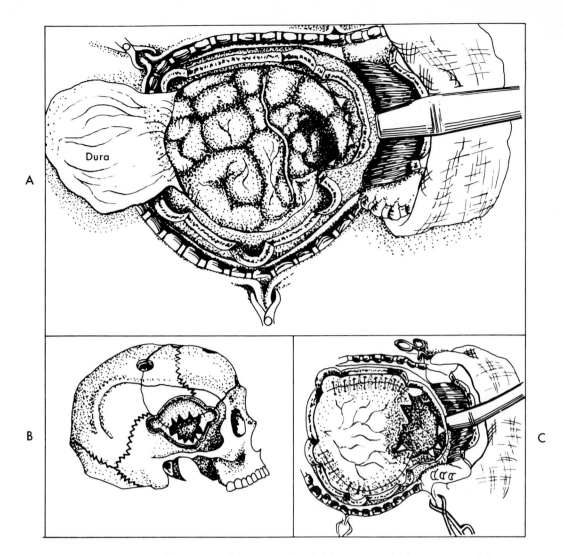

Fig. 23-42. Craniotomy with subtemporal decompression. **A,** Malignant cerebral tumor exposed. **B,** Bony defect. **C,** Dural defect. (From Carini, E., and Owens, G.: Neurological and neurosurgical nursing, ed. 6, St. Louis, 1974, The C.V. Mosby Co.)

hemostatic clips such as Weck Hemoclips, McKenzie clips, or Ligaclips. The brain surface is protected by moist cottonoid strips.

10. The surgeon places cottonoid strips and brain retractors, self-retaining (Fig. 23-43) and manual, appropriately while working toward visualizing the particular pathologic entity.

11. Brain spoons, Cushing pituitary spoons, and Ray curettes, as well as pituitary rongeurs or other tumor forceps, must be available for tumor removal. Also, a selection of dissectors, Cushing and Gerald forceps, and a bipolar coagulation unit are used. Completely filled irrigating syringes and a full range of moist cottonoid patties and strips must be within easy reach of the surgeon and the assistant. Following correction of the pathologic condition and control of bleeding,

the brain may be irrigated with an antibiotic solution of the surgeon's choice.

12. The dura mater may be left open, or it may be closed. If closure is done, it is usually by interrupted sutures of no. 4-0 silk, 4-0 Polyglactin suture, or 4-0 black braided nylon. Under some conditions, dural substitutes may be used. A drain may or may not be used.

13. The bone flap may or may not be replaced. If swelling is anticipated, it is usually not replaced. If the flap is free and replaced, holes may be drilled in it and the skull and suture material inserted to secure it in place. The craniotome or Midas Rex can be used for this purpose. During drilling, a dura protector is used on the skull side. A brain spoon can serve as a dura protector.

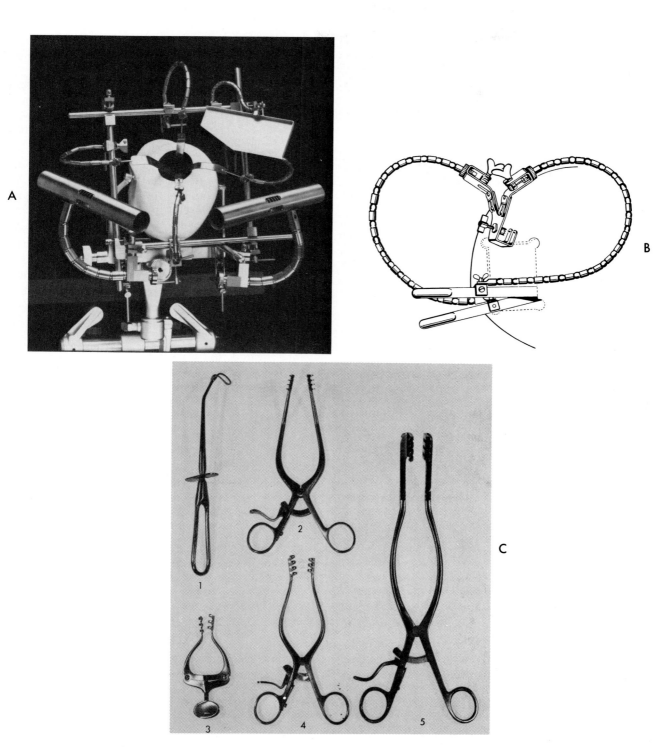

Fig. 23-43. A, Greenberg retractor with blades, poles, and adapters. **B,** Leyla-Yasargil self-retaining retractor. **C,** Retractors: *1,* Cushing subtemporal decompression retractor; *2,* Adson cerebellar retractor; *3,* Jansen mastoid retractor; *4,* Weitlaner retractor; *5,* Beckman laminectomy retractor. (**A** courtesy Codman & Shurtleff, Randolph, Mass.; **B** courtesy Holco Instrument Corp., New York.)

14. Periosteum and muscle are approximated with no. 2-0 or 3-0 Polyglactin synthetic absorbable suture or no. 2-0 or 3-0 silk or Surgilon. The galea is closed with the same sutures as above. Skin closure can be interrupted or continuous and of silk or synthetic suture material, such as nylon, or skin staples.

Craniotomy for cerebrospinal rhinorrhea

Cerebrospinal rhinorrhea is a rupture of the dura mater, with evagination of the torn arachnoid through the dura mater into a hole or fracture in the skull communicating with one of the nasal sinuses or the nasal cavity. This results in leakage of cerebrospinal fluid from the nose. Repairing the defect is necessary to prevent air from being trapped under pressure in the brain and to prevent intracranial infection.

Operative procedure

1. Usually, a frontal craniotomy is carried out, and the dura mater is opened. The frontal lobe is elevated until the defect can be visualized. The surgeon may elect to use the microscope.
2. The dura mater is dissected from the orbital and cribriform plates.
3. The defect in the bone is defined, and the bony defect may be filled with methyl methacrylate or covered with tantalum mesh.
4. The dural defect may be closed with sutures, but usually some type of patch is placed over it. A piece of muscle, pericranium, fascia, gelatin foam, silicone sheeting, or freeze-dried dura substitute may be used. These may be sutured or glued. Some surgeons do not fasten the patch into place.
5. The dural incision is sutured, and the wound is closed.

A similar procedure is carried out in the temporal or suboccipital region to repair a defect in cerebrospinal otorrhea.

Craniotomy for intracranial aneurysm

An aneurysm is a vascular dilation usually caused by a local defect in the vascular wall. Within the cranial cavity an aneurysm may impinge on the third nerve or the optic chiasm. Hemorrhage into the subarachnoid space, causing sudden, severe headache, is generally the first evidence of an intracranial aneurysm.

Modern neurosurgical techniques have made operations on intracranial aneurysms more feasible. Fatal hemorrhage is the greatest hazard of the condition and of the operation. To prevent this, control of blood pressure, as well as vascular supply to the region beyond the limits of the lesion, may be required. Occasionally control of the cerebral circulation at the level of the cervical carotid artery is desired. The artery may be exposed and controlled by means of preplaced ligatures or clamps that can be tightened to occlude the vessel if bleeding occurs at the aneurysm site

during the operation. This is a separate preliminary surgical procedure.

Procedural considerations. Aneurysm clips and appliers of the surgeon's choice must be included with the instrumentation. Figures 23-44 and 23-45 illustrate a few of the clips and appliers available. A minimum of two appliers for each type of clip must be included; both temporary and permanent clips must be available. Temporary clips include Mayfield, McFadden, Drake, Yasargil, Sugita, and Schwartz. Heifetz, Sundt-Kees, Olivecrona, Housepian, Scoville, Yasargil Phynox, and Sugita are types of permanent aneurysm clips. Today most clips have been updated with an alloy that is MRI compatible. Permanent clips can be removed from the vessel if necessary. The clip appliers serve as clip removers.

Aneurysm clips should never be compressed between the fingers. Clips should be compressed only when seated in their appliers. Once a clip has been compressed, it should be discarded. Clips that have been compressed may be sprung and may slip, causing complications such as bleeding or compression of another vessel or of a nerve.

The full armamentarium of aneurysm occlusion tools should be available for the surgeon. Besides clips, fast-setting aneuroplastic resinous material, a piece of temporal muscle, ligature carriers, or any other material requested by the surgeon should be in the room and ready to use. Fine silk ligatures and hemostatic clips, with or without bipolar coagulation of the neck of the aneurysm, have also been used successfully.

A basic craniotomy setup is required in addition to the special items mentioned. Supplementary suction must be immediately available on the field to prevent hemorrhage from obscuring the surgeon's vision if the aneurysm dome ruptures during operation and for removing smoke resulting from laser dissection.

Operative procedure

1. A frontal, frontotemporal, or bifrontal craniotomy may be done to approach an aneurysm in the area of the circle of Willis. The bifrontal approach requires extra scalp clips and hemostatic forceps. All aneurysm instruments preferred by the surgeon must be included.
2. After the dura mater has been opened, a self-retaining brain retractor is placed, and the optic nerve and subarachnoid cisterns are exposed. The olfactory nerve may be coagulated and divided with a long scissors for better exposure.
3. The operating microscope is positioned. Microinstruments, including a microbipolar bayonet, are used (Figs. 23-46 through 23-56).
4. Bridging veins are coagulated with bipolar coagulating forceps. Irrigation, which may be a part of the bipolar unit, is necessary during bipolar coagulation.
5. The covering arachnoidal webs are dissected away with microdissectors, hooks, elevators, scissors,

Text continued on p. 743.

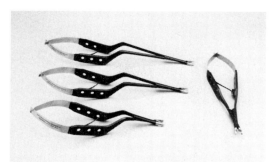

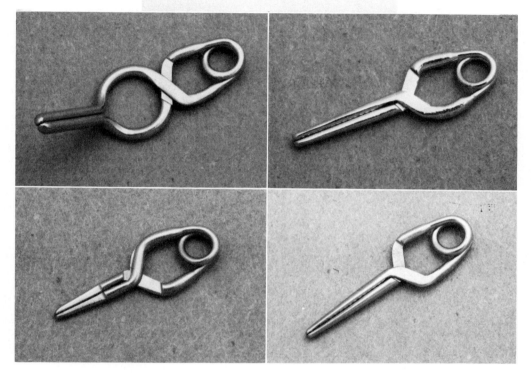

Fig. 23-44. Yasargil microaneurysm, standard aneurysm clips and appliers. (Courtesy Aesculap, Burlingame, Calif.)

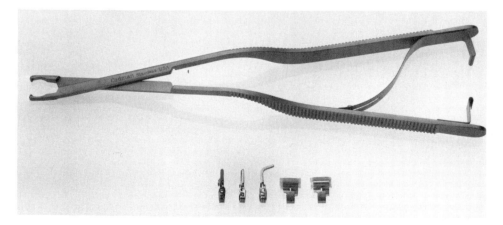

Fig. 23-45. Sundt aneurysm clips and applier. (Courtesy Codman & Shurtleff, Inc., Randolph, Mass.)

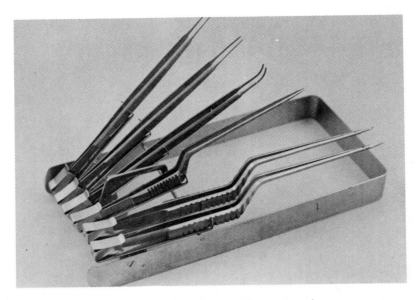

Fig. 23-46. Microscissors and forceps in rack.

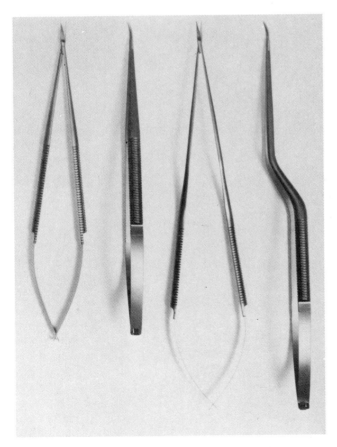

Fig. 23-47. Rhoton titanium microscissors. (Courtesy Codman & Shurtleff, Inc., Randolph, Mass.)

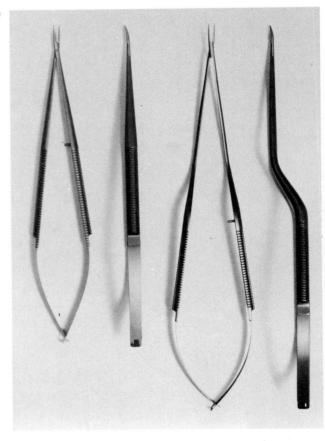

Fig. 23-48. Rhoton microsurgical needle holders. (Courtesy Codman & Shurtleff, Inc., Randolph, Mass.)

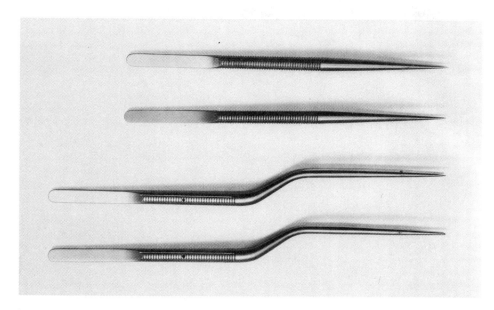

Fig. 23-49. Rhoton microsurgical forceps, straight and bayonet. (Courtesy Codman & Shurtleff, Inc., Randolph, Mass.)

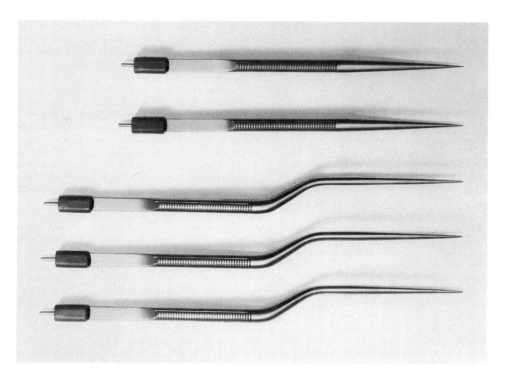

Fig. 23-50. Rhoton microsurgical bipolar forceps, straight and bayonet. (Courtesy Codman & Shurtleff, Inc., Randolph, Mass.)

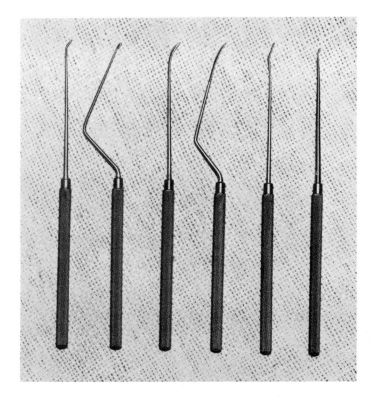

Fig. 23-51. Malis microsurgical instruments. *Left to right,* Semisharp dissector, curette, two elevators, sharp dissector, round dissector. (Courtesy Codman & Shurtleff, Inc., Randolph, Mass.)

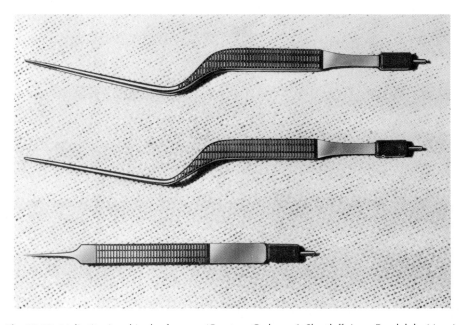

Fig. 23-52. Malis titanium bipolar forceps. (Courtesy Codman & Shurtleff, Inc., Randolph, Mass.)

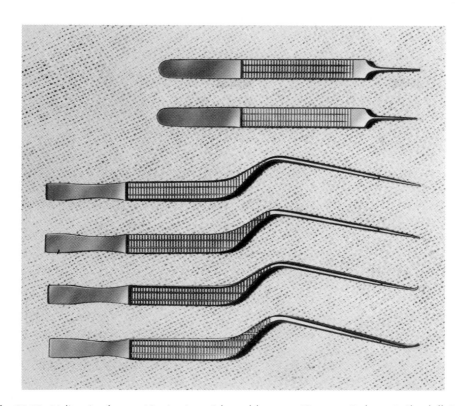

Fig. 23-53. Malis microforceps (titanium), straight and bayonet. (Courtesy Codman & Shurtleff, Inc., Randolph, Mass.)

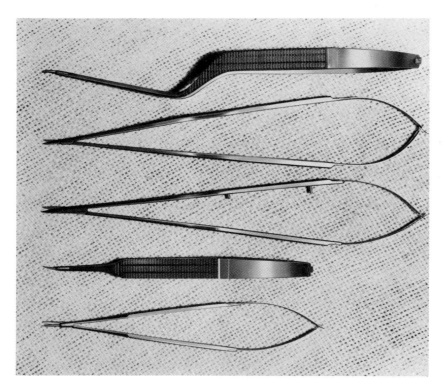

Fig. 23-54. Malis microsurgical scissors. (Courtesy Codman & Shurtleff, Inc., Randolph, Mass.)

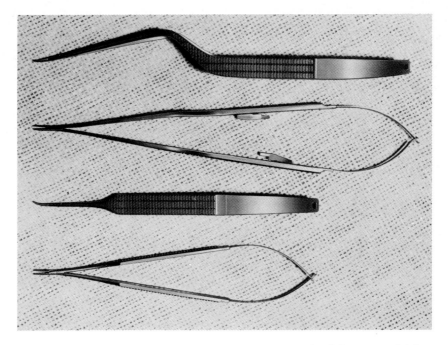

Fig. 23-55. Malis microsurgical needle holders. (Courtesy Codman & Shurtleff, Inc., Randolph, Mass.)

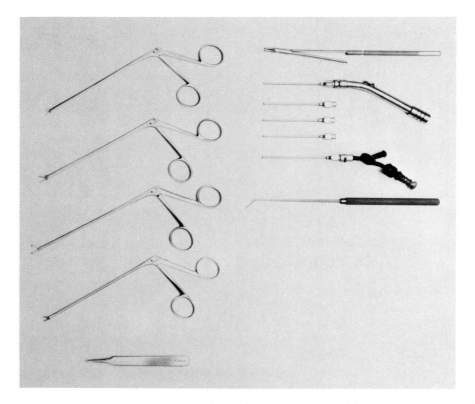

Fig. 23-56. Microinstruments for neurosurgical procedures. *Bottom to top: left,* Forceps, rongeurs, and scissors; *right,* arachnoid knife, Malis suction-coagulation handle and four tips, Cadac microsuction handle and tip, blade breaker and holder. (Courtesy Codman & Shurtleff, Inc., Randolph, Mass.)

knives, forceps, a micro diamond knife, and an irrigating bipolar.

6. Careful dissection of the arachnoid and clear visualization of the neck of the aneurysm without rupture of the dome are the aims of the surgeon.

7. The parent arteries are identified and freed so they can be occluded with a temporary clip if necessary. Other structures, such as the optic chiasma and optic nerves, are identified.

8. As the surgeon works slowly toward the dome and neck of the aneurysm, the patient's blood pressure is lowered for easier control of hemorrhage, should the aneurysm rupture.

9A. If the neck of the aneurysm can be isolated, a clip is placed across it. Clips such as the Sundt-Kees and Heifetz have Teflon linings and can be used to approach the aneurysm from a 180-degree angle to avoid excessive manipulation and traction of the parent vessel, if the neck is on the underside of the vessel. These clips support the vessel and serve as a clip graft.

9B. When clipping is not feasible, coating the aneurysm with fast-drying methyl methacrylate has good results. The chemicals are mixed, and, before the chemical hardens, it is applied to the surface of the aneurysm with a disposable plastic syringe and the plastic cannula from a large (16- or 14-gauge) Angiocath. All surrounding tissues must be walled off with cottonoid material before the acrylic substance is mixed and applied.

10. As soon as the aneurysm has been occluded, the blood pressure is returned to normal, and the aneurysm site is checked for bleeding. When the surgeon is satisfied that the operative field is dry, wound closure is begun.

Craniotomy for arteriovenous malformation

An arteriovenous malformation consists of thin-walled vascular channels that connect arteries and veins without the usual intervening capillaries. These vascular lesions may be microscopic or massive.

Malformations vary widely in size, area of involvement, and structure. Arteriovenous fistulas may be congenital or may result from trauma or disease. Vascular anomalies may also give rise to subarachnoid or intracerebral hemorrhage or may have extensive irritative effects and cause focal or generalized seizures.

These lesions are difficult to treat successfully. Feeding vessels can be clipped with or without partial removal of the lesion. Total removal, when possible, gives best results. Microsurgical techniques and the laser have made total removal without devastating injury to surrounding brain tissue and vessels possible in many cases.

Other methods of treating these malformations have been tried. One successful method has been with the Gamma knife. Only a few health care facilities offer this procedure.

Operative procedure

1. A supratentorial or infratentorial craniotomy is done, depending on the location of the lesion.

2. The feeding arteries are exposed a distance from the malformation, then traced toward it, and occluded a short distance before they penetrate its substance. This spares as many of the arteries to the brain as possible. The feeding arteries may be occluded by clipping, coagulation, ligation, or laser beam coagulation.

3. The malformation is dissected out with suction and bayonet forceps. Additional vessels are clipped or coagulated along the way. Usually one or more draining veins are left to be ligated as the last step in the removal.

4. Closure and dressing are as described for craniotomy.

Craniotomy for intracranial revascularization

Microbypass technique, developed in 1967, is used to shunt blood flow around an occluded portion of the internal carotid artery or the middle cerebral artery by anastomosing the superficial temporal artery to the middle cerebral artery distal to the occlusion. Today, the procedure is also used for revascularization for giant aneurysm, AVMs, and tumor.

Procedural considerations. Craniotomy for intracranial revascularization, although brief in description, is long and tedious; 7 hours is not unusual. Positioning is crucial to prevent pressure on superficial nerves, vessels, and vulnerable skin areas. Blood gas monitoring and arterial pressure readings are done routinely during the procedure. An arterial line may be placed before the patient's arrival in the surgery department or as a preliminary procedure in the operating room. Sterile and unsterile probes for the Doppler ultrasonic scanners should be available.

Operative procedure

The procedure occurs in two steps:

1. The *first stage* is reflection of the scalp flap on the operative side to expose the superficial temporal artery for dissection. Care must be taken in placing the hemostatic scalp clips to make sure they are farther apart than usual to prevent compromise of the scalp circulation following diversion of the flow of the temporal artery. Care also must be taken to prevent injury to the temporal artery as the scalp incision is made and the flap reflected.

2. After the superficial temporal artery is identified, the microscope is positioned, and the microinstrumentation is put to use.

3. The portion of the temporal artery to be used is freed but not occluded until the time of anastomosis. It may be supported and covered with Gelfoam or cottonoid material soaked in a papaverine solution. Papaverine helps prevent vessel spasm.

4. The temporal muscle is incised and retracted with fishhook retractors to begin the *second stage* of the procedure.

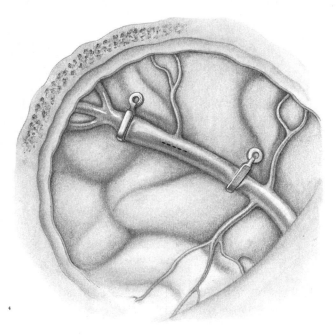

Fig. 23-57. Exposure of the middle cerebral artery with clips. (From Neurosurgery wound closure, Ethicon, Inc.)

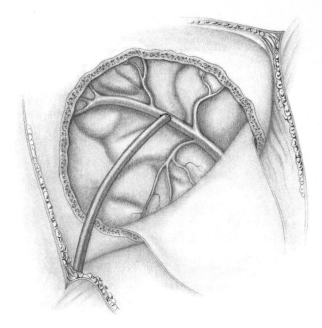

Fig. 23-58. The final anastomosis of the superficial temporal artery to the middle cerebral artery. (From Neurosurgery wound closure, Ethicon, Inc.)

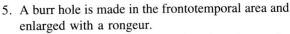

5. A burr hole is made in the frontotemporal area and enlarged with a rongeur.

6. The dura mater is opened and anchored over the bone edges with silk or black braided nylon sutures. The self-retaining brain retractor is used.

7. The middle cerebral artery is located, and a branch suitable for anastomosis is isolated. Flow is occluded by temporary microvascular clips, such as Heifetz, Sugita, or Yasargil (Fig. 23-57).

8. Flow also is occluded in the superficial temporal artery; the artery is cut, and an end-to-side anastomosis is completed with very fine suture material, such as no. 10-0 monofilament nylon (Fig. 23-58).

9. The temporary microvascular clips are removed. The vessels are observed for patency and flow.

10. The wound is closed, and dressings are applied.

Craniotomy for pituitary tumor (craniopharyngioma, optic glioma, and other suprasellar and parasellar tumors)

Procedural considerations. The setup is as for craniotomy with these additional pituitary instruments:

Ray curettes (ring, sharp)
Spinal needles, no. 22 or 24
Luer-Lok syringe, 10 ml
Angulated suction tips, right and left; large and small
Curettes, small, nos. 0 through 4-0

Operative procedure

1. Either a bifrontal or a unilateral incision is made in the frontal or frontotemporal region. Most unilateral approaches are carried out from the right side.

2. Wet brain retractors over moist cottonoids are inserted for exposure of the optic chiasma and the pituitary gland. The frontal and often the temporal lobes are retracted. The olfactory nerve may be coagulated and divided with scissors.

3. A DeMartel, Edinborough, Yasargil, or Greenberg self-retaining retractor is placed to maintain exposure. Aneurysm clips and applicators should be available to control unexpected bleeding from major vessels. The microscope may be moved into place.

4. Using a syringe with moistened plunger and a no. 22 or 24 spinal needle, the surgeon attempts to aspirate the contents of the tumor to guard against inadvertently entering an aneurysm or vessel.

5. The tumor capsule is coagulated for hemostasis and incised with a no. 11 blade on a long knife handle. With a pituitary rongeur or cup forceps, the tumor is removed.

6. Small stainless steel, copper, or Ray curettes, as well as suction, may be used during tumor removal.

7. A wide clip may be applied to the stalk of the pituitary, which may then be cut distally. A long angulated scissors is especially helpful for this.

8. If the tumor capsule is to be removed, bayonet forceps, cup forceps, nerve hooks, and suction aid in the dissection.

9. Closure and dressing are as described for craniotomy.

In case of pituitary adenoma with a prefixed chiasma, the surgeon may elect to remove the anterior wall of the sphenoidal sinus and sella turcica with an air drill to gain access to the tumor.

In the case of craniopharyngioma, extreme caution must be used in removing fluid from the capsule because the fluid is extremely irritating and may cause chemical leptomeningitis. Calcified pieces of tumor are dissected and removed in the same manner as the capsule of a pituitary adenoma. This is an extremely difficult procedure because of deposits on the carotid arteries, the optic nerves, and optic chiasma. The tumor capsule is often left behind on the hypothalamus to avoid stripping off blood vessels supplying this structure. Many moist cottonoid strips are used to protect the surrounding areas from the cystic contents.

Suprasellar meningiomas usually arise from the tuberculum sallae just anterior to the optic nerves and chiasma. Tumor removal is similar to that of a pituitary adenoma except that the electrosurgical cutting loop may be used to excavate the interior of the tumor. After the tumor has been removed, the site of its attachment to the dura is thoroughly coagulated to prevent recurrence. Other meningiomas arising at the base of the skull are treated by similar techniques.

Transsphenoidal hypophysectomy

Endocrine pituitary disorders, such as Cushing's syndrome, acromegaly, malignant exophthalmos, and hypopituitarism resulting from intrasellar tumors, as well as nonpituitary disorders, such as advanced metastatic carcinoma of the breast and prostate, diabetic retinopathy, and uncontrollable severe diabetes, have been successfully treated by transsphenoidal hypophysectomy.

Rapid access to the sella turcica is achieved. Complete extracapsular enucleation of the pituitary in cases of hypophysectomy and possible complete removal of small pituitary tumors, with the remaining normal portion of the gland left intact, can be obtained. Patients are relatively free of pain after surgery. No visible scar remains.

Procedural considerations. Transsphenoidal hypophysectomy is performed with the patient under light general endotracheal anesthesia, combined with a local anesthetic. The patient is placed in a semisitting position, with head against the headrest. A portable image intensifier is used. The horizontal beam is centered on the sella turcica. A subnasal midline rhinoseptal approach is used.

The face, mouth, and nasal cavity are prepared with an antiseptic solution. Infiltration of the nasal mucosa and the gingiva with a local anesthetic agent containing 1:2000 epinephrine is helpful in initiating submucosal elevation, as well as diminishing oozing from the mucosa. A sterile adhesive plastic drape is applied to the entire face with additional sterile drapes to ensure a relatively sterile operative field. Sterile sponges or cotton is placed in the patient's mouth so only the upper gum margin is exposed.

A biopsy setup is required, as well as special instruments (Fig. 23-59). The operating microscope is used for the cranial portion of the procedure.

Operative procedure

1. Using the biopsy setup on a separate small Mayo table, the surgeon may take a small piece of muscle from the previously prepared thigh to be used later in the procedure. This is kept in a moist sponge.
2. An incision is made in the middle of the upper gum margin. The soft tissues of the upper lip and nose are elevated from the bone with an elevator, and the nasal

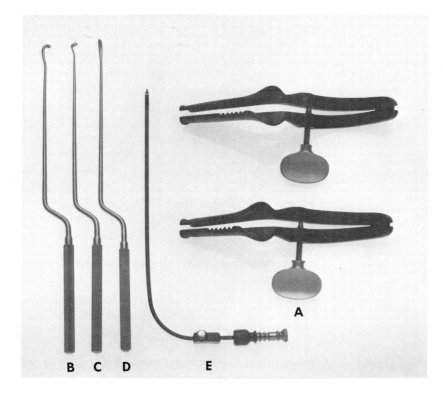

Fig. 22-59. Special instruments for transsphenoidal hypophysectomy. **A,** Hardy's modified Cushing bivalve speculum. **B,** Hardy's enucleator. **C,** Hardy's enucleator. **D,** Hardy's dissector. **E,** Hardy's suction tubes. (Courtesy Codman & Shurtleff, Inc., Randolph, Mass.)

septum is exposed. The nasal mucosa is elevated from either side of the nasal septum, which is flanked by the blades of a Cushing bivalved speculum. The inferior third of the anterior cartilaginous septum and osseous vomer are resected, as is the floor of the sphenoidal sinus, exposing the sinus cavity. The floor of the sella turcica can be identified.

3. The floor is opened with a sphenoidal punch, and the dura mater is incised. The hypophyseal cavity should be opened only in patients undergoing surgery for pituitary adenoma. In these patients the gland is explored, and the tumor is identified and removed.

4. The extracapsular cleavage plane is identified, and the superior surface of the pituitary is dissected until the stalk and the diaphragmatic orifice are found. Cotton pledgets are applied for exposure, hemostasis, and protection of structures.

5. The stalk is sectioned low with a sickle knife, and the lateral posterior and inferior surface of the pituitary is dissected with an enuclear.

6. The gland is removed in toto, and the sellar cavity may be packed with muscle obtained previously from the thigh. The floor is reconstructed with cartilage from the nasal septum.

7. Antibiotic powder may be used and nasal packing introduced for 2 days. The gingiva incision is closed with catgut.

Some surgeons prefer to perform this operation by means of a lateral rhinotomy with a transantral-transsphenoidal approach. An ear, nose, and throat (ENT) surgeon may be available to do the initial opening, depending on surgeon preference. If an ENT surgeon does assist, a separate setup is available.

Craniectomy

Craniectomy is incision into the skull and removal of bone by enlarging one or more burr holes, using rongeurs to gain access to the underlying structures.

A craniectomy procedure may be required to remove tumors, hematomas, scars, or infections of the bone. Craniectomy is also indicated as treatment for craniosynostosis in infants and to relieve pressure on the brain from depressed bone or internal hemorrhage resulting from trauma.

Craniectomy with evacuation of epidural or subdural hematoma

Following trauma, decompression of the brain, as well as removal and drainage of blood clots and collections of liquefied blood from outside or beneath the dura mater, is accomplished.

Operative procedure

1. A linear or small horseshoe incision is made over the site of the lesion. The initial procedure is similar to craniotomy. One or more burr holes are made. A bone flap is not turned.

2. If a blood clot or collection of bloody fluid is found outside or beneath the dura mater, the burr hole is further enlarged, with a Kerrison or double-action rongeur, until adequate exposure is obtained. Bone edges are waxed, and cottonoid strips are put in position along the edges.

3. Clot and fluid are evacuated, and hemostasis is accomplished with coagulation or the use of hemostatic clips.

4. In cases of chronic subdural hematoma the inner and outer membranes are stripped and coagulated.

5. The brain is irrigated, using catheters or directly employing an Asepto or bulb syringe. Large amounts of saline irrigating solution are used until the return appears clear.

6. A silver or a hemostatic clip may be placed on the cortex at the site of a small incision. Another clip is placed on the dura mater. These are tag clips that are visible on postoperative x-ray films to check the bleeding site.

7. A small drain or a polyethylene or red rubber catheter may be inserted subdurally for additional drainage, or a closed drainage system, such as the Jackson-Pratt, may be used through a separate stab wound in the skin posterior to the incision.

Additional burr holes are made during the course of the procedure to be sure clots in other areas do not remain undetected and untreated.

Craniectomy for craniosynostosis

Craniectomy for craniosynostosis is performed on infants whose suture lines have closed prematurely. If diagnosis is made shortly after birth, the condition can be corrected by surgically separating the two involved bones and treating the area to prevent resealing until most of the growth of the brain has occurred. The surgeon merely restores the patency of the suture and allows growth of the brain to correct the cosmetic deformity.

Operative procedure. After the scalp incision is made over the appropriate skull suture, the dura mater is stripped off the underside of the skull. A generous strip of the bone edges joining to form the fused suture is then removed with heavy scissors, a craniotome, a rongeur, or a Kerrison punch. The bone edges are waxed. Preformed Silastic sheeting can be inserted over the bone edges bordering the craniectomy and sutured or stapled in place. When sutures are used, holes must be placed in the bone edges bordering the craniectomy before the sheeting is placed.

Suboccipital craniectomy or posterior fossa exploration

Perforation and removal of the posterior occipital bone and exposure of the foramen magnum and arch of the atlas are done to remove a lesion in the posterior fossa (Fig. 23-60).

Procedural considerations. Depending on the type and size of the lesion, the exposure may be unilateral or bilateral. The operation may include the removal of the arch of the atlas. This approach gives the surgeon access to the fourth ventricle, the cerebellum, the brainstem, and the cranial nerves.

The sitting position may be preferred, but the park bench position is also utilized. An extra-high instrument table or two Mayo stands and standing stool are necessary for the nurse.

Operative procedure

1. Prior to the initial surgical incision, an occipital burr hole is done for placement of a ventricular catheter. This can be done as a separate procedure or concurrently with the procedure.

2. The incision may be made from mastoid tip to mastoid tip, in an arch curving upward 2 cm above the external occipital protuberance.
3. Scalp bleeding is controlled, and the skin flap is retracted with the Weitlaner retractors.
4. A periosteal elevator is used to free the muscles, which are then divided with an electrosurgical blade, using cutting current. The incision is deepened. A self-retaining retractor is used. The laminae of the first two or three cervical vertebrae may be exposed.
5. One or more holes are drilled in the occipital bone. If a Hudson brace is used, the cerebellar extension is attached. The Midas Rex or Anspach drill is very

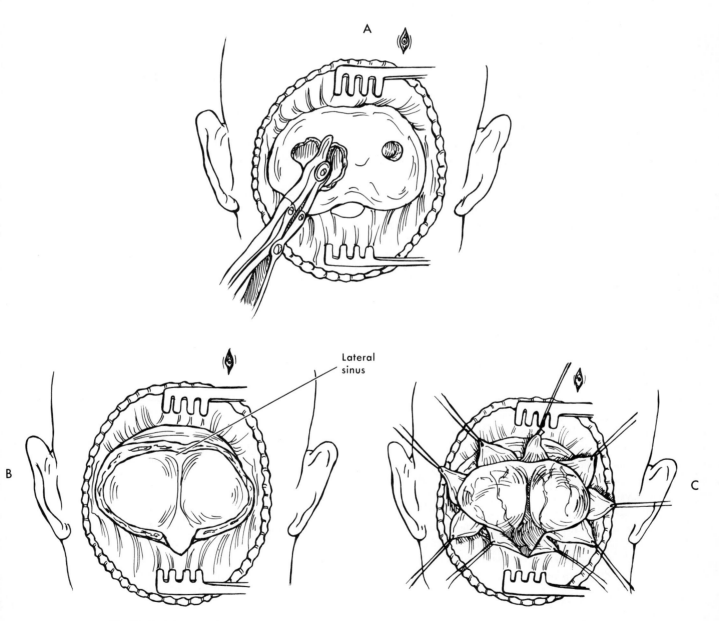

Fig. 23-60. Suboccipital craniectomy. **A,** Craniectomy being performed. **B,** Dura mater exposed. **C,** Dura mater incised and cerebellum exposed. (From Sachs, E.: Diagnosis and treatment of brain tumors and the care of the neurosurgical patient, ed. 2, St. Louis, 1949, The C.V. Mosby Co.)

beneficial for this approach because it reduces the time needed in making the opening.

6. The dura mater is stripped from the bone. A double-action rongeur, Raney punch, Kerrison punch, or Leksell rongeur is used to enlarge the hole and smooth the edges.

7. Osseous and cerebellar venous bleeding is controlled at each step with bone wax, Gelfoam, and electrocoagulation to prevent air embolism.

8. The dura mater is opened. A small brain spoon or cottonoid strip is used to protect the brain as the initial nick is extended with scalpel or scissors. The dural incision is continued until the cerebellar hemispheres, the vermis, and the tonsils can be visualized. Hemostatic clips are used on the dura mater as necessary. Dural traction sutures are placed.

9. The cisterna magna is opened, emptied of spinal fluid, and protected with a cottonoid strip.

10. The cerebellar hemispheres are inspected. Bleeding is controlled with the bipolar coagulator. A needle may be introduced through a small coagulated incision in the cerebellar hemisphere in an attempt to palpate or tap a deep lesion.

11. Brain retractors over cottonoid strips are placed for exposure. The handle of the retractor must be kept dry to avoid slippage in the surgeon's hand. However, the inserted edge should be wet to prevent damage or tears in the brain surface. These retractors may be positioned in areas that control respiration or other vital functions, so every effort must be made to avoid jarring these instruments in the operative field. When the pathologic entity is identified, a self-retaining retractor may be placed.

12. Long bayonet forceps, bayonet cup forceps, pituitary forceps, suction, and the electrosurgical loop tips may be used to remove the lesion. Clips may be used to aid in hemostasis. A nerve stimulator may be used to identify cranial nerves; evoked potentials for brainstem monitoring are becoming routine.

13. After the lesion has been removed and bleeding controlled, further checking for adequate hemostasis is required. Venous pressure in the patient's head is increased by the anesthesiologist.

14. The dura mater may be partially or completely closed. The muscle, fascia, and skin are closed. A dressing is applied.

15. The patient must remain anesthetized until the supine position is achieved and the prongs of the headrest are removed. Particular attention must be given to the patient's head when removing these prongs to prevent tearing the scalp or damaging the eyes.

Subtemporal craniectomy for trigeminal exploration/rhizotomy

Trigeminal neuralgia (tic douloureux, fifth cranial nerve pain) is a condition characterized by brief, repeated attacks of excruciating pain in the face. Temporary relief of trigeminal neuralgia may be obtained by interruption of branches of the nerve divisions (ophthalmic, maxillary, and mandibular) by means of alcohol injection or surgical sectioning. This approach may also be used for exploration for trigeminal neuromas.

Procedural considerations. The patient may be placed in the supine or sitting position, depending on the surgeon's preference.

Operative procedure

1. A vertical temporal incision extending from the zygomatic process and through the temporal muscles and periosteum is made.

2. The soft tissue is freed from the bone with a periosteal elevator. The bone exposure is maintained with a self-retaining retractor.

3. A burr hole is made. The dura mater is freed from the underside of the temporal bone.

4. The burr hole is enlarged, with a double-action rongeur, to a diameter of about 2½ inches.

5. With a moist brain retractor, the dura mater overlying the temporal lobe is retracted upward. By means of blunt dissection with cottonoids held in bayonet forceps, the dura mater is elevated from the bony floor of the middle fossa.

6. The brain retractor is replaced by a self-retaining brain retractor placed deeper into the wound to hold up the temporal lobe and dura mater. The microscope provides light as well as magnification.

7. As the dura mater is elevated, the middle meningeal artery is seen as it leaves the foramen spinosum to join the dura mater. It is coagulated with bipolar bayonet forceps and may be clipped before being divided. A cottonoid, wood, or wax plug is packed into the foramen spinosum.

8. Additional blunt dissection uncovers the mandibular division of the trigeminal nerve and finally the trigeminal (gasserian) ganglion within its own dural sheath (dura propria). Bleeding is controlled with cottonoids and a hemostatic material such as Gelfoam and thrombin.

9. Some surgeons terminate the procedure after stripping the ganglion and its dura mater from that of the overlying temporal lobe. (The ganglion may be injected with saline solution, and the dura mater may be split.)

10. If a root section is to be performed, a no. 11 blade on a long knife handle is used to make an incision into the lateral rim of the dura propria. The sensory and motor roots of the nerve are defined with a fine nerve hook. The mandibular and maxillary sections of the root are usually then divided. These are elevated with a nerve hook and divided with a fine scissors or a fine blade. The ophthalmic portion of the root is spared, as is the motor root.

11. Absolute alcohol may be injected into the affected divisions of the nerve just distal to the ganglion.

12. Saline solution is injected into the dura mater overlying the temporal lobe to distend it.
13. The incision is closed, and dressings are applied.

Some surgeons prefer to section the posterior root of the trigeminal nerve by the suboccipital route.

Suboccipital craniectomy and decompression for trigeminal rhizotomy

Procedural considerations. The position of the patient for suboccipital craniectomy is sitting, prone, or semilateral. To be prepared, the nurse must know during the planning phase (usually the day before the procedure is scheduled) which position the surgeon plans to use.

Operative procedure

1. The incision is made vertically behind the mastoid process. A trephine or burr hole is made and enlarged with a rongeur.
2. The dura mater is opened. The cisterna magna is pierced to empty the cerebrospinal fluid and permit backward retraction of the cerebellum. A brain spoon, brain spatula, or lighted retractor over moist strips of cottonoid is used to gently lift the cerebellar hemisphere. The eighth nerve is readily seen. The fifth nerve is approached by opening the arachnoid of the cisterna pontis and suctioning out the fluid. Veins are protected and bleeding controlled by pressure over cottonoid strips.
3. The nerve and the vessels around it are identified. The nerve is decompressed by coagulating the vessel over the nerve or separating the vessel from the nerve with a Teflon pledget. The microscope facilitates microvascular decompression. The motor root medial and anterior to the sensory root is preserved.
4. The wound is closed.

Suboccipital craniectomy and glossopharyngeal nerve section

Posterior fossa exploration for glossopharyngeal neuralgia is occasionally necessary. The same posterior fossa approach is used as for trigeminal neuralgia. The cerebellar hemisphere of the affected side is gently elevated upward and toward the midline. The ninth, tenth, and eleventh nerves are identified and defined with bayonet forceps, nerve hooks, and fine dissectors. The ninth nerve and a portion of the tenth are consecutively elevated with a nerve hook and divided with a fine-tipped scissors.

Suboccipital craniectomy for acoustic neuroma

Usually the acoustic neuroma arises from the vestibular portion of the eighth cranial nerve within the auditory meatus. It is desirable, although not always possible, to remove the complete tumor without damage to the facial nerve.

Operative procedure

1. The posterior fossa approach may be used. A unilateral straight paramedian incision is made.

2. The cerebellum is retracted gently upward with brain retractors and is cushioned with moist cottonoids. The lower cranial nerves are defined with a nerve or aneurysm hook. A cottonoid is placed over these nerves to protect them. Veins draining the tumor into the superior petrosal sinus are identified and either clipped or coagulated and cut.
3. The tumor is excavated and resected by methods similar to those employed to remove a pituitary adenoma.
4. A nerve stimulator may be used to identify the facial nerve. Use of the operating microscope is advantageous because of the many nerves and vessels in the area.
5. A high-speed air drill may be used to unroof the auditory canal and expose the remaining tumor. Constant irrigation is mandatory during drilling.

More recently, very small tumors confined to the auditory canal have been approached by drilling directly through the temporal bone to open the auditory canal within the bone and avoid the posterior fossa.

Suboccipital craniectomy for Ménière's disease

Ménière's disease is characterized by recurrent explosive attacks of vertigo associated with nausea, vomiting, tinnitus, and progressive deafness. It is usually unilateral. The cause is obscure, and in intractable cases surgical section or partial section of the eighth nerve (acoustic) may be performed for relief. However, surgery is not often performed for Ménière's disease.

Operative procedure

1. The cerebellum is approached through a lateral vertical incision behind the ear. The cerebellum on the affected side is retracted.
2. The eighth nerve is exposed with bayonet forceps and gentle manipulation. The nerve is freed from the arachnoid of the lateral cistern. It is separated from the underlying structures with a blunt nerve hook. Care is taken to prevent traction on the nearby seventh nerve (facial).
3. With fine scissors the vestibular fibers in the anterior half of the nerve are divided over a nerve hook. If the patient has useful hearing, the posterior auditory branches are preserved. Tinnitus may be relieved by section of the anterior fibers of the auditory portion of the nerve.
4. The dura mater and wound are closed.

Cranioplasty

Cranioplasty is performed for repair of a skull defect resulting from trauma, malformation, or a surgical procedure. Cranial defects covered by muscular areas need not be repaired. The purposes of cranioplasty are to relieve headache, vertigo, fear of injury, or local tenderness or throbbing; to prevent secondary injury to the underlying brain; and for cosmetic effect.

Procedural considerations. Many materials have been used to repair skull defects, including bone and cartilage;

celluloid; metals, such as Vitallium and tantalum; and the synthetic resins, such as methyl methacrylate and silicone rubber. All involve technical problems. The use of commercially prepared cranioplastic synthetics that supply the needed chemicals and mixing containers has simplified the procedures of shaping and molding the prosthesis. Sometimes heavy wire mesh is cut to the shape of the defect, and the methyl methacrylate is molded over the mesh.

Operative procedure

1. A scalp flap is turned, and the bony defect is exposed.
2. The edges of the defect are trimmed, and a ledge is formed to seat the prosthesis.
3. After the bone defect has been prepared so it is slightly saucerized, the methyl methacrylate is mixed by adding one volume of liquid monomer to one volume of the powdered polymer. When this has formed a doughy mass, it is dropped into a sterile polyethylene bag. The soft plastic is then rolled on a flat surface into the desired shape, leaving the thickness to the approximate depth of the skull edges. A sterile test tube, syringe barrel, or other round object can be used, although a stainless steel roller is preferred because of its weight and ease of use.
4. The soft cranioplastic material in the bag is placed over the skull defect and, through light pressing with the ends of the fingers, is fitted into the missing skull area. The plastic bag is stretched by assistants as the surgeon molds the plate into the defect and forms an overlapping bevel edge. This overlapping fringe keeps the plate from falling inside the skull, as does the skull saucerization.
5. When the heat of the chemical reaction begins, the plate is lifted out of the bony wound and removed from the polyethylene bag.
6. When cool enough to handle, the excess material is trimmed away with bone rongeurs or cut with a saw and placed in the cranial defect.
7. A sterile carborundum wheel attached to the electrical bone saw or craniotome is used to smooth the rough spots and bevel the edges so the plate will blend gradually with the skull.

Mixing and fitting the plate takes about 7 minutes, as does hardening. Sutures may be used to hold the plate in place, generally at three or more points.

Microneurosurgery

Adaptation of the operating microscope for neurosurgery has resulted in improvement of many neurosurgical procedures and made new procedures possible. For years neurosurgeons have worn magnifying loupes to see small structures. Loupes usually have a magnification of 2 or 2.8. The microscope has a variety of magnifications ranging from 6 to 40, providing flexibility and precision. The coaxial illumination overcomes the difficulties of lighting neurosurgical wounds.

Use of the microscope restricts the surgeon's field of vision and mobility; therefore, the scrub nurse must be proficient. The operative field, unless video monitoring is available, cannot be seen. The scrub nurse must understand the surgical procedure, know the anatomy, know the names and uses of all the microinstruments, and be able to place each instrument in the surgeon's hand without delay so the surgeon will be able to use the instrument without readjusting it. The nurse must make it possible for the surgeon to perform the operation without looking away from the operative field. Instruments must be kept free of blood and tissue during use because the microscope also magnifies debris on the instruments, occluding the structure the surgeon is about to approach. The nurse must understand the degree of stress these difficult procedures place on the neurosurgeon.

Microneurosurgical instruments are expensive and delicate. Instructions for handling, cleaning, sterilizing, and storing these instruments should be followed. An instrument that is sprung, bent, dulled, hooked, or in any way damaged must never be handed to a surgeon for use but must be repaired or replaced.

Existing microsurgical instruments have been modified and adapted to the requirements of neurosurgery. These instruments often possess the following characteristics: bayonet shape, so the surgeon's hand remains outside the line of vision and the beam of the microscope light; finely sprung and fluted grip; long length for access to deep structures; and slender and delicate tips that take up as little space as possible.

Very fine microsutures are available. The neurosurgeon may want to open the suture pack and ready the suture for use. However, the scrub nurse should be able to open and handle a delicate suture without damaging it. Each time the surgeon must look away and then back to the surgical field, open wound time and anesthesia time are increased while the surgeon becomes reoriented to the field. Therefore, any assistance the nurse gives the surgeon saves time and directly benefits the patient.

Microsurgical techniques have been applied to cranial, spinal, and peripheral nerve operations. Perhaps microneurovascular surgery is the area in which the most progress has been made. However, patient outcomes following microsurgical procedures on cranial nerves, spinal nerves, and cord tumors and especially for repair of peripheral nerve injuries have been enhanced.

Some procedures in which microsurgery is of value are posterior fossa explorations, especially for tumors of the fourth ventricle or cerebellopontine angle; translabyrinthine and transpetrosal removal of small acoustic neuromas, with resulting preservation of the facial nerve; and transsphenoidal hypophysectomy and transsphenoidal operations for small intracranial tumors, such as pituitary adenomas or even craniopharyngiomas. Transclival operations are also performed. Small vessel endarterectomy, cerebral arterial bypass, cerebral aneurysm surgery, and excision of arteriovenous malformations are done under the microscope. Microsurgery also has advantages in the treatment of tumors and arteriovenous malformations of the spinal cord.

Stereotaxic procedures

The use of complex mechanisms to locate and destroy target structures in the brain is known as stereotactics. Predetermined anatomic landmarks are used as guides. Special head-fixation devices have been developed by surgeons and engineers for use with radiography, fluoroscopy, CT scans, and MRI to permit accurate placement of a probe directed at the target area. Stereotaxic procedures can also be done on the spinal cord. Common target areas for the stereotaxic approach include tumors, the basal ganglia, the thalamus, the hypophysis, aneurysms, and anterolateral spinal tracts. Target areas undergo biopsy or are destroyed by chemical or mechanical means or electrically stimulated to control intractable pain. Stereotaxic procedures are also done to place electrodes in various regions of the brain to determine the site of origin of seizures. Lesions in target areas are made to perform biopsies and remove tumors; alleviate pain; abolish movement disorders; change endocrine balance to reverse such conditions as retinopathy, acromegaly, and endocrine-sensitive cancers; and obliterate aneurysms.

Operative procedure. The patient's head is placed in a special head holder, and the probe is introduced into the brain through a burr hole along one axis of the head holder. The probe is placed in position for insertion, and radiography, fluoroscopy, CT scans, or MRI is used to check the axis along which the probe is to be introduced. The position of the probe is checked by the same method after it is believed to rest on target (Fig. 23-61).

Hollow cannulae, coagulating electrodes, cryosurgical probes, wire loops, and other lesion-producing or biopsy instruments have been introduced for the destruction of areas in the brain. Temporary and permanent nerve-stimulator electrodes are also introduced to augment the pain-control function of the central nervous system. These instruments are introduced through a burr hole or twist-drill hole in the skull.

Continuing advancements in technology allow for the use of the laser with stereotaxic equipment. The numerous stereotaxic frames available include the BRW, CRW, Lehsell, Patel, Pelorsus, and Reichert Mundinger.

Surgery of the globus pallidus, basal ganglia, and thalamus

Pallidotomy is incision into the globus pallidus, usually by electrosurgery. *Chemopallidectomy* is introduction of a sclerosing solution through a rigid catheter or cannula to produce a lesion. *Thalamotomy* is incision into the thalamus. *Chemothalamectomy* is creation of a lesion in the region of the ventrolateral nucleus of the thalamus by means of a chemical solution such as alcohol with iophendylate. Surgical intervention is intended to interrupt the nerve pathways and alleviate the crippling locomotor symptoms of persistent, intractable tremor or rigidity associated with multiple sclerosis, severe brain trauma, Parkinson's disease, and various types of cerebellar degeneration. Studies are being conducted on fetal pituitary allografts and transcortical intraventricular adrenal medullary grafting in the treatment of Parkinson's disease. Some new treatment frontiers pose difficult ethical questions for neuroscience research; these will be an ongoing dilemma in the development of new treatment protocols. Operations of this type are also performed on the thalamus in an attempt to relieve pain.

Procedural considerations. The patient must be conscious and cooperative to permit careful examination and observation of response to the procedure and the effects on the symptoms. Local anesthesia is used. The patient may be in a supine or semisitting position.

Operative procedure

1. The patient's head is positioned and secured in the stereotaxic frame.
2. A skin incision and burr hole are completed as for ventriculography.
3. It may be necessary to take ventriculograms, in addition to viewing the position of the cannulae or needles.
4. When the correct position has been achieved, tests or reversible lesions may be attempted. The patient's response is observed. Finally, the definitive lesion is created at the selected site by means of electrosurgery, chemical solutions, or a cryogenic unit.
5. The dura mater and incision are closed.

Cryosurgery

Cryosurgery is the use of subfreezing temperatures in the treatment of disease to create a lesion. It is used in neurosurgery for transsphenoidal destruction of the pituitary gland in patients with acromegaly, diabetic retinopathy, and metastatic breast carcinoma. It can also be used for the destruction of the posterior portion of the thalamus for the treatment of Parkinson's disease or other involuntary movement disorders.

Transsphenoidal cryosurgery of the pituitary gland

Transsphenoidal cryosurgery is of special benefit to the patient suffering from metastatic carcinoma of the breast. These patients are most likely to respond if they have benefited from previous hormonal therapy or oophorectomy. In the patient with diabetic retinopathy, transsphenoidal cryosurgery is indicated when further laser beam coagulation of retinal lesions is considered useless. With acromegaly, if optic nerve or chiasma compression is present, a craniotomy is usually necessary.

Patients may undergo retrograde jugular venography

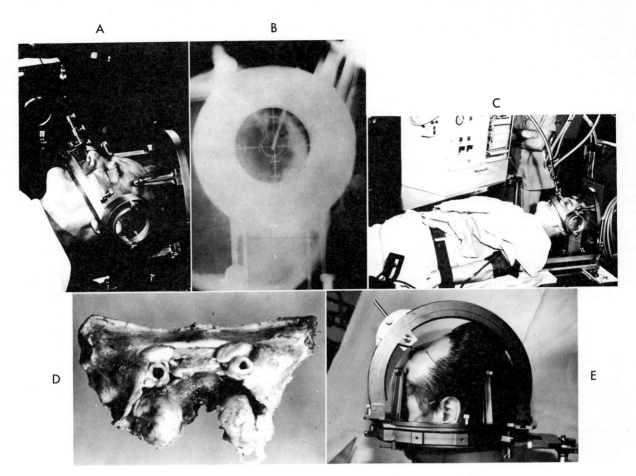

Fig. 23-61. Stereotaxic procedure. **A,** Patient's head is fixed to stereotaxic unit. Twist drill is inserted into anterior wall of sphenoidal sinus by way of left nostril into nasopharynx. **B,** Lateral x-ray film demonstrating freezing unit properly placed in target area (pituitary gland). Circle and cross-hairs are positioned at target point before insertion of cannula. **C,** Cannula in patient's left nostril is attached to freezing unit on table. X-ray equipment is seen in upper left background. Since procedure is performed with patient under local anesthesia, body straps are used to immobilize patient. **D,** Sella turcica viewed from above, demonstrating bone perforation at base through which cannula was inserted. To either side of sella turcica, internal carotid arteries are seen (*below,* siphon; *above,* with open lumen, cranial extension). Above sectioned arteries, optic nerves are seen passing into orbits. **E,** BRW stereotaxic frame. (**A** to **D** from Conway-Rutkowski, B.L.: Carini and Owens' neurological and neurosurgical nursing, ed. 8, St. Louis, 1982, The C.V. Mosby Co. **E,** Courtesy Radionics, Inc., Burlington, Mass.)

before surgery to outline the cavernous sinuses and carotid arteries. Patients with tumors must also have contrast CT scanning.

The advantages of transsphenoidal cryosurgery are:

1. Candidates in poor physical condition tolerate this procedure better than a craniotomy because it is less traumatic. Local rather than general anesthesia may be used.
2. Mortality and morbidity rates are low.
3. Complete destruction can be achieved with fair certainty in neoplastic glands and good certainty in normal glands.

Procedural considerations. The surgery is performed with fluoroscopic control. The patient is under local anesthesia supplemented with neuroleptanalgesia. Transtracheal anesthesia is used before insertion of an endotracheal tube for maintenance of a patent airway during the procedure. The patient is instructed to answer questions with hand signals.

Operative procedure

1. A topical local anesthetic administered with cotton applicators and 1% lidocaine injections through long needles are used to anesthetize the nasal and nasopharyngeal mucosa.
2. The head is placed in the stereotaxic head holder and

fixed after injection of local anesthetic in the skin at the points of fixation.

3. Preliminary x-ray films of the skull are taken to be sure that proper positioning has been achieved.

4. A guide is introduced, and a hole is drilled into the sphenoidal sinus and the floor of the sella turcica through the nasal vault. The guide is positioned fluoroscopically.

5. A cryoprobe is introduced through the guide into the pituitary gland, and its position is confirmed with x-ray films. The temperature of the probe is lowered to −18° to −19° C for 12 to 15 minutes. The probe can be used to feel the exact location of the dura mater surrounding the pituitary gland laterally and the diaphragm of the sella turcica superiorly.

6. The probe may be introduced to several depths of penetration into the sella turcica and additional lesions made. Additional holes may be drilled for further lesions.

7. The probe is withdrawn, and the nasal vault is inspected for bleeding. It can be packed with nasal packing. Antibiotics can be instilled before packing.

Patients are kept supine for 2 to 3 days and placed on a regimen of prophylactic antibiotics and cortisone replacement. Complications are meningitis secondary to cerebrospinal fluid leakage, extraocular palsy, damage to the optic nerve, and injury to cranial vessels such as the carotid and cavernous sinus. These can be prevented by an accurate preoperative evaluation and precise probe placement during surgery.

Shunt operations

Hydrocephalus is a pathologic condition in which there is an increase in the amount of CSF in the cranial cavity because of excessive production of, inadequate absorption of, or an obstruction that interferes with the flow of the fluid through the ventricular system.

Noncommunicating or internal hydrocephalus results from obstruction within the ventricular system. Ventricular fluid does not communicate with subarachnoid fluid.

Communicating or external hydrocephalus results from an obstruction outside the ventricular system. All the ventricles are enlarged, and ventricular and subarachnoid fluids freely communicate. Normal pressure hydrocephalus results from malabsorption of CSF.

Currently, the two most widely used methods to divert excessive CSF from ventricles to other body cavities from which it can be absorbed are ventriculoatrial (ventriculocardiac) and ventriculoperitoneal shunts. A catheter is inserted into the ventricular system (usually a lateral ventricle) and connected to a distal catheter that is placed in the right atrium of the heart or the peritoneal cavity (Fig. 23-62).

A valve system is used to direct the flow of CSF and regulate the ventricular fluid pressure by opening within a preset range and draining the excess fluid into the atrium or peritoneum. The valve system may be a separate unit, for example, the Holter valve, or Hakim or Denver system. The unit may be placed between the ventricular and distal catheters under the scalp just behind the ear (Fig. 23-63)

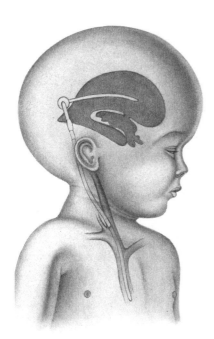

Fig. 23-62. Placement of ventriculoatrial shunt. (From Neurosurgery wound closure, Ethicon, Inc.)

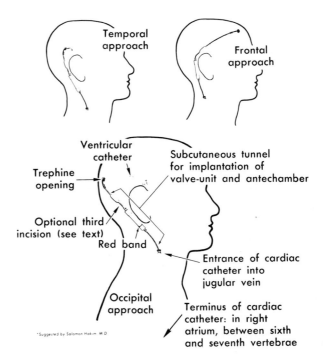

Fig. 23-63. Diagram of placement of Hakim ventriculoatrial shunt. (Courtesy Cordis Corp., Miami.)

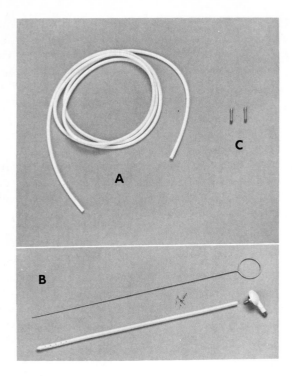

Fig. 23-64. Shunt is made from silicone tubing of special formula and consists of three parts: **A,** Peritoneal catheter. **B,** Ventricular with side perforations. **C,** Connector. Materials used in shunt can be sterilized in autoclave. (Courtesy Codman & Shurtleff, Inc., Randolph, Mass.)

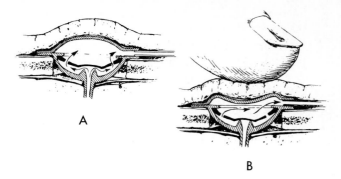

Fig. 23-65. Pudenz valve flushing device for ventricular shunts. **A,** Flanged silicone capsule and diaphragm valve shaped to fit into burr hole in skull. **B,** Pressure on capsule closes ventricular inlet and flushes shunt tube. (Courtesy Codman & Shurtleff, Inc., Randolph, Mass.)

or may be incorporated into the distal catheter (Fig. 23-64).

Usually a reservoir is inserted into the system between the ventricular catheter and the valve. The reservoir is also placed under the scalp just behind the ear or in a burr hole that was made to tap the lateral ventricle. The reservoir can be punctured through the scalp with a 25- or 26-gauge Huber needle to irrigate and clear an obstruction in the ventricular catheter, to introduce a contrast medium for an x-ray check of patency, to inject medication into the ventricle, or to serve as a flushing device when digital compression is applied (Fig. 23-65). Currently, the Ommaya reservoir is being utilized for the introduction of chemotherapeutic agents and for drainage of cystic brain tumors.

The valve assembly must be checked for patency and pressure before implantation. Each manufacturer provides specific instructions, which must be followed. As with all implantable devices, the shunt assembly must be kept free of lint, glove powder, or other potential foreign bodies that could cause a reaction by the patient's tissues.

Neurosurgeons and engineers frequently modify and improve shunt assemblies used today, as in the examples in Figs. 23-64 and 23-65. Valves are manufactured with pressure ranges of high, medium, low, and extra low. Slit-valve catheters have three pressure ranges: high, medium,

and low. All shunt systems and parts can be purchased sterile.

Other procedures that are sometimes done to correct hydrocephalus include cauterization of the choroid plexus of the lateral ventricles by placing a lensed ventriculoscope or laser into the ventricle through a burr hole to visualize and destroy the production site of CSF; ventriculoureteral shunts (requiring nephrectomy); lumbar subarachnoid shunt, in which a laminectomy is done and the cerebrospinal fluid is diverted into the peritoneal cavity; and ventriculocisternostomy, or Torkildsen procedure, in which a catheter is placed to shunt fluid from a lateral ventricle to the cisterna magna (Fig. 23-66).

Ventriculoatrial shunt

Procedural considerations. Insertion of a ventriculoatrial shunt is carried out with the patient in a modified supine position. The head is usually slightly elevated and turned to the left and may be supported on a doughnut. An x-ray film of the chest is taken to validate correct placement of the distal catheter, or the catheter can be placed under direct vision fluoroscopy with the image intensifier.

Operative procedure. When the distal slit-valve catheter is used, an incision is made in the neck to isolate the facial or the internal or external jugular vein. The atrial (distal) catheter is filled with normal saline solution, clamped with a bulldog clamp to prevent air from entering the circulatory system, and threaded into the right atrium through the isolated vein. Most catheters have a radiopaque tip for easy identification of placement during radiography. The catheter should lie at the T6 or T7 level.

Access is gained to the right lateral ventricle through a burr hole or twist-drill hole. The ventricular catheter is placed and connected to a reservoir. A tunnel is made under the skin from the burr hole to the neck incision with a uterine packing forceps or special tunneling device appropriate for the specific assembly being used. The atrial

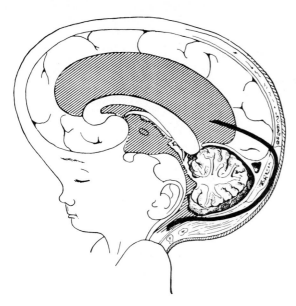

Fig. 23-66. Torkildsen operation (ventriculocisternostomy) showing catheter in place: one end in occipital horn of lateral ventricle, the other in cisterna magna. (From Conway-Rutkowski, B.L.: Carini and Owens' neurological and neurosurgical nursing, ed. 8, St. Louis, 1982, The C.V. Mosby Co.)

catheter is pulled through the tunnel to the burr hole and connected to the reservoir.

When a separate valve, such as the Holter, is used, the ventricular part of the procedure is carried out first. A special valve introducer and tube passer have been designed for use with the Holter assembly.

A single-catheter shunt system without a reservoir is also available. The distal end is a slit valve, and the proximal end is a ventricular catheter.

Ventriculoperitoneal shunts

The ventricular portion of this procedure is the same as for ventriculoatrial shunts. The distal catheter is much longer and is threaded from the ventricular puncture site under the scalp and superficial tissues of the neck, chest, and abdomen to the abdominal incision. The tip of the distal catheter may be placed under the liver.

Some precautions that must be taken during the valve implant procedures include the following:

1. Trapping of air in the valve assembly unit should be prevented.
2. Storage fluid surrounding the valve should be removed, pumped out of the valve, and replaced with Ringer's solution.
3. Extreme care should be used in handling the unit. It should never be placed on gauze or linen, to avoid lint or other foreign body. *The unit is always placed in a basin.*
4. Lubricants should never be used on the unit. The patient's body fluid adequately lubricates the device.

5. The valve must be properly oriented. It permits only one-way passage of fluid.
6. The valve system must not be pumped excessively immediately after surgery. This can cause too rapid a fluid loss, leading to a rapid decrease in ventricular size. This is poorly tolerated and may lead to subdural hemorrhage.

Frequently, shunts must be revised. Some shunts become obstructed. Others become disconnected or malfunction mechanically in some way. The growth of infants and children may require revision of distal tubings.

Operations on the back
Laminectomy

Laminectomy is removal of one or more of the vertebral laminae to expose the spinal cord. Laminectomy, hemilaminectomy, and interlaminar approach are performed to reach the spinal cord and its adjacent structures to treat compression fracture, dislocation, herniated nucleus pulposus, and cord tumor, as well as for spinal cord stimulation and insertion of infusion pumps for pain control. Section of the spinal nerves, including cordotomy and rhizotomy, requires similar surgical exposure. Laminectomy is also done to insert subarachnoid shunts for hydrocephalus or pseudotumor cerebri.

Procedural considerations. Laminectomy can be done with the patient in the prone, lateral, knee-chest, or sitting position. It is performed on the cervical, thoracic, or lumbar spine.

Laminectomy instruments include the basic neurosurgical set and the following:

2 Straight pituitary rongeurs, large and small
2 Angled pituitary rongeurs, large and small
1 Tower back retractor with blades
1 Scoville hemilaminectomy retractor
4 Beckman-Adson self-retaining laminectomy retractors, sharp, 12 inches, 2 regular and 2 large
4 Key periosteal elevators, ¼, ½, ¾, and 1 inch
2 Adson self-retaining cerebellum retractors, angled
1 Horsley bone cutter, large 10½ inches
2 Spurling-Kerrison laminectomy rongeurs, downbiting, 3 and 5 mm
2 Schlesinger cervical punches, thin-lipped rongeur, 3 and 5 mm
2 Love nerve root retractors
2 Angled curettes, nos. 3 and 4
2 Diamond-jawed needle holders, 9 inches
6 Cone ring curettes
5 Scoville curettes, nos. 1, 3, 4, 5, and 6
1 Penfield no. 4
2 Freer dissectors
1 Murphy ball probe

Operative procedures
Laminectomy for herniated disc (nucleus pulposus)
1. A midline vertical or transverse incision is made at the operative site.

2. Hemostatic forceps may be placed on the underside of the skin edge and everted for hemostasis. Deeper vessels are usually electrocoagulated.

3. Two self-retaining retractors (Cone, Weitlaner, or Adson) are inserted for exposure.

4. The fascia is incised in the midline with Mayo scissors, electrosurgical cutting tip, or a scalpel.

5. One side of the spinous processes is exposed by sharp dissection.

6. The paraspinous muscles and periosteum are stripped off the laminae with a knife and sharp periosteal elevators. Cutting current dissection with the electrosurgical unit may be used.

7. As each area is stripped, a gauze sponge is packed around the bony structures with a periosteal elevator to aid in blunt dissection and to tamponade bleeding. The paraspinous muscles are dissected from all the laminae (Fig. 23-67). In disc surgery this may be done only on one side, the side of the lesion.

8. A laminectomy retractor is then placed in position. Either a Scoville (a blade on the tissue side and a slightly shorter hook on the bone side), Tower, or Beckman-Adson retractor can be used.

9. Cottonoid strips or patties are placed in the extremes of the field for hemostasis.

10. The edges of the laminae overlying the interspace with the herniated disc are defined with a curette. A partial hemilaminectomy of these laminal edges extending out into the lateral gutter of the spinal canal is performed with a Schwartz-Kerrison rongeur. The bone edges are waxed.

11. The flaval ligament is grasped with a vascular bayonet forceps with teeth, and a no. 15 blade on a no. 7 knife handle is used to incise it as close to the midline as possible. Cottonoid strips or patties are passed through this incision to protect the underlying dura, and a window is cut in the flaval ligament with a no. 15 blade on a no. 7 knife handle (Fig. 23-68).

12. Additional ligaments out in the lateral gutter of the spinal canal may be removed with a large curette or a Cloward punch after first protecting the dural sac and nerve root with a cottonoid.

13. A dural elevator and a Love or copper nerve root retractor are used to retract the nerve root and dural sac to expose the disc space (Fig. 23-67).

14. Epidural veins are controlled by packing with narrow cottonoid strips and if necessary by careful coagulation with a bipolar bayonet.

15. Any herniated fragment of disc is removed with a pituitary rongeur.

16. After coagulation of its surface, an opening is cut into the posterior aspect of the interspace with a no. 11 or 15 blade on a no. 7 knife handle.

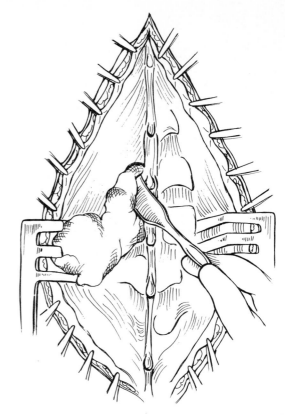

Fig. 23-67. Laminectomy: exposing vertebrae by dissecting muscle away from spine. (From Sachs, E.: Diagnosis and treatment of brain tumors and the care of the neurosurgical patient, ed. 2, St. Louis, 1949, The C.V. Mosby Co.)

17. Pituitary rongeurs, straight and angled, narrow and wide, are used to remove the disc material from the interspace.

18. Straight and angled Scoville and ring curettes help to further clean out the interspace. Disc material so loosened is removed with the pituitary rongeurs.

19. The area is irrigated with Ringer's or normal saline solution, and the interspace is explored with a suction tip.

20. The nerve roots and extradural space are explored with a blunt nerve hook.

21. If no further specimen is obtained, hemostasis is secured with cottonoid strips or patties. If possible, neither gelatin sponge nor gauze nor other hemostatic material is used.

22. The cottonoid strips are removed from the epidural space, the bed is unflexed, and the area is further irrigated. A change of position sometimes causes more disc material to protrude, and the interspace is reexposed with a nerve root retractor to rule out this possibility.

23. All cottonoid strips and patties, and retractors are removed, and the wound is closed.

A

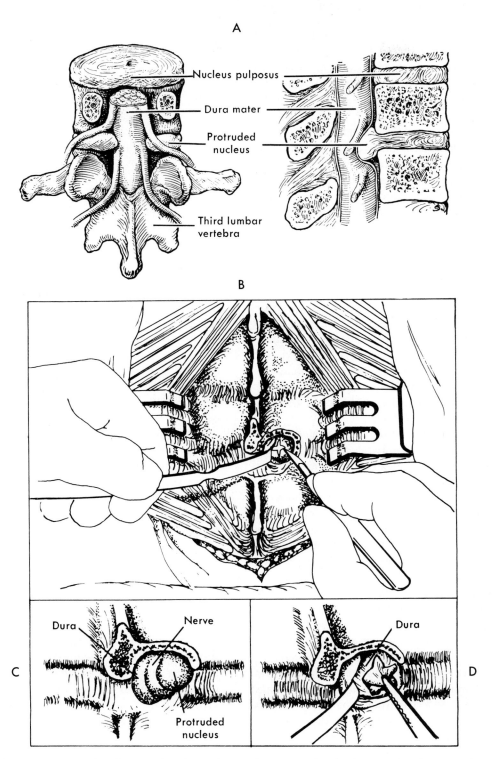

Nucleus pulposus

Dura mater

Protruded nucleus

Third lumbar vertebra

B

C

Dura

Nerve

Protruded nucleus

D

Dura

Fig. 23-68. A, Normal and herniated nucleus pulposus (disc). **B,** Window has been made in lamina, and ligament has been incised to expose underlying dura mater and nerve root. **C,** Relationship of dura mater, nerve root, and protruded nucleus pulposus (disc). **D,** Retraction of nerve root over dura mater and removal of disc. (From Carini, E., and Owens, G.: Neurological and neurosurgical nursing, ed. 6, St. Louis, 1974, The C.V. Mosby Co.)

For cervical or thoracic discs, only the protruding fragment is removed and limited if any exploration of the interspace is performed. This is because attempts of adequate interspace exploration require retraction of the dural sac, which contains the spinal cord at these levels. Such retraction would result in cord injury and paralysis. For thoracic discs, a costotransversectomy or chest approach is used.

Laminectomy for spinal cord tumors

1. The fascial incision is made in the midline, both sides of the spinous processes are dissected out, and the paraspinous muscles are taken down bilaterally, one side at a time.
2. One or more double-bladed Scoville or Beckman-Adson self-retaining retractors are placed to maintain the bony exposure.
3. A midline laminectomy is performed, with the spinous processes excised with a Horsley bone cutter. Various rongeurs (such as Leksell, double-action, Cloward) are used to remove the laminae after defining the edges with a curette. The Midas Rex drill may also be used. The bone edges are waxed.
4. The remaining flaval ligament is removed with scissors, scalpel, and Kerrison or Cloward rongeurs. Epidural fat is electrocoagulated and if necessary removed with dissecting scissors, so the dura mater is exposed fully.
5. A wide moist cottonoid is placed over the superficial soft tissues and muscle down to the bone bordering the exposed dura mater. This provides additional hemostasis.
6. The dura mater is elevated with a small hook and nicked with a no. 15 knife blade. A grooved director is inserted beneath the dura mater, and the dural incision is extended over it, using long forceps and fine scissors. Alternatively, the incision may be lengthened by pulling apart the two edges of the dural incision with bayonet forceps or by pushing at the ends of this incision with the edge of a dural elevator. Traction sutures of no. 4-0 silk or nylon on dura needles are placed in the dural edges, and the cord is exposed (Fig. 23-69).
7. The cord is explored for the pathologic area. Aspiration through a no. 22 needle on a plain-tipped syringe may be carried out. The tumor may be encountered extradurally or intradurally. Whenever possible, the tumor mass is dissected free and removed by suction, dissecting scissors, the cutting electrosurgical forceps, cottonoid, small (pituitary) scoops, curettes, pituitary rongeurs, or an ultrasonic aspirator (Fig. 23-28). Bleeding is controlled with a moist cottonoid, hemostatic clips, gelatin gauze, and topical hemostatics. Bipolar coagulation is used around the nerves and spinal cord. The spinal subarachnoid space may be explored with a small rubber catheter to detect blockage.
8. The wound is irrigated with normal saline or Ringer's solution, Asepto syringes, and suction.
9. Hemostasis is obtained; the dura mater is closed with a no. 4-0 or 5-0 silk, 4-0 black braided nylon, or 4-0 Polyglactin suture.
10. The incision is checked for further bleeding, and the paraspinous muscles are approximated with no. 0 Polyglactin synthetic absorbable suture or no. 2-0 silk. The remainder of the wound is closed.

In the case of extradural tumors, intradural exploration is omitted.

The operating microscope may be used, especially on intradural tumors and vascular anomalies. The laser also may be used and should be available, along with the intraoperative ultrasound and ultrasonic aspiration (Fig. 23-28).

Laminectomy for meningocele.

Malformations such as meningoceles are usually congenital. They are a threat to the life of the newborn infant because the defect may predispose to infection or spinal cord damage. Defects of the cord and spinal nerves are often associated with the condition. There also may be spina bifida, a congenital defect resulting from incomplete closure of the vertebral canal.

Operation for repair of meningocele is directed at preserving intact the neural elements involved and at closing the cutaneous, muscular, and dural defects.

For surgery on infants, small hemostats, retractors, and other instruments are provided. Large bone-cutting instruments may be omitted. The nerve stimulator may be needed.

Cervical cordotomy (Schwartz technique, thoracic cordotomy, rhizotomy)

Cervical cordotomy is division of the spinothalamic tract for the treatment of intractable pain. Pain management techniques, epidural administration of opiates, or percutaneous cordotomy may be initiated for pain management. High cervical cordotomy is an effective surgical procedure. Rhizotomy is interruption of the roots of the spinal nerves with the spinal canal. Anterior rhizotomy is division of the anterior or motor spinal nerve roots for the relief of spasm; posterior rhizotomy is division of the posterior or sensory spinal nerve roots for the relief of intractable pain.

Procedural considerations. Cervical cordotomy may be performed with the patient under general anesthesia, but, to permit intraoperative testing of the level of analgesia achieved, local anesthesia is preferred. The nurse should keep an accurate account of the amount of local anesthetic agent used. In a very ill or apprehensive patient, a drop

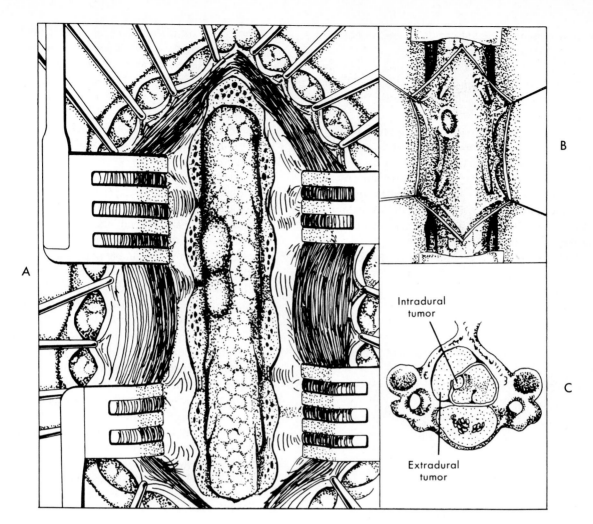

Fig. 23-69. A, Laminectomy completed: dura mater and tumor exposed. **B,** Dura mater incised and retracted, revealing pia arachnoid over spinal cord and part of tumor. **C,** Diagram of cross-section of tumor site and location of extradural and intradural pathologic areas. (From Carini, E., and Owens, G.: Neurological and neurosurgical nursing, ed. 6, St. Louis, 1974, The C.V. Mosby Co.)

in blood pressure or cardiac symptoms may develop if too much local anesthetic is injected.

The patient is placed in a prone position, with head slightly flexed to a level below the horizontal level of the cervical spine. It is essential to keep the patient as comfortable as possible and to offer reassurance frequently.

Operative procedure

1. The skin is infiltrated with a local anesthetic agent, the incision line is marked, and longer needles are used to block the second and third cervical nerves at their points of emergence from the spinal canal.
2. A midline incision is used. Hemostatic forceps are placed to control bleeding, and the Weitlaner retractor is inserted for exposure.
3. Using the electrosurgical unit (cutting current) with the spatula blade, the surgeon separates the muscles from one side of the arches and laminae of the first

and second cervical vertebrae. An angled periosteal elevator may be used for further dissection. A gauze sponge may be packed into the wound to enhance the dissection as well as to aid hemostasis.

4. A Scoville hemilaminectomy retractor with short hook and longer blade is inserted between the midline structures and the reflected paraspinous muscles. The flexion of the head is increased when the retractor is inserted.
5. The Schwartz self-retaining retractor (modified Gelpi) is placed, with the multitoothed end in the occipital bone and the sharp point penetrating the spinous process of C2 to widen the interlaminar space between C1 and C2 vertebrae. (For additional exposure it may be necessary to remove some of the laminae with a Kerrison rongeur.)
6. Large moist cottonoid strips are placed over the su-

perficial tissues and muscle down to the bone bordering the exposed dura mater.

7. With the use of a dural hook, the dural incision is made with a no. 7 knife handle and a no. 15 blade. A vascular or Metzenbaum scissors is used to lengthen the incision.

8. With no. 4-0 silk stay sutures on an ophthalmic needle, the dural edges are retracted and secured with curved or straight mosquito hemostats.

9. While suctioning is being performed on cottonoid strips to remove spinal fluid, the dentate ligament is identified at its dural attachment with bayonet forceps and followed to the cord and left attached to prevent distortion of the cord.

10. A fine bayonet forceps (Gerald) is used to elevate the dentate attachment to provide visualization of the anterolateral quadrant of the cord and the anterior nerve rootlets.

11. The cord is incised with a slightly curved cordotomy knife (Fig. 23-70).

12. After the incision is made, the patient is checked for adequacy of the level of analgesia. If the level is not satisfactory, the cord incision is deepened.

13. Hemostasis is obtained, the dural incision is closed, retractors are removed, and the wound is checked for bleeding and is closed.

As technology improves, the laser is being utilized in performing this procedure.

For *bilateral cordotomy*, the muscles are separated from both sides of the arches and laminae of the vertebrae. A double-bladed Scoville retractor is used, and the Schwartz retractor (modified Gelpi) is placed according to the side of the cord being approached. The cordotomy is performed on one side and then on the other. With bilateral high cervical cordotomy, falls in blood pressure and respiratory difficulty may occur.

High thoracic cordotomy is performed unilaterally or bilaterally in a similar manner, but a hemilaminectomy or total laminectomy at two levels must usually be performed to gain adequate exposure. The lateral or prone position may be used.

Rhizotomy is performed through a similar exposure with the appropriate nerve roots dissected free of any large radicular vessels, held up with a nerve hook, crushed with a hemostatic forceps, and divided with fine-tipped scissors. A silver clip may be placed on the distal ends of the roots before division. This aids in hemostasis and permits subsequent radiologic visualization of the extent and precise level of the root section (Fig. 23-71).

Removal of anterior cervical disc with fusion (Cloward technique)

This procedure is done to relieve pain in the neck, shoulder, and arm caused by cervical spondylosis or herniated disc. It entails removal of the disc and fusion of the vertebral bodies. Bone dowels for the fusion are obtained from the patient's iliac crest or from a bone dowel bank.

Procedural considerations. The patient is placed in the supine position, with the head turned very slightly to the left and with the right hip elevated for exposure of the iliac crest (if the bone dowel is to be taken from the iliac crest). The basic minor dissecting set is used, plus the following instruments (Fig. 23-72).

2 Cloward self-retaining retractors, 1 large and 1 small, with assorted blades (with and without teeth)
4 Drill guards (various sizes), cervical drill, and dowel cutters
1 Cloward bone graft holder
1 Cloward bone graft impactor, double-ended
2 Cloward hand retractors
2 Cloward vertebral spreaders, 1 regular and 1 self-retaining
1 Mallet
2 Adson cerebellum retractors, angled
3 Cloward rongeurs, 2, 3, and 5 mm
Spinal fusion curettes, straight and angulated, nos. 0, 00, and 3-0

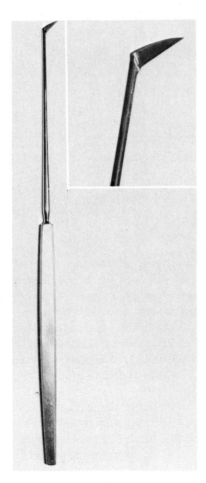

Fig. 23-70. Schwartz cordotomy knife. (Courtesy K. Cramer Lewis, Department of Illustrations, Washington University School of Medicine, St. Louis.)

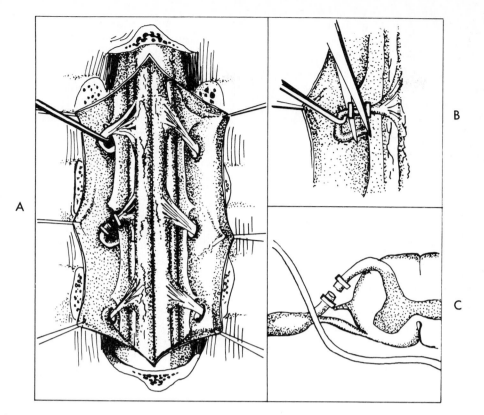

Fig. 23-71. Posterior rhizotomy after laminectomy. **A,** Spinal cord and roots exposed. **B,** Posterior root identified. **C,** Diagram showing cross-section of spinal cord and divided posterior root. (From Carini, E. and Owens, G.: Neurological and neurosurgical nursing, ed. 6, St. Louis. 1974. The C.V. Mosby Co

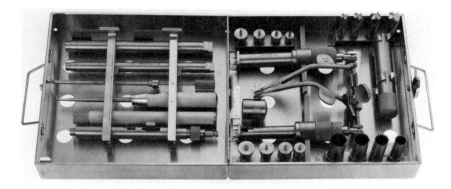

Fig. 23-72. Instruments for anterior cervical disc removal with fusion. *Left side:* Cloward dowel cutter shaft, dowel ejector, osteophyte elevator, depth gauge, guard guide (large, small). *Right side, bottom to top:* dowel ejector pins, dowel cutter pins, cervical drill guards (small and large), drill guard cap, drill shaft, cervical drills, crossbar handle, dowel cutter shaft guard, vertebra spreader, and spanner wrench. (Courtesy Codman & Shurtleff, Inc., Randolph, Mass.)

Operative procedure

1. A transverse skin incision is made on one side of the neck (usually the right) directly over the involved disc space; curved mosquito hemostats or Michel clips are placed on the skin edges for hemostasis.
2. A Weitlaner retractor is placed, and the platysma mus-

cle is divided with Metzenbaum scissors and tissue forceps with teeth or with the electrosurgical cutting blade.

3. The medial edge of the sternocleidomastoid muscle is defined with the scissors by blunt and sharp dissection.

4. A vertical plane of dissection between the carotid sheath laterally and the trachea and esophagus medially is created by blunt finger dissection. This plane is held open with Cloward hand retractors. Meyerding finger retractors, or U.S. Army retractors.

5. The anterior surface of the spine is identified, and the long muscles of the neck are peeled off the anterior surface of the spine with periosteal elevators. Bleeders are coagulated with a dural elevator or bayonet forceps.

6. A 20-gauge spinal needle is inserted a short distance into the disc space, and a lateral x-ray film is taken to determine the level of the exposure.

7. While x-ray films are being developed, the neck incision is covered, an incision is made over the iliac crest, and straight hemostats are applied and retracted.

8. Soft tissue is dissected until the crest is reached, using Mayo scissors, tissue forceps, electrosurgical cutting blade, and Richardson retractors for exposure.

9. A Hudson brace with the Cloward dowel cutter is used to remove the bone graft. (Care must be exercised to use dowel cutter, Cloward guide, and cervical drill guards matched for size.) The dowel should have cortex at both ends. The dowel hole is inspected and waxed if needed. The incision is packed with gauze sponges and covered.

10. The Cloward self-retaining retractors (two long and two short blades) are inserted into the neck incision. The right blade should be slightly longer than the left. Care is used to protect the carotid artery and the esophagus. A combination of sharp and dull blades is used to acquire the best retraction. If a toothed blade is used, the teeth are carefully hooked beneath the long muscle of the neck.

11. A no. 15 or 11 blade on a no. 7 knife handle is used to cut into the disc space; a fine pituitary ronguer is used to remove the disc material, which is saved and weighed as a specimen. A vertebral spreader is inserted into the vertebral space to widen the area, and further disc material is removed with the rongeur or small curettes (angled or straight, nos. 0 to 4-0) until the entire surfaces of both vertebrae are clean. A Surgairtome with small burr may also be used.

12. The Cloward bone guide is inserted into the disc space to measure its depth.

13. After the drill guard is adjusted so the drill can protrude no farther than the measured depth of the interspace, the cervical drill guard is inserted around the disc space, with the aid of a mallet, until the points catch the vertebral bodies above and below the interspace.

14. After the guard is in place, the vertebral spreader is removed or spread to a more limited degree.

15. The Cloward drill on a Hudson brace is inserted into the guard, and the hole is drilled. (The bone dust on

the drill point is inspected and saved in a medicine glass.) Cottonoid strips or topical hemostatics are used for active bleeders. Bone wax should not be used on the walls of the disc hole. Thrombin-soaked cottonoid pledgets may help control bleeding.

16. The bottom of the hole is checked for further disc or cartilaginous material, which is removed. The guide may be removed and replaced, and drilling may be done several times until the desired depth is reached. The drill and guide are then removed.

17. Further bone is removed by use of the Cloward cervical punch or curettes until complete anterior decompression of the nerve root or dural sac is obtained. Nerve hooks may be used here for demonstration of adequate dissection. The Air Drill 100 or Midas Rex may also be used.

18. The depth of the hole is measured and compared with the dowel. The dowel may be trimmed with a drill, rongeur, or rasp. The shaped dowel attached to the impactor is inserted into the hole and tapped into place. The double-edged impactor is used to drive the dowel in deeper if necessary. The spreader is removed, and bone dust may be applied.

19. Hemostasis is obtained and the wound irrigated; the vertebral spreader and retractors are removed, and both incisions are closed.

Carotid surgery of the neck
Carotid artery ligation

Carotid artery ligation is performed to occlude the internal carotid artery.

It may be done to control anticipated hemorrhage during intracranial surgery for vascular anomalies. A permanent occlusion may be necessary for the control of intracranial hemorrhage or small, repeated strokes from an intracranial lesion.

Procedural considerations. Special clamps, such as the Selverstone (Fig. 23-73) Selibi, and Crutchfield carotid artery clamps (Fig. 23-74) are available for gradual occlusion of the artery. Occlusion may protect the patient from debilitating or fatal intracranial hemorrhage from aneurysm and may be used to treat carotid-cavernous fistula.

Only a basic minor instrument set is used.

Operative procedure

1. The skin is incised, and a Weitlaner retractor is inserted for exposure.

2. The carotid artery is freed. A small Penrose tubing, umbilical tape, or vessel loop is passed around the vessel for retraction.

3A. *For temporary control* of the carotid artery (during procedures for very large aneurysms or arteriovenous anomalies): an umbilical tape is passed around the vessel and fixed, using the Roper-Rumel tourniquet in such a manner that occlusion can be accomplished immediately if necessary.

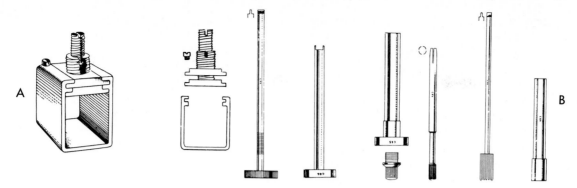

Fig. 23-73. A, Selverstone carotid artery clamp. **B,** Selverstone carotid artery clamp accessories. (Courtesy Codman & Shurtleff, Inc., Randolph, Mass.)

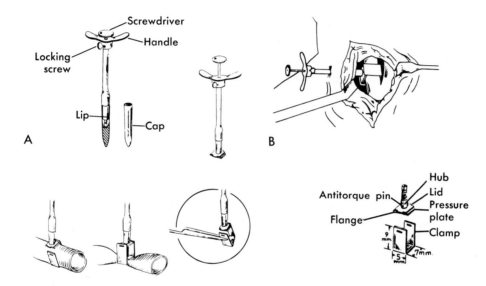

Fig. 23-74. Crutchfield carotid artery clamp. **A,** Control assembly. **B,** Clamp assembly. (Courtesy Codman & Shurtleff, Inc., Randolph, Mass.)

3B. *For permanent occlusion:* two heavy silk ligatures are used, and the artery may be divided between ligatures. Transfixing suture ligatures may be used as well if the artery is divided.

3C. *For gradual occlusion:*

    a. A carotid clamp, such as the Selverstone, Selibi, or Crutchfield, is placed in position around the artery.

    b. A small stab wound is made adjacent to the incision.

    c. The control assembly with cap is passed through the stab wound. By loosening the locking screw and pressing down on the screwdriver, the operator can remove the cap.

    d. The control assembly is snapped on the lid of the clamp, and with a hemostatic forceps holding the clamp, each flange is gently forced into position.

    e. Using the dot on the screwdriver as an indicator,

the number of turns for complete occlusion is noted. The clamp is then unscrewed a measured number of turns, and the screwdriver is locked. The control assembly is capped and left in place, protruding through the stab wound.

4. The incision is closed, and a dressing is applied.

After the procedure the carotid artery clamp accessories are packaged and sterilized. They are kept at the patient's bedside for daily adjustments and returned to the operating room or central service for resterilization after each use. They must be returned to the patient's bedside as soon as possible to be available if the patient cannot tolerate the occlusion and the clamp must be opened immediately.

Carotid surgery for carotid-cavernous fistula

Ligation of the common carotid artery is one mode of surgical treatment for a carotid-cavernous fistula. Another form of surgical treatment is to embolize the fistula with muscle or other material. The segment of external carotid artery just distal to the carotid bifurcation is occluded with vascular clamps and incised as a point of entry. A piece of muscle is labeled with a metal clip and attached to a length of silk so it can be visualized by radiography and withdrawn if necessary. It is introduced into the internal carotid artery through the arteriotomy in the external carotid artery after the internal and common carotid arteries are occluded and after the proximal external carotid artery clamp is removed. The internal and then common carotid artery clamps are released as the clamp is removed. The proximal external carotid artery clamp is reapplied, leaving a small proximal opening in the arteriotomy unclamped for the protrusion of the tag suture on the embolus. The blood flow in the common internal carotid artery system then pushes the embolus up to the fistula.

In either case, internal carotid ligation is usually done after satisfactory placement of the embolus. In some cases a frontotemporal craniotomy is also performed, and the internal carotid artery clipped intracranially as well.

Endarterectomy is another procedure involving the cerebral circulation, although not directly involving the brain and cranial nerves (Chapter 26). Endarterectomy consists of exposing the carotid artery in the neck at the site of occlusion, incising the vessel, and removing the associated sclerotic tissue. Electroencephalographic (EEG) or evoked response monitoring may be used intraoperatively.

Peripheral nerve surgery
Sympathectomy

Sympathectomy is excision of a portion of the sympathetic division of the autonomic nervous system. Most sympathectomies are performed on the paravertebral chain and are named for the region resected, for example, cervical, thoracolumbar, and lumbar. The periarterial sympathectomy, vagotomy, and presacral neurectomy are other procedures that are occasionally performed on the autonomic system.

The principal diseases treated by sympathectomy are vascular disorders of the extremities and intractable pain from certain nerve injuries, chronic abdominal conditions, and hyperhidrosis.

Procedural considerations. The position of the patient depends on the region to be resected.

Basic dissecting instruments and the microscope are used, plus the following:

For *retropleural and transthoracic approaches*, rib resecting instruments are added (Fig. 23-75).

For *thoracic and lumbar approaches*, the following are added:

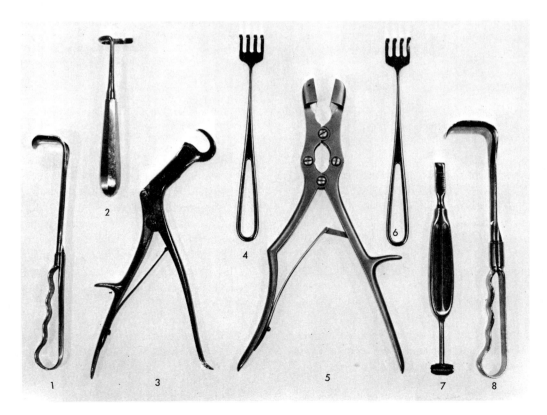

Fig. 23-75. Instruments for rib resection. *1*, Richardson retractor; *2*, Doyen rib raspatory; *3*, Stille rib shears; *4*, blunt rake retractor; *5*, Sauerbruch rib rongeur; *6*, blunt rake retractor; *7*, Alexander costal periosteotome; *8*, Richardson retractor.

2 Volkman rake retractors, large, eight-pronged, blunt
3 Malleable copper retractors
2 Richardson retractors, large
2 Weinberg retractors, large
2 Deaver retractors
2 Harrington retractors
2 Beckman retractors

For the *thoracic approach*, Beckman or Scoville laminectomy retractors are added.

For the *abdominal approach*, Balfour self-retaining retractors are added.

Cervicothoracic sympathectomy (dorsal)

Dorsal sympathectomy entails removal of the cervicothoracic chain, often from the fourth cervical to the third thoracic ganglion. Sympathetic denervation of the upper extremities and heart may be accomplished by cervicothoracic sympathectomy. The vasospastic phenomenon of Raynaud's disease is relieved by this procedure. It also may be beneficial in relieving intractable angina pectoris.

Procedural considerations. For the anterior approach, both the laminectomy set and rib instruments are used, plus deep retractors and a nerve stimulator. The setup for the posterior approach is as for the anterior approach, plus rib-resecting instruments, periosteal elevators, small rib retractors, a firm rubber pad, and operating room bed attachments for the posterolateral position.

Operative procedure
Anterior approach

1. The patient is placed in a supine position with head rotated to the opposite side, as in mastoidectomy (Chapter 19). General endotracheal anesthesia is necessary because there is a possibility of puncturing the pleura.
2. A transverse incision is made one fingerbreadth above the clavicle, the clavicular head of the sternocleidomastoid muscle is severed, and the deep cervical fascia is divided.
3. The phrenic nerve and the jugular vein are protected, and the anterior scalene muscle is divided to expose and isolate the underlying subclavian artery. The thyroid axis, one of its branches, is ligated and divided.
4. The stellate ganglion, deep against the vertebral body, is brought into view and lifted on a nerve hook. The sympathetic chain is traced upward to the middle cervical ganglion and divided. Deep dissection behind the pleura exposes the upper thoracic ganglia, which are removed to below the third thoracic ganglion. Clips may be placed on the sympathetic nerves before their division.
5. The wound is closed according to the surgeon's preference.

Posterior approach

1. The patient is placed in the lateral position, and a paravertebral incision is centered over the third rib. The trapezius muscle is divided, and the rhomboid is split in line with its fibers. The third and fourth ribs are isolated extrapleurally, and the posterior 4 to 5 cm is resected. The transverse processes may be removed to provide better exposure.
2. The sympathetic trunk, which lies on the anterolateral aspect of the vertebral body, is reached by carefully reflecting the pleura. The trunk is picked up on a nerve hook, traced up and down, and removed, usually from the stellate ganglion to the fourth thoracic ganglion. Clips may be applied to the nerve before severing the fibers.
3. A firm rubber tube may be left in the wound during closure. Suctioning apparatus is applied to this tube as the last deep fascial suture is drawn tight; all air is aspirated, and the tube is quickly withdrawn.
4. The subcutaneous tissue and skin edges are closed.

Nerve repairs

Peripheral nerve injuries are the most common indication for this surgery. Nerve tumors are rare in comparison. During wartime, injuries of nerves assume particular importance because of their frequency and disabling results.

When the continuity of a nerve is destroyed, function distal to the site of injury is lost. Recovery will occur only if regeneration of nerve axons take place from the healthy proximal segments. These axons must grow down the axis cylinders of the nerve beyond the injury if they are to reinnervate their end organs and allow function to return.

When a nerve is divided, the cut ends retract, become scarred, and form neuromas. Regenerating axons from the proximal segment cannot bridge such a gap or penetrate the scar tissue. An unobstructed path down the axis cylinder must be made available if nerves are ever again to move muscles or transmit sensation. All procedures are directed toward obtaining the best possible conditions for regeneration.

Procedural considerations. A basic dissecting instrument set is used, plus the following:

Nerve stimulator
Jeweler's nerve forceps
Microsutures
Loupes
Operating microscope
Intraoperative EMG recorder
Microforceps
Microscissors
Microneedle holders
Microdissectors
Tongue blades
Sterile double-edged razor blades (can be ethylene oxide sterilized in their paper wrappers)

For lesser procedures such as spinal-accessory-facial anastomosis in the neck, division of the volar carpal ligament for median nerve compression at the wrist, or repair

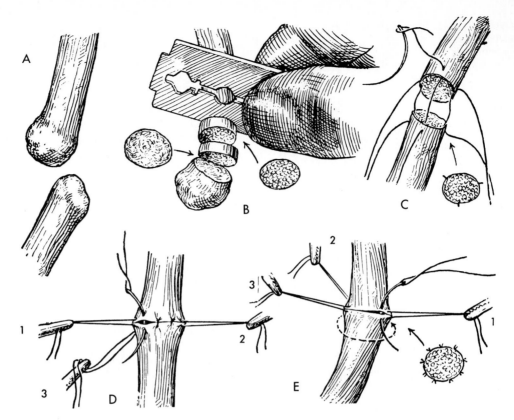

Fig. 23-76. Nerve repair. **A,** Divided nerve with neuroma. **B,** Serial resection of neuroma to healthy nerve fibers. **C,** Placement of sutures in epineurium. **D** and **E,** Approximation and tying of sutures. (From Sachs, E.: Diagnosis and treatment of brain tumors and care of the neurosurgical patient, ed. 2, St. Louis, 1949, The C.V. Mosby Co.)

of a small digital nerve, suitable modification may be made.

The positioning, skin prep, and draping of the patient depend on the site of the injury. A large area is prepped.

General anesthesia is usually preferred, with the patient positioned for maximum accessibility to the injured nerve. Exposure must be adequate because considerable mobilization of the nerve is often necessary. A dry field may be achieved by using a tourniquet on the involved extremity.

Operative procedure. The site of injury is explored, with careful attention to hemostasis. Nerve ends are dissected from surrounding scar tissue, and neuromas are excised. Moist umbilical tapes, vessel loops, or Penrose tubing may be passed about the nerve to handle it more easily and with less trauma.

The nerve repair (anastomosis) is made with multiple fine sutures placed only through the nerve sheath or epineurium (Fig. 23-76). Tension at the suture line is eliminated by such maneuvers as freeing up a long length of nerve on either side of the point of injury, transposition of the nerve in order to shorten its course, appropriate positioning of the extremity with plaster splinting during the postoperative period, and, rarely, use of a nerve graft.

Some surgeons apply a cuff of inert material such as silicone about the anastomosis.

Hypoglossal facial nerve anastomosis

Hypoglossal facial nerve anastomosis is performed to restore function to an injured facial nerve. With certain lesions in the posterior fossa and during some procedures on the posterior fossa, the facial nerve may be damaged.

Operative procedure. An incision is made over the anterior edge of the sternocleidomastoid muscle, extending from the mastoid process downward for a distance of approximately 11 to 12 cm. The fascia and muscles are divided, and further dissection is carried out until the hypoglossal nerve is exposed and divided distally. The facial nerve is exposed and divided close to its exit from the stylomastoid foramen deep to the front of the mastoid process. The proximal end of the hypoglossal nerve is anastomosed to the distal end of the facial nerve with fine arterial or nerve sutures, and the wound is closed.

Occasionally a surgeon uses the accessory or even the phrenic nerve instead of the hypoglossal. Microsurgical techniques and instruments are used.

Carpal tunnel syndrome

Carpal tunnel syndrome is a condition of the hand in which the median nerve is compressed by the transverse carpal ligament or by displacement of the lunate bone or a volar carpal ganglion. Decompression of the nerve is done by removing part of the roof of the fibrous sheath of the ligament or the offending bone or ganglion.

Procedural considerations. The patient is placed in the supine position with the operative arm extended on a hand table or armboard. Local, regional, or general anesthesia may be used.

Operative procedure

1. A longitudinal skin incision is made in the thenar palm crease. This runs prependicular to and stops at the most distal transverse skin crease in the wrist. This incision generally suffices but may be extended into an L or a T.
2. A Weitlaner, mastoid, or self-retaining spring-action retractor is placed.
3. The fibers of the carpal ligament are divided transversely in blunt fashion at the most proximal point of exposure. A hemostat is introduced through this opening in the ligament, pointed distally, and spread. This protects the underlying median nerve. The ligament is divided between the jaws of the hemostat with a Mayo or plastic Metzenbaum scissors.
4. After this incision has been carried well into the palm, the remaining proximal fibers of the ligament are divided in the same fashion. A small vein retractor is placed on the proximal skin edges to facilitate this step.
5. A biopsy of the ligament may be obtained.
6. The incision is closed with fine sutures, and a bulky dressing is applied, with the fingers visible.

Ulnar nerve transposition at the elbow

Because of traumatic or anatomic problems, the ulnar nerve may be predisposed to irritation resulting in chronic discomfort. In such instances the position of the nerve can be changed to provide protection and comfort.

Procedural considerations. The patient is placed in the supine position. The arm may be supported in a functional position, with Webril and elastic bandages to attach it to the anesthesia screen, or it may be left free for the surgeon to manipulate during the procedure. The inner, posterior aspect of upper and lower arm must be exposed for the operation.

Operative procedure. A long incision is made, and the nerve is dissected free from the surrounding soft tissues with Metzenbaum scissors and hemostatic forceps. Moist umbilical tapes, vessel loops, or Penrose tubing is passed around the freed segment of the nerve to aid in handling them for further dissection until a satisfactory length of nerve has been freed from above to below the elbow. The muscle and fascia entered by the nerve at each end of the field may be slit with a scissors to prevent tethering and kinking at these points after the nerve has been transposed. A fascial flap overlying the medial epicondyle of the humerus is cut and elevated, and the nerve is transposed beneath it. The fascia is then loosely reapproximated to the fascial edge remaining on the epicondyle with no. 3-0 silk or no. 2-0 Polyglactin synthetic absorbable suture. The wound is closed in layers.

An alternative procedure, medial epicondylectomy, is sometimes performed. In this case the nerve is not dissected out, but the medial epicondyle of the humerus is removed with a rongeur and the residual bone is waxed. The fascia and muscle tending to tether or kink the nerve, particularly distally, may be slit with a scissors, as in the transposition procedure.

BIBLIOGRAPHY

Barraquer, J.: The history of the microscope in ocular surgery, J. Microsurg. 1:288, 1980.

Camunas, C.: Transsphenoidal hypophysectomy, Am. J. Nurs. 80:1820, 1980.

Carpenter, M.B.: Human neuroanatomy, ed. 7, Baltimore, 1983, Williams & Wilkins.

Cottrell, J. and Turndorf, H.: Anesthesia and neurosurgery, ed. 2, St. Louis, 1986, The C.V. Mosby Co.

Eliasson, S.G., and others: Neurological pathophysiology, ed. 2, New York, 1984, Oxford University Press.

Guyton, A.C.: Basic human neurophysiology, ed. 3, Philadephia, 1981, W.B. Saunders Co.

Hoerenz, P.: The operating microscope. I. Optical principles, illumination systems, and support systems, J. Microsurg. 1:364, 1980.

Hoerenz, P.: The operating microscope. II. Individual parts, handling, assembling, focusing, and balancing, J. Microsurg. 1:419, 1980.

Hoerenz, P.: The operating microscope. III. Accessories, J. Microsurg. 2:22, 1980.

Kershner, D.D., and Claussen, J.A.: Craniofacial reconstruction, AORN J. 44:554, 1986.

Lamb, S.: Interstitial radiation for the treatment of brain tumors using the stereotactic method, J. Neurosurg. Nurs. 12:138, 1980.

LeMaitre, G., and Finnegan, J.: The patient in surgery: a guide for nurses, ed. 4, Philadelphia, 1980, W.B. Saunders Co.

Lenzi, G.L., and Pantano, P.: Symposium on neuroimaging, Neurologic Clinics, Philadelphia, 1984, W.B. Saunders Co.

Mitchell, S., and Yates, R.: Extracranial-intracranial bypass surgery, J. Neurosurg. Nurs. 17:5, 1985.

Mullaney, C.N.: Laser surgery in otolaryngology, Point of View 17:6, 1980.

Netter, F.H.: Nervous system, New York, 1983, Ciba Pharmaceutical Co.

Nolte, J.: The human brain: an introduction to its functional anatomy, ed. 2, St. Louis, 1988, The C.V. Mosby Co.

Nucleotome Surgical Protocol, San Leandro, Calif., 1987, Surgical Dynamics.

Pian, R.A., and others: Microsurgical treatment of 10 arteriovenous malformations in critical areas of the cerebrum, J. Microsug. 1:305, 1980.

Pincus, J.H., and Tucker, G. J.: Behavioral neurology, ed. 2, New York, 1985, Oxford University Press.

Poletti, C., and Ojemann, R.: Stero atlas of operative microneurosurgery, St. Louis, 1985, The C.V. Mosby Co.

Rand, R.: Microneurosurgery, ed. 3, St. Louis, 1985, The C.V. Mosby Co.

Ricci, M.: Core curriculum for neuroscience nursing, vol. I & II, Park Ridge, Ill., 1984, American Association of Neuroscience Nurses.

Scheithauer, B.W., and others: Pathology of invasive pituitary tumors with special reference to functional classification, J. Neurosurg. 65:733, 1986.

Shillito, J., and Matson, D.D.: An atlas of pediatric neurosurgical operations, Philadelphia, 1982, W.B. Saunders Co.

Sugita, K.: Microneurosurgical atlas, New York, 1985, Springer-Verlag.

Sundt, T., editor: J. Neurosurg. 71(4), 1989.

Tedesco, M.B., and others: Total nursing care of the vestibular nerve section patient, J. Neurosurg. Nurs. 12:2, 1980.

Thibodeau, G.A.: Anthony's textbook of anatomy and physiology, ed. 13, St. Louis, 1990, The C.V. Mosby Co.

Vaiden, R., and White, W.: Arteriovenous malformation of the brain, AORN J. 46(1), 1987.

Vogt, G., Miller, M., and Esluer, M.: Mosby's manual of neurological care, St. Louis, 1985, The C.V. Mosby Co.

Weck/Heifetz intracranial aneurysm clips, Long Island City, N.Y., 1975, Edward Weck & Co., Inc.

White, A., Rothman, R., and Ray, C.: Lumbar spine surgery, St. Louis, 1987, The C.V. Mosby Co.

Wilson, C.B.: A decade of pituitary microsurgery: The Herbert Olivecrona Lecture, J. Neurosurg. 61:814, 1984.

24 Plastic and reconstructive surgery

VIRGINIA L. FINNIE

The word *plastic* is derived from the Greek *plastikos,* which means "to mold, form, or contour." Plastic surgery deals with the healing, reconstruction, restoration of function, and/or correction of disfigurement or scarring resulting from trauma or acquired or congenital defects. Plastic and reconstructive surgery has the goals of restoring normal function and appearance and thus contributing to the patient's body image, self-esteem, and quality of life. Psychosocial integrity is often interwoven with the person's perception of his or her physical appearance. Fritz (1987) has suggested that cosmetic surgery improves self-image as well as mental health, which is as important as physical health. The effects of aging, cosmetically displeasing to some people may seriously affect their self-images; feelings of unattractiveness may diminish self-esteem and contribute to a negative body image. The perioperative nurse caring for the patient undergoing cosmetic plastic surgery and reconstruction needs to possess creativity, curiosity, insight, and an understanding of the human psyche. Because of its relationship to psychosocial integrity, plastic surgery has been called the surgery of the psyche.

Plastic and reconstructive surgery is not limited either to a single anatomic or biologic system or to a single operative technique. Rather, it relies on the basic techniques of surgery and a view of the patient as a "whole" biopsychosocial being. Only the anatomy of the hand is discussed in detail in this chapter (see Hand Surgery). Other anatomic relationships are described elsewhere in this book.

A wide variety of operations are standard parts of plastic and reconstructive surgery. The advancement of microsurgical techniques has expanded the repertoire of the surgeon to include sophisticated procedures in replantation of limbs and digits, microvascular free flaps, and the like to restore and retain functional use of aesthetic configuration. Breast augmentation, reconstruction, and reduction are included in this chapter. Tissue expanders are discussed with breast reconstruction, although they may be used in other areas of reconstruction. Recession and advancement of the mandible and maxilla and the treatment of hypertelorism and Crouzon's syndrome are included to demonstrate the perioperative nursing challenge of collaborating with a multidisciplinary health care team. The aesthetic problems, varieties of congenital and acquired defects, diversity of operative techniques, and the psychologic responses of patients offer unique learning experiences and challenges for providing perioperative nursing care.

PERIOPERATIVE NURSING CONSIDERATIONS

The nursing process is a deliberate, systematic method of individualizing nursing care. Through the nursing process, the perioperative nurse is able to focus on unique responses of the patient to the planned surgical intervention, with its attendant actual or potential health alterations. Each step of the nursing process is sequential in that the steps that follow it depend on information gathered and conclusions reached in each successvie step. It is an ongoing, dynamic process responsive to both the individual patient and changes within that patient's status.

Assessment/nursing diagnosis

During assessment, the perioperative nurse gathers and analyzes data and information that lead to the identification of actual or potential health problems or nursing diagnoses. The emphasis of this data collection is on preoperative, intraoperative, and postoperative events. In general, the perioperative nurse is concerned with the patient's ability to communicate, religious or cultural preferences, current health problems, risk factors, knowledge level, mobility limitations, skin integrity, sensory/perceptual status, emotional status, and overall physical condition (Seifert and Rothrock, 1989). Preoperative and postoperative visits by the perioperative nurse provide a sound basis for better understanding the patient, assessing his or her problems, and planning care that meets individual needs. Preoperative education helps to alleviate much of the fear and anxiety usually associated with a surgical intervention. Patients undergoing reconstructive plastic surgery often are experiencing a disturbance in their body image. The procedure may be elective or urgent as a result of trauma. The perioperative nurse must assess the patient for both physical and psychologic impacts from reconstructive and aesthetic surgery and incorporate patient findings into a plan of care. Nursing diagnoses that relate to the patient undergoing plastic and reconstructive surgery might include:

Sample Care Plan

NURSING DIAGNOSIS:

Body image disturbance

GOAL:

The patient will acknowledge feelings about altered structure/function.

INTERVENTIONS:

Assist patient to identify and express feelings and perception of physical deformity.

Provide environment (privacy, supportive listening) conducive to expression of feelings.

Help patient identify expectations regarding surgical correction and anticipated changes in body structure/function.

Determine whether expectations are realistic; clarify unrealistic expectations or misconceptions.

Convey sense of respect for abilities/strengths in coping with problems/concerns.

Refer the patient to other health professionals (clergy, social worker, psychiatric liaison) as appropriate.

NURSING DIAGNOSIS:

Anxiety related to surgical intervention, outcome

GOAL:

The patient's anxiety will be reduced.

INTERVENTIONS:

Broadly classify the patient's anxiety (mild, moderate, severe).

Introduce self and other members of the surgical team.

Determine the patient's normal coping patterns.

Communicate with the patient in a calm, unhurried, confident manner.

Encourage the patient to ventilate feelings and concerns.

Reduce distracting stimuli in the perioperative environment.

If the patient is awake, provide reassurance and information about the progress of the surgery.

Provide comfort measures (for example, warm blankets, soft music that the patient prefers).

Use touch as appropriate (for example, softly stroke hand).

Encourage and assist the patient to use personally effective coping strategies (for example, meditation, guided imagery, relaxation).

NURSING DIAGNOSIS:

Knowledge deficit related to perioperative events

GOAL:

The patient will verbalize an understanding of the sequence of perioperative events.

INTERVENTIONS:

Verify surgical consent with OR schedule and patient's statement of planned surgery.

Solicit the patient's questions; answer or refer questions as appropriate.

Explain the sequence of perioperative events and their purpose, as appropriate (holding area, operating room attire, insertion of lines and attachment of monitoring devices, type of anesthesia, postoperative recovery unit and protocols, and so on).

Provide sensory (what the patient will hear and feel) as well as factual information.

Whenever possible, provide printed material to reinforce patient education (preoperative routines, explanations of surgical intervention, discharge instructions).

- Body image disturbance
- Anxiety related to surgical intervention or outcome
- Knowledge deficit related to perioperative events
- Potential for injury related to surgical positioning
- Altered tissue perfusion related to surgical intervention

Planning

Once nursing diganoses are identified, the plan of care is designed for the specific patient. Planning involves setting priorities, establishing goals, identifying nursing interventions, and documenting the nursing care plan. Perioperative nurses often begin the early stages of planning as they are admitting the patient to the surgical suite. While assessing the patient, the nurse may be, at the same time, planning possible nursing interventions for identified patient problems. A Sample Care Plan for the patient undergoing plastic and reconstructive surgery might be as shown above.

Sample Care Plan—cont'd

NURSING DIAGNOSIS:
Potential for injury related to surgical positioning
GOAL:
The patient will be free of injury related to the surgical position.
INTERVENTIONS:
Determine whether the patient has any mobility limitations; adapt surgical position accordingly.
When possible, have patient assume surgical position prior to induction of general anesthesia; note areas of discomfort and adapt position accordingly.
Secure the patient to the operating room bed; reapply restraints following positional change.
Note the patient's nutritional status, body height and weight, skin integrity, and adequacy of protective tissue at dependent pressure sites.
Apply protective padding to operating room bed, dependent pressure sites, and vulnerable neurovascular bundles.
Prevent the compression of body parts against one another (such as crossed legs), the hard surface of the operating room bed, positioning accessories.
Maintain the patient in good body alignment; reassess body alignment following positional changes.
Keep sheets under patient dry and wrinkle-free
Provide adequate assistance to safely transfer the patient to and from the operating room bed.

NURSING DIAGNOSIS:
Potential for altered tissue perfusion related to surgical intervention (microvascular surgery, grafts)
GOAL:
The patient's tissue perfusion will be maintained and/or restored.
INTERVENTIONS:
Note any sensory/perceptual alterations in the affected body part; document them.
Maintain body temperature with thermia unit, reflective blankets, and the like.
Warm intravenous fluids, blood and blood products, and irrigating fluids.
Increase the temperature in the OR as indicated.
Monitor the patient's core temperature.
Provide intraoperative medications as prescribed for local irrigation (for example, heparinized saline); label all medications on the sterile field and document their administration.
Monitor tissue perfusion (for example, Doppler ultrasound) as prescribed and flap ischemic time; record results.
Note any swelling, change in color or temperature, or drainage from graft sites prior to discharge from the operating room.
Provide warm blankets for the patient at the conclusion of the surgical procedure.

Implementation

The planning and implementation phases of perioperative patient care are closely interrelated. Implementing a plan of care in the operating room involves gathering required patient care items, providing antimicrobial skin antisepsis, creating and maintaining a sterile field, initiating counts of surgical items, properly disposing of surgical specimens, classifying the patient's wound, dispensing medications, monitoring the patient, and collaborating with other members of the health care team to ensure a safe, efficient environment and outcome for the patient.

Preoperative skin preparation

Most surgical interventions require that the operative site and adjacent areas be cleansed prior to surgery. This treatment is prescribed by the physician and often carried out by the patient. Special attention is given to the fingernails for patients undergoing hand surgery; to hair for surgery of the head, face, or neck; and to oral hygiene for surgery in or near the mouth. The perioperative nurse should verify with the patient that the prescribed regimens have been carried out. The operative site should be inspected for any rashes, bruises, or other skin conditions. Shaving is avoided, if possible, as it creates an access for the entry of bacteria into the operative site. The eyebrows and eyelashes, in particular, are left intact to preserve facial appearance and expression. Either a povidone-iodine solution, an iodine-alcohol mixture, chlorhexidine, or Septisol may be selected for antimicrobial skin preparation. The use of chlorhexidine should be avoided around the ears and eyes; it has been reported to cause increased intraocular pressure, resulting in blindness.

Positioning and draping

The operating room bed must be positioned so that remaining space in the room can comfortably accommodate anesthetic equipment, members of the surgical team, instrument tables, and any adjunct equipment (hand table, drills, microscope, laser) to be used. The patient is carefully positioned on the operating room bed so that all operative sites may be appropriately exposed and the airway is easily observable and accessible.

Correct draping procedures depend on the location of the operative site or sites. Disposable drapes (Chapter 5) are strongly advocated because of their barrier qualities, ease of handling and storage, and versatility in adapting to a variety of plastic surgery procedures. Two of the most frequently used draping techniques in plastic surgery are the head drape and the hand drape. The latter can also be applied to other upper or lower extremities, as required by the surgical procedure. The advantage of these draping techniques is that each allows maximum mobility of the head or extremity. The following techniques represent one method of obtaining maximum accessibility and sterile coverage.

Head drape

The *head drape* (Fig. 24-1) consists of the following:

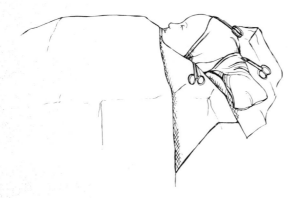

Fig. 24-1. Head drape

1. One barrier sheet folded in half, and two towels are placed beneath the patient's head with the towels uppermost. The folded half sheet covers the headrest or head portion of the operating room bed. One towel is brought around the patient's head on each side to cover all hair, leaving the entire face (and ears, as necessary) exposed, and the towel is then secured with two towel clamps. For craniofacial procedures, a towel folded lengthwise in quarters may be placed under the head to assist with moving the head from side to side.
2. Two towels are placed diagonally across the neck just under the chin and are secured to each other in the middle over the neck and on each side to the towel around the head with a total of three small towel clamps.
3. A full sheet is placed to cover the patient from neck to feet.

Hand drape

Before a hand drape is begun, a pneumatic tourniquet cuff is often applied to the upper arm over padding. The patient is supine on the operating room bed, with the affected arm extended and supported on a hand table. While an assistant on the other side of the operating room bed holds the patient's arm with both hands around the tourniquet cuff, the skin preparation solution is applied from fingertips to tourniquet cuff. Care is taken to keep the cuff dry and free of solution.

The following comprises the *hand drape* (Fig. 24-2):

1. Two folded barrier sheets are used to cover the hand table. The first sheet is placed with the folded edge nearest the patient (thus forming a cuff) and lies directly beneath the tourniquet.
2. Double-thickness, 4-inch stockinette is used to cover the extremity, and the edge is rolled over the tourniquet.
3. The upper arm and upper half of the body are covered by a folded sheet, with the folded edge placed across the part of the stockinette that covers the tourniquet cuff.
4. A small towel clamp that grasps the edge of the folded top sheet, the stockinette, and the edge of the cuff of the bottom sheet is placed on each side of the arm. This excludes the tourniquet cuff from the sterile field.
5. The remainder of the body is covered with one or two additional sheets.

Dressings

Dressings are an essential part of the operative procedure in plastic surgery and may determine the ultimate outcome of the surgical intervention. Dressings are usually applied while the patient is still anesthetized. In general, the dressing should accomplish the following five goals;

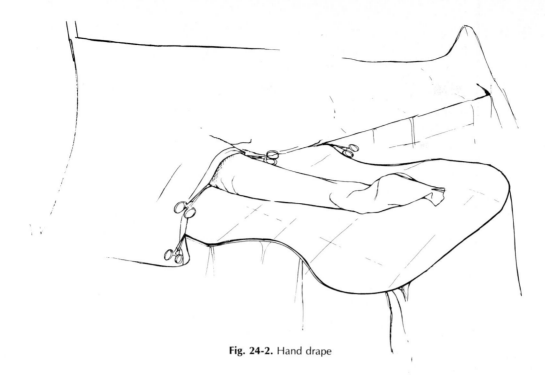

Fig. 24-2. Hand drape

(1) immobilize the part, (2) apply even pressure over the wound, (3) collect drainage, (4) provide comfort for the patient, and (5) protect the wound.

Pressure dressings are essential in the elimination of dead space, the prevention of hematoma formation, and the prevention of "third spacing" associated with liposuction and reconstructive procedures involving transfer of large muscle or tissue flaps. In some cases, pressure can be achieved by the use of catheters or drains placed within the operative site and connected to closed-wound suction devices, such as a Hemovac or Jackson-Pratt. In smaller wounds, a butterfly cannula may be inserted into the operative site, with the needle end placed in a "red top" tube.

The perioperative nurse should have the following general dressing supplies available in sterile form:

Nonadherent gauze (for example, Adaptic, NuGauze, Xeroform, Biobrane, Scarlet Red)
Petrolatum gauze, ½-inch (used for nasal packing)
Telfa
Fine mesh gauze
Interface
Gauze dressing sponges, 4 × 4 inches, 2 × 2 inches
Abdominal pads (most commonly used is 5 × 8 inches)
Cotton sheets and balls
Webril
Kling and Kerlix gauze rolls (2, 4, and 6 inches wide)
Steri-Strips, flesh colored and regular (⅛, ¼, ½, and 1 inch wide)

Also required are:

Tape (adhesive, plain and waterproof, paper, silk, and foam)
Ace bandages
Coban
Plaster supplies (as required for postoperative immobilization)

Anesthesia

Many plastic surgery interventions are performed after the administration of local, topical, or regional anesthesia, accompanied by intravenous sedation administered by either an anesthesia staff member or the perioperative nurse. All patients should have an intravenous line in place and appropriate monitors attached, including a blood pressure cuff, cardiac monitor leads, and a pulse oximeter (see Chapter 9). Emergency drugs, oxygen, and resuscitation equipment should be available prior to the administration of the anesthetic and/or sedation. All medications, including those on the sterile field, should be clearly labeled with drug name and strength. Medications administered from the sterile field or by the perioperative nurse should be appropriately documented in the patient record.

Patients receiving local anesthesia with or without sedation must have baseline data recorded on admission to the operating room and at prescribed intervals thereafter (for example, every 5 minutes during intravenous sedation; every 15 minutes during local anesthesia unaccompanied by sedation). The perioperative nurse who is monitoring the patient and/or administering the intravenous sedation should have no additional responsibilities such as circulating; attention should be focused on monitoring patient response to drug therapy.

Drugs most frequently administered for *local* anesthesia are lidocaine (Xylocaine) 0.5%, 1%, and 2%, and bupivacaine (Marcaine) 0.25%, 0.5%, and 0.75%. These drugs block the generation and conduction of impulses through nerve fibers. The patient's vital signs and state of consciousness should be closely monitored; early signs of central nervous system (CNS) toxicity include restlessness, numbness or tingling of the mouth, and light-headedness (Benson and Conte, 1989). Central nervous system stimulation may be followed by CNS depression; the patient may become drowsy or unconscious and hypotensive and demonstrate bradycardia and arrhythmias on the ECG monitor. Prior to administration of these drugs, the perioperative nurse should review the patient record and query the patient regarding hepatic impairment, cardiac or endocrine disease, and history of drug allergy.

Local anesthetics may be combined with epinephrine to slow vascular absorption at the site of injection, prolong the duration of anesthesia, and decrease bleeding in the operative field. Owing to its vasoconstrictive properties, epinephrine is contraindicated in surgery of the ears and digits of the feet or hands, where it may compromise blood supply in an area with already decreased vascularity; in regional anesthesia, including digital nerve blocks; in patients with hypertension or cardiac arrhythmias; and for patients receiving monoamine oxidase (MAO) inhibitors. The volatile anesthetics, halothane and enflurane, potentiate myocardial sensitivity to circulating catecholamines. Therefore, the anesthesiologist must be alerted prior to the injection of local anesthetics with epinephrine.

Drugs used for *topical* anesthesia include cocaine 4% and tetracaine (Pontocaine) 2%. With topical anesthesia, the agent is applied or sprayed to the surface as a solution. It is useful for certain plastic surgery procedures on the ear and nose; it is suitable for use on mucous membranes but not unbroken skin. Tetracaine has a duration of 1 to 3 hours. Cocaine, a vasoconstrictor, is a short-acting local anesthetic with a duration of 1 to 2 hours.

Drugs commonly prescribed for sedation accompanying the administration of local anesthesia include diazepam (Valium), midazolam (Versed), fentanyl (Sublimaze), and meperidine (Demerol). *Diazepam* is a CNS depressant; it provides sedation, light anesthesia, and anterograde amnesia during the surgical intervention (Benson and Conte, 1989). The CNS side effects are dose related; transient drowsiness, dizziness, ataxia, fatigue, and confusion may be observed. Apnea may occur, especially in the elderly surgical patient. Diazepam is contraindicated in any patient with respiratory depression or hypersensitivity. Intravenous diazepam should be administered slowly to avoid irritation, swelling, venous thrombosis, or phlebitis at the injection site. *Midazolam* is shorter acting than diazepam and less likely to cause pain or tissue irritation at the injection site. Its primary adverse reaction is respiratory depression; appropriate dosage and careful monitoring are essential with this agent. Elderly patients are particularly sensitive to midazolam-induced respiratory depression, which may be delayed for many hours. *Fentanyl* is a potent

synthetic narcotic analgesic, altering the perception of and response to pain. The patient must be closely observed for respiratory depression, depressed cough reflex, and skeletal muscle rigidity. Fentanyl must be administered slowly to avoid intercostal muscle rigidity. Extreme response may require the administration of a muscle relaxant and respiratory resuscitation. *Meperidine* produces analgesia as well as sedation. The patient should be closely observed for respiratory depression, hypotension, dizziness, and nausea. Narcotics, including meperidine, should not be administered to patients taking tricyclics or MAO inhibitors (within 14 days of MAO inhibitor use). Unpredictable and sometimes fatal complications such as cardiovascular collapse, seizures, and death may occur.

Implant materials

During surgical reconstruction, autogenous (autologous) tissue may be taken from one part of the patient's body and replanted in another part. This tissue has always been considered the most desirable implantation material. Homologous tissue is taken from the same species. Alloplastic materials are inert foreign substances that are readily available, leave no donor defect, are biodegradable, and do not undergo resorption. Implant materials should be noncarcinogenic, nontoxic, nonallergenic, nonimmunogenic, mechanically reliable, capable of resisting strain, biocompatible, sterilizable, and capable of being shaped into a desired shape or form.

Silicone is a frequently used implant material in plastic surgery. It is available in a variety of forms: sponges; blocks of varying firmness, which may be carved; adhesive; and gel. Medical-grade silicone has the advantages of heat and time stability, versatility, nonadherence, minimal tissue reaction, and lack of attack or alteration by the body. The disadvantages are encapsulation, which may

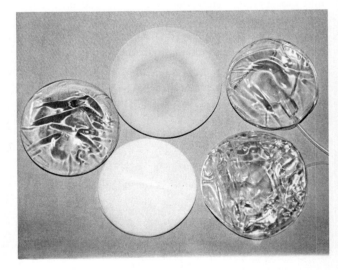

Fig. 24-3. Preformed silicone implants and gel-filled mammary prosthesis.

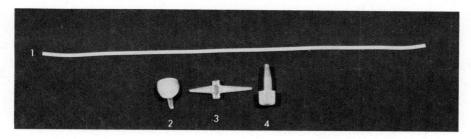

Fig. 24-4. Silicone rubber implants for hand surgery. *1,* Tendon rod; *2,* carpal lunate; *3,* Swanson finger joint prosthesis; *4,* carpal trapezium.

distort soft implants such as breast implants, and insufficient tensile strength for durability in weight bearing or stress. A variety of pre-formed silicone prostheses are available for surgical implantation to restore contour and function, including nose, chin, ear, breast, testicular, and penile implants (Fig. 24-3). Silicone rods can be implanted for formation of tendon sheaths prior to tendon grafting; bone and joint implants may be used for resection arthroplasty in hand surgery (Fig. 24-4).

Other implant materials used in plastic surgery include plastics such as Dacron, Marlex, and Teflon (Proplast); biologic materials such as collagen; metals such as stainless steel, Vitallium, titanium, and tantalum; and ceramics.

The perioperative nurse must exercise care when handling materials for implantation. Implant materials generally are prepackaged and sterile. They must be meticulously handled to prevent contamination. Powder must be wiped from surgical gloves, and the implant inspected for any defects and placed on a lint-free surface. Breast prostheses and tissue expanders should be placed in a container with sterile saline or antibiotic solution on the sterile field. If the implant needs to be sterilized, the manufacturer's directions must be followed. A basic procedure is as follows. The perioperative nurse should put on gloves (oil from the skin may cause an inflammatory response), wash the implant in a pure soap (such as Ivory), and rinse it with distilled water. The implant should then be placed on a lint-free surface and sterilized according to manufacturer's instructions. If the implant has an outer chamber or is a tissue expander, 10 cc of normal saline should be placed in the outer lumen with the fill tube. This tube should be kept in place during sterilization to allow for the exchange of pressures during the sterilization process. The implant should be rinsed thoroughly with normal saline before implantation in the patient. Silicone implants and tissue expanders should not be resterilized with ethylene oxide.

Special mechanical devices

Many special mechanical devices are used in plastic surgery. The perioperative nurse must be familiar with the operation and safety requirements of all equipment used. The manufacturer's instructions for proper sterilization methods and for special care after use must be followed. Each piece of equipment must be kept in working order. The following types of mechanical devices are used in plastic surgery.

Dermatomes

Used for removing split-thickness skin grafts from donor sites, dermatomes are of three basic types: knife, drum type, and motor driven.

1. Knife dermatomes
    a. Ferris-Smith (Fig. 24-5)—grafts obtained in freehand manner; sterile blades supplied by manufacturer
    b. Humby or Watson—has adjustable roller to control thickness of graft
    c. Weck (Fig. 24-6)—uses straight razor blades with interchangeable guards (0.008, 0.010, and 0.012 inch) to obtain small grafts; also used for debridement of burn wounds
2. Drum-type dermatomes—operate on the principle of fixing outer surface of skin to half of a metal drum and then moving rotating blade back and forth close to surface of the drum to obtain split-thickness skin graft
    a. Reese (Fig. 24-7)—tape containing adhesive is fixed to drum; dermatome cement is applied to skin in thin layer and allowed to dry for 3 minutes; distance between blade and drum (thickness of graft) is adjusted by inserting shim (0.008 to

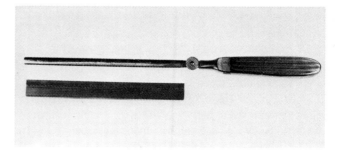

Fig. 24-5. Ferris-Smith knife dermatome handle and blade (straight razor).

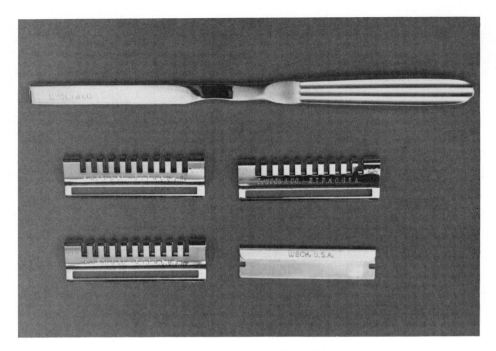

Fig. 24-6. Weck dermatome handle, guards, and blade (straight razor).

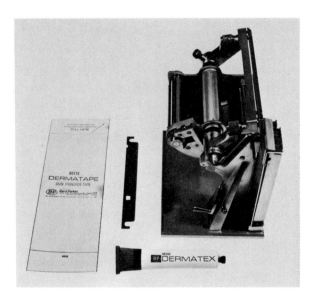

Fig. 24-7. Reese dermatome on stand, with tape, blade, and glue; shims are stored at lower right of dermatome stand.

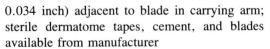

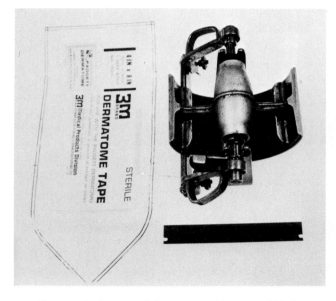

Fig. 24-8. Padgett-Hood dermatome with tape and blade.

0.034 inch) adjacent to blade in carrying arm; sterile dermatome tapes, cement, and blades available from manufacturer

  b. Padgett-Hood (Fig. 24-8)—grafts available in three sizes: baby model (3 × 8 inch), standard model (4 × 8 inch), and giant size (4 × 16 inch); cement applied to skin and directly to drum or used with dermatome tape; calibrated dial on dermatome can be adjusted to between 0.005 and

0.05 inch for desired level between knife blade, shim, and drum; sterile dermatome tapes, cement, and blades available from manufacturer

3. Motor-driven dermatomes—graft obtained with knife blade that moves back and forth like the blade of a hair cutter; power supplied by electricity or compressed gas; long sterile cable serves as drive shaft and runs between dermatome and its power source; motor activated by foot pedal or hand control

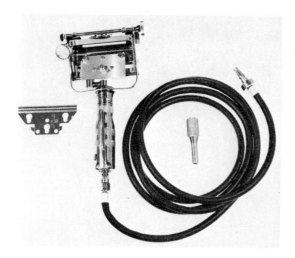

Fig. 24-9. Brown air dermatome and hose assembly with blade and check for securing blade.

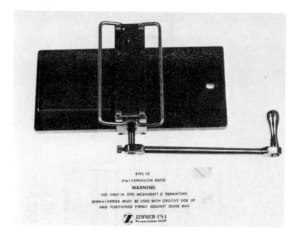

Fig. 24-10. Zimmer mesh graft II dermatome and dermacarrier with 3:1 skin expansion ratio.

a. Brown (Fig. 24-9)—available with electrical or pneumatic power source; thickness of graft adjusted by one or two calibrated knobs on dermatome (in thousandths of an inch); sterile blades supplied by manufacturer; may be gas or steam sterilized

b. Padgett—has the same operating mechanism as the Brown; motor located in the handle of the instrument; should be gas sterilized

4. Skin meshers (Fig. 24-10)—several types available, each designed to produce multiple uniform slits in a skin graft, approximately 0.05 inch apart, which allow for expansion of graft and multiple apertures in graft for drainage; graft placed on carrier and passed through mesher; sterile carriers for mesher supplied by manufacturer; usually in several sizes, which determine expansion ratio of skin graft (3:1 and 1.5:1 ratios most commonly used)

Insertion of the knife blade and guards of shims with any dermatome is done by the surgeon. It is also the surgeon's responsibility to remove the knife blade after obtaining a graft and before any instrument-cleansing procedures are begun by perioperative personnel. The blade should be disposed of in an appropriate puncture-resistant container.

Pneumatic-powered instruments (Fig. 24-11)

The power source is inert, nonflammable, and explosion-free compressed gas. The motor may be activated by a foot pedal or hand control. The various attachments may be gas or steam sterilized, as recommended by the manufacturer (*not* immersed in liquid). The following attachments are used in plastic surgery:

Kirschner wire driver and bone drill
Oscillating saw
Reciprocating saw
Sagittal saw
Roto osteotome, straight
Derma-Tattoo (used with reciprocating saw handpiece)
Dermabrader

Hall II air drill (Fig. 24-12). The Hall II air drill is pneumatic powered; the motor is activated by a pedal or a handpiece. Burrs and drill points of varied sizes are available for precision cutting and shaping of bone or for drilling holes in bone for wire passing. The drill may be steam or gas sterilized (*not* immersed in liquid).

Pneumatic tourniquet with inflatable cuff (Chapter 22). This tourniquet is used with most hand surgery procedures as well as other upper and lower extremity operations.

Bipolar coagulation unit. This unit is described in Chapter 23.

Fiberoptic instruments (Fig 24-13). Light source is described in Chapter 25. Attachments used in plastic surgery include a headlight for rhinoplasties, augmentation mammoplasties, and other procedures; a mammary retractor for augmentation mammoplasties; a rhytidectomy retractor; and a Dingman mouth gag attachment for cleft palate repairs.

Loupes (Fig. 24-14). Loupes are magnifying lenses used for microvascular surgery and nerve repairs.

Woods lamp (Fig. 24-15). The Woods lamp is an ultraviolet light used in determining viability of skin flaps in a darkened room after intravenous injection of 20 ml of 5% sodium fluorescein.

Instrumentation

Three types of sterile basic instrument trays are kept available in the plastic surgery operating room. With modification by addition of instruments for specific operations, these trays suffice for all plastic surgery operations:

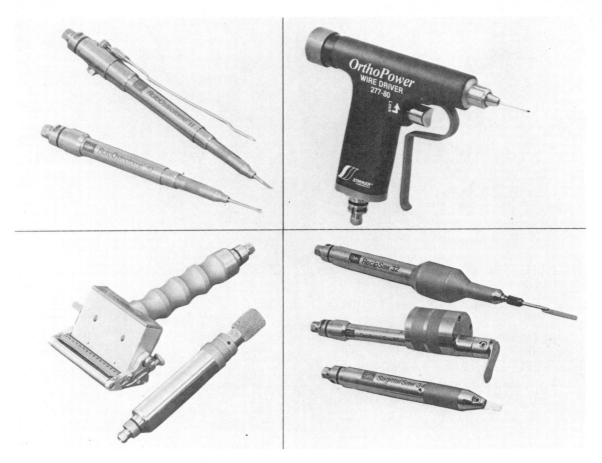

Fig. 24-11. Pneumatic-powered instruments.

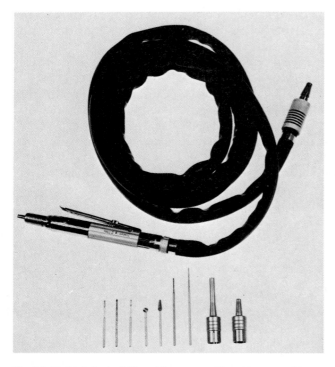

Fig. 24-12. Hall II air drill and hose assembly with assorted burrs and long and medium burr guards.

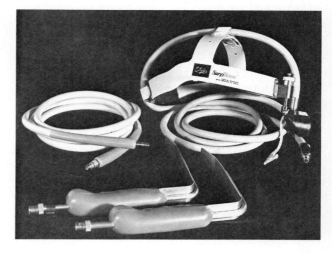

Fig. 24-13. Fiberoptic equipment: headlight, mammary retractors, and cord.

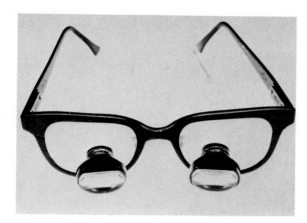

Fig. 24-14. Loupes, used for magnification.

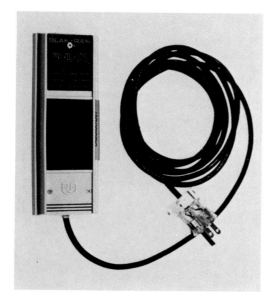

Fig. 24-15. Woods lamp and cord assembly.

Plastic local instrument set (Fig. 24-16)

Cutting instruments

2 Knife handles, no. 3, with blades, no. 15
  or 10
1 Stevens tenotomy scissors, curved
2 Iris scissors, 1 curved and 1 straight
1 Metzenbaum scissors, curved, 5¼ inches
1 Joseph dissecting scissors, curved, 5¾ inches

Holding instruments

1 Sponge-holding forceps, straight, 7 inches
10 Towel clamps, 3 inches
2 Adson tissue forceps, 2 × 1-inch teeth
1 Adson dressing forceps
1 Brown-Adson tissue forceps
1 Dressing forceps, 5 inches
2 Allis forceps
2 Skin hooks, single

2 Skin hooks, double, 10 mm
2 Skin hooks, double 2–3 mm

Clamping instruments

12 Mosquito hemostats, curved, 5¼ inches
6 Mosquito hemostats, straight, 5 inches

Exposing instruments

2 S-shaped retractors
2 Senn-Kanavel retractors

Suturing instruments

2 Brown needle holders, 6¾ inches
2 Webster needle holders

Accessory items

1 Joseph periosteal elevator
1 Freer septal elevator
2 Frazier-Ferguson suction tips, nos. 7 and 9
1 Ruler
1 Bowl, small
1 Luer-Lok syringe, 10 ml
2 Needles, 25 and 30 gauge
2 Medicine cups

Basic plastic instrument set (Fig. 24-17)

Cutting instruments

3 Knife handles, no. 3, with blades, nos. 10
  or 15
1 Knife handle, no. 3, long
1 Stevens tenotomy scissors, curved
    Iris scissors, 1 each straight and curved
2 Metzenbaum scissors, curved: 1 each 5¼ inches
    and 8 inches
1 Mayo scissors, straight, 6 inches
1 Wire suture scissors, 4¾ inches
1 Kaye dissecting scissors

Holding instruments

1 Sponge-holding forceps, straight, 7 inches
10 Towel clamps, 3 inches
4 Towel clamps, 5¼ inches
2 Adson tissue forceps, 2 × 1-inch teeth, fine
1 Adson dressing forceps
2 Brown-Adson tissue forceps
1 Dressing forceps, 5 inches
1 Tissue forceps with teeth, 5 inches
2 Bayonet dressing forceps: 1 each 5 and 7 inches
4 Allis forceps, 6 inches
2 Skin hooks, single
2 Skin hooks, double, 10 mm
2 Skin hooks, double, 2–3 mm

Clamping instruments

24 Mosquito hemostats, curved, 5¼ inches
12 Halsted forceps with teeth, straight, 5 inches
4 Ochsner forceps, 6½ inches
4 Kelly hemostats, curved, 5½ inches

Exposing instruments

2 S-shaped retractors
2 Senn-Kanavel retractors

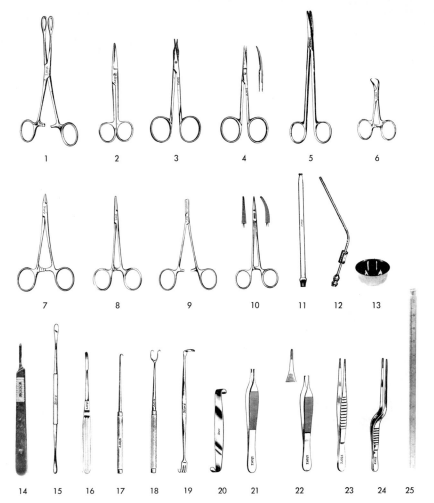

Fig. 24-16. Plastic local instrument set. *1*, Sponge-holding forceps; *2*, Brown dissecting scissors; *3*, Stevens tenotomy scissors; *4*, straight and curved iris scissors; *5*, Metzenbaum scissors; *6*, towel clamp; *7*, Brown needle holder; *8*, Webster needle holder; *9*, straight mosquito hemostat with teeth; *10*, straight and curved mosquito hemostats; *11*, Anthony suction tip; *12*, Frazier-Ferguson suction tip; *13*, small bowl; *14*, Bard-Parker knife handle no. 3; *15*, Freer septal elevator; *16*, Joseph periosteal elevator; *17*, single skin hook; *18*, double skin hook; *19*, Senn-Kanavel retractor; *20*, S-shaped retractor; *21*, Brown-Adson tissue forceps; *22*, Adson tissue and dressing forceps; *23*, dressing forceps; *24*, bayonet dressing forceps; *25*, ruler.

2 Cushing vein retractors
2 Army-Navy retractors
2 Rake retractors, four blunt prongs
5 Ribbon malleable retractors, assorted widths (4 to 7 inches)
6 Richardson retractors, assorted
2 Weider tongue depressors, 1 large and 1 small
2 Deaver retractors

Suturing instruments

2 Webster needle holders
2 Brown needle holders, 6¾ inches
2 Mayo-Hegar needle holders, 8 inches

Accessory items

1 Joseph periosteal elevator
1 Freer septal elevator

1 Ruler
1 Silver probe, 6 inches
2 Nasal specula, 1 short and 1 long
2 Bite blocks, 1 large and 1 small
1 Jaw hook
2 Anthony suction tips
3 Frazier-Ferguson suction tips, nos. 7, 9, and 11
1 Yankauer suction tube

Plastic hand instrument set (Fig. 24-18)

Cutting instruments

3 Knife handles, no. 3, with blades, no. 15
1 Stevens tenotomy scissors, curved
1 Metzenbaum scissors, curved, 5¼ inches
1 Iris scissors, straight
1 Mayo scissors, straight 6 inches

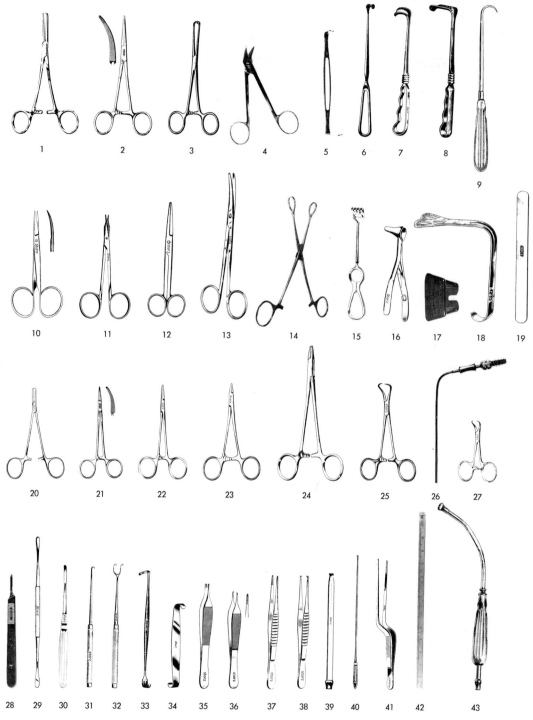

Fig. 24-17. Basic plastic instrument set. *1,* Ochsner forceps; *2,* straight and curved Kelly hemostats; *3,* Allis forceps; *4,* wire suture scissors; *5,* Army-Navy retractor; *6,* Cushing vein retractor; *7* and *8,* Richardson retractors; *9,* jaw hook; *10,* straight and curved iris scissors; *11,* Stevens tenotomy scissors; *12,* straight Mayo scissors; *13,* curved Metzenbaum scissors; *14,* sponge-holding forceps; *15,* rake retractor with blunt prongs; *16,* nasal speculum; *17,* bite block; *18,* Weider tongue depressor; *19,* ribbon malleable retractor; *20,* Halsted forceps with teeth; *21,* straight and curved mosquito hemostats; *22,* Webster needle holder; *23,* Brown needle holder; *24,* Mayo-Hegar needle holder; *25,* large towel clamp; *26,* Frazier-Ferguson suction tip; *27,* small towel clamp; *28,* Bard-Parker knife handle no. 3; *29,* Freer septal elevator; *30,* Joseph periosteal elevator; *31,* single skin hook; *32,* double skin hook; *33,* Senn-Kanavel retractor; *34,* S-shaped retractor; *35,* Brown-Adson tissue forceps; *36,* Adson tissue and dressing forceps; *37,* dressing forceps; *38,* tissue forceps with teeth; *39,* Anthony suction tip; *40,* silver probe; *41,* bayonet dressing forceps; *42,* ruler; *43,* Yankauer suction tube.

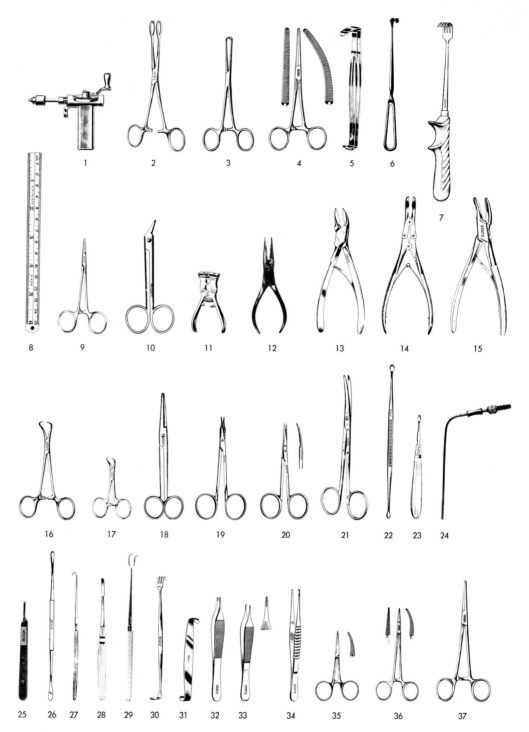

Fig. 24-18. Plastic hand instrument set. *1,* Bunnell hand drill; *2,* sponge-holding forceps; *3,* Allis forceps; *4,* straight and curved Kelly hemostats; *5,* Army-Navy retractors; *6,* Cushing vein retractor; *7,* rake retractor with blunt prongs; *8,* ruler; *9,* Webster needle holder; *10,* wire suture scissors; *11,* Kirschner wire cutter; *12,* needle-nose pliers; *13,* bone-cutting forceps; *14,* Ruskin rongeur; *15,* Lempert rongeur; *16,* large towel clamp; *17,* small towel clamp; *18,* straight Mayo scissors; *19,* Stevens tenotomy scissors; *20,* straight and curved iris scissors; *21,* curved Metzenbaum scissors; *22* and *23,* curettes; *24,* Frazier-Ferguson suction tip; *25,* Bard-Parker knife handle no. 3; *26,* Freer septal elevator; *27,* single skin hook; *28,* Joseph periosteal elevator; *29,* double skin hook; *30,* Senn-Kanavel retractor; *31,* S-shaped retractor; *32,* Brown-Adson tissue forceps; *33,* Adson tissue and dressing forceps; *34,* tissue forceps with teeth; *35,* straight and curved Hartmann mosquito hemostats; *36,* straight and curved mosquito hemostats; *37,* Ochsner forceps.

Bone-cutting forceps, 1 angular and 1 straight, 7 inches
1 Wire suture scissors, 4¾ inches

Holding instruments

2 Sponge-holding forceps, straight, 7 inches
2 Towel clamps, 5¼ inches
10 Towel clamps, 3 inches
2 Adson tissue forceps, 2 × 1-inch teeth
2 Adson dressing forceps
2 Brown-Adson tissue forceps
1 Tissue forceps with teeth, 5 inches
2 Allis forceps, 6 inches
2 Skin hooks, single
2 Skin hooks, double, 10 mm
2 Skin hooks, double, 2–3 mm

Clamping instruments

6 Hartmann mosquito hemostats, curved
12 Mosquito hemostats, curved, 5¼ inches
2 Mosquito hemostats, straight, 5¼ inches
2 Kelly hemostats, curved, 5½ inches
2 Ochsner forceps, 6½ inches

Exposing instruments

6 Senn-Kanavel retractors
2 S-shaped retractors
2 Cushing vein retractors
2 Army-Navy retractors
2 Rake retractors, four blunt prongs

Suturing instruments

3 Webster needle holders

Accessory items

1 Joseph periosteal elevator
1 Freer septal elevator
1 Ruler
1 Bunnell hand drill
2 Needle-nose pliers, 6¼ inches
2 Frazier-Ferguson suction tips, nos. 7 and 9
    Ruskin rongeurs, 1 large and 1 small
1 Lempert rongeur
1 Set Kirschner wires
1 Kirschner wire cutter
    Curettes assorted

Special supplies

In addition to the basic instrument sets, the following sterile supplies are available at all times and are added to instrument sets for nearly all procedures:

Marking pen
Epinephrine 1:200,000 for injection
X-ray film, unexposed (for pattern making)
Electrosurgical unit

Evaluation

During the surgical intervention, the perioperative nurse is constantly evaluating the patient's response to nursing interventions, anesthesia, and the surgery itself. Progress or lack of progress toward the identified patient

goals is constantly monitored. The results of this monitoring enable the perioperative nurse to reassess the patient, reorder priorities of patient care, establish new patient goals, and revise the perioperative care plan.

At the conclusion of the surgical intervention, the perioperative nurse reviews whether identified patient outcomes have been achieved. The patient's skin integrity is assessed; dressings are applied and their integrity established prior to discharge from the operating room. Any drains or tubes incorporated in the dressing should be noted. Infusion sites are inspected, and the type of infusing solution, flow rate, and amount infused are noted in the patient record. Documentation of local anesthetics, sedation, or other medications received by the patient is similarly performed. The patient's response during the perioperative period is noted; any unusual or untoward responses are reported to the nurse in the discharge unit. The transport vehicle is obtained; any special equipment needed during patient transport is also obtained and checked for proper functioning. Warm blankets may be provided, and the patient is gently moved to the transport vehicle. The patient who is recovering from general anesthesia is placed in a safe position on the vehicle; the awake patient should be assisted to a position of comfort.

The perioperative nurse should give the report to the nurse in the discharge unit. Areas requiring ongoing patient observation should be noted in this report; the patient's preoperative, intraoperative, and immediate postoperative status is reported also. Using the Sample Care Plan introduced earlier in this chapter, the perioperative nurse may give part of the report based on patient outcomes. If they were achieved, they may be stated as follows:

- The patient acknowledged feelings about altered body structure/function.
- The patient's anxiety was reduced.
- The patient verbalized an understanding of perioperative events.
- The patient was free of injury related to the surgical position.
- Tissue perfusion at the graft and surgical site was maintained and/or restored.

SURGICAL INTERVENTIONS
Replacement of lost tissue (skin graft)
Free skin graft

Skin grafting provides an effective way to cover a wound if vascularity is adequate, infection is absent, and hemostasis is achieved. Skin from the donor site is detached from its blood supply and placed in the recipient site, where it develops a new blood supply from the base of the wound. Color match, contour, and durability of the graft are all considerations in selection of an appropriate donor area.

Skin grafts can be either split-thickness or full-thickness

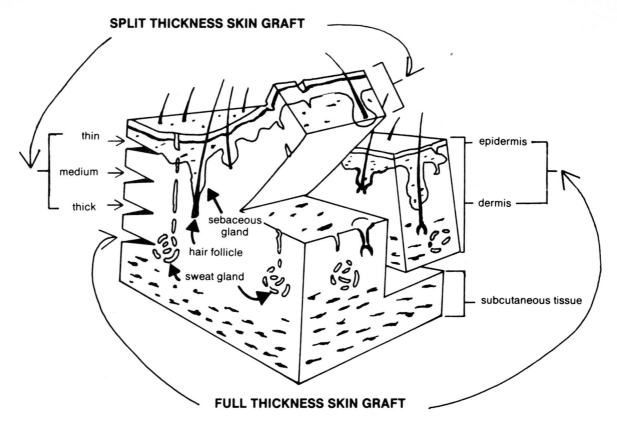

Fig. 24-19. Split-thickness and full-thickness skin grafts.

grafts (Fig. 24-19). A split-thickness (or partial-thickness) skin graft contains epidermis and only a portion of the dermis of the donor site; it varies from a thin graft to a thick graft. Although this type of graft becomes vascularized more rapidly and the donor site heals more rapidly than a full-thickness graft, it may exhibit postgraft contraction, be minimally resistant to surface trauma, and look the least like normal skin in texture, suppleness, pore pattern, hair growth, and other characteristics (Vasconez and Vasconez, 1988). A split-thickness skin graft (STSG) may be meshed; meshed grafts can expand to many times their normal size. Meshing allows the graft to be placed on an irregular recipient area; however, its appearance may be aesthetically undesirable. A full-thickness skin graft (FTSG) contains both epidermis and dermis. The advantages of this type of graft are that it causes minimal contracture, can be used in areas of flexion, has a greater ability to withstand trauma, can add tissue where there has been a loss or padding is required, and is aesthetically more acceptable than a STSG. The donor site can be closed primarily, leaving a minimal defect. Other types of grafts that are available are: bone, cartilage, nerve, tendon, and autologous fat grafts. Referred to as composite grafts, these are also free tissue grafts that must reestablish vascularity in the recipient area.

The donor site for a STSG heals by regeneration of epithelium from dermal elements that remain intact. Therefore, only a dressing is placed over this donor site. Because no dermal elements remain when an FTSG is taken, this donor site does not heal spontaneously. It heals only if another layer of skin is placed over it, either by suturing the wound edges of the donor site together or by applying a STSG over it. A scar remains at the donor site of a skin graft. Therefore, donor sites that are covered by clothing are generally chosen.

For a graft to survive, the vascularity of the recipient area must be adequate, contact between the graft and recipient bed must be maintained, and the graft-bed unit must be adequately immobilized. Postoperatively, the nurse must observe for signs of revascularization of the graft by ingrowth of blood vesels from the recipient bed. Accumulation of material betweeen the graft and the recipient site that increases the distance through which the new blood vessel must grow, such as hematoma or wound exudate, must be prevented. Color, temperature, signs of infection, blanching of the skin, pain and discomfort, edema, vasoconstriction, and venous congestion should be noted and any change reported to the surgeon. Documentation of any changes should be made. If the patient is discharged to home following surgery, patient and family education should include reportable signs and symptoms of potential complications.

A stent or tie-over dressing is often placed over a skin graft (Fig. 24-20). This exerts even pressure, ensuring good contact between graft and recipient site. It also eliminates potential shearing forces at the graft–recipient site interface that might disrupt new blood vessels growing into the graft.

Procedural considerations. A plastic local instrument set is required, plus a dermatome of choice, a skin mesher, a marking pen, and unexposed x-ray film.

The patient is positioned so that both donor and recipient sites are well exposed. Both areas are prepped and draped to maintain adequate exposure and mobility, as required.

Operative procedure

1. The recipient site is prepared as necessary. This step may involve excision of a benign or malignant skin tumor, debridement of an open wound, or release of a scar contracture.
2. Careful planning and marking before harvesting the graft from the recipient site are essential. When feasible, a pattern of the recipient site is made with unexposed x-ray film. This pattern is transferred to the donor site and outlined with a marking pen.
3. STSGs are harvested with a Weck knife or dermatome of the surgeon's choice.

4. Moist sponges soaked in 20 mg Neo-Synephrine per 1000 cc normal saline are applied to the donor sites to aid hemostasis. A small amount of methylene blue should be placed in the solution of Neo-Synephrine as a marker to identify it from other solutions on the sterile field. Topical thrombin may also be used to aid in hemostasis. It comes prepackaged and ready to attach to the sprayer. Topical thrombin is for *topical* use only and not for injection. These sponges are removed, and the donor site is covered with Biobrane or Opsite.
5. If the graft is to be meshed, it is now applied to specifically supplied carriers for use with certain skin meshers.
6. A graft that is not immediately applied to the recipient site dries quickly, particularly a meshed graft. Therefore, grafts should be kept in moist gauze sponges contained in a small basin to prevent inadvertent loss of the graft. Meshed skin should not be removed from its carrier until it is applied directly to the recipient site.
7. Whether applied as a sheet or meshed, STSG may be sutured or stapled with a skin stapler. Nonadherent gauze is usually applied as the first layer of dressing over a graft. Moist dressings should be applied to all meshed grafts to prevent desiccation and loss of the graft.

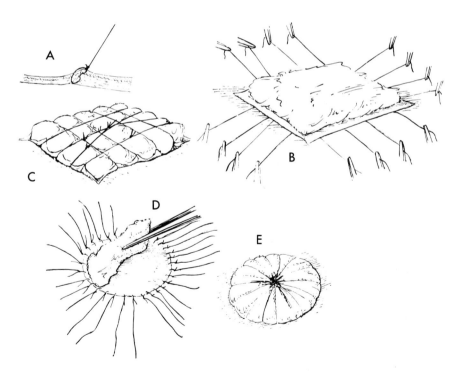

Fig. 24-20. A, Method of fixation of skin graft to edges of wound. **B,** Nonadherent dressing is applied over skin graft, and on this a generous pad of acrylic fiber. **C,** Long ends of suture are tied over fiber to produce area of pressure between graft and base. **D,** Similar dressing is applied to circular graft. **E,** Long suture ends are tied over circular graft (often called "stent" dressing). (From Wood-Smith, D., and Porowski, P.C., editors: Nursing care of the plastic surgery patient, St. Louis, 1967, The C.V. Mosby Co.)

8. Fat adherent to the graft is trimmed. The graft is applied to the recipient site and usually sutured at the edges, and these sutures are left long to tie over a stent dressing (Fig. 24-20). Blood clots beneath the graft are removed by saline irrigation before the dressing is applied.

Preservation of skin grafts

A skin graft may be harvested but not used immediately. Skin can be obtained from the patient on whom it is to be grafted (autograft) or from a donor (allograft). Skin that is obtained for future grafting must be preserved and stored in a safe, controlled environment until it is used.

Setup

The setup should include the skin specimen and the following items:

Sterile 3-inch rolled gauze
Basin with isotonic solution
Sterile container with screw cap
Adhesive tape for sealing and labeling container

Procedure

1. The skin should be kept on the instrument table until it is ready for storage.
2. The skin must be kept moist with an isotonic solution such as balanced salt solution or saline at all times.
3. The skin is gently flattened, smoothed out, and placed on a piece of roller gauze moistened with the isotonic solution, with its external surface facing downward.
4. The scrub nurse rolls the gauze and skin loosely, places the roll in the sterile container, and secures the cap.
5. The circulating nurse labels the jar with the donor's name and hospital number, location of donor site, date of collection, and size of graft.
6. If the surgeon anticipates using the preserved skin within 14 days, it may be stored in a refrigerator at between 1° and 10° C (34° and 50° F) until it is used. An alternative method is to place the skin in a tissue medium such as McCoy's; the tissue may then be stored in a refrigerator at between 1° and 10° C (34° and 50° F) for 30 days until it is used.
7. If the surgeon does not anticipate using the skin within 14 days, it can be maintained by one of several long-term storage methods. One method is to place the skin in a cryoprotectant (such as ethylene glycol) for 1 to 2 hours at 4° C (39° F), then gradually cool the skin to −70° C (−94° F), and store in a liquid nitrogen freezer.

Flaps

The term *flap* refers to tissue that is detached from one area of the body and transferred to the recipient area with either part or all of its original blood supply intact or reestablished (Fig. 24-21). The base or pedicle of the flap is that portion through which the blood supply enters or exits. Because flaps carry their own blood supply, they are usually used to cover recipient sites that have poor vascularity and full-thickness tissue loss. Flaps are used for reconstruction or wound closure. They are useful for covering exposed bone, tendon, or nerve. They may be used if operating through the wound may be necessary at a later date to repair underlying structures. Flaps containing skin and subcutaneous tissue retain more properties of normal skin and shrink less than skin grafts. Flaps, however, have some disadvantages, such as bulky appearance, failure to match tissue of the recipient site in texture or color, and the possibility of requiring multiple operations and prolonged hospitalization.

Flaps may be classified according to blood supply. *Random patten* flaps consist of skin and subcutaneous tissue vascularized by random perforators with limited length to width ratio. *Axial pattern* flaps have a well-defined arteriovenous supply along the long axis; they can be comparatively long in relation to width. Flaps may also be classified according to position or how they are rotated after elevaton. *Advancement* flaps are cut and advanced to reconstruct a nearby defect. *Transposition* flap are advanced along an axis that forms an angle to the flap's original position. *Rotation* flaps are similar to transposition flaps but are semicircular and rotate along a greater axis. *Island* flaps of isolated sections of skin and subcutaneous tissue are tunneled beneath the skin to new sites. *Pedicle* flaps were the forerunners of *muscle* and *musculocutaneous* flaps. These consist of skin and underlying muscle; they are very mobile and can be rotated into distant defects. *Free* flaps are actually a form of tissue transplantation. Using microsurgical techniques, a defined amount of skin, muscle, or bone can be isolated, detached, and reattached to recipient vessels near the new site. The vascular pedicle may contain functional nerves, yielding sensory flaps to provide protective sensation or motor flaps to restore function. Bone and joints may be transplanted as free flaps, as in the case of toe-to-thumb transfers.

Procedural considerations. A basic plastic instrument set is required, plus the following:

Electrosurgical unit
Extra hemostats
Dermatome of choice
Marking pen
X-ray film, unexposed
Skin mesher

Positioning, prepping, and draping of the patient are carried out to maintain adequate exposure and mobility of both the flap donor and recipient sites.

Operative procedure

1. The recipient site is prepared in the same manner as for a skin graft.
2. When feasible, a pattern of the recipient site is made and transferred to the donor area.
3. The flap is incised, elevated, and transferred to the

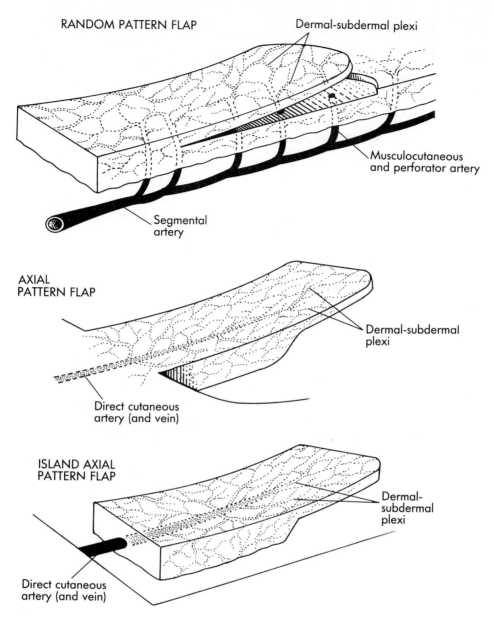

RANDOM PATTERN FLAP

Dermal-subdermal plexi

Musculocutaneous
and perforator artery

Segmental
artery

AXIAL
PATTERN FLAP

Dermal-subdermal
plexi

Direct cutaneous
artery (and vein)

ISLAND AXIAL
PATTERN FLAP

Dermal-
subdermal
plexi

Direct cutaneous
artery (and vein)

Fig. 24-21. Types of flaps.

recipient site. The edges of the flap are sutured to the periphery of the recipient site.

4. The flap donor site is repaired by approximating the skin edges directly or by covering the defect with a skin graft or another flap.
5. Drains are usually placed under flaps.
6. Dressings are applied with particular attention to immobilization of the flap, which may require stockinette, padding, or plaster of Paris.
7. When a pedicle flap is divided, the surgeon may want to check the adequacy of circulation within the flap. Checking can be done by placing rubber-shod clamps across the base of the pedicle and injecting 20 ml of 5% sodium fluorescein intravenously. After 10 minutes have elapsed, all lights in the operating room are turned off, and a Woods lamp is held over the flap to determine the presence or absence of fluorescence within the flap.

Composite graft

Composite grafts are composed of compound tissues that are completely separated from the blood supply of the donor site and transplanted to another area of the body. The survival of a composite graft depends on ingrowth of new blood vessels from the recipient site around the periphery of the graft. Therefore, composite grafts are usually small so that no portion of the graft is greater than 1 cm from its periphery. An example of compound tissues used as composite grafts is hair transplants, composed of skin, fat, and hair follicles. which are used to treat male pattern baldness.

Procedural considerations. A plastic local instrument set is required, plus the following:

Marking pen   X-ray film, unexposed

Positioning, prepping, and draping of the patient are such that adequate exposure of both donor and recipient sites is maintained.

Operative procedure

1. The recipient site is prepared by excising tissue, such as a scar or a benign or malignant skin lesion.
2. When feasible, a pattern of the recipient site is made and transferred to the donor site.
3. The composite graft is excised. The donor site is either closed by approximating its skin edges or left unsutured (such as in hair transplant donor sites).
4. Meanwhile, the composite graft is kept in a moist sponge until it is sutured to the edges of the recipient site.
5. Dressings of choice are applied to the composite graft and donor site.

Breast reconstruction

The loss of a breast due to cancer may have a devastating effect on many women. Breasts are symbolic of a woman's femininity and sexuality. They are also functionally necessary for nurturing children. Changes in body image resulting from mastectomy is one of the most difficult psychologic aspects of breast reconstruction. The patient must realize that following reconstructive surgery she will not be the same as her preoperative state. The breast will resemble a mound and will be as symmetrical as possible to the contralateral side.

Breast reconstruction can be performed immediately following mastectomy or delayed. The patient's physical condition and preference dictate this decision.

Contraindications to breast reconstruction may include metastasis to major organs such as liver, bone, or lung. The use of chemotherapy and radiation does not preclude reconstruction but may delay it somewhat due to the healing processes.

Reconstruction of the breast can be accomplished in three ways: available tissue and an implant, tissue expanders, and myocutaneous flaps. Use of available tissue is the easiest procedure; however, insufficient tissue remains after mastectomy in numerous patients. When sufficient tissue exists, an implant of the appropriate size is placed under the remaining skin flap and/or muscle, and the contralateral side is adjusted accordingly by either a reduction mammaplasty or mastopexy to achieve symmetry.

Breast reconstruction using tissue expanders

Tissue expansion is a means of stretching normal tissue adjacent to a defect in order to mechanically create re-dundancy of normal tissue to correct the defect. For breast reconstruction, the expander is basically the same shape as a breast prosthesis. The expander may have a metal-backed, self-sealing silicone valve at its dome or a small, dome-shaped reservoir that is positioned subcutaneously at a distance from the expander but connected to it. In either case, weekly percutaneous injections of normal saline are placed in the expander until the tissue has reached the desired maximum stretch, usually based on a 3:1 ratio. When the desired stretch has been accomplished, the temporary tissue expander is removed and a permanent implant placed.

A combination tissue expander and permanent prosthesis is also available. The procedure of expansion is the same as with a temporary tissue expander; however, when the tissue has reached desired maximum expansion, a portion of the saline fill is removed to achieve a size and "drooping" of the reconstructed breast comparable to the contralateral breast.

Procedural considerations. A basic plastic instrument set is used. The round breast shape expander is supplied in a sterile package from the manufacturer and is available in multiple sizes (Fig. 24-22). The care of the tissue expander is the same as for other implantable devices. The patient is positioned supine with the arms extended on armboards. Prepping and draping are carried out in the routine manner to expose the operative site.

Operative procedure

1. A submuscular pocket is created for the temporary expander. In addition, a tunnel and pocket are created at an adjacent site from the main sac for the placement of the injection dome and the connecting tube.
2. The tissue expander is tested before insertion for watertight integrity.
3. The expander is then inserted, the reservoir positioned subcutaneously and connected, the wound closed, and the expander filled with sterile saline solution until blanching of the skin is achieved. The amount is recorded on the patient record. Instillation of 3 to 5 cc of methylene blue into the expander can help to identify the proper location of the fill tube postoperatively.
4. Additional inflation of the tissue expander usually begins 2 to 3 weeks after initial placement and thereafter on an average of every 7 days. The time from implant insertion until complete fill varies according to the desired maximum stretch.
5. After the desired expansion has occurred, the temporary expander is exchanged for a permanent prosthesis.

Breast reconstruction using myocutaneous flaps

The latissimus dorsi myocutaneous flap is a single-stage reconstruction of the breast following mastectomy. It is used when significant tissue deficiency occurs following a radical or modified radical mastectomy. The latissimus dorsi muscle is a wide muscle extending over the mid-

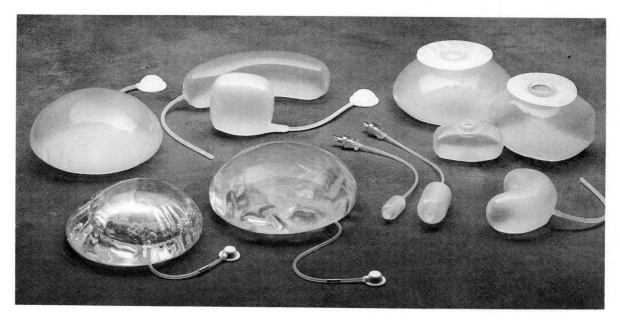

Fig. 24-22. Tissue expanders.

thoracic portion of the back and inserting into the humerus; its blood supply comes from the thoracodorsal artery and perforators from the upper lumbar arteries and the intercostal vessels. This rich vascularity allows the surgeon flexibility in orienting and positioning the flap to the pattern of the deficit on the anterior chest wall. Latissimus dorsi flaps for breast reconstruction may be used in conjunction with an internal breast prosthesis, with or without adjustment in the size of the contralateral breast.

Procedural considerations. The skin island and area of dissection for the latissimus dorsi flap are drawn on the patient's back before prepping and draping (Fig. 24-23).

The patient is placed in a lateral position with the arm on the operative side extended and elevated on a sling support. Pressure points are protected by the use of pillows and sheet rolls, and the patient is stabilized. The patient is prepped and draped, exposing the affected breast area and muscle.

A basic plastic instrument set is used, plus long Metzenbaum scissors, long DeBakey forceps, Deaver retractors, Freeman areolar markers, lighted breast retractors or a headlight, and a second electrosurgical unit.

Two surgical teams work simultaneously, one freeing the muscle flap and the other preparing the recipient site.

Operative procedure

1. Initially the island of skin is incised transversely across the back, with care being taken so that the scar will be covered by a bra or bathing suit.
2. The muscle is then freed from the overlying skin by undermining so that part or all of the muscle may be mobilized.
3. The skin island and the muscle are then tunneled

through the axilla to the chest wall (Fig. 24-23, *C*). The insertion of the muscle on the humerus and accompanying blood vessels are left undisturbed. The latissimus dorsi muscle fills the space left by the missing pectoralis muscle.

4. The island of skin is oriented to the recipient site, and both are sutured into place (Fig. 24-23, *D*).
5. A silicone implant is placed under the muscle before suturing to reconstruct the breast mound.
6. The wound is drained by closed wound suction catheters.
7. The nipple-areola complex may also be reconstructed by sharing the nipple on the unaffected side or by using groin or auricular tissue. It can be done at the time of reconstruction or at a later date as a minor procedure under local anesthesia (Fig. 24-23, *E*).

Trans-rectus abdominis myocutaneous flap (TRAM)

The TRAM is a single-stage reconstruction of a postmastectomy breast with the transverse rectus abdominis muscle. This flap gives the patient and plastic surgeon an alternative to the latissimus dorsi flap by taking the excess tissue from the lower abdomen to construct the breast, usually without the need for an implant (Fig. 24-24).

Procedural considerations. Markings on the patient are made preoperatively with the patient in an upright position. A basic plastic instrument set is used as for the latissimus dorsi flap. The patient is positioned supine with arms extended on armboards. Positioning the patient for this procedure is particularly difficult because of the need to promote closure of the abdominal wound, support cir-

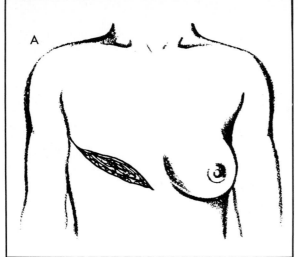

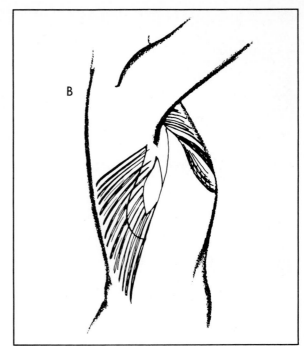

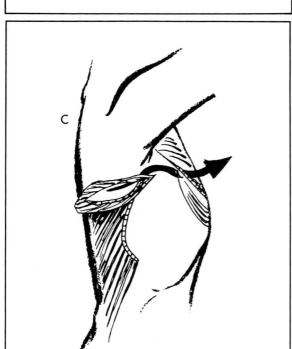

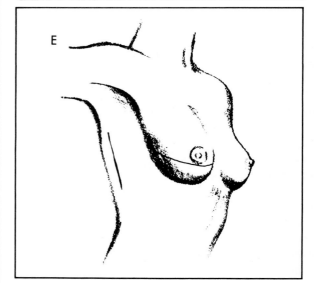

Fig. 24-23. Latissimus dorsi flap for reconstruction following mastectomy (see text for procedure).

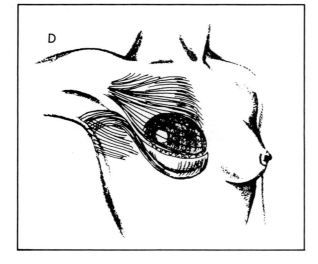

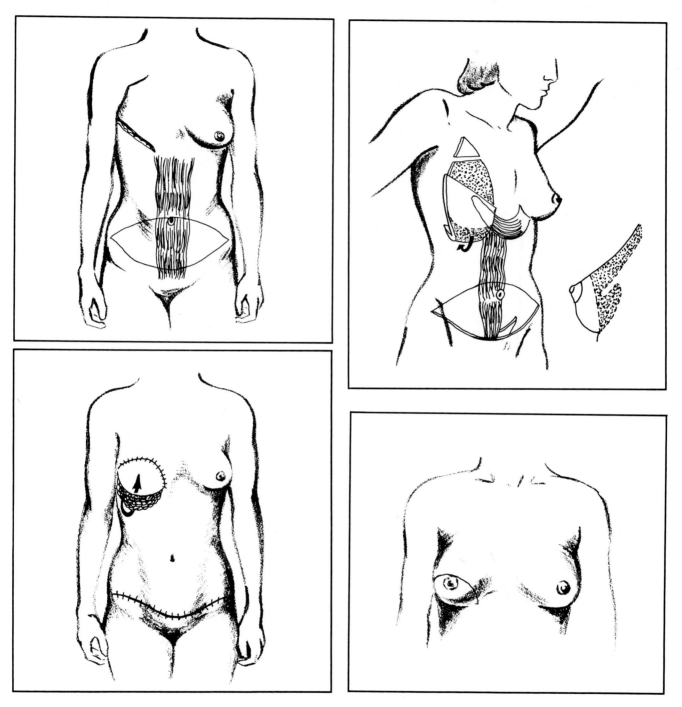

Fig. 24-24. TRAM flap for postmastectomy breast.

culation to the flap, and protect the patient from injury. The operating room bed is often flexed; additional padding of the lower extremities may be required. The chest and abdomen are prepped and draped simultaneously.

Operative procedure

1. The skin from the mastectomy scar is excised.
2. The transverse rectus abdominis muscle is dissected and tunneled subcutaneously to the midline.
3. The flap is brought to the chest wall and fixed medially; the thinnest portion of the flap is superior and medial, and the thickest portion is inferior and lateral.
4. Because of the amount of tissue available, an implant is often unnecessary.

Nipple reconstruction

This procedure may be done at the time of the original reconstruction, but most surgeons feel they have a better result if it is done as a secondary procedure after the reconstruction has healed and symmetry is achieved. Tissue may be harvested from the groin, auricular area, or contralateral nipple. Tattooing may complete the reconstruction.

Augmentation mammoplasty

Breast augmentation is done for hypomastia, to correct breast asymmetry, and to re-create the breast after mastectomy. A silicone breast prosthesis is inserted to enlarge or form the breast mound. Formation of a fibrous capsule after insertion of a silicone prosthesis is one of the associated problems. Postoperative exercises reduce capsule formation. Placing the implant under the pectoralis muscle also contributes to softness (Fig. 24-25).

Procedural considerations. A basic plastic instrument set is used, plus lighted fiberoptic retractors. The breast implants (Fig. 24-26) are packaged in sterile containers from the manufacturer and given to the scrub nurse when breast size is determined. The patient is placed in a supine position. The arms may be extended on armboards to approximately 60 degrees. Alternatively, the hands may be placed over the lower abdomen, then elbows protected with foam padding, and the arms gently secured with adhesive tape to the operating room bed. Prepping and draping are carried out in the routine manner to expose the operative site.

Operative procedure. Augmentation mammaplasty is done through areolar, inframammary, or axillary incisions. Either the underlying breast tissue or the pectoralis muscle from the chest wall is elevated. A pocket is dissected and the implant placed in the pocket. Electrocoagulation is used to achieve hemostasis. The pocket may be irrigated with an antibiotic solution before placement of the implant. The wound is closed in layers and a light gauze dressing applied. A bra or an Ace wrap may be used for support.

Reduction mammoplasty

Reduction mammoplasty is indicated for the patient with gigantomastia or macromastia resulting in back pain, intertrigo, or deep grooving in the shoulders from the weight of the breasts or to achieve symmetry following surgery on the contralateral side following a mastectomy. Excessive breast tissue and its overlying skin is excised, with reconstruction of the breast contour, size, shape, and symmetry (Fig. 24-27). Preoperatively, the patient needs

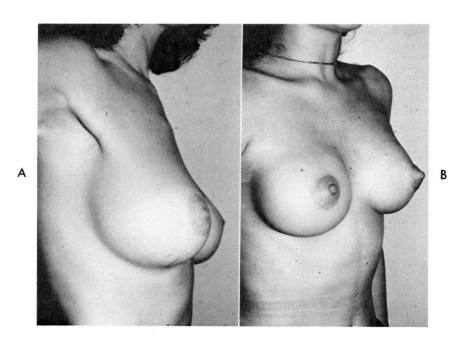

Fig. 24-25. A, Augmentation mammoplasty implant under muscle. **B,** Implant under breast tissue.

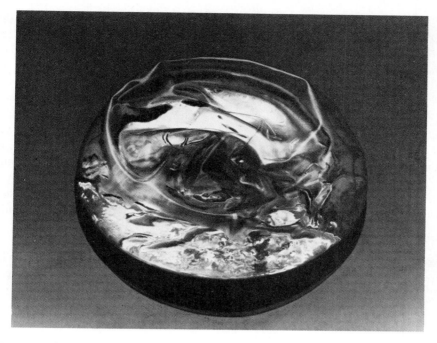

Fig. 24-26. McGhan double-lumen round mammary implant. (Courtesy McGhan Medical/3M, St. Paul, Minn.)

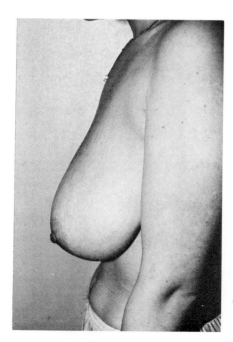

Fig. 24-27. Patient with pendulous breasts before reduction mammoplasty.

to be aware that the scars will be visible and that she may have a slight degree of asymmetry. Autologous blood should be available and the patient typed and cross-matched before undergoing anesthesia.

Procedural considerations. A basic plastic instrument set is used, plus the following:

"Cookie cutter" areola marker
Skin stapler
Electrosurgical unit
Marking pen
Tape measure
2 closed wound suction systems

A scale for weighing specimens should also be available, and tissue from each side should be carefully weighed and marked appropriately.

The patient is placed in a supine position with arms slightly extended on padded armboards. The hips should be positioned at the break in the operating room bed so that the patient may be raised to a sitting position if necessary. Standard prepping and draping are done. Care should be taken not to remove the preoperative markings.

Operative procedure
1. The skin to be excised, as well as the new site for the nipple, is marked (Fig. 24-28).
2. The skin between the new and the old nipple sites is incised and removed, the nipple remaining attached to the underlying breast tissue.
3. The redundant segment of breast tissue inferior to the nipple is excised through an inverted-T incision. Tissue from each breast is measured and kept separately.

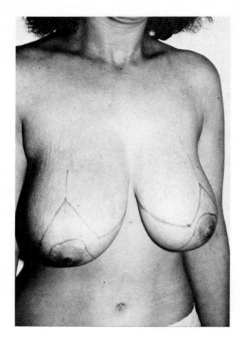

Fig. 24-28. Area of excision marked before surgery.

4. The nipple and adjacent tissue are mobilized and sutured in place.
5. The medial and lateral skin edges are approximated in a vertical suture line inferior to the nipple.
6. The inframammary elliptical incision is trimmed and closed transversely (Fig. 24-29). Closed wound suction catheters may be placed. The wound is dressed.

Reduction for gynecomastia

Gynecomastia is a relatively common pathologic condition that consists of bilateral or unilateral enlargement of the male breast. It occurs primarily during puberty or after the age of 40. Although it may be produced by a variety of diseases, it is usually related to excessive hormone production or alterations in hormonal balance. It may also be seen in elderly men and in men following excessive use of marijuana. All subareolar fibroglandular tissue is removed, and the resultant defect is surgically reconstructed. The patient may be positioned in a supine position or semi-Fowler's position, according to the surgeon's preference. Supplies and equipment needed are the same as for a simple mastectomy, plus a basic plastic instrument set. Because suction-assisted lipectomy (SAL) may be used for contouring, suction cannulae and an aspirator should also be available.

Operative procedure
1. A periareolar incision is made. Through this incision, the fibrous and ductal attachments of the underlying glandular tissue to the nipple are divided.
2. A cuff of fatty tissue is left attached to the underlying nipple surface to protect the blood supply.
3. The breast tissue mass is then gently dissected. Carrying the dissection to the pectoralis fascia is usually necessary to remove the entire mass.
4. Hemostasis is carefully achieved.
5. When all subcutaneous tissue has been mobilized, a three-layer closure is carried out. A small drain may be inserted to prevent hematoma formation. A firm pressure dressing is applied.

Correction of congenital deformities
Cleft lip repair

The normal upper lip is composed of skin, underlying orbicularis oris muscle, and mucosa. Two skin ridges near the midline outline the central philtrum of the lip. The vermilion (red portion of the lip) peaks at the philtral ridge

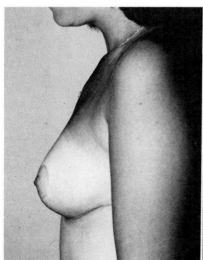
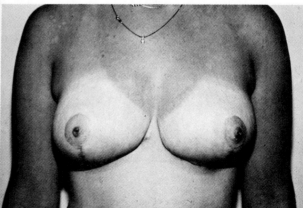

Fig. 24-29. Postoperative reduction mammoplasty.

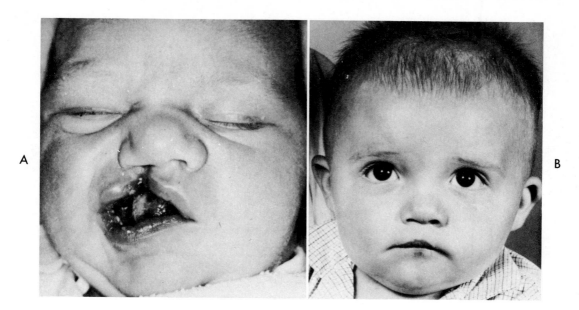

Fig. 24-30. **A,** Infant with complete unilateral cleft of lip. **B,** Repair 1 year later.

on each side and gently curves downward as it reaches the midline to form the Cupid's bow. A deficiency in tissue (skin, muscle, and mucosa) along one or both sides of the upper lip, or rarely in the midline, results in a cleft at the site of this deficiency. The deficiency of tissue present with a cleft lip results in distortion of the Cupid's bow, absence of one or both philtral ridges, and distortion of the lower portion of the nose. Cleft lip is usually associated with a notch or cleft of the underlying alveolus and a cleft of the palate.

Cleft lip repair is most often performed when the infant is about 3 months of age. Lip repair is directed toward rearrangement of existing tissues to approximate the nor-

mal lip as closely as possible (Fig. 24-30). Some consideration may also be given to correcting the nasal deformity at the time of cleft lip repair.

Procedural considerations. A plastic local instrument set is required, plus the following special instruments (Fig. 24-31):

2 Brown lip clamps
2 Calipers
1 Fomon retractor
2 Skin hooks, double, 5 mm
    Beaver scalpel handles and blades, no. 64 and no. 65
      Logan's bow
2 Knife blades, no. 11

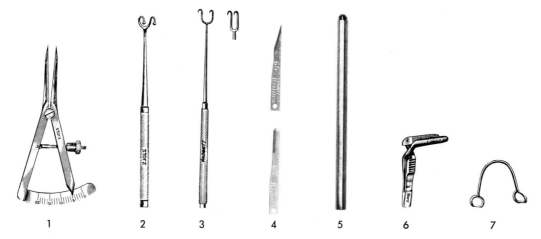

1   2   3   4   5   6   7

Fig. **24-31.** Special instruments for cleft lip repair. *1,* Caliper; *2,* Fomon retractor; *3,* 10-mm and 5-mm double skin hooks; *4,* Beaver scalpel blades nos. 64 and 65; *5,* Beaver scalpel handle; *6,* Brown lip clamp; *7,* Logan's bow.

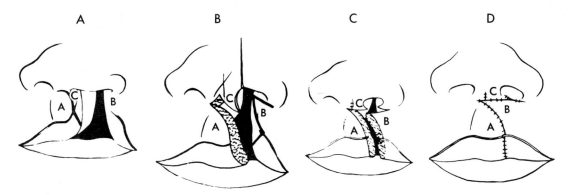

Fig. 24-32. Rotation-advancement method to correct complete unilateral cleft of lip. **A,** Rotation incision marked so Cupid's bow—dimple component A will rotate down into normal position; flap C will advance into columella and then form nostril sill. **B,** Flap A has dropped down, flap C has advanced into columella, and flap B has been marked. **C,** Flap B is being advanced into rotation gap, while skin roll flap is interdigitated at mucocutaneous junction line. **D,** Scar is maneuvered into strategic position where it is hidden at nasal base and floor and philtrum column and interdigitated at mucocutaneous junction. (From Millard, D.R.: In Grabb, W.C., and Smith, J.W., editors: Plastic surgery: a concise guide to clinical practice, Boston, 1980, Little, Brown & Co.)

1 Needle, 25 gauge, on straight hemostat
2 Cotton-tipped applicator sticks
1 Tongue depressor, disposable
  Marking pen
  Methylene blue
  Epinephrine 1:200,000 (for injection)

The patient is placed in the supine position, with the head at the edge of one end of the operating room bed. The head drape is used. The surgeon may stand or sit at the patient's side or just above the patient's head during the operation.

Operative procedure. Many types of cleft lip repair are in common use, one of which is illustrated in Fig. 24-32. The following steps are applicable to all lip repairs:

1. Normal landmarks are identified and marked or tattooed. Precise measurements, using calipers and a ruler, are made so that corresponding points can be marked along the cleft.
2. The lip may be infiltrated with epinephrine 1:200,000, or lip clamps may be used to aid hemostasis.
3. Incisions are made along the markings for the repair.
4. The abnormal musculature is dissected.
5. Additional dissection along the maxilla and nose may be performed.
6. Closure is done in three layers: muscle, skin, and mucosa.
7. A Logan's bow is applied to the cheeks with tape strips.

Cleft palate repair

The palate is made up of the bony or hard palate anteriorly and the soft palate posteriorly. The alveolus borders the hard palate. A separation or cleft of the palate occurs in the midline and may involve only the soft palate or both hard and soft palates. The alveolus may be cleft on one or both sides.

The major function of the soft palate is to aid in the production of normal speech sounds. An intact hard palate is necessary to prevent escape of air through the nose during speech and to prevent the egress of liquid and food from the nose.

Cleft palate repair is usually performed when a child is 12 to 18 months old. The various operations used to achieve surgical closure of the palate all employ tissue adjacent to the cleft (in the form of flaps) and shift it centrally to close the defect.

Procedural considerations. A basic plastic instrument set is required, plus the following special instruments (Fig. 24-33):

  Dingman mouth gag with assorted blades
1 Blair palate hook
2 Palate knives
2 Blair palate elevators, L-shaped, dull and sharp
2 Burlisher clamps, curved
2 Crile-Wood needle holders, 6 inches
1 Stratte needle holder, delicate
  Fomon lower lateral scissors, 1 short and 1 long
2 Cushing tissue forceps, 7 inches
2 Cushing dressing forceps, 7 inches
1 Brown forceps, 6 inches
12 Cottonoids, 1 × 1 inch, with strings
  Epinephrine 1:200,00 (for injection)
  Marking pen
  Bipolar electrosurgical unit
  Volumetric suction bottle

The patient is placed in the supine position, with the head at the edge of one end of the operating room bed. The head drape is used. Many surgeons sit just above the patient's head and cradle the head on their lap (with the patient's neck hyperextended).

Operative procedure. One of the most frequently used cleft palate repairs is illustrated in Fig. 24-34. The following steps are common to all palate repairs:

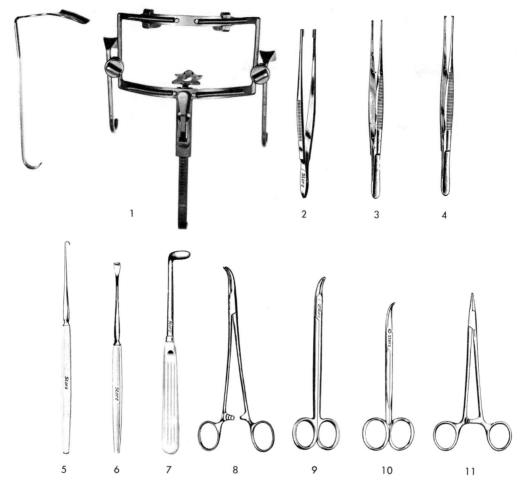

Fig. 24-33. Special instruments for cleft palate repair. *1,* Dingman mouth gag with assorted blades; *2,* Brown forceps; *3,* Cushing dressing forceps; *4,* Cushing tissue forceps; *5,* Blair palate hook; *6,* palate knife; *7,* Blair L-shaped palate elevator; *8,* curved Burlisher clamp; *9,* long Fomon lower lateral scissors; *10,* short Fomon lower lateral scissors; *11,* Crile-Wood needle holder.

1. The Dingman mouth gag is inserted. Maintenance of the position of the endotracheal tube is crucial at this point.
2. The outlines of the palatal flaps are marked.
3. The palate is injected with epinephrine 1:200,000 for hemostasis.
4. The flaps are incised and elevated.
5. Closure is in three layers: nasal mucosa, muscle, and palatal mucosa.
6. A large horizontal mattress traction suture is placed through the body of the tongue. If the patient experiences upper airway obstruction after extubation, traction is placed on this suture to pull the tongue forward, rather than inserting an airway that might harm the palate repair.

Pharyngeal flap

When abnormal speech (velopharyngeal insufficiency) results despite a cleft palate repair, a secondary surgical procedure may be necessary to improve speech. Typical "cleft palate speech" is characterized primarily by an excess of air escaping through the nose during speech. This hypernasality often results from insufficient bulk or movement of the muscles of the soft palate. To decrease or eliminate this problem, tissue from the pharynx, in the form of a pharyngeal flap, is added to the soft palate. This flap also reduces the size of the opening between the oropharynx and nasopharynx, thus decreasing or eliminating the nasal escape of air during speech.

A pharyngeal flap repair may be done at any age, but most are done before the patient is 14 years old. A pharyngeal flap also may be part of primary cleft palate repair.

Procedural considerations. The same instruments are needed as for cleft palate repair, plus two no. 14 Fr red rubber catheters.

Positioning and draping of the patient are as described for cleft palate repair.

Operative procedure

1. The Dingman mouth gag is inserted.
2. The palate and posterior wall of the pharynx are injected with epinephrine 1:200,000 for hemostasis.

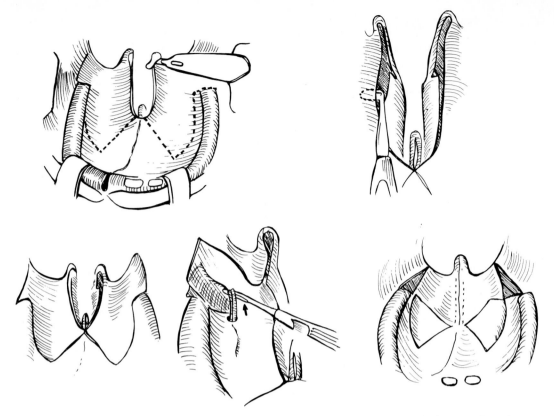

Fig. 24-34. Closure of cleft of soft palate by V-Y (Wardill-Kilner) palatoplasy. A V-shaped incision is made on oral side of palate; mucoperiosteal flaps are elevated on oral and nasal sides, with preservation of blood vessels; Y-shaped closure (in three layers) closes cleft and lengthens palate. (Redrawn from Randall, P.: In Grabb, W.C., and Smith, J.W., editors: Plastic surgery: a concise guide to clinical practice, Boston, 1980, Little, Brown & Co.)

3. The palate is incised, and the pharyngeal flap is incised and elevated.
4. The pharyngeal wall donor site may be sutured or left open.
5. The pharyngeal flap is sutured to the palate, and the palate is closed.
6. A traction suture is placed through the body of the tongue.

Ear reconstruction for microtia

Microtia refers to congenital total or subtotal absence of the external ear. The technique of ear reconstruction for microtia described here also may be applied to traumatic defects of the external ear. The external ear is a complex structure with numerous fine details. Its basic framework is cartilage with a thin layer of subcutaneous tissue and skin covering the cartilage. It is difficult to reproduce the fine detail of the normal ear. The general principles of ear reconstruction include placing a framework (carved costal cartilage) in a subcutaneous tissue pocket and, later, lifting this away from the side of the head. This requires several individual operations, or stages, to complete. Because the external ear has attained virtually full growth by age 6 years, ear reconstruction is usually started at age 4 years and completed by the time the child begins school.

Tissue expansion may also be employed in the treatment of microtia. It requires multiple stages to accomplish. Tissue expanders may be custom-made for the patient, or several styles and shapes are available to the surgeon.

Procedural considerations. A plastic local instrument set is required, plus calipers, a marking pen, and epinephrine 1:200,000 for injection.

If the operation includes obtaining an autogenous costal cartilage graft, the following separate setup is required in addition to a plastic local instrument set:

2 Knife handles, no. 3, with blades, no. 10
1 Key periosteal elevator
1 Duckbill rongeur
1 Rib shears, small
1 Alexander costal periosteotome
1 Teflon cutting board
  Bipolar electrosurgical unit
  Sterile x-ray film, unexposed

The patient is placed in the supine position on the operating room bed. The head drape is used, leaving both ears and postauricular areas well exposed. The lower costal cartilages on one side are also prepped and draped if a cartilage graft is to be used.

Operative procedure

1. During the first-stage operation, the ear remnants are excised or repositioned, as indicated.
2. Simultaneously, or during a second-stage operation, a costal cartilage graft (which must be carved to resemble the normal auricular cartilage framework) or a preformed silicone ear implant is placed in a subcutaneous pocket along the side of the head.
3. Several months later, the ear framework in its subcutaneous pocket is elevated from the side of the head and a split-thickness skin graft is used to cover the retroauricular defect.
4. Subsequent stages include various adjustments, often using split-thickness or full-thickness skin grafts, to make the ear appear more normal.
5. Use of a red-top tube with a butterfly cannula makes a convenient drain for the ear reconstruction and allows the subcutaneous pocket to adhere to the framework beneath.

Otoplasty

A congenital deformity, in which the ear protrudes abnormally from the side of the head, is generally the result of an absent or insufficiently pronounced antihelical fold of the external ear. The various methods of otoplasty attempt correction by creating an antihelical fold, which "pins" the ear back against the side of the head (Fig. 24-35).

Protruding ears may be unilateral or bilateral. Otoplasty is usually performed on children just before they start school. It is also performed on adults, in which case either general or local anesthesia may be used.

Procedural considerations. A plastic local instrument set is needed, plus the following:

Calipers
22-gauge needles or straight needles
Cotton-tipped applicator sticks
Methylene blue
Marking pen
Epinephrine 1:200,000 for injection
Mineral oil

The patient is placed in the supine position on the operating room bed, and a head drape is used, leaving both ears well exposed. The patient's head is turned with the affected ear up and with the lower ear well padded to avoid pressure injury.

Operative procedure

1. The antihelical fold is created by bending the external ear backward. The position of the antihelical fold is marked by placing 22-gauge or straight needles through the ear from anterior to posterior, applying methylene blue to the tip of the needles, and withdrawing them.

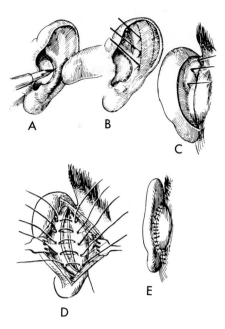

Fig. 24-35. Otoplasty for correction of protruding ears. **A,** Antihelix defined by applying pressure to ear. **B,** Position of antihelical fold marked by passing straight needles through ear. **C,** Needle points visible along posterior surface of ear with ellipse of skin to be excised marked. **D,** Section of ear cartilage incised and scored or excised with sutures placed to hold cartilage back. **E,** Posterior ear incision sutured. (Redrawn from Wood-Smith, D., and Porowski, P.C., editors: Nursing care of the plastic surgery patient, St. Louis, 1967, The C.V. Mosby Co.; and Converse, J.M., editor: Reconstructive plastic surgery, vol. 4, Philadelphia, 1983, W.B. Saunders Co.)

2. An ellipse of skin is excised from the posterior surface of the ear after it has been infiltrated with epinephrine 1:200,000 for hemostasis.
3. The ear cartilage is usually incised near the antihelical fold, and the anterior surface of the cartilage is scored to allow it to bend backward.
4. Sutures are usually placed to hold the cartilage in its new position.
5. The skin incision is closed.
6. A bulky dressing exerting moderate compression on the ears is applied. Cotton soaked in mineral oil and saline is usually placed behind the ear to avoid pressing the posterior ear surface against the side of the head.
7. A red-top tube with a butterfly cannula makes a convenient drain for the ear reconstruction and allows the subcutaneous pocket to adhere to the framework beneath.

Repair of syndactyly

Syndactyly refers to webbing of the digits of the hand or feet. The most common form of syndactyly is symmetrical webbing in two otherwise normal hands. It may, however, be associated with other abnormalities in the hand, such as extra fingers (polydactyly) or bony abnor-

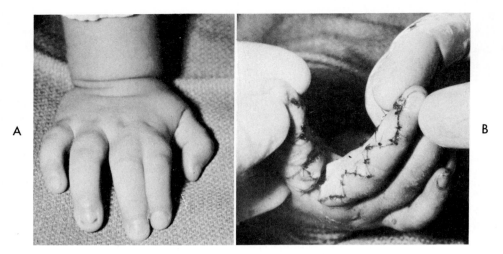

Fig. 24-36. A, Syndactyly involving index and long fingers. **B,** Skin web separated; triangular flaps and skin grafts visible along sides of both fingers.

malities. In syndactyly with normal digits, a web of skin joins adjacent fingers (Fig. 24-36, *A*); each finger, however, has its own tendons, vessels, nerves, and bony phalanges. Although the skin web may appear loose, a deficiency in skin is always present when surgical separation is undertaken. Plans for taking a skin graft (usually full thickness) should always be made. Surgical separation of syndactyly is performed at any time after the age of approximately 12 months.

Toe syndactyly is less often treated surgically than finger syndactyly because proper function of the foot does not require fine movements of individual toes. Although the setup and description that follow are for the repair of finger syndactyly, they can also be applied to the repair of toe syndactyly.

Procedural considerations. A plastic local instrument set is required, plus a marking pen, unexposed x-ray film, a pediatric pneumatic tourniquet, and an Esmarch bandage.

The patient is placed in the supine position on the operating room bed with the affected arm extended on a hand table. A pediatric pneumatic tourniquet is used. A hand drape is used, and both inguinal areas are prepped and draped (donor sites for full-thickness skin grafts).

Operative procedure

1. Skin incisions are marked, and the tourniquet is inflated.
2. The skin is incised, and small flaps at the sides of fingers and in the web are elevated.
3. After these flaps have been sutured into position, patterns of areas of absent skin on the sides of fingers are made and transferred to the skin graft donor site.
4. The skin graft is taken, and the donor site wound is dealt with appropriately.
5. Skin grafts are sutured to fingers (Fig. 24-36, *B*).
6. Stent dressings are placed over the skin grafts. The

entire hand is immobilized in a bulky dressing (see hand surgery section) or in a long-arm plaster cast.

Hypospadias repair

Hypospadias is a congenital anomaly in which the urethra ends on the ventral surface of the penile shaft or in the perineum. It is usually accompanied by a downward curvature of the penis, called *chordee,* especially during erection.

The goal of hypospadias repair is to allow for a normal urinary stream and for normal sexual function. This requires excision of the scar tissue that causes the chordee and construction of a urethra that extends to the distal end of the penis (Chapter 15). Hypospadias repair is usually performed between the ages of 1 and 2 years, so that psychosocial problems can be prevented.

Construction of a new urethra requires the addition of new tissue along the ventral surface of the penis. Most patients with hypospadias have not been circumcised. This is advantageous because the prepuce can be used to provide the extra tissue that is needed (usually in flap form). Some methods of hypospadias repair make use of free skin grafts.

More than 150 different operations have been described for the correction of hypospadias. The advances in the state of the art of hypospadias repair over the past decade have led to a one-stage procedure, usually with the technique of Horton and Devine. The Hodgson technique is an alternative for repair of the defect, depending on the choice of the surgeon and characteristics of the patient's deformity. It employs the establishment of an island of tissue from which a tube may be constructed to connect the urethra through an acceptable cosmetic channel to the tip of the penis. A transurethral plastic stent remains in place postoperatively for 7 days. Although the Hodgson method is a popular approach to repair of hypospadias, the Horton-Devine repair will be detailed here. The suggested readings at the end of the chapter include references for specific variations and alternatives for the one- or multiple-stage repair and the rationale for selecting each technique.

Procedural considerations. Instrumentation includes a plastic local instrument set, plus urethral sounds, nos. 8 to 22 Fr; Foley catheter of appropriate size, with a guide or stylet; a small feeding tube; a lubricant for the catheter and sounds; and a bipolar electrosurgical unit.

The patient is placed in the supine position on the operating room bed, with a folded sheet beneath the buttocks to elevate the hips slightly and with legs stabilized in a frog-leg position. The perineum is scrubbed with soap and water and is towel dried, followed by the routine skin prep.

Operative procedure. The Horton-Devine repair (Fig. 24-37) consists of the following steps:

1. Lidocaine with 1:200,000 epinephrine is injected for hemostatic purposes.
2. Incisions are made into the shaft and fibrous tissue beginning at the meatus and continuing to the coronal sulcus and encircling the glans penis. The chordee (scar tissue) is resected.
3. The dissection continues beneath the glans, a triangular flap is elevated, and lateral wings of the glans are freed with sharp dissection.
4. On the ventral surface of the penis a long penile flap, based distally on the urethral meatus, is outlined and elevated.
5. The glans flap is used to form the roof of the urethra using nos. 5-0 and 6-0 Dexon sutures.
6. The retrograde portion of the flap is flipped forward to form the ventral surface of the urethra, and multiple interrupted sutures complete the reconstruction of the glans.
7. The lateral wings are brought around the neourethra and sutured together at the midline.
8. The ventral skin deficit is closed with preputial flaps.

9. A small feeding tube or indwelling Foley catheter is left in place for 3 days after surgery.
10. Postoperative edema is controlled with a compression dressing of Elastoplast, which is placed snugly but not tightly around the shaft of the penis.

The two-stage operation described by Byars yields reproducible results and is described here.

First stage (Fig. 24-38, *A*)
1. An indwelling catheter is placed into the bladder through the existing urethral meatus.
2. A traction suture is placed through the glans penis.
3. The chordee (scar tissue) is excised from the urethral opening to the tip of the glans.
4. The prepuce is incised in the dorsal midline to create two folded flaps.
5. Both preputial flaps are unfolded and rotated ventrally to cover the defect between the meatus and tip of the glans left by excision of the chordee.
6. The flaps are sutured in placed with the ends of the sutures left long.
7. A dressing of nonadherent gauze and acrylic fiber is placed over the flaps, and the long ends of the sutures are tied over it. The entire penile shaft is encased in inch-wide strips of Elastoplast.
8. The catheter is taped to the patient's thigh, and open drainage is maintained by placing the end of the catheter within two folded abdominal pads held in place at the thigh by ties.

Second stage (Fig. 24-38, *B*)
1. A Foley catheter with a stylet in the lumen is inserted into the bladder through the existing meatus.
2. The stylet is rotated to permit palpation of its tip in the perineum; an incision is made over the prominence into the urethra.
3. The distal (flared) end of the catheter is pulled out through the perineal urethrostomy and sutured in place.
4. A traction suture is placed through the glans penis.
5. A rectangular area surrounding the urethral defect is

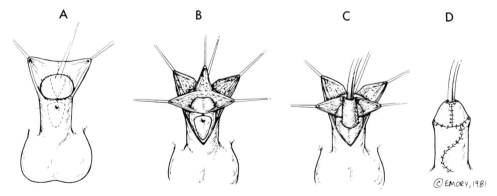

Fig. 24-37. Horton-Devine repair of hypospadias. **A,** Incisions from meatus to coronal sulcus. **B,** Triangular flap is elevated, and lateral wings of glans are freed. **C,** Urethral meatus is outlined and elevated. **D,** Functional and cosmetic closure is completed with small feeding tube or Foley catheter in place. (Courtesy Emory University School of Medicine, Atlanta.)

A

B

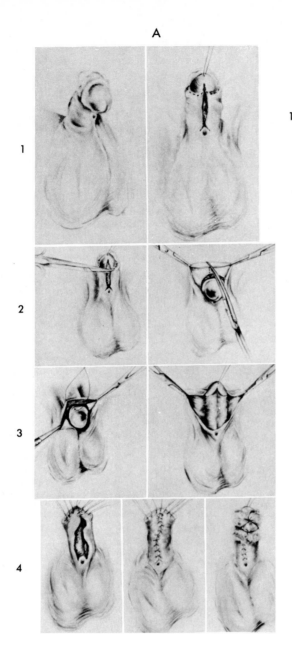

Fig. 24-38. Byars hypospadias repair. **A,** First stage. *1,* Midpenile shaft hypospadias with chordee at left; traction suture through glans and initial incision of first stage at right. *2,* Preputial incision at left; dorsal slit incision at right. *3,* Preputial flaps developed, and midline suture placed dorsally to stabilize known points at left; ventral surface presents large raw area where scar has been excised to straighten penis at right. *4,* Preputial flaps sutured over ventral penile shaft raw surface, and tie-over dressing placed over flaps. **B,** Second stage (perineal urethrostomy has been done). *1,* Rectangular incision from meatus to tip of glans; sides of this flap are elevated and inverted to form new urethral tube. *2,* Closure of subcutaneous tissue and skin in multiple tiers over new urethral tube. Operation depicted here was done in three stages; it is now done in two stages with new urethral tube and existing meatus connected at time of second-stage repair. (From Byars, L.T.: Surg. Gynecol. Obstet. *92:*149, 1951.)

incised from the meatus to the tip of the glans. This tissue is tubed by suturing the edges together to form the new urethra. The surrounding skin edges are undermined and sutured together over the new urethral tube.

6. The penile shaft is dressed with gauze and inch-wide Elastoplast strips.
7. Catheter drainage is the same as step 8 of the first-stage operation.

The major complication of these procedures is urethrocutaneous fistulas, which may require further surgery or heal spontaneously. Of note in the one-stage technique is the use of the Gittes and McLaughlin manner of injection to induce penile erection, thus indicating the degree of success of the removal of the constricting chordee.

Orbital-craniofacial surgery

A number of congenital anomalies involve the orbital-craniofacial skeleton. These include (1) hypertelorism (Fig. 24-39), in which the distance between the orbits is increased; (2) Crouzon's disease (Fig. 24-40), which includes premature closure of the cranial sutures, resulting in an abnormally shaped skull, exophthalmos and hypertelorism, parrot's beak nose, and maxillary hypoplasia; and (3) Apert's syndrome, which includes the same craniofacial deformities as Crouzon's disease plus syndactyly or other hand anomalies. Recent advances in plastic surgery make surgical correction of some of these deformities possible.

Binocular vision is normal in humans. It involves the coordinated use of both eyes to obtain a single mental impression of objects. Binocular vision is usually absent

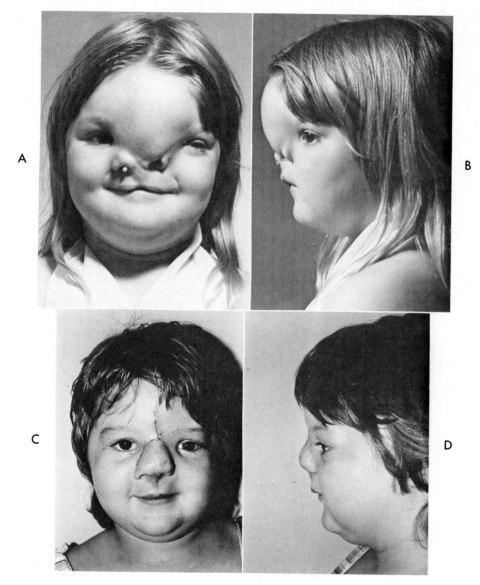

Fig. 24-39. Hypertelorism. **A,** and **B,** Before surgery, front and side views. **C** and **D,** After surgery, front and side views. (Courtesy Emory University School of Medicine, Atlanta.)

in the craniofacial anomalies because of the increased distance between the orbits. The purpose of orbital-craniofacial surgery is to provide the patient with binocular vision, by moving the orbits closer together, and to provide the patient with a more acceptable appearance, by moving the bones of the orbital-craniofacial skeleton into a more normal position. Correction of the deformity seen in Crouzon's disease and Apert's syndrome involves a surgically created LeFort III maxillary fracture (Fig. 24-41).

Although an extracranial approach may be used, an intracranial approach is used in most cases; therefore, a neurosurgeon and a plastic surgeon perform these operations through a bifrontal (coronal) craniotomy approach. A tracheostomy may be done before the start of the procedure. Bone grafts from hips or ribs are necessary to augment areas of bone deficit, which result from movement of the craniofacial skeleton.

Procedural considerations. These operations are usually performed on children. They are very extensive procedures, often lasting 12 to 14 hours. Blood loss is considerable. Postoperative complications, such as cerebral edema or meningitis, can be formidable. The perioperative nurse must pay particular attention to the following important details: (1) insertion of a Foley catheter into the patient's bladder before the operation is started, (2) positioning of the patient on the operating room bed so that all bony prominences are well padded, and (3) availability of accurate means for measuring blood loss (usually a volumetric suction bottle and scales for weighing sponges).

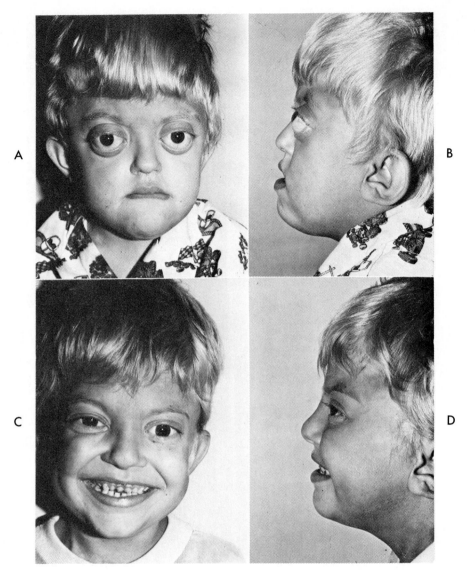

Fig. 24-40. Crouzon's disease. **A** and **B,** Before surgery, front and side views. **C** and **D,** After surgery, front and side views. (Courtesy Emory University School of Medicine, Atlanta.)

A basic plastic instrument set, craniectomy instruments and supplies (Chapter 23), and tracheostomy instruments and supplies (Chapter 21) are required, plus the following:

    Hall II air drill, Elane, or Midas Rex drill
    Oscillating and reciprocating bone saws
6 Osteotomes, assorted sizes, straight and curved
1 Mallet
3 Curettes, assorted
3 Rongeurs, assorted
2 Calipers
1 Brown fascia needle
1 Set coil arch bars
2 Rowe maxillary forceps
2 Polyethylene buttons
2 Foam rubber pads, small
    Volumetric suction bottle
    Scales for weighing sponges
    Marking pen

A separate setup is necessary for obtaining the bone graft. It includes a plastic hand instrument set, plus the following:

1 Weitlaner retractor
3 Curettes, assorted
6 Osteotomes, assorted
1 Mallet
    Hall II air drill
    Teflon cutting board

The patient is positioned, prepped, and draped as described for a bifrontal craniotomy (Chapter 23). The entire face is left exposed, however, and may temporarily be covered with a plastic drape until the portion of the operation requiring access to the face is reached. The bone graft donor site is also prepped and draped so that both iliac crests and the lower ribs are exposed.

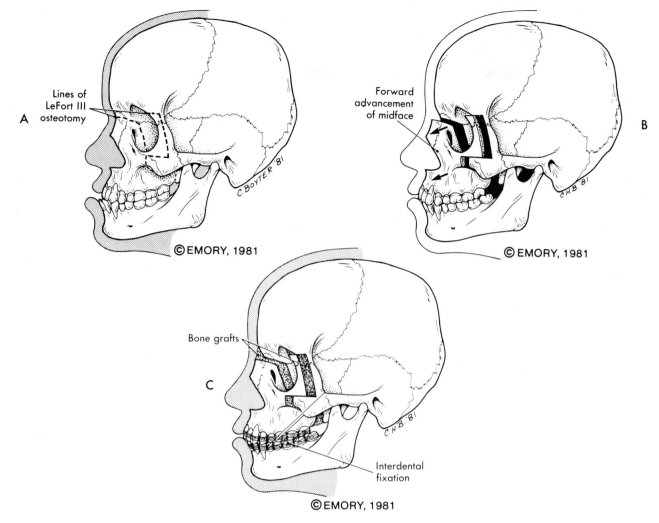

Fig. 24-41. Steps in surgical correction of Crouzon's disease deformities. (Courtesy Emory University School of Medicine, Atlanta.)

Operative procedure

1. Tracheostomy, if required, is performed first, followed by application of arch bars, when indicated (as in Crouzon's disease and Apert's syndrome).
2. The bifrontal craniotomy/craniectomy is performed.
3. Orbital osteotomies (Fig. 24-41, *A*) into the anterior cranial fossa are performed bilaterally.
4. Bilateral conjunctival (lower eyelid) and labiogingival sulcus incisions (for Crouzon's disease and Apert's syndrome) are made for other orbital and for maxillary osteotomies.
5. The bones of the orbital-craniofacial region are now moved (Fig. 24-41, *B*), based on measurement of the intercanthal distance (in hypertelorism) or occlusion of the teeth (in Crouzon's disease and Apert's syndrome).
6. Bone grafts may be taken from the calvarium, ribs, or hips to augment areas of bone deficit, which result from movement of the craniofacial skeleton.

7. Bone grafts are fixed in place with interosseous wires and by means of intermaxillary fixation applied to arch bars (for Crouzon's disease and Apert's syndrome) (Fig. 24-41, *C*).
8. The craniotomy, conjunctival, intraoral, and bone graft donor site incisions are closed.

Surgery for maxillofacial trauma
Reduction of nasal fracture

Usually a closed reduction of the bony nasal fragments is performed by digital and instrumental manipulation. Occasionally an open reduction with interosseous wire fixation of nasal bone fragments is necessary. A nasal fracture may involve a fracture of the nasal bones or cartilage (including the septum). Closed reduction of a nasal fracture is most often performed under topical and local anesthesia.

Procedural considerations. A plastic local instrument set is required, plus the following:

2 Nasal specula, 1 short and 1 long
1 Asch forceps or rubber-shod Kelly hemostats
4 Metal applicator sticks and wisps of cotton
1 Brown nasal splint
    Nasal packing of choice
    Topical and local anesthetic agents of choice

The patient is placed in the supine position. An intravenous infusion is started and a blood pressure cuff is applied. The head drape is used.

Operative procedure

1. Topical anesthesia for the nasal mucosa and nerve block anesthesia around the nose are administered.
2. The Asch forceps is introduced intranasally to elevate the bony fragments, while with digital pressure the surgeon's other hand molds the bones into position.
3. The nasal septum is inspected and realigned with the Asch forceps, if necessary.
4. Bilateral anterior nasal packs are placed.
5. Half-inch tape strips are applied over the skin of the nose, followed by application of the nasal splint and a nasal drip pad.

Reduction of mandibular fractures

The purpose of treatment for a mandibular fracture is to restore the patient's preinjury dental occlusion. With some types of fractures, a closed reduction with immobilization by means of intermaxillary fixation is sufficient for treatment. With a majority of mandibular fractures, however, an open reduction with wire fixation is necessary, plus supplemental intermaxillary fixation to achieve adequate immobilization for healing.

Intermaxillary fixation is most often accomplished by applying arch bars to the maxillary and mandibular teeth. Number 24 stainless steel wires are placed around the necks of the teeth and are ligated around the arch bars to hold the latter in place. Latex bands are attached to the tongs on the maxillary and mandibular arch bars to fix the teeth in occlusion (Fig. 24-42). If the patient is edentulous, arch bars are attached to dentures or specially fabricated dental splints. The dentures or splints are held in place by means of wires placed around the mandible (for the mandibular arch bar) and through the nasal spine and around the zygomatic arches (for the maxillary arch bar). Scissors or wire cutters must be sent with the patient to PACU to prevent aspiration, should the patient vomit.

Procedural considerations. A basic plastic instrument set, plus the following instruments and supplies, is needed for an open reduction of a fractured mandible:

1 Hall II air drill
2 Dingman bone-holding forceps (Fig. 24-43)
1 Concept nerve stimulator
    Stainless steel wires, nos. 24, 26, and 28
1 Marking pen
    Electrosurgical unit
    Epinephrine 1:200,000 for injection

For the application of arch bars or other types of interdental wiring techniques, a separate Mayo setup with the following instruments and supplies is required:

1 Set coil arch bars and latex bands
    Stainless steel wire, no. 25 or 26
2 Mayo-Hegar needle holders, 8 inches
1 Wire suture scissors, 4¾ inches
2 Weider tongue depressors, large and small
1 Yankauer suction tube
1 Freer septal elevator
6 Mosquito hemostats, curved, 5¼ inches
1 Brown fascia needle (if dentures or splints are used)
1 Drain, small

If arch bars are applied before the open reduction is performed, this latter setup must be kept completely separate from the instruments used for the open reduction. Because the mouth is a contaminated area, a complete change of gowns, gloves, and drapes is necessary after the intraoral procedure.

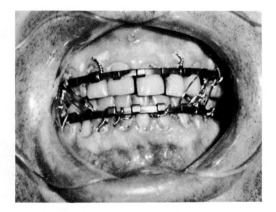

Fig. 24-42. Teeth in occlusion with arch bars in place. Tongs on arch bars will accept latex bands, which maintain occlusion for several weeks (wire around tongs are shown).

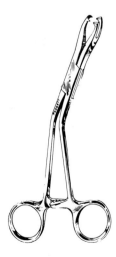

Fig. 24-43. Dingman bone-holding forceps used in reduction of mandibular fractures.

The patient is placed in the supine position on the operating room bed. The head drape is used.

Operative procedure

1. Arch bars may be applied before or after the open reduction.
2. A line inferior and parallel to the lower border of the mandible at the fracture site is marked, and the area is infiltrated with epinephrine 1:200,000 for hemostasis.
3. The incision is made so the inferior border of the mandible is exposed. The nerve stimulator may be used to aid in identification of the marginal mandibular branch of the facial nerve in fractures of the posterior body and angle of the mandible.
4. The fracture is reduced by manipulation. Holes are drilled into the mandible on each side of the fracture line with the Hall II air drill, while an assistant holds the reduced fracture with the aid of Dingman bone-holding forceps.
5. Stainless steel wire is inserted through the holes and twisted tightly to secure the fracture fragments in anatomic alignment.
6. A small drain is usually placed in the wound, and the wound is closed in layers (periosteum, platysma muscle, and skin).
7. The latex bands may be applied to the arch bars at this time but more frequently are applied later, after the patient is fully awake and reactive.
8. A moderate compression dressing is applied to cover the submandibular wound and drain.

Reduction of maxillary fractures

Maxillary fractures are usually classified as follows: (1) Lefort I, or transverse maxillary fracture; (2) LeFort II, or pyramidal maxillary fracture; and (3) LeFort III, or craniofacial disjunction, which includes fractures of both zygomas and the nose. A maxillary fracture produces malocclusion, as does a mandibular fracture. In addition, depending on the severity of the fracture, it may produce considerable deformity of the middle of the face, usually perceived as a flattening or "smashed-in" appearance of the middle of the face.

Closed reduction with intermaxillary fixation suffices for treatment of LeFort I and some LeFort II fractures. The more severe LeFort II and all LeFort III fractures require open reduction in addition to intermaxillary fixation.

Procedural considerations. The basic plastic instrument set is required, plus the following:

Hall II air drill or Elane drill
Stainless steel wires, nos. 25, 26, and 28
Rowe maxillary forceps, right and left
Brown fascia needle
Polyethylene buttons
Small foam rubber pad
Marking pen
Electrosurgical unit
Epinephrine 1:200,000 for injection

A separate Mayo setup for the application of arch bars is required, as described for reduction of mandibular fractures.

The patient is placed in the supine position on the operating room bed. The head drape is used.

Operative procedure. Arch bars are applied before or after the open reduction, or they may be the only mode of treatment in closed reduction. In addition to ligating the maxillary arch bar to the teeth, it must also be suspended from stable bones superior to the fractured maxilla (which is unstable). In LeFort I fractures, suspension may be around both zygomatic arches via passage of percutaneous wires. In LeFort II and III fractures, suspension wires are placed through holes drilled bilaterally in the zygomatic process of the frontal bone. This requires incisions in both lateral eyebrow areas. The following description pertains to open reduction of LeFort II and III fractures:

1. After injection of epinephrine 1:200,000 for hemostasis, bilateral incisions are made to expose the infraorbital rims and frontozygomatic suture lines.
2. The Rowe maxillary forceps are applied intranasally and intraorally to disimpact and reduce the maxilla.
3. Holes are drilled into bone on each side of fracture lines along the infraorbital rim (and frontozygomatic area for LeFort III fractures, after reducing the zygomatic fractures).
4. Stainless steel wires are passed through these holes and twisted down tightly to maintain the reduction.
5. Suspension wires are passed from the eyebrow incisions, behind the zygomatic arches, into the mouth with the Brown fascia needle. A pullout wire is looped through each suspension wire within the eyebrow incision, brought out through the skin near the hairline, and tied down over a polyethylene button and foam rubber padding. Self-tapping screws, mini-compression plates, and bone grafts may also be used, based on the surgeon's preference.
6. Incisions are closed.
7. When indicated, reduction of a nasal fracture is then performed.

Reduction of zygomatic fractures

Fractures of the zygoma (the cheek or malar bone) are corrected by either closed or open reduction. The two most common types of zygomatic fractures are depressed fractures of the arch and separation at or near the zygomaticofrontal, zygomaticomaxillary, and zygomaticotemporal suture lines, which constitutes a *trimalar* fracture. Although fractures of the zygoma can interfere with the ability to open and close the mouth properly, their chief consequence is a flattening of the cheek on the involved side, which results from a depressed trimalar or zygomatic arch fracture. Treatment is directed toward elevating the depressed fracture and maintaining the reduction. Closed reduction is the procedure used for treatment of zygomatic arch fractures, whereas most trimalar fractures are reduced by means of open reduction with internal fixation.

Procedural considerations. A plastic local instrument set, a Suraci zygoma hook-elevator, and a jaw hook are required for a closed reduction. A basic plastic instrument set, plus the following instruments and supplies, is required for an open reduction:

> Hall II air drill
> Stainless steel wires, nos. 26, 28, and 30
> 1 Suraci zygoma hook-elevator
> 1 Jaw hook
> 1 Kerrison rongeur
> 2 Blair retractors
> K-wire driver with set of assorted Kirschner wires and sterile cork (optional)
> Bipolar electrosurgical unit
> Marking pen
> Epinephrine 1:200,000 for injection

The patient is placed in the supine position on the operating room bed. The head drape is used.

Operative procedure. Closed reduction is performed by elevating the depressed fracture with a percutaneous bone hook. Stabilization of a trimalar fracture may then be achieved by inserting a transantral Kirschner wire from the fractures side to the normal side.

The technique of open reduction of a trimalar fracture is as follows:

1. Incisions are marked along the lateral eyebrow and lower eyelid over the zygomaticofrontal suture line and zygomaticomaxillary suture line (infraorbital rim) fractures, respectively.
2. After injection with epinephrine 1:200,000 for hemostasis, incisions are made down to bone, and suture lines are identified and exposed.
3. The depressed zygoma is elevated with a Kelly hemostat or periosteal elevator placed behind the body of the zygoma through the lateral eyebrow incision. Bone hooks placed percutaneously or at the fracture sites may be used instead.
4. Holes are drilled in bone on each side of the fracture lines. Stainless steel wires are passed through the hole and twisted down tightly to maintain the reduction. (Reduction and stabilization of two of the three fractures are sufficient.)
5. An alternative method of stabilization of the fractures is interosseous wiring of the zygomaticofrontal fracture and placement of a transantral Kirschner wire.
6. Incisions are closed.
7. An eye-patch dressing may be applied.

Reduction of orbital floor fractures

The orbital floor is the eggshell-thin bone on which the eye and periorbital tissues rest. It separates the orbit from the maxillary antrum. Orbital floor fractures usually occur in combination with fractures of the infraorbital rim (maxillary and zygomatic fractures). An isolated depressed orbital floor fracture with an intact infraorbital rim is called a "blowout" fracture.

Symptoms of orbital floor fractures are diplopia and enophthalmos. Diplopia is caused by entrapment of periorbital fat and extraocular muscles in the fracture line, which restricts movement of the eyeball. Enophthalmos usually results from a fracture extensive enough to allow herniation of periorbital fat into the maxillary antrum, which gives the eye a sunken appearance. Treatment is directed toward relief of these symptoms.

Because the orbital floor is so thin, comminuted fractures occur frequently and segments of bone may be irretrievably lost into the maxillary antrum. If the floor cannot be reconstructed by elevating the bony fragments, its integrity must be restored with an implant (cartilage graft, bone graft, or alloplastic material).

Procedural considerations. A basic plastic instrument set is required, plus the following:

> 2 Blair retractors
> Hall II air drill
> Alloplastic material of choice (Teflon or Silastic sheet) (Fig. 24-44)
> Marking pen
> Bipolar electrosurgical unit
> Epinephrine 1:200,000 for injection

In addition, instruments and supplies listed for reduction of maxillary and zygomatic fractures may also be needed because orbital floor fractures often occur in combination with these fractures.

Fig. 24-44. Sheets of alloplastic implant material: *left,* Teflon; *right,* Silastic. Small segments are cut to fit for reconstruction of fractured orbital floor.

The patient is placed in the supine position on the operating room bed. The head drape is used.

Operative procedure

1. A lower eyelid incision is marked and the eyelid injected with epinephrine 1:200,000 for hemostasis and incised down to the infraorbital rim.
2. Periosteum is elevated from the infraorbital rim and orbital floor.
3. The fracture is identified, and any entrapped periorbital tissues are reduced by gentle traction.
4. Continuity of the orbital floor is reestablished by reducing the fracture, replacing any bone chips if possible, or inserting an autogenous graft or alloplastic implant.
5. The orbital floor implant is secured anteriorly to the infraorbital rim with a suture after a hole has been drilled in the bone.
6. The incision is closed in one layer (skin).
7. An eye-patch dressing may be applied.

Elective orthognathic surgery

A large number of patients are afflicted with either acquired or congenital facial defects that affect the maxilla and/or mandible. The condition of many of these patients can be improved dramatically with orthodontic care; however, many also require surgical rearrangement of the maxilla or mandible.

Psychosocial and functional deficits are related to abnormalities of the maxilla and mandible. Surgical correction of these defects can improve the quality of life for these patients. Surgery is usually delayed until an adequate number of permanent teeth are in place for postoperative immobilization. Proper preoperative planning is of great importance to these patients.

Operative procedure

1. Arch bars are applied for postoperative immobilization.
2. Intraoral incisions provide exposure.
3. The maxilla or mandible is cut as indicated by the preoperative workup.
4. Bone is advanced or set back to a predetermined position.
5. Bones are wired in place with grafts in defects as needed.

Surgery for acute burns

A majority of burns result from exposure to high temperatures, which injures the skin. Thermal skin injury may be caused by flame, scald, or direct contact with a hot object. Similar destruction of skin can result from contact with chemicals such as acid or alkali or contact with an electrical current. The latter, however, often involves extensive destruction of the underlying tissue and physiologic systems in addition to the skin.

Intact skin provides protection against the environment for all underlying tissues and organs. It aids in heat reg-

RULE OF NINES	
Head & Neck	9%
Right upper extremity	9%
Left upper extremity	9%
Anterior trunk	18%
Posterior trunk	18%
Right lower extremity	18%
Left lower extremity	18%
Perineum	1%

ulation, prevents water loss, and is the major barrier against bacterial invasion. Burn patients are, therefore, some of the most acutely ill patients brought to the operating room. The greater the degree of injury to the skin, expressed in percent of total body surface area (TBSA) and depth of burn, the more severe the injury. The most common method of measuring TBSA is by employing the Rule of Nines, in which the body is divided into areas equal to multiples of 9 (see box).

Partial-thickness (first- and second-degree) burns heal by regeneration of skin from dermal elements that remain intact. Full-thickness (third-degree) burns require skin grafting to heal because no dermal elements remain intact. Both partial- and full-thickness burns may require debridement of necrotic tissue (eschar) before healing can occur by skin regeneration or grafting. Allograft may be used to cover the burned area during the initial healing process. However, the allograft must be carefully tested for immune deficiency diseases. Xenograft (for example, pig skin) may also be used for covering the burned area.

Procedural considerations. The essentials of skin grafting are discussed in the section on free skin grafts. This section therefore deals only with the procedure for debridement of burn wounds.

A basic plastic instrument set is required, plus a knife dermatome, an electrosurgical unit, topical thrombin solution, a pneumatic tourniquet for isolated extremity burns, and a topical antimicrobial agent of choice.

Because most burn wounds become infected within a few days, burns are contaminated, and appropriate operating room procedures are followed.

Most burn patients arrive in the operating room with dressings covering their wounds. These are removed after the patient has been anesthetized, to minimize pain and loss of body heat through the open burn wounds. The temperature in the operating room should be constantly monitored so that the patient's normal body temperature is maintained. The loss of heat from the body is increased by the lack of intact skin caused by a burn.

Operative procedure

1A. Nonviable tissue is excised down to underlying muscle fascia.

1B. An alternative method is tangential excision of the burn wound, which is performed with a knife dermatome. This type of excision is usually carried down only to subcutaneous fat, rather than to fascia.

2. Hemostasis is obtained with electrocoagulation or use of topical thrombin solution.

3. Dressings saturated with the topical antimicrobial agent of choice are applied.

Although skin grafting may be done at the time of wound debridement, it is usually performed several days later in burns that are extensive.

Aesthetic surgery

Aesthetic surgery is usually performed under local anesthesia with sedation. The perioperative nurse must be prepared to monitor the patient during the procedure. Baseline vital signs should be recorded on the operating room record. A blood pressure cuff, pulse oximeter, and cardiac monitor electrodes should be placed. Intravenous fluids should be started. The operating room should be kept quiet and patient privacy protected. Care should be taken to avoid conversation that could be misinterpreted by the patient.

Rhinoplasty

Deformities of the external nose and nasal septum may be congenital or secondary to previous trauma (Fig. 24-45). The goal of rhinoplasty is to improve the appearance of the external nose. This is accomplished by reshaping the underlying framework of the nose, which allows the overlying skin and subcutaneous tissue to redrape over the new framework. Reshaping the nasal skeleton usually includes rasping down of a dorsal hump, partial excision of lateral and alar cartilages, shortening of the septum, and osteotomy of nasal bones. A procedure to alter the nasal septum, *septoplasty* or *submucous resection* (SMR), often accompanies rhinoplasty.

The goal of SMR is to improve the nasal airway by resecting a segment of septal cartilage. Septoplasty reshapes the existing septal cartilage; it may aid in altering the appearance of the nose or in improving the airway.

Rhinoplasty is performed through incisions made inside the nose; it therefores leaves no visible scars. Small external incisions at the alar bases and near the nasal bridge are also used to narrow the nose.

Procedural considerations. A plastic local instrument set is required, plus the following special instruments (Fig. 24-46):

    1 Jansen-Middleton septal forceps
    4 Metal applicators and wisps of cotton
    1 Aufricht nasal retractor
    1 Formon retractor
    3 Pituitary rongeurs, assorted sizes, straight and upturned
    1 Nasal scissors, angled
    1 Kazanjian nasal forceps
    1 Fomon lower lateral scissors
    2 Joseph button-end knives, straight and angular
    1 Ballenger swivel knife, straight
    2 Joseph saws, 1 right and 1 left
    2 Chisels, 2 mm and 4 mm
    1 Cinelli double-guarded osteotome, straight
    2 Guarded chisels, straight, right and left
    1 Mallet

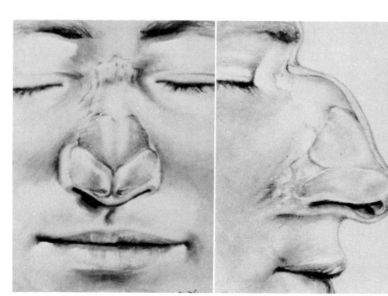
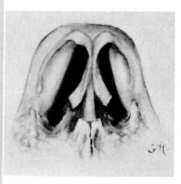

Fig. 24-45. Skeleton of abnormal nose with soft tissues superimposed. (From Brown, J.B., and McDowell, F.: Plastic surgery of the nose, ed. 2, Springfield, Ill., 1965, Charles C. Thomas, Publisher.)

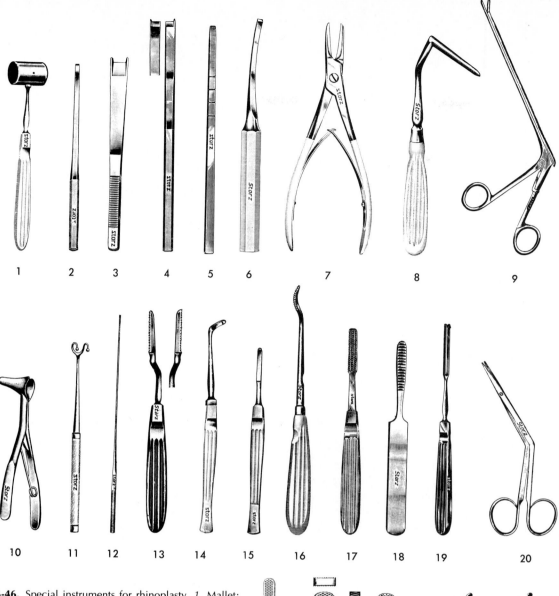

1 2 3 4 5 6 7 8 9

10 11 12 13 14 15 16 17 18 19 20

Fig. 24-46. Special instruments for rhinoplasty. *1*, Mallet; *2*, 2-mm chisel; *3*, Cinelli double-guarded osteotome; *4*, right and left straight-guarded chisels; *5*, 4-mm chisel; *6*, Blair chisel; *7*, Kazanjian nasal forceps; *8*, Aufricht nasal retractor; *9*, pituitary rongeur; *10*, nasal speculum; *11*, Fomon retractor; *12*, metal applicators; *13*, right and left Joseph saws; *14*, Joseph angular button-end knife; *15*, Joseph straight button-end knife; *16*, Aufricht rasp; *17*, Maltz nasal rasp; *18*, Brown nasal rasp; *19*, Ballenger straight swivel knife; *20*, angled nasal scissors; *21*, Fomon rasps; *22*, silver osteotomes.

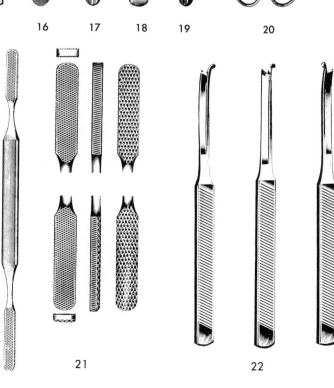

21 22

1 Brown nasal rasp (upward stroke)
1 Maltz nasal rasp (downward stroke)
1 Diamond rasp (optional)
  Fomon rasp
  Aufricht rasp
  Silver osteotomes
1 Nasal septum forceps (for SMR)
  Brown nasal splint
  Nasal packing
  Fiberoptic light source and headlight (optional)

Rhinoplasty may be performed under local anesthesia. A separate local anesthetic setup should contain the following:

Bayonet forceps
Sponges
Local anesthetic of choice, topical and local
Syringe, 10 ml
Needles, 30 gauge and 25 gauge × 1½
Petrolatum gauze for nasal packing
Atomizer (optional)

From this setup (before scrubbing), the surgeon can do the preliminary nasal preparation, inject the local anesthetic, and pack the nose with gauze or cotton soaked in 4% cocaine solution. With this procedure the local anesthesia can take effect while the surgeon is scrubbing. Intravenous fluids are started, and a blood pressure cuff, pulse oximeter, and cardiac monitor electrodes are placed.

The patient is placed in the supine position on the operating room bed. The head drape is used. The surgeon may use a headlight while performing the operation.

Operative procedure
1. Topical and local anesthetics are administered by the surgeon. The topical anesthetic is applied with applicator sticks or an atomizer.
2. Intranasal incisions are made, and the skin and soft tissues of the nose are elevated from the underlying nasal bones and cartilage.
3. The tip of the nose is reshaped by excising portions of the alar and lateral cartilages on each side.
4. The nasal dorsum (hump) is reduced by removing portions of the bone and septum.
5. The nasal bridge is narrowed by means of medial and lateral osteotomies of the nasal bones.
6. The intranasal incisions are sutured.
7. Bilateral anterior nasal packs are inserted, and a nasal splint and drip pad (moustache dressing) applied.

If an SMR is performed at the time of rhinoplasty, it usually immediately precedes step 2. Septoplasty may be performed at any time during the operative procedure.

Blepharoplasty

The aging process causes a sagging or relaxation of eyelid skin and the orbital septum. As the latter becomes weaker, it allows periorbital fat to bulge. These changes are perceived as baggy eyelids, which give the patient a chronically tired appearance. The goal of blepharoplasty is to improve the patient's appearance.

Loose skin and protruding periorbital fat of the upper and lower eyelids is removed. The upper eyelid skin can be so redundant that it encroaches on the patient's field of vision. Blepharoplasty is often performed with rhytidectomy.

Procedural considerations. A plastic local instrument set is required, as well as two Blair retractors, a bipolar electrosurgical unit, a marking pen, and a local anesthetic.

Blepharoplasty is usually performed under local anesthesia. Intravenous fluids are started, and a blood pressure cuff, pulse oximeter, and cardiac monitor electrodes are applied.

The patient is placed in the supine position on the operating room bed. The head drape is used.

Operative procedure (Fig. 24-47)
1. The local anesthetic is injected after the incision lines have been marked bilaterally.
2. An ellipse of excess skin is excised from the upper eyelids.

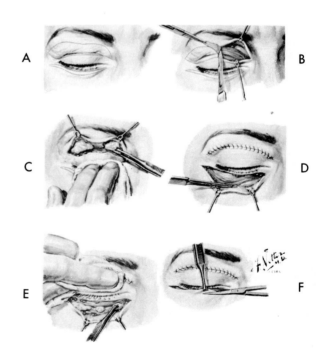

Fig. 24-47. Blepharoplasty for baggy eyelids. **A,** Areas of proposed skin excision marked with methylene blue or marking pen. **B,** Strip of skin excised from upper lid; fat pad shining through orbital fascia and orbicular muscle of eye. **C,** Orbital fascia opened in two places (medially and laterally). Pressure on eyeball causes fat pads to bulge. They are teased out meticulously. **D,** Upper lid incision sutured with continuous no. 6-0 silk. Orbicular muscle fibers are separated from skin. **E,** Orbital fascia opened; fat pads bulge because of digital pressure and are teased out meticulously. **F,** Skin tailored to fit and sutured. (Copyright 1967 Ciba-Geigy Corporation. Reproduced with permission from Clinical symposia, illustrated by Frank H. Netter, M.D. All rights reserved.)

3. After a strip of the orbicularis oculi muscle and orbital septum is incised or removed, protruding periorbital fat is excised and coagulated.

4. The upper eyelid incisions are sutured in one layer.

5. The lower eyelid incisions are made close to the ciliary margin or through a transconjunctival approach when only fat is to be excised.

6. A skin flap or skin-muscle flap is elevated away from the orbicularis oculi muscle.

7. Protruding periorbital fat is excised from beneath the orbicularis muscle.

8. The skin flaps are draped over the lower eyelids, and any excess skin is excised. Removal of too much skin from the lower eyelid can cause an ectropion.

9. The lower eyelid incisions are sutured in one layer.

10. Finely crushed ice on moist gauze 4 × 4 pads is applied to the eyes.

Rhytidectomy (facelift)

As the aging process progresses, the skin of the face and neck becomes loose and redundant. This is particularly noticeable in the "jowl" areas and just beneath the chin. A rhytidectomy is designed to improve the patient's ap-

pearance by removing some of the excess skin and sometimes the excess fat of the neck. Rather than excising the redundant skin directly, incisions adjacent to or within hairlines are used so that the scars are virtually indiscernible.

Procedural considerations. A basic plastic instrument set is required, plus the following:

1 Gorney or Kaye facelift scissors
2 Deaver retractors, 1 inch
2 Army-Navy retractors
2 Cushing tissue forceps, 7 inches
2 Brown-Adson forceps
2 Cushing dressing forceps, 7 inches
6 Burlisher clamps, curved
Rhytidectomy retractor (optional)
Metzenbaum scissors, long
Marking pen
Bipolar electrosurgical unit
Fiberoptic light source
Local anesthetic agent of choice
Skin stapler

A rhytidectomy is usually performed with local anesthesia. Intravenous fluids are started, and a blood pressure cuff, pulse oximeter, and cardiac monitor leads applied. The patient is placed in the supine position on the operating room bed. The head drape is used. Minimal or no hair is shaved.

Operative procedure (Figs. 24-48 and 24-49)
1. Bilateral incision lines are marked—from the temporal

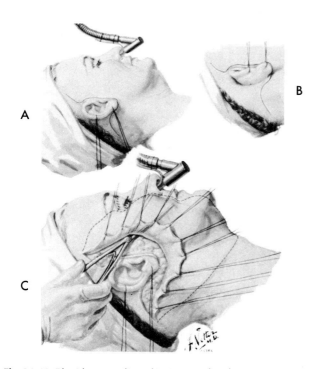

Fig. 24-48. Rhytidectomy: line of incision and undermining. **A,** Traction sutures of no. 4-0 silk placed in auricle; temporal incision curved posteriorly for better support of upward pull. **B,** Incision carried under earlobe and then curved posteriorly upward and then caudad toward midline. **C,** Skin undermined almost to nasolabial fold, to area of mental foramen, and to midline of neck as far down as thyroid cartilage. Care is taken to avoid injury to submandibular branches of facial nerve and facial artery. (Copyright 1967 Ciba-Geigy Corporation. Reproduced with permission from Clinical symposia, illustrated by Frank H. Netter, M.D. All rights reserved.)

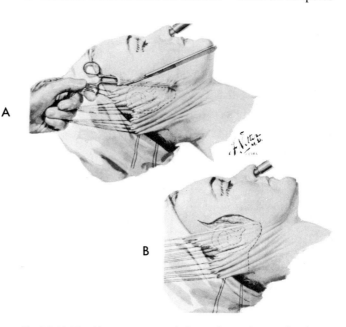

Fig. 24-49. Rhytidectomy: removal of superfluous skin. **A,** Skin drawn upward to proper degree of tension and incision made along posterior margin of clamp. **B,** Incision continued upward around posterior margin of auricle and then backward to excise skin specimen. (Copyright 1967 Ciba-Geigy Corporation. Reproduced with permission from Clinical symposia, illustrated by Frank H. Netter, M.D. All rights reserved.)

scalp, in front of the ear in a natural skin wrinkle line, around the earlobe, onto the posterior surface of the ear, and into the occipital scalp.

2. The incision lines, both temples, cheeks, upper neck, and the submental area are injected with the local anesthetic agent.

3. After the incisions are made, large flaps of skin and subcutaneous tissue are elevated from the face and upper third of the neck, meeting in the midline in the submental area and exposing the SMAS (superficial muscular aponeurotic system) and platysma. The SMAS and platysma are tightened, trimmed, and sutured behind and above the ears.

4. The edges of the flap are grasped with Allis forceps, and superior and posterior traction is placed on the flaps. The excess fat is removed, the platysma is plicated in the midline, and the neck is contoured. Suction may be used for the contouring.

5. Excess skin at the flap edges is excised, which pulls tight the tissue in the previously redundant areas.

6. Drains, if used, are inserted.

7. Incisions are closed in one or two layers.

8. A moderate pressure dressing is applied.

Dermabrasion

Sanding or planing of the skin is done primarily to smooth scars and surface irregularities of the skin. Dermabrasion is most commonly performed to improve the appearance of facial scars, especially the irregular scars resulting from acne vulgaris. It may also be used for the removal of foreign body tattoos. It is less successfully used for removal of professional body tattoos and to smooth fine wrinkle lines of the face.

The goal in treating irregular surfaces with dermabrasion is to sand or plane down the high points of elevations so that the low ones appear less deep. Dermabrasion removes epidermis and a portion of the dermis of the skin. Healing occurs from residual dermal elements, as in partial-thickness burns or split-thickness skin-graft donor sites.

Procedural considerations. Instrumentation includes a plastic local instrument set, dermabrader, marking pen, and protective goggles.

The operation may be performed under general or local anesthesia. The patient is positioned and draped so that the area to be dermabraded is well exposed.

Operative procedure
1. The bases of pitted scars and depressions are marked.
2. The skin is planed with the dermabrader.
3. A single layer of the dressing of choice is applied to the dermabraded area.

Scar revision

This involves the rearranging or reshaping of the existing scar by means of a scar revision procedure so that the scar is not as noticeable. The simplest form of scar revision is excision of an existing scar and simple resuturing of the wound. This may improve scars that are wide.

The Z-plasty is the most widely used method of scar revision. It breaks up linear scars, rearranging them so that the central member of the Z lies in the same direction as a natural skin line. Scars that are parallel to skin lines are less noticeable than scars that are perpendicular to skin lines. A contracted scar line also can be lengthened to a limited extent with a Z-plasty.

Procedural considerations. A plastic local instrument set and a marking pen are required.

The operation may be performed under local or general anesthesia. The patient is positioned, prepped, and draped so the scar that is to be revised is well exposed.

Operative procedure
1. The pattern for the planned revision is marked.
2. The scar is excised.
3. The surrounding tissue is undermined and the wound edges approximated according to the surgeon's markings.
4. Dressings may or may not be applied.

Abdominoplasty

Abdominoplasty is particularly useful in improving the appearance (and to a certain extent, function) of persons who have lost a great deal of weight. Obesity produces distention and stretching of the skin of the abdomen. Although weight loss reduces the volume of the underlying fat, it does not produce concomitant reduction in the excess surface area of the overlying skin, resulting from destruction or insufficiency of elastic fibers in the skin. The stretched skin remains as an apron that hangs from the lower abdomen, sometimes as far as the knees. The rectus abdominus fascia is also stretched in obese patients, and weight loss does not restore its integrity.

Abdominoplasty is usually performed to remove redundant skin and fat of the lower abdomen; it also repairs any laxity of the rectus muscle.

Procedural considerations. A basic plastic instrument set is required, as well as extra retractors and clamping instruments, an electrosurgical unit, and a marking pen. Antiembolism hose are usually in place or applied in the operating room.

The patient is placed in the supine position, with slight flexion at the hips. Draping is such that the entire abdomen, lower costal margins, upper thighs, and both anterior iliac spines are exposed.

Operative procedure
1. A low, transverse abdominal incision across both inguinal areas laterally and the superior border of the mons pubis in the midline is marked and incised down to fascia.
2. A large flap of skin and subcutaneous tissue is elevated away from the fascia of the anterior abdominal wall.

3. The umbilicus is left in its normal position.
4. The abdominal flap is elevated further until the xiphoid process of the sternum and the lower costal margins are reached.
5. If diastasis of the rectus abdominus fascia is present, plication is performed from the xiphoid process to the mons pubis.
6. The flap of abdominal skin and subcutaneous tissue is pulled inferiorly, and excess tissue is excised.
7. A small incision is made in the midline of the flap to accommodate the umbilicus, which is then sutured peripherally to the flap.
8. Drains may or may not be used, followed by closure of the lower abdominal incision in two layers.
9. Postoperatively the patient is placed in the hospital bed in high Fowler's position.

Suction lipectomy

In this body-contouring technique, a slender cannula is inserted into the subcutaneous layer and fat is aspirated by vacuum. Suction lipectomy may be used for body contouring on the buttocks, flanks, abdomen, thighs, upper arms, knees, ankles, and chin. Suction lipectomy is not a substitute for weight loss, and it is not a cure for obesity. Plastic surgeons prefer to do this procedure on relatively young patients, those under the age of 40, because the skin of younger patients readily contracts to the newly contoured frame. The procedure may be done in a hospital or an ambulatory surgery facility.

Immediate preoperative preparation includes asking the patient to stand while the area of deformity is outlined. Two lines are usually drawn on the skin surface, one delineating the major area of defect, the other placed a short distance outside the first area. These lines make it easier for the plastic surgeon to make a smooth transition toward the normal tissue by adjusting the amount of fat removed from the center to the periphery of the deformity. The patient may remain standing and be prepped circumferentially with a spray bottle of warm iodophor solution. Care should be taken to protect the patient's privacy.

Procedural considerations. A plastic local instrument set is used. A general anesthetic is administered.

Operative procedure

1. A small incision from ½ to 1 inch long is made in the area closest to the deformity that can best be concealed.
2. A suction curette or blunt cannula (Fig. 24-50) is inserted through the incision.
3. The curette is attached to a firm suction tubing and connected to the aspirating (suction) unit (Fig. 24-51).
4. The high vacuum pressure created by the unit causes the fat cells to emulsify so that they can be suctioned through the vacuum opening near the rounded tip of the curette.
5. The incision is closed by one or two sutures, and a bulky pressure dressing is applied to the area.

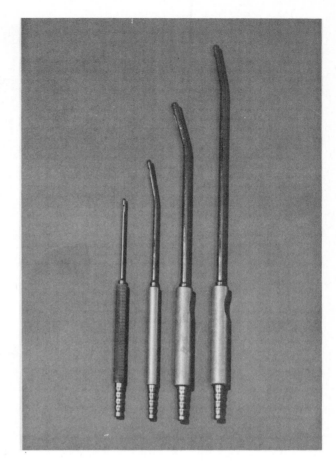

Fig. 24-50. Suction lipectomy curettes.

6. Compression garments may be applied to maintain even pressure. Taping may also be used, based on the surgeon's preference.

Excision of pressure sores

Pressure sores result from prolonged compression of soft tissues overlying bony prominences. *Decubitus ulcer* defines a type of pressure sore that is produced while the patient is lying down. Prolonged pressure causes thrombosis of small blood vessels and anoxia of soft tissues, with eventual necrosis. A person with normal sensation perceives discomfort in an area of prolonged or excessive pressure and changes position before irreversible soft tissue damage occurs. Pressure sores therefore occur in patients who lack normal sensation, such as paraplegics, or in patients who are too ill or weak to change their positions, even though they are uncomfortable.

The most common sites for the occurrence of pressure sores are over the sacrum, the greater trochanter, and the ischial tuberosity. The basic principals of the surgical repair of pressure sores are excision of the ulcer and underlying bony prominence, followed by adequate soft tissue coverage of the area (usually a local flap with a skin graft used to cover the flap donor site).

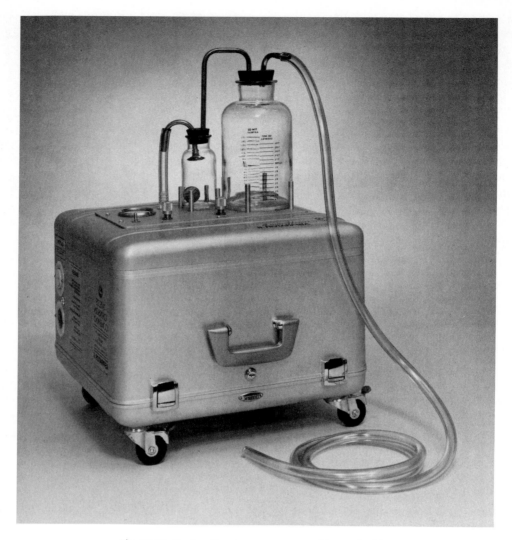

Fig. 24-51. Suction lipectomy vacuum machine and tubing.

Procedural considerations. A basic plastic instrument set is required, plus the following:

Osteotomes, assorted sizes, straight and curved
Mallet
Gigli saw and handle
Curettes, assorted
Key periosteal elevator
Duckbill rongeur
Bone wax
Dermatome of choice
Electrosurgical unit
Marking pen
Closed wound drainage system

The patient is positioned and draped so that the pressure sore, adjacent flap donor site, and a skin graft donor site are well exposed.

Operative procedure

1. The area to be excised and the local flap are outlined.
2. The ulcer is excised along with the underlying bony prominence.

3. Large suction catheters are placed into the defect left by excision of the ulcer and beneath the flap.
4. The flap is sutured in place.
5. A split-thickness skin graft is usually used to resurface the flap donor site.
6. A stent dressing is placed over the skin graft, and gauze dressings or a plastic spray dressing are applied over the suture lines of the flap.

Gender reassignment

Transsexualism defines the condition in which an individual with chromosomes and internal and external organs normal to one sex identifies psychologically and socially with attributes of the opposite sex. Reassignment of sex by means of surgery is the last step to be taken in treatment of transsexuals. It is performed only after the patient has been treated with hormones of the opposite sex, has experienced a period of cross-gender living, and has had intensive psychiatric evaluation. Most institutions performing this type of surgery have gender-identity teams who evaluate and treat transsexuals. These teams usually include a variety of professionals: psychiatrist, psychologist, endocrinologist, plastic surgeon, urologist, gynecologist, and social worker.

The surgical techniques for assignment of male to female are technically easier. A breast augmentation may be performed if hormone therapy has not sufficiently changed breast size. Construction of the neovagina includes radical penectomy, bilateral orchiectomy, urethroplasty, perineal dissection, creation of a neovaginal vault, vaginoplasty, and vulvoplasty.

The surgical technique for female to male is technically more difficult and requires multiple surgical procedures. Considerations that must be addressed are twofold: A neophallus that will allow the patient to stand to void must be constructed, as well as a phallus that will permit stimulation of a sexual partner during intercourse. This may require a radial artery forearm free flap with a later-stage surgical insertion of a prosthesis for "stiffening."

■ Hand surgery

Plastic surgery of the hand is directed toward restoration of function. It deals with the treatment of acute injuries, as well as reconstruction in established deformities. A systematic surgical approach for the restoration of hand function includes (1) replacement of lost tissue covering; (2) restoration of bony architecture; (3) repair of severed nerves; (4) restoration of the motor unit, either by tendon repair, tendon graft, or tendon transfer; and (5) replantation of severed digits.

Surgical anatomy

The functional unit in hand surgery consists of the hand, digits, wrist, and forearm. Each of these structures has a *radial* and an *ulnar* side, as determined by its position in relation to the radius and ulna of the forearm, rather than a lateral and medial side. Each also has a *dorsal* and *volar,* or *palmar,* surface. To avoid confusion, the digits of the hand are referred to as the thumb and the index, long, ring, and little fingers.

The skeletal framework of the hand and wrist consists of three distinct parts: (1) the metacarpals, or bones of the hand; (2) the phalanges, or bones of the digits; and (3) the carpals, or bones of the wrist (Fig. 24-52). The five metacarpals articulate distally with the proximal phalanges of each digit at the metacarpophalangeal (MP) joints. The two bones of the thumb are the proximal phalanx and the distal phalanx, which articulate at the interphalangeal (IP) joint. Each of the four fingers contains three bones: a proximal phalanx, a middle phalanx, and a distal phalanx. Each finger therefore has three joints: (1) the metacarpophalangeal joint, (2) the proximal interphalangeal (PIP) joint between the proximal and middle phalanges, and (3)

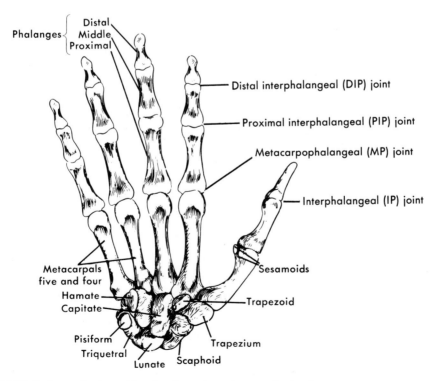

Fig. 24-52. Skeleton of wrist and hand, palmar view. (From Hollinshead, W.H.: Anatomy for surgeons. Vol. 3. The back and limb, ed. 2, New York, 1969, Harper & Row, Publishers.)

the distal interphalangeal (DIP) joint between the middle and distal phalanges.

The carpus (wrist) consists of eight bones arranged in two rows. The proximal row includes the scaphoid (navicular), lunate, triquetrum, and pisiform. The distal row includes the trapezium (greater multangular), trapezoid (lesser multangular), capitate, and hamate. The metacarpals articulate proximally with the distal row of carpal bones. The proximal row of carpal bones articulates with the radius and ulna of the forearm.

Motion of the thumb and fingers is achieved through the action of muscles intrinsic and extrinsic to the hand. The intrinsic muscles are those whose muscle bellies lie within the hand: (1) the interosseous and lumbrical muscles

of the hand, which flex the MP joints while extending the PIP and DIP joints and permit spreading and approximation of the fingers; (2) the muscles of the thenar eminence, which aid in adduction, abduction, flexion, and opposition of the thumb; and (3) the muscles of the hypothenar eminence, which aid in abduction, flexion, and opposition of the little finger.

The extrinsic muscles are so called because the muscle bellies are located in the forearm while the tendons pass into the hand, dorsally beneath the extensor retinaculum (Fig. 24-53), and volarly beneath the flexor retinaculum (Fig. 24-54) at the wrist, to insert on the phalanges of the thumb and fingers. The dorsal group consists of the extensor tendons, which extend the finger MP joints and the

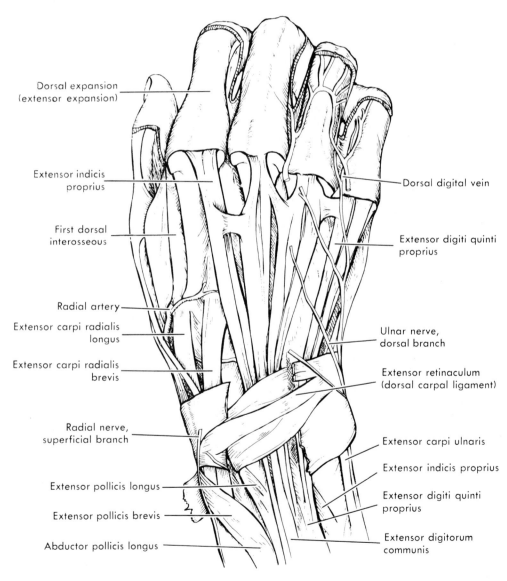

Fig. 24-53. Dorsum of hand and wrist; finger and long thumb extensor tendons pass under extensor retinaculum at wrist. (Reproduced by permission from J.C.B. Grant's atlas of anatomy, 6th ed., copyright © 1972, The Williams and Wilkins Co.)

thumb MP and IP joints. The volar group consists of the flexor tendons, one for the thumb and two to each finger. The paired finger flexors are the superficial (sublimis) flexor tendons, which flex the PIP joints, and the deep (profundus) flexor tendons, which flex the DIP joints. In addition to the finger and thumb flexors and extensors, other muscles of the forearm have tendinous insertions that work to abduct the thumb and flex and extend the wrist.

Although hand movements are achieved by the action of various muscles and their tendons, muscle function depends on adequate innervation of the muscle belly. The

motor nerves of the hand are (1) the radial nerve to the extensors, (2) the median nerve to a majority of the flexor tendons and a few intrinsic muscles, and (3) the ulnar nerve to a majority of the intrinsic muscles and the remaining flexors.

Sensation in the hand is provided by the same three nerves: (1) the radial nerve supplies the dorsal radial hand and fingers; (2) the median nerve, the volar (palmar) radial hand and digits (thumb, index, long, and radial side of the ring finger); and (3) the ulnar nerve, the remaining dorsal and volar ulnar hand and fingers. As the terminal

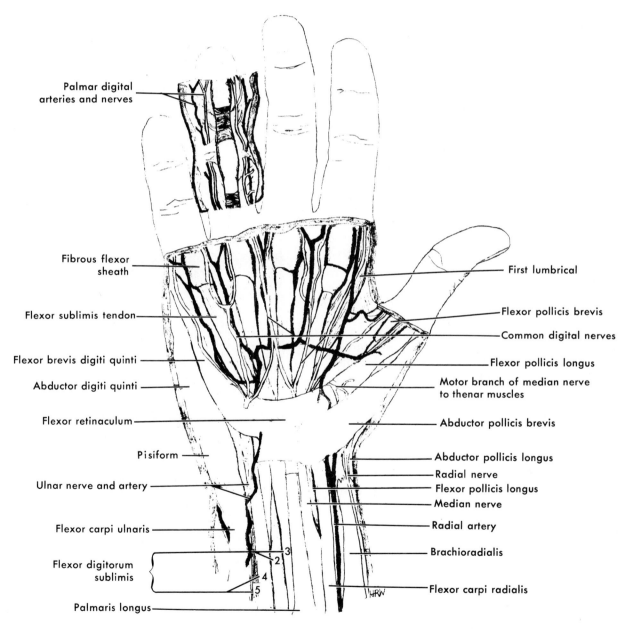

Fig. 24-54. Volar (palmar) surface of hand and wrist; median nerve, finger, and long thumb flexor tendons pass beneath flexor retinaculum (transverse carpal ligament) at wrist. (Courtesy Heather R. Weeks, The Jewish Hospital School of Nursing, St. Louis, Mo.)

sensory branches of the median and ulnar nerves enter the thumb and fingers, they are called digital nerves (Fig. 24-54).

The principal blood supply for the hand is from the radial and ulnar arteries that form a superficial and deep palmar arch in the hand, giving off terminal branches to both sides of each digit, called digital arteries after they enter the fingers and thumb (Fig. 24-55). A rich network of dorsal veins serves to return blood from the hand.

A minimum of skin and subcutaneous tissue covers the dorsum of the hand and digits. The skin covering the volar (palmar) surface is anchored to underlying fascia in areas of skin folds. Because of these fascial attachments, the skin and subcutaneous fat pads of the volar (palmar) surface do not move about during flexion and grasping of an object. The palmar fascia is a thick fibrous structure overlying the blood vessels, tendons, and nerves in the palm of the hand, to which skin is anchored, principally at the palmar skin creases. The palmar fascia sends extensions into each digit.

Special equipment
Pneumatic tourniquet (see also Chapter 22)

Because it renders the operative field relatively bloodless, a tourniquet is almost essential in dealing with the complex, delicate, and vital structures within the hand. The tourniquet should be the pneumatic type, inflated with compressed gas, the pressure of which can be determined with an accurate gauge. Each tourniquet must be checked at regular intervals against a tourniquet test gauge (Fig. 24-58, *B*) or a mercury manometer to maintain the accuracy of its gauge. The tourniquet can be a dangerous device when not in good working order and when improperly used.

The arm cuff of the tourniquet should be smooth and broad so pressure is distributed evenly over a wide area. Sheet cotton (Webril), stockinette, or a tourniquet cover may be wrapped smoothly around the limb where the tourniquet will be applied. It should be placed as far proximally on the arm as possible, where a greater amount of soft tissue provides padding for underlying nerves and blood vessels as they are compressed against bone when the tourniquet cuff is inflated. There should be no kinking of the tubing between the cuff and gas-regulating mechanism. To prevent a chemical burn, antimicrobial solutions used for skin preparation should not be allowed to run beneath the tourniquet cuff.

The arm is exsanguinated by progressively wrapping the arm from fingertips to tourniquet cuff (distal to proximal) with a 3-inch Esmarch rubber bandage. The tourniquet is quickly inflated to prevent filling superficial veins before occlusion of the arterial blood flow. The Esmarch bandage is removed after inflation of the tourniquet cuff. The amount of pressure used to inflate the tourniquet depends on the size of the extremity and the patient's age and systolic blood pressure.

Tourniquet time should be kept to a minimum. Times of inflation and deflation should be recorded. After completion of the surgical maneuver that required use of the tourniquet, deflation of the cuff should be accompanied by total removal of the tourniquet cuff from the arm. If the cuff is left on the arm after being deflated, it may cause some obstruction to the return of venous blood, which is perceived as increased bleeding at the operative site.

Boyes-Parker hand operating table (Fig. 24-55)

The hand table is used for most hand operations. Adjustable legs allow fitting to any standard operating room bed level. The legs also provide maximum stability of the operative field. The surgeon and assistants sit during the operation. A stainless steel pan with drain and plug may be placed in the hand table to facilitate irrigation of wounds.

Stryker SurgiLav (Fig. 24-56)

The SurgiLav is a sterile disposable system for lavage and debridement of tissue. It provides a pulsating jet stream of fluid when attached to a standard solution bag or bottle. Sterile disposable handpieces and tubing assemblies are available from the manufacturer, as well as several different types of irrigation tips and splash shields.

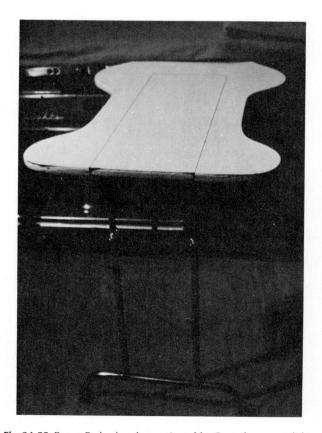

Fig. 24-55. Boyes-Parker hand operating table. Central segment slides out so stainless steel pan can be inserted during wound irrigation.

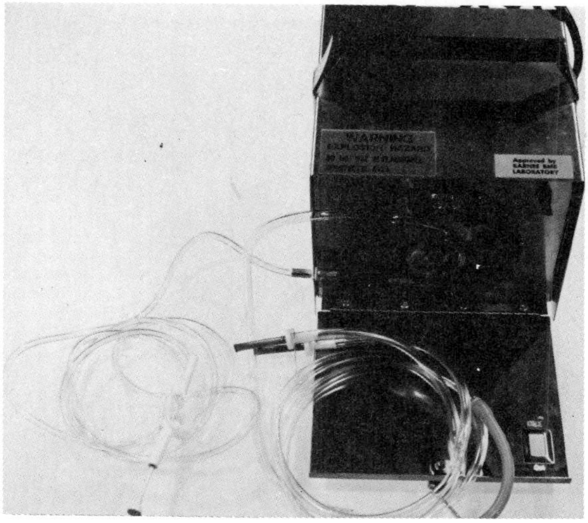

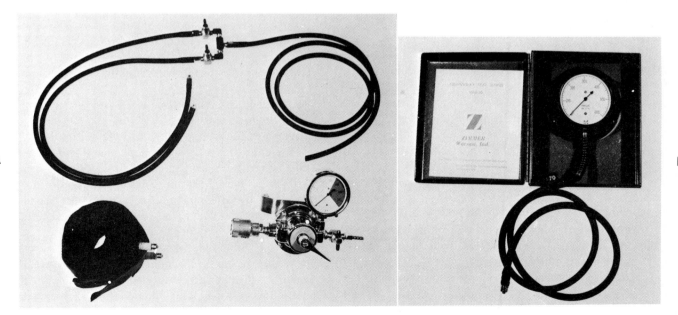

Fig. 24-56. Stryker SurgiLav for wound irrigation in hand surgery. Wheel at back of assembly is shown with tubing at bottom, which leads to solution bag or bottle; tubing at left delivers pulsatile flow of solution through multiple orifice irrigation tip shown here.

Intravenous regional anesthesia

Intravenous regional anesthesia (Chapter 9) is often used for hand operations and may be administered by the surgeon or an anesthesiologist. A pneumatic tourniquet with a double cuff plus dual control valves and tubing (Fig. 24-57) is used. A butterfly needle is inserted into a vein of the affected extremity and secured with tape. The position of the needle within the vein is verified by irrigating with sterile saline solution in a 10-ml syringe, which is left attached to the tubing of the butterfly needle. An Esmarch bandage is used to exsanguinate the extremity, and the *proximal* cuff of the tourniquet is inflated. After removal of the Esmarch bandage, 0.5% lidocaine is injected intravenously through the butterfly needle (usual dose is 3 mg/kg of body weight, not exceeding a total dose of 250 mg). The butterfly needle is removed, and pressure is applied at the venipuncture site for several minutes. Prepping and draping of the patient usually follow.

The advantage of a tourniquet with a double cuff is as follows: When the patient experiences moderate discomfort from the proximal cuff pressure (approximately 30 minutes after inflation of the cuff), the *distal* cuff may be inflated. The distal cuff lies over an anesthetized area of the arm, and the patient's discomfort should be reduced. After inflation of the distal cuff, the proximal cuff is deflated.

Dressings and immobilization

Basic conditions for good wound healing after hand surgery are immobilization and elevation. Adequate immobilization achieves support and splinting to protect against both active and passive motion. With most hand operations, because of many closely related movements, immobilizing the entire hand, fingers, wrist, and distal two thirds of the forearm is usually necessary. This immobilization is often maintained for 3 or 4 weeks after surgery. Application of the means of immobilization must therefore be performed with care while the patient is still anesthetized. Although plaster of Paris may be used to achieve immobilization, many surgeons prefer a soft, bulky hand

A

B

Fig. 24-57. Dual tourniquet cuff set for use with regional intravenous anesthesia. **A,** Dual cuff, dual control valves with tubing, and tourniquet pressure gauge (in mm Hg). **B,** Tourniquet test gauge.

dressing. Steps in the application of a hand dressing are as follows:

1. An assistant supports the hand, which is elevated by flexing the elbow and resting it on the hand table.
2. Nonadherent gauze is applied over incisions.
3. Gauze dressing sponges in thin layers are placed between the fingers to prevent maceration. These sponges must be uniform thickness from proximal to distal to prevent pressure on digital blood vessels.
4. A thicker layer of gauze is placed between the thumb and index finger to prevent an adduction contracture of the thumb. In addition to abduction, the thumb is also rotated into opposition as the dressing is applied.
5. Mechanic's waste or acrylic fiber is placed in the palm of the hand for bulk so that it can support the PIP and DIP joints of the fingers in extension. It may also be added to the thumb–index finger web space to maintain thumb abduction.
6. Folded abdominal pads are placed vertically across the dorsal and volar surfaces of the wrist for support.
7. Two Kling gauze rolls are wrapped around the hand and forearm so that the MP joints are in approximately 90 degrees flexion, the PIP and DIP joints are extended, the thumb is in abduction and opposition, and the wrist is in a neutral position. All fingertips must be exposed to permit inspection for determining viability.
8. Inch-wide strips of adhesive tape are applied vertically over the dressing (to avoid constricting bands).

Surgical interventions
Treatment of fractures

Fractures within the scope of hand surgery may involve the phalanges in the fingers, the metacarpals in the hand, and the carpals in the wrist. The basis for treatment of any fracture is reduction of the fracture and immobilization until healing occurs.

Reduction of a fracture may be closed or open. Closed reduction is performed by manipulating the fracture fragments beneath intact skin and subcutaneous tissue. X-ray studies verify the reduction. Open reduction is performed by making an incision, visualizing the fracture site, and then manipulating the fragments under direct vision. X-ray films are usually also obtained after open reduction.

Immobilization of a fracture may be external or internal. External methods include splinting and casting. Internal immobilization in hand fractures is usually accomplished by inserting Kirschner wires (Fig. 24-58). This may be the sole method by which a reduction can be stabilized. It has the additional advantage of allowing motion in a maximum number of hand joints while immobilizing only the injured part, thus preventing unnecessary joint stiffness.

Procedural considerations. A plastic hand instrument set, a Kirschner wire driver, an Esmarch bandage, and a marking pen are required.

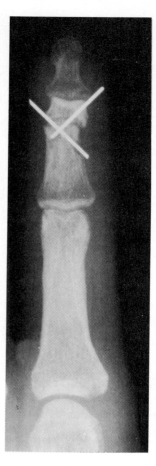

Fig. 24-58. Radiograph shows fracture of middle phalanx of index finger following open reduction, with internal fixation by means of crossed Kirschner wires across fracture site.

The patient is placed in the supine position on the operating room bed, with the arm extended on a hand table. The hand drape is used.

Operative procedure (open reduction, internal fixation)

1. The incision is marked.
2. The pneumatic tourniquet is inflated.
3. The incision is made, and the fracture is exposed.
4. The fracture is reduced by manipulating the fragments digitally or instrumentally under direct vision.
5. While an assistant holds the reduced fracture, Kirschner wires are driven into bone, usually across the fracture site. (Mini screws and plates may also be used as internal fixation.)
6. After x-ray films are obtained to verify the fracture reduction and immobilization, the Kirschner wires are cut off so that the ends are buried beneath skin or with a short segment protruding through skin. This segment is twisted down with needle-nose pliers.
7. The incision is sutured in one layer (skin).
8. A hand dressing is applied.

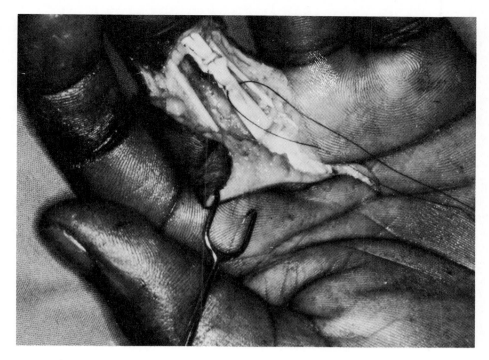

Fig. 24-59. Primary repair of flexor profundus tendon of long finger in distal palm.

Tendon repair

When continuity of a tendon is interrupted by avulsion or laceration, a specific active movement of one or more joints of the hand is lost. The treatment is tendon repair. Primary flexor or extensor tendon repair is usually performed at the time of injury or within several days of the acute injury. When adequate tendon length is present on each side of the laceration, repair is performed by suturing the tendon ends together (Fig. 24-59). When the laceration is near the bony insertion of the tendon, the distal tendon segment is too short to permit adequate purchase for a suture. In this case, tendon repair is performed by reinserting the proximal end of the tendon into bone.

Procedural considerations. A plastic hand instrument set, an Esmarch bandage, a marking pen, and no. 3-0 or 4-0, double-armed, nonabsorbable suture on Keith needles are required.

The patient is placed in the supine position on the operating room bed, with the arm extended on a hand table. The hand drape is used.

Operative procedure

1. The skin laceration is usually enlarged to permit adequate exposure of the tendon laceration, after the skin extensions for the laceration are marked and the tourniquet is inflated.
2. An additional incision in the hand or wrist or both may be necessary to identify the retracted proximal tendon end.
3. The tendon is repaired by placing a no. 4-0 or 5-0,

double-armed, nonabsorbable suture through the tendon ends and approximating the ends. A pullout suture may or may not be placed through the tendon suture.
4. If the repair involves reinsertion of the tendon into bone, a small bone flap is raised, a straight Keith needle is drilled through the bone with the hand drill, and the suture ends from the tendon are passed through the bone and are tied down over a foam-rubber padding and a polyethylene button.
5. Incisions are closed in one layer.
6. A hand dressing is applied.

Flexor tendon graft

A graft is used to restore function when the original tendon is incapable of so doing because of a large gap between ends of a lacerated tendon or because of a failed primary tendon repair. Although extensor tendon grafts are possible, the vast majority of free tendon grafts are flexor profundus and flexor pollicis longus tendon grafts. A gap large enough to preclude approximation by direct suturing of the tendon ends results from loss of a segment of tendon at the time of injury or from shortening of the proximal tendon end if too much time has elapsed since the original injury. A failed primary tendon repair is usually caused by scar tissue that inhibits adequate tendon gliding. Tendon gliding must be sufficient to produce appropriate joint movement when the muscle belly of the tendon contracts. If a great deal of scar tissue is present in the tendon bed, a free tendon graft also may fail to glide sufficiently to

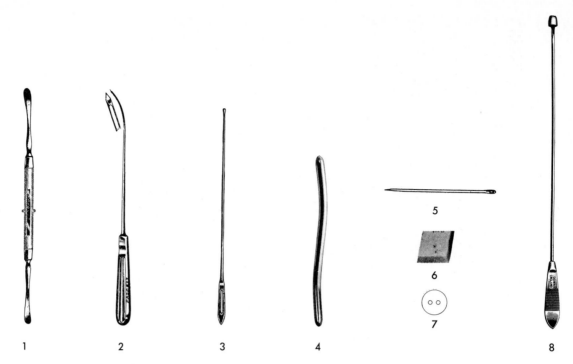

Fig. 24-60. Special instruments for flexor tendon graft. *1*, Freer septal elevator (with hole); *2*, Sanders-Brown fascia needle; *3*, silver probe; *4*, no. 6 Hegar dilator (with hole); *5*, Keith needle; *6*, foam rubber; *7*, polyethylene button; *8*, Brand tendon stripper.

produce adequate joint movement. In this case a silicone rod may be inserted into the tendon bed. The scar tissue that forms around the rod creates a pseudosheath through which a tendon graft is placed 6 to 8 weeks later. The pseudosheath often permits better tendon gliding.

The most commonly used donor tendon for a free graft is the palmaris longus tendon in the wrist and forearm. The plantaris tendon in the leg is also frequently used. Toe extensor tendons are used less commonly.

Procedural considerations. A plastic hand instrument set is required, plus the following special instruments (Fig. 24-60):

1 Brand tendon stripper
1 Sanders-Brown fascia needle
1 Silver probe, 9 inches
1 Hegar dilator, no. 6, with hole
1 Freer septal elevator with hole
1 Keith needle, straight
1 Polyethylene button
1 Foam rubber pad, small
1 No. 4 Lane needle, taper cut point
1 Goniometer
1 Esmarch bandage
  Marking pen
  Double-armed nonabsorbable suture, no. 3-0 or 4-0
  Silicone tendon rod, 3 mm (optional)

The patient is placed in the supine position on the operating room bed, with the arm extended on a hand table. The hand drape is used. If the plantaris tendon or a toe extensor tendon is to be used as the donor tendon, the lower extremity also must be prepped and draped. Use of a pneumatic tourniquet on the leg is optional.

Operative procedure
1. After marking incisions and inflating the pneumatic tourniquet, the surgeon makes a distal incision to expose the insertion of the flexor profundus tendon into the distal phalanx, and a proximal incision is made in the hand or wrist or both.
2. Scar tissue in the tendon bed is excised.
3. If the flexor tendon bed is not deemed suitable for a tendon graft, a 3-mm silicone rod is inserted and sutured distally to the profundus tendon remnant attached to the distal phalanx (Fig. 24-61).
4. If the tendon bed is suitable or a silicone rod has previously been inserted, a free tendon graft is obtained with the Brand tendon stripper.
5. Approximation of the proximal tendon end and graft is performed in the palm or wrist.
6. The graft is threaded through the tendon bed to the distal phalanx (Fig. 24-62), where it is inserted as described in step 4 of tendon repair, after the tension of the graft has been carefully adjusted.
7. The incisions are closed in one layer.
8. A hand dressing is applied.

Peripheral nerve repair and grafting

Nerve repair is done by direct approximation of nerve or severed nerve ends or by means of a nerve graft to

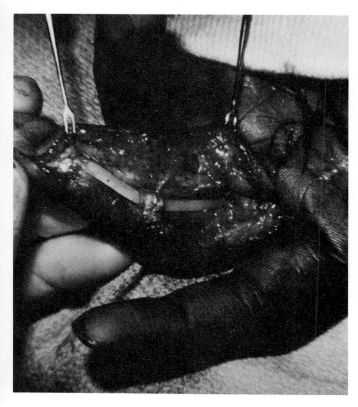

Fig. 24-61. Silicone rod placed into profundus tendon bed of long finger in preparation for flexor tendon grafting.

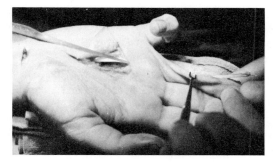

Fig. 24-62. Flexor tendon graft being threaded through profundus tendon bed of ring finger from palm to distal phalanx. Palmaris longus tendon has been obtained with Brand tendon stripper through small wrist incision.

attempt to restore continuity of a nerve in the hand, wrist, or forearm and regain sensation or motor function.

Procedural considerations. A plastic hand instrument set is required, plus the following special instruments (Fig. 24-63):

1 Jeweler's forceps
1 Castroviejo-Vannas scissors, curved
2 Castroviejo needle holders, straight, with and without lock
Nerve hook (von Graefe muscle hook)
Razor blade
Nerve stimulator

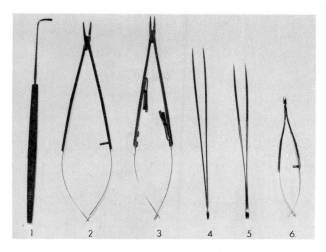

Fig. 24-63. Special instruments for nerve repair and grafting. *1,* von Graefe muscle hook; *2,* Castroviejo needle holder without lock; *3,* Castroviejo needle holder with lock; *4* and *5,* jeweler's forceps; *6,* Castroviejo-Vannas scissors.

Esmarch bandage
Marking pen
Loupes or operating microscope

The patient is placed in the supine position on the operating room bed, with the arm extended on a hand table. The hand drape is used. If a nerve graft is to be used, a lower extremity is also prepped and draped. Use of a pneumatic tourniquet on the leg is optional.

Operative procedure
1. After incisions are marked and the tourniquet is inflated, the proximal and distal nerve ends are exposed.
2. Devitalized nerve tissue or scar at the severed nerve ends is resected sharply with a razor blade, back to normal nerve tissue, where individual nerve bundles can be visualized.
3. With the aid of loupes or the operating microscope, individual nerve bundles are approximated (Fig. 24-64) with a fine, nonabsorbable suture (usually no. 7-0 to 10-0 nylon).
4. If a nerve graft is used, it is obtained through a series of short transverse incisions or one long vertical incision along the posterolateral aspect of the leg. Approximation of the nerve bundles between the graft and proximal and distal nerve ends is performed as in step 3.
5. The incisions are sutured, and dressings are applied. The hand dressing is applied so tension at the site of repair is prevented.

Implant arthroplasty

Destruction of the cartilage that forms the articular surface of a joint results in stiffness and pain during movement of the joint. Traumatic arthritis and rheumatoid arthritis are the most common causes of destruction of articular joint surfaces. Excision of the diseased joint surface af-

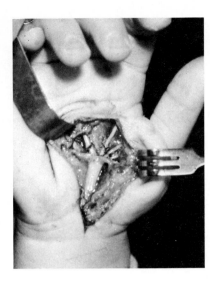

Fig. 24-64. Severed branches of median nerve have been reapproximated with fine sutures.

fords relief of pain and improves joint motion. Insertion of an implant is an adjunct to resection arthroplasty. The implant serves as a dynamic joint spacer, not a joint prosthesis. In severe cases, custom total joint prostheses may be used.

The most commonly used implants in hand surgery are flexible implants made of silicone rubber (Silastic). Flexible implants available for arthroplasty within the scope of hand surgery are finger joints (for MP and PIP joints), wrist joint, carpal trapezium, lunate, and navicular (scaphoid).

Procedural considerations. A plastic hand instrument set is required, plus the following:

Alloplastic rasps
Oscillating bone saw
Hall II drill with Swanson burrs
Alloplastic implant of choice (Fig. 24-4)
Esmarch bandage
Marking pen

The patient is placed in the supine position on the operating room bed, with the arm extended on a hand table. The hand drape is used.

Operative procedure
1. After the incision line is marked and the pneumatic tourniquet is inflated, the involved joint is exposed through an appropriate incision.
2. In finger joint resection arthroplasty, the joint surfaces are excised together with comprehensive soft tissue release of the joint capsule. In resection arthroplasty of a carpal bone, the involved bone is completely excised.
3. In finger joint arthroplasty, the medullary canals of the two adjacent bones are reamed with the Hall II drill with Swanson burrs. In carpal bone implant resection arthroplasty, holes are reamed in one appropriate adjacent bone.

4. The two stems of a finger or wrist joint implant or the single stem of a carpal bone implant is seated in adjacent bones.
5. Soft tissues of the joint capsule (ligaments, tendons) are repaired.
6. The skin incisions are closed.
7. A hand dressing is applied.

Palmar fasciectomy

Dupuytren's contracture is a progressive disease involving the palmar fascia and the digital extensions of the palmar fascia. It usually begins with a small nodular thickening in the palm, most frequently in line with the ring finger. With progression of the disease, additional nodules appear, usually with skin adherent to them. Subsequent contracted longitudinal bands of palmar fascia may appear beneath the skin. When the digital extension of the palmar fascia become involved in the disease process, flexion contractures of the finger MP and PIP joints result.

The cause of Dupuytren's contracture is unknown. One or both hands may be involved. The disease may also be present in the foot in the form of nodules and cords involving the plantar fascia. It does not result in contracture of the toes, however, because the plantar fascia has no digital (toe) extensions.

Surgery is the preferred treatment for Dupuytren's contracture, preferably at an early stage in the disease before irreparable joint damage occurs as the result of prolonged fixed flexion contracture. Surgical procedures include fasciotomy (simple division of contracted bands) or partial or total excision of the palmar fascia. In long-standing disease with irreversible joint changes, amputation of the finger may be the only treatment possible.

Procedural considerations. A plastic hand instrument set is required, plus an Esmarch bandage and a marking pen.

The patient is placed in the supine position on the operating room bed, with the arm extended on a hand table. The hand drape is used.

Operative procedure (Fig. 24-65)
1. Incision lines are marked, often with several Z-plasties to lengthen the involved skin of the finger and palm (as for scar revision).
2. The tourniquet is inflated.
3. After incisions are made, flaps of skin and subcutaneous tissue are carefully elevated to preserve their blood supply, exposing the fibrotic palmar fascia and its digital extensions.
4. Part or all of the palmar fascia and digital extensions is excised.
5. The tourniquet is usually released before skin closure so that hemostasis can be obtained.
6. Incisions are sutured. A shortage of skin is sometimes noted at this point, in which case coverage by means of a full-thickness skin graft is required.

A   B   C

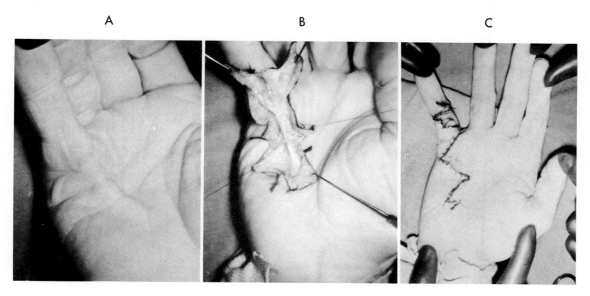

Fig. 24-65. Dupuytren's contracture involving palmar fascia and its digital extensions into little finger. **A,** Cord and nodules in palm with mild flexion contracture of little finger. **B,** Contracted band of palmar fascia exposed. **C,** Wound closure with multiple Z-plasties to lengthen contracted skin.

7. If skin grafts are used, they are stented, and then a hand dressing is applied.

Carpal tunnel release

The transverse carpal ligament is incised or excised, with or without synovectomy, to relieve the symptom complex produced by compression of the median nerve within the carpal canal at the wrist. The carpal tunnel is located along the volar surface of the wrist. Its rigid boundaries consist of carpal bones along three sides and the transverse carpal ligament along the fourth (volar) side. The median nerve, superficial and deep finger flexors, and the long thumb flexor tendon all pass through the carpal tunnel before entering the hand (Fig. 24-55). Any condition that decreases the size of the canal, such as fracture of a carpal bone, or increases its volume, such as the hypertrophic synovitis of rheumatoid arthritis, may cause pressure on the median nerve with resultant symptoms of carpal tunnel syndrome. However, in a majority of cases the cause of carpal tunnel syndrome is unknown.

The symptoms of median nerve compression at the wrist are usually pain and paresthesia in the thumb, the index finger, the long finger, and the radial half of the ring finger. Long-standing median nerve compression may result in hand weakness and thenar muscle atrophy. The condition may be unilateral or bilateral.

Procedural considerations. A plastic hand instrument set is required, plus an Esmarch bandage and a marking pen.

The patient is placed in the supine position on the operating room bed, with the arm extended on a hand table.

The hand drape is used. The operation may be performed under general, axillary block, or intravenous regional anesthesia.

Operative procedure

1. After appropriate skin marking and inflation of the pneumatic tourniquet, an incision is made across the volar wrist surface and base of the palm for adequate exposure of the transverse carpal ligament.
2. The transverse carpal ligament is incised along its entire length. A segment of it may be excised.
3. Synovectomy of structures within the carpal canal may or may not be performed.
4. The incision is closed in one layer.
5. A hand dressing is applied.

■ Microsurgery

Reconstructive microsurgery involves the use of an operating microscope and special instruments to reconstruct or replant tissue lost through injury or disease. Today's skilled microsurgeons can successfully anastomose the ends of a vessel measuring less than 1 mm in diameter. The success of microsurgery depends on several factors: (1) the individual and collective experiences of the surgical team and the members' ability to work together, relieving each other as necessary during long operations; (2) the surgeon's knowledge of the physiology of the microcirculation; (3) many hours of practice in the laboratory by the surgical team; and (4) the availability of proper microscopes (Fig. 24-66), microvascular instruments (Fig. 24-67), and microvascular suture.

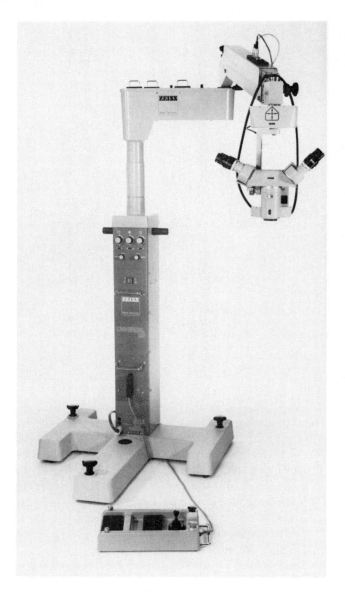

Fig. 24-66. Zeiss OPMI-6 operating microscope.

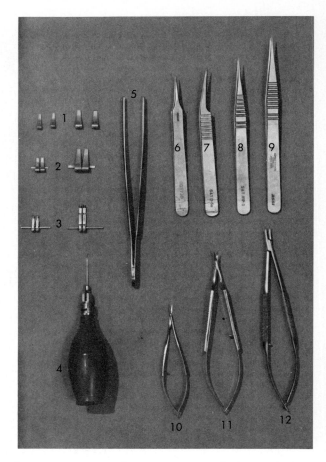

Fig. 24-67. Microvascular instruments. *1,* Single vessel clamps; *2,* approximator clamps; *3,* nerve approximator clamps; *4,* Bishop-Harmon irrigating bulb and cannula tip; *5,* clamp-applying forceps; *6,* jeweler's forceps; *7,* Acland vessel dilator; *8* and *9,* Pierse tissue forceps; *10,* Vannas scissors; *11,* Castroviejo-Vannas scissors; *12,* Barraquer needle holder.

Replantation of amputated body part

Replantation is an attempt to reattach a completely amputated digit or body part. Revascularization is the procedure performed on incomplete amputations, when the part remains attached to the body by skin, artery, vein, or nerve. Good candidates for replantation are those with the following amputations: (1) thumb, (2) multiple digits (Fig. 24-68), (3) through the palm, (4) wrist or forearm, (5) elbow and above the elbow, and (6) almost any body part of a child.

The success of digital replantation depends primarily on the microsurgical repair of one digital artery and two digital veins. Replantation of an amputated part is ideally performed within 4 to 6 hours after injury, but success has been reported up to 24 hours after injury if the amputated

part has been cooled. Proper care of the amputated body part(s) is vital to successful replantation (Fig. 24-69). The ultimate aim of replantation is the restitution of function beyond that provided by a prosthesis.

Procedural considerations. A regional anesthesia is usually given to replantation patients. Because of the length of these surgeries (12 to 16 hours), positioning is important. The operating room bed and armboards should be carefully padded with egg crate foam to support the supine patient. The surgeon may prefer the room temperature to be between 75° and 80° F before the patient arrives because the warm room will reduce vasoconstriction in the extremities. A K-thermia blanket may be placed between the sheet and the mattress of the operating room bed to keep the patient's body temperature between 98.6° and 101° F. The surgeon usually brings the amputated part to the operating room before the patient arrives to ensure ample time for preparation of the amputated part for replantation.

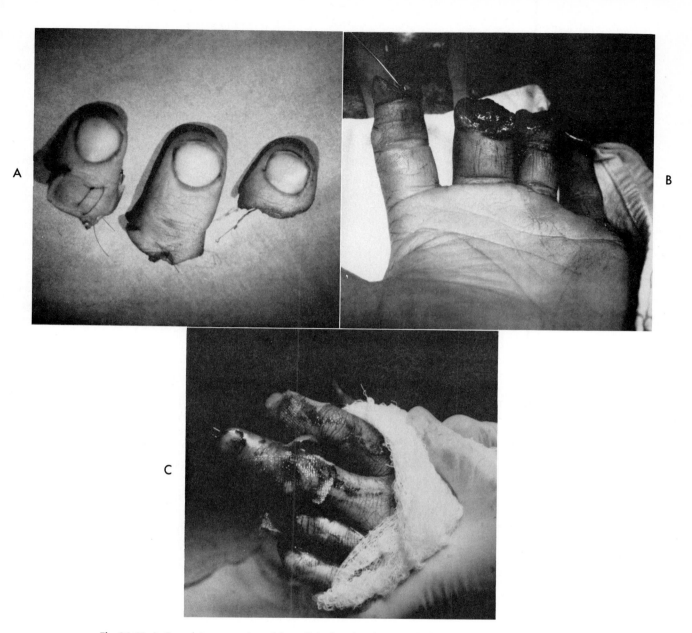

Fig. 24-68. A, Complete amputation of three digits from hand. **B,** Hand after amputation. **C,** Reattachment of three completely amputated digits to the hand.

Instrumentation includes a plastic hand instrument set, microvascular instruments, a Kirschner wire driver, Kirschner wires, an operating microscope, and a bipolar electrosurgical unit.

A pneumatic tourniquet cuff is placed on the patient's upper arm, and a hand drape is used.

Operative procedure

1. Bone ends are shortened to eliminate tension on vascular anastomoses to be done later; the bone is stabilized by means of internal fixation with Kirschner wires.

2. Flexor and extensor tendon repairs are usually performed next.

3. The digital nerves are repaired with the aid of loupes or the operating microscope.

4. With microsurgical instruments and techniques, two digital veins are repaired, followed by repair of one digital artery. If ischemic time has been prolonged, digital vessel repair may precede repair of tendons and nerves.

5. The skin is sutured.

6. A bulky supportive hand dressing is applied.

Toe-to-hand transfer

This reconstructive procedure involves surgical removal of a single or multiple toes and anastomosing of

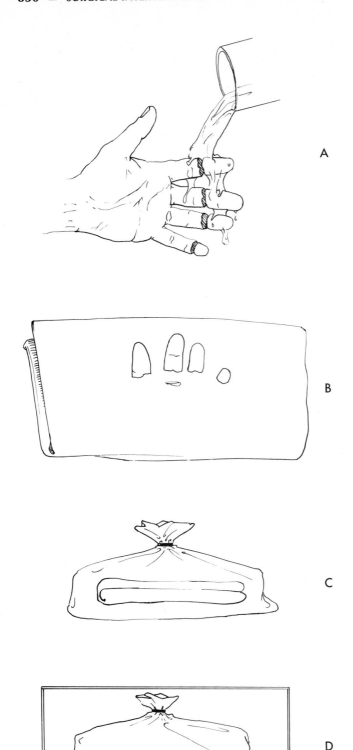

the vessels of the toes to those on the hand to restore finger and thumb functions. It is lengthy (12- to 16-hour) surgery, entailing a two-team approach, one at the foot for toe removal and one at the recipient site, the hand.

Procedural considerations. The patient is placed in the supine position on the operating room bed. The patient is placed on an anticoagulation regimen during the anastomosis procedure. Two tourniquets are needed, one on the thigh of the operative foot and one on the operative arm. Both extremities are separately prepped and draped. Instrumentation includes a plastic hand set, microvascular instruments, power Kirschner wire driver, and Kirschner wires. Additional equipment includes the operating microscope, two tourniquet power sources, two bipolar electrosurgical units, marking pen, and Esmarch bandage.

Operative procedure

1. The surgeon preparing the hand determines adequate blood flow and vessel location on the thumb or finger site (Fig. 24-70, *A*). This may prevent a needless amputation of the toe.
2. Appropriate skin flaps are incised to expose the veins on the dorsum of the hand and clamped with microvessel clips.
3. The radial artery or branches are dissected out and prepared for anastomosis.
4. The flexor and extensor pollicis longus tendons are located and transfixed.
5. The bone at the base of the thumb is prepared for the toe.
6. The nerves to the thumb are dissected out with adequate length for suturing without tension.
7. The toe is circumscribed with a racquet-shaped incision (Fig. 24-70, *B*), and the veins are isolated through the dorsal aspect and clamped with microvessel clips.
8. The extensor tendon is dissected proximally and transected over the base of the metatarsal.
9. The dorsalis pedis artery is dissected to the digital vessels with ligation of all branches of that vessel to prepare for the anastomosis.
10. On the plantar surface, the digital nerves and flexor tendons are transected at levels of adequate length for anastomosis (Fig. 24-70, *C*).
11. The toe is transected at the level previously determined for adequate length of the thumb.
12. The toe vessels are anastomosed microsurgically to the thumb vessels. The toe is attached to the thumb area by Kirschner wires (Fig. 24-70, *D*).

An aesthetic and functionally effective hand can be achieved through this procedure (Fig. 24-70, *E*).

Free jejunal tissue transfer

Reconstructive problems in patients undergoing laryngectomy and upper cervical esophagectomy can be adequately solved by free jejunal transfer. Modern micro-

Fig. 24-69. All severed body parts should be sought, including small pieces of mangled tissue. The following steps should be performed: **A,** Rinse; **B,** Wrap in moist towel; **C,** place towel in clean plastic bag and seal; **D,** cool on ice. The iced bag should be sent to the replantation center with the patient.

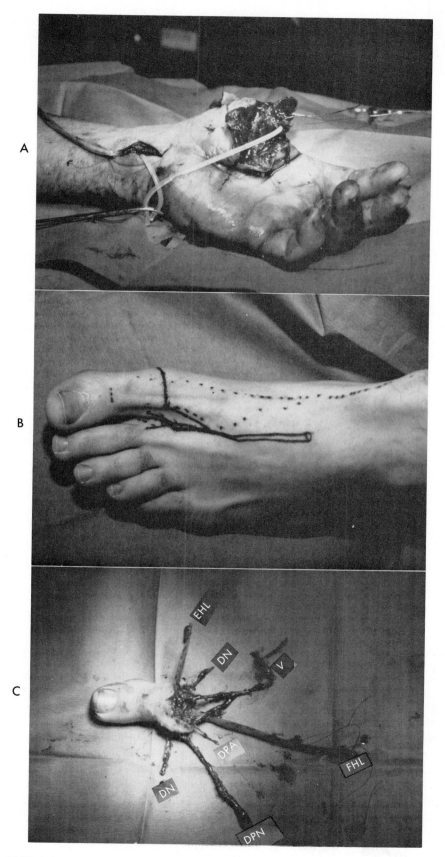

Fig. 24-70. A, Preparation of thumb site. **B,** Marking of toe. **C,** Identification of vessels. *DN,* Digital nerve; *DPN,* dorsalis pedis nerve; *DPA,* dorsalis pedis artery; *EHL,* extensor hallucis longus tendon; *FHL,* flexor hallucis longus tendon; *V,* vein.

Continued.

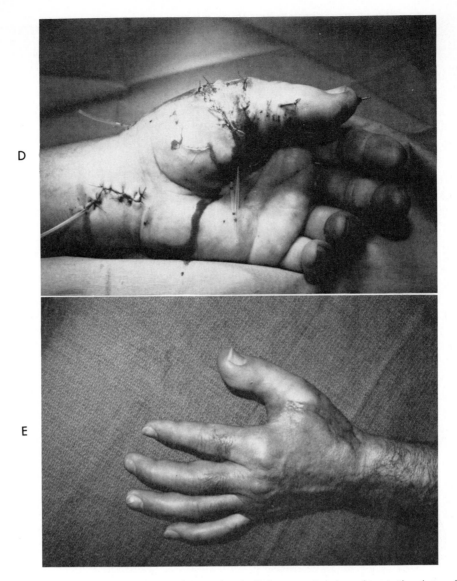

Fig. 24-70, cont'd. D, Attachment of toe to thumb. **E,** Postoperative view of toe-to-thumb transfer.

surgical techniques greatly improve the success rate. Free jejunal transfers have proved beneficial:

1. In patients with massive resection of the laryngopharynx when resection may extend into the oropharynx or even the lower nasopharynx and encompass a large portion of the cervical esophagus
2. In patients with radiation failure in whom laryngopharyngoesophagectomy is required
3. In patients with secondary reconstruction of the hypopharynx or cervical esophagus in whom other methods have failed because of flap necrosis or radiation
4. In patients in whom primary pharyngoesophageal radiation has resulted in hypopharyngeal stricture unresponsive to dilation

5. In isolated cases in which a large area of oral lining is lost

Procedural considerations. The patient is positioned, prepped, and draped for laryngectomy with the abdomen exposed. The abdomen is covered with sterile towels during laryngectomy. When laryngectomy is completed, all instruments and drapes are discarded after the wound has been covered with sterile towels. The patient is again prepped and draped for the free tissue graft.

The basic plastic instrument set is used, plus abdominal instruments for the graft and microsurgical and vascular instruments for the graft anastomosis. The operating microscope or loupes may be used for preparation of the graft and graft placement.

Operative procedure. A two-team approach is used. Neck dissection is carried out, at which time donor vessels are identified and preserved. The abdomen is opened, and the ligament of Treitz located. A suitable segment is identified in the first 2 feet of jejunum with a single dominant vascular pedicle. The segment with its pedicle is resected, and bowel continuity reestablished. The abdomen is closed as the microsurgeon prepares the bowel vessel for anastomosis. The donor-recipient vessels in the neck are prepared, using the microscope. The proximal bowel anastomosis is made, followed by the vascular anastomosis. When the microvascular clamps are removed, pulsation of the mesenteric vessels and peristalsis should begin. The distal bowel anastomosis is then done. The neck is closed, leaving a small Silastic window over the jejunal segment to allow for close, postoperative observation of the transplant.

REFERENCES

Benson, D.S., and Conte, R.R.: 89/90 Nursing Meds, Norwalk, 1989, Appleton & Lange.

Fritz, P.S.: Cosmetic surgery. In Wells, M. (ed.): Decision making in perioperative nursing, Philadelphia, 1987, B.C. Decker.

Seifert, P.C., and Rothrock, J.C.: Perioperative assessment tool. In Guzita, C.E., and others (eds.): Clinical assessment tools for use with nursing diagnoses, St. Louis, 1989, The C.V. Mosby Co.

Vasconez, L.O., and Vasconez, H.C.: Plastic and reconstructive surgery. In Way, L. (ed.): Current surgical diagnosis and treatment, Norwalk, Conn., 1988, Appleton & Lange.

BIBLIOGRAPHY

American Society of Plastic and Reconstructive Surgeons: Background information on suction lipectomy, developed for the media, Plast. Surg. News 8(1):12, 1983.

American Society of Plastic and Reconstructive Surgical Nurses, Inc.: Core curriculum for plastic and reconstructive surgical nursing, Pitman, NJ, 1989, Anthony J. Jannetti.

AORN: AORN standards and recommended practices for perioperative nursing, Denver, 1990, The Association.

Baptist, G.: Perioperative nursing roles. Plastic Surgical Nursing 5:86, 1985.

Black, J.: Nursing process for the craniofacial surgical patient. Plastic Surgery Nursing 5:18, 1985.

Bostwick, J.: Breast reconstruction following mastectomy. Contemporary Surgery 27:15, 1985.

Chang, W.H.: Fundamentals of plastic and reconstructive surgery, Baltimore, 1989, The Williams & Wilkins Co.

Cohen, B., and Aaronson, S.: Free tissue transfer, AORN J. 38:602, 1983.

Converse, J.M., editor: Reconstructive plastic surgery: principles and procedures in corrective reconstruction and transplantation, ed. 4, Philadelphia, 1983, W.B. Saunders Co.

Goin, J., and Goin, M.: Changing the body: psychological effects of plastic surgery, Baltimore, 1981, Williams & Wilkins.

Grabb, W.X., and Smith, J.W., editors: Plastic surgery: a concise guide to clinical practice, ed. 3, Boston, 1980, Little, Brown & Co.

Grazer, F.M., and Klingbeil, R., editors: Body image: a surgical perspective, St. Louis, 1980, The C.V. Mosby Co.

Grossman, J.A.: Abdominoplasty: indications and technique, AORN J. 44:582, 1986.

Gulanick, M., and others: Nursing care plans, St. Louis, 1986, The C.V. Mosby Co.

Harbal, M.B., and others: Advances in plastic and reconstructive surgery, Chicago, 1984, Year Book Medical Publishers.

Hester, R., and others: Reconstruction of cervical esophagus, hypopharynx and oral cavity using free jejunal transfer, Am. J. Surg. 140:487, 1980.

Hollinshead, W.H.: Anatomy for surgeons, vol. 3, ed. 3, New York, 1982, Harper & Row.

Holloway, N.M.: Medical Surgical Care Plans, Springhouse, Pa., 1988, Springhouse.

Horton, C.E.: Plastic and reconstructive surgery of the genital area, Boston, 1980, Little, Brown & Co.

Jacobs, S., and Stoldt, L.: Replantation for traumatic amputations, AORN J. 39:956, 1984.

Kaye, B., and Gradinger, G., editors: Symposium on problems and complications in aesthetic plastic surgery of the face. St. Louis, 1984, The C.V. Mosby Co.

Kutz, J., Thomson, C., and Klein, H.: Toe-to-hand transfers. In American Academy of Orthopaedic Surgeons: Symposium on microsurgery: practical use in orthopaedics, St. Louis, 1979, The C.V. Mosby Co.

Lindquist, J.: Psychological aspects of microsurgical replantation. Plastic Surgical Nursing 2:65, 1982.

Mangan, M.: Patient education with tissue expanders. Plastic Surgical Nursing 6:76, 1984.

Markland, A.: Nursing care of the suction lipectomy patient. Plastic Surgical Nursing 4:44, 1984.

Mathes, S.J., and Nahai, F.: Clinical atlas of muscle and musculocutaneous flaps, St. Louis, 1982, The C.V. Mosby Co.

Milford, L.: The hand, ed. 2, St. Louis, 1982, The C.V. Mosby Co.

Moncada, G.: Special nursing considerations for the craniofacial patient. Plastic Surgical Nursing 5:14, 1985.

Moncada, G.A.: Plastic and reconstructive surgery. In Rothrock, J. (ed.), Perioperative care planning, St. Louis, 1990, Mosby–Year Book, Inc.

Rees, T.D.: Aesthetic plastic surgery, Philadelphia, 1980, W.B. Saunders Co.

Tessier, P.: Plastic surgery of the orbit and eyelids, New York, 1981, Masson.

Woods, J.: Current state of the art in breast reconstruction, Plastic Surgical Nursing 4:85, 1984.

Woodward, J.R., and Cleveland, R.: Application of Horton-Devine principles to the repair of hypospadium, J. Urol. 127:1155, 1982.

25 Thoracic surgery

BRENDA S. GREGORY

Advances in clinical diagnostic methods and improvements in delivery of anesthesia have resulted in standardization of thoracic procedures over the last 30 years. Records reflect that until the present century, only small portions of the lung had been removed. As early as 1499 an unsuccessful excision of a herniation of the lung was recorded. In 1861, the French surgeon Péan removed part of a lung for tumor with recovery of the patient. During the late 1800s several successful procedures were completed; the conditions which required surgery included lung abscess, gangrene of the lungs, tumor, and trauma. The physiology of the lungs became less threatening as

sections or the entire lung were removed with complete recovery of the patient. The traumatic injuries, including gunshot and stab wounds, resulted in attempted successful and unsuccessful procedures. Treatment of tuberculosis, which has been attempted for centuries, also provided a reason for developments in thoracic procedures. Despite advances in treatment of other forms of cancer by chemotherapy or radiation therapy, lung resection remains the primary cure for malignancy of the lung. Indications for surgery of the lung and pleura include failure of conservative therapy, additional support of medical measures for the general disease, or treatment following trauma.

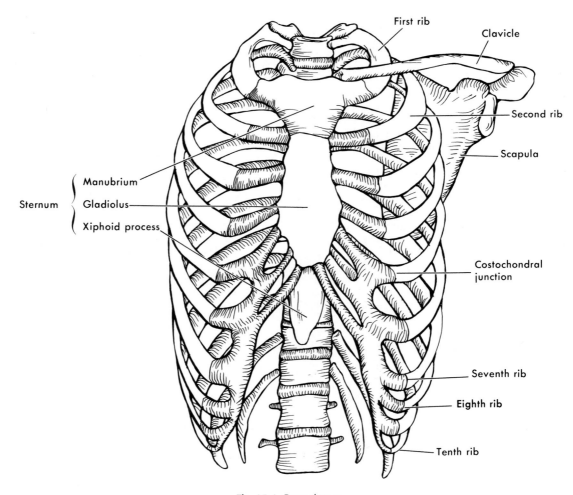

Fig. 25-1. Bony thorax.

SURGICAL ANATOMY

The skeletal framework of the thorax is formed anteriorly by the sternum and costal cartilages, laterally by the 12 pairs of ribs, and posteriorly by the 12 thoracic vertebrae (Figs. 25-1 and 25-2). This airtight compartment is enclosed in the root of the neck by Sibson's fascia and is separated from the abdomen by the diaphragm.

The sternum, or breastbone, forms the anterior thoracic wall in the midline. It consists of three parts: (1) the upper part, or manubrium; (2) the body, or gladiolus; and (3) the lower cartilage, or xiphoid process. The manubrium articulates with the clavicles and the first two ribs on each side; the gladiolus articulates with the remaining true ribs by separate costal cartilages; and the xiphoid fuses with the gladiolus in early development and is attached to the diaphragm by the substernal ligament (Figs. 25-1 and 25-3).

Normally, the lateral walls of the thorax are formed by the 12 pairs of ribs. Posteriorly, each pair of ribs articulates with its corresponding thoracic vertebra (Fig. 25-2). Anteriorly, the first seven ribs articulate with the sternum. The eighth, ninth, and tenth ribs articulate with the costal cartilages of the rib above; however, the eleventh and twelfth are not fixed to the costal arch (Fig. 25-1).

The muscles of each hemithorax (Figs. 25-3 and 25-4) include the 11 external and 11 internal intercostal muscles, which fill the spaces between the ribs.

An intercostal artery, vein, and nerve accompany each intercostal muscle. The arteries communicate with the internal thoracic artery anteriorly and arise from the aorta posteriorly. The intercostal veins follow the course of the arteries and communicate with the mammary veins anteriorly and with the azygos and hemiazygos veins posteriorly.

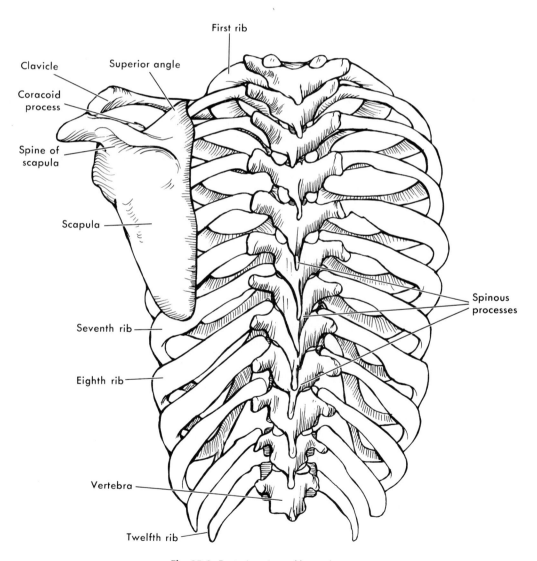

Fig. 25-2. Posterior view of bony thorax.

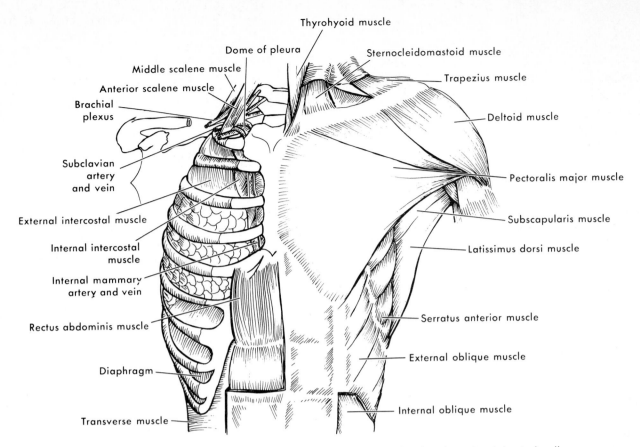

Fig. 25-3. Anterior view of thorax and contiguous portions of base of neck and anterior abdominal wall. *Right half,* Superficial layer of muscles and fascia; *left half,* relations of deep muscles of neck and abdomen to rib cage, intercostal muscles, diaphragm, and internal mammary vessels; relations of muscles, nerves, and vessels with first rib; and anterior relations of lung.

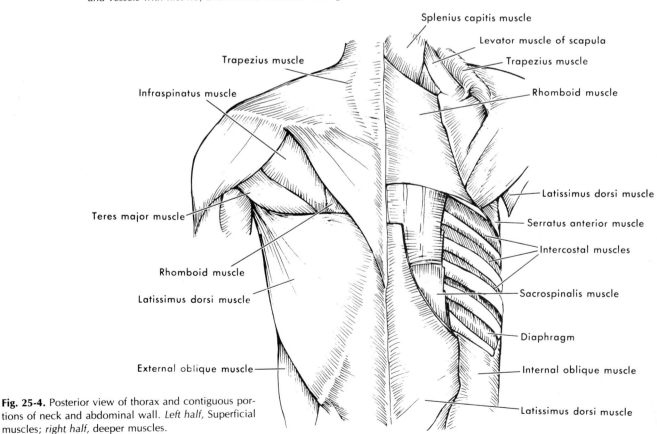

Fig. 25-4. Posterior view of thorax and contiguous portions of neck and abdominal wall. *Left half,* Superficial muscles; *right half,* deeper muscles.

During surgery, great care is taken to prevent injury to the intercostal nerve, which passes forward and alongside the posterior intercostal artery and which shares with the superior branch of the artery the intercostal groove on the inferior edge of the corresponding rib. When the nerve must be disturbed, an anesthetic agent may be injected to prevent postoperative pain.

The chest cavity is subdivided into the right and left pleural cavities, which contain the lungs and are separated by the mediastinum, which lies medially between the two pleural membranes. The *parietal pleura*, the membrane that lines the inner surface of each hemithorax, is adjacent to the inner surfaces of the ribs posteriorly and the mediastinum medially and covers the surface of the diaphragm except at the central portion. Part of the parietal membrane is reflected back at the root of each lung to form a sac around it. This reflection is called the *visceral pleura*. A serous secretion existing between these two membranes acts as a lubricant to minimize friction.

The lungs are the essential organs of respiration. The base of each lung rests on the diaphragm, whereas its apex (upper end) projects into the base of the neck at a level above the first rib. The bronchus, the nerves, the lymphatics, and the pulmonary and bronchial vessels enter and leave the lung on the mediastinal surface in a structure known as the hilum, or root, of the lung. Deep fissures

divide the spongy, porous lung into lobes. The primary bronchi divide, then subdivide in each lobe and eventually become bronchioles. The right lung has an upper, middle, and lower lobe, and the left lung has only an upper and lower lobe (Fig. 25-5). However, the lungs are similar in that each is composed of 10 major segments. Each segment extends to the pleural surface, expanding in volume from its center to its peripheral edges. Each segment also has its own bronchus and branches of the pulmonary artery and vein.

The bronchial arteries, arising from the aorta, supply nourishment to the lungs. They vary in their number and course. The arrangement may include two branches to the left lung and one branch to the right lung, which later branches into two, or there may be one branch for each lung or two branches for each lung. The pulmonary arteries carry the blood to the pulmonary parenchyma, and the pulmonary veins transport the oxygenated blood to the left atrium.

The nerves of the lungs are a part of the autonomic nervous system (Chapter 23). They regulate constriction and relaxation of the bronchi and of the blood vessels within the lungs.

Although the thoracic cavity is an airtight space, the lungs inspire outside air through the nasal passages, trachea, and bronchi. The main function of the lungs is to

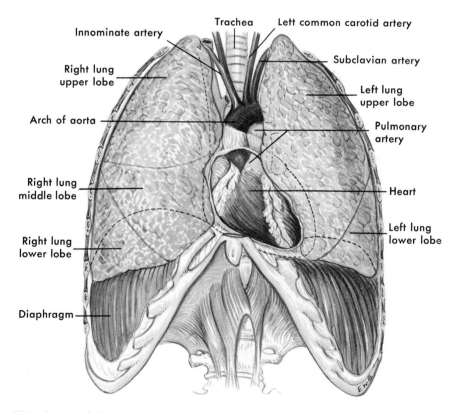

Fig. 25-5. Organs of thoracic cavity. Part of pericardium has been removed to expose heart. (From Schottelius, B.A., and Schottelius, D.D.: Textbook of physiology, ed. 18, St. Louis, 1978, The C.V. Mosby Co.)

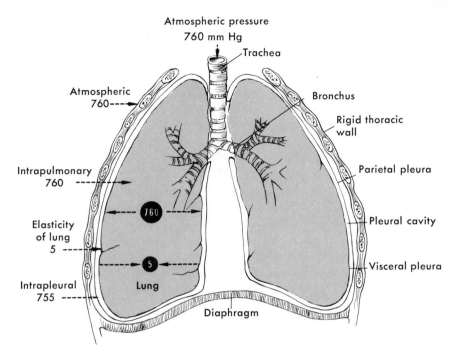

Fig. 25-6. Illustration of thoracic cavity structures showing intrapulmonary and intrapleural pressures with chest wall in resting position. (From Schottelius, B.A., and Schottelius, D.D.: Textbook of physiology, ed. 18, St. Louis, 1978, The C.V. Mosby Co.)

exchange carbon dioxide for oxygen. Normally, as the thorax expands, the lungs also expand and draw air in; as the thorax relaxes and compresses the lungs, air is forced out. Inspiration normally takes place when the intrathoracic pressure is slightly below atmospheric pressure (76 cm Hg or 760 mm Hg) and when a partial vacuum exists between the parietal and visceral pleural (intrathoracic) surfaces. As the muscles of inspiration contract to enlarge the chest cage, the lungs passively follow the diaphragm and chest wall because of decreased intrathoracic pressure. The acts of inspiration and expiration are the result of air moving in and out so the pressure is equal to that of the atmosphere at the end of expiration (Fig. 25-6).

The normal intrapleural pressure varies from -9 to -12 cm H_2O during inspiration and from about -3 to -6 cm H_2O during expiration. The greatest amount of air that can be expired after a maximum inspiration is termed the *vital capacity*. Size, age, gender, and pulmonary disease of the patient influence vital capacity. Any condition that interferes with the normally negative intrapleural pressure affects respiratory function.

PERIOPERATIVE NURSING CONSIDERATIONS
Assessment/nursing diagnosis

During assessment, the perioperative nurse gathers information (patient data) that is important to planning patient care. The perioperative nurse may begin data collection through a review of the patient's medical record, including results of the history, physical examination, laboratory and other diagnostic workups, and the nursing history and assessment. Important signs and symptoms that the patient has displayed are confirmed by the perioperative nurse during admission to the operating room, typically in the holding area. Part of the assessment focuses on the respiratory system. The nurse may question the patient or otherwise confirm the presence of an increased cough, increase in sputum production, recurrent hemoptysis, malaise, shortness of breath, substernal chest discomfort, weight loss, poor appetite, adequacy of nutrition, and hypoxia. The results of the physical examination of the chest should be reviewed; the perioperative nurse may auscultate the chest and confirm the presence of crackles or wheezes on inspiration or expiration. These respiratory sounds may be persistent if the disease state is advanced.

The results of diagnostic and laboratory tests should be reviewed. These tests may include the chest x-ray, which will be needed in the operating room. This film outlines the lesion, if any is present, and defines its shape and space-occupying nature (that is, tracheal shift). The presence of air in the hilar region, pleural effusion, or atelectasis may also be confirmed by radiological evidence. Sputum analysis for culture and sensitivity may alert the perioperative nurse to an infectious process; cytology may confirm a malignancy. The patient may have already undergone diagnostic bronchoscopy or mediastinoscopy; if so, the results should be reviewed for AFB smear, culture, bronchial washing, and biopsy results. Computed tomography (CT) scans of the chest, as well as the brain, liver, and abdomen, may reveal the presence or absence of metastasis; radioisotope scans may have been done for similar reasons. The results of pulmonary function tests and arterial blood gases should be reviewed; they assist the perioperative nurse in collaborating with the surgical team to maintain effective gas exchange during the surgical intervention. Patients hospitalized for surgery related to carcinoma may have received chemotherapy or radiation therapy prior to surgery; assessment of the skin and the patient's general condition is important in preventing perioperative complications.

Following a general and focused review of the patient's medical record and patient interview, the perioperative nurse formulates nursing diagnoses. These statements reflect actual or potential problems in which the perioperative nurse will intervene, either independently or collaboratively with the surgical team. Nursing diagnoses should be individualized and prioritized for each patient. Nonetheless, nursing diagnoses that might be common to the patient undergoing thoracic surgery include the following:

- Potential for impaired gas exchange related to the surgical intervention
- Potential for impaired skin integrity related to surgical positioning, length of the surgical intervention, and/or the use of chemical antimicrobial agents on the skin
- Potential for injury related to positioning, use of equipment, and length of the surgical intervention
- Potential for fluid volume excess related to decreased surface area of the lung for perfusion and administration of IV fluids during surgery
- Potential for infection related to inadequate secondary defenses (presence of existing disease process) and surgical disruption of tissues

Planning

The plan of nursing care includes goals derived from the nursing diagnoses. These goals need to be measurable; they will become part of the process of evaluation. The perioperative nurse needs to identify criteria by which goals will be measured. For example, for the goal "The patient will maintain adequate gas exchange," the perioperative nurse might select such criteria as pink skin, nailbeds, or mucusa; normothermia; adequate capillary refill; lung sounds clear to auscultation and percussion; normal chest excursion; and vital signs and pulse oximetry readings that are within normal ranges. Once goals are derived, nursing interventions are specified to achieve the goals. A Sample Care Plan for the patient having thoracic surgery might be as shown on pp. 840-841.

Implementation

During implementation of the plan of care, the perioperative nurse is concerned with both preparatory patient considerations (such as positioning, presurgical diagnostic interventions, draping) and the requirements of the surgical intervention (medications, instruments, equipment, and supplies). These patient care needs are coordinated with the other nursing interventions identified in the specific patient care plan.

Endoscopy
Medications

Topical, local, or general anesthesia may be used. The topical (or local) anesthetic setup should include:

1 Headlight
2 Laryngeal mirrors, various sizes
1 Lingual spatula
2 Sprays with straight and curved cannulae and anesthetic drugs, as ordered
1 Laryngeal syringe with straight and curved cannulae
1 Jackson cross-action forceps
1 Schindler pharyngeal anesthetizer, if desired
2 Medication cups
1 Emesis basin
1 Basin, small, with very warm water
1 Luer-Lok syringe, 10 ml, and needles, 20 and 22 gauge, for transtracheal injection
6 Gauze sponges, 4 × 4 inches
1 Box paper tissues
1 Adjustable stretcher
1 Footstool

The anesthetic drugs frequently used are lidocaine (Xylocaine), procaine (Novocain), and tetracaine (Pontocaine) with or without epinephrine. Cetacaine may be also used.

Pauses of 3 to 4 minutes are taken between applications of the anesthetic agent to the tongue, palate, and pharynx, and then to the larynx and to the trachea. The anesthetic agent is applied by means of a spray or laryngeal syringe with a straight or curved cannula.

Some physicians prefer to have the patient sit upright and gargle with the topical anesthetic mixture, rinse it around in the mouth, and then expectorate it, thereby producing a partial anesthesia of the buccal mucosa and pharynx.

For direct bronchoscopy a long metal cannula attached to a syringe is generally used to apply the anesthetic agent to the surface of the vocal cords; then the agent is injected through the anesthetized glottis into the trachea. This act causes the patient to produce a sharp, sudden cough.

For intrabronchial anesthesia a portion of the anesthetic agent is introduced through the bronchoscope.

Refer to Chapter 9 for perioperative nursing considerations when monitoring the patient receiving local or monitored anesthesia care.

Draping

Aseptic technique is used during an endoscopy. The principles of draping for other procedures are followed (Chapter 5).

Sample Care Plan

NURSING DIAGNOSIS:
Potential for impaired gas exchange related to surgical intervention
GOAL:
The patient will experience adequate gas exchange during the surgical procedure.
INTERVENTIONS:
Determine the preoperative status of gas exchange by laboratory results and assessing the patient; report deviations of studies.
Obtain chest x-rays for the intraoperative period.
Obtain the double-lumen endotracheal tube with a soft, inflatable cuff.
Obtain humidifier for ventilator gases.
Obtain equipment for and monitor arterial blood gases.
Obtain equipment for and assist with patient preparation for hemodynamic monitoring: ECG, CO_2 analyzer, pulse oximeter, arterial pressure, central venous pressure; evaluate results provided by these monitoring devices during procedure.
Obtain equipment for temperature monitoring; check temperature during procedure.
Obtain thermal blanket and place on operating room bed; check equipment prior to procedure; monitor during procedure.
Place ECG monitoring pads; monitor for arrhythmias.
Position the patient to provide access to the endotracheal tube, efficient ventilatory function, and prevention of injury.
Obtain and label specimens (ABG, blood count) to be sent to laboratory; evaluate results of tests and report abnormal values.

NURSING DIAGNOSIS:
Potential for impaired skin integrity related to position, length of surgical intervention and/or use of antimicrobial agents on the skin
GOAL:
The patient's skin integrity will be maintained.
INTERVENTIONS:
Note skin integrity preoperatively.

Determine presence of preexisting conditions that could compromise skin integrity (age, obesity, diabetes, allergies, radiation therapy).
Pad the operating room bed.
Apply principles of positioning for efficient circulatory function for lateral or supine position during the procedure; protect vulnerable neurovascular bundles.
Identify and pad pressure sites:
1. Lateral position: ear, acromion process, iliac crest, greater trochanter, medial and lateral condyles, malleolus
2. Supine position: occiput, scapula, olecranon, sacrum, ischial tuberosity, calcaneous
Stabilize the patient in lateral position on the operating room bed; check for tape sensitivity if adhesive tape is used.
If hair is removed from the operative site, use clippers or a depilatory (check patient sensitivity); shave the patient with wet shave if a razor must be used.
Prevent pooling of skin preparation solutions at the bedline, site of ECG electrodes, or electrosurgical dispersive pad.
Monitor temperature of thermal unit during the procedure.
Note skin integrity postoperatively; compare to preoperative status.

NURSING DIAGNOSIS:
Potential for injury related to positioning, use of equipment, and length of surgical intervention
GOAL:
The patient will be free from injury.
INTERVENTIONS:
Test equipment prior to procedure.
Position the patient in the best possible body alignment to allow visualization of the operative field.
1. Assess for preexisting conditions (joint implants, arthritis, restricted movement).
2. Stabilize the patient in lateral position (beanbag, sandbag, soft shoulder roll, pillows between knees).

Sample Care Plan—cont'd

3. Flex the upper arm slightly (not exceeding 90-degree extension) above the head on a raised padded armboard or supported on padding.
4. Use adequate number of individuals to position the patient for the lateral position.

Consider principles of placement when placing the electrosurgical dispersive pad; shave the area if necessary.

Decrease surgical time by anticipating needs of the patient and surgical team; use instruments and equipment properly.

Be familiar with the surgical intervention and its planned execution.

Complete sponge, sharp, and instrument counts.

Secure tubing from urinary and chest catheters; maintain tubing patency.

NURSING DIAGNOSIS:

Potential for fluid volume excess related to decreased surface area of the lung for perfusion and administration of IV fluids during surgery

GOAL:

The patient will maintain appropriate fluid balance.

INTERVENTIONS:

Insert indwelling urinary catheter; use aseptic technique.

Position drainage bag off floor, where it is readily observable.

Observe urinary output hourly during the procedure; report output less than 30 cc per hour.

Provide access for administration of IV fluids; assist with administration and insertion of lines.

Monitor results of hemodynamic parameters; report appropriately.

Monitor blood loss during the procedure; report appropriately.

Provide blood (including autologous) or blood products for fluid replacement; assist in replacement therapy and patient monitoring.

Observe for symptoms of shock (hypotension, abnormal ECG); report symptoms and initiate corrective nursing actions.

Observe for symptoms of excess blood loss (rapid, weak pulse, rapid respirations, cool, moist skin, and early, slight rise in blood pressure); report symptoms and initiate corrective nursing actions.

Observe for symptoms of fluid excess (tachycardia, increased blood pressure); report symptoms and initiate corrective nursing actions.

Have available and administer furosemide (Lasix) and other diuretic agents as prescribed; monitor for therapeutic results.

NURSING DIAGNOSIS:

Potential for infection related to inadequate secondary defenses (presence of existing disease process) and surgical disruption of tissues

GOAL:

The patient will be free of infection.

INTERVENTIONS:

Create and maintain a sterile field.

Wear proper operating room attire.

Utilize aseptic technique when opening supplies, moving about the sterile field, completing skin preparation, catheterizing the patient, and inserting intravenous lines.

Complete skin preparation at the incision site and point of insertion of monitoring lines to decrease microbial contamination.

Monitor traffic patterns; limit the number of individuals entering and leaving the operating room.

Administer antibiotic of choice for irrigation and intravenous administration; check for patient allergies; record all medications administered by the perioperative nurse or from the sterile field.

Decrease surgical time by anticipating patient needs.

Monitor sterile technique of team members; initiate corrective action for breaks in technique.

Obtain appropriate suture; consider whether patient is obese, malnourished, or presents with symptoms of a secondary disease process when selecting suture.

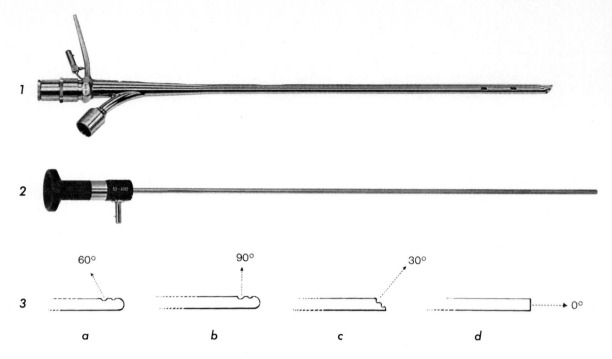

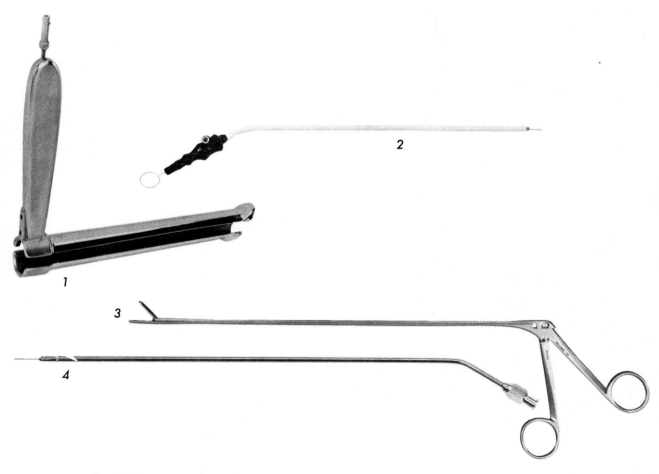

Fig. 25-7. Instruments for bronchoscopy. *1,* Holinger ventilating fiberoptic bronchoscope; *2,* fiberoptic light carrier; *3,* fiberoptic bronchoscopic telescopes: *a,* forward oblique 60°; *b,* lateral 90°; *c,* right angle 30°; *d,* forward 0°. (Courtesy Pilling Co., Fort Washington, Pa.)

Fig. 25-8. Instruments for mediastinoscopy. *1,* Carlens mediastinoscope; *2,* insulated suction tube; *3,* Jackson laryngeal forceps; *4,* aspirating needle. (Courtesy Pilling Co., Fort Washington, Pa.)

Instrumentation

Instruments are designed for direct inspection and observation of the larynx, trachea, bronchi, or mediastinum; to remove secretions; to obtain washings or tissue for bacterial and cytologic studies, or to remove tissue. They are also designed to remove foreign bodies.

Bronchoscope. The standard bronchoscope is a rigid speculum for visualizing the tracheobronchial tree. The rigid bronchoscope might be selected for biopsy of a large central mass, removal of a large foreign object, or biopsy of a vascular mass to provide a mechanism for hemorrhage control less possible with the flexible bronchoscope. The rigid bronchoscope remains the instrument of choice for removal of foreign bodies in infants and children. A fiberoptic light carrier is inserted into the bronchoscope to illuminate the distal opening. A side channel has been incorporated into the bronchoscope to permit aeration of the lungs with oxygen or anesthetic gases (Fig. 25-7). An additional device, the Sanders Venturi system, which is available to the anesthesiologist, provides adequate patient observation and ventilation during bronchoscopies and laryngoscopies. Fiberoptic telescopes permit visualization of the upper, middle, and lower lobe bronchi. They can be passed in patients with jaw deformity or rigid cervical spine with less difficulty than the rigid scope. Flexible fiberoptic bronchoscopes are being used with increased frequency, as is video endoscopy.

Mediastinoscope. The mediastinoscope is used to view lymph nodes or masses in the superior mediastinum. The instrument is a hollow tube with a fiberoptic light carrier (Fig. 25-8). A fiberoptic illuminator with a light intensity dial provides power and control of illumination (Fig. 25-9).

Lasers. The Nd:YAG laser might be used for endobronchial stenosis or photoradiation of bronchogenic cancer during a bronchoscopy. Use of laser equipment requires a thorough understanding of the equipment, responsibilities, and the procedure (Chapter 10).

Light carriers, cord, and illuminator. Each standard scope requires a fiberoptic light carrier, cord, and illuminator. Duplicates of each, along with the appropriate replacement light bulbs for the illuminator, should be available for immediate use.

The light source (Figs. 25-9 and 25-10) should be tested periodically and also immediately before use.

Sponge carriers and sponges. The metal sponge carrier (Fig. 25-11) consists of two parts: an inner rod, which has two jaws protruding from its distal end, and an outer band, which is screwed down on the inner rod so a sponge can be held securely within the jaws. Small gauze sponges are used to keep the field dry, remove secretions, or apply a topical anesthetic agent.

Specimen collectors. Cytologic specimen collectors, such as the Clerf (Fig. 25-11) or Lukens, are used to hold secretions as they are obtained.

Aspirators. Aspirating tubes of different lengths and designs (Fig. 25-11) are used to remove secretions and collect material for microscopic examination and cultures. The straight aspirating tube with one or two openings at the distal end is used to remove material from the pharynx, larynx, and esophagus. The curved aspirating tube with a flexible tip is used to remove secretions from the upper and dorsal orifices of the bronchi.

Forceps. Various types of forceps are designed to remove foreign bodies or tissues for histologic study. In bronchoscopy a biting tip forceps may be used to secure tissue for study. A forceps with jaws that veer laterally at about a 45-degree angle from the instrument's axis permits visualization during the biopsy maneuver. A bronchoesophageal forceps (Fig. 25-12) consists of a stylet, a cannula with a handle, a screw, a locknut, and a set screw. Forceps for laryngeal and bronchial regions are designed to remove tissue specimens.

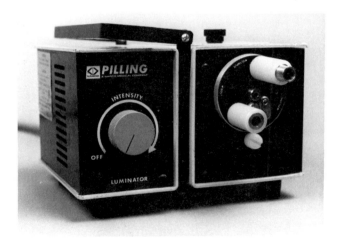

Fig. 25-9. Fiberoptic illuminator with multipurpose adaptor that accepts several types of fiberoptic light cords. (Courtesy Pilling Co., Washington, Pa.)

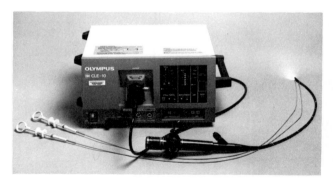

Fig. 25-10. Cold light source with flexible endoscope. (Courtesy Olympus, New Hyde Park, N.Y.)

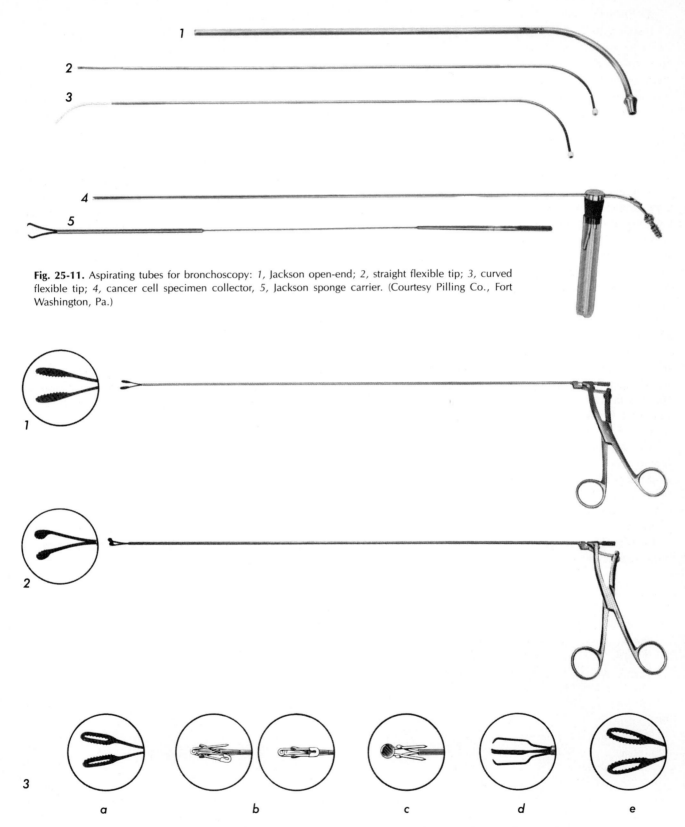

Fig. 25-11. Aspirating tubes for bronchoscopy: *1,* Jackson open-end; *2,* straight flexible tip; *3,* curved flexible tip; *4,* cancer cell specimen collector, *5,* Jackson sponge carrier. (Courtesy Pilling Co., Fort Washington, Pa.)

Fig. 25-12. Forceps for bronchoscopy. *1,* Jackson forward grasping forceps with serrated, cupped jaws; *2,* Jackson side-curved grasping forceps; *3,* forceps for foreign body removal: *a,* Jackson fenestrated peanut grasping, *b,* Clerf-Arrowsmith safety pin closer, *c,* Jackson approximation forceps, *d,* Gordon bead grasping, *e,* Jackson fenestrated meat grasping forceps. (Courtesy Pilling Co., Fort Washington, Pa.)

Handling, terminal disinfection, and care

Handling of instruments. To ensure long life of the optical system of endoscopes, each instrument should be kept straight at all times when not in use. Flexible endoscopes should never be severely bent.

Only the instrument manufacturer should replace a scope part. When a telescope is sent for repair, it must be properly packed in a padded instrument case and placed within a padded carton to ensure protection of the lens system during transportation. A direct blow can break the objective window or lenses of telescopic endoscopes. The junction of the flexible and rigid portions of the scope is the most vulnerable point.

During use, the patient might bite down while the flexible portion of the scope is being passed. A specially designed mouthpiece may be used to prevent damage to the scope. The sheath covering the flexible part may become perforated after contact. When a new covering is needed, the instrument should be sent to the manufacturer.

Cleaning endoscopes. Rigid endoscopes can be cleaned with soap and water. Terminal disinfection should be accomplished with activated glutaraldehyde or by steam sterilization if the scope is heat and pressure tolerant. The manufacturer's procedures for cleaning, terminally disinfecting, or terminally sterilizing flexible endoscopes should be followed. Usually, the flexible scopes can be washed with soap and water, then soaked in activated glutaraldehyde or an iodophor concentrate germicide. If feasible, they should be sterilized by ethylene oxide. In some facilities, specially designed washers, and in some cases sterilizers, may be available for terminal processing of endoscopes.

Cleaning a telescopic endoscope. The scope is held vertically by its ocular end and is wiped repeatedly with downward strokes, using gauze sponges or a soft brush saturated with surgical soap and water. Special attention is given to surface joints and crevices that may retain mucus. The scope is then dried thoroughly with clean gauze sponges.

Optical telescopes should never undergo boiling or steam sterilization. Sterilization can be accomplished with ethylene oxide. High-level disinfection is achieved by use of a noncorrosive microbicidal solution.

Cleaning aspirating tubes and sponge carriers. These instruments are cleaned and flushed with soap and water and are sterilized by steam or gas. Special care must be given to spiral-tipped aspirators. All bent or broken-tipped aspirators should be sent to the manufacturer for repair.

The sponge carrier collar must be unscrewed before it is cleaned. After sterilization the threads of the carrier are oiled. The carrier is reassembled and stored lying straight.

Cleaning forceps. The forceps may be placed in an ultrasonic cleaner. After cleaning, each forceps is taken apart, one at a time, by unscrewing the nut and removing the stylet. All parts are examined carefully, and noncorrosive solvent oil is applied to the crotch of the forceps.

Each forceps is reassembled and the action tested; then it is stored lying straight with jaws open. In perfect forceps (1) the jaws are close together in parallel position; (2) the handles just touch when the jaws are closed; (3) the jaws go into the cannula when the forceps is closed and protrude widely without expanding the spring when it is open; (4) the end nut, located in the stylet, is in place; (5) the side screw is tight; and (6) the distal end and jaws' edges are smooth on finger examination.

Setting and testing the illumination. To test the fiberoptic light carrier and telescope, the instrument should be held vertically by the ocular end. The endoscope should always be tested immediately before passage into the patient. The light intensity dial should be set at the proper level, as specified by the manufacturer. The light source should be switched on and off to test its function.

Postprocedure concerns

Patient safety during and following endoscopy under topical or local anesthesia is a concern due to medications administered. The gag reflex may not return for 2 to 3 hours. The patient should be restricted from any oral intake until the gag reflex has returned. During bronchoscopy, particularly rigid, teeth could be loosened or oral structures damaged. The lips, teeth, and oral mucosa should be examined to assure undisturbed integrity. Patients are also anxious to know the results of the procedure and benefit from openness and willingness to discuss feelings and perceptions.

Thoracotomy
Positioning

Thoracotomies can be performed with the patient commonly in one of three positions. The type of position is determined by the operative procedure planned. There are three basic approaches: (1) posterolateral thoracotomy, (2) anterolateral thoracotomy (Fig. 25-13), and (3) median sternotomy. The prone position can also provide access in some procedures.

Draping

The drapes are a fenestrated sheet or single sheets surrounding the incision site. A magnetic pad could be placed on the drapes below the incision site when the patient is placed in lateral position to prevent instruments from falling from the field.

Instrumentation

Instrumentation for thoracic surgery includes the laparotomy instrument set (Chapter 11), plus the following specialty items (Figs. 25-14 and 25-15).

Cutting instruments

  2 Nelson scissors, curved, 10 inches (Fig. 25-14)
  1 Potts tenotomy scissors, 7½ inches
  1 Potts dissecting scissors, angulated 60-degree, 7½ inches
  1 Wire cutter

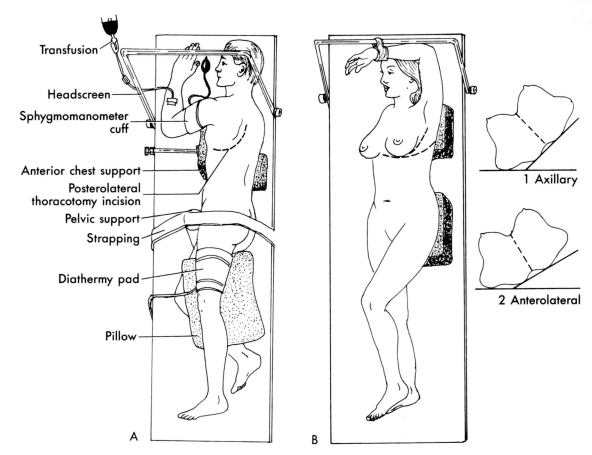

Labels (A): Transfusion, Headscreen, Sphygmomanometer cuff, Anterior chest support, Posterolateral thoracotomy incision, Pelvic support, Strapping, Diathermy pad, Pillow

Labels (B): 1 Axillary, 2 Anterolateral

Fig. 25-13. Positions for thoracotomy incisions. **A,** Lateral position for posterolateral incision. **B,** Semi-lateral position for axillary or anterolateral position.

Holding instruments

14 Backhaus towel clamps, 5 inches
2 Potts-Smith vascular forceps, smooth, 7 inches
2 Potts-Smith vascular forceps, fine-toothed, 7 inches
6 Rumel thoracic clamps, 9 inches (Fig. 25-14)
4 Duval lung-grasping forceps (Fig. 25-14)
1 Semb forceps, 9¼ inches

Clamping instruments

6 Right-angled clamps, assorted lengths and angulations
4 Sarot or Lees bronchus clamps, right and left (Fig. 25-14)

Vascular instruments

2 Crafoord coarctation clamps
4 Patent ductus clamps, 2 angulated and 2 straight
2 Satinsky clamps
2 Cooley clamps

Bone instruments (Fig. 25-15)

1 Alexander periosteotome
1 Overholt elevator
2 Doyen rib raspatories and elevators, 1 right and 1 left
1 Liston-Stille bone-cutting forceps
1 Bethune rib shears

1 Sauerbruch rib rongeur, double-action, square jaw
1 Stille-Luer bone rongeur, multiple action

Median sternotomy instruments

1 Sternal saw (Fig. 25-15)
1 Lebsche sternal knife (Fig. 25-15)
1 Mallet
1 Sternal spreader
1 Sternal approximator
2 Bone tenacula, single-hook
1 Bone punch or awl with fenestrated tip

Retractors

2 Volkmann rake retractors, blunt, six- or eight-pronged
2 Kelly retractors, large
1 Burford-Finochietto rib retractor with 2 sets blades (Fig. 25-15)
3 Finochietto retractors, assorted sizes (Fig. 25-15)
2 Bailey rib contractors (Fig. 25-15)
1 Davidson scapula retractor (Fig. 25-15)

Suturing instruments

6 Sarot needle holders, 10 inches and 12 inches
4 Hemoclip appliers
Bronchus or thoracic stapler

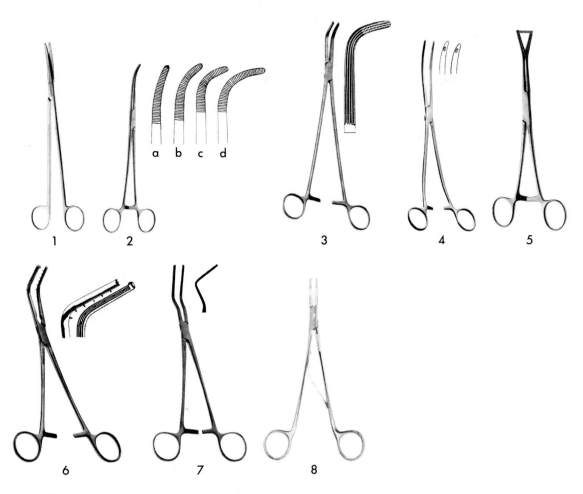

Fig. 25-14. Instruments for lobectomy and pneumonectomy. *1,* Nelson scissors; *2,* Rumel thoracic clamps, *a* to *d*; *3,* Harrington forceps; *4,* Willauer-Allis thoracic tissue forceps; *5,* Duval lung-grasping forceps; *6,* Sarot Bronchus clamp; *7,* Lees Bronchus clamp; *8,* hemoclip appliers. (*1* through *7,* courtesy Codman & Shurtleff, Inc., Randolph, Mass.; *8,* courtesy Zimmer, Inc., Warsaw, Ind.)

Accessory items

    Electrosurgical unit
2 Disposable chest catheters, selected sizes (with appropriate connectors)
1 Bone wax
2 Asepto syringes
1 Water-seal drainage system (Fig. 25-16)
2 Suction tubings, 6-foot lengths
6 Pieces umbilical tape, 18 inches

Nursing staff should determine the thoracic surgery arrangement of items on the instrument table and Mayo stand; this arrangement should be an effective standard method that applies principles of work simplification and thorough knowledge of procedures.

Chest tubes

In the presence of restrictive and obstructive pulmonary disease, the lung may not fully expand or contract, causing a reduction in alveolar ventilation with resultant hypoxia.

Other conditions that interfere with respiratory function are mucus, a foreign body in a bronchus, closed pneumothorax (simple and tension types), open pneumothorax, hemothorax, and multiple rib injuries that produce paradoxic motion of the thoracic cage (Fig. 25-17).

The normal function of the lungs is caused by elasticity and negative intrapleural pressure. Collapse of the normal lung follows any condition that reduces or eliminates the negative intrapleural pressure if the lung is not adherent to the chest wall. When the pleural space is filled with air, reducing the negative pressure, the lung collapses. This action may cause complete collapse if the pressure within the intrathoracic (pleural) space becomes positive.

A diminished negative pressure or occurrence of actual positive pressure in one pleural space may cause the mediastinum to shift toward the opposite side. When this happens, not only does the affected lung collapse because of a positive pressure in the pleural space but also the

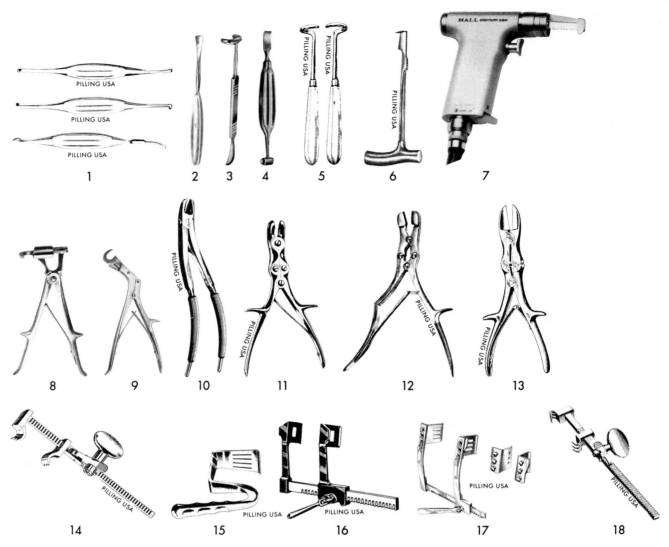

Fig. 25-15. Instruments for thoracotomy. *1,* Overholt elevators, nos. 1, 2, and 3; *2,* Langenbeck periosteal elevator; *3* Matson rib elevator and stripper; *4,* Alexander costal periosteotome; *5,* Doyen rib raspatories, right and left; *6,* Lebsche sternal knife; *7,* sternal saw; *8,* Sauerbruch rib shear; *9,* Giertz (first rib) rib guillotine; *10,* Bethune rib shears; *11,* Stille-Luer bone rongeur; *12,* Sauerbruch rib rongeur; *13,* Stille-Liston bone-cutting forceps, straight; *14,* Bailey rib spreader; *15,* Davidson scapula retractor; *16,* Finochietto rib retractor;*17,* Burford rib retractor with two sets detachable blades; *18,* Bailey rib retractor. (*1, 5, 6,* and *10* through *18,* courtesy Pilling Co., Fort Washington, Pa.; *2, 4, 8,* and *9,* courtesy Edward Weck and Co., Research Triangle Park, N.C.; *7,* courtesy Zimmer, Inc., Warsaw, Ind.)

function of the lung on the opposite side may be impaired as a result of compression by the shifted mediastinum. Tension pneumothorax can produce serious effects as air continues to escape from the lung into the intrapleural space. The air is unable to return to the bronchi to be exhaled, thereby increasing the intrapleural pressure. When a large opening in the chest wall allows direct communication of the pleural space with atmospheric pressure, it may cause death if the mediastinum becomes mobile. The exposure of the pleural space to atmospheric pressure collapses the affected lung. The positive pressure is also transmitted to the mediastinum, which in turn shifts toward

the opposite side and may cause the opposite lung to collapse.

Paradoxic motion of the chest results from severe instability of the chest wall because of multiple and often bilateral rib fractures; with inspiration, partial collapse of the thoracic space occurs. The blunt injury that caused the multiple rib fractures also causes severe contusion of the lung itself. This contusion contributes to impairment of lung function by affecting gas exchange, which may result in severe, life-threatening hypoxia.

One or more chest tubes may be inserted for postoperative closed chest drainage. The chest tubes provide a

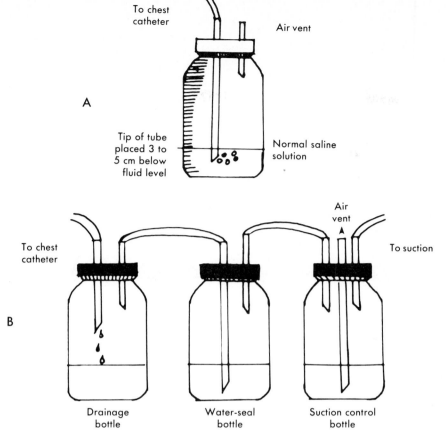

Fig. 25-16. Methods of draining pleural space, using bottle system as model. **A,** Single bottle used for water-seal drainage. **B,** Three-bottle system used for water-seal suction.

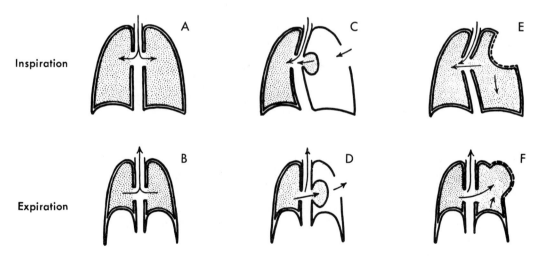

Fig. 25-17. Pathophysiology of severe chest injuries. **A** and **B,** Normal physiology of inspiration and expiration. **C** and **D,** Open (sucking) wound of thorax. On inspiration, air at atmospheric pressure rushes in through defect, **C,** collapsing lung. Next, positive pressure causes mediastinum to shift, compressing opposite lung. On expiration, **D,** air from lung on uninjured side reenters collapsed lung and is rebreathed in next inspiration. Impaired cardiopulmonary function in presence of sucking wound of chest is caused by (1) collapse of lung on injured side; (2) partial collapse of opposite lung; (3) increased functional dead space caused by rebreathing of unoxygenated air from collapsed lung; and (4) diminished venous return to right side of heart. **E** and **F,** Primary effect of paradoxical motion resulting from flail or stove-in chest is diminution of pulmonary ventilation and extensive rebreathing from one lung to the other. Venous return to right side of heart is impaired. Appropriate treatment requires intubation of trachea and use of volume-limited ventilator. (From Johnson, J., and Kirby, C.K.: Surgery of the chest, ed. 4, Chicago, 1970, Year Book Medical Publishers, Inc.)

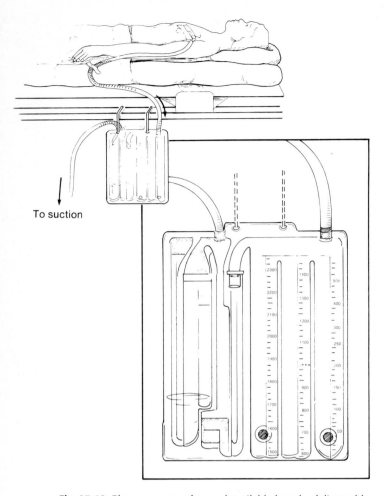

Fig. 25-18. Pleurevac, one of several available brands of disposable chest drainage systems. The system functions like a three-bottle system in that the unit collects drainage, maintains a seal to prevent air from entering the pleural cavity, and prevents excessive buildup of negative pressure. (From Abels, L.F.: Mosby's manual of critical care, St. Louis, 1979, The C.V. Mosby Co.)

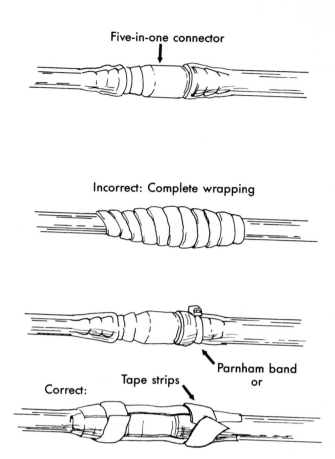

Fig. 25-19. Method of securing chest tubes after connected to water-seal drainage system.

conduit for drainage of air, blood, and other fluid from the intrapleural or mediastinal space and reestablishment of negative pressure in the intrapleural space. The chest tubes are clamped until connected to a sterile, water-seal drainage system. Water-seal suction may be necessary when a persistent air leak cannot be controlled by drainage alone. Historically, a two- or three-bottle system was used to accomplish this. Several compact, disposable units are available (Fig. 25-18). These units are preferable because they are easier and safer to use. The principles of operation remain the same and can be described more easily by using the bottle system model (Fig. 25-16). The first bottle collects the drainage from the intrapleural space, the second bottle provides the water seal, and the third provides the suction control determined by the level of water. The disposable units have only two compartments; one for water

seal and the second for drainage. These units can also be used with suction.

If two chest tubes are inserted, they may be connected by a Y connector to a single drainage unit or attached individually to two separate units. All connections should be banded or otherwise secured to ensure an intact system (Fig. 25-19). The drainage system must be sterile and maintained in a position lower than the patient's body to prevent air and fluid from reentering the chest cavity. Clamps for the tubing should always be available as a precautionary measure in the event of accidental interruption of the closed system. These clamps should be prominently attached to the patient's gown or bed and sent to the patient's room.

Monitoring

During a thoracotomy, the patient requires constant monitoring of laboratory results (ABG), temperature, blood loss, and urine output. The results are communicated with other team members for continuity of care.

Blood replacement

A procedure requiring extensive tissue dissection and removal in a highly vascular area could result in the need for replacement of blood during or following the procedure. A patient may have autologous blood ordered; often the diagnosis may prohibit patient donation of his or her own blood. The blood type and amount of blood ordered prior to the procedure should be noted and its availability determined. During the procedure, every effort should be made to control and monitor bleeding. If blood collection and/or reinfusion systems are used, manufacturer's instructions and institutional protocols should be followed.

Postprocedure concerns

Patients are transferred to PACU using care not to dislodge the chest catheter, urinary catheter, or monitoring equipment. The endotracheal tube usually remains in place to maintain an adequate air exchange. Air exchange and effective ventilation are two immediate needs of the patient after thoracotomy. Functional capacity may be altered due to muscle injury, which can cause the patient to experience discomfort turning or moving the shoulder and arm. Patients are often anxious about their limitations, the environment, and the results of the procedure. They benefit from information shared and from being allowed to discuss their feelings and needs. Family members should be informed of the status of the patient following the procedure.

Documentation

Documentation of perioperative care includes assessment of the patient upon admission to the operating room, nursing interventions, and postoperative evaluation. Documentation for a patient undergoing a thoracotomy specifically addresses positioning aids, position of the patient, medications administered, results of laboratory tests completed, equipment used such as a thermia blanket, urine output, blood replacement, insertion of chest tubes and drainage systems, and postoperative evaluation of skin integrity and injury.

Discharge information

The patient is discharged from the operating room to PACU following thoracotomy. The report to the PACU nurse is often a collaborative effort of the nurse and anesthesiologist. The perioperative nurse reports the patient's preoperative status, including anxiety level and understanding of the procedure, to assist the PACU nurse in meeting the emotional needs of the patient. A description of the position of the patient during the procedure provides criteria for assessment and evaluation of mobility. Results of immediate postoperative assessment including skin integrity, location and type of dressing applied, location and type of drains, blood loss, fluid replacement, medications administered, and laboratory results obtained during the

procedure are reported as a baseline for assessment in the PACU. The PACU nurse must be informed of the procedure completed, particularly if it varies from the anticipated procedure. The perioperative care plan should be reviewed and patient outcomes reported.

Evaluation

As part of the care planning process, the perioperative nursing goals are evaluated. They may be restated as brief outcomes. For the goals identified for the patient undergoing thoracic surgery, they would be:

- The patient's gas exchange was unimpaired; laboratory results and vital signs were normal; skin, nailbeds, or mucosa were pink; lung fields were clear bilaterally; and chest excursion was normal.
- The patient's skin integrity was maintained.
- The patient sustained no injury from the surgical position.
- Fluid balance was maintained; there were no fluid excesses or deficits.
- The patient will not experience a postoperative wound infection; the incision site will remain approximated and dry, without redness, drainage, or undue tenderness. (This is a long-term goal, and its evaluation will require the collaboration of the nurse in the patient care unit.)

SURGICAL INTERVENTIONS
Endoscopy (diagnostic or therapeutic)

Endoscopy refers to examination of hollow body organs or cavities with instruments that permit visual inspection of the contents and walls of organs or cavities. The endoscopic procedures pertinent to thoracic surgery are bronchoscopy and mediastinoscopy. Each endoscopist has preferences regarding the type of endoscope, positioning of the patient, type of anesthetic, and equipment. Invasive diagnostic or therapeutic measures enhance the decision to pursue surgical intervention by providing information related to the disease process including histology, location of the lesion, and lesion extent. Therapeutic endoscopy provides treatment by removal of the lesion or foreign body.

Standard bronchoscopy using rigid bronchoscope

Standard bronchoscopy is the direct visualization of the mucosa of the trachea, the main bronchi and their openings, and most of the segmental bronchi and removal of material for microscopic study if necessary.

Bronchoscopy is an integral part of the examination of patients with pulmonary symptoms such as persistent cough or wheezing, hemoptysis, obstruction, or abnormal roentgenographic changes. Common causes of bleeding (hemoptysis) are bronchiectasis, carcinoma, and tuberculosis. Congenital anomalies and suspected presence of a foreign body, especially in infants and children, are responsible for emergency examination of the respiratory tract.

Bronchoscopy is done to determine whether a lesion is in the tracheobronchial passages, to identify and localize that lesion accurately, and to observe periodically the effects of therapy. In suspected carcinoma the aspirated secretions obtained by bronchoscopy may contain malignant cells.

Procedural considerations. Bronchoscopy on an adult patient may be completed under local anesthesia; a child should receive general anesthesia. The adult patient receiving local anesthesia may experience discomfort and anxiety. To reduce anxiety, personnel should be introduced, intraoperative activities explained, and reassurance provided to the patient. The oral structures, including the teeth and lips, should be assessed for integrity. Loose teeth may require removal prior to or during the procedure.

Intravenous sedatives or analgesics may be administered during the procedure. See Chapter 9 for perioperative nursing considerations when monitoring the patient receiving local or monitored anesthesia care.

The patient may be positioned either in dorsal recumbent, with the shoulders elevated on a small roll or a sandbag to gently extend the head and neck, or in the sitting position.

The setup includes the following:

1 Bronchoscope (Fig. 25-7)
  Telescopes, desired types
  Fiberoptic light cords
  Fiberoptic light source
1 Suction tubing
2 Aspirating tubes (Fig. 25-11)
2 Specimen collectors (Fig. 25-11)
  Sponge carriers (Fig. 25-11)
2 Forceps, desired types (Fig. 25-12)
1 Bronchial spray and cannula
1 Lubricating jelly tube
1 Topical anesthesia set, if desired
1 Emesis basin
6 Gauze sponges
1 Round basin with sterile saline solution

The bronchoscopist risks contamination in the presence of communicable diseases. For this reason the endoscopist and assistants should wear face masks and eyeglasses, goggles, or a transparent shield attached to a headband. Aseptic technique is used to prevent any possibility of cross-contamination.

Operative procedure (Fig. 25-20)

1. The head is placed in position for visualization of the bronchus, to the left when the right main bronchi are inspected, and to the right when the left bronchi are inspected. The head is lowered for inspection of the middle lobe.
2. The bronchoscope is inserted over the surface of the tongue, usually through the right corner of the mouth. The patient's lip is retracted from the upper teeth with a finger of the endoscopist's left hand. The epiglottis is identified and elevated with the tip of the bronchoscope.
3. The distal end of the scope is passed through the true vocal cords of the larynx, and the upper tracheal rings are viewed. A small amount of anesthetic solution may be sprayed through the tube on the carina of the trachea and into the bronchus with the bronchial atomizer or spray. The patient's head is moved to the left to obtain a view of the right bronchi. The right-angle telescope is inserted with the light adjusted into the bronchoscope. The optical system should be kept free of precipitated moisture.
4. The segmental bronchial orifices of the upper right lobe bronchi are viewed and the telescope removed. Suction and aspirating tubes are introduced to clear the field of vision.
5. The middle lobe branches are inspected by inserting an oblique 45-degree angle telescope or right-angle telescope and advancing it. The patient's head is lowered to view the right middle lobe or turned to the right to view the left main bronchus.
6. Secretions are aspirated for study. Forceps for biopsy are inserted if desired; foreign bodies are removed with forceps.
7. The bronchoscope is removed. The patient's face is cleansed. If able, the patient is encouraged to sit on the edge of the operating room bed prior to transfer to the stretcher. An emesis basin and sponges should be provided for the patient's use. Assistance and support should be provided to the patient to prevent a fall.

Bronchoscopy using flexible bronchoscope

Flexible bronchoscopy is done to view structures that cannot be observed with a rigid scope. Flexible bronchoscopy may be performed in addition to a standard rigid bronchoscopy or as an independent procedure. If performed separately, the patient may remain on the transporting stretcher during the procedure. The bronchoscopy is completed for the same reasons as a rigid bronchoscopy.

Procedural considerations. Patient considerations are as described for rigid bronchoscopy.

The setup for flexible bronchoscopy includes the following:

Fiberoptic light source
Flexible bronchoscope
Flexible biopsy forceps
Flexible brush (optional); if used, slides and alcohol are necessary to collect specimen
Saline solution
Specimen container
Syringe for wash
Suction tubing with collection tube attached to collect wash specimen
Lubricant
Gauze sponges

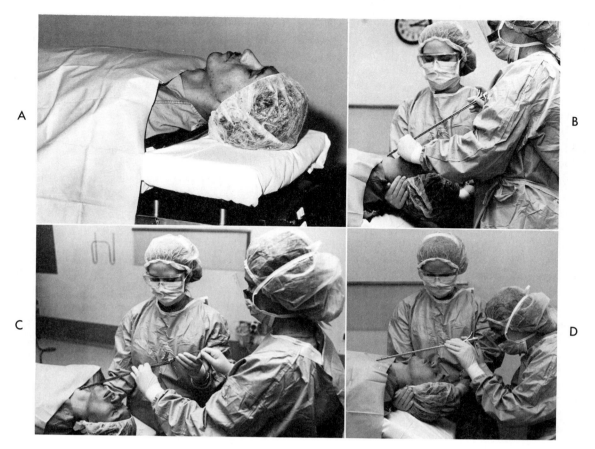

Fig. 25-20. A, Patient positioned with shoulder at table break for bronchoscopy. A shoulder roll or sandbag can be placed beneath the patient's shoulders. **B,** Initial position with head held high and supported. **C** Assistance is provided as the forceps or suction is guided while the head is supported. **D,** Position assumed as the endoscope is inserted; the head will be raised or lowered as the anatomy is viewed.

Operative procedure

1. The lubricated bronchoscope is passed through the adapter on the endotracheal tube, which is held secure by the anesthesiologist.
2. The suction tube is positioned with the specimen collector attached for collection of bronchial washings. When indicated, the suction tubing is connected to the bronchoscope; the container for collection is held securely in an upright position to prevent loss of the specimen through the suction.
3. Approximately 5 cc of saline solution is injected into the channel. Suction is quickly reapplied. This procedure may be repeated.
4. Following completion of the procedure, specimen containers are labeled and sent to the laboratory.

Mediastinoscopy

Mediastinoscopy is the direct visualization and possible biopsy of lymph nodes or tumors at the tracheobronchial junction, under the carina of the trachea, or on the upper lobe bronchi or subdivisions.

Mediastinoscopy may precede an exploratory thoracotomy in known cases of lung carcinoma. Patients with positive findings may be treated with radiation or chemotherapy, as indicated.

Procedural considerations. The setup for mediastinoscopy includes the following:

    Minor set of instruments
2 Mediastinoscopes, desired type
    Fiberoptic light cords
    Fiberoptic light source
1 Suction tubing
2 Aspirating tubes
1 Biopsy forceps
    Electrosurgical unit
    Endocardiac needle, 20 gauge, 8 inches

The patient is placed under endotracheal anesthesia and positioned as for a tracheostomy.

Operative procedure

1. A short transverse incision is made above the suprasternal notch and the pretracheal fascia exposed.
2. The pretracheal fascia is incised.
3. Tunneling is accomplished alongside the trachea by blunt (digital) dissection into the mediastinum.
4. The mediastinoscope is introduced under direct vision deep to the fascial plane and advanced along the side of the trachea toward the mediastinum.
5. The scope is manipulated to visualize the tracheal bifurcation, bronchi, aortic arch, and associated lymph nodes.
6. Lymph nodal tissue is located for biopsy and aspirated with a small-gauge needle and syringe for positive identification of a nonvascular structure.
7. Biopsy forceps are inserted through the scope and a tissue specimen excised. Pressure can be applied to the excision site with a bronchus sponge on a holder. The mediastinum is reinspected for bleeding.
8. The mediastinoscope is withdrawn.
9. Subcutaneous tissue is sutured with absorbable sutures. The skin is approximated and sutured with ligature on a cutting needle.
10. A small dressing is applied.

Operations involving the lung
Pneumonectomy

Pneumonectomy is removal of an entire lung, usually to treat malignant neoplasms. Other reasons for removal include an extensive unilateral bronchiectasis involving the greater part of one lung, drainage of an extensive chronic pulmonary abscess involving portions of one or more lobes, selected benign tumors or treatment of any extensive unilateral lesion. Other resections are often combined with pneumonectomy such as resection of mediastinal lymph nodes, resections of portions of the chest wall or diaphragm, or removal of parietal pleura.

Procedural considerations. The basic thoracic instrumentation is used. The patient is placed in the lateral position for a posterolateral incision.

Operative procedure

1. The skin, subcutaneous tissue, and muscle are incised using scalpel, suction, and electrocoagulation. Hemostasis is attained. If a rib is to be excised, the procedure discussed later is implemented.
2. The ribs and tissue are protected with moist sponges; the rib retractor is placed (Fig. 25-21) and opened slowly.
3. The lung is mobilized by freeing peripheral adhesions and dividing the pulmonary ligament. Dissection to the hilum of the involved lobe is carried out.
4. The superior pulmonary vein is gently retracted and the pulmonary artery dissected.
5. The branches of the pulmonary artery and vein of the involved lobe are clamped, doubly ligated, and di-

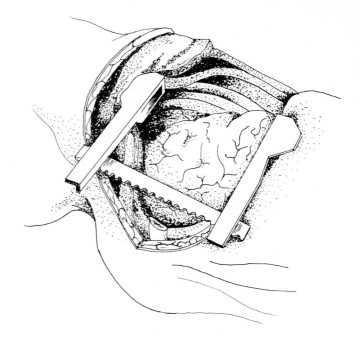

Fig. 25-21. Rib retractor placed for thoracotomy.

vided with fine right-angled vascular clamps, scissors, and nonabsorbable suture.
6. The inferior pulmonary vein is exposed by incising the hilar pleura and retracting the lung anteriorly. The inferior pulmonary vein is clamped, doubly ligated, and divided.
7. The bronchus clamp is applied and the bronchus near the tracheal bifurcation is divided. The stump is closed with atraumatic nonabsorbable mattress sutures or bronchus staples. If staples are applied, the scalpel is used to complete division of the bronchus. The lung is removed from the chest.
8. The pleural space is irrigated with normal saline to check for hemostasis and air leaks during positive pressure inspiration.
9. A pleural flap is created and sutured over the bronchial stump. Other methods of securing the bronchus might be used.
10. Hemostasis is assured in the pleural space.
11. Chest tube(s) are inserted (28–30 Fr) in the pleural space and brought through a stab wound at the eighth or ninth interspace near the anterior axillary line (Fig. 25-22). An upper tube is inserted through a second stab wound if indicated to evacuate leaking air.
12. The rib approximator (Fig. 25-23) is placed and closure begun with interrupted suture.
13. The muscle, subcutaneous tissue, and skin are closed. Drains are anchored to the chest wall with suture.
14. The dressing is applied.
15. Chest tube connections are secured with Parham bands or tape (Fig. 25-19), connected to water-seal drainage

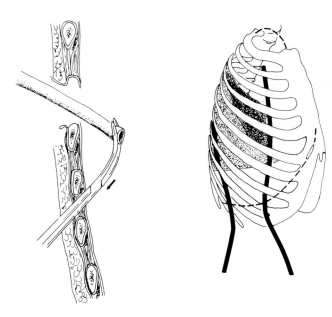

Fig. 25-22. Introduction of chest drainage tube through a stab wound; placement of apical and basal drainage tubes following upper and middle lobectomy.

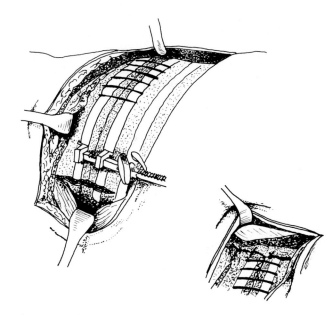

Fig. 25-23. Rib approximator placed for closure of incision. Heavy gauge suture used for closure of ribs.

following closure of the pleural space, and labeled (anterior/posterior).

Lobectomy (left upper)

Lobectomy is excision of one or more lobes of the lung. It is performed to remove metastatic involvement when the tumor is peripherally located and hilar nodes not involved. Other conditions affecting the lung and resulting in lobectomy might be bronchiectasis, giant emphysematous blebs or bullae, large centrally located benign tumor, fungal infections, or congenital anomalies.

Procedural considerations. The basic thoracic instrumentation is used. The patient is placed in a lateral position for posterolateral incision; the supine position may be used for upper and middle lobe resections. The procedure varies with the specific lobe to be removed due to anatomic structure.

Operative procedure

1. The skin, subcutaneous tissue, and muscle are incised using scalpel, suction, and electrocoagulation. Hemostasis is attained. If a rib is to be excised, the procedure discussed is implemented.
2. The ribs and tissue are protected with sponges. The rib retractor is placed and opened slowly.
3. The pleura is entered, and peripheral adhesions are freed with scissors, blunt dissection, or sponge on a sponge-holding forceps.
4. The hilar pleura is incised and separated.
5. The branches of the pulmonary artery(s) and vein(s) are isolated, clamped, doubly ligated, and divided

with fine, right-angled vascular clamps, scissors, and nonabsorbable suture.

6. The main trunk of the pulmonary artery is identified as is the fissure between the lobes.
7. The bronchus clamp is applied. The remaining lung is inflated to identify the line of demarcation. The bronchus is divided with a scalpel or heavy scissors.
8. Bronchial secretions are suctioned.
9. The bronchus is closed with atraumatic, noabsorbable mattress sutures or bronchus staples. If staples are applied, the scalpel is used to complete division of the bronchus.
10. Incomplete fissures are divided between hemostats with fine Metzenbaum scissors. Edges may be sutured closed.
11. A pleural flap is created and sutured over the bronchial stump. Other methods of securing the bronchus might be used.
12. The pleural cavity is thoroughly irrigated with normal saline and hemostasis is assured. The remaining lobes are inflated to check for air leaks and the degree of expansion of the remaining lobes is assessed.
13. The procedure is completed as for a pneumonectomy (steps 11 to 14).

Decortication

Decortication of the lung is removal of fibrinous deposit or restrictive membrane on the visceral and parietal pleura that interferes with pulmonary ventilatory function. The

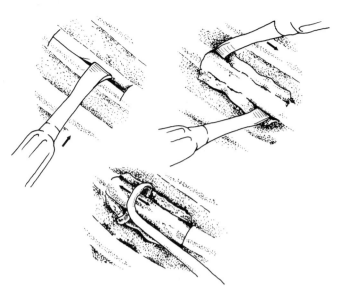

Fig. 25-24. Separation of muscles of rib with a periosteal elevator and rib stripper.

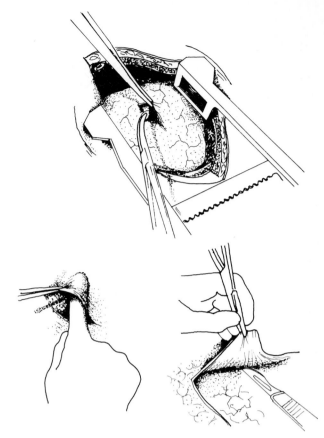

Fig. 25-25. Decortication. Methods of separating fibrous membrane from visceral pleura.

procedure results in blood loss and trauma and should be used only if the underlying lung is healthy. The objective is to return the lung to near normal function.

Procedural considerations. The basic thoracic instrumentation is used. The patient is placed in a lateral position for a posterolateral incision.

Operative procedure
1. The skin, subcutaneous tissue, and muscle are incised with the scalpel, suction, and electrocoagulation.
2. A rib, usually the fifth or sixth (Fig. 25-24), is stripped and resected.
3. The ribs and tissue are protected with moist sponges. The rib retractor is placed and slowly opened.
4. Parietal adhesions are divided to the margins of the lung, mediastinal surface and pericardium with thoracic scissors, forceps, and moist sponge on a sponge-holding forcep.
5. The fibrous membrane is incised and separated from the visceral pleura using blunt and sharp dissection and handling the tissues gently (Fig. 25-25).
6. The procedure is completed as for pneumonectomy (steps 11 to 14).

Drainage of empyema

Drainage of empyema is treatment for purulent effusion associated with acute or chronic infection. Empyema must be drained to prevent fibrothorax and further treatment with decortication. Acute empyema could be the result of lung abscess, pneumonia, or infection after thoracotomy. The procedure can be accomplished with the patient receiving local anesthesia when the infection is not extensive. Prolonged intrapleural infection results in chronic empyema,

which can create additional complications such as mediastinal shift, difficulty in swallowing, respiratory limitations, erosion into the bronchus, or deformity of the chest.

Procedural considerations. If the patient is anesthetized, the basic thoracic instrumentation is used. The patient is placed in a lateral position for an anterolateral incision. The chest cavity is irrigated profusely during and upon completion of the procedure.

Operative procedure
1. The skin and tissues are incised with a scalpel to expose the affected area of the lung. Suction is used to prevent spillage of drainage from the chest.
2. The pleural space is obliterated and an inflammatory response created by stripping the parietal pleura from the visceral pleura by sharp or blunt dissection and by inserting a catheter and instilling a sclerosing substance (unbuffed tetracycline, nitrogen mustard).
3. The incision site is closed as for other thoracotomy procedures.
4. A dressing is applied.

Segmental resection

Segmental resection is removal of one or more anatomic subdivisions of the pulmonary lobe. It conserves healthy, functioning pulmonary tissue by sparing remaining segments. Segmental resection is indicated for any benign lesion with segmental distribution or diseased tissue affecting only one segment of the lung with compromised cardiorespiratory reserve. The most common cause for removal is bronchiectasis. Other conditions requiring removal include chronic, localized inflammation or congenital cysts or blebs.

Procedural considerations. The basic thoracotomy instrumentation is used. The patient is placed in lateral position for an incision appropriate for the area removed.

Operative procedure

1. The skin, subcutaneous tissue, and muscle are incised with scalpel, suction, and electrocoagulation.
2. The parietal pleura is incised with a scalpel and scissors. Adhesions are divided with sharp or blunt dissection.
3. The segmental artery is identified to provide accurate identification of the bronchus of the diseased segment.
4. The segmental pulmonary vein and branches are ligated.
5. The bronchus is clamped with the bronchus clamp and the remaining lung is inflated. The intersegmental boundary is confirmed and proper placement of the clamp is assured.
6. The visceral pleura is incised around the diseased segment, beginning anterior to the hilum and progressing toward the periphery. Exposure is facilitated with malleable or other type of retractors. The intersegmental vessels are clamped with thoracic hemostats and ligated.
7. The segmental bronchus is transected. The stump is closed with atraumatic, nonabsorbable mattress sutures or bronchus staples (Fig. 25-26).

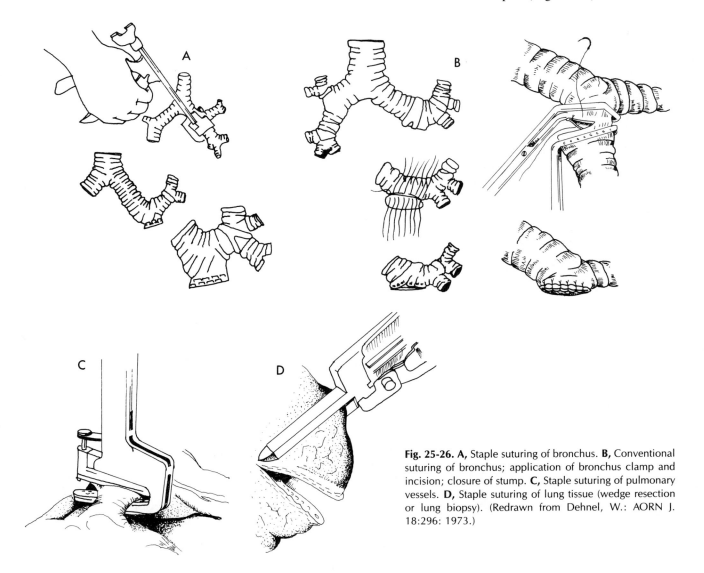

Fig. 25-26. A, Staple suturing of bronchus. **B,** Conventional suturing of bronchus; application of bronchus clamp and incision; closure of stump. **C,** Staple suturing of pulmonary vessels. **D,** Staple suturing of lung tissue (wedge resection or lung biopsy). (Redrawn from Dehnel, W.: AORN J. 18:296: 1973.)

8. Dissection is continued to separate segmental surfaces, and vessels are ligated as needed. The segment of the lung is removed.

9. A pleural flap is created and sutured over the bronchial stump. Other methods of securing the bronchus may be used.

10. The lung is reinflated and irrigated with normal saline. Bleeding is controlled with ligature or hemoclips.

11. The procedure is completed as for pneumonectomy (steps 11 to 14).

Wedge resection

Wedge resection is removal of a wedge-shaped parenchyma that includes the identified lesion, without regard for intersegmental planes. The resection is used for removal of small, peripherally located benign primary tumors of the lung.

Procedural considerations. Thoracic instrumentation is used. The patient is positioned to allow access to the operative site, with consideration of the area of lung to be removed.

Operative procedure

1. The skin, subcutaneous tissue, and muscle are incised using a scalpel, suction, and electrocoagulation.
2. The rib retractor is placed.
3. Bleeding is controlled, and small bronchi are secured with clamps and ligature. Large bronchi are ligated or sutured to prevent persistent air leak.
4. The wedge is outlined for excision, with a margin of normal tissue left, using one of the following techniques.
   a. Long hemostatic clamps are applied in three rows to outline the wedge. Excision is accomplished with a scalpel. The tissue is sutured with a running absorbable suture behind the clamps before removal. The edges of the tissue are oversewn with a continuous or interrupted suture (Fig. 25-27).

   b. The lobe is grasped with a lung clamp and the thoracic stapling instrument applied to the parenchymal portion of the lung. Staples are applied and the wedge excised with the scalpel. Staples are reapplied to the opposite side of the lesion adjoining the staple lines.
5. The specimen is removed. Air leaks are checked by irrigating. Bleeding is controlled with ligation or hemoclips.
6. The procedure is completed as for pneumonectomy (steps 11 to 14).

Lung biopsy

Lung biopsy is resection of a small portion of the lung for diagnosis. The biopsy allows removal of relatively large specimens for microscopic examination of the lung tissue. Indications include failure of closed methods (needle biopsy) for diagnosis or the presence of small localized lesions that can be removed by biopsy.

Procedural considerations. The basic instrument set and the following instruments are used:

1 Dissecting scissors
4 Duval lung grasping forceps
1 Rib retractor, small

The patient is positioned in a semilateral position for anterolateral incision.

Operative procedure

1. A short incision (approximately 5 cm) is made at the fifth intercostal space.
2. The pleura is incised; the ribs are retracted.
3. The lung is secured and pulled out the opening with the Duval lung clamp.
4. One or more segments of the lung are biopsied with application of a Satinsky clamp or application of staples with a stapling device. The tissue to be removed is excised with a scalpel. Following application of the

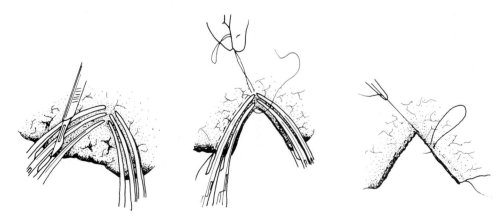

Fig. 25-27. Clamps applied to edge of lung tissue to be excised with scalpel. Sutured with a running suture and oversewn.

clamp, tissue edges are approximated with absorbable suture.

5. Bleeding is controlled by applying a moist sponge at the incision site. The area is irrigated and inspected for air leaks.
6. The chest tube (28 to 30 Fr) is inserted and connected to suction.
7. The incision is closed; drains are anchored to the chest wall.
8. The dressing is applied.

Open thoracostomy (partial rib resection)

Partial rib resection is removal of a portion of selected rib(s) through an open thoracostomy incision to allow healing and reinflation of an infected lung. The procedure is performed for treatment of chronic empyemic lesions to establish a mechanism for continuous drainage.

Procedural considerations. The basic thoracic instrument set and bone-cutting instruments are used. The patient is placed in a lateral position for a posterolateral incision. The surgical procedure can be completed under local anesthesia.

Operative procedure

1. The skin, subcutaneous tissue, and muscle are incised using scalpel, suction, and electrosurgery.
2. The rib is resected.
3. The pleura is incised. Suction is used to control anticipated drainage.
4. Aerobic and anaerobic swabs for culture and sensitivity are obtained.
5. The chest cavity is irrigated.
6. A large chest tube is inserted through the pleural opening.
7. The incision is closed or packed open (depending on the extent of disease process).
8. The tube is secured with a suture of heavy-gauge material on a cutting needle by passing through the incision and tying around the tube.
9. The chest tube is connected to a water-seal drainage system, and connections are secured.
10. A dressing is applied. An increased number of layers of dressing to absorb drainage may be necessary.

Closed thoracostomy (intercostal drainage)

Closed thoracostomy is insertion of a catheter through an intercostal space for establishment of closed drainage. The procedure provides continuous aspiration of air, blood, or infectious fluid from the pleural cavity. Indications are treatment of spontaneous pneumothorax, traumatic hemothorax, pleural effusion, or acute empyema.

Procedural considerations. The basic instrument set is used, with the following instrumentation added:

1 Local anesthesia set including syringes, needles, and anesthetic

2 Disposable chest catheters
1 Luer-Lok syringe, 30 cc
2 Aspirating needles, 16 gauge, 3½ inches
2 Culture tubes
1 Water-seal drainage system

The patient is placed in a lateral or sitting position (Chapter 6). The procedure may not take place in an operating room setting.

Operative procedure

1. The correct depth of insertion is gauged; the catheter is marked.
2. The operative site is anesthetized. An aspirating needle attached to a syringe is introduced into the chest cavity to verify presence of purulent drainage, air, or blood.
3. The skin is incised and a clamp introduced through the incision into the intercostal space and pleural cavity.
4. A catheter that fits the incision site without space around the circumference is inserted. The catheter is clamped to prevent egress of air as it is inserted in the cavity.
5. The incision site is sutured and the catheter secured.
6. The catheter is attached to water-seal drainage and the tubing secured. The clamp is removed.
7. A dressing is applied.

Excision of mediastinal lesion

This procedure entails the removal of a lesion from the mediastinum, which is divided into superior, anterior, middle, or posterior sections. A mediastinoscopy could determine the diagnosis of an anterior mediastinal lesion. Indications for excision of a mediastinal lesion include cystic hygroma, thymoma, lymphoma, or neurogenic tumor.

Procedural considerations. The thoracic instrumentation is used. A procedure on the superior mediastinum might require use of thyroid instruments (Chapter 16). The patient is in a supine position for a median sternotomy incision (lateral position may alternatively be used).

Operative procedure (for thymoma)

1. The skin and subcutaneous tissue are incised with scalpel, suction, and electrosurgery.
2. The sternum is transected with a power saw or sternal knife. Bleeding is controlled at the bone edges with bone wax (Fig. 25-28).
3. The thymus gland is dissected; vessels are clamped, ligated, and divided. The gland is removed.
4. The incision is closed. The sternum is reapproximated and closed with heavy wire. The skin is sutured closed.
5. A dressing is applied.

Correction of pectus excavatum and pectus carinatum

Pectus excavatum (funnel chest) and pectus carinatum (pigeon chest) are visually obvious defects. The procedure may be cosmetic or for correction of abnormalities re-

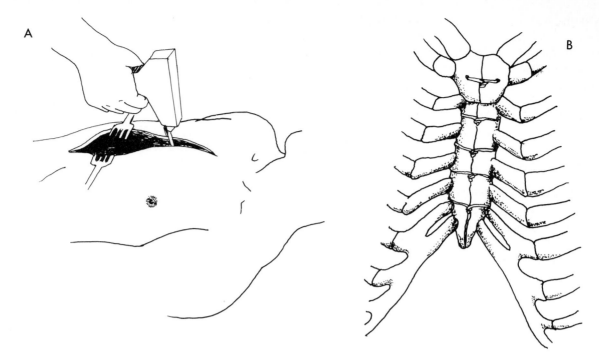

Fig. 25-28. Median sternotomy. **A,** Incision with power saw; **B,** closure with heavy gauge wire.

sulting from the defect that compromise the respiratory or circulatory system.

Procedural considerations. The thoracic instrument set is used. Instruments for lung resection and long instruments are not necessary. The following are added:

　　2 Gigli saws and handles
　　　Osteotomes or chisel
　　2 Bone hooks
　　2 Bone-holding forceps

Pectus excavatum is corrected for children aged 2 to 6 years. Pectus carinatum usually does not present until the teen years following completion of the growth spurt. Smaller instruments may be required for children. (See Chapter 29 for a discussion of the care of the pediatric surgical patient.)

The patient is positioned with a portion of the upper chest elevated on a soft roll or sheets. The incision is a median sternotomy or a bilateral inframammary incision.

Operative procedure

1. The skin and subcutaneous tissue are incised to the fascia with scalpel, suction, and electrosurgery.
2. The edges of the incision are protected and the rib retractor placed.
3. The fascial insertions of the greater pectoralis muscle into the sternum are incised and retracted using dissecting scissors, Pean forceps, and suture ligature.
4. A transverse incision (Fig. 25-29) is made.
5. The xiphoid process is separated from the sternum, and the substernal ligament and extension of the ab-

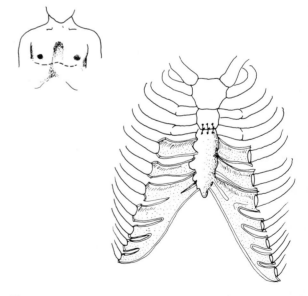

Fig. 25-29. Transverse incision for correction of pectus deformity. Closure of sternum with heavy gauge wire or suture.

dominal muscle divided using a scalpel, periosteal elevator, sternal knife, or Gigli saw and heavy scissors.

6. The posterior cartilages are cut with heavy scissors to free the depressed bone to allow the pleura and pericardium to drop back posteriorly and the heart to shift to a normal position.

7. The edges of the sternum are cut with the rongeur. Cartilages are shortened or resected to approximate the surfaces against each other. The sternum is bent to a normal position.

8. The corrected position of the sternum is maintained with mattress sutures across the osteotomy (Fig. 25-29). The pectoral and intercostal muscles are sutured. The xiphoid remains free.

9. Pleural drainage is accomplished and the incision closed.

10. A dressing is applied.

BIBLIOGRAPHY

Association of Operating Room Nurses: Standards and recommended practices for perioperative nursing, Denver, 1990, The Association.

Clemente, C.: Gray's anatomy, ed. 30, Philadelphia, 1985, Lea & Febiger.

Fishman, N.H.: Thoracic drainage: a manual of procedure, Chicago, 1983, Year Book Medical Publishers.

Fox, V., and Sherroll, A.N.: Thoracotomy for esophageal leiomyoma: preoperative, intraoperative and postoperative care, AORN J. 45:1136, 1987.

Fraulini, K.E.: After anesthesia: a guide for PACU, ICU and medical surgical nurses. Norwalk, Conn., 1987, Appleton and Lange.

Golanowski, M.: Thoracoscopy, an endoscopic look into the thorax, AORN J. 50:80, 1989.

Holloway, N.M.: Nursing the critically ill adult, ed. 3, Reading, Mass., 1988, Addison-Wesley.

Kirk, R.N., and Williamson, R.C.N.: General surgical operations, ed. 2, Edinburgh, 1987, Churchill-Livingstone.

Mackety, C.J.: Perioperative laser nursing, Thorofare, N.J., 1984, Charles B. Slack.

Meade, R.H., and others: History of thoracic surgery, Springfield, Ill., 1961, Charles C Thomas.

Nohl-Oser, H.C., and others: Surgery of the lung, Stuttgart, 1981, Georg Thieme Verlag.

Potter, P., and Perry, A.G.: Fundamentals of nursing, concepts, process and practice, ed. 2, St. Louis, 1989, The C.V. Mosby Company.

Schwartz, S., and others: Principles of surgery, ed. 4, New York, 1984, McGraw-Hill.

Waldenhausen, J.A., and Pierce, W.S.: Johnson's surgery of the chest, ed. 5, Chicago, 1985, Year Book Medical Publishers.

Welsh, S., Myre, L., and Gatch, G.: Pediatric bronchoscopy, special considerations, AORN J. 46:864, 1987.

26 Vascular surgery

ROSEMARY ANN ROTH

Vascular surgery in the 1990s is often indicated for either trauma (blunt or penetrating or the complication of displaced fractures) or alterations in tissue perfusion (emboli and occlusive disease). Early in the history of surgery, most traumatic wounds were treated by amputation; today, the indications for amputation are far more limited. Not until the seventeenth century did Harvey describe blood circulation as a closed system in which blood was pumped, and a century later did Lavoisier perceive the importance of oxygen to living tissue (Foss, 1989). Despite these discoveries, phlebotomy was a preferred treatment for a number of medical disorders; patients were often repeatedly "bled" to relieve symptoms attributed to offensive circulating substances. Mortality rates from traumatic vascular injury and acute arterial occlusion were high, even in the early part of the twentieth century. Following the introduction of the Fogarty embolectomy catheter in 1963, mortality rates for acute arterial occlusion dropped by 50%; as surgery progressed, limb salvage rates improved by 25% (James and others, 1987).

Vascular surgery is performed in most hospitals today and is no longer limited to major medical centers. The complexity and diversity of the procedures performed vary, however. Technologic advances, such as the use of the laser and the ultrasound scalpel, have proven valuable in vascular surgery (McCredie and others, 1986). Patients with acute arterial embolism or dissecting aneurysms often arrive at the hospital as surgical emergencies; other patients undergo lengthy elective limb salvage procedures that require precise, delicate vascular reconstruction. Despite the nature of the patient's vascular physiologic alteration, all patients require the attention of the perioperative nurse who cares for them.

SURGICAL ANATOMY
Arteries

Arteries are composed of three layers of tissue. The *tunica intima* is the smooth internal endothelial layer that is in contact with the blood, the *tunica media* is the muscular middle portion, and the *tunica adventitia* is the outer layer, composed of connective tissue.

Arteries successively divide into arterioles, which then further subdivide into capillaries, which connect with the venous system. At the capillary level, blood supplies oxygen to body tissues. Arteries can also form *anastomoses*, or connections with other arteries. These anastomoses tend to equalize blood distribution and pressure and also to form collateral circulation. *Collateral circulation* is important in vascular disease and often provides alternative pathways around occluded vessels.

Vasomotor nerves, which control vascular tone, arise from the sympathetic portion of the autonomic nervous system and are categorized as vasoconstrictor or vasodilator fibers.

Normal arterial function depends on the properties of elasticity and distensibility, which enable the vessels to compensate for changes in blood volume and pressure.

Atherosclerosis is the most common cause of occlusive vascular disease. The probable cause of peripheral vascular disease is initial damage to the intima of the artery with subsequent activation and aggregation of the body's platelets. Inflammation follows, with the deposition of lipoproteins forming an atheroma. Calcification of this vascular lesion leads to the development of an atherosclerotic plaque. Many factors, such as sex, age, hypertension, increased cholesterol, diabetes, cigarette smoking, and obesity, are thought to contribute to atherosclerosis.

Peripheral vascular disease generally occurs gradually. A localized lesion is usually an indication of more systemic disease. The body's network of collateral blood vessels is an adaptive mechanism to supply oxygenated blood as a compensatory mechanism in the development of vascular disease. Not until the end stages of vascular occlusion does gangrene develop.

Abdominal aortic aneurysms occur primarily below the renal arteries. An aneurysm involves intimal damage of the aorta and weakening of the media or elastic portion of the arterial wall. Gradually the vessel wall in the damaged area expands, and atheroma develops within the aneurysm sac. An abdominal aortic aneurysm has minimal symptoms and is generally discovered on routine history and physical examination. Mortality is low with elective resection of the aneurysm. Dissection and rupture of the aneurysm dramatically increase operative mortality.

The initial symptom of vascular disease in the aortoiliac vessels and distal arteries is intermittent claudication. This indicative symptom occurs distal to the arterial obstruction and occurs with exercise. The increased muscle demand for oxygen with exercise cannot be met distal to the arterial obstruction. Anaerobic metabolism occurs, and muscle cramping develops. As soon as the patient stops walking, the cramps disappear. The second symptom, rest pain, develops as the vascular disease progresses. Rest pain occurs without exercise and is a constant discomfort, primarily at night. The body is now unable to meet the oxygen needs of distal tissues even at rest. Unless the vascular disease is corrected, gangrene can develop. Gangrene occurs when the arterial vessels are unable to meet the oxygen needs of distal tissues even at complete rest.

Vascular lesions in the carotid artery occur primarily at the bifurcation of the common carotid artery into the internal and external carotid artery. The internal carotid artery supplies the brain with its oxygen needs. Obstruction in this arterial vessel leads to cerebrovascular insufficiency. Clinical conditions that generally indicate the need for a carotid endarterectomy are transient cerebral ischemia, asymptomatic bruits, stable strokes, and chronic cerebral ischemia.

Veins

Veins are thin-walled vessels that return the blood to the heart. They are composed of the same three basic layers as arteries, but the tunica media is thin; veins can contract only minimally.

The intimal layer of a vein contains semilunar folds of tissue, or valves. These valves prevent the backflow of blood. Because little pumping pressure from the heart carries across the capillary beds, one-way valves are necessary to overcome the pull of gravity and prevent backflow of blood in the venous system. The negative pressure created by the relaxed right ventricle helps venous return by its sucking effect, and the contraction of visceral and skeletal muscles helps propel venous blood toward the heart.

Capillaries enlarge into venules, which in turn enlarge into successively bigger veins, returning the deoxygenated blood to the heart.

PERIOPERATIVE NURSING CONSIDERATIONS
Assessment/nursing diagnosis

A preoperative assessment is necessary for an adequate understanding of the patient's disease, the patient's response, and the proposed surgical procedure. Knowledge of vascular disease and its development assists the perioperative nurse in performing a comprehensive assessment and developing a plan of care for patients undergoing surgical procedures involving the aortoiliac, femoral, popliteal, and carotid arteries.

The perioperative nurse should assess the patient for the development and extent of vascular symptoms. Identification of related medical conditions, such as diabetes, hypertension, and heart disease, are also important considerations in the development of a plan of care. The patient's nutritional status, use of alcohol and cigarettes,

caffeine intake, and any existing skin lesions should also be identified. Preoperative location, grading, and marking of distal peripheral pulses can assist the nurse with intraoperative assessment of tissue perfusion. After reviewing the results of the patient's physical examination, the perioperative nurse should verify signs and symptoms of vascular disease that need to be considered during intraoperative care. Muscle and skin atrophy, the presence of ulceration or necrosis in distal tissues, pain, neurovascular status, skin color and temperature, and other integumentary changes should be noted.

The nurse should assess the patient's understanding of and anxiety over the proposed surgical procedure and the surgical routine. Reinforcement or correction of misunderstandings is possible only if the nurse identifies the patient's current level of knowledge. Identification of the patient's fears and concerns helps the nurse with planning appropriate nursing interventions. In addition, the patient should be able to identify the location and nature of the surgical procedure.

Vascular surgery can be lengthy. Attention to the maintenance of the patient's tissue and skin integrity as well as body temperature is important, especially considering the air-conditioned environment of the operating room.

The perioperative nurse must be familiar with the location and presence or absence of peripheral pulses. These should be graded (that is, 0 = absent to 4+ = normal) per institutional grading scales. The perioperative nurse can evaluate the patient's extremities for color, temperature, and strength of pedal pulses during the surgical procedure. This assessment indicates tissue perfusion distal to the arterial obstruction. When the perioperative nurse knows such assessment will be required, it should be performed during the initial preparation of the patient to provide for baseline comparisons.

Invasive diagnostic tests are performed preoperatively to identify the extent and location of the patient's peripheral vascular disease. The introduction of contrast media through a catheter into the vascular or venous system of the patient facilitates this visualization. Angiography also involves the injection of contrast media into the patient's arterial system and the taking of serial radiographic pictures of the movement of the dye through the arteries (Fig. 26-1). Digital subtraction angiography is one such technique that uses a computer to make the image along with contrast injection (Fig. 26-2). These arteriograms should be available in the operating room for the surgical team's reference throughout the surgical procedure.

Based on the perioperative nurse's assessment, the identification and prioritization of nursing diagnoses aid in the development of an individualized plan of care. Potential nursing diagnoses for a patient undergoing vascular surgery would include:

· Anxiety related to the surgical intervention and its outcomes

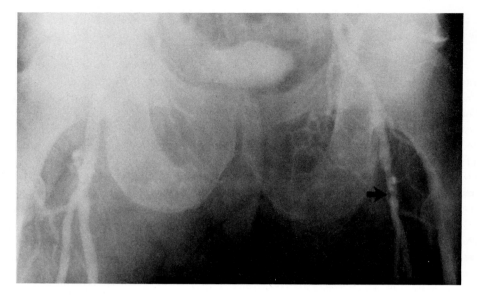

Fig. 26-1. Femoral angiogram. *Arrow* indicates stenosis of the left femoral artery. (Courtesy of The Genesee Hospital, Rochester, N.Y.)

- Potential altered body temperature (hypothermia) related to surgical exposure
- Potential fluid volume deficit related to loss of body fluids
- Potential for impaired skin integrity and altered tissue perfusion related to surgical positioning
- Potential for infection related to contamination of the wound and the surgical field

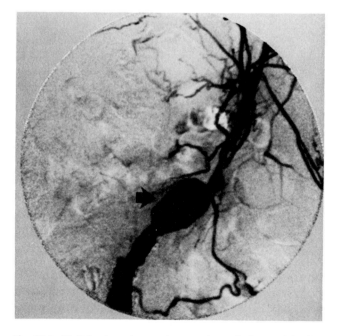

Fig. 26-2. Digital subtraction angiogram. *Arrow* indicates right iliac aneurysm. (Courtesy of The Genesee Hospital, Rochester, N.Y.)

Planning

Once nursing diagnoses are identified and prioritized for the individual patient, the perioperative care plan is developed. Based on nursing diagnoses, goals are identified for the patient. Nursing interventions are identified that will assist the patient toward goal achievement. Because perioperative nursing practice is collaborative, the perioperative nurse develops a plan of care that extends from the admission to the surgical suite through safe recovery from surgery. Some patient goals are measured immediately on discharge from the operating room; others require the collaboration of the PACU or unit nurse for final evaluation. The perioperative nurse thus develops and contributes to a comprehensive, holistic plan of patient care. Such care planning provides evidence of quality patient care and provides a mechanism of communication and continuity of care with other health care professionals. A Sample Care Plan for the patient undergoing vascular surgery, utilizing the suggested nursing diagnoses, is shown on p. 865.

Implementation

Before the patient is brought into the operating room, the perioperative nurse should procure the necessary medical and surgical supplies and equipment for the intended surgical intervention.

Intraoperative arteriography provides the surgeon with information and documentation of the patency of a vessel or graft. If intraoperative arteriograms are anticipated, an appropriate operating room bed with x-ray capabilities should be available. Laser-assisted peripheral angioplasty requires the use of image intensification to visualize the location of the laser probe and angioplasty catheter at the

Sample Care Plan

NURSING DIAGNOSIS:
Anxiety related to the surgical intervention and its outcomes
GOAL:
Patient will verbalize decreased anxiety.
INTERVENTIONS:
Include the family, significant other, or both, in explanations of perioperative routines.
Allow time for patient's questions; provide explanations or make appropriate referral.
Note verbal and nonverbal indications of anxiety; assist the patient with anxiety-reducing techniques such as rhythmic breathing and relaxation.
Encourage ventilation of concerns and fears.
Provide emotional support and supportive nursing measures (for example, touch).
Demonstrate warmth, calmness, and acceptance of the patient's anxiety.
Maintain a quiet environment.
Document patient's reactions.

NURSING DIAGNOSIS:
Potential altered body temperature (hypothermia) related to surgical exposure
GOAL:
The patient's body temperature will remain within normal limits during the intraoperative phase.
INTERVENTIONS:
Limit the patient's physical exposure; expose only those body surfaces required for skin preparation.
Use warmed skin preparation solutions.
Place a warming device (such as a padded hyperthermia blanket) on the operating room bed.
Provide the anesthesiologist with a fluid warmer.
Monitor the patient's temperature.
Use warm saline for irrigation.
Provide warm blankets at the end of the surgical procedure.

NURSING DIAGNOSIS:
Potential fluid volume deficit related to loss of body fluids
GOAL:
The patient will maintain fluid balance.
INTERVENTIONS:
Determine the availability of replacement blood and/or blood products.
Assist with the insertion of intravenous lines and fluid replacement therapy. Keep IV lines patent.
Estimate blood loss on sponges and drapes.
Initiate autotransfusion as required.

Record the amount of irrigation used.
Document the contents of the suction canisters.
Monitor and document hourly urine output; communicate results of all outcome measurements.
Monitor vital signs and oxygen saturation; assist with the collection and interpretation of intraoperative blood analyses.

NURSING DIAGNOSIS:
Potential impaired skin integrity and altered tissue perfusion related to surgical positioning
GOAL:
The patient will maintain skin integrity and tissue perfusion.
INTERVENTIONS:
Document the patient's preoperative skin condition and tissue perfusion.
Position the patient on a cushioning device (gel-filled or eggcrate mattress) on the operating room bed.
Keep OR bed sheets dry and wrinkle-free.
Pad all bony prominences.
Maintain body alignment.
Place restraining straps snugly but not tightly.
Protect vulnerable neurovascular bundles from compression.
Check and record tissue perfusion (color, temperature, pulses) as required.
Elevate drapes off the patient's toes; use appropriate positioning accessories.
Reassess and document the patient's postoperative skin condition and tissue perfusion.

NURSING DIAGNOSIS:
Potential for infection related to contamination of the wound and the sterile field
GOAL:
The patient will not develop a postoperative wound infection.
INTERVENTIONS:
Maintain surgical asepsis.
Monitor traffic in the operating room throughout the procedure.
Assure that personnel are appropriately attired.
Document the classification of the surgical wound.
Follow appropriate implant precautions; record implanted devices.
Secure, prepare, and administer antibiotic therapy as prescribed. Note patient allergies.
Record any medications administered by the perioperative nurse or from the sterile field.

site of the vascular lesion. An appropriate operating room, capable of image intensification, must be used. The perioperative nurse needs to coordinate the availability of x-ray personnel with the surgical procedure. Appropriate contrast dye, catheters, and impermeable sterile x-ray covers must be available. Radiation-protection devices, such as aprons and shields, should also be used for the patient, when possible, and for the surgical team members. Team members should wear photographic film badges.

The electrocardiogram and direct arterial lines are used for monitoring and assessment. The intraarterial line is usually placed in the patient's radial artery. Continuous assessment of the patient's arterial pressure is a critical part of the surgical procedure. Left atrial pressure (LAP) through a Swan-Ganz catheter also may be monitored, depending on the patient's physiologic status. A general anesthetic may be administered, and the patient intubated; local or regional anesthesia may also be used, depending on the surgical intervention. Because many patients undergoing vascular surgery have generalized arteriosclerotic disease, the nurse should be constantly alert for cardiac arrhythmias and blood pressure changes.

A urinary catheter should be inserted, especially if the proposed procedure involves the renal arteries or clamping the aorta above the renal arteries, if considerable blood loss is anticipated, or if the planned procedure time is lengthy. Urinary catheterization facilitates accurate hourly measurements of urine during and after the surgical procedure and assists in the assessment of renal perfusion and fluid status.

Positioning of the patient undergoing vascular surgery is of particular importance because of restricted circulation distal to the area of arterial obstruction and a generalized state of poor circulation. For most surgeries the patient is placed supine on the operating room bed. A foot board may be applied to the operating room bed to prevent the weight of drapes resting on the patient's lower extremities. For a carotid endarterectomy, the patient's head is supported on a doughnut or a head support. A roll may be placed between the scapulae. For surgical procedures involving a lower extremity, the patient's thigh is externally rotated and abducted with the knee flexed. A small bolster may be used under the knee to support the patient's leg.

In addition, the patient's age and medical problems, such as diabetes, can necessitate extra attention to positioning. Proper skeletal alignment during surgery prevents injury to the neuromuscular system. Attention to the skin overlying bony prominences, especially the heels and elbows, and the use of proper supports and pads prevent injury to the patient. Owing to the lengthy nature of these procedures, an eggcrate mattress or gel-filled pad can be placed on the operating room bed to help prevent patient injury. For the same reasons, members of the scrubbed team should also be cognizant of heavy instruments and drapes resting on the patient's body and take measures to avoid pressure injuries.

Skin preparation for vascular surgery is extensive. For abdominal aortic surgery, the patient's skin is prepared from the nipple line to the midthigh area. For peripheral vascular surgery on the extremities, the patient is prepped from the umbilicus to the feet. The patient's legs are prepared circumferentially. For carotid surgery, the patient is prepped from the ear and chin on the affected side to below the clavicle.

Draping should permit the surgeon free access to involved areas. For example, abdominal surgery may also require exposure of the groin region for possible exploration of the femoral arteries. A femoral-popliteal bypass on one leg may require access to the other leg for harvesting of the saphenous vein. Impervious drapes should be used to prevent contamination of the surgical field from blood and irrigation fluids.

Vascular monitoring equipment

Assessing blood flow through diseased vessels by palpation is often difficult. Physical assessment of the patient's hemodynamic status during surgery can be further complicated by spasms of the vessel walls, the cool environment of the operating room, and alterations in blood pressure caused by hemorrhage. Vascular monitoring equipment can be used by the surgeon in the operating room to evaluate tissue perfusion.

A Doppler device uses ultrasonic, high-frequency sound waves to assess the movement of blood through a vessel. The Doppler device is critical when pulses cannot be palpated. When the sound waves encounter dissimilar tissues, such as red blood cells moving through an artery, some of the sound is reflected back to the probe. The pitch of the sound is directly related to the velocity of blood flow. Using a coupling gel, the unsterile Doppler probe can be placed on the patient's skin distal to the surgical site. Some probes can be sterilized and used directly in the surgical wound. Besides providing an audible signal, the Doppler can provide a permanent record of the sound if a recorder is attached. The unit is inexpensive and easily transported. Surgical personnel can use the Doppler after minimal training.

An electroencephalogram (EEG) accurately determines reduced cerebral perfusion during a carotid endarterectomy. With appropriately selected patients, the EEG can obviate the use of an external shunt. Trained personnel are necessary to operate this expensive equipment.

Sutures

Most vascular sutures are made of synthetic, nonabsorbable materials such as Dacron, polyester, polytetrafluoroethylene, and polypropylene. Occasionally, silk may be used. These sutures are sometimes converted to monofilament by the impregnation of other synthetics such as Teflon.

Vascular sutures have swaged-on needles of various sizes and are available in sizes 0 to 8-0. The suture may be single armed or double armed (that is, a needle on one or both ends). The size and curve of the needle depend on the vessel and its location.

Prostheses

Arterial prostheses are synthetic, tubular conduits that are designed to replace or bypass diseased vessels. They are available as straight or bifurcated grafts and are usually made of Teflon or Dacron.

Most prostheses are commercially sterilized. If they are sterilized in the hospital, the manufacturer's recommendations should be followed. Repeated autoclaving of a prosthesis is inadvisable because the integrity of the fiber may be destroyed. Ethylene oxide sterilization, with adequate aeration, is usually recommended.

Teflon and Dacron grafts are available in woven or knitted form. Woven grafts do not ordinarily require preclotting, but they tend to fray on cut edges. Knitted grafts, other than needing preclotting with the patient's own blood, are softer and easier to suture and provide for tissue ingrowth.

A knitted graft is usually prepared before insertion, according to the surgeon's preference. This graft preparation minimizes blood loss from seepage through the graft interstices. Sometimes the surgeon prefers to preclot the graft with the patient's blood or, after inserting the graft, to open the occluding clamps individually and momentarily to fill the graft with blood to accomplish the same purpose.

Expanded polytetrafluoroethylene (PTFE) is used as an alternative material for vascular prostheses. It is pliable, does not fray, sutures well, and needs no preclotting. This graft can also come with internal rings to aid in graft patency and is available in various lengths and diameters.

Grafts are available in various sizes. The sizes commonly used for abdominal procedures are 14 to 22 mm; for the extremities, the sizes are usually 4 to 10 mm.

Instrumentation

For abdominal vascular surgery, the instrument setup includes the basic laparotomy set (Chapter 11), plus the following vascular instruments:

Cutting instruments

2 Knife handles, no. 7 with blades nos. 11 and 15
2 Potts-Smith vascular scissors, 1 straight and 1 angled

Holding instruments

4 Potts-Smith tissue forceps, 2 smooth and 2 with teeth
4 DeBakey vascular forceps, 2 long and 2 short

Clamping instruments

4 Angled peripheral vascular clamps
4 Aortic occlusion clamps

3 Satinsky clamps, various sizes
4 DeBakey ring-handled bulldog clamps
4 DeBakey cross-action bulldog clamps
2 Fogarty occlusion clamps

Suturing instruments

4 Needle holders (narrow diamond jaw)

Retractors

2 Kelly retractors, extra large
2 Deaver retractors, extra large
2 Harrington retractors, wide and narrow
2 Weitlaner or Garrett retractors (for extension of incision into the legs)

Accessory items

2 Heparin flushing needles
  Tissue occlusion clips and appliers (for example, Hemoclips)
  Dacron tape or vessel loops
  Nerve hook
  Submucous elevator
  Fogarty arterial catheters
  Fogarty clamp inserts

For peripheral vascular surgery on the extremities, the instruments include a basic minor set with the following vascular instruments:

Cutting instruments

2 Knife handles, no. 7 with blades nos. 11 and 15
2 Potts-Smith vascular scissors, 1 straight and 1 angled

Holding instruments

4 Potts-Smith tissue forceps, 2 smooth and 2 with teeth
4 DeBakey vascular forceps, 2 long and 2 short

Clamping instruments

2 Satinsky clamps
2 Aortic cross-clamps
4 Angled peripheral vascular clamps
4 DeBakey ring-handled bulldog clamps
4 DeBakey cross-action clamps
2 Fogarty occlusion clamps
1 Henley clamp

Suturing instruments

4 Needle holders (narrow diamond jaw)

Retractors

2 Weitlaners or Garrett retractors

Accessory items

2 Heparin flushing needles
  Tissue occlusion clips and appliers (for example, Hemoclips)
  Dacron tape or vessel loops
  Submucous elevator
  Nerve hook
  Fogarty arterial catheters
  Fogarty clamp inserts

In situ procedure instruments

Vascular dilators
Microvascular scissors
Mills valvulotome
Leather in situ valve cutter kit

Heparinization

Heparin may be used locally or systemically to prevent thrombosis during the operative procedure. When a vessel is completely occluded during the operation, heparin can also be injected directly into the distal artery before the clamp is secured. Heparinized saline irrigation, usually 5000 units in 500 ml of normal saline, is often used. The dosage and concentration of heparin in saline solution may vary according to the surgeon's preference.

Documentation

Documentation of patient problems and nursing actions addressing these identified problems is important. For a patient undergoing vascular surgery, possible areas to document include the integrity of the patient's skin, the presence or absence of peripheral pulses, the surgical position and positioning devices used, fluid intake and output, and the achievement of patient goals. During surgery, various local anesthetic drugs and irrigating solutions, such as thrombin, antibiotic, and heparin solutions, may be used. The scrub nurse should label each container with the solution type and strength. The circulating nurse maintains an accurate record of the solutions used and the amounts administered. The type, size, and serial and lot numbers of vascular implants should be documented according to institutional policy and procedure.

Evaluation

Evaluation is an ongoing process during which the perioperative nurse determines the extent to which the patient goals are met. This phase is continuous throughout the implementation of the nursing process. Assessing, observing, and appraising are actions of the perioperative nurse for this phase.

The conclusion of the intraoperative phase is the transfer of the care of the peripheral vascular patient to colleagues in the PACU or the intensive care unit. A nursing report should be given when the perioperative nurse transfers the care of the patient to other individuals. The report should include the surgical procedure performed, the patient's fluid status, any allergies, and the achievement of patient goals. The care provided in the operating room should complement the patient's care preoperatively and postoperatively.

Specific evaluation of the five nursing diagnoses and their goals mentioned for a patient undergoing peripheral vascular surgery may be stated as patient outcomes. Some of the outcomes will have been achieved at the end of the intraoperative phase. Others require ongoing evaluation during the postoperative phase. Patient outcomes may be phrased as follows:

- The patient demonstrated a reduction in anxiety as evidenced by relaxed facial expression, verbalization of feeling less anxious, and verbalization of an understanding of the surgical intervention and perioperative routines.
- The patient maintained a normal body temperature as evidenced by postoperative temperature equitable to preoperative level and absence of postoperative shivering.
- The patient maintained normal fluid volume as evidenced by postoperative pulses equitable to the preoperative level, hourly urine output of at least 30 cc, and good skin turgor.
- The patient demonstrated skin and tissue integrity; there were no skin lesions except those evident on preoperative assessment, and skin temperature and color were adequate.
- The patient will experience no postoperative wound infection as evidenced by absence of redness and swelling at the incision site and normal white blood cell count.

SURGICAL INTERVENTIONS
Abdominal aortic aneurysmectomy

Abdominal aortic aneurysmectomy is surgical obliteration of the aneurysm, which may or may not include the iliac arteries, with insertion of a synthetic prosthesis to reestablish functional continuity. The majority of abdominal aortic aneurysms begin below the renal arteries, and many extend to involve the bifurcation and common iliac arteries. Severe pain, along with symptoms of hypotension, shock, and distal vascular insufficiency, usually indicates rupture or dissection and represents a true emergency condition. The prime surgical consideration when a rupture or dissection (longitudinal splitting of arterial wall) occurs is the control of hemorrhage by occluding the aorta proximal to the point of rupture.

Procedural considerations. The patient is placed in the supine position. The skin is prepped for a midline abdominal incision, and draping is completed to permit access to the groin region for possible exploration of femoral arteries. The pedal pulses should be marked before the beginning of the procedure so they may be located immediately if the surgeon requests a check of the pulses. This assessment of pulses can be done manually or with an ultrasonic instrument (Doppler).

Operative procedure
1. The abdomen is opened through a midline incision (Fig. 26-3, A) from the xiphoid process to the symphysis pubis. Hemostasis is accomplished, and exploration is completed as described for laparotomy (Chapter 11).

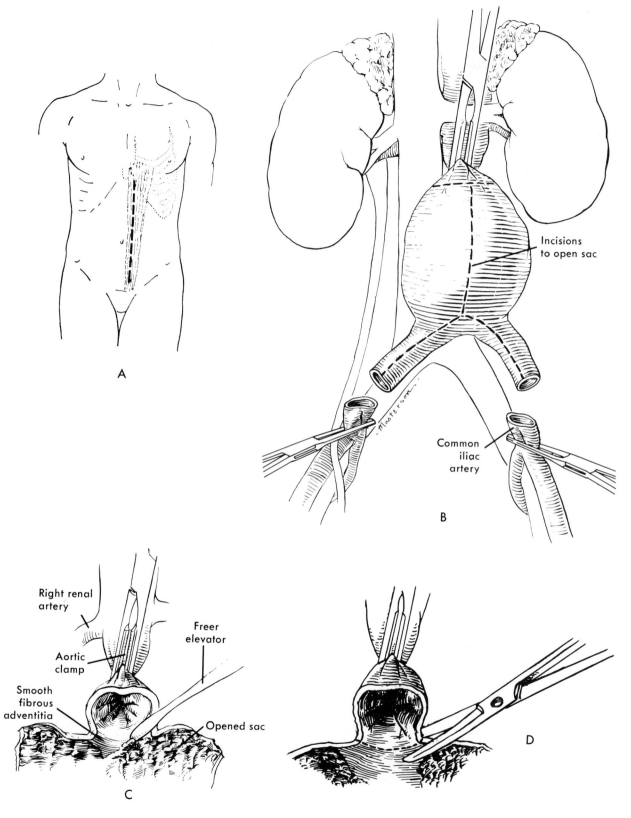

Fig. 26-3. Resection of abdominal aneurysm: end-to-end anastomosis. **A,** Initial incision. **B,** Sac is opened after obtaining proximal and distal control. **C,** Endarterectomy at cuff of aorta. **D,** Posterior wall is divided, or, if posterior wall is adherent, anastomosis is performed.

Continued.

2. Kelly and Deaver retractors are inserted in the wound. If necessary for exposure, a portion of the small bowel can be placed outside the abdomen and covered with moist laparotomy packs or a Lahey bag.

3. The parietal peritoneum is incised over the aorta and extended superiorly to expose the aneurysm and also inferiorly over the bifurcation and beyond the iliac arteries. Metzenbaum scissors, smooth forceps, and hemostats are used.

4. Careful blunt and sharp dissection is continued to expose the aorta above the aneurysm to permit application of moist umbilical tapes or vessel loops and loose placement of an aortic clamp. The renal artery and ureters are protected.

5. The iliac vessels and bifurcation are inspected for evidence of small aneurysms, thrombosis, and calcification. Moist tapes or vessel loops are placed around the iliac arteries, and vascular clamps are applied.

6. An aortic clamp such as the Crafoord, Cooley, or Satinsky is applied and closed. Opening of the aneurysm is undertaken with a scalpel or electrosurgical blade and heavy scissors.

7. The aneurysm is completely opened, and all atheromatous and thrombotic material is removed. The aneurysm walls may be excised but usually are left in place for eventual reinforcement of the prosthesis. In either case the posterior aspect of the aorta is left intact. Bleeding is controlled, especially from the lumbar vessels that enter posteriorly.

8. A bifurcated prosthetic graft of appropriate size is prepared for insertion. Occasionally, if the aneurysm does not involve the aortic bifurcation, a straight tubular graft is used. Preclotting of a knitted graft may be accomplished by immersing the graft in a small quantity of the patient's own blood, as previously described.

9. The aortic cuff is prepared for anastomosis by irrigating it with heparinized saline solution and by re-

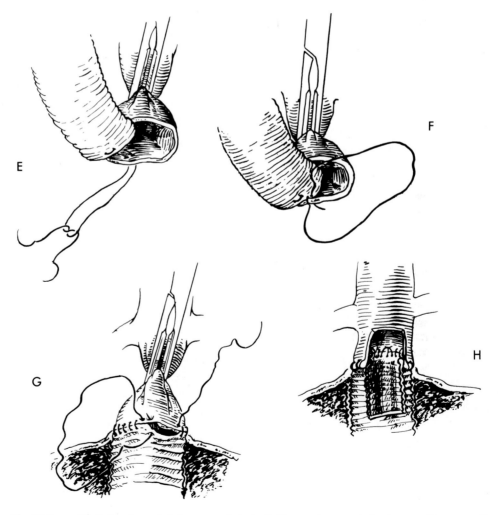

Fig. 26-3, cont'd. E, Anastomosis is begun posteriorly. **F,** Over and over suturing from graft to aorta. **G,** Complete anastomosis in front. **H,** Cutaway view.

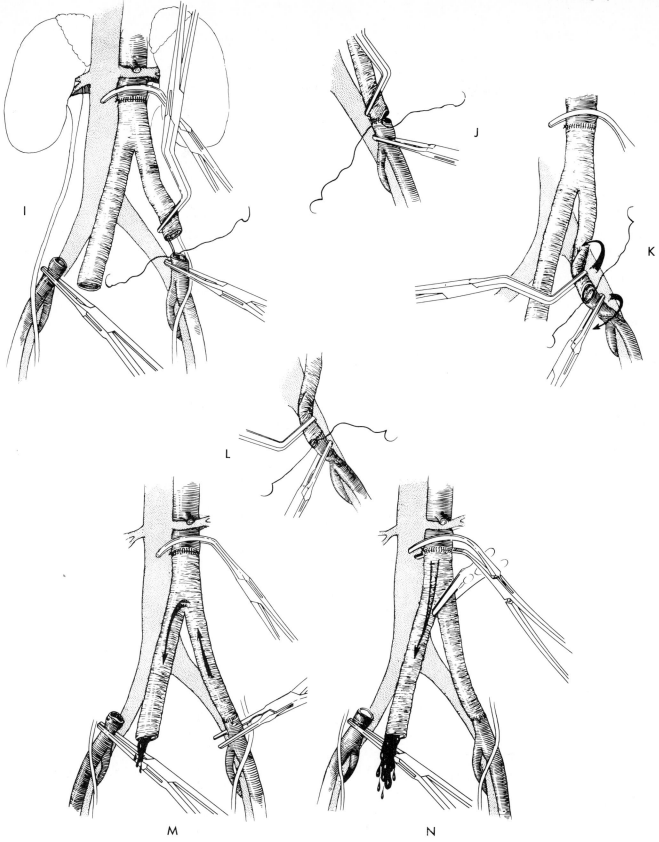

Fig. 26-3, cont'd. I to L, First iliac anastomosis: **I,** placement of mattress suture; **J,** medial row; **K,** medial row completed; rotation for lateral row; **L,** lateral row. **M** and **N,** Restoration of flow to first leg: **M,** backflow is checked; **N,** proximal aorta is flushed. (From Hershey, F.B., and Calman, C.H.: Atlas of vascular surgery, ed. 3, St. Louis, 1973, The C.V. Mosby Co.)

moving all fibrotic plaques. One or two vascular sutures (double armed) are used to accomplish the anastomosis by a through-and-through continuous suture. Additional interrupted sutures may be needed if the anastomosis leaks on completion.

10. The distal vessels are opened and inspected for back-bleeding, and heparinized saline solution may be injected to prevent clotting.

11. Each limb of the graft is anastomosed to the iliac artery, using a smaller vascular suture and similar technique. After the first side of the anastomosis has been completed, blood is permitted to circulate, and the remaining limb of the graft is clamped gently to prevent trapping of air and leaking during the last part of the anastomosis. Bleeding is controlled.

12. The parietal peritoneum is closed.

13. The abdominal wound is closed.

Aortoiliac endarterectomy

Aortoiliac endarterectomy is the surgical removal of intraluminal atheromatous obstructive plaques and the restoration of arterial flow to the leg or foot. Aortoiliac endarterectomy is usually accomplished through a vertical arteriotomy with a primary closure. Synthetic patch material may be used, if necessary, to restore the normal caliber of the artery. The surgeon may choose simply to bypass the obstructed segment, in which case the procedure for abdominal aortic aneurysmectomy would be followed.

Procedural considerations. The setup required is as described for abdominal aortic aneurysmectomy, plus endarterectomy instruments and bifurcated and straight tubular synthetic prostheses if endarterectomy is not feasible.

Operative procedure

1. The first five steps of the procedure for aortic aneurysmectomy are followed.

2. An aortic clamp such as the Crafoord or Satinsky is applied, and the arteriotomy is begun. Heparin solution may be injected, and the clamp closed immediately.

3. The arteriotomy incision is completed, and plaques are removed.

4. Arteriotomies are closed with fine, nonabsorbable vascular sutures.

5. A sympathectomy may be performed. The ganglia are identified and grasped with a nerve hook, and occlusion clips are used to clip the nerve. The nerve is then divided with Metzenbaum scissors.

6. The procedure is completed as in steps 12 and 13 for aneurysmectomy.

Femoral-popliteal bypass

Femoral-popliteal bypass is the restoration of blood flow to the leg with a graft bypassing the occluded section of the femoral artery. The bypass may be a saphenous vein or straight synthetic graft. The patency of the popliteal artery must be demonstrated by angiography for a suc-

cessful bypass procedure. If popliteal patency is doubtful, artery exploration is necessary as the first procedure. Involvement of the popliteal artery may necessitate the exposure and use of the tibial vessels for the lower anastomosis. If this occurs, the procedure could require the use of microvascular instruments and technique.

Procedural considerations. The patient is placed in a supine position. The thigh is externally rotated and abducted with the knee flexed. Prepping and draping include the entire groin and leg. The instrument setup includes the basic minor and vascular sets plus the following: Gelpi retractors, Garrett or Weitlaner retractors, a Crawford-Cooley tunneler, and supplies and equipment for operative arteriograms.

Operative procedures
Exploration of common femoral artery

1. A vertical incision, extending downward about 6 inches along the medial aspect of the thigh, is made over the femoral artery below the inguinal area, and a Garrett or Weitlaner retractor is inserted.

2. The common femoral artery is located, the sheath of the artery is bluntly dissected in both directions, and the artery is dissected free for complete exposure.

3. Moist umbilical tapes or vessel loops are passed around the common femoral, the superficial femoral, and the deep femoral arteries.

Exploration of upper popliteal artery

1. A vertical incision, extending down just past the patella, is made along the medial aspect of the lower thigh. If the popliteal artery is diseased, an incision below the knee is necessary to expose the tibial vessels.

2. The saphenous vein and nerve are retracted with small retractors.

3. A Weitlaner retractor is used to retract the muscles after blunt dissection or the exploration of the upper and lower artery. However, in exploring the midportion, the gastrocnemius muscle must be divided to expose the artery.

4. The popliteal vein is bluntly dissected from the artery and retracted with umbilical tape or a small, blunt vein retractor.

5. The popliteal artery is dissected free, the knee is flexed, and a moist umbilical tape is passed around the popliteal artery. It may be desirable at this time to perform arteriograms if doubt exists about the patency of the popliteal and distal arterial tree.

6. The saphenous vein is exposed by joining the femoral and popliteal incisions the length of the thigh or through multiple short incisions along the medial thigh. If the vein is suitable, the necessary length is resected. If a prosthesis is used, the length and size are determined, and the graft may be preclotted as previously described.

7. The saphenous vein is prepared for use by carefully ligating side branches with fine silk and dissecting all fibrous bands from the adventitia. Finally, because of venous valves, the vein *must* be reversed so the end originally in the groin is anastomosed to the popliteal artery.

8. The tunneler is passed beneath the sartorius muscle from the popliteal fossa to the groin.

9. The graft is carefully pulled through the tunnel and positioned to prevent kinks or twists.

10. Heparin solution is injected into the common femoral artery, and the vessels are occluded with an angled vascular clamp.

11. An incision is made into the femoral artery with a no. 11 knife blade and extended with a Potts-Smith angulated scissors.

12. The graft is anastomosed to the artery with fine vascular sutures (two single-armed or one double-armed suture).

13. The knee is flexed, and a vascular clamp is placed on the popliteal artery at the graft site.

14. An incision is made into the popliteal artery as explained for the femoral arteriotomy.

15. The graft is sutured to the popliteal artery, and, before completion, the femoral occluding clamp is momentarily opened to eliminate clots.

16. All occluding clamps are removed, and a check for leaks is made before closure.

17. The incision is closed as described previously.

Femoral-popliteal bypass in situ

Femoral-popliteal bypass in situ is the restoration of blood flow to the leg, bypassing an occluded portion of the femoral artery with a patient's transected saphenous vein, which remains in place. The procedure includes incising the venous valves and interrupting the venous tributaries. The adequacy of the patient's saphenous vein can be validated before the surgical procedure by a saphenous phlebogram. Varicose veins or a previous saphenous vein ligation and stripping are contraindications to the in situ procedure. The advantages of the in situ procedure include increased graft availability and improved patency. A disadvantage is the time-consuming aspect of this technique. Valves can be incised with microvascular scissors, a Mills valvulotome, or a Leather in situ valve cutter kit.

Operative procedure

1. The procedure is as for femoral-popliteal bypass. The groin incision is extended downward over the course of the saphenous vein. A skin bridge may be left between the groin and popliteal incisions. The skin bridge is thought to decrease the severity of lymphedema postoperatively.

2. The saphenous vein is exposed and divided at its proximal and distal ends. Venous tributaries are occluded with arterial clips, such as Hemoclips, or fine nonabsorbable sutures.

3. The first valve at the femoral junction is incised with a microvascular scissors or a Mills valvulotome. The disposable internal valve cutter is introduced into the proximal end of the vein and passed down to the popliteal area. This disposable cutter is used to incise the internal valve.

4. The saphenous vein is distended with heparinized saline, papaverine, or heparinized blood to identify any valvular obstruction or open venous tributary. Another pass of the valve cutter alleviates the obstruction. Open branches of the saphenous vein can also be ligated with arterial clips or fine nonabsorbable sutures.

5. The incompetent saphenous vein is used to bypass the occluded segment of the femoral artery (see steps 11 to 17 of the femoral-popliteal bypass procedure).

Laser-assisted balloon angioplasty

Laser-assisted balloon angioplasty is the surgical treatment of a diseased artery with laser energy and balloon catheters to restore the internal patency of the vessel. This technique has increased the options for patients undergoing vascular surgery. The perioperative nurse must be prepared for additional invasive surgery if the laser procedure fails or a vessel perforation occurs.

Procedural considerations. Laser safety precautions are necessary for this procedure (Chapter 10). In addition, the perioperative nurse must be knowledgeable about and have available a variety of balloon catheters and laser probes. An instrument setup similar to that used for a femoral-popliteal bypass is used. Image intensification is necessary for this procedure. A radiopaque ruler placed along the patient's leg validates the site of the lesion during image intensification.

Operative procedure

1. The first three steps of the procedure for femoral-popliteal bypass are followed.

2. A longitudinal arteriotomy in the superficial femoral artery is made.

3. A guidewire is introduced into the arteriotomy down to the lesion. The laser probe can then be advanced over the guidewire. Some laser probes do not require the initial placement of a guidewire. The placement of the probe at the site of the lesion is verified with image intensification and the radiopaque ruler.

4. Depending on the type of guidewire being used, the surgeon may remove the guidewire prior to activating the laser. The laser is activated. The probe is deliberately advanced back and forth through the lesion slowly. The laser energy allows the surgeon to create a channel through the lesion.

5. Once the channel is created in the lesion, a balloon catheter is introduced through the arteriotomy. The dilating balloon is inflated with fluid consisting of a dilute solution of the contrast media. This use of contrast media allows visualization of the balloon on fluroscopy.

The surgeon repeatedly inflates and deflates the balloon in the area of the lesion with a handheld syringe or inflation device until the normal diameter of the vessel is achieved. The inflation pressure should be monitored with a pressure gauge to prevent rupture of the vessel.

6. An intraoperative arteriogram can be done to visualize the outcome of the procedure.

7. The arteriotomy is closed with a continuous nonabsorbable suture. The incision is closed with absorbable sutures and the skin closed with staples.

Femorofemoral bypass

Femorofemoral bypass is an extraanatomic bypass that is performed when the surgical risk for the patient is high because of a complicated medical condition or technical problems with the procedure. Severe cardiac or pulmonary disease may prevent the patient from undergoing a more definitive procedure. Also, an infection in a previously placed graft precludes its replacement with another prosthesis. Subcutaneous vascular grafting is an option in these conditions because the procedure bypasses normal vascular anatomy and can be done under local anesthesia with adjunct sedation. Another extraanatomic procedure that can be done in these instances is an axillofemoral bypass involving the subcutaneous placement of a prosthesis from the axillary artery to the femoral artery on the same side.

Procedural considerations. The patient is positioned on the operating room bed in a supine position. For a femorofemoral bypass, a small pad is placed under each knee. The area prepared for surgery extends from the umbilicus to midthigh. The genitalia are covered with a sterile towel.

Operative procedure

1. A longitudinal incision is made over each femoral artery from the inguinal ligament to just below the femoral bifurcation (Fig. 26-4).

2. Each common femoral, superficial femoral, and deep femoral artery is dissected free, mobilized, and secured with umbilical tapes or vessel loops.

3. The graft tunnel between the two femoral arteries is created across the pubic symphysis in the subcutaneous tissue. This tunnel is created with digital dissection, scissors dissection, or the passage of a clamp or tunneler across the preperitoneal space.

4. A Dacron vascular graft is passed through the subcutaneous tunnel with care to prevent kinking of the graft.

5. Vascular clamps are placed on the common femoral, superficial femoral, and deep femoral arteries. A longitudinal arteriotomy is made in the common femoral artery.

6. An end-to-side anastomosis using nonabsorbable vascular sutures is performed to join the graft with the common femoral artery. A similar anastomosis is done on the other side.

7. After the clamps are released and flow is restored, the

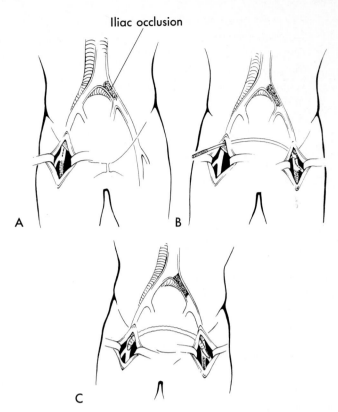

Fig. 26-4. Femorofemoral bypass. **A,** Iliac occlusion with femoral incision. **B,** Incisions exposing bilateral femoral arteries with tunneler in place between two incisions. **C,** Femorofemoral bypass in place. (From Haimovici, H., editor: Vascular surgery: principles and techniques, Norwalk, Conn., 1984, Appleton-Century-Crofts.)

patient's pulses are checked; the circulating nurse may be asked to inspect the patient's feet.

8. The femoral incisions are closed with absorbable sutures and the skin closed with staples.

Arterial embolectomy

Arterial embolectomy entails an incision made in the affected artery to remove thromboembolic material. Emboli may be clot particles, a foreign body, air, fat, or a tumor that circulates through the bloodstream and becomes lodged as the vessel decreases in size. More often the direct source is a mural thrombus, associated with cardiac or vascular disease. Pain or numbness distal to the obstruction is the initial symptom, followed by other signs of vascular occlusion, such as pallor or absence of pulses.

Procedural considerations. The patient is placed in the supine position, the skin area is prepped, and draping is completed to permit access to the affected area.

The instrument setup includes the basic minor and vascular sets, including Fogarty arterial and irrigating catheters.

Operative procedure

1. The initial incision is completed, and the artery is carefully exposed to permit the application of vascular clamps (Fig. 26-5).
2. An incision is made into the artery with scalpel blade no. 15 or 11. A Fogarty catheter is carefully inserted beyond the point of clot attachment. The balloon is inflated, and the catheter is withdrawn along with the detached clot.
3. As backflow is obtained, a vascular clamp is applied below the arteriotomy.
4. The artery may be flushed by injection of heparinized saline solution through a small irrigating catheter.
5. The arterial closure is completed with vascular sutures. The wound closure is accomplished in the usual manner, and dressings are applied.

Carotid endarterectomy

Carotid endarterectomy is the removal of an atheroma at the carotid artery bifurcation. Lessening the likelihood of any transient or permanent neurological deficit is a major concern during a carotid endarterectomy. The use of a temporary carotid artery shunt, such as the Javid shunt, allows for a continuous blood flow through the carotid artery and to the brain. Some disadvantages in using this temporary device are the additional dissection necessary for its placement and the possibility of dislodging debris when inserting the shunt.

Two techniques that facilitate continual assessment of cerebral perfusion are the use of cervical block anesthesia or electroencephalography. A conscious patient under cervical block anesthesia can be observed for neurologic deficits encountered during the procedure. In addition, the patient under general anesthesia can be monitored with an electroencephalogram (EEG). If either method demonstrates reduced cerebral perfusion, the surgeon may decide to use a temporary carotid artery shunt. The shunting device should always be available and sterile during the procedure.

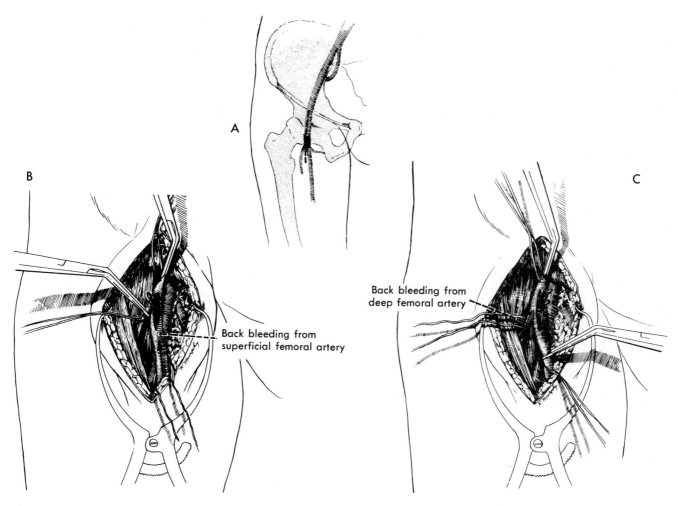

Fig. 26-5. Femoral embolectomy. **A,** Incision. **B,** Backflow from superficial femoral artery is checked. **C,** Backflow from deep femoral artery (profunda femoris) is checked.

Continued.

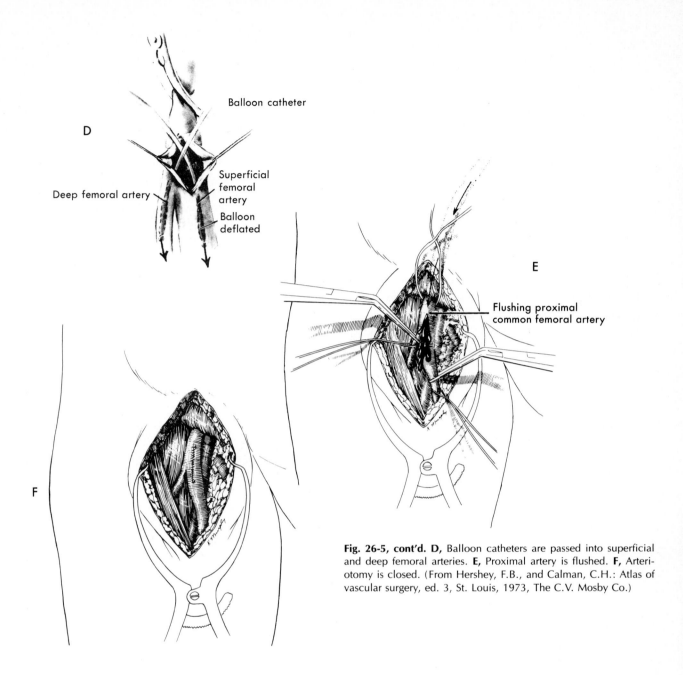

Fig. 26-5, cont'd. D, Balloon catheters are passed into superficial and deep femoral arteries. **E,** Proximal artery is flushed. **F,** Arteriotomy is closed. (From Hershey, F.B., and Calman, C.H.: Atlas of vascular surgery, ed. 3, St. Louis, 1973, The C.V. Mosby Co.)

Procedural considerations. The patient is placed on the operating room bed in a supine position with the head supported on a doughnut or head support. A roll may be placed between the scapulae.

Operative procedure

1. A longitudinal incision is made over the area of the carotid bifurcation. The Weitlaner self-retaining retractor may be placed for exposure (Fig. 26-6).
2. With Metzenbaum scissors, the soft tissue is dissected for exposure of the carotid artery and its bifurcation.
3. Blunt dissection with vascular tissue forceps and a small, right-angle clamp is used to dissect and free the carotid artery, including the bifurcated portion. A

moistened umbilical tape or vessel loop is passed around the vessel for ease of handling.

4. The external, common, and internal carotid arteries are clamped.
5. With DeBakey tissue forceps and a no. 11 scalpel blade, an arteriotomy is made over the stenotic area. The incision is lengthened with a Potts-Smith angulated scissors to expose the full extent of the occluding plaque.
6. With a blunt dissector, the plaque or plaques are dissected free from the arterial wall. Heparin solution is used as an irrigant to clean the intima.
7. Arteriotomy is closed with fine vascular sutures. A

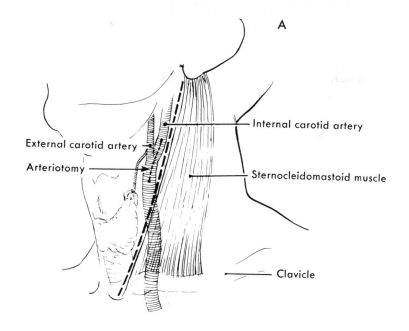

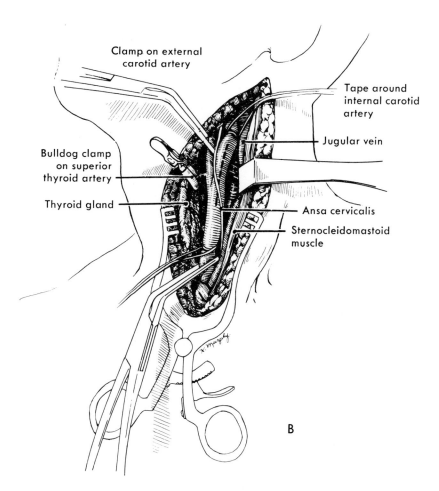

Fig. 26-6. Carotid endarterectomy. **A,** Incision. **B,** Exposure of carotid bifurcation. (From Hershey, F.B., and Calman, C.H.: Atlas of vascular surgery, ed. 3, St. Louis, 1973, The C.V. Mosby Co.)

synthetic or autogenous patch graft may be used to restore the arterial lumen if it appears to be narrowed. Before complete closure, blood flow is temporarily restored through the arteries to wash away any free plaques, air, or thrombi. To do this, the occluding clamps are opened and closed individually: first the external artery, then the internal artery, and last the common carotid artery clamps. The closure of the arteriotomy is completed.

8. The occluding clamps are removed from the external and common carotid arteries; *the internal carotid artery clamp is removed last.* This ensures that any minor debris missed will be flushed harmlessly into the external rather than the internal carotid artery.

9. Additional interrupted sutures may be needed to control leakage.

10. The wound closure is accomplished in the usual manner, and dressings are applied.

Carotid endarterectomy with temporary bypass
Operative procedure

1. The first five steps as described for carotid endarterectomy are followed.

2. A piece of tubing (polyethylene or Silastic) with a suture tied around its center or a commercially prepared shunt device is inserted in the common carotid artery and the internal carotid artery to maintain cerebral blood flow and is held with tourniquets or ring clamps (Fig. 26-7).

3. The plaque is removed as described for carotid endarterectomy.

4. Before the arteriotomy closure is completed, the ring

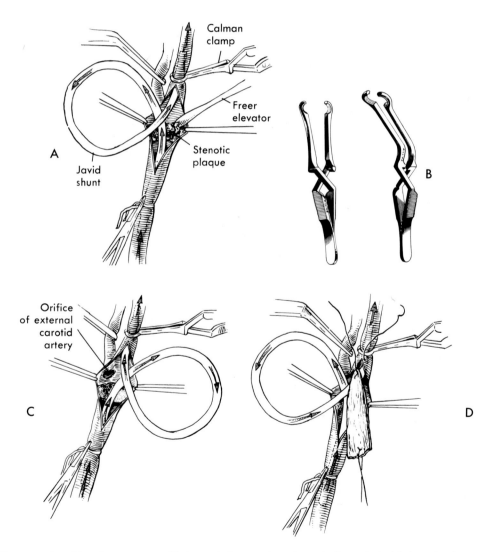

Fig. 26-7. Carotid endarterectomy with internal shunt and patch angioplasty. **A,** Javid shunt in place. Stenotic plaque peeled away. **B,** Calman ring clamps to hold internal shunts in place. **C,** Shunt rotated for completion of endarterectomy. **D,** Patch angioplasty begun.

clamp or tourniquet on the internal carotid artery is released, and the shunt is removed from the internal carotid artery, which is then momentarily reclamped. The shunt is removed from the common carotid artery, and a partial occlusion clamp, incorporating only the unclosed suture line, is applied. The external carotid occluding clamp is removed, followed by the common carotid artery clamp, and last, the internal carotid artery occluding clamp.

5. The closure of the arteriotomy is completed, and the partial occlusion clamp removed.

6. The wound is closed in the usual manner.

Shunt operations for portal hypertension

Obstruction of the portal system, which may be intrahepatic or extrahepatic, is the direct cause of portal hypertension. Intrahepatic obstruction, which is more common, may result from cirrhosis or infectious hepatitis. Extrahepatic obstruction, which represents about 15% of the total, may be caused by thrombosis, compression, or congenital abnormalities. The most important indication for surgery is hemorrhage of esophageal or gastric varices. An effective shunt between the hypertensive portal and lower caval circulation produces a fall in portal pressure, with subsequent disappearance of varices and protection against further hemorrhage.

Preoperatively, a portal venogram usually is obtained by percutaneous splenic puncture or the venous phase of mesenteric arteriography.

Portacaval anastomosis

Through an abdominal incision, an anastomosis is established between the portal vein and the inferior vena cava (Fig. 26-8).

Procedural considerations. The patient is placed on the operating room bed in a supine position with a pad under the patient's right side. The instrument setup includes the basic laparotomy and vascular sets, plus the following for measuring portal pressures: a manometer, a three-way stopcock, polyethylene tubing, and a syringe and needles.

Operative procedure

1. The abdominal incision is completed with instruments and materials as previously described. Abdominal exploration is carried out.

2. A jejunal mesenteric vein is isolated and cannulated with polyethylene tubing by a simple cutdown technique, using a no. 11 scalpel blade and fine plastic or vascular scissors, Adson forceps, two curved mosquito hemostats, and silk ligatures. With a three-way stopcock, a spinal manometer is attached to the tubing, and intravenous saline solution is injected into the manometer.

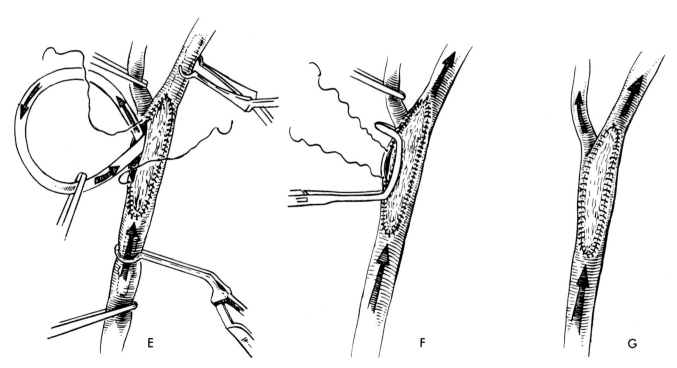

Fig. 26-7, cont'd. E, Shunt being withdrawn from internal carotid artery. **F,** Flow restored to internal carotid artery during completion of patch angioplasty. **G,** Patch angioplasty completed. (From Hershey, F.B., and Calman, C.H.: Atlas of vascular surgery, ed. 3, St. Louis, 1973, The C.V. Mosby Co.)

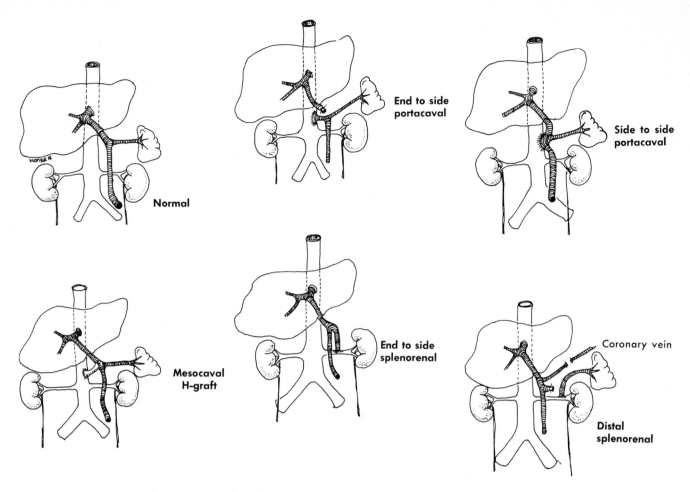

Fig. 26-8. Types of portal-systemic venous shunts used to relieve portal hypertension.

3. The portal pressure is measured and determined by the height of the saline solution meniscus above the right atrium when it comes to rest. Normal limits range from 45 to 150 mm. The abdominal range is from 200 to 600 mm.

4. As the portal vein and inferior vena cava are dissected free, extreme caution is exercised to prevent injury to important surrounding structures, for example, the duodenum, gallbladder, cystic and common bile ducts, and the hepatic artery and its branches.

5. Moist umbilical tapes are applied to the portal vein and the vena cava, both above and below the prepared sites for anastomosis.

6. Noncrushing vascular clamps are placed on the portal vein. If an end-to-end anastomosis is contemplated, the vein is ligated. If a side-to-side anastomosis is to be established, the vein is incised. Small clots are carefully removed, and the lumen may be irrigated with saline solution.

7. A Satinsky or other suitable partial occluding clamp is placed on the vena cava. An elliptical section of the vessel wall that is secured within the inner aspect

of the clamp is excised with vascular scissors. The size of the section removed should correspond to the lumen of the portion of the portal vein that has been prepared for anastomosis.

8. The anastomosis is completed with a continuous vascular suture, fine vascular forceps, and long fine needle holders.

9. The portal pressure is retaken to determine functioning of the shunt.

10. The peritoneum is closed. Closure of the muscle, fascia, and skin is completed. Dressings are applied.

Splenorenal shunt

Through a left midline or subcostal incision, an anastomosis is established between the proximal splenic and the left renal veins (Fig. 26-8).

Operative procedure

1. A midline or subcostal incision is made.

2. The spleen and splenic artery are mobilized, and the pancreas is separated from the splenic pedicle; the phrenocolic ligament is divided.

3. The spleen is removed with angular and curved artery forceps and silk sutures.
4. The renal vein is dissected free, and vascular clamps are applied.
5. An anastomosis of the splenic vein to the left renal vein is carried out in a manner similar to that for the portacaval anastomosis.
6. The wound is closed as described for the portacaval shunt operation.

Distal splenorenal shunt (Warren shunt)

A distal splenorenal shunt is an anastomosis between the distal end of the splenic vein and the left renal vein (Fig. 26-8).

Operative procedure
1. A long transverse or bilateral subcostal incision is made, and a limited abdominal exploration is carried out.
2. The splenic vein lying at the upper border of the pancreas is approached through the lesser omental bursa.
3. The distal end of the pancreas and splenic vein is carefully separated. Multiple fine suture ligatures are required.
4. The gastrocolic ligament is freed from the greater curvature of the stomach, and the gastrocolic vein is ligated.
5. The left renal vein is dissected free.
6. The splenic vein is divided near its junction with the mesenteric vein, and the proximal end is closed with a fine continuous vascular suture.
7. The distal (splenic) end of the splenic vein is swung to the renal vein, and an end-to-side anastomosis with a fine vascular suture is accomplished in a manner similar to that for a portacaval anastomosis.
8. The coronary vein is ligated.
9. The wound is closed as described for a portacaval anastomosis.

Mesocaval interposition shunt (Drapanas shunt)

A mesocaval interposition shunt is placement of a short Dacron prosthetic graft between the superior mesenteric vein and inferior vena cava (Fig. 26-8).

Operative procedure
1. Incision and pressure measurements are done as in portacaval anastomosis steps 1 to 3.
2. The superior mesenteric vein is identified and isolated through an incision at the base of the transverse mesocolon.
3. The inferior vena cava is approached through the mesenteric reflection of the right colon, and about 4 cm of vein is exposed.
4. A Satinsky clamp is placed partially occluding the vena cava, and an ellipse of vein wall is removed.
5. A short (about 6 to 8 cm) section of an 18- to 20-mm Dacron graft is sutured end to side to the vena cava with a fine vascular suture.
6. The superior mesenteric vein is occluded between vascular clamps, and the graft is sutured end to side to the vein. Appropriate flushing of the graft is carried out before completion of the anastomosis.
7. All vascular clamps are removed, and pressures are again taken, as in portacaval anastomosis.
8. The abdomen is closed as in portacaval anastomosis.

Access procedures

Access procedures are performed on patients in acute or chronic renal failure to facilitate hemodialysis. The surgeon may elect to insert a shunting device or to create an arteriovenous fistula. The radial artery and the cephalic vein in the arm are most often used for access procedures. Other vessels, such as the saphenous vein and posterior tibial artery in the leg, can be used as necessary.

Arteriovenous shunt

The arteriovenous shunt is used mainly for patients in acute renal failure. Once in place, the shunt can be used immediately for dialysis. A shunt can also be used to treat a patient during evaluation for arteriovenous fistula.

Procedural considerations. The patient is placed in a supine position with the arms extended on a wide armboard. An arteriovenous shunt is usually performed with local or local standby anesthesia (monitored anesthesia care). A basic minor instrument set is required, plus the following:

4 DeBakey ring-handled bulldog clamps
2 Johns Hopkins bulldog clamps
4 Arteriovenous fistula clamps
2 Vascular forceps
1 Potts-Smith vascular scissors
2 Needle holders
  Arteriovenous fistula tunneler
  Arterial dilators

Operative procedure
1. After skin cleansing, sterile drapes are applied around the site. A local anesthetic is infiltrated, and a small incision is made over the venous site. Bleeding vessels are clamped and ligated. The vein is dissected free of the fascia, and two heavy silk ties are placed around the vessel and held with clamps. A vascular clamp is applied to the proximal end of the vein, which is then cut and ligated distally.
2. A small incision is made at the selected arterial site after it is infiltrated with local anesthetic. Bleeding vessels are ligated. The artery is exposed and dissected free. Two heavy silk ties are placed around the artery. A vascular clamp is applied to the proximal end of the artery, and the distal end is incised and ligated.
3. Vessel tips are inserted into the open ends of the vein and artery and are tied securely with the heavy silk sutures. A small amount of heparin solution is injected.

The selected appliance is then connected to the vessel tips linking the vein and artery. The vascular clamp is removed from the vein and then from the artery, and the shunt has been accomplished.

4. The fascia and skin are closed carefully over the vessel tips and ends of the appliance to prevent twisting or occluding in any way.

5. Sterile dressings are applied and held securely in place with a gauze roller bandage.

Arteriovenous fistula

The surgeon may elect to create a direct arteriovenous fistula between the radial artery and the cephalic vein. These vessels would then be used for direct cannulation with large-bore needles for hemodialysis. This method is preferable to an external shunt, which carries a high risk of thrombosis and infection.

Other alternatives are to use a saphenous vein or a prosthetic graft, such as a polytetrafluoroethylene (PTFE) graft, to join the brachial artery and cephalic vein.

Inferior vena cava interruption
Transperitoneal approach

A transperitoneal approach may be used to ligate the vena cava, creating total or partial occlusion. Ligation or interruption of the vena cava is performed to prevent pulmonary embolism when anticoagulant therapy fails or cannot be initiated. In the female patient, a transabdominal

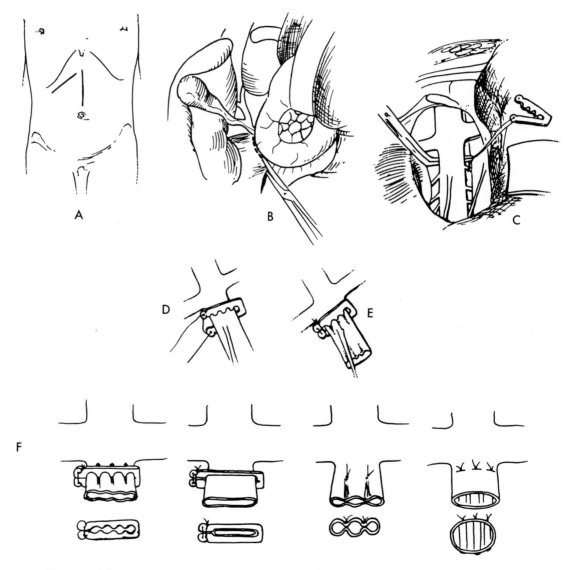

Fig. 26-9. Inferior vena cava interruption, transperitoneal approach. **A,** Incision. **B,** Mobilization of duodenum. **C,** Passage of clip. **D,** Closure of clip. **E,** Positioning of clip. **F,** Other methods of partial interruption. (From Haimovici, H., editor: Vascular surgery: principles and techniques, Norwalk, Conn., 1984, Appleton-Century-Crofts.)

incision may be used to permit ligation of the ovarian veins.

Operative procedure

1. A straight or curved paramedian incision is employed (Fig. 26-9).
2. The muscles are split in line with their fibers. Deep retractors are placed for adequate exposure.
3. The peritoneum and abdominal contents are bluntly dissected anteriorly, and sponge-holding forceps are used to expose the vena cava.
4. Deep in the wound, the vena cava is dissected free with sharp and blunt dissection.
5. With a Mixter forceps, two heavy silk ties are passed around the vena cava and tied approximately ½ inch below the renal arteries. The vena cava is not cut. A Teflon clip may be used instead of ligatures. Several types of clips are available commercially (Fig. 26-9, F) and allow for partial flow of venous blood to reduce vascular congestion in the lower extremities.
6. The incision is closed in layers as for lumbar sympathectomy.

Vena cava filter insertion

Vena cava filter insertion entails the partial occlusion of the inferior vena cava with an intravascular umbrella filter, such as a Mobin-Uddin or Kimray-Greenfield (Fig. 26-10) inserted under fluoroscopy with local or standby anesthesia. The Mobin-Uddin device must be inserted through the jugular vein, whereas the Greenfield device offers the option of jugular or femoral vein insertion.

Procedural considerations. The patient is placed in the supine position with the head turned to the left. Instruments are the same as for arteriovenous shunts. A fluoroscopy unit and equipment are needed, as well as the filter setup.

Operative procedure (for insertion of Mobin-Uddin filter in jugular vein)

1. The filter is loaded and prepared for use according to manufacturer's instructions before an incision is made.
2. The incision and approach to the right internal jugular vein are made (Fig. 26-10).
3. The vein is isolated between tapes, and a venotomy is made.
4. The loaded filter is inserted into the vein and threaded under fluroscopy to the appropriate place in the inferior vena cava.
5. The filter is opened into position, and the stylet removed.
6. The venotomy is closed with a vascular suture.
7. The incision is closed.

High ligation of saphenous veins with or without excision

The saphenous trunk may be ligated and divided with or without subsequent stripping and excision. A series of

cup-shaped valves maintains the venous blood flow in a direction toward the heart. Disease may disturb the normal functioning of these valves, resulting in distention or back pressure. The veins gradually become dilated. Those in the lower extremities are most frequently affected. Dilation of the saphenous vein produces venous stasis, which may be followed by secondary complications.

The objective of surgical intervention is to interrupt or remove the diseased veins, thus preventing ulceration, secondary edema, pain, and fatigue in the extremity.

Procedural considerations. The patient is placed on the operating room bed in a supine position with the legs slightly abducted. Ligation or stripping of the lesser saphenous veins may require placing the patient in the prone position. Drapes are placed to enable flexing and lifting at the knee. Instruments include the basic minor instrument setup (Chapter 11), plus the following:

2 Weitlaner self-retaining retractors
6 Mosquito hemostats, 5½ inches
   Vein strippers with various tips available
   Elastic bandages

Operative procedure

1. The incision is made in the upper thigh, parallel to the crease in the groin. Bleeding vessels are clamped and ligated.
2. The saphenous vein is identified and isolated. Margins of the wound are separated with a Weitlaner self-retaining retractor.
3. The saphenous vein and branches are doubly ligated with black silk ties or transfixed, clamped, and divided. The proximal stump is dissected upward to the point at which it enters the femoral vein, where it is carefully religated.
4. If the saphenous vein is to be excised, an incision is made at its distal, pedal portion at the ankle, and the vein is identified, ligated, and divided.
5. A vein stripper is inserted and advanced to the proximal end of the vein in the groin, where it is secured with a heavy suture, and the tip is attached.
6. As the stripper is pulled up the leg, external compression is applied.
7. Tributaries may be ligated through numerous small incisions along the course of the vein.
8. The groin wound is closed in layers with interrupted sutures, and other small incisions are similarly closed. Dressings and circular compression bandages are applied.

Peritoneovenous shunt

A peritoneovenous shunt is the establishment of a shunt to allow unidirectional flow of fluid from the abdomen through a valve into the venous system, with a resulting increase in intravascular volume and renal perfusion. A peritoneovenous shunt is performed on patients with intractable ascites resulting from cirrhosis or malignancy.

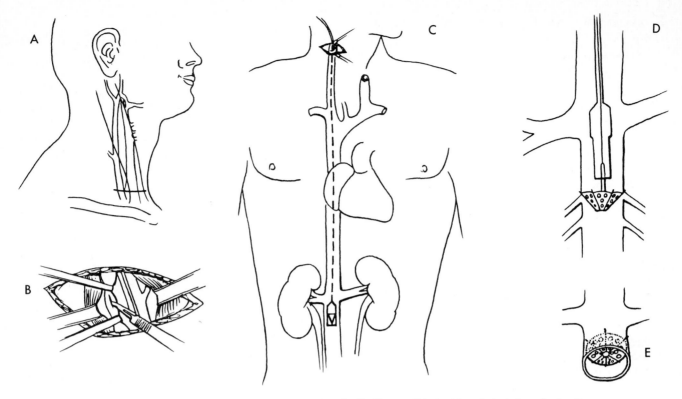

Fig. 26-10. Inferior vena cava interruption with umbrella filter. **A,** Skin incision. **B,** Isolation of vein. **C,** Passage of catheter. **D,** Insertion of umbrella. **E,** Fixation of umbrella. (From Haimovici, H., editor: Vascular surgery: principles and techniques, Norwalk, Conn., 1984, Appleton-Century-Crofts.)

Procedural considerations. The patient is placed in a supine position with the shoulders elevated and the head turned toward the left. Prepping and draping include the right side of the neck, clavicular area, anterior thorax, and upper outer quadrant of the abdomen. The instrument setup includes the basic minor setup, plus the vascular instruments.

The shunt is prepared and sterilized according to the manufacturer's instructions.

The procedure can be performed with local or standby anesthesia.

Operative procedure

1. A transverse supraclavicular incision is made. Hemostasis is achieved. The external or internal jugular vein is exposed and isolated with moist umbilical tapes.

2. A transverse incision is made through the anterior rectus sheath to expose the posterior rectus sheath. Hemostasis is achieved.

3. The subcutaneous tunnel is prepared from the abdominal to the neck incision, remaining anterior to the ribs and the clavicle.

4. A tunneler is used to pass the catheter from the abdominal to the neck incision. The outlet tubing of the shunt is ligated to the blunt end of the tunneler with a heavy silk suture.

5. The pointed end of the tunneler is advanced through the superior flap of the abdominal incision, exiting through the supraclavicular incision. Care is taken to prevent rotational tension of the tubing. All clamps applied to the tubing must be shod with rubber.

6. The tubing is cut flush with the tunneler.

7. Two purse-string sutures of a nonabsorbable vascular material are placed in the posterior rectus sheath and peritoneum. An incision of 1 cm is made through the tissues into the abdomen.

8. The flexible cannula of the shunt is placed into the fluid-filled abdomen. The purse-string sutures are secured around the valve stem to prevent leakage of peritoneal fluid.

9. Valve function is demonstrated by free flow of ascitic fluid through the outlet tubing in the neck.

10. All air bubbles are removed from the outlet tubing, and the tubing is clamped with a rubber-shod clamp at the entrance into the supraclavicular incision.

11. A venotomy is made in the jugular vein with a no. 11 scalpel blade. The outlet tubing is advanced into the vein and placed in the superior vena cava.

12. The tubing is secured to the wall of the jugular vein with two encircling nonabsorbable vascular sutures. The cephalic segment of the vein is ligated. Every

precaution is taken to prevent air emboli during the venotomy and catheter placement.

13. The rubber-shod clamps are removed from the outlet tubing, and the shunt function is established.
14. The tubing is secured to the fascia and muscle.
15. The neck and abdominal incisions are closed, and the wounds are dressed.

Venous access procedure

The venous access procedure entails the placement of an indwelling catheter in the superior vena cava or right atrium for total parenteral nutrition. The Broviac and Hickman catheters are primarily used for this procedure. The perioperative nurse should be familiar with the access technique and catheter used. Special attention should be given to maintaining the patient's skin integrity during positioning. The cephalic vein or the external jugular vein is the preferred catheter insertion site.

Procedural considerations. The procedure is usually done with local anesthesia and fluroscopy. The patient is placed in the supine position with arms at sides and head turned away from the operative side. A pad can be placed under the patient's shoulders to facilitate exposure of the operative area. The skin is prepped according to the surgeon's preference.

Operative procedure

1. The local anesthetic solution is injected into the selected venous cutdown site.
2. For a jugular vein cutdown, a transverse incision is made over the vein in the neck. For a cephalic vein cutdown, an incision is made inferior to the coracoid process in the area of the deltopectoral groove.
3. The vein is identified and isolated with moist umbilical tapes or fine nonabsorbable sutures.
4. With a long alligator forceps a subcutaneous tunnel is made from the cutdown site to the identified exit site of the catheter, usually medial to the breast.
5. A small incision is made over the exit site.
6. The catheter is introduced into the exit site and advanced through the subcutaneous tunnel to the cutdown incision. The Dacron felt cuff of the catheter should be in the subcutaneous tunnel. The catheter is filled with heparinized saline.
7. The vein is ligated distally. A venotomy is made with a no. 11 scalpel blade, and the catheter is introduced into the vein and advanced to its full length.
8. A ligature is placed around the vein to secure the catheter. The catheter is aspirated. Dark venous blood should be present.
9. Radiographic documentation of the catheter's correct position is obtained with fluoroscopy.
10. The venotomy and skin incisions are closed. The catheter is affixed to the skin with a nonabsorbable suture.
11. A sterile dressing is applied, and the catheter is taped to the chest.

REFERENCES

Foss, J.: A history of trauma care: from cutter to surgeon. AORN J. *50*:21, 1989.
James, E.C., and others: Principles of basic surgical practice, Philadelphia, 1987, Hanley and Belfus.
McCredie, J.A., and others: Basic surgery, New York, 1986, Macmillan.

BIBLIOGRAPHY

Adams, J.T., and DeWeese, J.A.: Venous interruptions. In Haimovici, H., editor: Vascular surgery: principles and techniques, Norwalk, Conn., 1984, Appleton-Century-Crofts.
Bender, J.M., and Faubion, J.M.: Total parenteral nutrition, AORN J. *40*:354, 1984.
Bensen, J., and Karmondy, A.: In situ artery bypass: surgery for leg salvage, AORN J. *45*:40, 1987.
Butler, S.: Carotid endarterectomy: care in the OR, AORN J. *32*:42, 1980.
Cox, J., and Jacobs, C.: Laser-assisted angioplasty: treating peripheral vascular disease, AORN J. *46*:835, 1987.
Cimochowski, G.E., and others: Greenfield filter vs. Mobin-Uddin umbrella, J. Thoracic Cardiovasc. Surg. *79*:358, 1980.
Connolly, J.E.: In situ saphenous vein bypass. In Haimovici, H., editor: Vascular surgery: principles and techniques, Norwalk, Conn., 1984, Appleton-Century-Crofts.
Czapinski, N., and others: Nursing plan for abdominal aortic aneurysms, AORN J. *37*:205, 1983.
DeWeese, J.A.: Vascular surgery—what's new in surgery, Bull. Am. Coll. Surg. *71*:58, 1986.
Fernsebner, B., and Baum, P.: Teaching the patient with a vena cava filter, AORN J. *39*:65, 1984.
Fernsebner, B., and others: Surgical prevention of pulmonary emboli, AORN J. *39*:56, 1984.
Gould, D.: Vascular access procedures for hemodialysis, AORN J. *36*:704, 1982.
Haimovici, H., editor: Vascular surgery: principles and techniques, Norwalk, Conn., 1984, Appleton-Century-Crofts.
Hallett, J.W., and others: Manual of patient care in vascular surgery, ed. 2, Boston, 1987, Little, Brown & Co.
Hardy, J., editor: Hardy's textbook of surgery, ed. 2, Philadelphia, 1988, J.B. Lippincott Co.
Hinnant, J., and Stallworth, J.: Simplified surgery for varicose veins, AORN J. *34*:135, 1981.
King, S.: Patient care in vascular surgery, AORN J. *33*:843, 1981.
Leather, R.P., and others: Instrumental evolution of the valve incision method of in situ saphenous vein bypass, J. Vasc. Surg. *1*:13, 1984.
Moore, W.: Vascular surgery: a comprehensive review. ed. 2, Orlando, 1986, Grune & Stratton, Inc.
Rutherford, R.: Vascular surgery, ed. 2, Philadelphia, 1984, W.B. Saunders Co.
Schwartz, S., editor: Principles of surgery, ed. 5, New York, 1989, McGraw-Hill.
Sigley, D.: Nursing roles in vascular access surgery, AORN J. *38*:811, 1983.
Webster, M.: Carotid endarterectomy indications and techniques, Surg. Rounds *8*:57, 1985.
Wilson, S.E., and others: Current status of vascular access techniques, Surg. Clin. North Am. *62*:531, 1982.

27 Cardiac surgery

PATRICIA C. SEIFERT

The treatment of congenital and acquired heart disease has been positively affected by a greater understanding of the natural history of the disease, more precise diagnostic techniques, improvements in perioperative management, and an expanding array of surgical interventions. These achievements are reflected in new procedures for the treatment of coronary artery disease, valvular dysfunction, thoracic aneurysms, and congenital abnormalities. Patients with conditions hitherto considered hopeless, such as idiopathic cardiomyopathy and hypoplastic left heart syndrome, can benefit from cardiac transplantation.

Mechanical ventricular support devices are presently available for patients with end-stage ischemic heart disease to bridge the period until a suitable organ donor can be found. Future trends will include refinements in laser technology and implantable biomaterials as well as clinical applications of microcellular engineering and heterograft organ replacements.

Cardiac disease is commonly divided into acquired and congenital lesions. The timing of surgery is dependent on the appearance of dysfunctional symptoms. A number of congenital lesions, such as atrial septal defect (ASD) and the bicuspid aortic valve, may not require surgical intervention until adulthood. Selection of the procedure is based on the underlying pathology, the skill and experience of the surgical team, and the availability of ancillary support and equipment.

SURGICAL ANATOMY

The *heart* (Fig. 27-1) is a four-chambered muscular organ that acts as a power pump for the circulatory system. It is enclosed in a pericardial sac within the mediastinum, which lies between the lungs, posterior to the sternum, and anterior to the vertebrae, esophagus, and the descending portion of the aorta. The diaphragm is positioned below the heart (Fig. 27-2). The cardiac wall is composed of three layers: the epicardium, the outer lining; the myocardium, or muscular layer, which is the important functional layer; and the endocardium, the inner lining (Fig. 27-3).

Two thirds of the heart is located to the left of the midline, and the remaining third to the right. Although functionally divided into right and left halves, the heart is rotated to the left, with the right side located anteriorly and the left side relatively posterior.

Each half of the heart contains an upper and a lower communicating chamber: the atrium and the ventricle. The right atrium receives desaturated blood from the inferior and superior venae cavae, and from the coronary circulation via the coronary sinus. The left atrium receives oxygenated blood from the lungs via the pulmonary veins. From the atria, blood flows through the atrioventricular valves into the ventricles.

The left ventricle pumps blood into the major vessels of the *systemic* circulatory system: the aorta and its main branches to the head, upper extremities, abdominal organs, and lower extremities. The right and left internal (thoracic) mammary arteries, used as grafts during bypass surgery, branch off the subclavian arteries in the neck and course behind and parallel to the edges of the sternum. The arteries of the circulatory system subdivide into arterioles and eventually into capillaries, where internal respiration and metabolic exchange occur. From the capillary beds, desaturated blood flows into the venules and veins and finally returns to the right atrium.

In the *pulmonary* circulatory system, blood is pumped from the right ventricle through the pulmonary valve into the main pulmonary artery. It divides into the right and left pulmonary arteries, which further subdivide into arterioles and the capillaries of the lungs. External respiration occurs in the capillary beds, where carbon dioxide is exchanged for oxygen. Freshly oxygenated blood from the lungs flows through the pulmonary veins into the left atrium.

Although in *fetal* circulation there is normally a mixing of blood from the right and left sides of the heart (Fig. 27-4), extrauterine mixing of arterial and venous blood is not normal and eventually produces hemodynamic derangements. It is demonstrated not only in infants with congenital defects but also in adult patients with acquired ventricular septal defects, for example, resulting from an infarcted interventricular septum. Because blood flows from an area of higher pressure, the left atrium or ventricle, to an area of lower pressure, the right atrium or ventricle, blood is shunted through these defects, increasing pulmonary blood flow and the workload of the right ventricle.

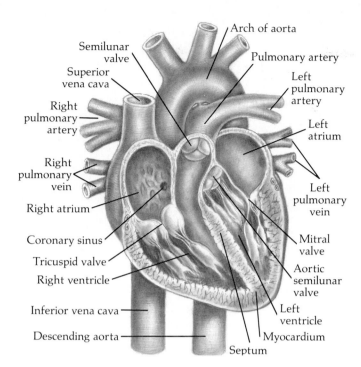

Fig. 27-1. Frontal view of the heart. Systemic venous blood returns to the heart via the inferior and superior venae cavae. It enters the right atrium, flows through the tricuspid valve into the right ventricle, and is ejected through the pulmonic valve into the pulmonary circulation. The blood is oxygenated in the lungs and returns to the left atrium through the pulmonary veins. From the left atrium, it flows through the mitral valve into the left ventricle, where it is ejected through the aortic valve into the aorta and the systemic circulation. (From Thompson, J.M., and others: Clinical nursing, ed. 2, St. Louis, 1989, The C.V. Mosby Co.)

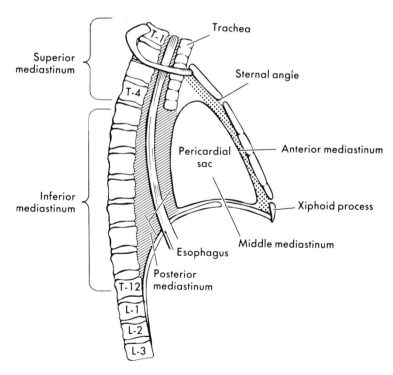

Fig. 27-2. Regions of the mediastinum. (Modified from Brantigan, O.C.: Clinical anatomy, New York, 1963, McGraw-Hill.)

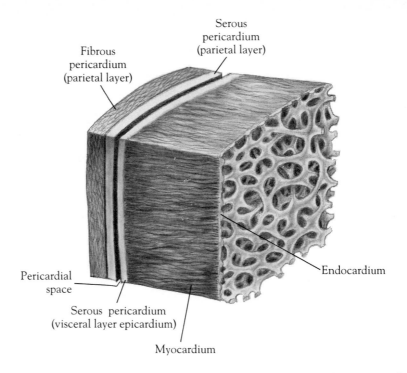

Fibrous
pericardium
(parietal layer)

Serous
pericardium
(parietal layer)

Endocardium

Pericardial
space

Serous pericardium
(visceral layer epicardium)

Myocardium

Fig. 27-3. Cross-section of cardiac muscle showing its three layers (endocardium, myocardium, and epicardium) and pericardium. (From Thompson, J.M., and others: Clinical nursing, ed. 2, St. Louis, 1989, The C.V. Mosby Co.)

The *coronary* circulation (Fig. 27-5) supplies oxygen and nutrients to the myocardium. The heart receives its blood supply from the left and right coronary arteries, which originate in the sinuses of Valsalva behind the cusps of the aortic valve in the ascending aorta. The left main coronary artery divides into the left anterior descending coronary artery and the circumflex coronary artery; along with the right coronary artery, these arteries represent the three main vessels of the coronary arterial system. Atherosclerotic plaques within these arteries jeopardize myocardial blood flow and produce ischemic pain (in most cases) and irreversible damage if untreated. The main coronary arteries are situated in the epicardium, which facilitates their accessibility during coronary bypass procedures. From these arteries arise the septal perforators and other branches that penetrate the entire myocardium. The cardiac veins empty into the right atrium via the coronary sinus (Fig. 27-1); the thebesian veins, prominent in the walls of the right atrium and the right ventricle, open directly into these chambers.

Nerve impulses to the heart travel from the medulla oblongata (Chapter 23) along the middle cervical nerve, which is composed of sympathetic fibers, and the vagus nerve, composed of parasympathetic fibers. The sympathetic nerves promote an increase in the force and rate of contraction, and the parasympathetic fibers cause a decrease in the heart rate. Running vertically along the right and left sides of the pericardium are major branches of the phrenic nerve, which innervate the diaphragm and stimulate it to contract. Identifying this nerve is important for protecting the diaphragm in procedures in which the lateral pericardium is incised or excised.

Within the myocardium itself, certain areas of tissue are modified to form a *conduction* system (Fig. 27-6). The process of excitation and contraction originates in the *sinoatrial (SA) node,* located at the junction of the superior vena cava and the right atrium. The impulse spreads to the *atrioventricular (AV) node,* located medial to the entrance of the coronary sinus in the right atrium, close to the tricuspid valve. From the AV node, the impulse spreads to the *bundle of His,* which extends down the right side of the interventricular septum. The bundle divides into the right and left *bundle branches,* which terminate in a network of fibers called the *Purkinje system.* The Purkinje fibers are spread throughout the inner surface of both ventricles and the papillary muscles, which when stimulated produce contraction of the heart muscle. The location of conduction tissue is clinically significant during surgical repair of atrial or ventricular septal defects.

During myocardial contraction and relaxation, unidirectional blood flow is maintained by the four cardiac *valves* (Fig. 27-7). The *atrioventricular* valves are located between the atrium and the ventricle. The right atrioventricular valve is called the *tricuspid valve* and contains three leaflets. The left atrioventricular valve, called the *mitral valve,* consists of two leaflets. Each of these valves

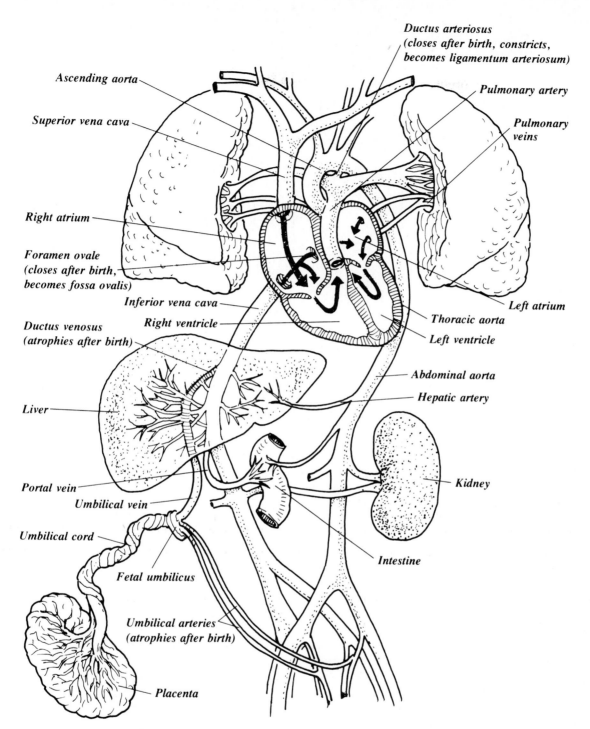

Fig. 27-4. Fetal circulation. The mother's blood is circulated to the placenta, where nutrients and oxygen are exchanged for the fetus's metabolic products. From the placenta, blood flows through the umbilical vein to the fetus's ductus venosus and inferior vena cava to the right atrium. The major portion of the blood in the right atrium flows through the foramen ovale into the left atrium, thereby bypassing the fetal lungs. From the left atrium the blood flows into the left ventricle, which pumps it into the aorta and the umbilical arteries back to the placenta. Venous return from the superior vena cava enters the right atrium, where part of it passes through the foramen ovale and the rest enters the right ventricle, which pumps it into the pulmonary artery. The pulmonary blood flow is shunted through the ductus arteriosus into the aorta. A small amount of pulmonary flow enters the lungs and returns to the left atrium via the pulmonary veins. (From Seifert, P.C., and Lefrak, E.A.: Atrial septal defect: the adult patient, AORN J. 39:617, 1984, Reprinted with permission from © The Association of Operating Room Nurses, Inc, 10170 E. Mississippi Avenue, Denver, Colo. 80231.)

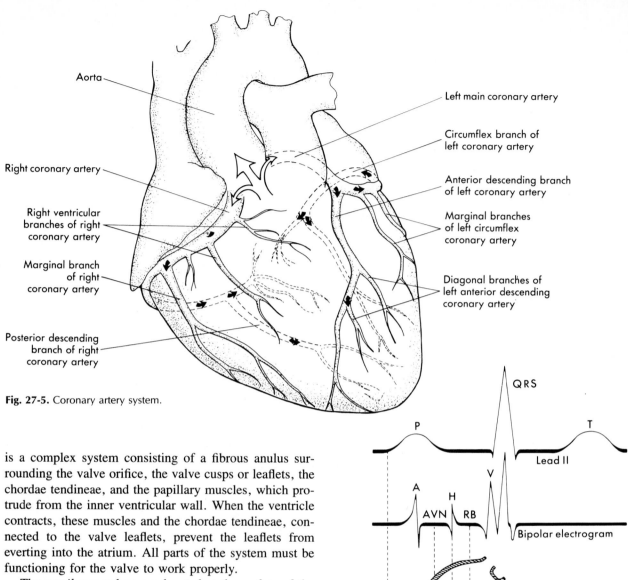

Fig. 27-5. Coronary artery system.

is a complex system consisting of a fibrous anulus surrounding the valve orifice, the valve cusps or leaflets, the chordae tendineae, and the papillary muscles, which protrude from the inner ventricular wall. When the ventricle contracts, these muscles and the chordae tendineae, connected to the valve leaflets, prevent the leaflets from everting into the atrium. All parts of the system must be functioning for the valve to work properly.

The *semilunar* valves are located at the outlets of the left and right ventricles. These valves are known as the *aortic* and *pulmonic valves*, respectively. They are less complex than the atrioventricular valves, and they open and close passively with the cyclic fluctuations in the blood pressure that occur during systole and diastole.

Abnormalities such as stenosis, insufficiency, or a combination of both impair the mechanical function of the valves. Stenosed valves have leaflets that are fibrous and stiff, with uneven and adherent margins. Insufficient or incompetent valves, such as those with leaflet degeneration or perforations, dilated anuli, or ruptured chordae tendineae, produce regurgitation of blood into the originating chamber. These conditions, or a combination of stenosis and insufficiency, strain the myocardium by increasing intracardiac pressure, volume, and workload. Any of the four valves may be congenitally deformed; acquired valvular heart disease most commonly affects the mitral and aortic valves and is thought to be due to the increased

Fig. 27-6. Conducting system of heart muscle tissue. *Top,* Limb lead; *middle,* His bundle electrogram; *bottom,* sites of origin of various complexes. *SAN,* Sinoatrial node; *AVN,* atrioventricular node; *H,* His deflection; *V,* ventricular deflections; *RB,* right bundle; *LB,* left bundle; *PI,* posteroinferior ramus of *LB; AS,* anterosuperior ramus of *LB.* (From Effler, D.B.: Blades' surgical diseases of the chest, ed. 4, St. Louis, 1978, The C.V. Mosby Co.)

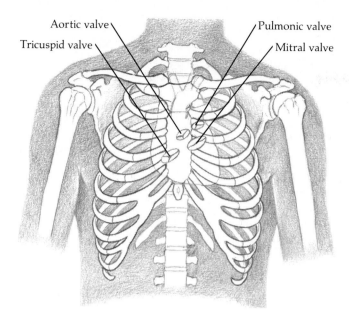

Fig. 27-7. Anatomic position of cardiac valves. (From Thompson, J.M., and others: Clinical nursing, ed. 2, St. Louis, 1989, The C.V. Mosby Co.

stress associated with the higher pressures within the left chambers of the heart.

PERIOPERATIVE NURSING CONSIDERATIONS

Specialized nursing considerations that are indicated for thoracic operations (Chapter 25) also apply to cardiac surgery.

Assessment/nursing diagnosis

Because the severity of the pathologic changes varies among patients, knowledge of the physical derangements, psychosocial concerns, and functional health patterns enables the nurse to plan care and manage the patient perioperatively (Guzzetta and others, 1989). The nursing data base should include the patient's biopsychosocial history, the physical examination, and results from laboratory tests.

History

The history includes information about the patient's health status as well as perceptions and expectations of the disease and the recommended intervention. Patients with cardiac disease may display symptoms of ischemic chest pain (angina pectoris), undue fatigue, dyspnea, and syncope. Depending on their severity, these symptoms affect the patient's functional status and the ability to engage in activities of daily living (see the box).

A cardiovascular disease *risk factor profile* (Table 27-1) is helpful in planning care for hospitalization and discharge by focusing on areas that might require further

---

NEW YORK HEART ASSOCIATION FUNCTIONAL CLASSIFICATION SYSTEM (NYHA CLASS)

Class I
Patients with cardiac disease do not display symptoms of syncope, undue fatigue, dyspnea, or anginal pain with ordinary physical activity.

Class II
Patients with cardiac disease are comfortable at rest but display the above symptoms during ordinary physical activity.

Class III
Patients with cardiac disease, although comfortable at rest, are markedly limited functionally and display symptoms with less than ordinary exercise.

Class IV
Patients with cardiac disease are unable to engage in any physical activity without discomfort and may have symptoms of cardiac insufficiency even at rest.

Adapted from the New York Heart Association: Diseases of the heart and blood vessels: nomenclature and criteria for diagnosis, ed. 6. Boston, 1964, Little, Brown & Co.

Table 27-1. Risk factors for cardiovascular disease

Nonmodifiable	Modifiable
Age	Elevated serum lipids
Sex	Hypertension
Family history	Cigarette smoking
Race	Impaired glucose tolerance
	Diet high in saturated fat, cholesterol, and calories
	Sedentary life-style
	Psychologic stress
	Personality type

Adapted from Matthews, K.A., and others, eds.: Handbook of stress, reactivity, and cardiovascular disease. New York, 1986, John Wiley & Sons; and Price, S.A., and Wilson, L.M.: Pathophysiology: clinical concepts of disease processes, ed. 2, New York, 1982, McGraw-Hill.

patient education. A history of rheumatic fever or frequent tonsillitis as a child is significant because the sequelae of rheumatic fever and streptococcal infections can lead to damage of the cardiac valves. The presence of diabetes is notable because this disease affects the vascular system and may retard healing and predispose the patient to infection. Hypertension and obesity increase the workload of the heart; the latter may also increase the risk for postoperative infection because adipose tissue is poorly vascularized. Mental stress has been increasingly implicated in the development of myocardial ischemia (Rozanski and others, 1988).

Risk factors associated with postoperative infection include previous cardiac surgery, duration of surgery and cardiopulmonary bypass, blood transfusion, postoperative blood loss, and length of preoperative hospitalization (Cruse and Foord, 1980; Ottino and others, 1987).

The patient's knowledge and understanding of the disease process and its effect on his or her functional, physiologic, and psychologic status should also be part of perioperative nursing assessment. The patient's personal strengths, external resources, and coping strategies should be determined. The nurse should note any cultural or religious beliefs that are relevant to perioperative patient care.

Physical examination

The physical assessment provides the perioperative nurse with baseline data and information about potential problems that might require intervention. The appearance of the skin offers clues to the cardiovascular status. Dryness, coolness, diaphoresis, paleness, edema, poor capillary refill, bruising, and petechiae can reflect impaired cardiovascular function. Visual problems and headaches

may be related to inadequate cardiac output, atherosclerotic disease, or medications such as digitalis. The presence of chronic or local infection should be identified; if untreated, these may become potential sources of postoperative infection.

Nutritional status is assessed to determine increased potential for infection, skin breakdown, or other complications.

The patient's level of consciousness, memory, comprehension, and emotional status should be assessed. Confusion, restlessness, slurred speech, numbness, or paralysis can signal impaired perfusion. Their presence preoperatively should be noted by the perioperative nurse.

During respiratory assessment, the perioperative nurse should note the use of accessory muscles or nostril flaring, and auscultate breath sounds. Adventitious sounds such as rales, wheezes, and rhonchi may point to pulmonary edema. Orthopnea, shortness of breath, or dyspnea may require elevation of the head of the stretcher and assistance during transfer onto the operating room bed. If the patient is receiving oxygen, flow rate and method of administration should be noted.

Alleviating pain is a prime consideration in the care of the cardiovascular patient because pain is a myocardial stressor. A patient with angina should come to the operating room with nitroglycerin tablets or transdermal patches. Cold is another stressor because the shivering that accompanies chilling elevates the metabolic rate; the patient should be kept warm.

Heart sounds, murmurs, and friction rubs provide clues to congenital, ischemic, or valvular heart disease or pericarditis. The patient may complain of palpitations. Apical, radial, and/or femoral pulses also reflect cardiac function; their rate, rhythm, and quality should be determined. The presence of cyanosis or peripheral edema should be noted.

The blood pressure may be high, normal, or low. The hypertensive patient may have left ventricular hypertrophy and the hypotensive patient may display changes in neurologic, gastrointestinal, and renal function. Blood pressures should be checked bilaterally. Unequal pressures in the arms may be a contraindication for the use of the internal mammary artery as a bypass graft on the side of the lower blood pressure, where perfusion may not be optimal. Patients with coarctation of the aorta demonstrate unequal blood pressures of the upper extremity, and patients with dissecting aneurysms may have unequal carotid, femoral, brachial, or radial artery blood pressures when the dissection occludes one or more of these vascular branches (Fig. 27-8). Normal changes in the very elderly heart should be differentiated from pathologic conditions (see the accompanying box).

Patient education and preparation for home care maintenance should begin on the patient's admission. The perioperative nurse acts to reinforce, review, clarify, and add to important information and instructions the patient and

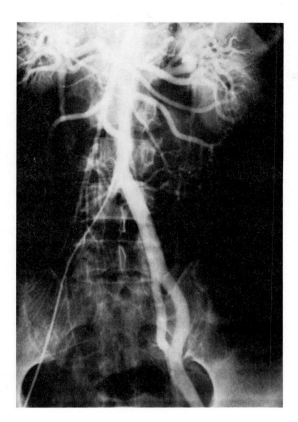

Fig. 27-8. Occluded right iliac and femoral arteries due to compression of the false lumen of dissecting aortic aneurysm against the vessels. (From Seifert, P.C.: Dissecting aortic aneurysms: A problem in Marfan's syndrome, AORN J. 43:445, 1986. Reprinted with permission from © The Association of Operating Room Nurses, Inc, 10170 E. Mississippi Avenue, Denver Colo. 80231.)

CHANGES IN THE NORMAL VERY ELDERLY HEART

1. **Myocardial Walls**
   Increased subepicardial fat
   Increased heart weight

2. **Chambers**
   Decreased left ventricular cavity
   Increased left atrial cavity

3. **Valves**
   Fibrous thickening at contact points
   Mitral valve anular calcification
   Protrusion or buckling of mitral leaflets toward left atrium

4. **Epicardial Coronary Arteries**
   Tortuous
   Calcific deposits
   Increased cross-sectional luminal area (dilated)
   Mild atherosclerosis
   Atherosclerotic plaques composed of fibrous tissue and calcific deposits (hard lesions)

5. **Aorta**
   Dilated ascending aorta with rightward shift
   Elongated, tortuous thoracic aorta
   Calcific deposits

Adapted from Waller, B.F.: Contemporary issues in cardiovascular pathology. Philadelphia, 1988, F.A. Davis.

---

family or significant other need in planning for discharge. The patient's ability to cough and breathe deeply should be determined; the patient should be taught to use a cough pillow or splinting techniques. Required life-style changes should be reviewed, and the patient's feelings about these modifications elicited. The nurse should verify that the patient knows reportable signs and symptoms associated with the specific procedure and understands prescribed medications, dosages and times, potential side effects, and signs and symptoms. Any misconceptions should be clarified or referred to an appropriate source. The family or significant other's ability and willingness to assist the patient in home care maintenance should be queried; referrals to an agency for assistance at home may be required.

Because cardiac function affects all the body's organ systems, assessment of the patient should be comprehensive whenever possible. A thorough assessment also alerts the physician and the nurse to the need for special diagnostic tests and laboratory procedures.

Diagnostic studies

Most patients referred for surgery have had complete clinical evaluations including both invasive and noninva-

sive studies. After the history and physical assessment, a resting *electrocardiogram (ECG)* is ordered. Even if the resting ECG is normal in a patient suspected of having coronary artery disease (CAD), an *exercise ECG* (stress test) may be performed because ST segment changes indicating myocardial ischemia are often apparent only during or after exercise. In patients with intractable arrhythmias, electrophysiology (EP) studies may be performed to locate the site of irritable ventricular foci that can be surgically removed or controlled with an implantable defibrillator (Platia, 1987).

Chest roentgenography provides information about the size of the cardiac chambers, thoracic aorta, and pulmonary vasculature, as well as the presence of calcium in valves, pericardium, coronary arteries, and aorta. Lateral chest x-ray films of patients with prior sternal operations demonstrate the chest wires and extent of pericardial adhesions (Fig. 27-9). In patients with coarctation of the aorta,

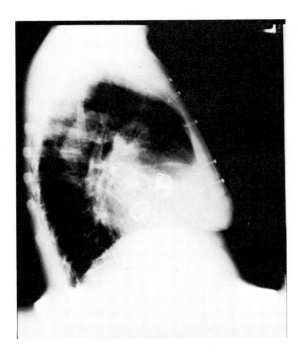

Fig. 27-9. Anterior-posterior chest x-ray film. Note chest wires and pericardial adhesions from previous median sternotomy. (Courtesy Edward A. Lefrak, MD, Annandale, Va.)

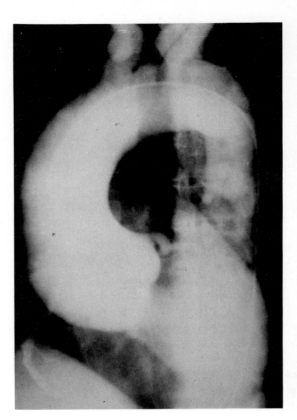

Fig. 27-10. Aortogram of dissecting ascending aortic aneurysm, with aortic insufficiency. (From Seifert, P.C.: Dissecting aortic aneurysms: A problem in Marfan's syndrome, AORN J. 43:445, 1986. Reprinted with permission from © The Association of Operating Room Nurses, Inc, 10170 E. Mississippi Ave, Denver Colo. 80231.)

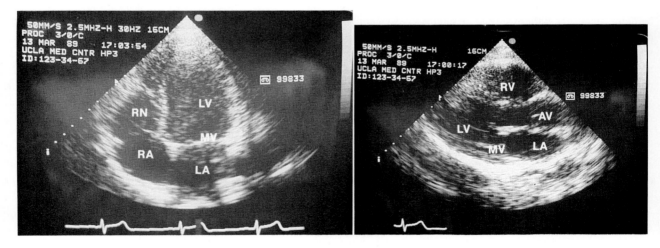

Fig. 27-11. Two-dimensional echocardiography. Note that labels have been added to identify the structures. *RA,* Right atrium; *RV,* right ventricle; *LA,* left atrium; *LV,* left ventricle; *MV,* mitral valve. (From Canobbio, M.M.: Cardiovascular disorders: Mosby's clinical nursing series, St. Louis, 1990, The C.V. Mosby Co.)

rib notching is evident on the left side of the thorax due to the tortuous path of hypertrophied intercostal arteries. In patients with suspected thoracic aneurysms, *arteriography* with radiographic dye is performed to determine the size and location of the aneurysm and the site of the intimal tear in dissecting aneurysms (Fig. 27-10).

Echocardiography is a noninvasive test that evaluates both the structure and function of the heart by transmitting sound waves to the heart and measuring those sound waves reflected back to the transducer (Fig. 27-11). They are processed by the transducer, which creates visual images of the structure's movements. This test is commonly used to assess valvular function and to determine the degree of valvular stenosis or regurgitation. It can also demonstrate a tumor or thrombus in the atrial cavity.

Radionuclide imaging is employed to illustrate wall motion and blood flow through the heart and to quantify cardiac function. These noninvasive techniques are generally well tolerated by patients, especially when they may be too unstable to withstand a cardiac catheterization. They may also be used as a complement to catheterization. The most common radionuclide tests are the multiple-gated acquisition (MUGA) scan (also known as blood pool imaging) and exercise thallium perfusion scintigraphy. In the MUGA, multiple images are viewed to evaluate regional and global wall motion of the heart and to determine the ejection fraction (Barkett, 1988). Exercise thallium perfusion scintigraphy provides additional information about the function of the heart by reflecting deficits in myocardial perfusion at rest and after exercise. The procedure is similar to a MUGA except that there is an exercise portion of the study (performed on a bicycle).

The integration of computer analysis in imaging techniques has improved quantification of acquired and congenital heart disease and refined the diagnostic accuracy of these tests. Newer techniques include duplex scanning, digital subtraction angiography, computed tomography, and magnetic resonance imaging.

Cardiac catheterization provides the most definitive information about the extent and location of ischemic, valvular, and congenital heart disease. A radiopaque plastic catheter is inserted retrogradely through the aortic valve into the left side of the heart by a percutaneous puncture or a cutdown to the vessels of the brachial artery (Sones technique) or the femoral artery (Judkins technique). The right heart is approached via a venous route. To perform coronary angiography that demonstrates coronary anatomy, contrast media is injected into the coronary ostia. Obstructions (Fig. 27-12), flow, and distal perfusion can be assessed. Ventriculography illustrates contractile weaknesses of the ventricles as well as shunting and regurgitation of blood. These studies are used to assess the degree of myocardial dysfunction in acquired and congenital lesions and to plan interventions such as coronary artery bypass grafting or cardiac transplantation if cardiac function is irreversibly compromised. The cardiologist can

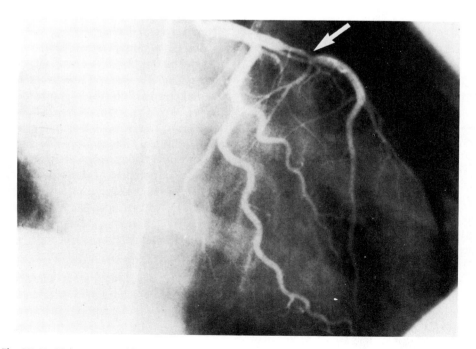

Fig. 27-12. Right anterior oblique (RAO) view of left coronary artery injection demonstrating high-grade stenosis of the left anterior descending coronary artery *(arrow)* at the lead of the first septal perforator. (From Andreoli, K.G., and others: Comprehensive cardiac care, ed. 6, St. Louis, 1987, The C.V. Mosby Co.)

HEMODYNAMIC CONCEPTS

Cardiac Output
The amount of blood (in liters) ejected by the left ventricle per minute; product of heart rate times the stroke volume

Cardiac Index
The cardiac output corrected for differences in body size

Preload
The volume of blood in the ventricle at the end of diastole; the pressure of blood in the ventricle at the end of diastole. Central venous pressure (CVP) measures right heart preload; pulmonary capillary wedge pressure (PCWP) indirectly measures left heart preload

Afterload
The impedance, or resistance, the heart must overcome to pump blood into the systemic circulation; the left ventricular wall tension during systole; systemic vascular resistance

Contractility
The inotropic state of the heart; the ability of the ventricle to pump

Ejection Fraction
The percentage of end-diastolic volume ejected into the systemic circulation; indicator of ventricular function

Adapted from Hurst, J.W., ed.: The heart, arteries and veins, ed. 6, 2 vols. New York, 1986, McGraw-Hill.

---

compute the orifice of a stenosed valve, or determine the degree of regurgitation of an incompetent valve.

Ventricular, atrial, and pulmonary pressures are recorded and cardiac output and ejection fraction estimated (see the box on Hemodynamic Concepts and Table 27-2). Oxygen saturation of cardiac chambers and the ratio of pulmonary to systemic blood flow (Qp/Qs) are calculated in patients with shunts and congenital or acquired defects. Cinearteriograms record the movement of the heart, and cut films from these cines may be displayed in the OR during surgery.

The cardiac catheterization laboratory has also become the site for more aggressive interventional therapies related to evolving and acute myocardial infarctions. Coronary thrombolysis with streptokinase and tissue plasminogen activator can dissolve fresh blood clots and reopen, or recanalize, the artery. Percutaneous transluminal coronary angioplasty (PTCA) may be performed to dilate the artery, and laser angioplasty is becoming more popular. In many instances these interventions may obviate the need for surgical bypass grafting, although restenosis is not uncommon, and eventually the patient may require an operation (Kereiakes and others, 1986). To maintain patency after PTCA, some researchers are using intracoronary stents (Palmaz, 1988).

Laboratory tests

Preoperative laboratory tests are used to assess various organ systems (Table 27-3). Hematologic tests include a detailed coagulation profile to uncover hemorrhagic disorders. In patients who have been on aspirin or dipyridamole, a low platelet count may alert the perioperative nurse to anticipate prolonged bleeding necessitating replacement of this blood product. The patient's blood type is also determined, and the appropriate order placed with the blood bank. Precautions are taken to test the blood for viral contamination and for cold antibodies that could produce agglutination of the patient's blood during surgery when the patient is cooled to hypothermic temperatures.

Liver and kidney function test results may be abnormal in patients with chronic heart failure, possibly owing to congestion related to right heart failure in the former and reduced blood flow in the latter. Progressive improvement in hepatic and renal function is anticipated with successful operative intervention.

Additional perioperative laboratory examinations may include arterial blood gases and enzyme markers of myocardial damage (such as the creatine-kinase MB isoenzyme, known as MB bands), especially in the presence of persistent angina. Pulmonary function tests are performed to determine baseline data and to plan postoperative care when respiratory function may be impaired owing to the use of extracorporeal circulation and stasis of lung secretions that accompany prolonged surgery (Hurst, 1986).

After a comprehensive review of individual patient data, the perioperative nurse identifies relevant nursing diagnoses, from which the perioperative plan for patient care will be derived. For the patient undergoing cardiac surgery, the nursing diagnoses might be as follows:

- Decreased cardiac output related to mechanical factors (altered preload, afterload, contractility, heart rate)
- Potential for infection (wound) related to surgical disruption of tissues
- Potential for injury related to surgical position
- Knowledge deficit related to perioperative events
- Potential impaired tissue integrity related to cardiopulmonary bypass and hypothermia

Table 27-2. Cardiac catheterization data

Hemodynamic data	Normal values		
FLOW			
Cardiac output (CO)	4.0-8.0 L/min		
Cardiac index (CI)	2.5-4.0 L/min/m²		
Ejection fraction (EF)	60%-70%		
Left ventricular end-diastolic volume (LVEDV)	90-180 ml		
Stroke volume (SV)	60-130 ml/beat		
Stroke volume index (SVI)	35-70 ml/beat/m²		
PRESSURES (mm Hg)	**SYSTOLIC**	**DIASTOLIC**	**MEAN**
Venae cavae			0-5
Right atrium (RA)			2-6
Right ventricle (RV)	20-30	0-5	
Pulmonary artery (PA)	20-30	10-20	10-15
Pulmonary capillary wedge pressure (PCWP)			4-12
Left atrium (LA)			4-12
Left ventricle (LV)	120	0-5	
Left ventricular end-diastolic pressure (LVEDP)			5-12
Aorta	120-140	60-80	70-90
Brachial artery	120	70	
Femoral artery	125	75	
RESISTANCES			
Systemic vascular resistance (SVR)	<20 Wood units		
Total pulmonary resistance	<3.5 Wood units		
Pulmonary vascular resistance (PVR)	<2.0 Wood units		
SHUNTS (Qp/Qs)			
Pulmonary flow/systemic flow	1:1		
OXYGEN SATURATIONS			
Venae cavae	70%		
Right atrium	70%		
Right ventricle	70%		
Pulmonary artery	70%		
Pulmonary veins	97%		
Left atrium	97%		
Left ventricle	97%		
Aorta	97%		
VALVE ORIFICES (ADULT)			
Aortic	2–4 cm²		
Mitral	4–6 cm²		
Tricuspid	10 cm²		
ANGIOGRAPHIC DATA	**FINDINGS**		
Coronary arteries	Anatomy/function coronary vascular bed; distal coronary flow; AV fistula; atherosclerosis; anomalous origin of coronary arteries		
Ventriculography	Anatomy/function of ventricles and associated structures; LV aneurysm; congenital abnormalities; valvular stenosis/regurgitation; shunts		
Valvular angiography	Intact mitral/tricuspid complex; valvular incompetence/stenosis/regurgitation		
Pulmonary angiography	Pulmonary embolism; congenital abnormalities		
Aortography	Patency of aortic branches; normal mobility, competence, and anatomy of aortic valve; aneurysms: saccular, fusiform, dissecting; origin of aortic dissection; shunts or anomalous connections; congenital defects or obstructions		

Adapted from Sabiston, D.C., and Spencer, F.C.: Gibbon's surgery of the chest, 2 vols., ed. 4. Philadelphia, 1983, W.B. Saunders Co.

Table 27-3. Laboratory data

Test	Normal values	Test	Normal values
Arterial Blood Gases (ABGs)		Creatinine (urine, 24 hour)	
pH	7.38–7.44	Male	20–26 mg/kg/24 hr
PO_2	95–100 mm Hg	Female	14–22 mg/kg/24 hr
PCO_2	35–40 mm Hg	Electrolytes	
Blood chemistry		Potassium (K)	3.8–5.0 mEq/L
Glucose (fasting)	70–110 mg/100 ml	Sodium (Na)	136–142 mEq/L
Protein (total)	6.8–8.5 g/100 ml	Chloride (Cl)	95–103 mEq/L
Blood urea nitrogen (BUN)	8.0–25 mg/100 ml	Magnesium (Mg)	1.5–2.0 mEq/L
Uric acid	3.0–7.0 mg/100 ml	Lipids	
Cardiac enzymes		Cholesterol	<200 mg/dl
Creatine phospho-kinase (CPK)	<70 IU/L	Triglycerides	10–190 mg/dl
		Phospholipids	150–380 mg/dl
CPK–MB (isoen-zyme)	0–7 IU/L	Free fatty acids	9.0–15.0 mM/L
Coagulation profile		Liver function	
Platelet count	150,000–400,000/μL	Albumin (serum)	3.5–5.0 g/dl
Prothrombin time (PT)	Depends on thromboplastin reagent used; typically 9.5–12.0 sec	Alkaline phospha-tase	20–90 IU/L
		Globulin (serum)	2.3–3.5 g/dl
Thrombin time	Depends on concentration of thrombin reagent used; typically 20–29 sec	Serum bilirubin (total)	0.2–1.4 mg/dl
		Pulmonary Function	
Partial thromboplastin time (PTT)	Depends on phospholipid reagent used; typically 60–85 sec	*Normal values vary depending on the patient's age, sex, weight, and race. The following are generally calculated:*	
		Residual volume (RV)	
Activated PTT	Depends on activator and phospholipid reagents used; typically 20–35 sec	Tidal volume (TV)	
		Expiratory reserve volume (ERV)	
		Inspiratory reserve volume (IRV)	
Complete blood count (CBC)		Total lung capacity (TLC)	
Hemoglobin (Hgb)		Vital capacity (VC)	
Male	13.5–18.0 g/dl	Urinalysis	
Female	12.0–16.0 g/dl	Color	Amber, yellow
Hematocrit (Hct)		Clarity	Clear
Male	42%–52%	pH	4.6–8.0
Female	35%–47%	Specific gravity (SG)	1.002–1.035
Red blood cells (RBC)		Protein	0.0–8.0 mg/dl
Male	$4.6–6.2 \times 10^6/\mu L$	Sugar, ketones, RBC, WBC, casts	Negative
Female	$4.2–5.4 \times 10^6/\mu L$		
White Blood Cells (WBC)	$4.5–11.0 \times 10^3/\mu L$		

Adapted from Henry, J.B.: Todd-Sanford-Davidson clinical diagnosis and management by laboratory methods, ed. 17. Philadelphia, 1984, W.B. Saunders Co.

Planning

Nursing diagnoses are the framework around which the plan of care is devised. Each nursing diagnosis should have a corresponding goal statement. The goal should be measurable, with criteria by which to evaluate its achievement. For example, for the goal "The patient will demonstrate adequate cardiac output," the perioperative nurse might identify criteria such as vital signs and hemodynamic status consistent with or better than preoperative parameters; fluid and electrolyte balance consistent with preoperative levels; absence of rate, rhythm, or conduction defects; absence of iatrogenic injury to the heart; and normal clotting parameters. Each of these criteria becomes evidence that the goal was achieved. When goals are evaluated, they may be noted in the perioperative record as outcome statements. Some outcomes will have been achieved at the conclusion of the surgical procedure; others require ongoing evaluation in the postoperative period to be adequately measured. The evaluation section on p. 917 indicates the requirement for ongoing goal measurement by the use of "will" rather than stating the outcome goal as having been achieved. A Sample Care Plan for the patient having cardiac surgery is shown on pp. 900-901; the perioperative nurse will need to identify criteria specific to the patient for each of the stated goals.

Implementation

Some considerations, other than those previously mentioned, can be useful in implementing the nursing care plan for patients undergoing cardiac surgery.

Special facilities

The operating room must be large enough to accommodate bulky, highly specialized equipment while maintaining aseptic technique. Multiple electrical outlets, auxiliary lighting, and additional suction outlets should be available.

Instrumentation and equipment

The basic setup described for thoracic procedures (Chapter 25) is used, along with some specialized cardiovascular instruments and equipment.

Vascular clamps, which are designed to occlude blood flow partially or completely, must be maintained in good condition if they are to prevent fracture of the delicate intima of the blood vessels and still retain their specific holding qualities. There are many variations in construction of vascular instruments (Chapter 26). The jaws may consist of single or double rows of fine, sharp, or blunt teeth or special cross-hatching or longitudinal serrations. The working angles of the clamps also vary. All clamps are designed to hold the vessels securely and without trauma (Fig. 27-13).

A variety of sternal retractors are available to meet specific needs. With the increased use of the internal mammary artery (IMA), exposure of the retrosternal artery bed has been made easier with retractors that elevate the sternal border (Fig. 27-14). Some sternal retractors have attachments that provide improved exposure of the left atrium during mitral valve replacement (Fig. 27-15). Pediatric multipurpose retractors (Fig. 27-16) can be used for surgery requiring midline sternotomy or lateral thoracotomy incisions. Exposure of the left atrium or the aortic root may also be accomplished with handheld retractors (Fig. 27-17).

Special equipment may also be required:

Sternal saw and motor
Autotransfusion system
Cell processor
Electrical fibrillator
DC defibrillator and internal paddles (Fig. 27-18)
External and internal pulse pacemaker generator (single and dual chamber)
Epicardial pacemaker leads (temporary and permanent)
Fiberoptic headlight and light source
Thermia unit
Pump oxygenator
Intraaortic balloon pump
Mechanical assist pumps

Suture materials

A variety of nonabsorbable cardiovascular sutures with atraumatic needles are available from most suture manufacturers. Synthetic sutures of Teflon, Dacron, polyester, or polypropylene are usually selected for insertion of prostheses and for vascular anastomoses. Most sutures are double armed with a needle on each end. Because of the number of stitches required for prosthetic valve placement, alternately colored suture may be helpful to avoid confusion. Vessel loops and umbilical tapes are commonly used to identify and to retract blood vessels and other structures. Wire (or heavy suture in children) is used to approximate the sternum, with plastic or nylon bands occasionally added to reinforce fragile bone (Fig. 27-19). Skin staplers may be used to close skin incisions.

Supplies

The following supplies are generally used in most cardiac procedures. Depending on surgeon preference, other items may be added or substituted.

Rubber-shods
Pill sponges
Various size Silastic or polyvinyl chloride tubing
Adaptors, connectors, stopcocks
Tourniquet catheters
Disposable drapes
Foot-control and hand-control electrosurgical pencils
Extra syringes and needles for injections, infusions, and blood samples
Marking pen to identify anastomotic sites and mark grafts
Irrigation cannulae
Disposable vascular (bulldog) clamps
Autotransfusion supplies
Chest tubes, chest drainage system

Text continued on p. 905.

Sample Care Plan

NURSING DIAGNOSIS:
Decreased cardiac output related to mechanical factors (altered preload, afterload, contractility, heart rate)
GOAL:
Patient will demonstrate an adequate cardiac output.
INTERVENTIONS:
Check clotting function, coagulation profile, and electrolyte values.
Monitor blood pressures (arterial, CVP, PCWP) and ECG.
Measure and report blood loss (such as suction and sponges).
Maintain adequate supply and assist with administration of replacement blood and/or blood products.
Follow institutional protocol for allergic blood reaction.
Have topical hemostatic agents available.
Have inotropic and antidysrhythmic medications available; assist with administration.
Prepare (or have available) autotransfusion system.
Monitor, report, and record urine output and chest tube drainage; keep tubes and catheters patent.
Have available defibrillator (with appropriate internal and external paddles), fibrillator, external pacemaker, temporary epicardial pacemaker leads, and appropriate ECG cables for cardioversion and intraaortic balloon pump.

NURSING DIAGNOSIS:
Potential for wound infection related to surgical disruption of tissues

GOAL:
Patient will be free of wound infection.
INTERVENTIONS:
Verify that prescribed preoperative prophylactic antibiotic has been administered.
Dress all invasive arterial and venous lines.
Use depilatories or electric clippers to remove hair at the surgical site; avoid razors if possible.
Routinely, prepare anatomic area to knees (or lower if leg vein needed) with antimicrobial antiseptic agent.
Monitor aseptic technique; correct breaks.
Have available prescribed topical antibiotics.
If the operating room bed is raised, lowered, or turned from side to side, take measures to maintain sterility of field.
Confine and contain instruments used in groin or leg; change gloves when moving from lower extremities to chest.
Protect sterility of closed urinary drainage system.
Maintain sterility of instrument setup until patient discharged from operating room.
Document lot and serial numbers of all implants.

NURSING DIAGNOSIS:
Potential for injury related to surgical position
GOAL:
Patient will be free of injury from surgical position.
INTERVENTIONS:
Obtain and prepare appropriate positioning accessories.

Sample Care Plan—cont'd

Maintain proper body alignment.
Pad and protect vulnerable neurovascular bundles and dependent pressure areas.
Prevent pooling of skin preparation agents at bedlines.
Pad thermia blanket.
Keep all surfaces dry and wrinkle-free.
Ensure patency/security of peripheral and central lines, catheters, and electrosurgical dispersive pad on positional changes.
Have adequate personnel to assist with positional changes; lift (do not pull) patient during all positioning maneuvers.
Safely secure patient to operating room bed; ensure patient stability.

NURSING DIAGNOSIS:
Knowledge deficit related to perioperative events
GOAL:
Patient will describe perioperative events.
INTERVENTIONS:
Explain/describe the following events:

NPO status
Administration and effects of preoperative medication
Transport to operating room
Holding area
Insertion of peripheral, arterial, and venous lines
Operating room environment (temperature, staff, attire, equipment)
Induction of anesthesia
Skin preparation

Anticipated length of surgery
Surgical intensive care unit and patient status (for example, unable to talk while intubated and plans for alternate methods of communication)

Determine patient's desire for additional knowledge (respect denial).
Answer questions; clarify misperceptions.
Know where family or significant other will be waiting during surgery; provide communication per institutional protocol.

NURSING DIAGNOSIS:
Potential for impaired tissue integrity related to cardiopulmonary bypass or hypothermia
GOAL:
Patient's tissue integrity will be maintained.
INTERVENTIONS:
Place thermia blanket on OR bed.
Preoperatively, provide warm blankets as required.
Expose only those body areas required for surgical intervention.
Monitor patient's temperature (esophageal, rectal, bladder, and/or ventricular septal).
Adjust room temperature as needed.
Inspect cardiopulmonary bypass lines for patency and presence of particulate matter; alert surgeon as indicated.
Avoid excessive ice particles on heart.
Use solutions of appropriate temperature when irrigating the heart (cold during arrest; warm before and after arrest).

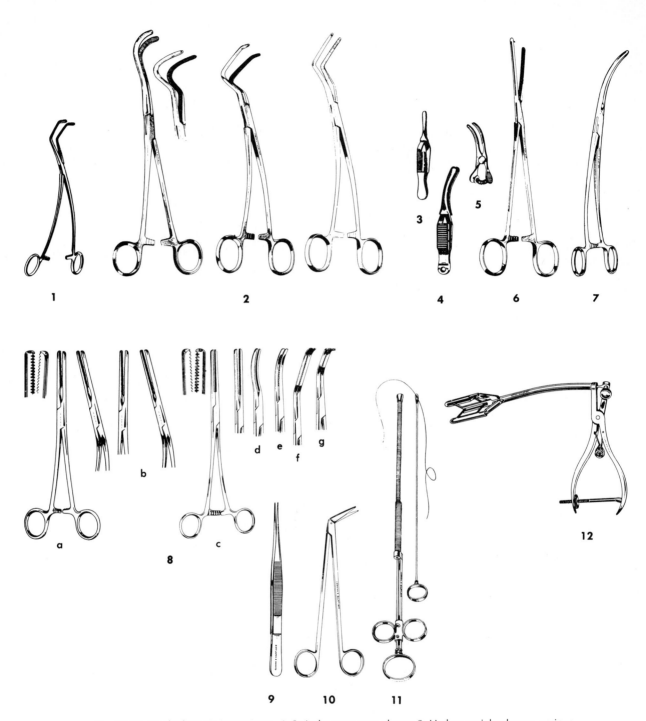

Fig. 27-13. Cardiothoracic instruments. *1,* Satinsky vena cava clamp; *2,* Harken auricle clamps, various sizes; *3* to *5,* bulldog clamps, straight, curved, and adjustable spring type; *6,* Gross coarctation occlusion clamp; *7,* Crafoord coarctation clamp; *8,* vascular clamps: *a,* patent ductus, straight and curved; *b,* coarctation, straight and curved; *c,* anastomosis, straight; *d,* spoon; *e,* curved; *f,* aortic; *g,* appendage; *9,* Potts thumb forceps, fine; *10,* Potts 60-degree angled scissors; *11,* Rumel tourniquet; *12,* Gerbode mitral valvulotome. (Courtesy Codman & Shurtleff, Inc., Randolph, Mass.)

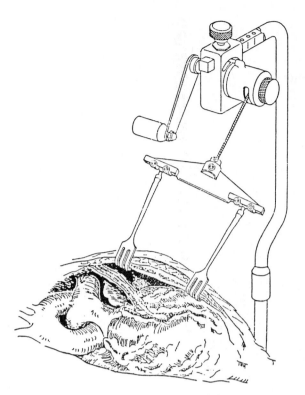

Fig. 27-14. Retractor used to elevate sternal border for exposure of the internal mammary artery. (Courtesy Rultract, Inc., Cleveland, Ohio.)

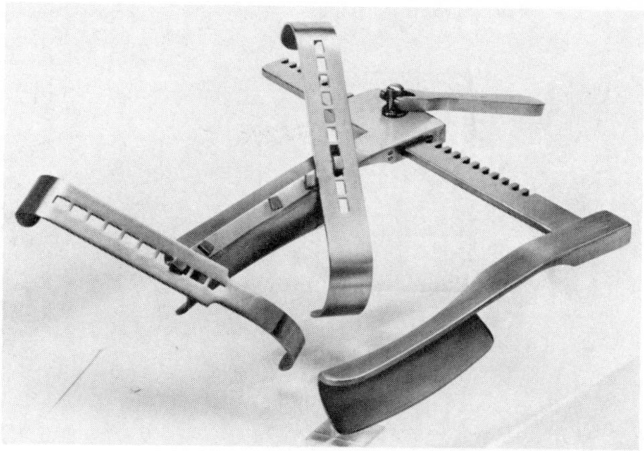

Fig. 27-16. Pediatric cardiac self-retaining retractor with detachable blades. Retractor can be used for midline sternotomy or lateral thoracotomy. (Courtesy Pilling ® Company, Fort Washington, Pa.)

Fig. 27-15. Sternal self-retaining retractor with attachments for left atrial retraction during mitral valve replacement. (Courtesy Pilling ® Company, Fort Washington, Pa.)

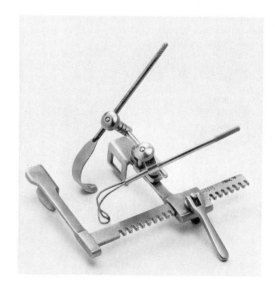

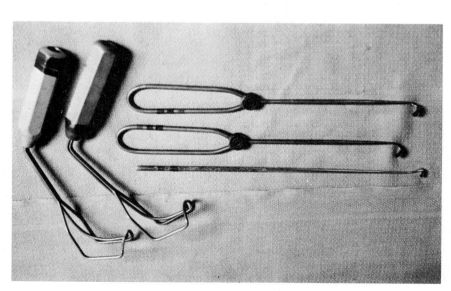

Fig. 27-17. Atrial retractors *(left)*, aortic valve leaflet retractors *(right)*.

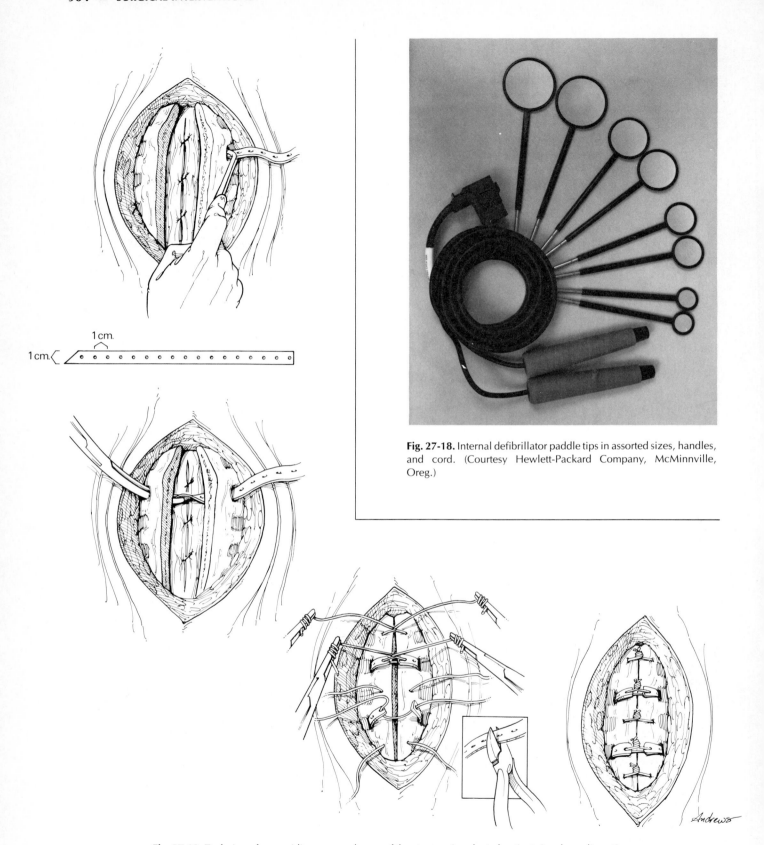

1 cm.
1 cm.

Fig. 27-18. Internal defibrillator paddle tips in assorted sizes, handles, and cord. (Courtesy Hewlett-Packard Company, McMinnville, Oreg.)

Andrews

Fig. 27-19. Technique for providing secure closure of the sternum in selected patients in whom disruption may be anticipated, for example, obese, elderly individuals with chronic obstructive pulmonary disease. A perforated heavy band of nylon is passed around the sternum and secured by a twisted stainless steel wire. Two bands are usually sufficient. Additional encircling wire sutures should be inserted. (From Cooley, D.A.: Techniques in cardiac surgery, ed. 2, Philadelphia, 1984, W.B. Saunders.)

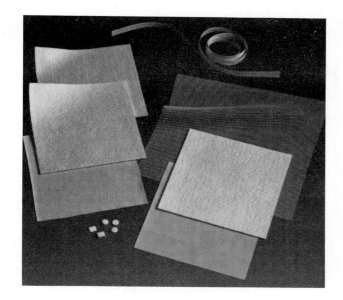

Fig. 27-20. Assorted prosthetic materials to repair intracardiac and extracardiac defects: tapes, Teflon and Dacron patches, and pledgets. (Courtesy Meadox Medicals, Inc., Oakland, N.J.)

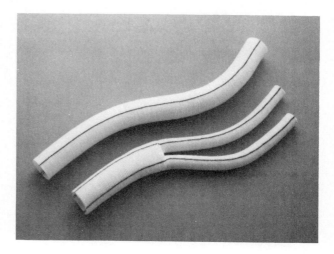

Fig. 27-21. Straight and bifurcated arterial tube grafts. (Courtesy Meadox Medicals, Inc., Oakland, N.J.)

Prosthetic material

In addition to these general supplies, special supplies are needed for repair or replacement of cardiovascular structures.

Intracardiac patches, heart valves, and synthetic grafts should be handled with care to prevent damage or the introduction of foreign materials.

Teflon, a fluorocarbon fiber, and Dacron, a polyester fiber, are available in a variety of meshes, fabrics, felts, tapes, and sutures and are also combined with other materials in prosthetic heart valves (Fig. 27-20).

Teflon patches are made in a variety of forms for intracardiac and outflow tract use. Varying degrees of firmness, thickness, and porosity are available for specific uses. Low reactivity, strength retention, and tissue acceptance are important properties to be considered in selecting such patches.

Dacron arterial grafts are usually used in cardiac surgery, although reinforced expanded polytetrafluorethylene (PTFE) is being used with increasing frequency. There are two types of Dacron grafts: knitted and woven. Woven prosthetic grafts are usually employed when the patient has been given heparin because the interstices are tighter and bleeding is usually reduced. Knitted grafts do not fray as readily as woven grafts when cut. The grafts are available in sizes suitable for straight arterial grafts, as well as for aortic bifurcated grafts (Figs. 27-21 and 27-22).

Tube grafts reinforced at one or both ends with metal rings have been used in surgery for thoracic and abdominal aneurysms; the intraaortic device is anchored in place with nylon tapes tied around the rings. Some surgeons may elect to insert a few interrupted stitches to further secure

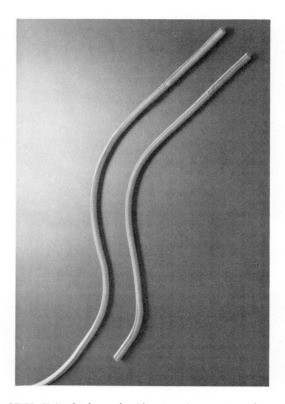

Fig. 27-22. Knitted tube graft with external support; used in areas where compression of the prosthesis may jeopardize blood flow. (Courtesy Bard Cardiosurgery Division, C.R. Bard, Inc., Billerica, Mass.)

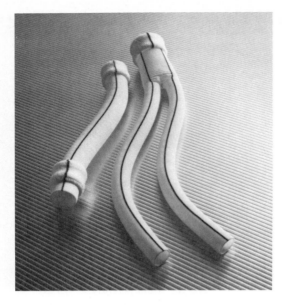

Fig. 27-23. Ringed intraaortic prosthesis, straight and bifurcated, for emergency repair of dissecting aneurysms. (Courtesy Meadox Medicals, Inc., Oakland, N.J.)

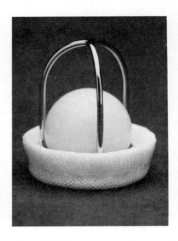

Fig. 27-24. Starr-Edwards ball-cage aortic valve prosthesis. (Courtesy Baxter Healthcare Corp., Edwards CVS Division, Santa Ana, Calif.)

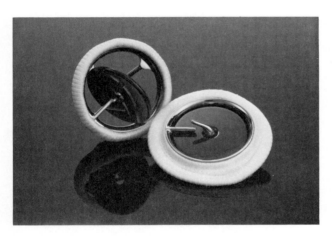

Fig. 27-25. Medtronic-Hall tilting disk valve prosthesis. (Courtesy Medtronic, Inc., Minneapolis, Minn.)

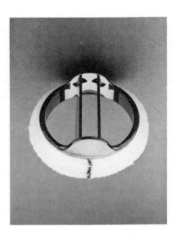

Fig. 27-26. St. Jude Medical bileaflet tilting disk valve prosthesis. (Courtesy St. Jude Medical, Inc., St. Paul, Minn.)

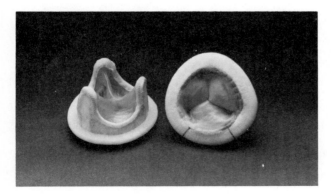

Fig. 27-27. Carpentier-Edwards porcine valve prosthesis. (Courtesy Baxter Healthcare Corp., Edwards CVS Division, Santa Ana, Calif.)

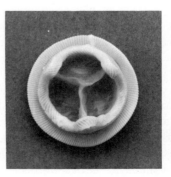

Fig. 27-28. Hancock porcine valve prosthesis. (Courtesy Medtronic, Inc., Minneapolis, Minn.)

the prosthesis. If one end of the graft has no ring or the ring has been cut, routine anastomotic techniques are used (Fig. 27-23). Graft sizers are available for these grafts.

Valve prostheses

Valve prostheses are selected according to their hemodynamics, thromboresistance, and ease of insertion. Most mechanical prostheses employ a ball and cage or tilting disk design. These valves allow complete closure with slight regurgitation to prevent stasis of blood (Figs. 27-24 through 27-26).

In addition, porcine heterograft prostheses (Figs. 27-27 and 27-28) are used. The valve consists of an aortic valve from a pig, which is sutured to a Dacron-covered stent. The advantage of using this valve is that long-term anticoagulants are then not necessary in most patients (Edmunds, 1987). Obturators for sizing prosthetic valves as well as valve holders are shown in Fig. 27-29. Table 27-4 compares biologic and mechanical prosthetic heart valves.

Aortic valve homografts are being used with increasing frequency due to their advantages: little or no risk of thromboembolism, optimal hemodynamic function, no need for anticoagulation drugs, and no risk of sudden catastrophic failure. Moreover, they demonstrate a lower incidence of infective endocarditis than mechanical or biologic valves, and their long-term durability is superior to bioprostheses (Graf and Gonzalez-Lavin, 1988; Yankah and others, 1988). The entire ascending aorta and valve (Fig. 27-30) or the valve alone (Fig. 27-31) may be inserted. Homografts are cryopreserved and must be thawed according to strict protocol prior to implantation (Lange and Hopkins, 1989).

Conduits consisting of mechanical or biologic aortic valves attached to a tube graft (Fig. 27-32) are used in procedures such as repair of dissecting aneurysms requiring replacement of the aortic valve and ascending aorta. If vein grafts must be inserted into the conduit or if a direct coronary ostial anastomosis is required, an eye cautery is used to make the opening into the graft and at the same

Table 27-4. Prosthetic heart valves

Biologic		Mechanical		
DESCRIPTION		**DESCRIPTION**		
Heterograft	*Homograft*	*Ball & cage*	*Tilting disk*	
Carpentier-Edwards Hancock		Starr-Edwards	Medtronic-Hall	St. Jude Medical
Porcine aortic valve	Cadaveric/organ donor aortic valve (with and without stent)	1260 aortic 6120 mitral	Spherical monodisk	Bileaflet
ADVANTAGES		**ADVANTAGES**		
Anticoagulation not needed unless history of AF	Anticoagulation not needed unless history of AF	Long-term durability Good hemo-dynamics	Good hemodynamics in all sizes	Excellent hemodynamics in all sizes
Low incidence of TE	Excellent hemodynamics in un-stented form	Slight valve noise	Slight valve noise Long-term durability	Slight valve noise Popular in children
Inaudible Minimal hemolysis	No hemolysis			Long-term durability
DISADVANTAGES		**DISADVANTAGES**		
Late failure; failure rate increased in children	? Late failure Placement of un-stented valve technically more difficult	Anticoagulation required Some hemolysis	Anticoagulation required Some hemolysis Small incidence of thrombotic occlusion	Anticoagulation required Some hemolysis
Suboptimal hemo-dynamics in smaller sizes (19 mm, 21 mm aortic)	Limited availability			

AF = atrial fibrillation; TE = thromboembolism
From Austen, W.G.: Choosing a valve substitute (pp. 360–363). In Grillo, H.G. and others (eds.): Current therapy in cardiothoracic surgery, Philadelphia, 1989, B.C. Decker.

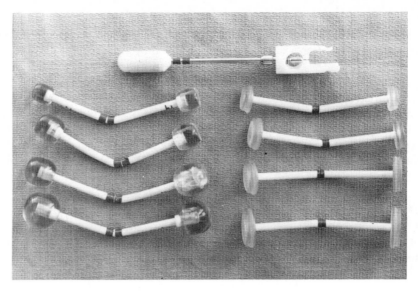

Fig. 27-29. Assorted valve sizers and holder.

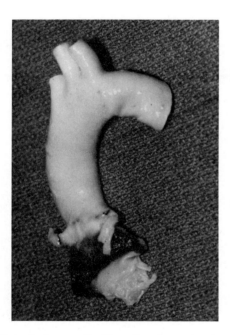

Fig. 27-30. Aortic homograft with aortic valve and arch vessels attached. (Courtesy CryoLife, Inc., Marietta, Ga.)

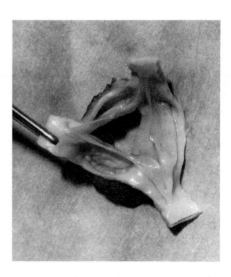

Fig. 27-31. Aortic valve homograft. (Courtesy CryoLife, Inc., Marietta, Ga.)

time heat-seal the cut edges of the prosthesis. In neonates, conduits with valves interposed between tube graft material (Fig. 27-33) are used to reconstruct right ventricle–pulmonary artery continuity. Homograft conduits may be used for these procedures as well (Turley and others, 1989).

In addition to the use of allografts to avoid the complications associated with prosthetic valve replacement,

valve repair rather than replacement has received widespread interest, resulting in greater use of mitral and tricuspid *annuloplasty rings* (Fig. 27-34) to restore valvular competence (Frater, 1987; Sand and others, 1987). Special obturators with a holder are used to size the anulus.

Safety considerations include storing prosthetic materials in a clean, protected environment and utilizing them according to manufacturers' instructions. Prior to implantation, biologic valves must be rinsed with saline to remove the formaldehyde storage solution. During insertion they should be kept moist with saline. Mechanical valves should be protected from scratching or other injury.

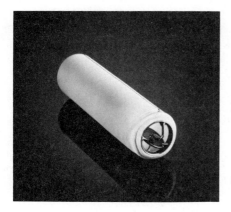

Fig. 27-32. Valved conduit with Medtronic-Hall tilting disk valve prosthesis. (Courtesy Medtronic, Inc., Minneapolis, Minn.)

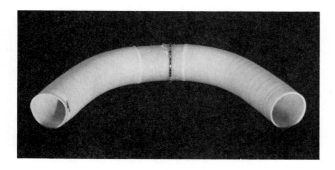

Fig. 27-33. Valved conduit with Hancock porcine valve prosthesis within tube graft. (Courtesy Medtronic, Inc., Minneapolis, Minn.)

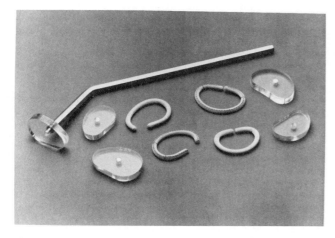

Fig. 27-34. Annuloplasty rings, sizers, and sizer handle. The tricuspid rings are notched to avoid suturing in conduction tissue. (Courtesy Baxter Healthcare Corp., Edwards CVS Division, Santa Ana, Calif.)

Preinduction

The patient is brought to the operating room suite, where a peripheral arterial pressure line and venous infusion lines are inserted. A local anesthetic may be used at the insertion sites and a sedative such as Valium injected intravenously. In neonates and infants, premedication may be omitted if the child is relaxed, but heavy premedication may be indicated when a right-to-left shunt exists and the child's struggling would aggravate the cyanosis (Beynen and Tarhan, 1989). A cutdown may be required to insert arterial pressure lines. If an umbilical artery catheter is in place, it is used.

A preoperative assessment is performed, and the nurse reviews the chart for completion and documentation of laboratory results, diagnostic data, and other pertinent information. Preoperatively, cardiac surgical patients are likely to exhibit more stress and anxiety than other types of patients. Nurses should anticipate and prepare for this reaction because anxiety increases myocardial oxygen consumption; Slogoff and Keats (1989) have demonstrated that postoperative myocardial infarction after coronary bypass was consistently related to the appearance of new myocardial ischemia.

Children are encouraged to bring a favorite toy or security blanket to the operating room. Efforts to reduce the family's anxiety level result in less emotional stress being transmitted to the patient.

Admission to the operating room

Depending on the amount of sedation received preoperatively, the patient may require assistance onto the operating room bed. Warm blankets can be provided while the patient is still awake for comfort and to reduce shivering. Infants are especially susceptible to hypothermia because of their relatively large surface area, less adipose tissue, and limited ability to generate heat. The environmental temperature should be maintained as close as possible to the skin temperature.

Padding of the arms, hands, and feet can be performed while the pressure lines are attached to transducers and the ECG cables are inserted into the monitors.

Anesthesia induction

The choice of anesthetic agent(s) depends on the cardiovascular effects of the anesthetic and the patient's hemodynamics and general health (Warner and Warner, 1989). Because the period of induction is one of the most critical during the procedure, close monitoring of the patient is required, especially for patients with ventricular ischemia from congenital or acquired disease. Anesthetic management focuses on keeping myocardial oxygen demand low and the oxygen supply high (Kaplan, 1987; Tarhan, 1989).

Table 27-5. Perioperative patient monitoring

Monitoring device	Location	Measures

Arterial line	Peripheral
	  Radial artery
	Central
	  Femoral artery
	  Aorta (with needle attached to
	    pressure tubing, or with sensor
	    in bypass circuit)
		Arterial blood pressure (direct)

Blood pressure (B/P) cuff	Arm	Arterial B/P (indirect)
Central venous pressure (CVP) line	Right atrium (RA)	RA pressure (e.g., CVP)
Pulmonary artery (PA) catheter	RA (proximal port)	RA pressure (e.g., CVP)
(Swan-Ganz)	Right ventricle (RV) (midline port)	RV pressure

	Distal PA (distal port)	PA and pulmonary capillary wedge
		  pressure (PCWP)
		Indirect measure of left atrial and
		  left ventricular (LV) pressure
		Cardiac output

Left atrial (LA) line	Left atrium	LA, LV pressure
Pulse oximeter	Finger cot	Oxygen saturation of arterial hemo- globin
Urinary drainage catheter	Urinary bladder	Urine output, renal perfusion/ function
Temperature probes	Esophagus Urinary bladder Rectum Ventricular septum Bypass circuit	Temperature (core and peripheral)

Monitoring

Maximal monitoring of hemodynamic and other variables is indicated during cardiac surgery (Table 27-5). After intubation, additional pressure lines may be inserted to measure central venous pressure and pulmonary artery pressures. Although the need for routine pulmonary artery pressure monitoring has been questioned (Tuman and others, 1989), its use is still widespread. Peripheral and central arterial and venous pressures are usually monitored directly by means of a transducer and oscilloscope. Perioperative nurses may be required to assist with the preparation and placement of central lines; they should observe the ECG monitors for signs of ventricular irritability, such as ectopy or tachycardia, and be prepared to assist with defibrillation of the patient if necessary.

A urinary drainage catheter is inserted for monitoring renal function, especially during and after cardiopulmonary bypass. It may contain a thermistor temperature probe. Other temperature probes may be placed, usually in the esophagus, nasopharynx, or rectum. Ventricular septal temperatures may be recorded while the patient's heart is arrested.

The skin is carefully inspected before ECG and electrosurgical dispersive pads are placed. Bony prominences, especially at the back of the head, are padded to prevent pressure necrosis resulting from hypoperfusion and hypothermia during bypass. Because infants and children are especially vulnerable to skin breakdown, additional precautions to avoid pressure injuries are recommended.

Drugs

Numerous medications are used during surgery (Table 27-6). They may be stocked by the anesthesia department or nursing personnel and should be readily available.

Positioning

The supine position provides optimum exposure for the institution of cardiopulmonary bypass and the surgical repair of the heart and great vessels. In addition, there is less respiratory impairment and discomfort with this approach (Harlan and others, 1980). The arms and hands are padded and placed at the patient's side. The legs may be slightly everted to provide access to the femoral arteries for insertion of pressure lines or intraaortic balloon pump lines or to excise the saphenous vein.

The lateral position (Chapter 25) may be used in operations on the descending thoracic aorta and in certain

Table 27-6. Medications used during cardiac surgery

Type/Name	Purpose
ANALGESICS AND ANESTHETICS	
Morphine	Narcotic anesthesia/analgesia
Fentanyl (Sublimaze)	Synthetic narcotic anesthesia/analgesia
Sufentanil (Sufenta)	Synthetic narcotic anesthesia/analgesia
Halothane (Fluothane)	Inhalation anesthesia
Enflurane (Ethrane)	Inhalation anesthesia
ANTIBIOTICS	
Cefazolin (Ancef)	Broad-spectrum prophylaxis
Tobramycin (Nebcin)	Aerobic gram-negative and gram-positive bacteria
Vancomycin	Serious or severe endocarditis
ANTICOAGULANTS/COAGULANTS	
Heparin sodium	Systemic anticoagulation
Protamine sulfate	Reverse heparin
CARDIOVASCULAR MEDICATIONS	
Antidysrhythmics	
Amiodarone (Cordarone)	Controls life-threatening dysrhythmias, slows AV conduction
Bretylium (Bretylol)	Controls life-threatening dysrhythmias, prolongs refractory period
Lidocaine (Xylocaine)	Reduces ventricular ectopy
Nifedipine (Procardia)	Reduces coronary artery spasm
Procainamide (Pronestyl)	Slows AV conduction, suppresses ventricular dysrhythmias
Quinidine	Slows AV conduction
Inotropic agents	
Amrinone (Inocor)	Increases force and velocity of contraction
Dobutamine (Dobutrex)	Increases force of contraction
Dopamine (Intropin)	Increases force of contraction
Isoproterenol (Isuprel)	Increases rate and strength of contraction, vasoconstriction
Peripheral vasoconstrictors	
Epinephrine	Increases rate and strength of contraction, blood pressure
Norepinephrine (Levophed)	Increases force and velocity of contraction
Phenylephrine (Neo-Synephrine)	Increases blood pressure
Vasodilators	
Nitroglycerine (Tridil)	Dilates coronary arteries, reduces afterload
Phentolamine (Regitine)	Reduces afterload
Sodium nitroprusside (Nipride)	Reduces preload and afterload
DIURETICS	
Furosemide (Lasix)	Decreases renal reabsorption of sodium and chloride
Mannitol	Reduces cerebral edema
ELECTROLYTES	
Calcium chloride	Increases force of contraction, corrects acid-base balance
Potassium chloride	Corrects acid-base balance, improves myocardial contraction
Sodium bicarbonate	Corrects acidosis
MISCELLANEOUS	
Aminophylline	Bronchodilator
Atropine	Prevents reflex bradycardia caused by surgery
Diazepam (Valium)	Reduces anxiety-induced stress, provides sedation
Ephedrine (Bronkaid)	Clears bronchial passages
Papaverine	Smooth muscle relaxant, reduces blood vessel spasm (IMA)
Potassium cardioplegia	Produces almost immediate diastolic arrest of the heart, myocardial protection
Propranolol (Inderal)	Decreases heart rate, blood pressure, contractility, and cardiac output

Adapted from Guzzetta, C.E., and Dossey, B.M.: Cardiovascular nursing. St. Louis, 1984, The C.V. Mosby Co.

pediatric procedures. The presence of severe mediastinal adhesions may necessitate this approach as well.

Prepping and draping

For procedures requiring excision of the saphenous vein, the prep extends from the jaw to the feet and includes the anterior chest, abdomen, groin, and legs. The legs are prepped circumferentially and the chest and abdomen from bedline to bedline.

In procedures not requiring saphenous vein excision, the prep extends to the knees to give the surgeon access to the femoral artery and/or saphenous vein, should the need arise. In the lateral position, the patient is prepped anteriorly and posteriorly to the knees. To retard heat loss in infants, prep solutions should be warmed first.

After the prep, the patient is draped so that the anterior chest, abdomen, and inguinal area are accessible. The perineum is covered and a towel may be placed across the umbilicus to connect the side drapes. When the saphenous vein is to be excised, both legs remain exposed, with only the feet covered. When draping, the nurse should consider the placement of bypass lines so that they remain securely attached and do not become contaminated. A small drape or towel may be placed over the groin area when access to it is not immediately necessary. If later the femoral artery needs to be accessed, the drape can be discarded.

Median sternotomy

The skin incision extends from the sternal notch to the linea alba below the xiphoid process. The sternum is divided with a saw, and a sternal retractor inserted. If the internal mammary artery and/or the saphenous vein will be used, they are made available at this time. The pericardium is incised and retracted.

In repeat sternotomies, adhesions from a previous cardiac operation must be dissected. The sternum may be split with a vibrating saw and the retrosternal tissue cut free. Increased risk of bleeding and laceration of the ventricle, in addition to the presence of dense adhesions,

should alert the nurse to the possibility of instituting femoral vein–femoral artery bypass (discussed later). Because of the amount of surgical manipulation involved in dissecting the adhesions, the patient may fibrillate. Internal-external paddles may be needed if two internal paddles cannot be inserted into the scarred pericardium. An external paddle is placed behind the patient prior to the prep; one internal paddle is placed on the anterior surface of the heart, and the patient defibrillated. Occasionally, two internal paddles can be used if one of these has a pediatric-sized paddle tip that can be inserted laterally through an opening in the pericardial adhesions. Anterior-posterior and lateral chest x-ray films are useful to determine the extent of retrosternal adhesions and to count the number of chest wires for removal (Fig. 27-9). On occasion a patient presents for repeat mitral valve surgery. If the initial operation was performed through a thoracotomy incision, sternal adhesions may be minimal or nonexistent, and the special precautions associated with repeat sternotomy may not be necessary.

Cardiopulmonary bypass

The temporary substitution of a pump oxygenator for the heart and lungs provides the surgeon sufficient time to complete complicated and lengthy procedures under direct vision in a relatively dry, motionless field. Systemic venous return to the heart flows by gravity drainage through cannulae (Fig. 27-35) placed in the superior and inferior venae cavae (or through a single cannula in the right atrium) into tubing connected to the bypass machine. Here blood is oxygenated, filtered, warmed or cooled, and pumped back into the systemic circulation through a cannula placed in the ascending aorta or occasionally in the femoral artery (Fig. 27-36). Because blood is oxygenated by the machine, the lungs do not need to function and can be deflated to provide better exposure of the mediastinal structures.

A percutaneous method of instituting cardiopulmonary bypass employs large-bore, thin-walled sheaths inserted

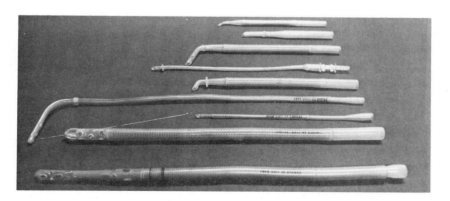

Fig. 27-35. Arterial and venous perfusion cannulae. (Courtesy Harvey Cardiopulmonary Division, C.R. Bard, Inc., Santa Ana, Calif.)

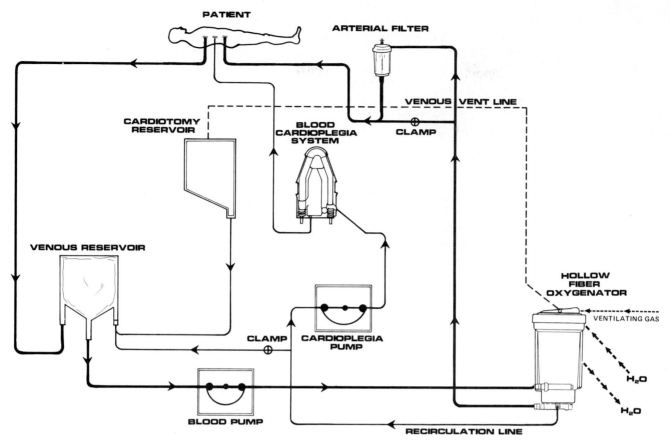

Fig. 27-36. Extracorporeal circuit. This diagram illustrates a typical extracorporeal blood circuit used during open heart bypass surgery. Venous blood exits the patient and drains by gravity into a venous reservoir. The blood is then pumped into the hollow-fiber membrane oxygenator. The oxygenator's heat exchanger controls the temperature of the blood during surgery. The ventilating gas flowing into the oxygenator removes carbon dioxide and adds oxygen to the blood. The oxygenated bloods then flows through the arterial filter and back to the patient. Oxygenated blood is also taken from the hollow-fiber oxygenator and mixed with a cardioplegia solution before being pumped through the blood cardioplegia system heat exchanger, where it is cooled. The blood is then periodically infused into the coronary arteries in order to nourish the heart while it is arrested during bypass. (Courtesy Shiley, Inc., Irvine, Calif.)

into the femoral artery and veins. It is gaining popularity in emergency situations in which the environment is not conducive to the more traditional methods, such as the cardiac catheterization laboratory and the emergency department (Phillips and others, 1989; Phillips, 1986).

By diverting blood away from the heart, cardiopulmonary bypass also decompresses the ventricles, thereby reducing myocardial wall tension, a significant determinant of myocardial oxygen demand. This principle is evident when cardiopulmonary bypass or other means of ventricular support are employed to "rest" the heart. Further decompression is achieved by venting the left ventricle to remove air and accumulated thebesian and bronchial venous return, as well as systemic return flowing around the venous cannulae. The venting catheter is inserted into the left ventricle via the right superior pulmonary vein, or

occasionally through the left ventricular apex. The venting line is connected to the suction lines of the bypass machine. A small venting catheter may also be inserted into the ascending aorta.

Prolonged extracorporeal membrane oxygenation (ECMO) provides circulatory assistance for infants and children with reversible pulmonary insults, such as persistent fetal circulation, and for right ventricular assistance when right heart failure or pulmonary hypertension exists (Spray, 1987).

Improvements in filtration methods have substantially reduced the incidence of gaseous and particulate emboli.

Many types of pump-oxygenators are available. Generally, one of the following two methods of gas exchange (that is, removal of carbon dioxide and subsequent oxygenation) is used:

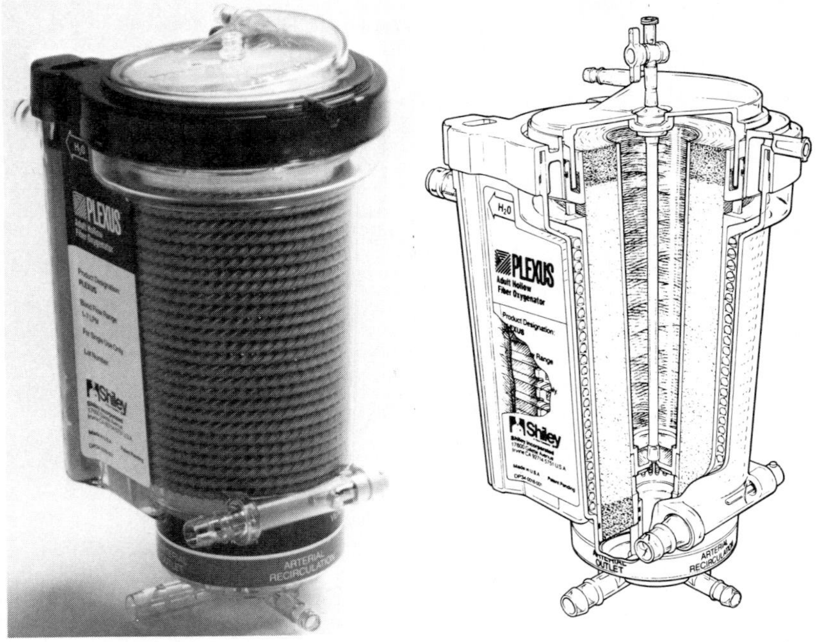

Fig. 27-37. Hollow-fiber oxygenator and cutaway showing internal design. (Courtesy Shiley, Inc., Irvine, Calif.)

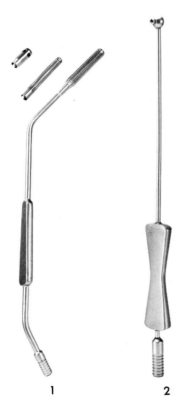

1. *Bubble method*, in which oxygen is bubbled through a column of venous blood
2. *Membrane method*, in which the oxygen is diffused through a gas-permeable membrane that separates the oxygenating gas and the venous blood

Although bubble oxygenators are more commonly used due to their simplicity of design, cost, and ease of use, hollow fiber membrane oxygenators (Fig. 27-37) are increasing in popularity because of better platelet preservation, less use of bank blood, and better postoperative renal function (Hill and others, 1985). The trend may be toward this method also because it is the only one that does not employ a direct blood-gas interface, which is inherently destructive to the formed elements of the blood.

The roller pump has important basic features and is commonly used. It propels the blood through flexible plastic tubing and, with careful calibration and judicious use, can provide relatively atraumatic blood flow. Arterial blood flow with any roller pump, however, is "nonpulsatile" and will be manifested by a "mean" arterial wave form on the oscilloscope during total cardiopulmonary bypass.

Two or more suction lines are ordinarily used during cardiopulmonary bypass to return lost blood directly to the oxygenator (Fig. 27-36). These lines usually combine conventional handheld suction tubes (Fig. 27-38) and ventricular decompression lines or sumps.

Before the initiation of cardiopulmonary bypass, the entire extracorporeal circuit, as well as the tubing and

Fig. 27-38. *1,* Intracardiac suction tube with interchangeable tips; *2,* coronary perfusion cannula with malleable shaft, size 4, 5, or 6 mm diameter for ¼-inch tubing. (Courtesy Sarns, Inc., Ann Arbor, Mich.)

cannulae, must be "primed," or rendered free of air, to prevent air emboli. The priming solution is usually a combination of colloid and crystalloid fluids. The colloid component may be blood, albumin, or plasma fraction, and the crystalloid component is usually lactated Ringer's solution or 5% dextrose and water. Most, if not all, institutions today employ the technique of hemodilution, meaning that crystalloid solutions are predominantly used to prime the pump in an attempt to reduce the amount of bank blood being used. It has the advantage of reducing cost, the number of homologous serum reactions, and the incidence of hepatitis and human immunodeficiency virus (HIV), as well as providing better perfusion of the capillary beds because of reduced blood viscosity.

The amount and kind of drugs used in the priming solution vary among institutions, but heparin is routinely added to reduce clot formation in the bypass circuit.

Arterial blood flow rates are calculated according to the patient's height, weight, and body surface area and are adjusted during bypass, depending on the arterial and venous pressure values and the result of blood gas determinations.

Once the patient is on bypass, systemic cooling is begun via the heat exchanger incorporated into the oxygenator. When sufficient cooling is achieved, the surgeon will prepare to perform the repair. The aorta is cross-clamped, and the heart is arrested.

Myocardial protection

Improvement in the results of cardiac surgery are due in great part to progress made in the protection of the myocardium. Circulatory interruptions, ischemia, and hypoperfusion are required to permit the surgeon sufficient time to repair cardiac lesions under direct vision. Unless measures are taken to protect the myocardium during these periods, irreversible damage can result. Protection is achieved by cooling the heart (and the rest of the body) and by rapidly arresting the heart so that myocardial energy resources are preserved (Siwek and Dagget, 1989).

Hypothermia

Most cardiac surgical procedures performed today employ some degree of hypothermia. This is especially true in the field of pediatric cardiac surgery, in which total circulatory arrest in conjunction with profound hypothermia ($14°$ C [$57.2°$ F] to $18°$ C [$64.4°$ F]) may be used. Hypothermia may be generally defined as the deliberate reduction of body temperature for therapeutic purposes. A moderate degree of hypothermia, to $28°$ C ($82.4°$ F), permits reduction of oxygen consumption by 50%. At $20°$ C ($68°$ F) there is a further reduction of about 25%. Total body hypothermia can be achieved by surface cooling, application of a cooling blanket, or the heat exchanger of the heart-lung machine. Except for patients undergoing very complex procedures, in whom surface cooling may

be accomplished before the surgical procedure, the cooling and rewarming processes are performed during cardiopulmonary bypass.

In addition to systemic hypothermia, local hypothermia is used to further cool the heart. The topical application of saline slush or the continuous irrigation of the pericardial well with chilled saline accomplishes this. Insulation pads placed behind the heart reduce heat conduction from relatively warmer organs. Transmural cooling is achieved with cardioplegia (discussed later).

Two principal dangers are inherent in the use of hypothermia. First, frostbite can occur with surface cooling during which the patient is covered with plastic bags of ice. Wrapping the extremities is usually effective in preventing frostbite, and providing additional padding can reduce pressure injuries. Potential injury to the phrenic nerve and cardiac tissue from ice chips should be considered (Daily and others, 1987; Robicsek and others, 1989).

Second, ventricular fibrillation can occur during the cooling process. This is usually not a problem when the patient is on cardiopulmonary bypass. It can be a real concern with patients who are undergoing surface cooling before surgery. Ventricular fibrillation is unusual at temperatures above $32°$ C ($89.6°$ F), but in children with cyanosis it can occur at higher temperatures.

Cardioplegic arrest

Rapidly arresting the heart during diastole is beneficial because an arrested heart uses less energy than a fibrillating or beating heart. Cardioplegia with hypothermia reduces energy requirements even further.

Cold cardioplegic arrest is accomplished by infusing the coronary arteries with a $4°$ to $10°$ C ($39.2°$ to $50°$ F) solution containing potassium (5 to 50 mEq/L) and various buffering agents to counteract ischemic acidosis.

Cardioplegia solution is delivered, under pressure, to the coronary circulation at frequent intervals to maintain the hypothermic arrest. Potassium is routinely used as the cardioplegic, or paralyzing, agent, causing cardiac arrest by depolarizing the myocardial cell membrane. Potassium can be added to cold blood or crystalloid solution.

The coronary circulation is entered by direct cannulation of the coronary ostia (Fig. 27-38, 2) or indirectly via the aortic root proximal to the aortic cross-clamp. Direct infusion into available vein grafts enhances transmural cooling, as does retrograde infusion through the coronary sinus (Kalmbach and Bhayana, 1989; Diehl and others, 1988). When the heart is sufficiently arrested, the ECG reflects a straight line; when electrical activity is noticed on the monitor (fine fibrillation), cardioplegia is reinfused when continued cooling is desired (approximately every 15 to 20 minutes).

During this period, the surgical repair is completed. The heart is allowed to rewarm, and the perfusionist rewarms the body with the heat exchanger. Air is evacuated from the left ventricle. The cross-clamp is removed. The heart has begun to fibrillate and converts spontaneously or may require internal defibrillation. Temporary epicardial pacing wires may be sutured to the right atrial appendage and the right ventricle, to be used if needed postoperatively.

When the surgeon is satisfied that the heart is performing adequately, termination of cardiopulmonary bypass is initiated. Venous flow is gradually reduced by clamping the venous line(s), and a commensurate reduction in arterial flow is made by the perfusionist. When heart action is sufficient and systemic and pulmonary blood pressures stabilized, bypass is terminated and the cannulae removed.

Closing

After hemostasis is achieved, catheters are inserted into the pericardium for mediastinal drainage. If either or both pleura have been entered, chest tubes are inserted as well. The tubes are connected to straight or Y connectors to a water-seal drainage system (Chapter 25) or an autotransfusion drainage system.

For chest closure in *median sternotomy,* corresponding holes may be punched or drilled on each side of the sternum to facilitate placement of wire sutures; wires with heavy, cutting, atraumatic needles may also be used. The wire sutures are twisted, cut, and buried into the sternum (Fig. 27-19). A layer of sutures is placed to approximate the

---

PATIENT TRANSFER REPORT

1. Procedure (include source of autogenous grafts): _____

2. Monitoring devices: type, location
   CVP line(s) _____ Arterial line _____
   Swan-Ganz _____ Peripheral lines _____

3. Intraoperative problems:
   Excessive blood loss _____
   Dysrhythmias _____
   Blood pressure _____
   Bypass problems _____

4. Blood
   Given _____
   Available in blood bank _____
   Components given (and time) _____

5. Urine output _____

6. Drugs:
   Used _____
   Required in ICU:
   nitroprusside _____ lidocaine _____
   dopamine _____ dobutamine _____
   nitroglycerin _____ other _____

7. Tubes/drains:
   mediastinal _____ pleural _____

8. Epicardial pacemaker leads (single, dual) _____

9. Weight (Kg) _____

10. Allergies _____

11. Electrolyte levels: K _____ Na _____

12. Patient problems/concerns _____

13. ICU bed number _____

14. Estimated time of patient arrival _____

Reported by _____ Date/time _____

Reported to _____

CVP = central venous pressure; ICU = Intensive Care Unit; K = potassium; Na = sodium

fascia over the sternum. The subcutaneous tissue is closed with absorbable suture. Continuous or interrupted synthetic sutures or skin staples may be used for skin closure.

Prior to transferring the patient, the nurse telephones a report to the recovery area, usually the intensive care unit (ICU). The box on p. 916 lists information commonly supplied. In addition, the patient's special concerns and fears as well as significant physiologic alterations should be communicated.

Perioperative documentation follows the standard protocol and should include a complete description of the procedure performed and identification of medications and all implanted material (with lot and serial numbers).

Evaluation

Evaluation of perioperative care includes the determination of whether the patient met the goals of the care plan. Such evaluation assists perioperative nurses in determining if the nursing interventions designed for a specific patient were successful in goal achievement. This type of data collection becomes the basis of the development

of future plans of care for similar patients. Evaluation may be documented in the perioperative record as outcome statements. For the nursing diagnoses and the subsequent plan of care presented in this chapter for the cardiac surgery patient, those outcome statements might be as follows:

- The patient demonstrated adequate cardiac output.
- The patient will be free of wound infection.
- The patient was free of injury related to the surgical position.
- The patient described perioperative events.
- The patient's skin integrity was maintained.

SURGICAL INTERVENTIONS

The following section will deal with operations for acquired and congenital forms of heart disease. Unless otherwise noted, they are performed through a median sternotomy incision using aortocaval cardiopulmonary bypass (Fig. 27-39) and cardioplegia with routine chest drainage and closure as described.

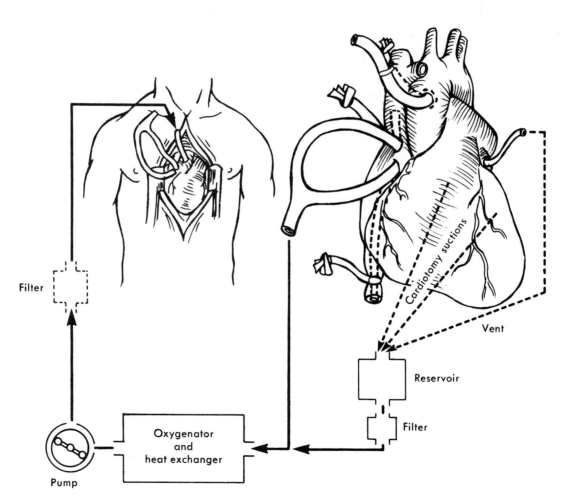

Fig. 27-39. Diagram of extracorporeal circuit showing placement of aortic and caval cannulae.

Extracorporeal circulating procedures

Procedure for cannulation

1. A longitudinal pericardial incision is made, and the pericardial edges are retracted by suture to the chest wall.
2. The aorta, if it is to be cannulated for arterial blood return to the patient, is dissected free, as are the venae cavae.
3. Each vena cava is encircled with an umbilical tape, the loose ends of which are threaded with a stylet through a ¼ × 4 inch red rubber or plastic tubing tourniquet and held taut by a hemostat.
4. Purse-string sutures are placed in the aorta and right atrium or venae cavae for the eventual placement of the perfusion cannulae.
5. The ascending aorta is cannulated for the arterial blood return. A partial occlusion clamp is used to isolate a segment of the aortic wall. The wall is incised, the cannula is inserted, and the purse-string suture is secured with a tourniquet. It is important to have the distal end of the cannula clamped before it is inserted into the aorta. The arterial cannulation is generally performed before the caval cannulations so that direct access for blood replacement is available if needed.
6. For the venous return to the pump-oxygenator, the inferior and superior venae cavae are cannulated. An incision is usually made in the atrial appendage for the inferior caval cannula, and a transverse incision through the atrial wall is made for the superior caval cannula. Each incision is made over a curved partial occlusion vascular clamp, and the cannula is inserted. The purse-string suture is secured with a tourniquet, and the catheter is permitted to fill partially with blood before being connected to the venous line. With double cannulation, compression on the venae cavae (by tightening the tourniquets around each cannula) forces all venous return into the cannulae, producing total cardiopulmonary bypass (CPB). Partial CPB exists when the cavae are not compressed with tapes; it allows some venous return to flow around the cannulae into the heart.
7. Often only the right atrium is cannulated for the venous return to the pump in procedures in which the heart need not be completely empty of blood, such as an aortic valve replacement or coronary artery bypass procedures.

Procedure for femoral cutdown for arterial cannulations. To save time, a second team may simultaneously prepare the arterial return site if the femoral artery is selected for cannulation.

A vertical or oblique incision is made in the femoral triangle, and the femoral artery is exposed. Umbilical compression tapes are passed around the vessel above and below the proposed arteriotomy. (Two vascular clamps may also be applied to the vessel.) An incision is made into the vessel, and the perfusion catheter is inserted retrogradely into the artery as the proximal clamp or tourniquet is released. After the cannula is in place, the proximal tourniquet is tightened to prevent bleeding from the arteriotomy. A clamp must be on the distal end of the perfusion cannula before it is inserted into the artery.

Procedure for pump-oxygenator preparation. While the surgical team prepares the cannulations for connection to the pump-oxygenator, the perfusionist tests and completes assemblage of the equipment.

1. Before the incision is made, the tubing is passed to the perfusionist after the proximal ends have been secured to the drapes.
2. After the venous and arterial lines are connected to the pump-oxygenator, blood is pumped through the lines to displace air in the tubing. To prevent air emboli, caution is exercised, particularly as the arterial connection is completed. This connection is usually made under a saline drip.
3. When all connections are properly secured and the pump-oxygenator is ready, partial bypass is begun. After the flow is in balance, the tapes around the venae cavae are tightened, and total cardiopulmonary bypass is achieved. The perfusion rate is adjusted as the operation proceeds.

Procedure for bypass termination

1. After the intracardiac procedure has been completed, all air is evacuated from the left ventricle.
2. Defibrillation may be spontaneous with removal of an aortic cross-clamp, if used, or rewarming, if hypothermia was induced. If not, electrical defibrillation will be necessary.
3. Compression tapes around the venae cavae are released, and venous flow to the pump is reduced. Arterial flow is also reduced to equal the venous return. When heart action is sufficient and systemic arterial blood pressure is stabilized, venous return is further reduced, and the patient is taken off bypass by clamping all lines and stopping the pump.
4. As the cannulation catheters are removed, the purse-string sutures are tightened and tied. Additional sutures may be required for tight closure.
5. Protamine sulfate, a heparin antagonist, is administered.
6. The pericardium is usually left open for drainage.

Closure of femoral incision

1. The femoral catheter is removed, and the arteriotomy is closed with nonabsorbable cardiovascular suture. Compression tapes and bulldog clamps, if used, are removed.
2. The wound is closed with absorbable sutures, and

the skin is closed with interrupted or continuous sutures.

3. Dressings are applied to all wounds.

In infants and children, the technique is modified. Due to the greater pliability of the aorta, insertion of the aortic cannula is more difficult. A double purse-string is placed around the location of the aortotomy for retraction. Venous cannulae are usually placed directly into the superior and inferior venae cavae, keeping the cannulae out of the right atrium and improving exposure. A venting catheter may be placed into the left atrium near the right superior pulmonary vein; the stab wound can be used to insert pressure tubing to monitor left atrial pressure postoperatively.

Surgery for acquired heart disease
Pericardiectomy

Pericardiectomy is the partial excision of the adhered, thickened fibrotic pericardium to relieve constriction of compressed heart and large blood vessels.

Myocardial contractility is restricted by the adhered portions of the scarred, thickened pericardium. As the pericardial space is obliterated and calcification of the pericardium occurs, the heart is further compressed. Ascites, elevated venous pressure, decreased arterial pressure, edema, and hepatic enlargement result. This condition is usually caused by chronic pericarditis, which may be of tubercular, rheumatic, viral, or neoplastic origin.

Procedural considerations. Occasionally cardiopulmonary bypass may be requested on a standby basis, but usually the supplies and instruments for bypass are not needed.

Operative procedure

1. The lungs are displaced laterally, and the phrenic nerves are identified and carefully protected. The pericardium is incised.
2. The atria and the ventricles are freed. The outer thickened pericardium is removed as indicated. The cartilage scissors may be used. The fibrous adherent portions are carefully dissected with dry dissectors and Metzenbaum scissors. Caution is exercised to prevent perforation of the atria and right ventricle; thus small areas of adherent pericardium may be retained.
3. Dissection is continued, and the large blood vessels are exposed and freed as indicated.
4. Drainage catheters are placed near the heart or through the pleural spaces. Connections to the water-seal drainage system are established as described in Chapter 25.

Operations for coronary artery disease

Treatment of coronary artery disease includes revascularization of the ischemic myocardium with coronary artery bypass grafting (CABG) using autogenous saphenous vein and the internal (thoracic) mammary artery (IMA), and repair of left ventricular aneurysm. Also included are surgery for ischemia-related mitral valve regurgitation (MR) and repair of ischemia-related ventricular septal defects (VSD), which are covered under mitral valve surgery and congenital repairs, respectively. Although the efficacy of CABG remains controversial, it does alleviate angina pectoris and prolongs life in patients with left main coronary disease and triple-vessel disease (Virmani and others, 1988). The IMA demonstrates excellent long-term patency (Marker, 1989; Loop and others, 1986). In addition, the increasing number of reoperations for coronary artery disease has stimulated the search for alternative conduits such as the gastroepiploic artery (Pym and others, 1987) and synthetic grafts.

Procedural considerations. Coronary artery instruments (Fig. 27-40) are added to the basic setup for cardiac surgery.

Coronary artery bypass grafting (CABG) with saphenous vein and internal mammary artery (IMA)
(Figs. 27-41 and 27-42)
Operative procedures

1. A median sternotomy is performed as described; the necessary length of saphenous vein is harvested from one or both legs, and/or the internal mammary artery is dissected free.
2. The distal end of the vein is identified to place the vein in a reversed position so that the semilunar valves do not interfere with the flow of blood. The vein is kept in heparinized blood.
3. A special retractor, such as the one in Fig. 27-14, can be used to expose the internal mammary artery which is dissected, subcostally, until the necessary length is obtained. Clips are used for hemostasis.
4. Cardiopulmonary bypass is instituted as previously described. Usually, mild to moderate hypothermia is employed.
5. Coronary anastomosis
   a. The aorta is cross-clamped. The affected coronary artery is identified and the anastomotic site prepared. Small bulldogs may be placed proximal and distal to the site of the anastomosis to prevent bleeding during suturing.
   b. A small incision is made into the coronary artery, and the vein is beveled to approximate the incision (side-to-side jump grafts may be performed as well).
   c. The anastomosis is made with fine cardiovascular sutures. Before the anastomosis is completed, the distal coronary artery may be probed to ensure patency.
   d. A small bulldog clamp is placed on the proximal portion of the vein before blood flow is reestablished through the coronary artery.
   e. Steps b through d are repeated for each subsequent anastomosis.

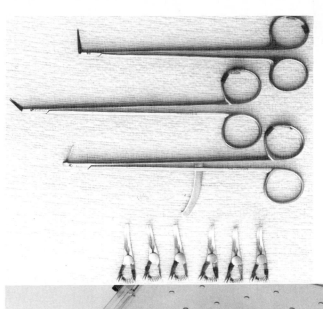

A

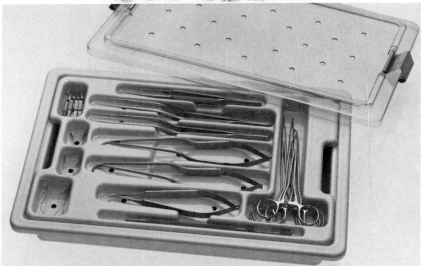

B

Fig. 27-40. A, Diethrich coronary artery instruments. **B,** Internal mammary artery instruments. (Courtesy Codman & Shurtleff, Inc., Randolph, Mass.)

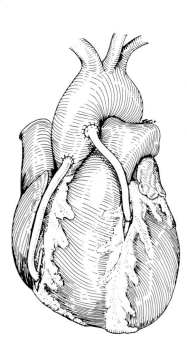

Fig. 27-41. Coronary artery bypass grafts with reversed saphenous vein to the left anterior descending coronary artery and the right coronary artery.

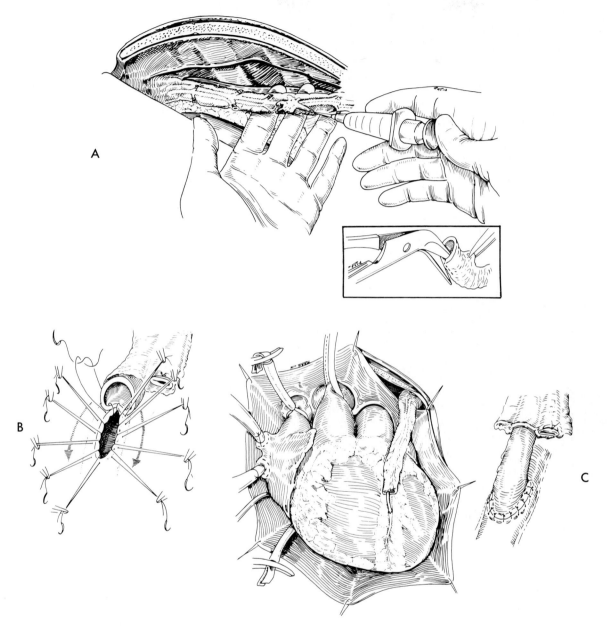

Fig. 27-42. Internal mammary artery (IMA)—coronary artery anastomosis. **A,** Left IMA is dissected from chest wall as pedicle containing mammary vein. Mobilizing artery in this manner is extremely safe, and side branches are controlled by stainless steel clips. Dilute solution of papaverine is sprayed vigorously into adventitia to effect dilation of small artery. Pedicle is then wrapped in gauze soaked with papaverine and stored until pump cannulation is performed. *Inset,* Iris scissors is used to divide isolated IMA and slit inferior wall. **B,** End-to-side anastomosis is constructed by interrupted 7-0 silk technique, inserting and tying each suture before next one is placed. This technique allows clear visualization of intimal suture line as grafting progresses. **C,** Artist's conception of left IMA graft to anterior descending branch of left coronary artery. Grafting is performed without any dissection or mobilization of coronary artery. (From Blades, B., editor: Surgical diseases of the chest, ed. 3, St. Louis, 1974, The C.V. Mosby Co.)

6. The anastomosis of the internal mammary artery to the coronary artery is done as described for the anastomosis of the saphenous vein graft to the coronary artery. No aortic anastomosis is required because the internal mammary artery remains intact at its takeoff from the subclavian artery.

7. The cross-clamp is removed and the heart defibrillated.

8. Aortic anastomosis (may be performed while the aorta is clamped).

   a. The aorta is partially occluded with an angled vascular clamp, such as a Beck, Reynolds, or Cooley clamp, and a small segment is resected, approximately the diameter of the vein graft. An aortic punch may be used for this.

   b. The vein is anastomosed, end to side, to the aorta with fine vascular sutures. The partial occlusion clamp is removed, allowing the proximal portion of the vein to fill with blood.

9. The aortic anastomoses of the vein grafts are usually marked with clips or rings for future identification.

10. Cardiopulmonary bypass is discontinued, and the sternum is closed.

Ventricular aneurysmectomy

Ventricular aneurysmectomy is the excision of an aneurysmic portion of the left ventricle and reinforcement with synthetic patch material (Fig. 27-43).

An aneurysm of the left ventricle (LV) occasionally develops after a severe myocardial infarction in which part of the myocardium is replaced by thin scar tissue. The scar may stretch as a result of the left ventricular pressure, thus forming an aneurysm. The aneurysm is usually adherent to the pericardium, and it may not be possible to

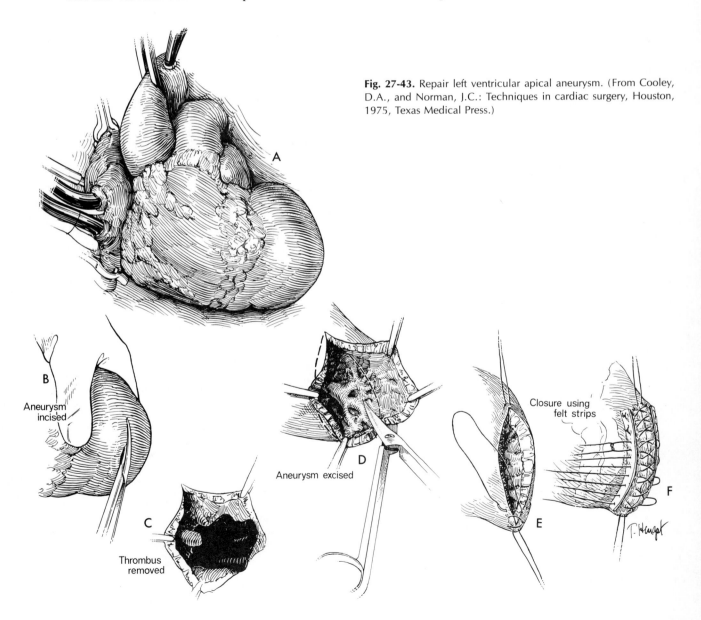

Fig. 27-43. Repair left ventricular apical aneurysm. (From Cooley, D.A., and Norman, J.C.: Techniques in cardiac surgery, Houston, 1975, Texas Medical Press.)

dissect it free until cardiopulmonary bypass has been established.

Procedural considerations. The patient is placed in the supine position. The setup is as described for open heart surgery, plus Teflon felt strips, pledgets, and no. 0 cardiovascular sutures on a large needle.

Operative procedure

1. A median sternotomy is performed, and cardiopulmonary bypass is begun as described.
2. The scar tissue of the ventricle is excised and any clot removed carefully.
3. A cuff of scar tissue is left, through which heavy cardiovascular sutures reinforced with Teflon felt pledgets are passed.
4. The LV is vented with an apical catheter; after the ventricle is de-aired, the catheter is removed and closure of the incision completed.

Operations on the mitral valve

Mitral stenosis, the most common acquired valvular lesion, is usually caused by rheumatic fever. The normal opening in the valve is about 5 cm². As the disease progresses, the mitral valve becomes a narrow slit in a fibrotic plaque, severely limiting blood flow into the left ventricle (Fig. 27-44). Mitral stenosis causes a rise in pressure and dilation of the left atrium. This pressure is transmitted throughout the pulmonary vascular bed, with subsequent pulmonary hypertension, right ventricular hypertrophy, and possibly tricuspid valve regurgitation.

The major symptoms are dyspnea, fatigue, and orthopnea. A characteristic diastolic murmur is heard, and atrial fibrillation is not unusual. An embolism may result from clots in the atrial appendage. Later findings are severe pulmonary congestion and right ventricular failure.

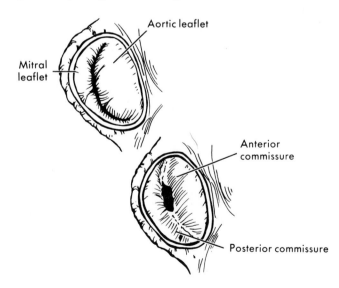

Fig. 27-44. Normal mitral valve *(left)*; fusion and thickening of valve leaflets in center and surrounding area *(right)*.

Mitral regurgitation may accompany mitral stenosis or be due to leaflet perforation, anular dilation, or elongated or ruptured chordae. Ischemic heart disease may produce papillary muscle dysfunction. Symptoms are similar to stenosis. Late findings are severe pulmonary congestion and right ventricular failure (Schakenbach, 1987).

The surgeon's selection of the procedure (repair or replacement) is determined by the stage of disease, presence or absence of calcification, history of thromboembolism and heart rhythm, and any associated pathologic defects.

A number of reparative procedures that preserve the native valve are gaining popularity because the complications associated with prosthetic replacement and anticoagulation can be avoided (Sand and others, 1987). The technique selected must be tailored to the unique pathophysiologic findings; therefore, the surgeon carefully evaluates the leaflets and related structures prior to deciding which procedure to employ. Because there is always a possibility that the valve may have to be replaced, instruments (and prostheses) for replacement as well as repairs should be available (Seifert, 1987). Also included are atrial handheld or self-retaining retractors (Figs. 27-15 and 27-17), obturators for sizing prosthetic rings and valves, sizer or prosthesis handles, and special suture if requested.

Mitral valve repairs
Open commissurotomy of the mitral valve for mitral stenosis

Open commissurotomy is the separation of fused, adherent leaflets of the mitral valve under direct vision.

Procedural considerations. The patient is placed in a supine position for a median sternotomy. The setup is as described for open heart procedures, with mitral valve instruments.

Operative procedure

1. A median sternotomy is performed, and cardiopulmonary bypass begun as described.
2. The left atrium is incised, and the valve is inspected.
3. Fused leaflets are separated with vascular forceps and scissors and/or a knife. The mitral valve dilator may be used.
4. The valve is again inspected for any resultant insufficiency and, if necessary, anular plication may be performed (Fig. 27-45, *A*).
5. The left atrium is closed with a continuous cardiovascular suture.

Mitral annuloplasty for mitral regurgitation

Mitral annuloplasty is the reduction of a dilated anulus using a suture technique or inserting a prosthetic ring (Fig. 27-45).

Operative procedure

1. The left atrium is incised, and sump suctions are inserted into the atrial cavity to remove blood.

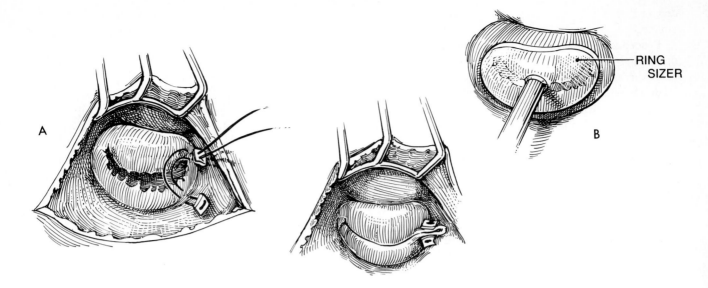

Fig. 27-45. Mitral annuloplasty. **A,** Commissural plication; **B,** Carpentier ring annuloplasty. (From Walhausen, J.A., and Pierce, W.S.: Johnson's surgery of the chest, ed. 5, Chicago, 1985, Year Book Medical Publishers.)

2. The anulus, leaflets, chordae, and the rest of the mitral complex are inspected.

3A. If part of the anulus is dilated, a nonabsorbable mattress suture is used to plicate the commissure adjacent to the posterior portion of the mural leaflet. The suture is buttressed with a felt pledget (Fig. 27-45, *A*).

3B. If there is generalized anular dilation, a Carpentier (1983) ring technique may be used. An obturator is used to determine the appropriate size ring. Interrupted sutures are placed around the circumference of the anulus and then into the ring. When the stitches are tied, the excess anular tissue is evenly drawn up against the prostheses (Fig. 27-45, *B*).

4. The valve is inspected for residual insufficiency, and the left atrium is closed.

Mitral valvuloplasty for mitral regurgitation

Mitral valvuloplasty is the repair of the valve leaflets or related structures. Selection of the appropriate repair for perforated or redundant valve leaflets or for shortened or elongated chordae tendineae requires careful assessment and evaluation of the abnormalities present (Carpentier, 1983; Frater, 1987; Galloway and others, 1988).

Operative procedure

1. Perforated leaflets can be patched with pericardium.

2. Redundant leaflet tissue can be resected. The cut edges are sewn together, and the corresponding anular segment plicated (Fig. 27-46). An annuloplasty ring also may be inserted as described previously.

3. Shortened, fused chordae tendineae can be lengthened and mobilized by their division into secondary chordae or by incising the tip of the papillary muscles.

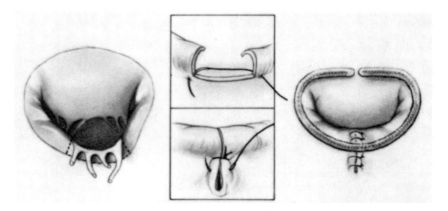

Fig. 27-46. Repair of mural leaflet prolapse by rectangular resection and plication, with insertion of annuloplasty ring. (From Carpentier, A.: Cardiac valve surgery: the French correction, J. Thorac. Cardiovasc. Surg. 86:323, 1983.)

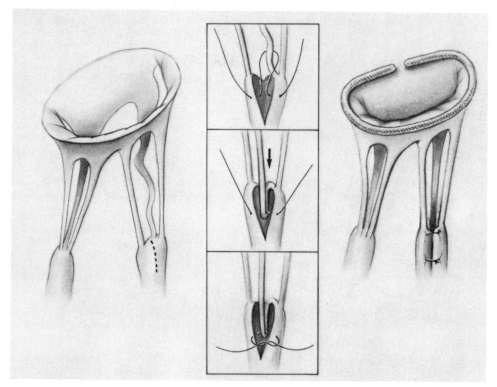

Fig. 27-47. Repair of anterior leaflet prolapse due to chordal elongation, by a shortening plasty of the chordae. (From Carpentier, A.: Cardiac valve surgery: the French correction, J. Thorac. Cardiovasc. Surg. 86:323, 1983.)

4. Redundant tissue of elongated chordae may be implanted into the papillary muscle head or folded over itself and secured with a suture (Fig. 27-47).

Mitral valve replacement (MVR)

Mitral valve replacement is the excision of the mitral valve leaflets, chordae tendineae, and papillary muscles and replacement with a mechanical or biologic prosthesis (Fig. 27-48). Some researchers recommend retaining the mural leaflet and associated chordae and papillary muscles to enhance postoperative ventricular function (Spencer and others, 1985).

Procedural considerations. Although the surgeon may intend to implant a specific type of prosthesis, patient-related factors (see box) or prosthetic valve complications (see box), may force a change in plans. A complete range of valves should be available, as well as saline to rinse the formaldehyde storage solution from biologic prostheses, should they be used. A small catheter may be inserted through the orifice of a mechanical valve to allow air to exit from the left ventricle.

Operative procedure

1. The aorta is cross-clamped with a curved vascular clamp such as a Crafoord or DeBakey, and cardioplegia infused through the aortic root.
2. The left atrium is incised, blood is suctioned away, and the incision is enlarged to expose the mitral valve for subsequent replacement (Fig. 27-48, *A* and *B*).
3. The pathologic condition is determined, and the valve leaflets are excised with the papillary muscles and chordae tendineae. Selection of the cutting instrument depends on the degree of calcification present and the method of excision. Rongeurs may be used to debride calcium particles. A small margin of the valve anulus is retained to insert fixation sutures to the valve. The ventricle is inspected, and all loose debris is removed.
4. The valve sizer is used to determine the correct size of the prosthesis.
5. Nonabsorbable cardiovascular sutures (about 20) are first placed in the retained margin of the valve; the ends are tagged with mosquito hemostats and then placed into the sewing ring of the prosthesis.
6. The sutures are held taut as the prosthesis is guided into position (Fig. 27-48, *D*) and secured, and the sutures are tied and cut.
7. Continuous nonabsorbable sutures are used to close the atriotomy. The patient is placed in reverse Trendelenburg's position. Air is aspirated from the left ventricle through a hypodermic or vent needle or a catheter placed through the prosthetic orifice (Fig. 27-48, *E*), and the atrial closure is completed. It is important to evacuate the air completely before the heart resumes beating and the cross-clamp is removed.

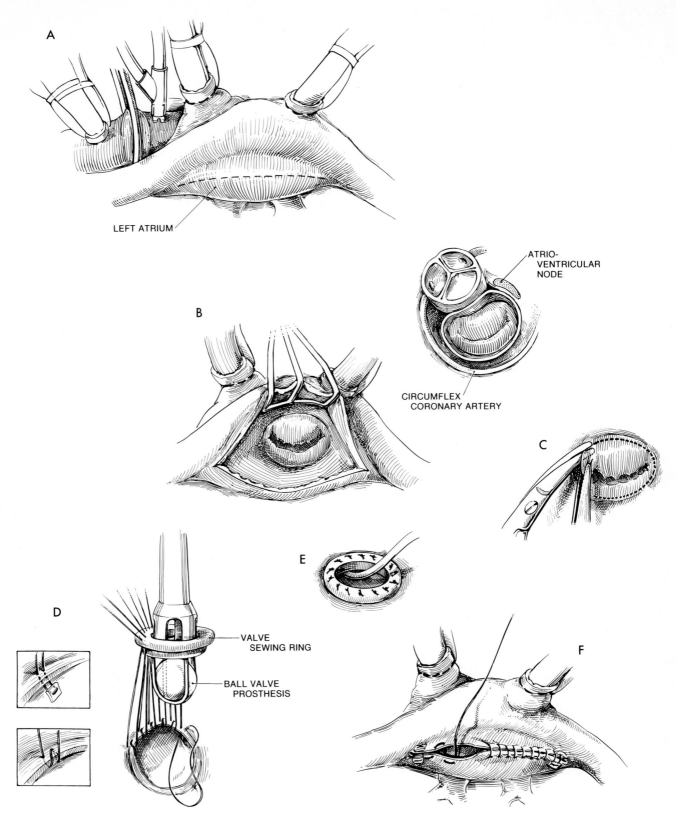

A

LEFT ATRIUM

ATRIO-
VENTRICULAR
NODE

CIRCUMFLEX
CORONARY ARTERY

B

C

D

E

VALVE
SEWING RING

BALL VALVE
PROSTHESIS

F

Fig. 27-48. Mitral valve replacement. **A,** Line of incision, surrounding anatomy; **B,** atrial retractor in left atrium exposing mitral valve; **C,** valve excision; **D,** insertion of stitches into prosthesis and anulus; **E,** catheter inserted through prosthetic orifice to maintain incompetence, thus allowing air to exit left ventricle; **F,** closure of left atrial incision. (From Waldhausen, J.A., and Pierce, W.S.: Johnson's surgery of the chest, ed. 5, Chicago, 1985, Year Book Medical Publishers.)

PATIENT-RELATED FACTORS AND RISKS

Age

Sex

Residence

History of atrial fibrillation

Endocarditis (preoperative)

Connective tissue disorders (e.g., myxomatous changes)

Congenital anomalies (e.g., bicuspid aortic valve)

Enlarged left atrium

Left atrial thrombus

Left ventricular function (e.g., functional class, myocardial infarction, congestive heart failure)

Syncope

Anticoagulation compliance

Preexisting medical problems (e.g., diabetes mellitus, hypertension, hepatic or renal disease)

Valve lesion

Previous cardiac surgery

Adapted from Mitchell, R.S., and others: Significant patient-related determinants of prosthetic valve performance, J. Thorac. Cardiovasc. Surg. 91:807, 1986; and Salomon, N.W., and others: Patient-related risk factors as predictors of results following isolated mitral valve replacement, Ann. Thorac. Surg. 24:519, 1977.

VALVE-RELATED RISKS AND COMPLICATIONS

Thromboembolism

Anticoagulation-related hemorrhage

Prosthetic valve endocarditis

Perioprosthetic leak

Prosthetic failure

Adapted from Bodnar, E., and others: Assessment and comparison of the performance of cardiac valves, Ann. Thorac. Surg. 34:146, 1982; and Oyer, P.E., and others: Valve replacement with the Starr-Edwards and Hancock prosthesis: comparative analysis of late morbidity and mortality, Ann. Surg. 186:301, 1977.

Operation on the tricuspid valve
Tricuspid valve annuloplasty

Tricuspid valve annuloplasty is the reduction of a dilated anulus with a suture technique or a prosthetic ring. Tricuspid valve regurgitation in the adult is often the functional result of mitral valve disease. (Congenital tricuspid lesions are discussed later.) If the tricuspid valve does not regain competence after mitral valve correction or if tricuspid anular dilation occurs, repairs similar to mitral annuloplasty may be performed. Caution is taken to avoid injury to the atrioventricular (AV) node.

Operative procedure

1. Double venous cannulae are inserted so that they do not cross one another in the right atrium, and occluding tapes are tightened around the cavae and cannulae to prevent venous return from entering the right atrium and obscuring the surgical site.
2. The right atrium is opened longitudinally to expose the tricuspid valve. Sump suctions are inserted to remove coronary sinus drainage.
3A. In the DeVega (Rabago and others, 1980) technique (Fig. 27-49), a double-armed, felt-pledgeted suture is placed in the valve anulus, beginning at the anteroseptal commissure and continued around to the level of the coronary sinus orifice. The remaining arm is similarly placed. The suture is tied over a pledget with sufficient tension to reduce the anular area to the size desired.
3B. In the Carpentier (1983) technique (Grondin and others, 1975), a prosthetic ring is inserted in a manner similar to mitral valve ring annuloplasty (Fig. 27-45, B). To avoid potential injury to the AV node, tricuspid valve rings often have an interruption in that portion corresponding to the area of the nodal conduction tissue.
4. Saline may be injected into the ventricle to test the competence of the repair.
5. The right atrium is closed.

Operations on the aortic valve

Aortic stenosis produces obstruction of the left ventricular outflow. Whether caused by rheumatic fever, a congenital bicuspid valve, or calcific degeneration, the fused valve leaflets present an increasing pressure load on the ventricle. To compensate, the ventricle hypertrophies so that it can generate sufficient pressure to eject blood through the narrowed opening. Large pressure gradients are often measured during cardiac catheterization, with differences in systolic pressures between the ventricle and the aorta reaching 50 mm Hg or greater. In the early stages of the disease, a systolic aortic murmur may be heard, but patients are rarely symptomatic; eventually fatigue, exertional dyspnea, angina pectoris, syncope, and congestive heart failure may develop, presenting a grave prognosis. Sudden death is not uncommon.

Although balloon valvuloplasty has been performed in elderly patients for whom surgery poses too great a risk (Isner and others, 1987), total valve excision and replacement with a prosthesis or a homograft are often necessary.

Diastolic regurgitation of blood into the left ventricle

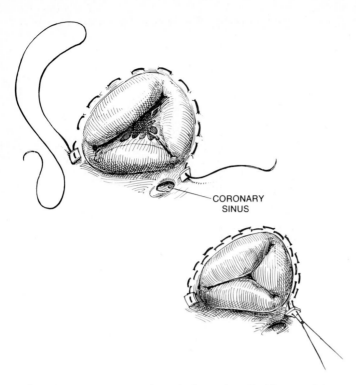

CORONARY
SINUS

Fig. 27-49. DeVega tricuspid annuloplasty. (From Waldhausen, J.A., and Pierce, W.S.: Johnson's surgery of the chest, ed. 5, Chicago, 1985, Year Book Medical Publishers.)

is caused by aortic insufficiency. Rheumatic fever, connective tissue disorders, and infective endocarditis may be responsible (Fig. 27-50). As this volume load increases, the left ventricle compensates by dilation and, later, hypertrophy. Symptoms of coronary insufficiency, cerebral hypoperfusion, and congestive failure are later findings.

Aortic valvulotomy

In aortic valvulotomy, the fused leaflets are sharply divided.

Procedural considerations. This procedure is commonly performed in children with congenital aortic stenosis. Positioning, incision, bypass, and aortotomy are similar to that described later for aortic valve replacement. Another reparative procedure is being used in patients with calcified valves. A high-speed drill is used to remove the calcium deposits from the leaflets and results in a more pliable valve and a lower pressure gradient (Mindich and others, 1988).

Aortic valve replacement

The aortic valve is excised and replaced with a mechanical or biologic prosthesis or an aortic valve homograft (Fig. 27-51).

Procedural considerations. To the basic setup are added:

Aortic valve instruments
Aortic valves, sizers, and holders

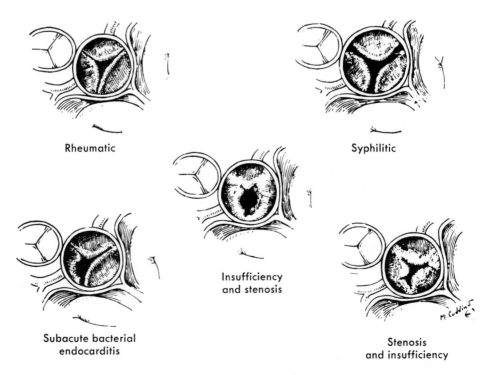

Rheumatic

Syphilitic

Insufficiency
and stenosis

Subacute bacterial
endocarditis

Stenosis
and insufficiency

Fig. 27-50. Pathologic patterns of aortic stenosis, insufficiency, and combined lesions. (From Blades, B., editor: Surgical diseases of the heart, ed. 3, St. Louis, 1974, The C.V. Mosby Co.)

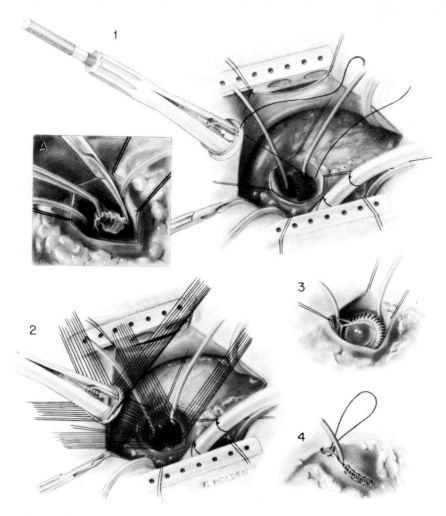

Fig. 27-51. Diseased aortic valve is completely excised, and overlapping fixation sutures are placed before valve is lowered into place. Silastic ball poppet is not replaced until valve chassis is firmly seated. (From Harken, D.E.: Mitral and aortic valve surgery. In Cooper, P., editor: Craft of surgery, ed. 2, Boston, 1971, Little, Brown & Co.)

Coronary artery perfusion cannulae (surgeon's preference)
Saline to rinse biological prostheses or homografts

Operative procedure

1. After the institution of CPB, a left ventricular vent is inserted.

2. The aorta is cross-clamped. If aortic insufficiency is present, the aorta is incised transversely and perfusion cannulae are inserted directly into the coronary ostia to infuse cardioplegia. If aortic stenosis is present, the initial bolus of cardioplegia may be infused into the aortic root. Once the heart is arrested, the aorta is opened.

3. The native valve is inspected, and the extent of the pathologic defect confirmed. If calcium deposits are present, they are debrided with scissors or rongeurs. The valve is carefully excised to avoid injury to the anulus and underlying structures. Narrow packing may be used in the left ventricle to confine small,

loose, calcified fragments that could subsequently embolize. Instruments should be wiped clean frequently.

4. The anulus is sized, and the proper prosthesis selected.

5A. If a biologic valve is selected, it is delivered to the field and rinsed in saline baths.

5B. If a homograft is used, it is delivered to the field and thawed in saline baths according to protocol.

5C. If a mechanical valve is chosen, it may be placed in an antibiotic solution until inserted. (Antibiotic solutions should not be poured directly onto biologic valves.)

6A. The new valve is implanted using a technique similar to that previously described for mitral valve replacement.

6B. If the aortic anulus is too small to accept a prosthesis of adequate size, a Konno procedure can be used to

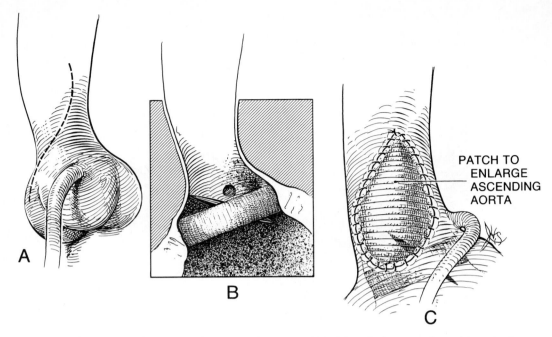

Fig. 27-52. Konno technique to enlarge ascending aorta. **A,** Incision; **B,** the aorta above the anulus is too small for a disk (or a ball-cage) valve to open properly; **C,** patch inserted. (From Waldhausen, J.A., and Pierce, W.S.: Johnson's surgery of the chest, ed. 5, Chicago, 1985, Year Book Medical Publishers.)

enlarge the anulus and proximal portion of the ascending aorta (Waldhausen and Pierce, 1985). A diamond-shaped patch of bovine pericardium or Dacron graft is placed longitudinally in the proximal anterior ascending aorta where the aortic anulus has been cut. The valve prosthesis desired is sutured to the natural anulus and then to the patch. The patch is sutured to the remaining edges of the aortotomy (Fig. 27-52).

7. The aorta is closed with nonabsorbable sutures, and the cross-clamp removed.
8. The left side of the heart is de-aired (by vent, by moving the operating room bed side to side, or by other maneuvers chosen by the surgeon). The patient is placed in the Trendelenburg's position, and the heart is not allowed to contract and eject blood until the surgeon is satisfied that no air remains within the left ventricle. The heart is defibrillated.
9. Rewarming of the heart continues, the venting catheter(s) are removed, and the chest is closed in the routine manner.

When *CABG* is to be performed in conjunction with *AVR*, the procedure is done in the following order:

1. The diseased valve is excised, the anulus sized, and the prosthesis selected.
2. Distal coronary anastomoses are performed.
3. The prosthetic valve is inserted.

4. The aorta (or left atrium in MVR) is closed.
5. The aortic cross-clamp is removed.
6. The proximal coronary anastomoses are inserted into the aorta with a partial occlusion clamp.

When the *aortic and mitral valves are both replaced,* the valves are first excised and the anuli sized. Then the mitral valve is implanted, followed by the aortic valve. The aorta is closed, and after sufficient de-airing of the left ventricle the left atrium is closed.

Operations on the thoracic aorta
Thoracic aortic aneurysmectomy

Thoracic aortic aneurysmectomy is excision of an aneurysmal portion of the ascending arch or descending thoracic aorta and replacement with a prosthetic graft, valve-graft conduit, or intraaortic prosthesis. Graft material placed in the thoracic aorta is usually preclotted to reduce bleeding. Aneurysms may be caused by atherosclerosis, arteriosclerosis, trauma, infection, or medial degeneration (Crawford, 1989a and 1989b). *Atherosclerosis* is a lesion of large and medium arteries, with deposits in the intima of yellowish plaques containing cholesterol, lipoid material, and lipophages. *Arteriosclerosis* is defined as a condition marked by loss of elasticity, thickening, and hardening of the arteries (Chapter 26). Further degeneration and destruction may lead to aneurysm formation. Any artery may become involved.

Surgical intervention becomes necessary when presenting symptoms indicate a compromise in circulation or danger of rupture; generally, medical management with hypotensive agents to reduce stress on the vessel is the preferred initial treatment.

Aneurysms can be characterized morphologically as follows: (1) saccular—a sac type of formation with a narrowed neck projecting from the side of the artery, (2) fusiform—a spindle-shaped formation with complete circumferential involvement of the artery, and (3) dissecting—a splitting of the intima of the aorta, permitting blood to pass between the layers of the wall to form a false channel; as the channel extends and enlarges, the blood flow is obstructed (Fig. 27-53).

Procedural considerations. Several methods of surgical treatment are available. In situations where ascending aneurysms produce anular dilation with subsequent aortic valve insufficiency, a Bentall-Bono procedure with a valved conduit (Fig. 27-32) may be performed to replace the aortic valve and the aneurysmal aorta (Fig. 27-54). This procedure necessitates reimplanting the right and left coronary ostia into the prosthetic graft. In patients with coronary artery disease, vein grafts may be inserted and anastomosed proximally to the prosthesis.

The type of cardiopulmonary bypass (CPB) depends on the location of the aneurysm. Femoral vein–femoral artery bypass is often instituted initially, as the enlarged and weakened aorta cannot be safely cannulated (Seifert, 1986). Because femoral bypass cannot adequately drain venous return from the upper body, an atrial venous cannula is Y'd into the femoral venous line after the aneurysm is controlled. Profound hypothermia with exsanguination may be needed in particularly complex lesions of the aortic arch where the aneurysm extends into the arch vessels, making placement of a cross-clamp difficult. Blood is drained from the body into the venous reservoir, and the bypass machine is turned off. When the repair is sufficiently completed, the pump is turned on and the body refilled with blood. Because this technique prolongs the procedure and imposes additional risk, the body is cooled to very low temperatures (15° C) to protect the heart and other organ systems (Waldhausen and Pierce, 1985).

In descending thoracic aortic aneurysms, the heart is not arrested; it continues beating to perfuse the upper body. Femoral bypass is instituted to perfuse the kidneys and lower extremities; normothermia is maintained.

Repair of ascending thoracic aortic aneurysm

Procedural considerations. To the basic setup are added aneurysm instruments. Valve instruments, coronary instruments, and an array of tube grafts, valves, and/or valved conduits should be available.

Operative procedure
1. The patient is positioned for a median sternotomy.
2. Cannulation of the femoral vein and femoral artery is performed.

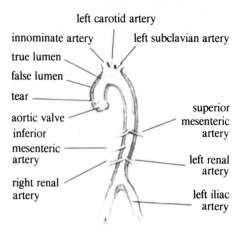

left carotid artery
innominate artery — left subclavian artery
true lumen
false lumen
tear
aortic valve — superior mesenteric artery
inferior mesenteric artery
right renal artery — left renal artery
left iliac artery

DeBakey Type I: Dissection of the ascending aorta. Usually begins as an intimal tear just above the aortic valve and extends to the distal portions of the aorta.

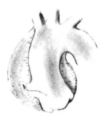

DeBakey Type II: Dissection is limited to the ascending aorta and usually terminates just proximal to the origin of the innominate artery.

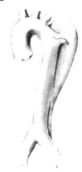

DeBakey Type III: Dissection of the descending aorta originating just distal to the origin of the left subclavian artery and extending distally for a varying distance.

Fig. 27-53. Types of dissecting thoracic aneurysms. (From Seifert, P.C.: Dissecting aortic aneurysms: a problem in Marfan's syndrome, AORN J. 43:443, 1986. Reprinted with permission from © The Association of Operating Room Nurses, Inc, 10170 E. Mississippi Avenue, Denver, Col. 80231.)

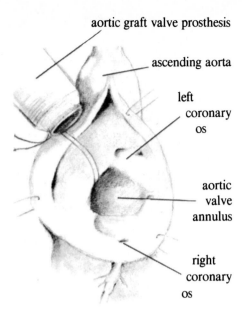

The proximal end of the prosthesis (valve prosthesis end) is inserted in the aortic valve annulus. Then the left and right coronary ostia are anastamosed to openings made in the graft.

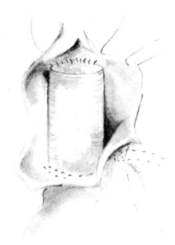

The distal end of the prosthesis is anastomosed to the distal aorta and the aneurysmal remnant is trimmed and approximated around the graft.

Fig. 27-54. Bentall-Bono procedure. (From Seifert, P.C.: Dissecting aortic aneurysms: a problem in Marfan's syndrome, AORN J. 43:443, 1986. Reprinted with permission © from The Association of Operating Room Nurses, Inc, 10170 E. Mississippi Avenue, Denver, Colo. 80231.)

3. The sternum is opened and the aneurysm inspected. If the right atrium is accessible for cannulation of venous return, drainage catheters are inserted.

4A. If the aortic anulus is not involved, the aneurysm is incised longitudinally, and a woven graft is anastomosed proximally and distally to healthy aorta.

4B. If the aortic anulus is involved, the ascending aorta is incised to the anulus. The leaflets are excised and the anulus measured. The proximal end of a valved conduit is inserted. An eye cautery is used to create openings in the graft at the location of the right and left coronary ostia, which are anastomosed to the graft. (If the patient has concomitant coronary artery disease, saphenous vein grafts are inserted.) The distal end of the conduit is sutured to healthy aorta, and the aneurysmal remnant is wrapped around the conduit (Fig. 27-54).

5. Bypass is discontinued and all incisions closed.

Repair of aortic arch aneurysm

Procedural considerations. Aneurysm instruments and woven grafts are available. If profound hypothermia is to be used, the patient may be covered with bags of ice at the beginning of the case. Precautions to prevent frostbite are instituted. The patient is positioned for a median sternotomy.

Operative procedure

1. Cannulation of the femoral vein and femoral artery is performed; if the superior and inferior venae cavae are accessible, they are cannulated for venous drainage.

2. Once the patient is cooled to the desired temperature, the arch vessels are individually cross-clamped (Fig. 27-55, A). (If exsanguination is indicated, cross-clamps are not used.) The aneurysm is incised, a tube graft selected, and the anastomosis to the descending aorta performed.

3. An opening is made into the side of the graft and is anastomosed to the common origin of the innominate, left carotid, and left subclavian vessels. The graft is cross-clamped proximally to the arch and de-aired (Fig. 27-55, B).

4. The proximal aorta is anastomosed to the graft while the patient is rewarming. The graft is de-aired and the patient weaned from bypass (Fig. 27-55, C).

5. All incisions are closed.

Repair of descending thoracic aortic aneurysm

Procedural considerations. Thoracotomy instruments and supplies are added to the basic setup; additional long aortic cross-clamps may be needed. Prosthetic grafts are available. The patient is positioned for a left posterolateral thoracotomy.

Operative procedure

1. Cannulation for femoral vein–femoral artery bypass is performed.

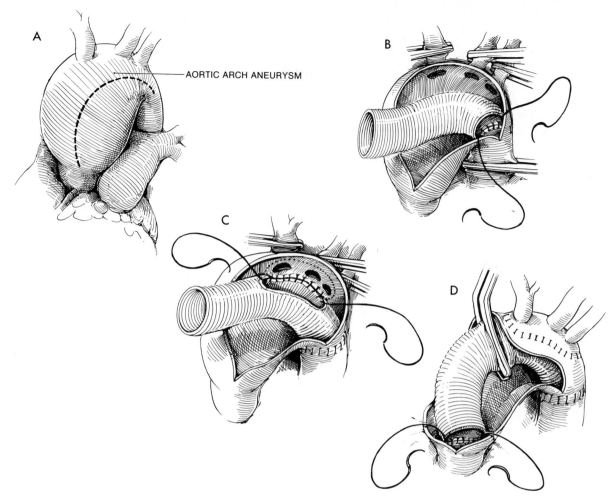

Fig. 27-55. Repair aortic arch aneurysm. **A,** Incision; **B,** distal anastomosis; **C,** anastomosis of graft to common origin of arch vessels; **D,** proximal anastomosis. (From Walhausen, J.A., and Pierce, W.S.: Johnson's surgery of the chest, ed. 5, Chicago, 1985, Year Book Medical Publishers.)

2. A thoracotomy incision is made, and the aneurysm is exposed and surrounding structures inspected. (Occasionally the surgeon makes two thoracotomy incisions for better access to and control of the aorta.) Renal involvement is assessed; if indicated, measures to protect the kidneys are instituted (for example, local cooling).

3. Normothermic femoral bypass is initiated.

4. The aneurysm is incised longitudinally, and the aorta is sized.

5A. A woven graft (Fig. 27-21) is inserted, and the aneurysmal remnants are wrapped around the graft.

5B. If an intraaortic prosthesis (Fig. 27-33) is used (in a dissecting aneurysm), it is inserted into the true aortic lumen and the aorta wrapped around the prosthesis. Dacron tapes are used to encircle the aorta and the proximal and distal rings. The tapes are tied, securing the prosthesis. Stay sutures may be inserted to secure further the prosthesis.

Mechanical circulatory assistance

A small percentage of patients cannot be weaned from CPB after open heart operations, even with the use of inotropic and vasodilator drugs. Various mechanical devices are available to support the circulation while the heart recovers or while the patient awaits cardiac transplantation.

Intraaortic balloon pump (IABP)

The IABP is a technique that employs the principle of counterpulsation. It can increase the cardiac output by as much as 0.5 L/min/m² and may permit separation of the patient from CPB (Fig. 27-56).

Operative procedure

1A. A flexible guidewire is passed through a percutaneous sheath into the femoral artery. The sheath is removed, and graduated dilators are inserted over the guidewire to dilate the overlying tissue and the artery wall.

1B. If the percutaneous route is not feasible, the femoral

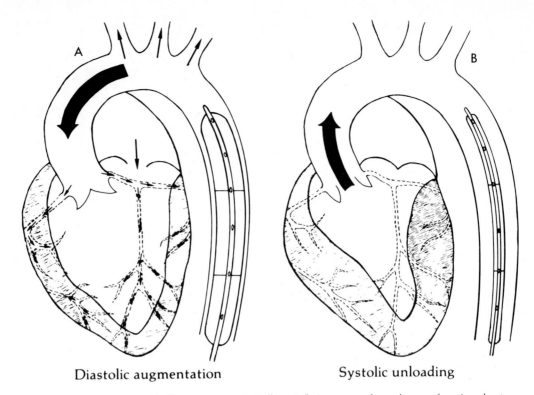

Diastolic augmentation   Systolic unloading

Fig. 27-56. Two phases of balloon pumping. **A,** Balloon inflation occurs from closure of aortic valve to end of diastole. Inflation causes retrograde flow of blood in aorta, increasing coronary perfusion pressure without increasing myocardial work or oxygen demand. Inflation also causes antegrade flow, increasing mean arterial pressure, renal flow, and cerebral flow. **B,** Balloon deflation occurs from just before opening of aortic valve to closure of aortic valve. Deflation encourages antegrade flow, decreasing afterload or resistance to left ventricular ejection. Deflation also decreases oxygen required by left ventricle, shortens systolic ejection, and increases stroke volume. (From Michaelson, C.R.: Congestive heart failure, St. Louis, 1983, The C.V. Mosby Co.)

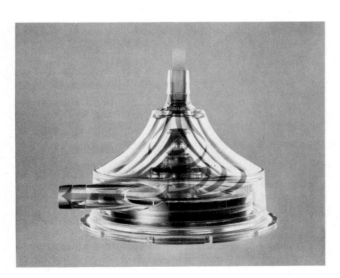

Fig. 27-57. Centrifugal pump. The Bio-Medicus pump can be used for extracorporeal circulation during cardiac surgery or as a ventricular assist device. (Courtesy Bio-Medicus, Inc., Eden Prairie, Minn.)

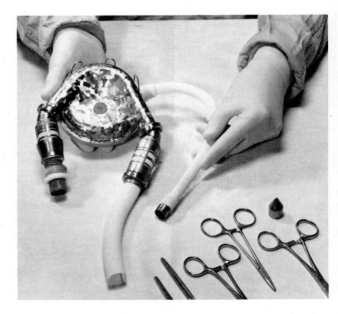

Fig. 27-58. Ventricular assist device (VAD). The pump is placed in the intraabdominal cavity. (Courtesy of Thermo Cardiosystems, Inc., Woburn, Mass.)

artery is exposed and a short segment of tube graft anastomosed to the artery. The IABP catheter is inserted into the artery through the graft, and a tape is tied around the graft surrounding the catheter. (For removal, the balloon is removed and the graft rimmed and oversewn.)

2. The furled balloon catheter is advanced to a position just distal to the left subclavian artery.
3. The balloon is unfurled and activated.

Ventricular assist pump

Ventricular assist pumps are designed to decrease the workload of the heart by diverting blood from the ventricle to an artificial pump that maintains systemic perfusion (Ruzevich, and others, 1988; Marchetta and Stennis, 1988).

Procedural considerations. If patients cannot be weaned from CPB with IABP, an assist system can be used. Cardiac support devices include centrifugal pumps (Fig. 27-57) and pneumatic (Fig. 27-58) or electric power assist devices. The pumps may be located internally (Fig. 27-59) or externally. In the device described below, bioprosthetic valves are incorporated into the circuit to maintain unidirectional blood flow.

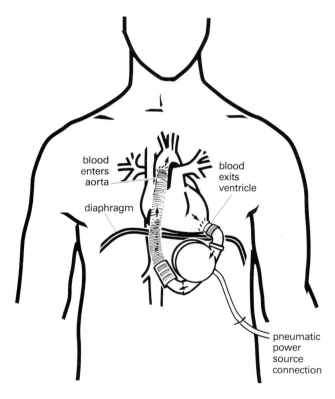

Fig. 27-59. Placement of ventricular assist device. Blood flows from the ventricle into the mechanical ventricle located below the diaphragm and is pumped into the ascending aorta. (Courtesy of Thermo Cardiosystems, Inc., Woburn, Mass.)

Left ventricular assist device (LVAD)

Operative procedure (Thermedics LVAD)

1. A median sternotomy and midline laparotomy are made in preparation for placement of ventricular and aortic cannulae and the intraabdominal pump.
2. The right atrium and femoral artery are cannulated for CPB.
3. The graft is preclotted, and the valves rinsed.
4. The pump and fittings are washed and assembled.
5. The pump is placed in the left upper quadrant of the abdomen intraperitoneally, and the drive line passed through a stab wound in the lower abdomen and connected to the power source.
6. Bypass is instituted.
7. The inlet tube of the pump is passed through an incision in the lateral diaphragm and inserted into the left ventricular apex.
8. The aortic (outflow) graft is anastomosed to the aorta and then to the outflow tube. The pump is filled with blood.
9. The pump, left ventricle, and aorta are de-aired, and the pump is started.
10. All connections are secured.
11. Bypass is discontinued, and the cannulae removed. To remove the pump the patient is returned to the operating room, the sternotomy reopened, and the cannulae removed.

If a centrifugal pump is used, the left atrium is cannulated for inflow to the pump, and the ascending aorta is cannulated for outflow from the pump. (Prosthetic valves are not required as the rotating pump maintains forward blood flow.)

These assist devices may be used for right ventricular failure or bilateral ventricular failure as well.

Total artificial heart (TAH)

The total artificial heart has not demonstrated great success as a permanent cardiac replacement, due to thromboembolism and infection. Along with right and/or left VADs (May and Adams, 1987), the TAH has been increasingly employed as a bridge to cardiac transplantation by supporting the circulation while a suitable donor heart can be found (Davis and others, 1989; Bolman and others, 1989; Pae and others, 1988; Hill, 1989).

Among the newer trends in providing ventricular support is the use of latissimus dorsi muscle for *cardiomyoplasty*. This technique uses electrostimulated skeletal muscle to reinforce or partially replace the heart muscle (Chachques and others, 1989; Acker and others, 1986; Carpentier and Chachques, 1987; Gardner, 1988).

The Nimbus *hemopump* (Fig. 27-60) is a mechanical assist device under investigation. It is based on the principle of Archimedes' screw and uses an axial flow pump inserted retrogradely into the left ventricle. The pump rotates as fast as 25,000 revolutions per minute to draw blood

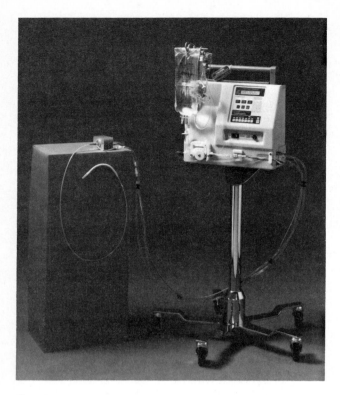

Fig. 27-60. Hemopump ventricular assist device (VAD). The tip of the catheter lies in the left ventricle. The axial flow pump, housed within the distal portion of the catheter, draws blood from the ventricle and propels it into the aorta. (Courtesy of Nimbus Medical, Inc., Rancho Cordova, Calif.)

from the left ventricle and propel it into the aorta and the distal vascular beds (Ferguson and others, 1988).

Heart and heart-lung transplantation

Heart transplantation (Fig. 27-61)

Cardiac transplantation is now a clinical reality. It has been surgically feasible since 1960, when the surgical method was developed (Emery and Pritzker, 1988). Orthotopic transplantation is most commonly performed, but heterotopic ("piggyback") and combined heart-lung procedures are done as well (Sutor and others, 1988). With the introduction of the immunosuppressive agent cyclosporine A, results have improved dramatically (Wallwork, 1989; Reitz, 1989). Important considerations continue to focus on recipient selection, the immune response, and control of infection (Rudolphi and others, 1987).

Procedural considerations. Individual instrument set-ups are necessary for the donor and the recipient.

Operative procedure

Donor heart. The donor heart is exposed through a median sternotomy. The aorta, pulmonary artery, and venae cavae are dissected. The venae cavae are occluded, the left atrium is opened to decompress the ventricle, and the heart is rapidly cooled and arrested.

The heart is excised by incising the left atrium circumferentially at the level of the pulmonary veins and by severing the aorta and pulmonary artery. The donor heart is immediately placed in cold saline and transported to the site where it will be inserted into the recipient.

Recipient heart. The recipient is placed on bypass with cannulation of the inferior vena cava and the superior vena cava; caval tapes are placed around the cavae. The patient is cooled to approximately 25° C and the caval tapes tightened. The pulmonary trunk and aorta are dissected immediately above their respective semilunar valves; the atria are incised to leave intact portions of the right and left atrial walls and the atrial septum of the recipient. The recipient heart is then removed.

The donor heart is placed in the pericardial well. The interatrial septum and the left and then the right atrial walls are approximated with running cardiovascular sutures. The donor and recipient aortas are similarly joined. Air is removed from the left side of the heart.

The aortic clamp is removed, and a clamp is placed across the donor pulmonary artery. The caval tape is removed, and vigorous ventricular fibrillation of the donor heart commences. Local cooling of the heart is discontinued at this point, and, before the pulmonary artery is sutured, all atrial suture lines are carefully inspected for significant bleeding areas. The pulmonary arteries are united, and the clamp removed. Defibrillation of the ventricles is usually effected with a single DC shock. A needle hole is established at the apex of the ascending aorta, so that residual air is expelled. The patient is then removed from extracorporeal bypass after a period of partial bypass. Cannulae are removed from the venae cavae or the peripheral veins. The incisions are closed as described previously.

Heart-lung transplantation (Fig. 27-62)

A three-anastomosis technique for combined heart-lung transplantation has been devised. This technique ensures preservation of the donor's sinus node and preservation of the recipient's recurrent laryngeal, vagus, and phrenic nerves.

Operative procedure. The recipient's diseased heart and lungs are excised separately or en bloc, with care taken not to injure the major nerves listed previously. The recipient's right atrium is saved to create a large atrial cuff for attachment to the donor heart. The bronchi are transected and the stumps clamped to prevent contamination. The trachea is transected just above the carina. The donor heart and lungs are brought onto the field. The right lung is placed in the right pleural space and the left lung positioned in the left pleural space. The tracheal and the right atrial anastomoses are performed, and rewarming is begun. The aortic anastomosis is performed, the aorta is de-aired, and the cross-clamp is removed.

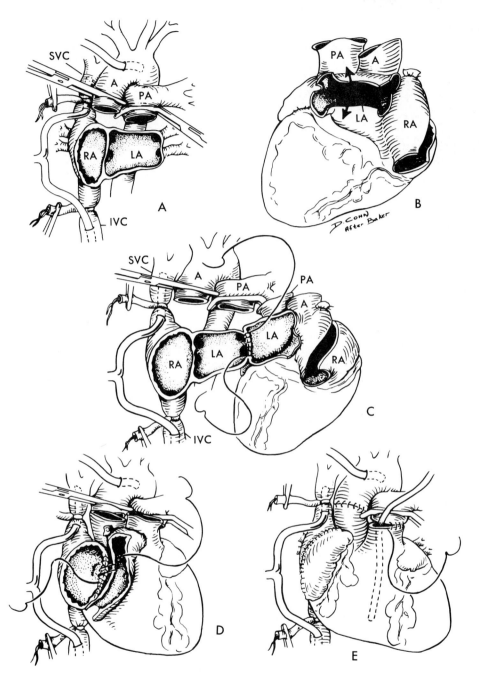

Fig. 27-61. Heart transplantation. **A,** Diagram of remaining cuff of recipient heart. Venae cavae and aorta are cannulated in chest to avoid additional incisions, which add to possibility of infection. **B,** Diagram of posterior surface of donor heart. Left atrium is opened through pulmonary veins, and excess removed. **C,** Suturing is started on lateral aspect of left atria. **D,** Right atria are then sutured. This technique avoids interatrial tracts. **E,** Aortae are anastomosed first so coronary circulation can be reestablished. Pulmonary arteries are joined last, and all air is carefully removed from heart. Cardiopulmonary bypass support is weaned off as function is restored. Support with cardiotonic agents is often required temporarily. (Modified from Effler, D.B.: Blades' surgical diseases of the chest, ed. 4, St. Louis, 1978, The C.V. Mosby Co.)

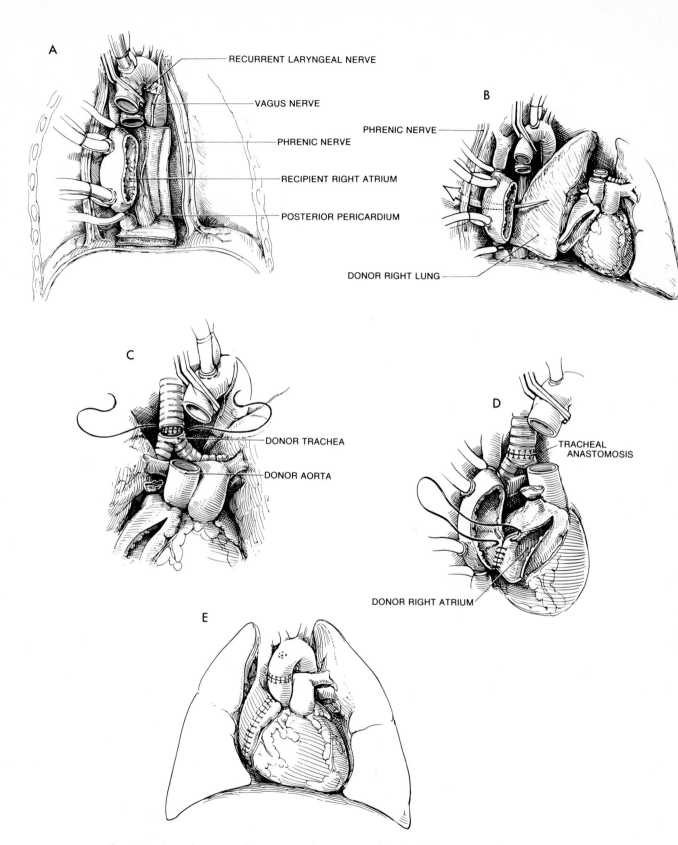

Fig. 27-62. Heart-lung transplantation. **A,** The recipient's heart and lungs are removed; **B,** the donor organs are placed in the field; **C,** the tracheal anastomosis; **D,** the right atrial anastomosis; **E,** completed procedure. (From Waldhausen, J.A., and Pierce, W.S.: Johnson's surgery of the chest, ed. 5, Chicago, 1985, Year Book Medical Publishers.)

Surgery for congenital heart disease

Congenital cardiac abnormalities occur in 1% to 2% of live-born infants (Turner and others, 1988) and are differentiated on the basis of whether they are cyanotic or acyanotic lesions. The cyanosis-producing abnormalities carry a graver prognosis.

Cyanosis is present because of a failure of delivery of pulmonary venous return to the systemic circulation (for example, transposition of the great vessels) or reduction in the volume of pulmonary blood flow (for example, tetralogy of Fallot or tricuspid atresia). The degree of cyanosis is affected by the amount of pulmonary blood flow or the extent of intracardiac mixing of blood through a shunt (Bojar, 1989).

Among the acyanotic group are the obstructive lesions (for example, aortic or pulmonary stenosis or coarctation of the aorta) that place an extra burden on the associated ventricle and can lead to heart failure. (Cyanosis may be apparent if the lesion is severe.) Shunt lesions (such as patent ductus arteriosus, ventricular septal defect, or atrial septal defect) increase pulmonary blood flow. If a large shunt is present, congestive heart failure can ensue (Turner and others, 1988).

Palliative procedures (described later) attempt to increase or decrease pulmonary blood flow or to increase intracardiac mixing of blood (Rashkind, 1982).

Repair of an atrial septal defect

Congenital defects in the atrial septum are closed, under direct vision, by a simple suture technique or by inserting a synthetic prosthetic patch or pericardial patch.

An atrial septal defect is a common congenital abnormality, and its classification is based on anatomic location and associated abnormalities (Fig. 27-63).

The *ostium secundum defect* is located in the superior and central portion of the septum. The *ostium primum defect* is in the lower portion of the atrial septum and is associated with other defects in the atrioventricular canal, usually with a cleft of the mitral valve or occasionally of the tricuspid valve. An accompanying ventricular septal defect may also be present. The *sinus venosum defect* is located at the atriocaval junction and is associated with partial anomalous pulmonary venous return.

An atrial septal defect results in a left-to-right atrial shunt that may be well tolerated in early life if the opening is small. However, if the defect is large or of the ostium primum type, with a marked shunting of blood, the workload of the right side of the heart is increased. The right side of the heart and the pulmonary artery and its branches become enlarged. The vascularity of the lung field is increased, with resulting pulmonary hypertension and subsequent failure of the right side of the heart. At this point the shunt may reverse (Fig. 27-64).

In early life the patient may be asymptomatic. The initial symptoms may include fatigue, retardation of normal weight gain, and increased susceptibility to respiratory infections. Later symptoms include those of failure of the right side of the heart and cyanosis with a reverse shunt.

A systolic murmur is heard with greatest intensity over the base of the heart.

Procedural considerations. The patient is placed in the supine position for a median sternotomy or in a right anterior oblique position for an anterolateral thoracotomy.

The instrument setup is as described for basic open heart

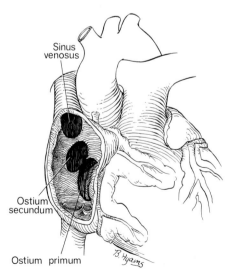

Fig. 27-63. Atrial septal defects are common congenital anomalies occurring in the sinus venosus, ostium secundum, and ostium primum. (From Cooley, D.A., and Norman, J.C.: Techniques in cardiac surgery, Houston, 1975, Texas Medical Press.)

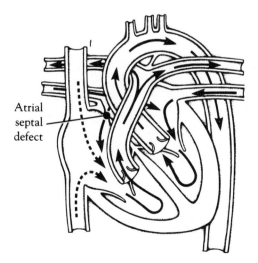

Fig. 27-64. Atrial septal defect. (From Whaley, L.F., and Wong, D.L.: Nursing care of infants and children, ed. 3, St. Louis, 1987, The C.V. Mosby Co.)

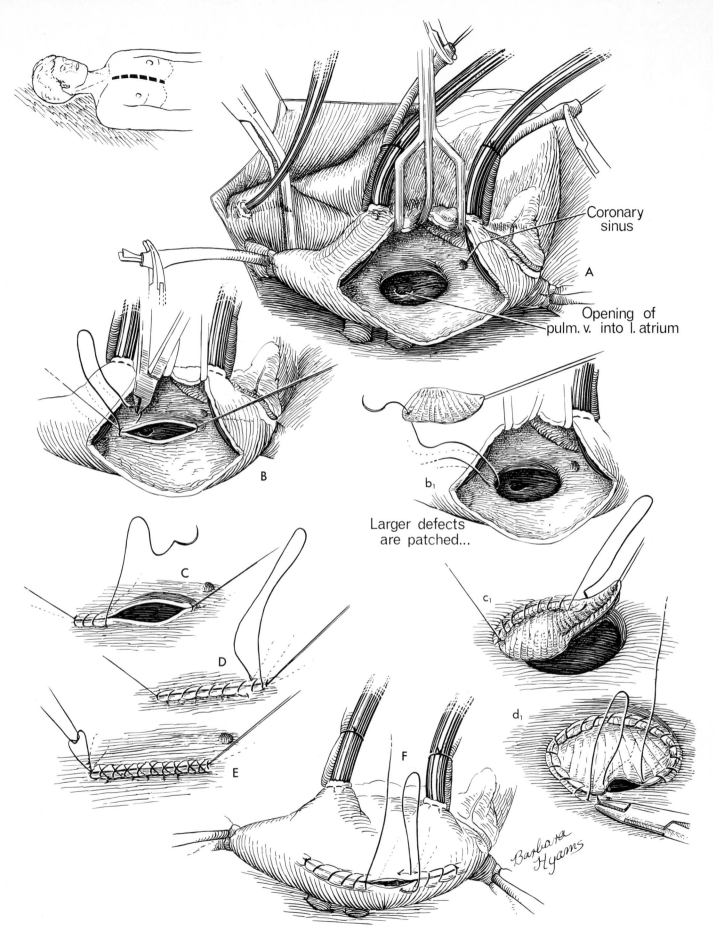

Coronary
sinus

Opening of
pulm. v. into l. atrium

A

B

b₁

Larger defects
are patched...

C

D

c₁

E

d₁

F

Barbara
Hyams

Fig. 27-65. Repair of ostium secundum defect. Patch closures (**b₁** through **d₁**) are done for larger defects. (From Cooley, D.A., and Norman, J.C.: Techniques in cardiac surgery, Houston, 1975, Texas Medical Press.)

surgery, with consideration given to the age and size of the patient, plus intracardiac patch material, 2 × 2 inches or larger.

Operative procedure (Fig. 27-65)

1. A right anterolateral or median sternotomy incision is made, and cardiopulmonary bypass begun as described.
2. The right atrium is incised, and the pathologic defect determined.
3. The defect is closed with a continuous suture, or a patch of pericardium or prosthetic material may be used. By filling the atrium with blood before the atriotomy is completely closed, air can be expressed from the atrium.

For the ostium primum defect with a cleft mitral valve, repair of the cleft is accomplished by approximation, using interrupted sutures.

Repair of a ventricular septal defect

Under direct vision, a congenital defect in the ventricular septum (Fig. 27-66) is closed by a simple suture technique or, in most instances, by inserting a synthetic prosthetic or pericardial patch. One of the most common congenital cardiac anomalies, a ventricular septal defect (VSD) is of little physiologic importance if small. The murmur is evident, but the patient is otherwise asymptomatic, and the heart is normal in size. Larger defects with a significant left-to-right shunt, high right ventricular pressure, increased pulmonary blood flow, and enlarged heart are repaired by surgery (Fig. 27-67). If left uncorrected, pulmonary volume overload results in pulmonary hypertension with subsequent reversal of the shunt to right-to-left and in cyanosis.

In adults, VSDs complicating myocardial infarction can be repaired with the technique described below. Depending on the location and extent of the interventricular rupture, various procedures can be performed using bovine pericardium or synthetic graft and buttressed sutures to patch the defect (Jones and others, 1987).

Operative procedure (Fig. 27-68)

1. A median sternotomy is performed, and cardiopulmonary bypass begun as described.
2. The right ventricle is opened and the defect is repaired, taking care to avoid damaging branches of the bundle of His.
3. Cardiopulmonary bypass is discontinued, and the sternum is closed.

Correction of tetralogy of Fallot

Tetralogy of Fallot is the most common congenital cardiac anomaly in the cyanotic group. Cyanosis, as seen in the superficial vessels of the skin, is the result of shunting unoxygenated blood into the systemic circulation.

The essential features of this condition are pulmonary stenosis, high ventricular septal defect, and overriding of the septal defect by the aorta, with resulting hypertrophy of the right ventricle—all of which may be subdivided into more complex variations (Fig. 27-69). The *infundibular* form of pulmonary stenosis is a long, localized constricture in the pulmonary outflow tract of the right ventricle. It is the most common type of this anomaly. *Valvular stenosis* and infundibular stenosis, however, may occur independently.

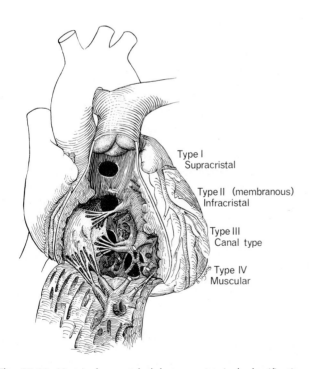

Fig. 27-66. Ventricular septal defects: anatomical classification. (From Cooley, D.A., and Norman, J.C.: Techniques in cardiac surgery, Houston, 1975, Texas Medical Press.)

Type I
Supracristal

Type II (membranous)
Infracristal

Type III
Canal type

Type IV
Muscular

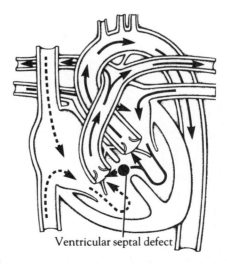

Ventricular septal defect

Fig. 27-67. Ventricular septal defect. (From Whaley, L.F., and Wong, D.L.: Nursing care of infants and children, ed. 3, St. Louis, 1987, The C.V. Mosby Co.)

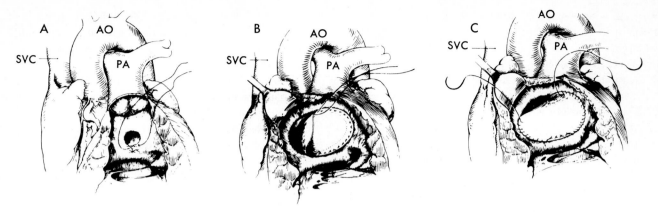

Fig. 27-68. Techniques for closing ventricular septal defects. **A,** Simple interrupted suture may be used if defect is small and has fibrous margins. **B,** Patch closure of ventricular septal defect with interrupted mattress sutures. **C,** Patch closure of ventricular septal defect using interrupted sutures at bottom of defect and continuous suturing technique for remainder of defect. (From Effler, D.B.: Blades' surgical diseases of the chest, ed. 4, St. Louis, 1978, The C.V. Mosby Co.)

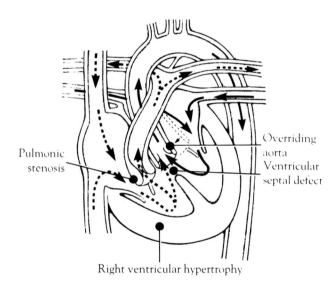

Fig. 27-69. Tetralogy of Fallot. (From Whaley, L.F., and Wong, D.L.: Nursing care of infants and children, ed. 3, St. Louis, 1987, The C.V. Mosby Co.)

In tetralogy of Fallot, blood flow into the lungs decreases as a result of pulmonary obstruction, and a right-to-left shunt of venous blood from the right ventricle to the left ventricle and aorta occurs.

Symptoms of tetralogy are cyanosis, dyspnea, episodes of acute dyspnea with cyanosis, retarded growth, clubbing of extremities, and reduced exercise tolerance. A systolic murmur and secondary polycythemia are usually present. Cardiac catheterization and angiocardiography aid in determining the diagnosis and plan of surgical treatment.

The selection of a palliative or corrective procedure is based on the age and general condition of the patient and the severity of the pulmonary stenosis.

Shunt for palliation

The shunt for palliation is one of several palliative procedures designed to divert poorly oxygenated blood from one of the major arteries back through one of the pulmonary arteries to the lungs for reoxygenation, thereby increasing the total blood flow in the pulmonary circulation.

Shunt procedures that increase pulmonary flow are described in Fig. 27-70, along with procedures to reduce pulmonary blood flow (pulmonary artery banding) and to increase intracardiac mixing of blood (Blalock-Hanlon ASD, and Rashkind septostomy).

The *Blalock-Taussig* procedure consists of an end-to-side anastomosis between the proximal end of the subclavian and pulmonary arteries. The procedure is performed on the side opposite the aortic arch. This shunt may be dismantled or ligated if a future operation for full correction is anticipated; however, the shunt has a tendency to decrease in size as the child grows.

In order to save the subclavian artery, a PTFE graft can be inserted between the subclavian artery and the pulmonary artery.

The *Potts-Smith* procedure consists of a side-to-side anastomosis directly between the aorta and left pulmonary artery. This procedure may be selected for infants because the size of the anastomosis is not limited by the lumen of the subclavian artery, as it is in the Blalock technique. However, it is more difficult to dismantle if future surgery is anticipated.

The *Waterston* procedure consists of anastomosis of the ascending aorta and the right pulmonary artery. It is advantageous for infants with very small pulmonary arteries. A possible complication is kinking of the pulmonary artery, forcing the major portion of blood flow to the right lung.

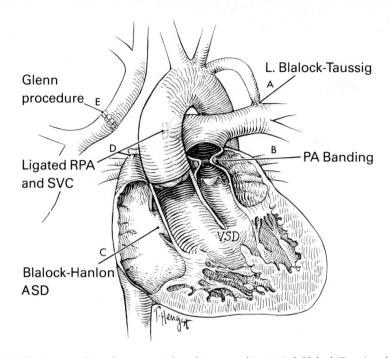

Fig. 27-70. Palliative procedures for congenital cardiac anomalies. **A,** Left Blalock-Taussig subclavian to pulmonary artery shunt applicable for tetralogy of Fallot and also for other congenital anomalies associated with insufficient pulmonary arterial flow. (A modification of the Blalock-Taussig procedure consists of interposing a PTFE graft between the left subclavian artery and the pulmonary artery, thereby preserving the subclavian artery.) **B,** Pulmonary artery banding used for anomalies associated with excessive pulmonary blood flow due to a large intracardiac left-to-right shunt. These include ventricular septal defect, truncus arteriosus, and others. **C,** Blalock-Hanlon creation of interatrial septal defect used predominantly for transposition of the great vessels but also for anomalies such as mitral or tricuspid atresia in which a large opening is advantageous to reduce intraatrial pressure. Dilation of a patent foramen ovale may be done with a balloon-tipped catheter (Rashkind technique). **D** and **E,** The Glenn procedure is used primarily for tricuspid atresia but is also used for transposition of the great vessels. In **D** the superior vena cava is anastomosed to the right pulmonary artery to direct approximately 35% of the systemic venous return to the right lung for oxygenation. This technique cannot be used if the pulmonary vascular resistance is elevated, as often occurs in transposition. The Glenn procedure **(E)** is usually performed by implanting the distal end of the pulmonary artery into the side of the superior vena cava. The cava is then ligated at the atriocaval junction. Ligation of the azygos vein may enhance the flow through the cavopulmonary anastomosis but may also increase the pressure in veins draining the upper half of the body. Techniques of delayed azygos ligation have been described in infants and children. (From Cooley, D.A.: Techniques in cardiac surgery, ed. 2, Philadelphia, 1984, W.B. Saunders Co.)

The *Glenn* procedure consists of anastomosis of the superior vena cava to the right pulmonary artery. This operation is employed infrequently in the treatment of tetralogy of Fallot (Fig. 27-70, *E*).

Procedural considerations. The patient is placed in a position that is specific for each procedure (supine or right or left lateral). Instruments are as previously described for open heart surgery, plus the following, with appropriate sizes for infants and children:

2 Potts-Smith aortic occlusion clamps
2 Johns Hopkins modified Potts clamps
2 Hendrin ductus clamps
2 Cooley anastomosis clamps

Operative procedures
Blalock-Taussig procedure (Fig. 27-70, *A*)

1. An anterolateral incision is made from the sternal margin to the midaxillary line. The chest cavity is opened and the lung retracted, as described previously.
2. The mediastinal pleura is incised and retracted with a stay suture.
3. The pulmonary artery is dissected from the surrounding tissue, with vascular forceps, dry dissector sponges, and Metzenbaum scissors. As the artery and branches are mobilized, heavy ligatures, moistened umbilical tapes, or fine silicone tubing is placed about them.
4. Branches of the vagus nerve are protected and retracted.

5. The subclavian artery is dissected completely from its origin to where it produces the internal mammary and costocervical branches. Its distal end is marked with a silk suture.

6. The subclavian artery is occluded with a vascular clamp, a ligature is placed at the distal segment, and the vessel is divided.

7. The pulmonary artery is occluded temporarily with a curved vascular clamp.

8. An incision of sufficient size to accommodate the subclavian artery is made with a scalpel with a no. 11 knife blade and Potts scissors.

9. An end-to-side anastomosis is completed with cardiovascular suture.

10. The clamps are released, and the suture line is inspected for hemostasis.

11. The mediastinal pleura is closed.

12. Closed chest drainage is established, and the chest wound is closed.

Potts-Smith procedure. A left posterolateral incision is made in the fourth intercostal space. The pulmonary artery is dissected from its surrounding tissue, and the descending aorta is mobilized. Occluding tapes and Blalock or Potts-Smith clamps are applied. A longitudinal incision is made in each artery, and a side-to-side anastomosis is completed with cardiovascular sutures. The pulmonary artery is released, and the suture line is inspected for hemostasis. The aortic clamps are then removed.

Waterston procedure. A right anterolateral incision is made in the fourth interspace. The pericardium is opened, and the ascending aorta is exposed. The right pulmonary artery is dissected as it passes beneath the ascending aorta. A heavy suture is passed around the right pulmonary artery and is used to occlude the artery temporarily. A curved vascular clamp is placed so one blade is behind the pulmonary artery and the other occludes a posterolateral portion of the ascending aorta. On closure of the clamp, both

the right pulmonary artery and a posterior portion of the ascending aorta are occluded. Parallel incisions are made in the aorta and the right pulmonary artery. An anastomosis is then made between the ascending aorta and right pulmonary artery.

Open corrective repair

The open corrective repair is done under direct vision and is the complete repair of the infundibular stenosis or pulmonary valve stenosis and closure of the ventricular septal defect.

Procedural considerations. The patient is placed on the operating room bed in a supine position. The setup is as described for open heart surgery, with consideration given to the age and size of the patient. Additional items to be added to the basic open heart setup include the following:

1 Intracardiac patch, 2 × 2 inches
1 Outflow cardiac patch, 2 × 2 inches
1 Felt patch, 4 × 4 inches

Operative procedure

1. A median sternotomy is performed, and cardiopulmonary bypass with hypothermia begun as described.

2. A vertical ventriculotomy over the infundibular area is performed (Fig. 27-71).

3. The ventricular septal defect is identified. Closure requires an intracardiac patch in almost all instances. This can be of a synthetic material or a piece of pericardium.

4. The hypertrophied infundibular muscle is excised, as completely as possible, from the right ventricular outflow tract. If the pulmonic valve is stenosed, the fused commissures are incised.

5. Interrupted or continuous cardiovascular sutures are placed in the septum with caution because of the danger of suturing a branch of the neuroconductive system.

6. After closure of the ventricular septal defect, an esti-

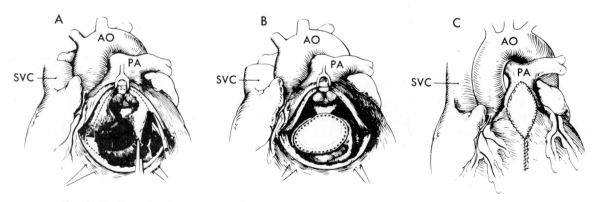

Fig. 27-71. Operation for correction of tetralogy of Fallot. **A,** Infundibulectomy or removal of outflow tract obstruction to right ventricle by sharp dissection. **B,** Closure of ventricular septal defect. **C,** If pulmonary anulus is too narrow, or if infundibulectomy does not open outflow obstruction adequately, patch in outflow tract may be necessary. (From Effler, D.B.: Blades' surgical diseases of the chest, ed. 4, St. Louis, 1978, The C.V. Mosby Co.)

mate is made whether the right ventricle can be closed primarily or whether a patch is necessary. If the pulmonic stenosis cannot be relieved adequately by valvulotomy and infundibulectomy, an outflow patch may be needed to enlarge the outflow tract. If the pulmonary artery or valve anulus is quite small, it may be necessary to extend the patch across the valve ring to the proximal portion of the pulmonary artery.

7. Cardiopulmonary bypass is discontinued, and the sternum is closed.

Operation for tricuspid atresia

Absence of communication between the right atrium and right ventricle is always accompanied by a second defect, an atrial septal defect, or a patent foramen ovale. Other abnormalities are also present in tricuspid atresia (Fig. 27-72). The infant displays cyanosis, periods of dyspnea, easy fatigability, and growth retardation. Congestive failure progresses rapidly.

Palliative operations consist of the Blalock-Hanlon procedure (Fig. 27-70, C), which enlarges the atrial septal defect, or anastomotic procedures for shunting the circulation to relieve the cyanosis, including the Blalock-Taussig, Potts-Smith, and Glenn procedures, which have been described previously.

Alternatively, a Fontan procedure may be performed, employing a valved conduit (Fig. 27-33). This allows for redirection of venous blood flow from the right atrium to the main pulmonary artery around the atretic tricuspid valve and right ventricle.

Operations for transposition of the great arteries

In the anomaly in which the aorta arises from the right ventricle and the pulmonary artery from the left ventricle, circulation is reversed (Fig. 27-73). However, to sustain life, there must be a communication between the two sides of the heart or major vessels: a patent foramen ovale, patent ductus arteriosus, atrial septal defect, ventricular septal defect, or partial transposition of the pulmonary veins, which permits oxygenated blood to enter the systemic circulation.

The newborn with this condition is cyanotic at birth and becomes severely incapacitated, with an enlarged heart that rapidly increases in size and progresses to congestive failure.

Palliative procedures that tend to improve intracardiac mixing, thereby increasing the oxygen content of the systemic blood, are done to sustain life until the infant has attained sufficient growth to tolerate a long corrective procedure. Palliative procedures include the Blalock-Hanlon and the Rashkind atrial septostomy (Fig. 27-70, C).

Corrective procedures include the Mustard atrial switch and the Senning atrial switch procedures, the Rastelli procedure, and the arterial switch procedures.

Rashkind atrial septostomy

The Rashkind atrial septostomy is the creation of an atrial septal defect to allow mixing of blood.

Procedural considerations. The Rashkind atrial septostomy is performed in the cardiac catheterization labo-

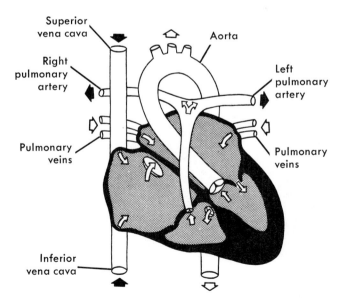

Fig. 27-72. Tricuspid atresia is characterized by small right ventricle, large left ventricle, and diminished pulmonary circulation. Atrial septal or other congenital defect is necessary to sustain life. (From Nursing Education Service: General signs and symptoms of congenital heart abnormalities, Columbus, Ohio, 1961, Ross Laboratories.)

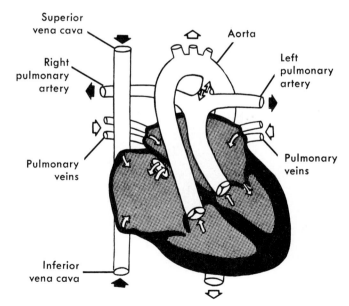

Fig. 27-73. Complete transposition of great vessels produces two separate circulations. Since aorta originates from right ventricle and pulmonary artery from left ventricle, abnormal communication between two chambers must be present to sustain life. (From Nursing Education Service: General signs and symptoms of congenital heart abnormalities, Columbus, Ohio, 1961, Ross Laboratories.)

ratory. A balloon-tipped catheter is advanced into the right atrium through a peripheral vein and is passed through the foramen ovale into the left atrium. The balloon is then inflated, and the catheter is pulled back into the right atrium, creating a large septal defect.

Blalock-Hanlon procedure

The Blalock-Hanlon procedure is the creation of an opening between the right and left atria at the interatrial groove. Cardiopulmonary bypass is not required.

Procedural considerations. The setup is similar to that for shunt operations.

Operative procedure

1. Through a right anterolateral thoracotomy incision, the interatrial groove is exposed.
2. Compression tapes are placed about the right pulmonary artery and the right pulmonary veins.
3. Occlusion of these vessels is completed, and a curved Cooley clamp is applied to include a portion of the right and left atria.
4. The segment, along with a section of the septum, is excised. The edges of the atrial walls are sutured together. Compression tapes are released.
5. Closure is completed.

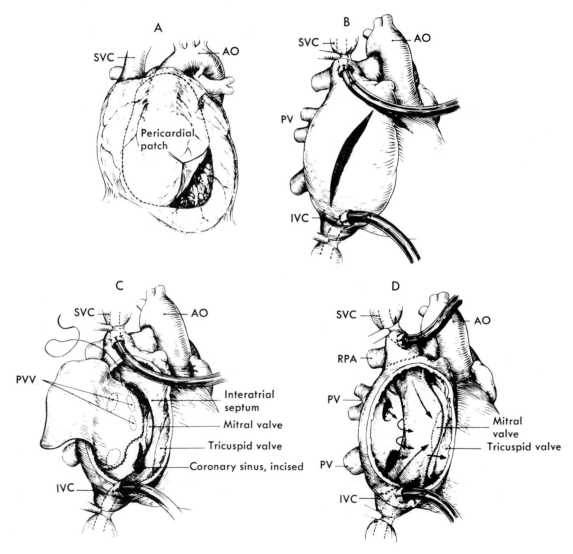

Fig. 27-74. Mustard procedure. **A,** Rectangular patch of pericardium or synthetic material is harvested with its long axis vertically. Length is from diaphragm to reflection onto aorta. Width leaves one comfortably away from phrenic nerves. **B,** Caval cannulae are inserted at junction of venae cavae and right atrium. Superior part of atriotomy goes toward atrial appendage. **C,** Patch is sutured between pulmonary veins and mitral valve, dividing the atrial septal defect in half. Incising the coronary sinus will commit coronary sinus flow into the new systemic venous atrium. **D,** Completed repair. Vena cava flow is now directed to mitral valve, and pulmonary venous blood to tricuspid valve. *SVC,* Superior vena cava; *AO,* aorta; *PV,* pulmonary vein; *IVC,* inferior vena cava; *PVV,* pulmonary veins; *RPA,* right pulmonary artery.

Mustard procedure

Under direct vision, the Mustard procedure excises the remaining segments of the atrial septum; a pericardial or synthetic patch is sutured in place in the atrial cavities creating a baffle so that the venous inflow is reversed. This permits the pulmonary venous return to be redirected into the right ventricle and the systemic venous return to be redirected into the left ventricle (Fig. 27-74).

Previous creation of an atrial septal defect may serve as a first stage for this procedure. Pericardium or synthetic patch is used as a baffle (Mustard and others, 1954).

Patients with an intact ventricular septum are candidates for an atrial switch type of operation.

Procedural considerations. The patient is placed on the operating room bed in a supine position. The setup is as described for open heart surgery, with consideration given to the age and size of the patient.

Operative procedure

1. A median sternotomy incision is completed as described.
2. A section of pericardium 2 × 3 inches is excised and placed in a heparin solution (Fig. 27-74, *A*).
3. Extracorporeal circulation is established as previously described.
4. A curved incision is made in the wall of the right atrium (Fig. 27-74, *B*).
5. The entire atrial septum is excised. The orifice of the coronary sinus is enlarged (Fig. 27-74, *C*).
6. A double-armed suture is placed three fifths of the way along the long margin of the pericardial graft.
7. The pericardial graft or synthetic intracardiac patch is sutured in place, excluding the coronary sinus and the left atrial appendage (Fig. 27-74, *C* and *D*).
8. An additional section of pericardium or synthetic patch is placed in the wall of the right atrium that enlarges the new left atrium.
9. Extracorporeal circulation is discontinued, and closures are completed.

Senning procedure

This alternative inflow procedure redirects venous flow. The Senning (1959, 1975) operation is preferred to the Mustard procedure by many surgeons because it is technically easier to perform and does not require the use of a patch that can eventually cause venous obstruction (Bender and others, 1989; Bove, 1987; Harlan and others, 1981).

Operative procedure (Fig. 27-75)

1. A median sternotomy is made and CPB instituted.
2. A right atrial incision is made longitudinally, extending to the insertion of the eustachian valve at the orifice of the inferior vena cava.
3. A lateral atrial septal flap is made and sutured above the left pulmonary veins.
4. The new systemic venous atrium is completed by su-

turing the edge of the original right atrial incision to the remnant of atrial septum between the mitral and tricuspid valves. This step creates a tube of right atrium containing the venae cavae at each end.

5. Pulmonary venous blood flows around this tube from an opening in front of the right pulmonary veins to the tricuspid valve.

Rastelli procedure

In patients with VSD and subpulmonary stenosis, the atrial switch operations have not demonstrated favorable results. The Rastelli (Rastelli and others, 1969) procedure is an anatomic correction that has the advantage of converting the left ventricle to the systemic pumping chamber (Waldhausen and Pierce, 1985). Either a valved conduit (Fig. 27-33) or an aortic valve homograft (Fig. 27-30) may be used to connect the right ventricle and the pulmonary artery.

Operative procedure

1. Median sternotomy and CPB are instituted.
2. The pulmonary artery is divided, and the proximal stump oversewn.
3. The right ventricle is incised high in the outflow tract.
4. A tunnel is created using Dacron prosthetic material to direct blood through the VSD into the aorta.
5. An outflow conduit is placed between the right ventricle and distal pulmonary artery.

Arterial switch procedure

Anatomic repair of the transposition is performed by switching the pulmonary artery to the right ventricle and the aorta to the left ventricle. Use of a prosthetic graft is avoided. The left ventricle must have developed sufficient contractile force to maintain systemic pressure once the procedure is completed. It occurs in patients with VSD and reversible hypertension; in patients without these defects, pulmonary artery banding (Fig. 27-70, *B*) is first performed to strengthen the left ventricle. Transfer of the coronary arteries must be accomplished without kinking, torsion, or tension (Yacoub, 1979; Yacoub and others, 1976; Jantene and others, 1976; Lecompte and others, 1981).

Operative procedure (Fig. 27-76)

1. Median sternotomy and CPB are performed as described.
2. The aorta is dissected away from the main and branch pulmonary arteries.
3. The coronary arteries are inspected, and the site for their transfer into the pulmonary artery is marked.
4. The aorta is cross-clamped and transsected above the sinuses and aortic valve; the pulmonary artery is transsected above the pulmonic valve.
5. The orifices of the coronary arteries with a rim of adjacent aortic wall are excised.
6. The corresponding sinuses of the pulmonary arteries

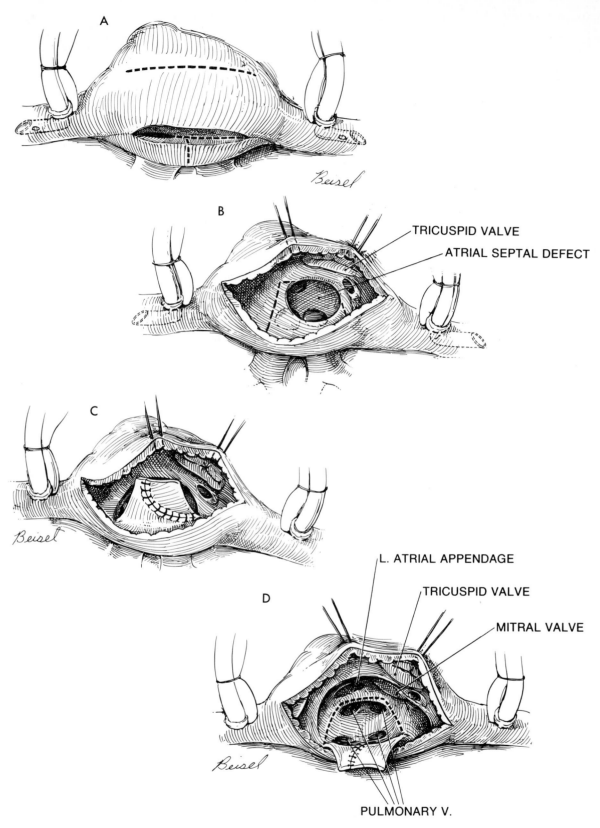

Fig. 27-75. Senning procedure for transposition of the great arteries. **A,** Right atrial incision extended to eustachian valve at orifice of inferior vena cava. **B** and **C,** A septal flap is developed, and a piece of pericardium sutured in the area of absent septum secundum. **D,** The flap is sutured around the left pulmonary vein orifices.

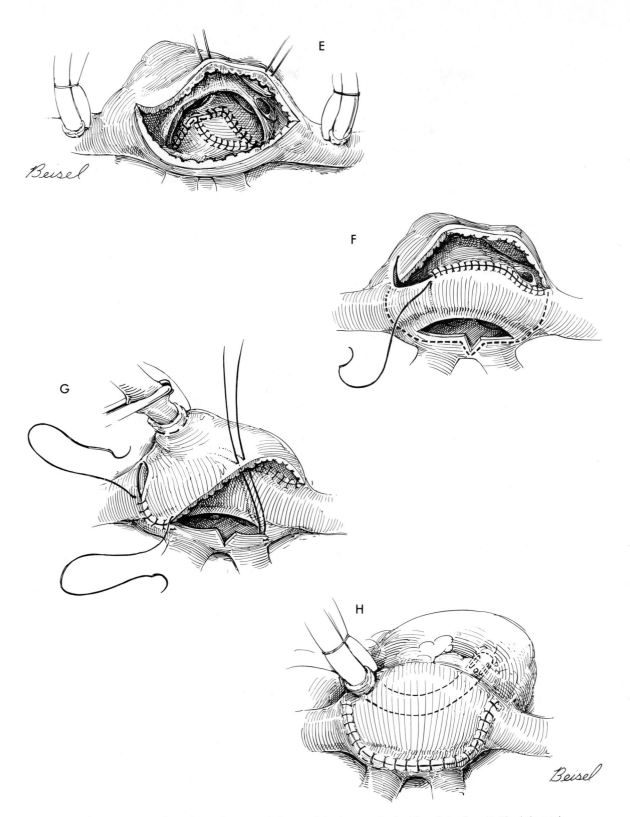

Fig. 27-75, cont'd. E, The ends are carried toward the base on both sides of the flap. **F,** The left atrial wall is incised and the free edge of the right atrium is sutured to the remnant of the atrial septum and the eustachian tube. **G** and **H,** The atrial flap is sutured across the venae cavae so as not to constrict them. (From Waldhausen, J.A., and Pierce, W.S.: Johnson's surgery of the chest, ed. 5, Chicago, 1985, Year Book Medical Publishers.)

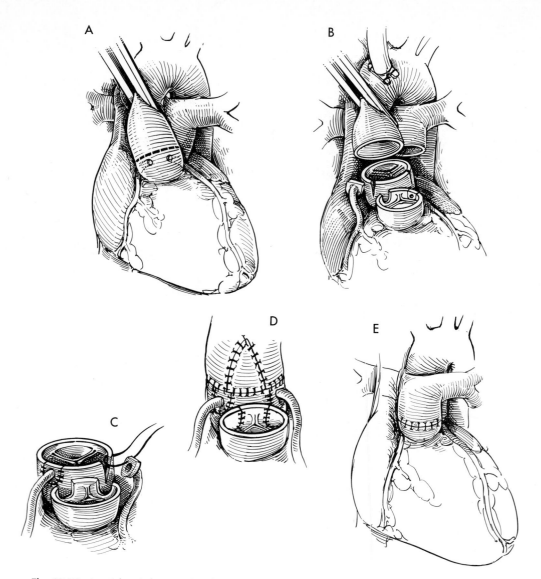

Fig. 27-76. Arterial switch operation for transposition of the great arteries. **A** and **B,** The aorta and pulmonary artery are transected; **C,** coronary arteries are transposed to the proximal pulmonary artery cuff; **D,** the distal aorta is anastomosed to the proximal pulmonary artery (patch enlargement may be required); **E,** the distal pulmonary artery is brought anterior to the aorta and sutured to the proximal aortic stump. (From Waldhausen, J.A., and Pierce, W.S.: Johnson's surgery of the chest, ed. 5, Chicago, 1985, Year Book Medical Publishers.)

are incised where previously marked. The cuff and coronary artery are then sutured into place. Care is taken not to kink the coronary arteries.

7. The distal pulmonary artery is brought anterior to the aorta. The distal aorta is anastomosed to the proximal pulmonary artery.

8. Bovine pericardium may be used to enlarge the aorta and patch the defects created by the excision of the coronary ostia.

Repair of truncus arteriosus

Truncus arteriosus is a retention of the embryological bulbar trunk. It results from failure of normal septation of this trunk into an aorta and pulmonary artery. In this anomaly a single great vessel leaves the base of the heart through a single semilunar valve. This vessel is situated just above the VSD and receives blood from both ventricles. It gives rise to the coronary arteries and supplies the entire pulmonary and systemic circulations (Fig. 27-77).

Total correction is quite successful even though replacement of the conduit will be required two to three times as the child grows (Waldhausen and Pierce, 1985).

Small (12 or 14 mm) extracardiac valved conduits are used (Fig. 27-33) to create a main pulmonary artery in small infants.

Infants who do not undergo repair show severe congestive heart failure with cyanosis and failure to thrive.

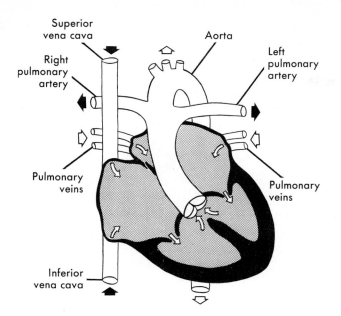

Fig. 27-77. Truncus arteriosus is retention of embryological bulbar trunk. This single arterial trunk overrides ventricles and receives blood from them through ventricular septal defect. Entire pulmonary and systemic circulation is supplied from this common arterial trunk. (From Nursing Education Service: General signs and symptoms of congenital heart abnormalities. Reprinted with permission of Ross Laboratories, Columbus, Ohio 43216, from Clinical Education Aid, vol. 7, © 1970, Ross Laboratories.)

Procedural considerations. The patient is placed in the supine position. The basic setup for a sternotomy is used, with consideration given to the age and size of the patient. A valved conduit, intracardiac patch material, 2 × 2 inches, and a ½ × 4 inch strip of Teflon felt are used.

Operative procedure

1. A median sternotomy is performed, and cardiopulmonary bypass is begun as previously described.
2. A cross-clamp is placed on the aorta, the pulmonary artery is excised from the aorta, and the aortic defect is closed with a double layer of continuous cardiovascular suture. The cross-clamp is removed.
3. A right ventriculotomy is made and the VSD repaired (Fig. 27-78, A).
4. The distal end of the valved conduit is anastomosed to the pulmonary artery.
5. The proximal end of the valved conduit (Fig. 27-33) is anastomosed to the right ventriculotomy using a Teflon felt buttress, which prevents sutures from cutting through the ventricular wall and enhances hemostasis (Fig. 27-78, B).
6. Cardiopulmonary bypass is discontinued, and chest closure is completed.

Open valvulotomy and infundibular resection for pulmonary stenosis

Open valvulotomy is the separation of the stenosed leaflets under direct vision; infundibular resection for pul-

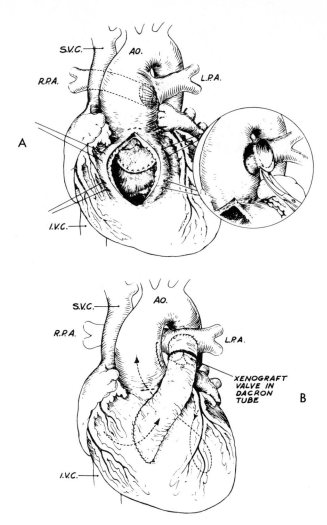

Fig. 27-78. Repair of truncus arteriosus. A, Ventricular septal defect has been closed with a patch, and the left ventricle is committed to the aorta. The only outlet for the right ventricle is the ventriculotomy. The inset shows the pulmonary artery of this type II lesion being disconnected from the truncus. B, Completed repair has a valve in a Dacron graft connecting the ventriculotomy site and the pulmonary artery. (From Effler, D.B.: Blades' surgical diseases of the chest, ed. 4, St. Louis, 1978, The C.V. Mosby Co.)

monary stenosis is excision of the hypertrophied infundibulum.

Procedural considerations. The patient is placed in the supine position. The basic setup for a sternotomy is used, with consideration given to the age and size of the patient.

Operative procedure

1. A median sternotomy is performed, and the cannulations are made for cardiopulmonary bypass as previously described.
2A. For *open valvulotomy,* the pulmonary artery is opened longitudinally, and the stenotic valve is incised with a scalpel or scissors (Fig. 27-79).
2B. For *infundibular resection,* the outflow tract of the

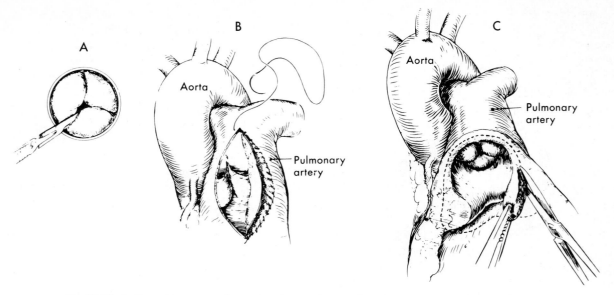

Fig. 27-79. A, Commissurotomy of stenotic valve. Knife is used, and care is taken to incise exactly on commissures. **B,** Diamond-shaped patch being used to enlarge pulmonary outflow tract and pulmonary valve anulus. If vertical pulmonary artery incision is made directly through anterior commissure of valve, the three valve cusps remain intact, and some valve competence is retained. **C,** Excision of obstructing infundibular tissue. (From Effler, D.B.: Blades' surgical diseases of the chest, ed. 4, St. Louis, 1978, The C.V. Mosby Co.)

right ventricle is opened, and the resection is performed, as described for tetralogy of Fallot.

Other procedures. Some surgeons use a valved conduit for the more severe forms of pulmonary stenosis and atresia. The Rastelli procedure (described previously) may be used to suture the conduit to the right ventricle and to the pulmonary artery, thus bypassing the atretic valve.

Closure of patent ductus arteriosus

Closure of the patent ductus arteriosus, an abnormal communication between the aorta and pulmonary artery, is achieved by suture ligation or by division of the ductus. The patent ductus arteriosus is an important fetal vascular communication whereby blood is shunted from the pulmonary artery into the aorta during intrauterine life. During fetal life the lungs are inactive, and the blood is oxygenated in the placenta. Normally the muscular coats of the ductus begin to contract soon after birth; the lumen is subsequently obliterated and blood flow through the shunt ceases (Fig. 27-4).

When the ductus remains patent after birth (Fig. 27-80), it creates a shunt from the aorta through the ductus into the pulmonary circulation. This increases the work of the heart and causes subsequent enlargement and hypertrophy of the left atrium and ventricle. However, when persistent patency of the ductus is associated with other malformations such as tetralogy of Fallot and extreme stenosis of the pulmonary orifice, it is a means of maintaining

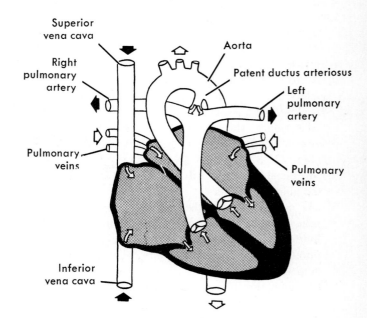

Fig. 27-80. Patent ductus arteriosus. Ductus fails to close after birth. (From Nursing Education Service: General signs and symptoms of congenital heart abnormalities, Columbus, Ohio, 1961, Ross Laboratories.)

life. Surgery is not performed if the patent ductus arteriosus is serving in a compensatory capacity.

Many children have few symptoms because of the small size of the shunt. A frequent clinical sign associated with this condition is a harsh, continuous murmur. Because the blood is oxygenated passing through the shunt, there is no cyanosis, clubbing, or reduction in peripheral arterial oxygen saturation. However, growth is retarded in children who have a large ductus. Other symptoms may include dyspnea, frequent upper respiratory infections, palpitation, limited exercise tolerance, and cardiac failure.

Procedural considerations. For newborn infants the surgeon and anesthesiologist may elect to perform this procedure in the intensive care nursery bed because the operation is a short one. The infant is placed in a right lateral position. The setup is as described, without items for cardiopulmonary bypass, but with special patent ductus clamps.

Generally a left posterolateral approach is used; in some cases, however, a left anterolateral approach is used.

Operative procedure

1. The incision is carried through the muscles over the fourth interspace. The chest wall is entered through the third or fourth intercostal space, using items as described for thoracotomy (Chapter 25). The wound edges are protected and retracted with a Finochietto rib spreader.
2. The pleura is incised with Metzenbaum scissors, and the left lung is protected and retracted with a moist pack and a malleable retractor.
3. The mediastinal pleura is opened between the phrenic and vagus nerves over the region of the ductus. The pleura is retracted by insertion of stay sutures. The recurrent laryngeal nerve is identified and protected. The aortic arch and pulmonary artery are dissected with fine scissors and dry dissectors. Fine arterial branches are divided and ligated with curved Crile or mosquito hemostats and nonabsorbable ligatures and cardiac suture ligatures.
4. The parietal pleura overlying the ductus is dissected with fine vascular forceps and scissors. Stay sutures are inserted to facilitate retraction.
5. The adventitial layer of the ductus is dissected free. A small portion of the obscure posterior ductus is carefully freed to admit a right-angle clamp. Tapes are passed around the aorta and below the ductus.
6A. For the *suture-ligation method* (Fig. 27-81), two ligatures are placed around the ductus, one near the aorta and the other near the pulmonary artery side, both of which are tied in place. Between these two ligatures, two transfixion sutures are inserted.
6B. For the *division of the ductus method,* the patent ductus clamps are applied as close to the aorta and pulmonary artery as possible. The ductus is divided halfway through and partially sutured with mattress cardiovascular sutures and continued back over the free

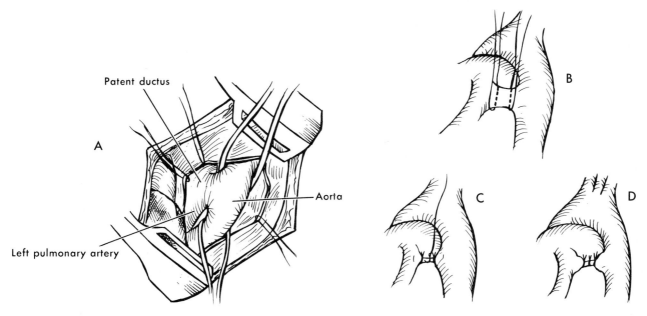

Fig. 27-81. Suture ligation of patent ductus arteriosus. **A,** Potts-Smith aortic clamp and ductus clamp in place. **B,** Ductus arteriosus partially divided. **C,** Closure of ductus arteriosus begun before the division completed to permit better control of bleeding should one clamp slip. **D,** Clamps removed showing completed suture lines.

edge with an over-and-over whip suture. After both openings are sutured, a sponge is held on the area for compression while the patent ductus clamps are removed.

7. The mediastinal pleura is closed with interrupted sutures. The lung is reexpanded, and a chest catheter is inserted to establish closed drainage.

8. The chest wall is closed in layers, and dressings are applied.

Repair of coarctation of the aorta

Coarctation of the aorta (Fig. 27-82) is repaired by excising a constricted segment of the aorta, plus an end-to-end anastomosis—with or without a graft—to reestablish continuity. In some instances a woven Dacron or PTFE patch may be used to enlarge the aortic diameter at the site of the coarctation, or a subclavian flap is used.

The lesion that narrows or constricts the lumen of the aorta may be classified as *infantile* or *adult*. In the infantile type the constriction is long and usually located in the aortic arch proximal to the junction of the aorta and ductus arteriosus. The ductus usually remains patent and may be associated with other cardiac defects. In the adult type the coarctation consists of a constricted area at or just distal to the junction of the aorta and left subclavian artery and the ductus, which is generally closed. This type is compatible with life for a considerable period of time.

Coarctation of the aorta is a fairly common congenital

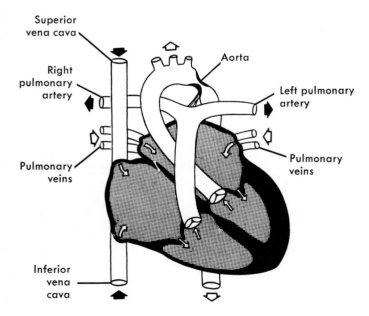

Fig. 27-82. Coarctation of aorta is characterized by narrow aortic lumen and exists as preductal or postductal obstruction, depending on position of obstruction in relation to ductus arteriosus. (From Nursing Education Service: General signs and symptoms of congenital heart abnormalities, Columbus, Ohio, 1961, Ross Laboratories.)

malformation, and the adult patient suffers from hypertension and complains of dyspnea, palpitation, vertigo, headache, epistaxis, and weakness. However, when the aorta is almost obstructed, hypertension is manifested in the upper part of the body with hypotension in the lower extremities. With hypertension above the constriction, the collateral blood supply, which unites the blood vessels of the shoulder, the upper extremities, and the lower extremities, increases markedly. In so doing, the intercostal vessels dilate, allowing their branches to carry blood from the subclavian arteries downward. Occasionally the vessels erode the lower margins of the ribs.

Procedural considerations. The patient is placed in the right lateral position. Instrumentation is as described for basic cardiac surgery, plus Teflon or Dacron woven or knitted vascular prostheses in assorted sizes (Fig. 27-20 and 27-21), to be used as necessary when primary anastomosis is not possible. Items for cardiopulmonary bypass are not needed.

Operative procedure (Fig. 27-83)

1. A left posterolateral incision is carried through the chest wall with resection of the fourth rib, as described for thoracotomy. As previously stated, the collateral blood vessels are somewhat enlarged, and bleeding may be profuse. Dry sponges are used throughout and weighed to determine accurate blood replacement. A Burford or Finochietto retractor is used.

2. The pleura is incised and the lung is retracted. The mediastinal pleura is incised over the constricted portion of the aorta, and the edges are sutured to the chest wall.

3. Careful dissection with fine vascular forceps and dry dissectors is continued to mobilize the aorta and the surrounding intercostal vessels. The laryngeal nerve is identified and protected. The ductus arteriosus is ligated and divided between ductus clamps.

4. *Resection with graft replacement* (Fig. 27-83, *C*)
   a. The curved or angled vascular clamps are applied, and the constricted segment is divided between them. A second set of clamps may be applied above and below, as a safety factor, in fashioning the cuffs for reapproximation.
   b. End-to-end anastomosis is accomplished with a continuous, everting mattress technique for the posterior wall and interrupted, everting mattress sutures for the anterior row. If the stricture is long, a synthetic aortic prosthesis is used to bridge the defect, or a gusset type of patch is used to enlarge the defect.
   c. The clamps are released slowly, the distal one first and then the proximal one. The blood pressure is noted at this time. Removal of clamps is not completed until the blood pressure is stabilized.

5. *Patch repair*
   a. The curved or angled vascular clamps are applied,

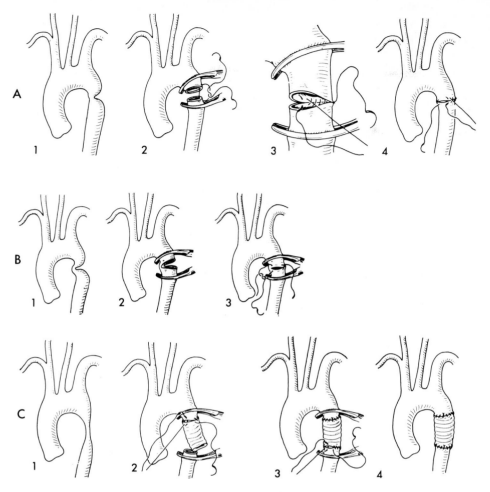

Fig. 27-83. Diagrams showing coarctation of aorta: types with methods of correction. **A,** Short narrow obstruction and steps in end-to-end anastomosis. **B,** Wedge excision with partial anastomosis completed, **C,** Segmental excision with graft replacement. (From Blades, B., editor: Surgical diseases of the chest, ed. 3, St. Louis, 1974, The C.V. Mosby Co.)

and a longitudinal aortotomy is performed with a no. 11 knife blade, a Potts scissors, and vascular forceps.

   b. A piece of graft material is inserted, large enough to widen the aorta, using a continuous cardiovascular suture.

   c. The clamps are removed, one at a time, as described in step 4c.

6. *Subclavian flap repairs* (Figs. 27-84 and 27-85)

   a. The aorta above and below the patent ductus is dissected out, as is the subclavian artery. The subclavian artery is ligated at the origin of the vertebral artery, which is also ligated.

   b. The aorta is incised distal to the area of narrowing, through the coarctation to the subclavian artery.

   c. The aorta is opened and the coarctation excised.

   d. The tip of the subclavian flap is brought down into the aorta and sutured with absorbable running sutures or nonabsorbable interrupted sutures.

   e. *The reverse subclavian flap procedure* (Fig. 27-85) is used in infants with coarctation of the aortic arch. The subclavian artery is ligated and transected at the origin of the vertebral artery. An incision is made in the aorta through the coarctation and into the subclavian artery. The subclavian flap is then sewn into the incision as in steps b through d above.

7. The parietal pleura is closed, leaving a small opening at the lower point. Closed drainage is established, and the chest wall is closed in layers. A dressing is applied.

Pulmonary artery banding

Pulmonary artery banding is the constriction of the pulmonary artery to reduce its diameter, thereby decreasing pulmonary blood flow (Fig. 27-70, *B*).

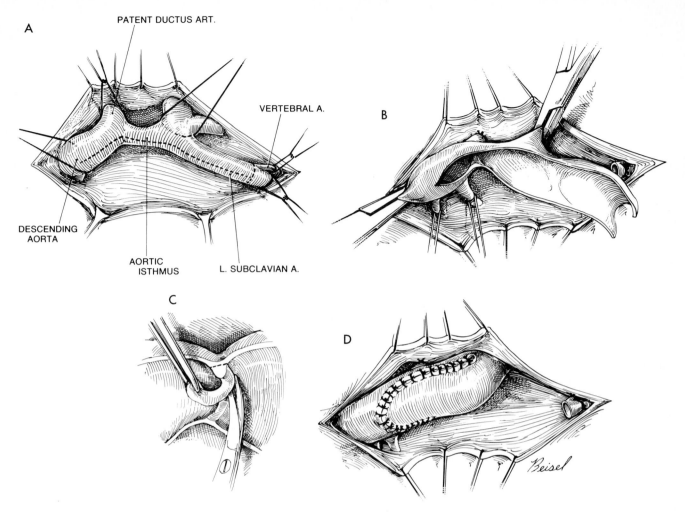

A
PATENT DUCTUS ART.

VERTEBRAL A.

B

DESCENDING
AORTA

AORTIC
ISTHMUS   L. SUBCLAVIAN A.

C

D

Beisel

Fig. 27-84. Subclavian flap procedure for coarctation of the aorta. **A,** Retraction stitches around the transverse arch, the descending aorta, and the left subclavian artery; the patent ductus arteriosus is ligated; **B,** aorta incised; **C,** coarctation shelf removed; **D,** subclavin flap anastomosed to descending aorta. (From Waldhausen, J.A., and Pierce, W.S.: Johnson's surgery of the chest, ed. 5, Chicago, 1985, Year Book Medical Publishers.)

An infant with an enlarged heart in intractable failure and a large left-to-right shunt may be treated effectively by a palliative pulmonary artery banding operation. This procedure is designed to reduce the flow of blood through the pulmonary artery to approximately one half to one third of the existing rate. A tape is looped about the artery and secured in place by a simple suture technique. Pressures are measured by direct needle puncture and before and after banding. A reduction of the distal pulmonary artery pressure by 50% to 70% is sought. Repair of the interventricular septal defect may be postponed until the child has been clinically stabilized and can withstand an open heart procedure (Bojar, 1989).

Procedural considerations. The patient is placed in the left lateral position if an anterolateral incision is to be used or in the supine position if a median sternotomy is to be used. Eight-inch pieces of various width tapes (sur-

geon's preference), with appropriate sizes for children, are used.

Hypoplastic left heart syndrome (HLHS)

Hypoplastic left heart syndrome consists of an absent or diminutive left ventricle and mitral atresia or stenosis, aortic valve atresia or stenosis, and a hypoplastic aorta. The right ventricle hypertrophies because it must carry the entire heart load. Without intervention, the infant rarely lives to be over 2 weeks old (Jonas and others, 1986). Hypoplastic left heart syndrome is one of the most challenging congenital anomalies. Norwood and colleagues (1980) were among the first to describe their operative procedures. They devised a two-staged physiologic repair that makes the right atrium the pulmonary conduit, and the right ventricle the systemic pump (Smith and Vernon-Levett, 1989).

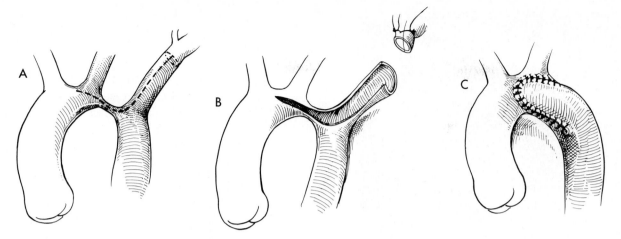

Fig. 27-85. Reverse subclavian flap procedure for coarctation of the aorta. **A,** Coarctation of aortic arch (left subclavian artery is ligated and transected); **B,** aortic incision; **C,** subclavian flap sewn to aorta. (From Waldhausen, J.A., and Pierce, W.S.: Johnson's surgery of the chest, ed. 5, Chicago, 1985, Year Book Medical Publishers.)

In 1984, Bailey and colleagues (1986) performed a heterograft cardiac transplantation on a neonate. Although the heterograft (baboon) heart was rejected, this procedure stimulated greater research into the mechanisms of immunologic responses to heterograft organs. Allograft cardiac transplantation is being employed with increasing success for this condition. The procedure is similar to that for adult transplantation.

Surgery for conduction disturbances

Disturbances of the conduction system can affect the rate and/or rhythm of the contracting heart. Surgical techniques have been developed to treat most types of supraventricular dysrhythmias and both ischemic and nonischemic ventricular tachydysrhythmias.

Cryosurgical ablation of accessory pathways

Cryoablation of accessory conduction pathways is the destruction of these pathways through freezing. Patients with Wolff-Parkinson-White (WPW) syndrome have accessory conduction pathways that bypass the normal AV node–His bundle system. Patients have frequent, recurring, symptomatic tachydysrhythmias that overstimulate the heart (Regas and others, 1986).

Operative procedure. Prior to surgery, the patient's accessory pathways are mapped in the electrophysiology laboratory to determine the origin of the pathway, its role in the tachydysrhythmia, the existence of additional pathways, and the effects of medication on the dysrhythmia. At operation, the surgeon initiates cardiopulmonary bypass and attaches electrodes to each atrium and ventricle. Intraoperative mapping is performed to verify the accessory system. When the pathway is located, the surgeon dissects down to it and cryoablates the tissue. After termination of

bypass and the achievement of hemostasis, the chest is closed in the routine fashion.

Insertion of permanent pacemaker

A permanent pacemaker (pulse generator and electrode) initiates atrial or ventricular contraction or both. Complete heart block and bradyarrhythmias are the most common indications for pacemaker implantation (Harthorne, 1989). The development of multiprogrammable and physiologic pacemakers has made possible the treatment of many forms of dysrhythmias and neuroconductive disturbances, even in neonates. A temporary pacemaker may also be used for acute forms of heart block and dysrhythmias that occasionally occur during cardiac surgery.

The three basic methods of placing electrodes for permanent cardiac pacing are transvenous, epicardial, and subxiphoid. The transvenous and subxiphoid approaches are most commonly used because they do not require a major thoracotomy or a general anesthetic and are therefore safer for high-risk patients. Epicardial electrodes are placed during cardiac operations when the chest is opened and the heart is exposed.

Pulse generators (Fig. 27-86) are typically powered by lithium, which lasts 5 to 10 years. The generators are classified into three groups: fixed rate (or asynchronous), ventricular demand, and physiologic. The asynchronous was the first type implanted and fires at a fixed rate, independent of the electrical activity of the heart. A major disadvantage of this type of pacing is competition between the heart's intrinsic beat and the paced beat, possibly resulting in ventricular fibrillation if the paced beat occurs during the T-wave period of the electrocardiogram. Ventricular demand pacemakers were developed in response to this problem and only fire at a fixed rate if spontaneous

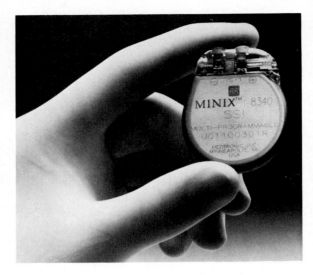

Fig. 27-86. Pacemaker generator. (Courtesy of Medtronic, Inc., Minneapolis, Minn.)

ventricular activity fails. Adding a sensing mechanism to the existing stimulating mechanism makes this type of pacing possible. "Physiologic" pacemakers maintain atrioventricular synchrony, taking advantage of atrial systole and enhancing cardiac output by as much as 20%.

There are two types of electrodes: myocardial (epicardial), which are attached to the heart muscle under direct vision, and endocardial, which are inserted transvenously. The stimulating and sensing electrodes are located at the tip of the lead, which attaches to the pulse generator (Fig. 27-87).

Pacing systems are also available as unipolar or bipolar. A pacemaker with one stimulating electrode at the tip of the lead is unipolar. The electrical current flows between the electrode and the pulse generator. A bipolar pacemaker has two stimulating electrodes at the tip of the lead. Electrical current flows between the two electrodes.

Insertion of transvenous (endocardial) pacing electrodes

Procedural considerations. The patient is placed in the supine position. Continuous electrocardiographic monitoring is essential, so the electrodes must be carefully placed. The patient should be made as comfortable as possible because this procedure can sometimes be lengthy and is frequently performed using local or local standby anesthesia (monitored anesthesia care).

Fluoroscopy is required; thus either a portable image intensifier is needed or the procedure is done in the special studies section of the radiology department.

A defibrillator and emergency drugs should be available because dysrhythmias can occur during catheter insertion.

The majority of these procedures are performed with local anesthesia, but monitored anesthesia care may be requested.

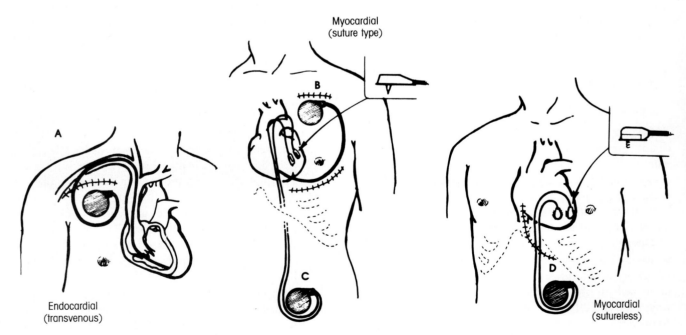

Fig. 27-87. Positions of pulse generator and leads. **A,** A transvenous endocardial system using the subclavian vein; **B,** an epicardial system with the pulse generator pocket on the anterior chest wall. The leads are the suture type. **C,** An epicardial system with an abdominal wall pocket. **D,** An abdominally placed pulse generator connected to suture screw-in leads. (From Guzzetta, C.E. and others: Cardiovascular nursing: bodymind tapestry, St. Louis, 1984, The C.V. Mosby Co.)

A minor set of instruments is used, plus the following:

1 Potts vascular scissors
2 Potts vascular forceps
2 Vascular needle holders
1 "Tunneling" instrument, such as a sponge-holding forceps or vaginal packing forceps
  Sterile pacemaker, electrodes, and connecting cable
  External pacemaker (for testing) or a pacing analyzer

Operative procedure (Fig. 27-87, A)

1. The skin and subcutaneous tissue are infiltrated with a local anesthetic, and the patient placed in Trendelenburg's position.
2. A cutdown is performed to isolate the subclavian vein, and the vessel is encircled with heavy sutures or umbilical tapes.
3. A venotomy is performed, usually with a no. 11 scalpel blade, and the pacing electrode is inserted through a dilator sheath, which is withdrawn after the lead insertion.
4. The electrode is advanced, under direct fluoroscopic vision, into the right atrium, through the tricuspid valve, and into the right ventricle.
5. The surgeon attempts to entrap the tip of the electrode in the *trabeculae carneae* of the right ventricular apex to stabilize it (Fig. 27-87). (If a dual chamber pacemaker is inserted, the second lead is entrapped in the right atrial appendage.)
6. The electrodes are attached, by appropriate cables, to an external pulse generator or a pacing analyzer for testing.
7. A pocket is created for the implantable pulse generator. The incision is carried down to fascia and a tunnel is formed, subcutaneously with a blunt instrument, to the subclavian incision.
8. The electrode is brought down through the tunnel and is attached to the pulse generator.
9. The pulse generator is placed in the pocket, and both incisions are irrigated with an antibiotic solution.
10. The incisions are closed in layers with absorbable sutures.

Insertion of myocardial (epicardial) pacing electrodes (Fig. 27-87)

Subxiphoid process approach

Procedural considerations. The setup is as described for placement of endocardial electrodes.

Operative procedure

1. If local anesthesia is used, the subxiphoid process and left upper quadrant area are infiltrated with the anesthetic.
2. A small, transverse incision is made below the xiphoid process and is carried down to the linea alba. A tunnel is created under the xiphoid process to the pericardium, which is incised to expose the heart.

3. The pacing electrode, mounted on its carrier, is screwed into the ventricular myocardium, and the carrier is removed.
4. The remainder of the procedure is as described for insertion of the endocardial electrode.

Sternotomy approach

Operative procedure

1. The mediastinum is opened, and an area of myocardium is chosen for placement of the pacing electrodes.
2. The electrode tips are screwed into or are sutured to the myocardium and are attached, by an appropriate cable, to an external pulse generator or pacing analyzer for testing.
3. The pocket and subcutaneous tunnel are created, as described for insertion of the endocardial electrode.
4. A chest drainage catheter is inserted, and the thoracotomy incision is closed.

Insertion of automatic implantable cardioverter defibrillator (AICD)

The AICD is an electronic device designed to monitor cardiac electrical activity and deliver prompt defibrillatory shocks (Fig. 27-88). Sudden cardiac death from malignant ventricular dysrhythmias (ventricular fibrillation and ventricular tachycardia) annually strikes an estimated 400,000 persons in the United States (Fonger and others, 1988).

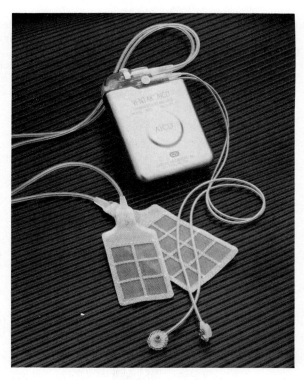

Fig. 27-88. Automatic implantable cardioverter defibrillator: generator *(top)*, ventricular patch leads *(middle)*, screw-in sensing leads *(bottom)*. (Courtesy C.P.I., Cardiac Pacemakers, Inc., St. Paul, Minn.)

Many of these patients cannot be helped by surgery or pharmacologic intervention. The AICD differs from a pacemaker in that the former senses ventricular tachycardia or fibrillation and the latter senses asystole. The AICD device consists of a generator, myocardial patches, and sensing electrodes.

Operative procedure. One of three approaches may be selected by the surgeon: a lateral thoracotomy, a subxiphoid, or a median sternotomy incision (Moss and others, 1984). The thoracotomy approach is often used for patients who have mediastinal adhesions from previous surgery. The subxiphoid approach is indicated when there is no history of cardiac surgery and none is planned. The median sternotomy approach is used when a concomitant cardiac operation is performed.

The sensing leads may be inserted via a transvenous or epicardial route to the right ventricle. The ventricular patches are sewn to the epicardium anteriorly and posteriorly. The generator is housed in a subcutaneous pocket near the umbilicus. The free ends of the lead system are tunneled to the generator and inserted. The device is tested, and the incisions are closed.

REFERENCES

Acker, M.A., and others: An autologous biologic pump motor, J. Thorac. Cardiovasc. Surg. 92:733, 1986.

Bailey, L. and others: Method of heart transplantation for treatment of hypoplastic left heart syndrome, J. Thorac. Cardiovasc. Surg. 92:1, 1986.

Barkett, P.A.: Cardiac MUGA scan: taking first-rate pictures of the heart, Nursing 88, October 1988, p. 76.

Bender, H.W., and others: Ten years' experience with the Senning operation for transposition of the great arteries: physiological results and late follow-up, Ann. Thorac. Surg. 47:218, 1989.

Beynen, F.M., and Tarhan, S.: Anesthesia for the surgical repair of congenital heart defects in children. In S. Tarhan: Cardiovascular anesthesia and postoperative care, ed. 2, Chicago, 1989, Year Book Medical Publishers.

Bojar, R.M.: Manual of perioperative care in cardiac and thoracic surgery, Boston, 1989, Blackwell Scientific Publishers.

Bolman, R.M., and others: Circulatory support with a centrifugal pump as a bridge to cardiac transplantation, Ann. Thorac. Surg. 47:108, 1989.

Bove, E.L.: Senning's procedure for transplantation of the great arteries, Ann. Thorac. Surg. 43:678, 1987.

Carpentier, A.: Cardiac valve surgery: the french correction, J. Thorac. Cardiovasc. Surg. 86:323, 1983.

Carpentier, A., and Chachques, J.C.: Latissimus dorsi cardiomyoplasty to increase cardiac output. In G. Rabago and D.A. Cooley, editors, Heart valve replacement and future trends in cardiac surgery, Mount Kisco, N.Y., 1987, Futura Publishing Co.

Chachques, J.C., Grandjean, P.A., and Carpentier, A.: A latissimus dorsi dynamic cardiomyoplasty, Ann. Thorac. Surg. 47:600, 1989.

Crawford, E.S.: Acute and chronic aortic dissection. In Grillo, H.C., and others: Current therapy in cardiothoracic surgery, Toronto, 1989, B.C. Decker.

Crawford, E.S.: Replacement of the thoracic aorta. In Grillo, H.C., and others: Current therapy in cardiothoracic surgery, Toronto, 1989, B.C. Decker.

Cruse, P.J., and Foord, R.: The epidemiology of wound infection: a ten-year prospective study of 62,939 wounds, Surg. Clin. N. Amer. 80:27, 1980.

Daily, P.O., and others: Clinical comparisons of methods of myocardial protection, J. Thorac. Cardiovasc. Surg. 93:324, 1987.

Davis, P.K., and others: Current status of permanent total artificial hearts, Ann. Thorac. Surg. 47:172, 1989.

Diehl, J.T., and others: Efficacy of retrograde coronary sinus cardioplegia in patients undergoing myocardial revascularization: a prospective randomized trial. Ann. Thorac. Surg. 45:595, 1988.

Edmunds, L.H.: Thrombotic and bleeding complications of prosthetic heart valves, Ann. Thorac. Surg. 44:430, 1987.

Emery, R.W., and Pritzker, M.R., editors: Cardiothoracic transplantation, Philadelphia, 1988, Hanley & Belfus.

Ferguson, J.J., and others: Animal and human application of the Nimbus Hemopump: a catheter-mounted ventricular support device (Abstr). Cardiology and Cardiovascular Surgery: Interventions 1988. 18th Annual Symposium of the Texas Heart Institute, 1988, page 60.

Fonger, J.D., and others: Impending sudden cardiac death: treatment with myocardial revascularization and the automatic implantable cardioverter defibrillator. Ann. Thorac. Surg. 46:13, 1988.

Frater, R.W.: Mitral valvuloplasty. In A.J. Roberts and C.R. Conti, editors: Current surgery of the heart, Philadelphia, 1987, J.B. Lippincott Co.

Galloway, A.C., and others: Current concepts of mitral valve reconstruction for mitral insufficiency, Circulation 78:1087, 1988.

Gardner, R.: Muscle-powered cardiac assist: a new alternative on the horizon, J. Cardiovasc. Nurs. 2:76, 1988.

Graf, D., and Gonzalez-Lavin, L.: The homograft: a new dimension in cardiac valve replacement, AORN J. 48:911, 1988.

Grondin, P., and others: Carpentier's annulus and DeVega's annuloplasty: The end of the tricuspid challenge, J. Thorac. Cardiovasc. Surg. 70:852, 1975.

Guzzetta, C.E., and others: Assessment tools for use with nursing diagnoses, St. Louis, 1989, The C.V. Mosby Co.

Harlan, B.J., Starr, A., and Harwin, F.M.: Manual of cardiac surgery, 2 vols., New York, 1980–1981, Springer-Verlag.

Harthorne, J.W.: Cardiac pacing. In Grillo, H.C., and others, editors: Current therapy in cardiothoracic surgery, Toronto, 1989, B.C. Decker.

Hill, A.G., and others: Hollow fiber membrane oxygenation and bubble oxygenation: a contrast. Proc. Amer. Acad. Cardiovasc. Perf. 6:51, 1985.

Hurst, J.W., editor: The heart, arteries and veins, ed. 6, 2 vols., New York, 1986, McGraw-Hill.

Isner, J., and others: Treatment of calcified aortic stenosis by balloon valvuloplasty, Am. J. Cardiol. 59:313, 1987.

Jantene, A.D., and others: Anatomic correction of transposition of the great vessels, J. Thorac. Cardiovasc. Surg. 72:364, 1976.

Jonas, R.A., and others: First-stage palliation of hypoplastic left heart syndrome: the importance of coarctation and shunt size, J. Thorac. Cardiovasc. Surg. 92:6, 1986.

Jones, M.T., and others: Surgical repair of acquired ventricular septal defect, J. Thorac. Cardiovasc. Surg. 93:680, 1987.

Kalmbach, T., and Bhayana, J.N.: Cardioplegia delivery by combined aortic root and coronory sinus perfusion, Ann. Thorac. Surg. 47:316, 1989.

Kaplan, J.A.: Cardiac anesthesia, ed. 2, 2 vols., Philadelphia, 1987 W.B. Saunders Co.

Kereiakes, D.J., and others: Emergent coronary bypass following intravenous recombinant tissue plasminogen activator therapy for acute myocardial infarction: results from a multicenter randomized trial. Circulation 74: Sup. II-368, 1986 (abstract).

Lange, P.L., and Hopkins, R.A.: Allograft valve banking: techniques and technology. In Hopkins, R.A.: Cardiac reconstructions with allograft-valves, New York, 1989, Springer-Verlag.

Lawrance, P.A., and Wieczorek, B.H.: Congenital valvular heart disease, J. Cardiovasc. Nurs. 1:18, 1987.

Lecompte, Y., and others: Anatomic correction of transposition of the great arteries, J. Thorac. Cardiovasc. Surg. 82:629, 1981.

Little, R.C., and Little, W.C.: Physiology of the heart and circulation, ed. 4, Chicago, 1989, Year Book Medical Publishers.

Loop, F.D., and others: Influence of the internal-mammary-artery graft on 10-year survival and other cardiac events, N. Engl. J. Med. 314:1, 1986.

Marchetta, S., and Stennis, E.: Ventricular assist devices: applications for critical care, J. Cardiovasc. Nurs. 2:39, 1988.

Marker, L.: Coronary artery bypass: internal thoracic artery bypass procedure, AORN J. 49:1533, 1989.

Matthews, K.A., and others, editors: Handbook of stress, reactivity, and cardiovascular disease, New York, 1986, John Wiley & Sons.

May, D.R., and Adams, M.A.: Ventricular assist devices: a bridge to cardiac transplantation, AORN J. 46:633, 1987.

Mindich, B., and others: Aortic valve salvage utilizing high frequency vibratory debridement, J. Am. Coll. Cardiol. 11:3A, 1988.

Moss, P.M., Chavez, B.B., and Prostko, J.M.: An implantable defibrillator: help for ventricular arrhythmias, AORN J. 40:551, 1984.

Mustard, W.T., and others: A surgical approach to transposition of the great vessels with extracorporeal circuit, Surgery 36:39, 1954.

Norwood, W.I., Kirklin, J.K., and Sanders, S.P.: Hypoplastic left heart syndrome: experience with palliative surgery, Am. J. Cardiol. 45:87, 1980.

Ottino, G., and others: Major sternal wound infection after open-heart surgery: a multivariate analysis of risk factors in 2,579 consecutive operative procedures, Ann. Thorac. Surg. 44:173, 1987.

Pae, W.E., and others: Staged cardiac transplantation: total artificial heart or ventricular assist pump? Circulation 78: Sup. III (5), III-66, 1988.

Palmaz, J.C.: Balloon-expandable intravascular stent, Am. J. Roentgenol. 150:1263, 1988.

Phillips, S.J.: Percutaneous cardiopulmonary bypass and innovations in clinical counterpulsation, Crit. Care Clin. 2:297, 1986.

Phillips, S.J., and others: Percutaneous cardiopulmonary bypass: application and indication for use, Ann. Thorac. Surg. 47:121, 1989.

Platia, E.V.: Management of cardiac arrhythmia: the nonpharmacologic approach, Philadelphia, 1987, J.B. Lippincott Co.

Pym, J., and others: Gastroepiploic-coronary anastomosis, J. Thorac. Cardiovasc. Surg. 94:256, 1987.

Rabago, G., and others: The new DeVega technique in tricuspid annuloplasty, J. Thorac. Cardiovasc. Surg. 21:231, 1980.

Rashkind, W.J.: Historical aspects of surgery for congenital heart disease, J. Thorac. Cardiovasc. Surg. 84:619, 1982.

Rastelli, G.C., McGoon, D.C., and Wallace, R.B.: Anatomic correction of transposition of the great arteries with ventricular septal defect and subpulmonary stenosis, J. Thorac. Cardiovasc. Surg. 58:545, 1969.

Regas, M.L., Hill, S.B., and Schmidt, C.V.: Wolff-Parkinson-White syndrome: cryosurgical ablation of accessory pathways, AORN J. 44:742, 1986.

Reitz, B.A.: Cardiac transplantation. In Grillo, H.C., and others, editors: Current therapy in cardiothoracic surgery, Toronto, 1989, B.C. Decker.

Roberts, A.J., and Conti, C.R., editors: Current surgery of the heart. Philadelphia, 1987, J.B. Lippincott Co.

Robicsek, F., and others: Experiments with a bowl of saline: the hidden risk of hypothermic-osmotic damage during topical cardiac cooling, J. Thorac. Cardiovasc. Surg. 97:461, 1989.

Rozanski, A., and others: Mental stress and the induction of silent myocardial ischemia in patients with coronary artery disease, N. Engl. J. Med. 318:1005, 1988.

Rudolphi, D.M., Nagy, K.M., and Verne, D.J.: Cardiac transplantation: organ procurement to patient discharge, AORN J. 45:80, 1987.

Ruzevich, S.A., Swartz, M.T., and Pennington, D.G.: Nursing care of the patient with a pneumatic ventricular assist device, Heart & Lung 17:399, 1988.

Sand, M.E., and others: A comparison of repair and replacement for mitral valve incompetence, J. Thorac. Cardiovasc. Surg. 94:208, 1987.

Schakenbach, L.H.: Physiologic dynamics of acquired valvular heart disease, J. Cardiovasc. Nurs. 1:1, 1987.

Seifert, P.C.: dissecting aortic aneurysms, AORN J. 43:443, 1986.

Seifert, P.C.: surgery for acquired valvular heart disease, J. Cardiovasc. Nurs. 1:27, 1987.

Senning, A.: Correction of the transposition of the great arteries, Ann. Surg. 182:287, 1975.

Senning, A.: Surgical correction of transposition of the great vessels, Surgery 45:966, 1959.

Siwek, L.G., and Daggett, W.M.: Myocardial protection. In H.C. Grillo and others, editors: Current therapy in cardiothoracic surgery, Toronto, 1989, B.C. Decker.

Slogoff, S., and Keats, A.S.: Randomized trial of primary anesthetic agents on outcome of coronary artery bypass operations, Anesthesiology 70:179, 1989.

Smith, J.B., and Vernon-Levett, P.: Hypoplastic left heart syndrome: treatment options, Matern. Child Nurs. 14:180, 1989.

Spencer, F.C., Galloway, A.C., and Colvin, S.B.: A clinical evaluation of the hypothesis that rupture of the left ventricle following mitral valve replacement can be prevented by preservation of the chordae of the mural leaflet, Ann. Surg. 202:673, 1985.

Spray, T.L.: Pediatric cardiac surgery. In Roberts, A.J., and Conti, C.R., editors: Current surgery of the heart, Philadelphia, 1987, J.B. Lippincott Co.

Sutor, S., and others: Domino transplants: sequential heart and heart-lung transplantation, AORN J. 48:876, 1988.

Tarhan, S.: Cardiovascular anesthesia and postoperative care, ed. 2, Chicago, 1989, Year Book Medical Publishers.

Tuman, K.J., and others: Does choice of anesthetic agent significantly affect outcome after coronary artery surgery? Anesthesiology 70:189, 1989.

Turley, K., Turley K., and Ebert, P.: Aortic allografts: reconstruction of right ventricle–pulmonary artery continuity, Ann. Thorac. Surg. 47:278, 1989.

Turner, T.L., Douglas, J., and Cockburn, F.: Craig's care of the newly born infant, ed. 8, London, 1988, Churchill Livingstone.

Waldhausen, J.A., and Pierce, W.S.: Johnson's surgery of the chest, ed. 5, Chicago, 1985, Year Book Medical Publishers.

Waller, B.F., editor: Contemporary issues in cardiovascular pathology, Philadelphia, 1988, F.A. Davis Co.

Wallwork J., editor: Heart and heart-lung transplantation, Philadelphia, 1989, J.B. Lippincott Co.

Warner, M.A., and Warner, M.E.: Anesthetic agents for cardiac surgery. In S. Tarhan, cardiovascular anesthesia and postoperative care, ed. 2, Chicago, 1989, Year Book Medical Publishers.

Yacoub, M.H.: The case for anatomic correction of transposition of the great arteries, J. Thorac. Cardiovasc. Surg. 78:3, 1979.

Yacoub, M.H., Radley-Smith, R., and Hilton, C.J.: Anatomical correction of complete transposition of the great arteries and ventricular septal defect in infancy, Brit. Med. J. 1:1112, 1976.

Yankah, A.C., and others, editors: Cardiac valve allografts 1962–1987, New York, 1988, Springer-Verlag.

BIBLIOGRAPHY

American Nurses' Association Division on Medical-Surgical Nursing Practice and American Heart Association Council on Cardiovascular Nursing: Standards of cardiovascular nursing practice, Kansas City, 1981, The Association.

Andreoli, K.G., and others: Comprehensive cardiac care, ed. 6, St. Louis, 1987, The C.V. Mosby Co.

Arciniegas, E.: Pediatric cardiac surgery, Chicago, 1985, Year Book Medical Publishers.

Bernhard, V.M., and Towne, J.B., editors: Complications in vascular surgery, ed. 2, New York, 1985, Grune & Stratton.

Bodnar, E., Wain, W.H., and Haberman, S.: Assessment and comparison of the performance of cardiac valves, Ann. Thorac. Surg. 34:146, 1982.

Cooley, D.A.: Techniques in cardiac surgery, ed. 2, Philadelphia, 1984, W.B. Saunders Co.

Cumberland, D.C., Starkey, I.R., and Oakly, G.D.G.: Percutaneous laser-assisted coronary angioplasty, Lancet 1:214, 1986.

Detre, K., and others: Percutaneous transluminal coronary angioplasty in 1985–1986 and 1977–1981, N. Engl. J. Med. 318:265, 1988.

Dillard, D.H., and Hillet, D.W.: Atlas of cardiac surgery, New York, 1983, Macmillan.

Eugene, J., and others: Comparison of continuous-wave lasers for end-arterectomy of experimental atheromas, J. Thorac. Cardiovasc. Surg. 93:494, 1987.

Grillo, H.C. and others, editors: Current therapy in cardiothoracic surgery, Toronto, 1989, B.C. Decker.

Guzzetta, C.E., and Dossey, B.M.: Cardiovascular nursing: bodymind tapestry, St. Louis, 1984, The C.V. Mosby Co.

Hazinski, M.F.: Nursing care of the critically ill child, St. Louis, 1984, The C.V. Mosby Co.

Henry, J.B.: Todd-Sanford-Davidson clinical diagnosis and management by laboratory methods, ed. 17, Philadelphia, 1984, W.B. Saunders Co.

Hill, J.: Bridging to cardiac transplantation, Ann. Thorac. Surg. 47:167, 1989.

Hopkins, R.A.: Cardiac reconstruction with allograft valves, New York, 1989, Springer-Verlag.

Little, R.C., and Little, W.C.: Physiology of the heart and circulation, ed. 4, Chicago, 1989, Year Book Medical Publishers.

Mitchell, R.S., and others: Significant patient-related determinants of prosthetic valve performance, J. Thorac. Cardiovasc. Surg. 91:807, 1986.

Morganroth, J., Parisi, A.F., and Pohost, G.M., editors: Noninvasive cardiac imaging, Chicago, 1983, Year Book Medical Publishers.

Price, S.A., and Wilson, L.M.: Pathophysiology: clinical concepts of disease processes, ed. 2, New York, 1982, McGraw-Hill.

Rabago, G., and Cooley, D.A., editors: Heart valve replacement and future trends in cardiac surgery, Mount Kisco, N.Y., 1987, Futura.

Rapp, J.H., and others: "Angiography" by magnetic resonance imaging: detailed vascular anatomy without ionizing radiation or contrast media, Surgery 105:662, 1989.

Rothrock, J.C.: Perioperative care planning, St. Louis, 1990, The C.V. Mosby Co.

Sabiston, D.C., and Spencer, F.C.: Gibbon's surgery of the chest, 2 vols., ed. 4, Philadelphia, 1983, W.B. Saunders.

Seifert, P.C., and Lefrak, E.A.: Atrial septal defect: the adult patient, AORN J. 39:617, 1984.

Seifert, P.C., and Speir, A.M.: Left ventricular rupture: a collaborative approach to emergency management, AORN J. 51:714, 1990.

Virmani, R., Atkinson, J.B., and Forman, M.B.: Aortocoronary saphenous vein bypass grafts. In Waller, B.F., editor: Contemporary issues in cardiovascular pathology, Cardiovascular Clinics, Philadelphia, 1988, F.A. Davis Co.

Part Three

SPECIAL CONSIDERATIONS

28 Practice and principles of ambulatory surgery

CHERYL A. SANGERMANO

Ambulatory surgery has grown dramatically as trends in health care delivery shift toward the outpatient population. As a result of government regulations, cost containment, consumer awareness, and the competitive environment in the health care arena, the evolution of ambulatory surgery has become one of the most successful alternatives in the health care delivery system today. Health care professionals and patients alike praise the convenience, cost effectiveness, and quality of care provided in this setting.

Today's current health care system requires fewer patients to be admitted to the hospital prior to their scheduled day of surgery. Ambulatory surgery patients are admitted to the ambulatory surgery facility or designated hospital unit, have their surgery, and return home the same day, thereby eliminating the need for hospitalization. *Short-stay, in-and-out, same-day,* and *one-day surgery* are a few of the terms used to describe ambulatory surgery. Whatever the term, the concept remains the same: safe, convenient, and cost-effective surgery administered to basically stable, healthy individuals who will assume responsibility for postoperative self-care at home.

No textbook today on perioperative nursing would be complete without a chapter on ambulatory surgery. This alternative health care delivery system has progressed from a concept to a fully implemented program in many hospitals across the country. The number of hospital-based and freestanding facilities has increased significantly since the infancy stage of ambulatory surgery in the early 1970s. Statistics show that ambulatory surgery comprised 20% of all surgeries in 1983 compared with 44% of surgeries in 1987. By 1995 an average of 60% of hospital-based surgeries are predicted to be performed on an outpatient basis (AHA, 1989).

The concept of ambulatory surgery was not designed as a panacea. Certain procedures cannot be performed unless the patient is admitted to the hospital for further observation and treatment. However, many predictable, uncomplicated procedures can safely be performed on people who are basically healthy and stable and have few potentially incapacitating disease entities. Over the years the number of procedures being performed on an ambulatory basis has paralleled the growth of cost-containment efforts and advances in technology. Many of the surgical procedures described in the preceding chapters may be performed on an ambulatory basis. Although some patients are not truly "ambulatory," the majority have physical and emotional coping mechanisms that are strong and flexible.

Many new concepts and techniques have evolved to meet the challenges of ambulatory surgery. One of these is in the area of anesthesia, with the introduction of short-acting anesthetic agents. For ambulatory surgical procedures, various anesthetic techniques may be utilized. These include general and regional anesthesia, intravenous sedation, and the administration of unsupplemented local anesthetics. The choice of anesthesia is dependent on the condition of the patient, the operative procedure and its duration, and surgeon preference.

This chapter does not describe operative procedures because the standards and recommended practices that apply to perioperative nursing and the perioperative setting are applicable whether the patient is ambulatory or an inpatient. The reader is referred to the specialty chapters for procedure information and to appropriate chapters for anesthesia and the managerial and safety concepts of perioperative nursing. The history of ambulatory surgery, organizational structures, conceptual principles, and perioperative nursing in the ambulatory surgery setting are discussed in this chapter.

HISTORY

The concept of ambulatory surgery undoubtedly precedes recorded history. Outpatient surgery is interwoven with the history of medicine and nursing and is referred to in the Bible, in early Indian writings, and in Greek history and Egyptian scrolls. Houses and temples were sites for outpatient surgery in ancient Greece and Rome. Ambulatory surgery made great strides during times of war, simply because there was no alternative.

Church-sponsored hospitals provided both inpatient and outpatient care during the Middle Ages. The nineteenth century, the age of medical discovery, was the time of Vesalius, Harvey, Lister, Pasteur, Florence Nightingale, and other pioneers in health care and infection control. The discovery of anesthesia in 1846 heralded a new era of surgery.

In this country the Massachusetts General Hospital established an outpatient department in the early 1800s and

964

helped to initiate the ambulatory surgery concept. In the early 1900s outpatient procedures were being performed on children in Glasgow, Scotland. The Waters Anesthesia Clinic in Indianapolis (1919), the Cohen and Dillon UCLA OP Clinic (1966), and the "Come-and-Go" Surgery Unit at George Washington University in Washington, D.C. (1966) were a few of the early outpatient surgery departments. The Phoenix Surgicenter, founded in 1970 by Drs. Wallace Reed and John Ford, was the first independently owned and operated, freestanding center. This well-known facility continues to operate. It is a prototype for other centers and has originated many concepts and practices that influence the field of ambulatory surgery today.

The rebirth and substantial growth of ambulatory surgery in this country since 1970 can be attributed to:

1. Prohibitive costs of inpatient hospitalization
2. Growing climate of cost containment coupled with prudent use of resources
3. Legislative and public scrutiny of government health care spending, notably Medicare and Medicaid
4. Transformation of the reimbursement system with the introduction of the prospective payment system and contractual agreements with third-party payers
5. Technologic advances in surgical and diagnostic equipment
6. Improved anesthesia technology, including development and administration of new short-acting anesthetic agents
7. Public's increased awareness of health care needs and alternatives
8. Pronounced benefits of early postoperative ambulation
9. Proven advantages of ambulatory surgery over traditional inpatient surgery for appropriately selected patients
10. Enthusiastic, pronounced satisfaction of patients, families, professional health care personnel, and third-party payers

SETTINGS AND ORGANIZATIONAL STRUCTURES

The settings in which ambulatory surgery takes place are as varied as the patterns of ownership, control, and operation of outpatient facilities. An ambulatory surgery facility may function as a hospital-integrated, a hospital-affiliated, or an independently owned and operated unit. Whatever the structure, most facilities have an organizational scheme and ambience that distinguish them from inpatient facilities. Emphasis is placed on ease of access to the unit, attractive surroundings, comfort, convenience, and efficiency.

Hospital-integrated facility

Approximately 70% of outpatient surgery is performed in traditional hospital operating rooms in hospital-integrated facilities (Gruendemann, 1987). In such facilities outpatients are integrated into the flow of inpatients throughout all three phases of the perioperative experience. Scheduling of outpatients is usually done using the same protocols as for inpatients and may be done on a block-scheduling or time-available basis. Outpatient procedures may either be interspersed with inpatient procedures on any given day or done on a day reserved solely for outpatients. The admitting process for these patients may be handled by the hospital's admitting department or by the ambulatory unit itself. Some hospitals have distinct preoperative and postoperative areas that are specifically designated for outpatients while integrating the flow of inpatients and outpatients into common surgical suites. Hospitals may also utilize designated areas for admission of preoperative patients in the morning and as postoperative recovery areas in the afternoon, with a blend of preop and postop patients at midday. Family members of both inpatients and outpatients in a hospital-integrated unit usually share a common waiting area. In addition to outpatients, hospital-integrated facilities may also handle the processing of patients who are to be admitted to the hospital following surgery. These patients are referred to as *day of surgery* (DOS) patients. Instead of being admitted 1 to 2 days prior to surgery for preoperative laboratory and diagnostic tests, these patients have the necessary tests done on an outpatient basis or on the day of surgery and are admitted after surgery. It is done in an effort to decrease hospital costs to both patients and third-party payers. The length of stay in the hospital depends on the procedure and recovery time.

Hospital-affiliated facility

The hospital-affiliated unit is a separate ambulatory surgery department with designated preoperative, intraoperative, and postoperative areas. This facility may be located within the hospital complex, adjacent to the hospital, or at a satellite location some distance from the hospital but still under the auspices of the hospital. The term *dedicated* is used to differentiate ambulatory surgery units that have separate staff, equipment, and policies and procedures. The hospital-affiliated unit is physically and organizationally separate from the main hospital operating room suites and caters exclusively to the outpatient population.

Freestanding facility

The freestanding facility is independently owned and operated and is not affiliated with a hospital or medical center. Independently operated ambulatory surgery centers comprise a growing segment of the industry. Spurred by the success of the Phoenix Surgicenter, the freestanding, independently owned facilities have shown that ambulatory surgery need not be performed in the traditional hospital setting to be safe and efficient. This type of facility operates under several different types of ownership: corporate, joint venture, or independent. Physicians have generally owned and operated these facilities but an increasing trend has been for health care corporation chains to own and operate such facilities.

Physician's office

Some types of ambulatory surgery can safely and effectively be performed in a physician's office. Surgical procedures vary with the surgeon's specialty and are limited to those in which complex equipment, specially trained personnel, a large inventory of supplies and instrumentation, or additional resources from a hospital are not needed. This type of ambulatory surgery requires its own policies and procedures as well as quality assurance criteria and is not addressed in this text.

APPEAL OF AMBULATORY SURGERY

The growth of ambulatory surgery since its inception has been phenomenal. Today a majority of procedures that were once performed on an inpatient basis are done safely in the ambulatory surgery arena. Patients are generally low-risk, physical status I (healthy), physical status II (mild systemic disease), or physical status III (severe systemic disease that is not incapacitating) according to anesthesia classifications (Apfelbaum, 1988). These patients have accepted the responsibility of self-care postoperatively at home.

With safety, efficiency, and cost-effectiveness well established, third-party payers not only support but encourage the use of ambulatory surgery facilities by their subscribers. This encouragement takes the form of monetary incentives and higher reimbursements for procedures performed on an outpatient basis. Government agencies, especially those associated with Medicare and Medicaid, are actively involved in discussion and legislation relating to the balance between acceptable care and decreased cost. Ambulatory care is a focal point and a prime topic of consideration in the health care system today.

Ambulatory surgery is appealing to patients and families. Disruption of normal daily activities, separation from family, time away from the workplace, and worry about financial outlays are minimized. Patients become active participants in their plan of care both before and after surgery.

For professionals in medicine and nursing, the advantages of ambulatory surgery are clear. For the surgeon there is convenience and less time away from the office. For the anesthesiologist there is opportunity to enter into and specialize in a different arena, one in which anesthetic agents and administration techniques may be altered to fit outpatient care and in which the use of preoperative medications can be almost eliminated. For the perioperative nurse there are boundless opportunities to condense and refine traditional nursing skills and to develop a mind-set that is specifically tuned to wellness, safety, comfort, patient education, and continuity of care. The emphases

on professional nurse cross-training, productivity, versatility, and independence are appealing to a motivated nurse. Because an ambulatory surgery center uses fewer preoperative tests and drugs, patients are active, awake, and involved in the preoperative period. The chances for an expanded nursing role are numerous in this setting.

The advent of ambulatory surgery has caused a rethinking of many traditional beliefs and myths related to surgery. For example, we now know that patients can assume considerable responsibility for their own recuperation and do so with ease when properly instructed. We also know that, within the limits of certain strict criteria, patients recover best in the comfort of their homes, rather than in hospital beds with overnight stays. Moreover, we realize that early, assisted ambulation is beneficial rather than detrimental to a patient's health.

Ambulatory surgery facilities are small in comparison to the entire organizational structure and makeup of a hospital. This unique feature has been one of the many reasons for the overwhelming success and acceptance of the ambulatory surgery concept. When patients are selected according to specific established criteria and well prepared and informed about their impending surgical experience, and professionals are properly educated, ambulatory surgery becomes a satisfying, successful way of delivering high-quality patient care.

COMMON ELEMENTS OF SUCCESSFUL AMBULATORY SURGERY PROGRAMS

The ambulatory surgery setting and the nature of the patients themselves mandate a new look and a fresh attitude toward the alternative of surgery without overnight hospitalization. In the traditional medical model, outpatients are minor cases to be treated at the end of the day's schedule and are considered inconsequential in terms of complications and possible lengthy followups; these beliefs are of course untrue. At first glance it would seem that ambulatory surgery patients might be treated as second-class patients, requiring much less time and trouble than complex trauma patients or others who are undergoing complicated surgical procedures. This is indeed the case when ambulatory units are hastily planned and rapidly constructed or converted from other facilities for the sole purpose of becoming competitive with other ambulatory surgery centers in the community. Ambulatory surgery patients should receive the same quality of care as inpatients.

Successful surgery centers, whether operated independently or by a hospital, have introduced a new setting and environment for the care of selected surgical patients. Managers have planned and organized ambulatory surgery services that strike an optimal balance between safety and quality, compromising neither.

Practices and principles of successful ambulatory surgery programs and settings include the following:

1. Well-defined, written patient selection criteria
2. Consideration of ambulatory surgery patients as distinct and primary recipients of care that integrates wellness philosophies, teaching and learning concepts, and self-care responsibilities
3. Attractive units with ambience, comfort, color, peace, and quiet
4. Facilities that are easily accessible and convenient for patients, staff, and physicians.
5. Thorough preoperative preparation of patients by physicians and office staff, use of brochures, and telephone interveiws by perioperative nurses from the facility
6. Streamlined, convenient admission process
7. Flexibility in hours of operation and scheduling for the convenience of physicians and patients
8. Fee schedules that are available to physicians' offices and patients when requested
9. Only the necessary preoperative laboratory, electrocardiography, and x-ray testing is done, with reliance instead on clinical judgment and assessment of the patient's condition
10. Emphasis on selection of staff who display effective interpersonal communication skills, positive attitudes, and willingness to be cross-trained and who are results oriented
11. Professional nurses, physicians, and anesthesiologists who incorporate a collaborative team concept in the delivery of high-quality patient care and are oriented to outpatient care
12. Minimal paperwork, with only essential chart forms and documentation that address patient care and outcomes
13. Replacement of preoperative sedation with skillful nursing preparation of the patient and anesthesia techniques that lead to rapid, comfortable postoperative recovery
14. Acceptance of family members and support persons as active participants and an integral part of patient education, both preoperatively and postoperatively
15. Effective patient and family teaching methods
16. Policies and procedures that adhere to standards and recommended practices of the perioperative setting
17. Managers and leaders who are attuned to budgeting, efficient staffing, time management and productivity, credentialing processes, public relations, marketing, and role modeling in communications and patient care
18. High-quality continuing education programs for all staff members
19. Quality assurance programs that identify patient problems, nursing interventions, and expected patient outcomes
20. Evaluation tools that measure the quality of care given by the health care team

Standards and recommended practices for the perioperative setting are applicable in both the inpatient and outpatient setting. Ambulatory care must meet the same standards of quality that apply to inpatient care.

PERIOPERATIVE NURSING IN THE AMBULATORY SURGERY SETTING

Perioperative nursing in the ambulatory surgery setting incorporates all components of the nursing process. Instead of the entire process occurring over several days, the time span is shortened to 3 to 4 hours. Although the time is compressed, the process is not diminished. The nursing process has to be instituted prior to admission if possible and be continued through discharge. The plan of care for each individual must be organized and efficient. Documentation of care must reflect assessment of patient needs, plan of care for positive patient outcomes, implementation of nursing interventions, and evaluation of care given.

As a result of the increasing number of complex surgical procedures being done on an outpatient basis, ambulatory surgery centers are beginning to care for more acutely ill patients. This change challenges the perioperative nurse who once cared for generally low-risk patients to assess and care for patients with a higher acuity level.

The rapport between nurse, patient, and family must be established at the time of initial contact. Establishing an effective positive nurse-patient relationship is a key factor in fostering patient satisfaction. The nurse is the patient's advocate. Patients and family members are active participants in the surgical experience. The role of the family in both the preoperative and postoperative areas cannot be underestimated. The success of the ambulatory surgery center relies heavily on effective patient and family interaction throughout the perioperative period.

The perioperative nurse in the ambulatory surgery center assumes a teacher-practitioner role. Patient education is an integral part of ambulatory surgery and must be adjusted to the patient population. It should be a continuous process beginning preoperatively and proceeding through discharge. The provision of patient education and emotional support during the surgical experience ensures that the patient engages in safe self-care postoperatively at home.

The ambulatory surgery center setting provides the distinct advantage of cross-training nursing personnel to be competent in all three phases of the perioperative setting. Although the nurse may be highly skilled in only one of the three phases, he or she can learn key practices and skills of another area to the point of being a safe, competent practitioner. Cross-training in ambulatory surgery is the hallmark of flexibility in perioperative nursing.

Preoperative phase

The physician must first determine the appropriateness of performing the surgical procedure on an ambulatory basis for each individual patient. The patient must be informed that the time spent in the ambulatory surgery center will be short. Information detailing the features of the center, nature of the staff, and level of services offered are given to the patient prior to the scheduled day of surgery, either verbally or in an explanatory brochure (Fig. 28-1).

A perioperative nurse calls the patient 1 to 7 days before the day of surgery to verify the time and nature of the surgery, time of arrival at the center, any restrictions on oral intake of food and liquids, type of attire to wear on the day of surgery, location of facility and parking, and items to bring, such as glasses, contact lenses, hearing aids, and insurance papers. The patient is instructed to leave all valuables including money and jewelry at home and is asked to identify the person who will assume responsibility for driving the patient home. Patients are also informed that someone should remain with them for the first 24 hours after surgery. Information given and acquired is documented (Fig. 28-2). The patient is encouraged to read the brochure and preoperative instructions carefully (Fig. 28-3).

To aid the preoperative nursing and medical assessment, the patient may be asked a series of health questions that describe pertinent physical disabilities, previous surgeries and anesthetics with associated responses, and vital information such as height, weight, allergies, and current medications. This assessment may be completed in various manners: preoperative phone interview, at the time of admission to the unit, or via written questionnaire that is returned to the center by mail prior to admission (Fig. 28-4).

The admission and registration process takes place 1 to 2 hours before the scheduled time of surgery. When preadmission information has been obtained before the day of surgery, the interview is short and well organized. It is important that the facility's reception personnel project a positive image and be skillful, pleasant communicators (Fig. 28-5).

The first impression of the facility is lasting. The style, decor, ambience, color, physical arrangement, and traffic flow should be positive and bring to mind the comforts of home rather than giving the impression of confinement and austerity. Staff attitudes greatly influence the patient's degree of satisfaction.

Following correct identification of the patient and admission to the unit, the patient and family member should be given an orientation to the facility and expected sequence of events. The patient then changes into the appropriate surgical attire, and provisions are made for the safekeeping of clothing and any valuables the patient may have brought. Preoperative nursing care and responsibilities include the following:

- Observation and assessment of general physical and psychosocial behavior, sensory/perceptual alterations, emotional status, interaction with family, and compliance with instructions
- Recording of vital signs
- Verification of signed informed surgical consent and patient's knowledge of surgeon, procedure, and expected outcomes (informed consent is the responsibility of the surgeon)
- Obtaining appropriate laboratory tests and x-rays as ordered
- Verification of required chart contents to include recent history and physical, lab, and x-ray results
- Administration of medication if ordered (traditional preoperative medications are not routinely given)
- Insertion of intravenous lines (may be done by anesthesia personnel)

What is Outpatient Surgery?

Technical advances in surgery and anesthesiology now permit many surgical procedures which formerly required hospitalization to be routinely performed on an outpatient basis. Experts estimate that nearly 40% of all surgeries can be performed safely, conveniently and at much lower cost without an overnight stay. Some of these procedures are:

- Ear, nose and throat (removal of tonsils and adenoids, insertion of ear drainage tubes)
- Gynecology (laparoscopy, tubal ligation, diagnostic D & C)
- Orthopedics (arthroscopy, fracture repair, tendon repair)
- Oral surgery (wisdom teeth extraction, dental restoration)
- General surgery (hernia repair, biopsy, removal of lesions and cysts)
- Plastic surgery (face lifts, rhinoplasty, eyelid surgery, breast augmentation)
- Urology (cystoscopy, vasectomy, circumcision)
- Ophthalmology (removal of cataracts, lens implants)
- Neurology (hand surgery, nerve repair)

Fig. 28-1. Information about ambulatory surgery can be disseminated to patients by use of brochures. (Courtesy Mountain States Surgery Center, Boise, Idaho.)

- Concise and complete documentation of observations and care given
- Frequent interaction with family or support person

Family members or support persons should be permitted to stay with the patient in the preoperative area, and provision made for their comfort (Fig. 28-6). Ambulatory surgery nurses should accept these people as integral to the patient's well-being. Colorful surroundings, such as wall or ceiling murals, promote relaxation of patients before surgery. Maintaining privacy and confidentiality is of utmost importance throughout the patient's stay. A perioperative nurse is in constant attendance in the preoperative area and may assist the surgeon and/or anethesiologist during examination of the patient.

When the equipment, supplies, and instrumentation for the procedure are ready and the surgeon has arrived, the patient may be transported to the surgical suite by several means: ambulatory, wheelchair, or stretcher. The mode of transportation depends on the patient's abilities, the effects of any medication given, and the policies of the facility.

Family members are directed to the waiting room, informed approximately how long the procedure will take, and made comfortable with coffee, soft drinks, snacks, magazines, or health information reading materials.

Intraoperative phase

Intraoperative nursing care of an ambulatory surgery patient is consistent with the standards and recommended practices utilized for an inpatient. Nursing care and responsibilities include the following:

- Identifying the patient, introducing self, and reviewing chart contents
- Assisting in transferring the patient to the operating room bed, properly positioning, and maintaining correct body alignment of patient
- Assisting anesthesiologist during induction
- Performing the same scrub and circulating nurse functions as in the inpatient setting
- Monitoring safety precautions and aseptic practices
- Completely and concisely documenting on the patient record

Text continued on page 973.

Within a few hours following outpatient surgery, patients are able to go home to recuperate, avoiding the unnecessary expense of hospital room and board.

How does a Surgery Center differ from a hospital?

Both hospitals and freestanding surgery centers offer outpatient surgery services. However, hospitals must have the staff, equipment and protocols necessary to manage a broad and complex range of surgeries. This complexity is unnecessary for outpatient surgery, and can compromise convenience and cost effectiveness.

The Mountain States Surgery Center was designed, equipped, and staffed exclusively for outpatient surgery. Although MSSC contains fully equipped operating suites and recovery rooms that meet the most stringent standards, the warmer, more relaxed atmosphere makes the surgical experience less frightening, particularly for our very young patients. Our commitment to personalized care also helps minimize the anxiety often associated with surgery.

Your comfort and convenience are important to us. MSSC is located in the new St. Luke's Medical Office Plaza which features covered parking for more than 100 cars. Admitting and laboratory procedures can often be completed the day of surgery, eliminating additional trips.

Individualized attention and sunny, comfortable patient areas help make your stay as pleasant as possible while your family relaxes in the spacious lobby.

Certainly, cost reduction is of critical importance. Because MSSC specializes exclusively in outpatient surgery, costs are far less than for comparable hospital inpatient surgery.

As different as MSSC is from a hospital, there are important similarities. Your surgeon is supported by a physician anesthesiologist and a skilled team of registered nurses and technicians specially trained in surgical and recovery care. Facilities and equipment meet the highest hospital standards.

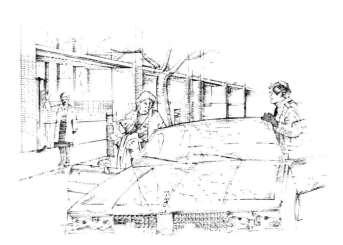

Fig. 28-1, cont'd. For legend see opposite page.

PREOPERATIVE CALLS

Date call made_____ Surgery date_____

Patient_____ Age _____ Phone _____

Person spoken to _____ Phone _____

Surgeon _____ Anesthetic _____ Procedure time _____

Procedure _____

MSSC brochure received?_____ (Instructions to patient: Read carefully, complete forms.
Bring name, address, phone number of insurance, name of policy holder, policy number,
and/or group number. We would like to have a deposit at admission to cover the amount
insurance will not pay.)

Tests ordered _____ Completed _____

Current health problems? _____

_____ Pregnant? _____

Reinforce knowledge of: NPO, shower, no jewelry, valuables, glasses, contact lenses;
limit number of people accompanying patient; apparel; parking area.

Person to transport_____ Responsible person _____

Arrival time _____

If child: stuffed animal or blanket? _____

Comments _____

_____ Signed _____RN

POSTOPERATIVE CALLS

Person spoken to _____ Call made date _____

Level of discomfort _____ Not reached _____

Any postoperative problems? _____

Action taken? _____

Activity tolerated at home _____

Home care instructions adequate? _____

General comments (include "care you received here"). _____

_____

_____

_____ Signed _____RN

Fig. 28-2. Form for documentation of preoperative and postoperative telephone calls by perioperative
nurse. (Courtesy Mountain States Surgery Center, Boise, Idaho.)

Ambulatory Surgery Centers

Grant Medical Center's Ambulatory Surgery Centers serve those patients who need surgery but do not require overnight hospitalization.

This allows you to have surgery in comfortable, safe, sterile surroundings, and to return home the same day of the surgery.

The Ambulatory Surgery Centers provide you the finest care at a low cost. Costs are kept to a minimum because you will not be required to stay overnight in the hospital.

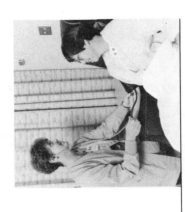

Outpatient Surgery

Grant Medical Center

Pre-Surgery Instructions

For your safety and comfort, you must follow these instructions:

- Eat only a light meal at dinner the night before your surgery.
- Do not drink any alcoholic beverages during the 24 hours before your surgery.
- Do not eat or drink anything, not even water or gum, after 12 midnight the night before surgery. It is important that your stomach be empty when your surgery is performed. If not, your surgery may be cancelled.
- Brush your teeth without swallowing.
- Wear as little jewelry as possible; all jewelry must be removed before going to the operating room.
- Wear little or no make-up. The doctors must be able to see your true color.
- Remove all nail polish before coming to the center.
- Bring the cases in which you place your eye glasses or contact lenses. Storing lenses in their case will help prevent their loss.
- Wear casual, comfortable, loose-fitting clothing.
- Remove your dentures before surgery. They will be placed in a denture cup and returned to you after surgery. Should you have a partial plate denture, please leave it at home.
- Bring to the hospital all medications that you currently take.
- Your physician will notify you of any other special instructions.

Center Facts

Location: Grant Medical Center has two Ambulatory Surgery Centers: one is located on the third floor of the main hospital; the other is located on the second floor of the Grant Eye & Ear Hospital.

To get to the main hospital's Ambulatory Surgery Center, enter the hospital at the corner of State Street and Grant Avenue. From the main lobby, take the elevator to the third floor. When you get off the elevator, please sign in and take a seat in the waiting area.

To get to the Grant Eye & Ear Hospital's Ambulatory Surgery Center, enter through the lobby at 323 East Town Street, take the elevator to the second floor, and follow the signs to the center.

Parking: Parking is available in the garage at 111 South Grant Avenue for the main hospital's Ambulatory Surgery Center and in the garage at 393 East Town Street for the Grant Eye and Ear Hospital's Ambulatory Surgery Center.

Your companion may drop you off at the appropriate hospital entrance before going to the parking garage.

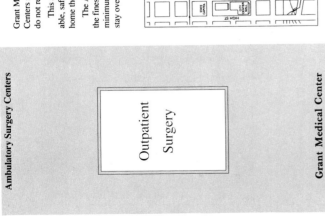

Scheduling

Your physician will schedule your surgery for you. A Grant Medical Center "liaison nurse" will contact you one to two days before your surgery. The nurse will confirm the date and time of arrival for your surgery and ask for necessary pre-admission information.

Pre-Admission Tests

Unless your physician requests pre-admission testing, any testing or lab work will be done at the Ambulatory Surgery Center on the day of your surgery.

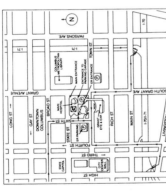

Day of Surgery

Please note: Outpatient surgery patients will not be permitted to leave the hospital unaccompanied.

Surgery will be cancelled for patients who have not made arrangements to be accompanied home before being admitted to the center.

Upon arriving at Grant Medical Center or Grant Eye & Ear Hospital, go to the Ambulatory Surgery Center. You will be greeted at the reception desk, and asked to verify pre-admission information.

All patients will be asked to sign a consent form when admitted to the center. When surgery is to be performed on a minor, the consent form must be signed by a parent or legal guardian who is present at the time of admission.

A waiting area is available for your escort, should he or she wish to wait. Your escort may also arrange to pick you up following the operation. If your escort chooses this option, they must leave a telephone number with the liaison nurse where they may be reached.

Before Surgery

- You will be given a hospital gown, robe, and slippers. A locker will be provided for your clothes and personal belongings.
- You will be taken to the operating room in a wheelchair or on a stretcher.

Anesthesia: Decisions about the choice of anesthesia will be made together with your surgeon.

"Local" anesthesia involves only the area of the body on which the surgery is to be performed. It will be administered by your surgeon.

"General" anesthesia is the type in which you will go to sleep. It is administered by physician specialists called "anesthesiologists." If you are having general anesthesia, you will be seen by an anesthesiologist before surgery.

After Surgery

Following your surgery, you will be returned to the Ambulatory Surgery Center if you had local anesthesia; or to the Post Anesthesia Care Unit for a period of time before returning to Ambulatory Surgery Center if you had general anesthesia. At both places, you will be closely observed by specially trained nurses.

You will receive written instructions about what to expect after surgery, such as information about when you should be able to stand up and move around. You will also receive specific instructions for your care after the operation.

Following your brief recovery period in the Ambulatory Surgery Center, and when your vital signs are stable, you will be discharged by your escort(s).

Remember, it is normal to feel a little dizzy or drowsy for several hours after your surgery. This is due to the action of the medicine used during anesthesia.

Therefore, you should not drive, operate any equipment, sign important papers, or make any

significant decisions during the first 24 hours after your surgery. Please arrange for a responsible adult to stay with you following surgery.

Post-Surgery Diet

Your surgeon will tell you about specific diet restrictions if necessary. If you have tolerated liquids well, you may gradually and slowly add other foods to your diet, until you are back on your normal diet.

Fig. 28-3. Explanatory brochure given to patient prior to admission, detailing preoperative instructions. (Courtesy Grant Medical Center, Columbus, Ohio.)

MOUNTAIN STATES SURGERY CENTER

Health History of			Date
YES	**NO**		
		1. Have you had surgery before? If yes, list operations and dates.	
		2. Did you have any problems with anesthesia? If yes, please explain.	
		3. Has any relative had problems with anesthesia? If yes, please explain.	
		4. Do you take any medication? If yes, what do you take and how often?	
		5. Are you allergic to anything? If yes, please list your allergies.	
		6. Have you ever had any problem with your blood pressure? If yes, please explain.	
		7. Have you ever had a heart murmur?	
		8. Does your heart ever skip beats, or beat irregularly?	
		9. Have you ever had angina, chest pain?	
		10. Do you get short of breath doing normal things?	
		11. Do you smoke? If yes, how much do you smoke?	
		12. If you don't smoke, have you ever smoked? When did you stop?	
		13. Have you had any wheezing, asthma, bronchitis, emphysema?	
		14. Do you have a cough? If yes, what do you cough up and how much do you cough up?	
		15. Have you had a cold, sore throat or the flu in the past two weeks?	
		16. Have you ever had tuberculosis?	
		17. Have you ever had any liver problems such as hepatitis, yellow jaundice or cirrhosis?	
		18. Have you ever had kidney problems such as blood in the urine, kidney stones, nephritis?	
		19. Are you a diabetic? If yes, list treatment.	
		20. Have you had any thyroid problems?	
		21. Have you had any nervous system problems such as seizures, unusual headaches, dizziness, blackout spells, stroke, paralysis, numbness? If yes, please explain.	
		22. Do you have any bleeding tendencies or problems such as anemia or blood disease?	
		23. Have you ever had thrombophlebitis (blood clots in the legs)?	
		24. Do you have any loose teeth, false teeth or caps? If yes, which ones?	
		25. Are you wearing contact lenses?	
		26. What is your height? Weight?	
		27. What was the date of your last menstrual period?	

Patient Signature

X

Examination By Anesthesiologist

Anesthesiologist Signature

X

Fig. 28-4. Health history, completed by patient before admission to ambulatory surgery unit. (Courtesy Mountain States Surgery Center, Boise, Idaho.)

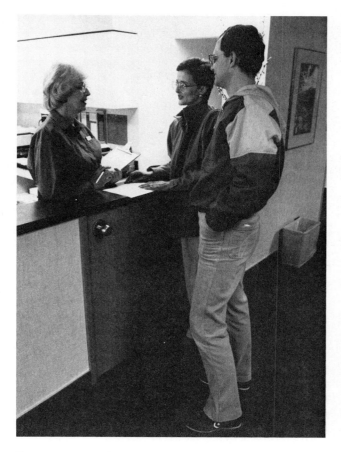

Fig. 28-5. Patient's first impression of ambulatory surgery facility is gained from initial contact with reception and admitting personnel.

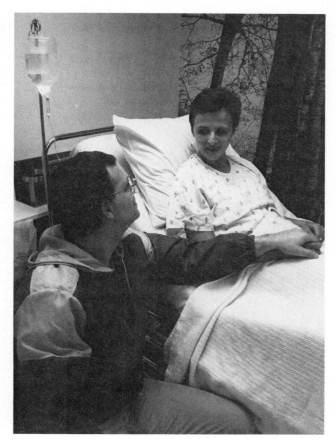

Fig. 28-6. Family and support people are integral part of preoperative area.

If the procedure is performed with either unsupplemented local anesthesia or surgeon-administered sedation, the circulating nurse is responsible for monitoring the patient throughout the procedure. The patient's vital signs are monitored by use of electrocardiogram, pulse oximetry, and noninvasive blood pressure monitor, as well as by general observation. The nurse must be familiar with the various types of monitoring equipment and have a basic understanding of normal and abnormal cardiac rhythms. Because of the constant monitoring the nurse must do throughout the procedure, a second circulator should be assigned to the room. This person is then responsible for anticipating and meeting the needs of the surgical team. The nurse monitoring the patient must not be expected to assume other circulating duties. Instead, the nurse must remain with the patient, be alert to changes in the patient's condition, and be ready to respond appropriately. Throughout the procedure the patient is made comfortable with pillows, supports, audiotapes, and explanations by the registered nurse.

After completion of the surgical procedure, the patient is transferred to the postanesthesia care unit (PACU) when general, regional, or supplemented local anesthesia has

been administered. A complete report on the status of the patient, procedure performed, medications given, dressings, and any allergies is given to the PACU nurse by the operating room circulating and/or monitoring nurse or anesthesiologist. The patient who required only unsupplemented local anesthesia may be transferred directly back to the ambulatory unit.

Postoperative phase

Ambulatory surgery is usually followed by a rapid recovery phase, especially if the patient has not been sedated preoperatively. Postoperative nursing care and responsibilities include the following:

- Assessment of patent airway, vital signs, potential for fluid volume deficit, wound dressings, and altered comfort states
- Knowledge of appropriate and prescribed actions for deviations from the norm
- Knowledge of effects of anesthesia and drugs commonly used intraoperatively
- Active encouragement of early ambulation and progressive fluid ingestion

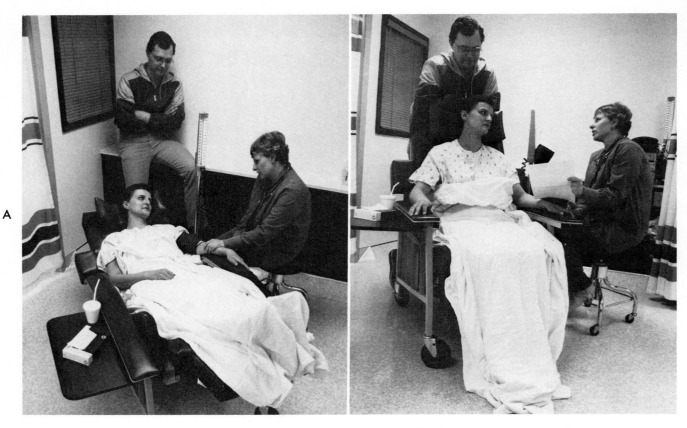

Fig. 28-7. After short recovery period in bed, patient is assisted to recliner by recovery area nurse. Recliner can be adjusted to several positions from **A,** reclining to **B,** upright.

- Patient and family education related to home care instructions
- Concise and complete documentation of care given and progress of patient
- Discharge of patient according to preestablished criteria

After phase one emergence from anesthesia, the patient is assisted to an upright position for phase two recovery. Recliner chairs that can be adjusted to several positions are often used in phase two (Fig. 28-7). Some ambulatory surgery units may have distinct, physically separate phase one and phase two recovery areas. Depending on the type of anesthesia administered, the patient may be taken directly from the operating room to a phase two recovery area. For patients who have received only unsupplemented local anesthesia, the phase two recovery area may be used as a place to take postoperative vital signs, review postoperative and home care instructions, and change from surgical attire to street clothes.

The patient is usually discharged 1 to 3 hours after the procedure when established criteria have been met. Written and verbal instructions for home care (Fig. 28-8) are given

to the patient and family member. A responsible adult must accompany the discharged patient who has received any anesthesia other than an unsupplemented local; the patient is instructed not to drive, sign any important legal papers, or make any important decisions for at least 24 hours.

Patients should be informed that their recovery and convalescence are not complete upon discharge. Most patients do not feel "normal" for at least a day following general anesthesia and should not plan to resume their usual activities when discharged. Safe recuperation can continue at home in familiar surroundings.

Upon discharge from the facility, the patient may be provided with a questionnaire that is to be returned via mail. This questionnaire provides the facility feedback about its services, any postoperative complications the patient may experience, and any additional comments or suggestions from the patient. It is an excellent way to measure the quality of services provided by the facility. In addition a perioperative nurse calls the patient at home 1 to 7 days after the surgery to evaluate recovery and general condition. For problems related to the surgical procedure, the patient is advised to consult the surgeon. The telephone call is important to determine patient satisfaction and effectiveness of care.

ARTHROSCOPY

G R A N T   H O S P I T A L
HOME CARE INSTRUCTIONS

The following instructions have been prepared to help you care for yourself, or be cared for, upon your return home today. These are guidelines for the immediate post-surgery period.

Medications

———— No medications, including nonprescription medications, unless ordered by the surgeon for twenty-four (24) hours.

———— Resume own medications.

Wound Care and Hygiene

———— Apply ice pack to knee the first twenty-four (24) hours while awake.

———— You may remove the pressure dressing after forty-eight (48) hours and apply bandaids to wounds.

———— You may shower or bathe after forty-eight (48) hours.

Activity

———— Limited activity for two (2) days, then resume activity as tolerated, keep the knee elevated as often as possible.

———— You may use crutches or a walker for several days, if you need them for comfort.

———— May return to school/work on ——————————————————————

Diet

———— Drink liquids and eat a light meal on the day of surgery, resume regular diet tomorrow.

———— Regular diet.

Anesthesia Precautions

———— No special precautions.

———— Do not operate a vehicle (automobile, bicycle, motorcycle), machinery, or power tools, make any important decisions or drink alcoholic beverages for twenty-four (24) hours.

———— Arrange for a responsible adult to remain with you for twenty-four (24) hours. You may be drowsy and lightheaded.

Expectations of Surgery

———— Mild pain.

Call your doctor for

———— Temperature above 100 degrees.

———— Severe pain or swelling.

———— Bleeding through bandage.

Additional Instructions ——————————————————————

——————————————————————

Call your doctor's office for an appointment on ——————————————

Physician's signature: ————————————————————————

Office ————————————————— Home —————————————

I have received and understand the above instructions ————————————
(Patient, Parent or Guardian)

Ambulatory Surgery Center Nurse's Signature ——————————————

Ambulatory Surgery Center Number ——————————————————

Addressograph

Fig. 28-8. Home care instructions. Patient signs the form to indicate that the instructions have been received and understood. A copy is given to the patient and the carbon copy becomes a permanent part of the medical record. (Courtesy Grant Medical Center, Columbus, Ohio.)

CONTINUING EDUCATION

Continuing education and staff development for all staff members must be relevant, ongoing, and documented. Staff should annually attend educational programs on CPR, fire and safety, and infection-control practices. Other educational opportunities may include programs related to the latest in technologic advances, new procedures, updated standards and recommended practices, and quality assurance activities. Observation and assessment skills are paramount in ambulatory surgery nursing and should be updated periodically.

Quality assurance in conjunction with continuing education assures high-quality patient care. Standards utilized in quality assurance activities include structure standards (how the unit is managed), process standards (what the nurse does for the patient), and outcome standards (what the patient can expect from the care given). The unit's quality assurance program must identify the scope of service provided by the unit as well as important aspects of care. For effective monitoring and evaluation of care given, quality assurance activities must identify indicators that will monitor the important aspects of care. Quality assurance activities are an important part of the care delivered in the ambulatory surgery setting.

DOCUMENTATION

Principles of documentation along with legal considerations guide the manager and staff of an ambulatory surgery unit in developing or refining patient record forms. At a minimum the patient record should contain the following:

1. Face sheet (demographics and insurance information)
2. Consent for treatment and surgical procedure
3. History and physical examination reports
4. Health history
5. Laboratory test results
6. Preoperative and postoperative instruction sheets
7. Preoperative nursing assessment flow sheet (Fig. 28-9)
8. Physician's order sheet
9. Anesthesia record
10. Intraoperative record
11. Postoperative record
12. Report of operation
13. Pathology report

All forms are reviewed periodically and revised as needed. Efficiency and conciseness, often stated as advantages of ambulatory surgery, must be reflected in the amount and quality of required documentation. Medical record dictums, accreditation standards, regulations, hospital policies, and physician requests are all considered in a policy for documentation.

Criteria for documentation include legal and professional considerations and standards, validation of the level of medical and nursing care provided, degree of teaching and learning, and policies of the institution. Charting should be concise and appropriate.

POLICIES AND PROCEDURES

Policies and procedures for an ambulatory surgery program or facility are developed according to the principles described in Chapter 2. Policies may differ in form and content from institutional hospital regulations. Variations also occur from one ambulatory surgery setting to another according to governing body, ownership, medical staff, accrediting and licensing bodies, and management.

Policies and procedures for ambulatory surgery may include statements of or information on the following:

1. Philosophy and mission statement
2. Goals for patient care
3. Scope of service
4. Anesthesia guidelines
5. Medical staff privileges and bylaws
6. Patient appointment system
7. Medical records
8. Patient selection criteria
9. Types of elective procedures
10. Regulations concerning unemancipated minor patients
11. Location, storage, and procurement of medications, supplies, and equipment
12. Responsibility for maintaining integrity of emergency drug supply
13. Means of securing assistance in an emergency
14. Cancellation policy
15. Operational hours
16. Surgical authorization
17. History, physical and preoperative lab studies, and any additional preoperative requirements
18. Preoperative patient education
19. Preoperative and postoperative transportation
20. Preoperative assessment
21. Preoperative telephone interview with patient
22. Handling and safekeeping of patient valuables
23. Infection control measures
24. Traffic control
25. Aseptic practices
26. Registered nurse as circulator
27. Monitoring of patients receiving local anesthesia
28. Sponge, sharp, and needle counts
29. Discharge criteria
30. Postoperative followup of patient
31. Admission of patient to hospital
32. Safety practices
33. Disaster plans
34. Quality assurance

GSH
THE GOOD SAMARITAN HOSPITAL
4TH & WALNUT STS.
LEBANON, PA 17042

The
Hyman S. Caplan
Pavilion GSH
THE GOOD SAMARITAN HOSPITAL

AMBULATORY PROCEDURE UNIT
PREOPERATIVE FLOW SHEET

SCHEDULED FOR: GENERAL ☐   LOCAL PLUS ☐
BLOCK ☐   LOCAL ☐   OTHER ☐

DIAGNOSIS:
SCHEDULED SURGERY

O.R. CHECKLIST	YES	NO	N/A
History & Physical On Chart			
Permit Signed			
CBC/U/A on Chart			
Chest X-Ray Report on Chart			
EKG on Chart			
Anes. Questionnaire on Chart			
Name Band - Arm/Leg R or L			
Dentures Out			
Jewelry/Hairpins - Off			
Voided Pre-Op			
Pre-Op Given			
Other Labs			
Other:			

DATE ___ ARRIVAL TIME: ___   AMBULATORY ☐ WHEELCHAIR ☐ STRETCHER ☐

ACCOMPANIED BY: ___   CALL FOR RIDE: YES ☐ NO ☐

DRIVER: (SAME ☐)   PHONE

HEIGHT: ___   WEIGHT: ___   NPO SINCE: ___

ADMITTING VS.: T _____ P _____ R _____ BP _____

SORE THROAT: YES ☐ NO ☐   COLD: YES ☐ NO ☐   FAMILY DOCTOR: ___
CONGESTION: YES ☐ NO ☐   COUGH: YES ☐ NO ☐

HISTORY OF PROBLEMS

HEART	YES ☐ NO ☐	KIDNEY	YES ☐ NO ☐
BP	YES ☐ NO ☐	HEPATITIS	YES ☐ NO ☐
LUNG:	YES ☐ NO ☐	GALL BLADDER	YES ☐ NO ☐
SEIZURES:	YES ☐ NO ☐	DIABETIC	YES ☐ NO ☐

OTHER: YES ☐ EXPLAIN

INITIALS ___   INITIALS ___

MEDICATIONS

TIME ORDER COMPLETED	ORDERS/MEDS/TREATMENTS
	IF DIABETIC: CHEMSTRIP ☐ FBS ☐
	RESULTS:
	IV ORDERED: YES ☐ NO ☐
	IF YES: SOLUTION/AMT.:
	SITE:
	CATH. SIZE: TIME:
	SIGNATURE:

ALLERGIES:

TIME	NURSES NOTES PLEASE SIGN ALL ENTRIES	

PREOP TEACHING DONE   YES ☐ NO ☐
SIDE RAILS UP POST MEDICATION   YES ☐ NO ☐ NA ☐
INSTRUCTED TO CALL FOR NURSE: YES ☐ NO ☐

VITAL SIGNS

TIME	T	P	R	BP	INITIALS	FULL SIGNATURES OF R.N. INITIALS

TIME TO O.R. ___   APU
R.N. SIGNATURE ___

Fig. 28-9. Preoperative nursing assessment and documentation form. (Courtesy The Good Samaritan Hospital, Lebanon, Pennsylvania.)

35. Departmental orientation
36. Continuing education

SUMMARY

Perioperative nursing care is the most constant and pervasive part of ambulatory surgical services. Nursing in the ambulatory setting demands judgmental and clinical skills. Nursing care that was formerly spread over a period of several days now is done in a few hours. Patient education takes on supreme importance.

Many surgical procedures can be done on an outpatient basis, in a nonaustere operating room setting, with selected patients. Patients benefit by having minimal separation from significant others and the home, and little disruption of daily living and job responsibilities.

The success of ambulatory surgery has dispelled several myths: (1) that an overnight hospital stay for postoperative observation and pain relief is necessary for every surgical patient, (2) that it is dangerous to administer general anesthesia and to intubate a patient in a setting other than a traditional inpatient operating room, (3) that all surgical patients must receive preoperative medications to reduce anxiety and dry secretions, (4) that patients must be taken to and from an operating room on a stretcher with the side rails up, (5) that family members should be allowed in the PACU only when the patient is fully awake and free of nausea and discomfort, (6) that parents are too emotionally involved with their children to be relied on to follow postoperative instructions or observe for complications, and (7) that most postoperative instructions are not followed because they are too complicated to be understood by patients and family members.

Many myths and ritualistic practices accompanying surgery have been discarded because of the acceptance and practices of ambulatory surgery. As innovative ways to provide low-cost, high-quality health care are expanded, ambulatory surgery will continue to be one of the most valuable and successful.

REFERENCES

AHA predicts ambulatory surgery will be 60% of all operations, Same Day Surgery, 13:71, 1989.

Apfelbaum, J.L.: Anesthesiologist's role in SDS changes to primary caretaker, Same Day Surgery, 12:5, 1988.

Gruendemann, B.J.: Ambulatory surgery: impact on nursing. In Association of Operating Room Nurses: Ambulatory Surgery Anthology, Denver, 1987, The Association.

BIBLIOGRAPHY

Ambulatory surgery and patient attire, AORN J. 41:1018, 1985.

Association of Operating Room Nurses: AORN standards and recommended practices for perioperative nursing, Denver, 1990, The Association.

Becker, A.: Same day surgery, a psychological approach, Todays OR Nurse 5:8, 1983.

Berkowitz, E.: Marketing gives ambulatory surgery units competitive edge, Same Day Surgery 6:13, 1982.

Brandon, J., and Radoszewski, P.H.: Ambulatory surgery centers must compete for customers—both patients and physicians, AORN J. 39:1036, 1984.

Burns, L.A.: Ambulatory surgery, developing and managing successful programs, Rockville, Md., 1984, Aspen Systems.

Curtin, L.L.: Ambulatory surgery: organization, finance, and regulation, Nurs. Management 15:22, 1984.

Curtin, L.L.: Packaging the professional for success (editorial opinion), Nurs. Management 16:7, 1985.

Curtin, L.L.: Survival of the slickest (editorial opinion), Nurs. Management 16:7, 1985.

Dean, A.F.: Free-standing surgery: what's in it for you, Todays OR Nurse 7:32, 1985.

Detmer, D.E.: Sounding board: ambulatory surgery, N. Engl. J. Med. 305:1406, 1981.

Earnhart, S.W.: Alternative solutions for common ambulatory surgery problems, AORN J. 45:30, 1987.

Edwards, B.J.: Insurer's policies for reimbursement boost day surgery, AORN J. 38:582, 1983.

Evolving patient education methods must reach changing population, Same Day Surgery 13:78, 1989.

Franz, J.: Challenge for nursing: hiking productivity without lowering quality of care, Mod. Healthcare 14:60, 1984.

Garlington, D.: How to turn down time into productive time in your OR, Hosp. Topics 62:4, 1984.

Gilbert, R.N.: Competition spurs ambulatory choice, Hospitals 57:67, 1983.

Gruendemann, B.J.: Dare to excel in ambulatory surgery (guest editorial), AORN J. 41:330, 1985.

Hoffman, G.L.: Quality control in ambulatory surgery, Bull. Am. Coll. Surg. 66:6, 1981.

House, M.W., and Wilkins, G.K.: A forward movement in medicine—ambulatory care, Nurs. Management 20:88Q, 1989.

Icenhour, M.L.: Quality interpersonal care: a study of ambulatory surgery patients' perspectives, AORN J. 47:1414, 1988.

Jackowitz, D.S., and Caron, J.P.: A price methodology for maintaining hospital outpatient surgery services in a competitive environment, J. Amb. Care Management 7:40, 1984.

Joel, L.A.: DRGs and RIMs: implications for nursing, Nurs. Outlook 32:42, 1984.

Johnson, S.: Preoperative teaching: a need for change, Nurs. Management 20:80B, 1989.

Kasdan, A.S., Kasdan, M.L., and Janes, C.: Taking the extra step: the nursing role in same day surgery, Todays OR Nurse 6:18, 1984.

Kempe, A.R.: Patient education for the ambulatory surgery patient, AORN J. 45:500, 1987.

Kuperwasser, B., and Dierckman, D.: Quality assurance in ambulatory surgery: "how to do it," Nurs. Management 19:72A, 1988.

McNeal, P., and Duncan, M.L.: Assessing patients in the holding area, Todays OR Nurse 7:16, 1985.

Mathias, J.M.: Ambulatory surgery meeting stresses quality of care, AORN J. 45:1191, 1987.

Mauldin, B.C., editor: Ambulatory surgery: a guide to perioperative nursing care, New York, 1983, Grune & Stratton.

Noon, B.E., and Davero, C.C.: Patient satisfaction in a hospital-based surgery setting, AORN J. 46:306, 1987.

Nursing specialty touted for ambulatory surgery, Hospitals 59:58, 1985.

O'Donovan, T.R.: Hospital ambulatory surgery units, Int. Anesth. Clin. 20:125, 1982.

Palmer, P.N.: Ambulatory surgery means business, AORN J. 38:470, 1983.

Poland, V.: Strategies for ambulatory surgery, AORN J. 39:1245, 1984.

Radoszewski, P.H.: Hospital-based outpatient surgery: planning the facility, AORN J. 47:746, 1988.

Radoszewski, P.H.: Strategies to meet increased competition for out-patients, AORN J. 42:666, 1985.

Radoszewski, P.H., and Brandon, J.A.: The ambulatory surgery center nurse, Nurs. Management 17:34J, 1986.

Roth, R.A.: Nursing interventions in an ambulatory surgery unit. Operating Room Nursing Forum, 1:2, 1987.

Roth, R.A., and Gruendemann, B.J.: Use of recommended practices, applications in ambulatory surgery, AORN J. 43:991, 1986.

Same-day surgery conference updates participants on legislation, risk management, accreditation, marketing, AORN J. 45:1461, 1987.

Shibe, J.: Justifying RNs in the OR, Todays OR Nurse 6:33, 1984.

Wetchler, B.V.: Ambulatory surgery: the future is now. In Association of Operating Room Nurses: Ambulatory Surgery Anthology, Denver, 1987, The Association.

Wetchler, B.V.: Patient selection criteria for 1987, AORN J. 45:30, 1987.

Wetchler, B.V.: Postanesthesia scoring system, AORN J. 41:382, 1985.

Wong, K.C., and Pace, N.L.: Ambulatory surgery and the basics of emergency surgical care, ed. 5, Philadelphia, 1981, J.B. Lippincott.

29 Pediatric surgery

JUDITH J. STELLAR

The highly specialized field of pediatric surgery began its dramatic development in the first half of this century. Prior to this, little distinction was made between the surgical treatment of children and that of adults. Pediatric surgery is now recognized as a separate subspecialty of surgery with board certification status.

The successful and rapid advancements in pediatric surgery can be attributed to the following:

1. Improved diagnostic procedures and techniques
2. A better understanding of physiologic, psychologic, and sociologic problems affecting infants, small children, preteeners, and adolescents
3. Improved knowledge about fluid and electrolyte balance, pharmacology, and nutrition and their effects on various pediatric age groups
4. Increased knowledge about the cause and physiology of congenital malformations
5. Improved anesthetic agents and techniques, along with better understanding of their effects on pediatric patients
6. Improved surgical techniques with more appropriate instrumentation and support equipment
7. Implementation of more effective medical and nursing care before, during, and after surgery

The development of high-risk pregnancy centers for mothers with problem pregnancies has resulted in earlier detection of malformations in fetuses as well as of other problems. Earlier detection has led to development of lifesaving operative procedures that can be performed in utero or immediately after delivery.

Pediatric patients are classified according to the following age groups in most hospitals:

1. Premature infant: less than 37 weeks of gestation
2. Neonate, or newborn: birth to 1 month of age; however, a premature infant may remain in this category until about 3 months of age
3. Infant: up to 1 year of age
4. Toddler: 1 to 3 years of age
5. Preschooler: 3 to 6 years of age
6. School-aged child: 6 to 11 years of age
7. Adolescent: 11 to 18 years of age; many hospitals consider 16 years as the upper age limit, with patients over this age considered as adults

Pediatric patients may also be hospitalized in mixed age units or according to clinical specialty.

PERIOPERATIVE NURSING CONSIDERATIONS
Assessment/nursing diagnosis

The nursing process is the basis for perioperative nursing care of pediatric patients.

The perioperative assessment is the first phase of the nursing process. The goal of a comprehensive nursing assessment is to gather sufficient data to formulate nursing diagnoses from which care is planned, implemented, and evaluated. The unique aspects of care of the pediatric surgical patient center on the fact that the child is a growing organism. Normally, infants and children have higher metabolic rates and different physiologic makeup than those of adults. Their oxygen, fluid, and caloric requirements are greater; add to these the stress of illness and/or surgery, and these requirements climb even higher. The perioperative nurse first must have a good understanding of the normal physical and psychologic parameters for pediatric patients. Then, the nurse will be able to recognize deviations from these parameters. In addition, the nurse must be familiar with normals for each age group. During any given day the perioperative nurse may care for all age groups of children—neonates through adolescents.

The preoperative visit is the first step in assessment. For children undergoing a procedure as ambulatory patients, the child and family visit the surgical suite and ambulatory surgical area 1 to 2 weeks prior to surgery, depending on the developmental level of the child. For children who are inpatients, the nurse visits the child and family in the unit. First the patient's chart is reviewed with particular attention given to the patient's age and developmental level, the seriousness of the physical condition, size including height and weight, and a review of the current nursing diagnoses and care plan. A discussion with the primary nurse facilitates data collection, assists in providing continuity of care, and provides the perioperative nurse with information regarding preoperative education done thus far.

The nurse then interviews the child and family. The purpose of the interview is to gather data, educate, and provide emotional support to both patient and family. The focus of this visit is a discussion of the perioperative process, not necessarily to provide preoperative education regarding the surgical procedure. In most hospitals, preoperative education is the responsibility of the primary nurse, child life therapists, and/or clinical nurse specialists. During the preoperative visit, the nurse discusses how the child progresses through the immediate preoperative, intraoperative, and postoperative phases of care. If any questions do arise concerning the surgical procedure, the family is referred to the surgeon, primary nurse, and/or anesthesiologist for further clarification or reinforcement of previous teaching. The perioperative nurse may briefly describe the roles of staff members and alleviate anxiety to a certain extent by allowing the parents and child to identify a real person behind the mask, gloves, and gown. The family is informed that the child may bring a favorite security object to the operating room and at what point after the operation the child can see the parents. Teaching is always done within a developmental framework, taking into account the cognitive and psychosocial abilities of the child. Medical play items, audiovisual aids, puppets, and photographs are all used in the education process.

Assessment continues when the child arrives in the surgical suite. Because the focus of operative preparation is psychologic rather than pharmacologic, the child usually arrives awake and alert. The nurse performs an abbreviated physical assessment, focusing on vital signs, cardiopulmonary status, integumentary system, nutritional/metabolic status, and psychologic state. The preoperative checklist is completed, which includes positive patient identification, verification of NPO status, a check of preoperative laboratory data, and communication of deviations from normal, noting the presence of an informed consent on the chart, and labeling the child's personal belongings. Throughout this process, the nurse provides emotional support to the child and family and helps to alleviate fear by administering care with a gentle, calm, trusting approach.

Assessment data, combined with knowledge of the planned surgical procedure, allow the perioperative nurse to anticipate requirements for surgical positioning, instrumentation, equipment and supplies, medications, and activities necessary to prevent injury to the pediatric patient. At the completion of the assessment phase, the perioperative nurse identifies nursing diagnoses. Five nursing diagnoses that apply to pediatric patients might be as follows:

- Knowledge deficit related to perioperative events
- Ineffective thermoregulation
- Potential for impaired skin integrity
- Potential for fluid volume deficit
- Potential for injury related to use of electrosurgical unit

Planning

Based on information about developmental levels and on additional information specific to the individual child's physical and psychosocial status, the medical diagnosis, and planned surgical intervention, the perioperative nurse develops a plan for patient care during surgery. Nursing care is predicated on relevant nursing diagnoses. For each nursing diagnosis, a goal is derived. Goals should be measurable with criteria by which to judge their attainment. Thus, for the goal "The patient and family will demonstrate knowledge of perioperative events and the role of various perioperative team members," criteria such as the child and family's ability to describe preoperative preparation and the perioperative routine on the day of surgery, the child's ability to locate the planned site of the surgical incision on a doll, and the child's ability to draw a picture of what he or she expects the surgical site to look like postoperatively might be identified. The demonstration of these behaviors or abilities then becomes the evaluative criteria by which the perioperative nurse measures goal achievement. For the five nursing diagnoses identified above, a Sample Care Plan has been developed. For each of the goals, the perioperative nurse needs to identify criteria appropriate to the child and surgical setting. A Sample Care Plan for the pediatric patient might be as shown on pp. 982-983.

Implementation

Age-appropriate communication is important in implementing the pediatric nursing care plan. Implementation begins during the perioperative nursing assessment and continues through discharge to the PACU or other discharge area. The *toddler* often fears parental separation and abandonment; separation or the surgical intervention may be perceived as a form of punishment. Toddlers fear, among other things, strangers, the dark, and machines. They attribute lifelike qualities to inanimate objects, believing that they, like the toddler, have feelings. Thus, a blood pressure cuff that squeezes the child's arm may be perceived to be doing so because it is angry with the toddler. Toddlers may also believe that their body is held together by their skin; anything that violates the skin integrity is feared. For this reason, Band-Aids are very important. Toddlers react with the environment using their senses. The perioperative nurse should allow the toddler to touch and feel objects as appropriate. Sensory information should be provided in a soft, gentle voice: what things will look like and feel like and what the toddler will touch and hear. A security object is extremely comforting. The operating room should be quiet; background noise should be controlled. Instruments, which are frightening to the toddler, should be covered. The toddler should be brought into the room when everything is ready to allow quick induction of anesthesia.

The *preschool* and *school-age* child may still perceive hospitalization or surgery as a punishment; there may be feelings of guilt associated with something the child thinks he or she said or did. The school-age child still fears painful

Sample Care Plan

NURSING DIAGNOSIS:
Knowledge deficit related to perioperative events
GOAL:
The child and family will demonstrate knowledge of perioperative events and the role of various perioperative team members.
INTERVENTIONS:
Perform preoperative visit and interview; educate the child and family, and provide emotional support.
Utilize audiovisual aids such as photographs, drawings, items for medical play, and/or a tour of the surgical suite.
Provide explanations on the child's level and at the parent's level of understanding.
Refer to nursing and other interdisciplinary team members to review, reinforce, or supplement preoperative education.

NURSING DIAGNOSIS:
Ineffective thermoregulation
GOAL:
The child's body temperature will be maintained at an appropriate level during the surgical intervention.
INTERVENTIONS:
Adjust room temperature approximately an hour before arrival of the child: 26° to 27° C (78.8° to 80.6° F) for infants and newborns; 23° to 24° C (73.4° to 75.2° F) for older children.

Place hyperthermia blanket on operating room bed; adjust blanket temperature to 38° to 40° C (100.4° to 104° F).
Provide radiant heat lamp for use during placement of monitoring lines, induction of anesthesia, positioning, skin preparation, and draping.
Warm blankets, skin preparation solutions, irrigation, and other solutions to body temperature prior to use.
Use warmers during administration of intravenous fluids and blood products; temperature settings should not exceed 38° C (100.4° F).
Monitor body temperature by rectal, esophageal, tympanic membrane, or other automatic temperature-monitoring device.
Document temperature at prescribed intervals; take appropriate action for temperature extremes.

NURSING DIAGNOSIS:
Potential for impaired skin integrity
GOAL:
The patient's skin integrity will be maintained.
INTERVENTIONS:
Prevent skin preparation solutions from pooling at bedline or under child.
Utilize body supports that conform to the size of the child (rolled diapers, towels, sheets, flexible sandbags, foam rolls); use inflatable bag or rolled sheet in place of kidney rest; use rolled towel for neck or shoulder elevation or support.

---

procedures; death may also be a fear at this age. Simple explanations in familiar terms are helpful at this developmental stage; a book or other teaching aid is useful during explanations. This child should be given as many choices as possible (for instance, letting the child decide into which hand the intravenous line will be inserted).

Adolescents may fear peer rejection, disability, loss of a body part, loss of control and status, and perhaps death. They need as much privacy as possible, and their attempts to be independent should be respected. The adolescent may

not wish to show any fear. Questions may not be asked while the parents are present. The perioperative nurse should provide explanations and answer questions as reasonably and truthfully as possible. If appropriate, some choices should be allowed, such as wearing underwear to the operating room. Patient care procedures that violate privacy, such as hair removal, skin preparation, and insertion of an indwelling urinary catheter, should be conducted after anesthesia is induced.

Key points in providing perioperative care to pediatric

Sample Care Plan—cont'd

Maintain all bed sheets and positioning supports dry and wrinkle-free.

Provide infant armboards or use padded tongue depressors to stabilize limbs containing intravenous lines.

Position Mayo stand over child's legs and lower part of operating room bed to support weight of drapes off child's body.

Use nonwoven, lightweight drapes (when possible) to reduce drape weight.

Determine any skin sensitivity to adhesive prior to application of self-adhering drapes or adhesive tape.

Have available, and use, nonallergenic or paper tape as indicated.

NURSING DIAGNOSIS:
Potential for fluid volume deficit
GOAL:
The patient will remain normovolemic.
INTERVENTIONS:
Maintain and protect patency of intravenous lines.
Review laboratory analyses for results of total blood volume.

Calculate estimated total blood volume using formula of 85 to 90 ml/kg of body weight if total blood volume has not been determined by laboratory tests.

Provide gram scales for weighing sponges discarded from operative field; weigh sponges and report estimated loss.

Provide suction units with reservoirs that measure in 5- to 10-ml increments.

Measure and record quantity of irrigating fluid used.

Provide appropriate amounts of intravenous fluid replacement (such as 250-ml containers).

Measure and record urinary output and output from other drainage tubes.

Send laboratory specimens for analyses as indicated; review results indicating fluid status.

NURSING DIAGNOSIS:
Potential for injury related to use of electrosurgical unit
GOAL:
The patient will be free from injury.
INTERVENTIONS:
Select appropriate size of adhesive electrosurgery dispersive pad; pad should be able to be molded or contoured to fit application surface yet provide sufficient body mass coverage.

Select pad application site with good tissue mass, as close to operative site as possible; shoulder, buttocks, thigh, or lengthwise on extremity may be selected.

Note condition of skin at dispersive pad placement site prior to placement and on pad removal.

Apply dispersive pad with firm but gentle pressure.

Verify that child is not lying on cord or pad connection.

Protect dispersive pad site from pooling of solutions.

Check dispersive pad contact after any positional changes.

---

patients include never leaving the child unattended, keeping the room quiet during induction, allowing the child to express fear and fearful behaviors (such as crying), using simple words without double meanings, allowing security objects to remain with the child until induction has been completed, and not being dishonest. If the child asks if something will hurt, explain that it will hurt like something they are familiar with (a bee sting, mosquito bite, and so on). The way children fall asleep during induction is likely to be the way they will wake up; thus, all attempts should be made to calm and reassure the child. Parents should be alerted to delays in the surgery schedule; in some instances, the child may be sent back to the pediatric unit.

Implementing the nursing care plan includes continual assessment and reassessment, as well as the initiation of activities that facilitate the surgical intervention and anticipate patient needs. In addition to positioning, surgical skin preparation, creating and maintaining a sterile field, collecting, dispensing, and recording specimens, administering medications, and providing a safe environment, special instruments and sutures must be provided for the pediatric patient.

Instrumentation

The same types of instruments are used in pediatric surgery as in adult surgery; however, pediatric instruments are usually shorter, have more delicate or less pronounced curves, and are lighter. A complete range of instrument sizes is necessary to make the appropriate size available for each child. Fewer instruments are normally required because incisions in children are shorter and more shallow. Use of basic instrument sets, grouped according to types of surgery performed (for example, minor or major), facilitates instrument counts. These sets are easily adapted to the patient's needs, as well as the surgeon's preferences, yet eliminate unnecessary instruments from the sterile field.

The following sets are examples of instrumentation used in pediatric surgery. The minor set is used for procedures such as inguinal hernia repair or pyloromyotomy. The major set is used for major chest and abdominal cases such as tracheo-esophageal fistula (TEF) and diaphragmatic hernia repair, omphalocele repair, and resection and pull-through for Hirschsprung's disease.

Smaller and larger instruments should be packaged separately and added to the surgical field as required.

Minor pediatric instrument set

2 Regular needle holders, 6 inch
1 Fine needle holder, 6 inch
1 Metzenbaum scissors, 7½ inch
1 Metzenbaum scissors, 5½ inch
1 Suture scissors
1 Straight strabismus scissors
1 Curved strabismus scissors
2 Fine mosquito or Halsted hemostats
4 Regular curved mosquito or Halsted hemostats
6 Regular straight mosquito or Halsted hemostats
2 Curved hemostats
2 Babcock forceps
3 Sponge-holding forceps, 9½ inch
6 Towel clamps, 3½ inch
2 Thymus/Lukens retractors
2 Phrenic retractors
2 Cushing vein retractors
2 Richardson retractors, ¾ inch
2 Knife handles, no. 3
2 Adson forceps with teeth
4 Debakey forceps, 6 inch

Major pediatric instrument set

2 Regular needle holders, 7 inch
2 Fine needle holders, 6 inch
1 Regular needle holder, 6 inch
1 Metzenbaum scissors, 7½ inch
1 Metzenbaum scissors, 5½ inch
1 Lincoln scissors
1 Curved Mayo scissors
1 Suture scissors
1 Straight strabismus scissors

1 Curved strabismus scissors
2 Fine curved mosquito or Halsted hemostats
10 Regular curved mosquito or Halsted hemostats
6 Regular straight mosquito or Halsted hemostats
2 Curved hemostats
2 Straight hemostats
6 Pean forceps
2 Allis forceps
4 Babcock forceps
1 Fine Schnidt clamp
3 Regular Schnidt clamps
1 Right-angle clamp, 7 inch
1 Lahey gall duct forceps
3 Sponge-holding forceps, 9½ inch
1 Towel clamp, 3½ inch
2 Army-Navy retractors
2 Thymus/Lukens retractors
2 Phrenic retractors
2 Cushing vein retractors
2 Small Deaver retractors
1 Set of Richardson retractors (2 of each size)
2 Adson forceps with teeth
1 Tissue forceps with teeth
2 Debakey forceps, 6 inch
2 Debakey forceps, 7½ inch
2 Tuttle forceps
1 Knife handle, no. 7
1 Knife handle, no. 3
1 Grooved director
1 Tonsil suction tube
1 Frazier suction tip, no. 11
1 Small Poole suction tube

Sutures

Small sizes of absorbable and nonabsorbable sutures are appropriate for the delicate and fragile tissues of infants and children. Sutures should have attached needles (atraumatic) to reduce tissue damage. The most common sizes are nos. 000 to 5-0 with ½- and ⅜-circle needles. Staples, both pediatric and regular sizes, are often used. Many skin incisions are closed with subcutaneous suture using subcuticular techniques; paper adhesive dressing strips or collodion is then applied.

Evaluation

The perioperative nurse evaluates care provided throughout the perioperative period. At the conclusion of the surgical intervention, the skin is inspected, especially at dependent pressure points and at the site of the electrosurgical dispersive pad. Inspection is carried out to detect any reddened, irritated areas or evidence of compression injury. The temperature of the skin is noted, as is the core temperature. The cardiopulmonary status is closely monitored as the child emerges from anesthesia; the perioperative nurse assists anesthesia personnel during emergence and protects the child from injury. Dry, warm blankets are provided. Hydration status is determined, replacement fluids administered, and fluid output noted. The child is transferred to and positioned on the PACU stretcher. The airway is protected, as are tubes, drains, and drainage devices.

The perioperative nurse provides an oral report to the nurse in PACU, focusing on the condition of the child, the response to surgery and anesthesia, presence of catheters and drains, the quality and amount of wound drainage, and a description of the dressings applied. Part of this report should focus on the goals established in the perioperative care plan. These goals may be reported as outcome statements. For the care plan presented in this chapter, they might be as follows:

- The child and family demonstrated knowledge of perioperative events and the roles of perioperative team members.
- The child's body temperature was maintained at an appropriate level during the surgical intervention.
- Skin integrity was maintained.
- The child remained normovolemic.
- There was no evidence of injury related to use of the electrosurgical unit.

The perioperative nurse may receive further feedback on the child's progress after the child is discharged from PACU; this information may be relayed by the surgeon, unit nurse, or clinical nurse specialist. This type of informal feedback helps "close the loop" of information. It allows the perioperative nurse to collect informally additional data regarding effectiveness of the care plan and provides the nurse with information about the outcomes of the perioperative care provided.

SURGICAL INTERVENTIONS

Pediatric surgery encompasses all specialties but, in general, can be divided into three major areas: congenital malformations or defects, acquired diseases of infancy and childhood, and trauma. A discussion of pediatric trauma is beyond the scope of this chaper. Several surgical procedures that may be designated pediatric have been presented in previous chapters of this text under particular specialty headings. Surgical interventions presented here include procedures that are commonly and uniquely performed in the area of pediatric general surgery.

Central venous catheter placement

The exposure and cannulation of a major vessel for the purpose of inserting and positioning a catheter in the vena cava just above the atrium are indicated for infants and children who require total parenteral nutrition (TPN) because feeding through the gastrointestinal (GI) tract is impossible, inadequate, or hazardous. Common conditions necessitating TPN are bowel fistulas, inadequate intestinal length, chronic diarrhea, extensive burns, and multiple trauma. The TPN fluids are delivered through a central venous catheter to avoid peripheral inflammation and thrombosis. Occasionally, a central venous catheter is indicated

for infants or children who require chemotherapy, antibiotic therapy, or other long-term IV medical treatment.

The preferred site of placement is the external jugular. The internal jugular may be chosen if the external jugular has been used or is too small. From the cannulation site, the catheter is tunneled under the skin about 5 to 10 cm. This is done to inhibit contamination of the blood stream from frequent dressing changes. In cases where the internal or external vein sites are unavailable, the catheter may be placed in the external iliac vein by way of a cutdown in the greater saphenous vein. In these cases the catheter is tunneled out into the abdominal wall.

Procedural considerations. The manufacturer's instructions for handling, preparing, and sterilizing the catheter must be followed. The catheter must not contact linty materials, glove powder, or other foreign matter.

Before insertion the catheter is flushed and filled with the infusion solution, special formula, or dextrose 10% in water to prevent air bubbles from entering the circulatory system and to eliminate blood clots in the catheter lumen. The catheter is connected to the pump, and infusion should begin as soon as the catheter is secured.

The child is appropriately positioned as dictated by the site chosen for cannulation. The area is prepped and draped.

Operative procedure
Catheter insertion into external jugular

1. A transverse incision is made over the lower portion of the medial border of the sternocleidomastoid muscle.
2. The external jugular vein is exposed and prepared for cannulation.
3. Using a long, hollow needle with an obturator, a subcutaneous tunnel is created, extending from the neck incision to the chest wall medial to the nipple.
4. The obturator is withdrawn, and the catheter is passed through the needle. The needle is removed, and the catheter then lies in the subcutaneous tunnel.
5. The external jugular vein is ligated distally, and the catheter is passed into the vein through an incision and advanced so that it lies at the point where the superior vena cava enters the atrium.
6. This position of the catheter is then confirmed by radiography in the operating room.
7. The catheter is secured at the exit site on the chest wall with nonabsorbable sutures.
8. Antimicrobial ointment is applied to the exit site, and an occlusive, transparent dressing is placed over this. The catheter is coiled under this dressing to avoid tension on the line and accidental displacement.
9. The infusion pump is connected to the infusing solution before the child is moved from the operating room bed.

Repair of atresia of the esophagus

Atresia of the esophagus is repaired, through a right retropleural thoracotomy, by closure of the tracheoesophageal fistula and anastomosis of the segments of the esophagus.

This congenital anomaly may arise between the third and sixth weeks of fetal life. Several types are recognized, the most common being an upper segment of esophagus ending in a blind pouch and a lower segment of esophagus communicating by a fistula with the trachea. Ideally this defect is recognized in the first hours of life, but more often the diagnosis is made in the first 36 to 48 hours of life. Prompt surgical intervention allows the child to breathe and eat without the danger of aspirating mucus, saliva, feedings, or stomach contents.

Procedural considerations. A gastrostomy may be done first to decompress the air-distended stomach, thus facilitating chest movement and ventilation and preventing reflux of stomach contents into the trachea. The patient is then positioned for a right thoracotomy, prepped and draped. The major instrument set is required, with the addition of the following:

Baby chest retractors
Baby T-malleables
Regular malleables
Infant malleables
Senn retractors
Gemini mixters
Neuromastoid retractors
Baker dilators
Vessel loops
Ligaclips
Cotton tip applicators
Umbilical tape
Chest tube (check size)
Infant Pleurevac
Malecot catheter (check size)
Fogarty catheters
Mineral oil

Operative procedure

1. The chest is entered through the fourth intercostal space. Removing the rib is not necessary (Fig. 29-1, *A*).
2. The pleura is gently dissected off the chest wall (Fig. 29-1, *B*).
3. As the dissection proceeds posteriorly, the azygos vein is encountered, which is divided to expose the fistula beneath (Fig. 29-1, *C*).
4. Tape or silk is passed under the fistula to apply traction gently (Fig. 29-1, *D*).
5. The fistula is clamped and transected, leaving a 3-mm cuff of tissue on the trachea to avoid compromising the lumen of the airway (Fig. 29-1, *E*).
6. To close the fistula, 3 or 4 interrupted sutures of 5-0 silk are used.
7. The fibrotic end of the distal pouch is excised, and the pouch is opened.
8. The upper pouch is then identified. This is made easier by the presence of a Replogle tube. A traction suture is placed in each pouch, and the distance between the

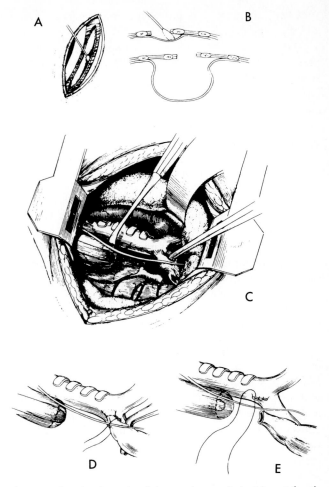

Fig. 29-1. Repair of atresia of the esophagus. **A,** Incision at fourth intercostal space. **B,** Dissection of pleura off chest wall. **C,** Identification and division of azygos vein to expose fistula beneath. **D,** Traction applied to fistula. **E,** Transection of fistula leaving 3-mm cuff on trachea. (Reprinted with permission from Coran, A.G., and others: Surgery of the neonate, Boston, 1978, Little, Brown and Co.)

proximal and distal portions of the esophagus is estimated. At this point the surgeon makes the decision to attempt primary anastomosis. If primary anastomosis is impossible, the distal esophagus is closed and tacked high on the prevertebral fascia. Infrequently, the gap between the proximal and distal portions of esophagus are so long that esophageal replacement is required. In these cases the upper pouch is brought out to the neck in the form of a cervical esophagostomy. When the child reaches 1 year of age, esophageal replacement is attempted through colon interposition or construction of a reverse gastric tube.

9. Primary anastomosis is performed with 5-0 or 6-0 silk, taking full thickness bites along anterior and posterior borders (Fig. 29-2). Some surgeons prefer the Haight or two-layer anastomosis (Fig. 29-3). The inner layer

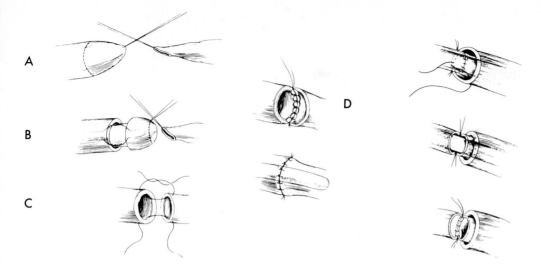

Fig. 29-2. Primary repair of atresia of the esophagus: single layer repair. **A,** Traction applied to proximal and distal esophagus. **B,** Blind proximal pouch transected. **C,** Full thickness bites of anterior and posterior borders. **D,** Repair completed with replogle tube in place to allow adequate lumen of esophagus. (Reprinted with permission from Coran, A.G., and others: Surgery of the neonate, Boston, 1978, Little, Brown and Co.)

Fig. 29-3. The Haight anastomosis. Mucosal layer of proximal pouch sutured to full thickness of distal esophagus. Muscular sleeve of upper pouch pulled down over inner anastomosis and sutured to muscle of distal esophagus. (Reprinted with permission from Coran, A.G., and others: Surgery of the neonate, Boston, 1978, Little, Brown and Co.)

is comprised of the upper pouch mucosa sutured to the full thickness of the distal esophagus. The muscular sleeve of the upper esophagus is then pulled down over the inner anastomosis and sutured to the muscular layer of the inferior esophagus. The incision is irrigated with saline.

10. Some surgeons place a no. 14 or 16 Fr extrapleural chest tube through a posterior stab wound. It is secured with absorbable sutures to prevent it from putting direct pressure on the anastomosis.

11. Muscle layers are closed with interrupted 5-0 or 6-0 silk or running 3-0 chromic suture.

12. Skin is closed with a running 5-0 suture, and a collodion dressing or dressing of gauze and tape is applied.

13. The extrapleural chest tube is water-sealed, and a chest x-ray is obtained.

Repair of congenital diaphragmatic hernia

A congenital diaphragmatic hernia is repaired by replacement of the displaced viscera into the abdominal cavity with surgical correction of the defect (Fig. 29-4).

The conventional surgical repair is through the abdomen. The concurrence of intraabdominal abnormalities is somewhat high in babies with diaphragmatic hernia; therefore, treatment is facilitated with an abdominal approach. It is technically easier to extract the viscera from below than to push them out of the thorax. The abnormal intrathoracic intrusion of the abdominal viscera usually causes severe compromise of intrathoracic pulmonary and vascular activities. Therefore, urgent restoration of more normal intrathoracic and intraabdominal relationships is the rule in these newborns. The lung may be hypoplastic because of prolonged compression in utero by the displaced abdominal viscera. A residual intrapleural space usually remains for a few days after surgery.

Procedural considerations. A chest tube can be inserted and connected to water-seal drainage. Insertion of a gastrostomy tube minimizes postoperative distention and facilitates feeding. Direct suturing of the margins of the defect is usually possible. Insertion of a prosthetic Silastic sheeting is occasionally required, and the sheeting should be available.

The major instrument set is required, plus the following:

Medium Ligaclips
Baby malleables
Baby Deavers
Chest tube (check size)
Infant Pleurevac (may fill to either 3.5 or 5 cm of water)
Umbilical tape
Red rubber catheter
Mineral oil

Have available

Neuromastoid retractors
Chest retractors
Bone wax
Marlex mesh or Silastic sheet

The infant is positioned supine on a hyperthermia blanket.

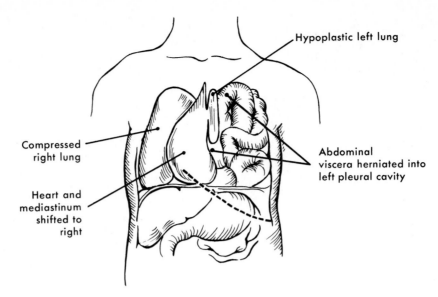

Fig. 29-4. Diaphragmatic hernia.

Operative procedure

1. A contralateral chest tube is placed in the anterior axillary line of the second intercostal space to prevent tension pneumothorax during surgery.
2. A subcostal incision going through all muscle layers is made on the side of the defect.
3. The abdominal viscera are withdrawn from the chest and held downward through the abdominal wound. Because abnormalities of abdominal viscera such as malrotation are associated with diaphragmatic hernia, the surgeon performs careful inspection of the organs at this time. If a malrotation is found, some surgeons prefer to repair it if the clinical condition of the infant allows it.
4. The defect is then carefully inspected including a search for a hernia sac, which is present in less than 5% of cases. If a sac is identified, it is excised. An ipsilateral chest tube is placed before the diaphragm is closed.
5. The posterior and anterior rims of the diaphragm are identified, and primary closure is performed with mattress sutures of 2-0 nonabsorbable material. If the rim of tissue is too small for mattress sutures, ample sutures of 2-0 or 3-0 silk are used. Occasionally, reinforced Silastic sheeting may be needed if sufficient diaphragm is not available for primary closure.
6. Gastrostomy is then performed in most cases.
7. The abdominal wall is then closed. If the musculature cannot accommodate the abdominal viscera, they are left open and skin is closed to leave a ventral hernia. The infant is returned to the operating room within 7 days for repair of the ventral hernia.

Nissen fundoplication

Nissen fundoplication is the wrapping of the fundus of the stomach around the esophagus at the gastric-esophageal junction. Nissen fundoplication is indicated for infants and children who suffer from severe gastroesophageal reflux (GER). The cause of GER in these patients is thought to be an inadequate antireflux barrier. The antireflux barrier consists of a combination of anatomic and physiologic factors, including sufficient amount and strength of muscle fibers located in the lower esophageal sphincter, adequate length of the abdominal esophagus, and a high-pressure zone in the lower esophagus. The combination of these factors forms the antireflux barrier and thus prevents GER. An incompetent antireflux barrier can result in life-threatening complications of GER, including obstructive apnea, aspiration pneumonia, esophagitis, and failure to thrive. The goal of the Nissen fundoplication is to re-create a competent antireflux barrier.

Procedural considerations. The major instrument set is required, plus the following:

Medium Ligaclips
Drain (¼ inch to ⅜ inch—check size)
Sterile specimen cup
Malecot catheter (check size)

Have available

Deaver retractors
Long instruments
Iron intern retractor
Balfour retractor
Bookwalter retractor
Maloney dilators (surgeon will place prior to scrubbing)

The patient is positioned supine. An appropriate-sized dilator is passed into the esophagus to prevent the wrap from impinging on the lumen of the esophagus (Fig. 29-5).

Operative procedure

1. A left subcostal incision is performed to allow exposure

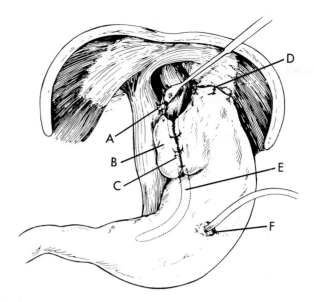

Fig. 29-5. Salient features of Nissen fundoplication in infants. **A,** Crural sutures to reduce hiatus. **B,** Generous loose, adequate tissue in the wrap. **C,** Sutures placed through seromuscular depth of both gastric and esophageal walls. **D,** Sutures to fix the fundus to the diaphragm. **E,** Appropriate-sized mercury-filled dilator to ensure adequate lumen. **F,** Gastrostomy in all infants and whenever there is any question of gastric outlet problems. (From Randolph, J.G.: Ann. Surg. 198:579–584, 1983. Reprinted with permission.)

of the lower esophagus to create adequate intraabdominal length.

2. The esophagus is mobilized to create adequate intraabdominal length.
3. The stomach is mobilized to allow loose wrap of fundus around esophageal junction; it is used as the lower edge of the wrap.
4. Sutures of 3-0 or 4-0 silk are placed through the seromuscular layers of both stomach and esophagus to fix the wrap.
5. Sutures are then placed to tack the fundus to the diaphragm.
6. Some surgeons place clips at the level of the GE junction and the wrap to aid in follow-up radiographic studies.
7. A gastrostomy is done in most cases.
8. The incision is closed in layers, and a collodion dressing is applied.

Ramstedt-Fredet pyloromyotomy for pyloric stenosis

The Ramstedt-Fredet pyloromyotomy for pyloric stenosis is the excision of the muscles of the pylorus to treat congenital hypertrophy of the pyloric sphincter that is obstructing the stomach. Signs and symptoms of high gas-

trointestinal obstruction appear at 2 to 6 weeks of age. The first sign is projectile vomiting that is free of bile. There may be a severe loss of body fluids and electrolyte imbalance.

Procedural considerations. The stomach is emptied just before induction of anesthesia, and the nasogastric tube is removed to guard against reflux of gastric contents around the tube during induction. A minor instrument set and a pyloric spreader are used.

The patient is prepped in the usual manner.

Operative procedure

1. The abdomen is opened through a right subcostal transverse skin incision. The rectus muscle is split vertically with spreading clamps, and the peritoneum is opened.
2. After the hypertrophied pylorus is delivered into the wound with a small vein retractor, the prepyloric area is grasped and rotated to expose the anterior superior border of the mass. An incision is made in the pyloric mass through the serosa and partially through the circular muscle throughout the length of the mass (Fig. 29-6, A).
3. The circular muscle is spread with the pyloric spreader on the submucosal base, so that all muscle fibers are completely divided (Fig. 29-6, B).
4. After completion of the separation, the pyloric end of the stomach is returned to the abdomen, and the peritoneum and posterior rectus sheath are closed with a continuous, absorbable no. 3-0 suture. The anterior rectus sheath is closed with a no. 4-0 absorbable suture.
5. The skin is closed with fine subcuticular sutures. Small adhesive strips or collidon is applied as dressing.

Emergency gastrointestinal procedures
Gastrostomy

Gastrostomy is establishment of a temporary or permanent channel from the gastric lumen to the skin to permit gastric emptying, liquid feeding, or retrograde dilation of an esophageal stricture.

Gastrostomy, done through an abdominal incision, is often performed with other surgical procedures to facilitate care of the infant or child after surgery.

Procedural considerations. A minor instrument set is required, plus a mushroom or Malecot catheter (no. 14 or 16 for infants and no. 18, 20, or 22 for older children) and a no. 11 knife blade on a knife handle.

Routine prepping of the patient is done.

Operative procedure

1. A short incision is made over the outer border of the left rectus muscle (Fig. 29-7, A).
2. The subcutaneous tissues and rectus fascia are exposed with two small retractors (Fig. 29-7, B).
3. The anterior rectus fascia is opened, and the rectus muscle is split with clamps, exposing the posterior rectus sheath (Fig. 29-7, C).
4. The peritoneum is opened, exposing the liver edge

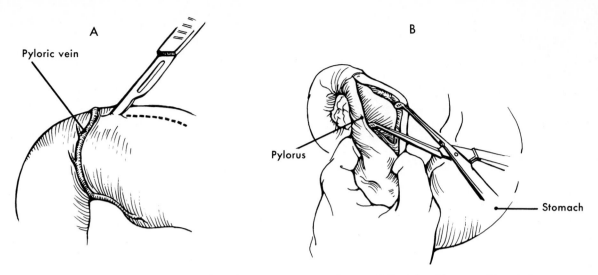

Fig. 29-6. Operative technique for pyloric stenosis. (From Benson, C.D.: Infants' hypertrophic pyloric stenosis. In Mustard, W.T., and others, editors: Pediatric surgery, 2nd edition. Copyright © 1969 by Year Book Medical Publishers, Inc., Chicago. Used by permission.)

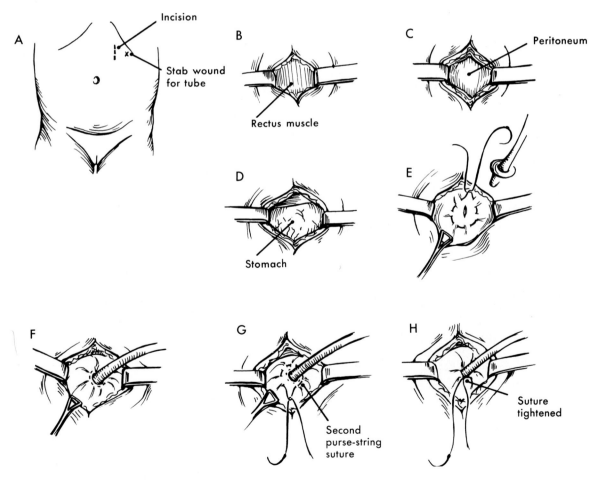

Fig. 29-7. Gastrostomy, **A,** Incision. **B,** Rectus muscle exposed. **C,** Posterior rectus sheath exposed. **D,** Peritoneum opened. **E,** Purse-string suture placed. **F,** Mushroom catheter inserted. **G,** Second purse-string suture placed. **H,** Suture tightened. (Modified from Gross, R.E.: An atlas of children's surgery, Philadelphia, 1970, W.B. Saunders Co.)

and the greater curvature of the stomach (Fig. 29-7, *D*).

5. The stomach is pulled out through the wound with a Babcock forceps. A circular purse-string suture of no. 4-0 silk is placed; in the center of this, a stab wound is made through the gastric wall (Fig. 29-7, *E*).

6. A mushroom catheter, often with the tip cut off, is inserted into the stomach, and the purse-string suture is tied (Fig. 29-7, *F*).

7. A second purse-string suture is placed outside the previous one, and the same needle is then taken through the peritoneum and the posterior rectus fascia to place the stomach against the peritoneum and thus prevent leaks (Fig. 29-7 *G*, and *H*).

8. The catheter is brought out through a left lateral stab wound (Fig. 29-7, *A*).

9. The stomach wall adjacent to the gastrostomy site is tacked to the undersurface of the peritoneum with interrupted sutures of 4-0 silk.

10. Routine abdominal closure is performed.

Omphalocele repair

Omphalocele is the protrusion of abdominal viscera outside the abdomen into a sac of amniotic membrane and peritoneum at the base of the umbilical cord. There is no skin covering. Omphalocele occurs during the eleventh week of fetal life when the viscera fail to withdraw from the exocoelomic position and occupy the peritoneal cavity. The resulting abdominal wall defect can vary in size from 2 cm to 15 cm. The sac may contain only a few loops of bowel to nearly all the intestines plus liver and spleen.

Associated anomalies include malrotation and abnormal fixation of the bowel.

Treatment at birth consists of applying warm saline packs on the sac surface and inserting a nasogastric tube to prevent distention. Surgical intervention is necessary to prevent rupture of the sac, infection, or both. If intrauterine rupture of the sac has occurred, the newly delivered child is kept warm, the bowel is inspected for perforation and torsion, and moist, warm dressings are applied.

An omphalocele is repaired by replacement of the viscera in the abdominal cavity, with reconstruction of the abdominal wall (Fig. 29-8).

Procedural considerations. Particular attention to maintaining body temperature is essential because of the massive exposed surface area from which body heat can be lost. The use of nitrous oxide as an anesthetic agent is avoided during this procedure as it causes increased gas in the intestine, which in turn makes the reduction of abdominal contents into the peritoneal cavity more difficult. The major instrument set is required, with the addition of the following:

Baby malleables
Ligaclips
Red rubber catheter

Have available

Silastic sheeting
Foley catheter with urimeter
Replogle tube
Malecot catheter

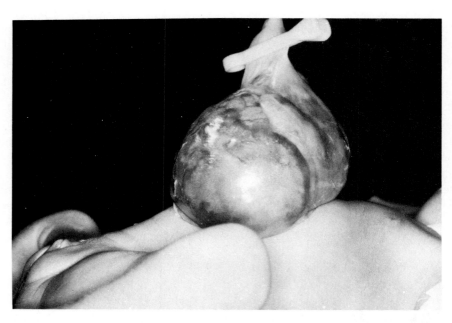

Fig. 29-8. Omphalocele containing liver. (Courtesy John R. Campbell, University of Oregon Health Sciences Center, Portland, Ore; from Jensen, M.D., and Bobak, I.M.: Maternity and gynecologic care: the nurse and the family, ed. 3, St. Louis, 1985, The C.V. Mosby Co.)

The infant is positioned supine and the abdomen, umbilical cord, and sac are prepped with an iodophor solution.

Operative procedure

1. In the presence of small defects, primary closure is attempted. The skin edges are freed, and the sac is excised. Abdominal contents are gently relocated into the peritoneal cavity. The abdominal cavity is closed in layers using 3-0 silk.

2. In certain cases where the defect is of medium to large size, a primary closure may not be accomplished. In these situations a staged procedure is done utilizing prosthetic reduction. In the first stage the infant is brought to the operating room and positioned and prepped as previously described.

2A. The sac is excised, and the umbilical vein and arteries ligated.

2B. Gastrostomy may be performed at this time.

2C. A silo is then created with Silastic mesh (Fig. 29-9). The mesh is secured through all layers of the edge of the defect utilizing a continuous locking suture of 2-0 Polydek (Fig. 29-9, *A*). The open end of the silo is closed in the same manner, thus creating a cylinder of mesh extending upward from the abdomen (Fig. 29-9, *B*).

2D. The open end of the cylinder is tied closed with umbilical tape (Fig. 29-9, *C*).

2E. The mesh silo suture line and edge of the defect are wrapped with Kling dipped in an iodophor solution to prevent infection. The infant is transferred to an open isolette, and the silo is suspended from the top of the isolette. Plastic wrap is applied to the silo to prevent heat loss.

2F. The infant is then transported to the neonatal intensive care unit, where daily reduction of abdominal contents is performed by adding a lower tie of umbilical tape. The abdominal viscera are completely reduced within 5 to 10 days, at which time the infant is returned to the operating room for the second stage of repair (Fig. 29-9, *D*).

2G. In order to avoid an appendectomy in the future on a child with a malrotated colon, an appendectomy may be performed at this time.

2H. The silo is removed, and the fascia is closed with interrupted sutures of 2-0 or 3-0 silk.

2I. The skin is closed with interrupted 4-0 silk. In an attempt to create an umbilicus, a purse-string suture is utilized in closing the inferior 2 cm of incision.

3. Another technique for treating large omphaloceles is painting the sac and surrounding skin with a 2% solution of merbromin (Mercurochrome) until an eschar forms to add strength to the sac and resist infection, or the sac may be treated with moist 0.5% silver nitrate dressings. The sac membrane gradually contracts, and skin closes the abdominal wall defect. Later surgery then repairs the abdominal musculature.

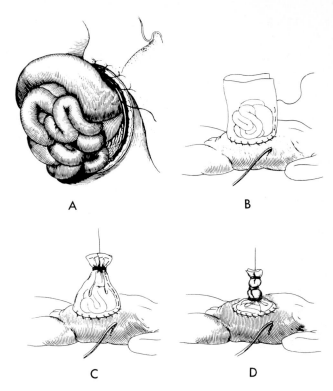

Fig. 29-9. Staged repair of omphalocele. **A,** Silastic mesh secured to all layers of edge of defect. **B,** Silo closed creating cylinder of mesh. **C,** Open end of silo tied with umbilical tape. **D,** Lower ties of umbilical tape applied to silo to gradually reduce viscera. (Reprinted with permission from Coran, A.G., and others: Surgery of the neonate, Boston, 1978, Little, Brown and Co.)

Umbilical hernia repair

An umbilical hernia is corrected by repair of the part of the intestine protruding at the umbilicus. An umbilical hernia is always covered by skin. Small umbilical hernias may be left untreated. They usually close within a few months to a year. Normally these defects are not closed surgically until the child is at least 2 years of age with some surgeons delaying repair until 4 years of age.

Procedural considerations. A minor instrument set is required. The child is prepped as discussed previously.

Operative procedure

1. An incision is made below the umbilicus through the skin and subcutaneous tissue.

2. Flaps of skin and subcutaneous tissue are mobilized and held back with small retractors to expose the rectus fascia and hernial protrusion.

3. The hernial sac, which is between the rectus muscle sheaths in the midline, is completely freed from all surrounding structures.

4. The sac is excised.

5. The peritoneum is closed with a continuous suture.

6. The two edges of the rectus fascia are brought together with interrupted no. 3-0 nonabsorbable sutures.

7. Subcuticular closure of the skin with a continuous, fine, absorbable suture is performed, and a pressure dressing is applied.

Inguinal hernia repair

An inguinal hernia is corrected by repairing a protrusion of a hernial sac, containing the intestine, in the inguinal canal. The testis develops high on the posterior wall of the abdomen. It gradually descends into the scrotum. Before the testis enters the inguinal canal, the processus vaginalis projects downward but retains a communication with the peritoneal cavity. The upper part of the processus does not; the remaining sac constitutes an indirect inguinal hernia. In the female, a similar hernial sac is contiguous with the round ligament.

Procedural considerations. A minor instrument set is used, and routine prepping is done.

Operative procedure

1. An incision is made over the inguinal area in the direction of the skin crease.
2. The subcutaneous tissue is opened, and hemostats are placed on bleeding vessels, which are then ligated.
3. Right-angle retractors are placed inferiorly and medially.
4. The external ring is identified, and the external oblique fascia is cleaned and freed with small Metzenbaum scissors.
5. The exernal oblique fascia is opened with a no. 15 knife blade on a knife handle, and the upper flap is freed. The lower flap is freed to expose the inguinal ligament.
6. Cord structures are opened at the upper end of the cord. Two forceps are used to grasp tissues at the same level and separate them.
7. The hernial sac is grasped with a hemostat, and structures of the cord are peeled downward and away from the sac with forceps until the sac is freed.
8. After the sac is opened and the surgeon's index finger inserted, the sac is pulled upward. The upward traction is maintained with two or three hemostats.
9. The sac is ligated with silk no. 3-0, and excess sac is removed. Repair of the inguinal canal may be done with silk sutures.
10. The subcutaneous tissue is closed with interrupted, fine sutures; closure of the skin is with fine, nonabsorbable subcuticular sutures. Collodion or paper adhesive dressing strips are applied.

Repair of intestinal obstruction

Repair of intestinal obstruction includes (1) untwisting of a volvulus, (2) division of a congenital band, (3) release of an internal hernia, (4) resection of bowel with anastomosis, or (5) creation of an intestinal stoma. Intestinal obstruction is the most frequent gastrointestinal emergency requiring surgery in the newborn. Early recognition is essential. Surgical intervention is usually within the first few hours after birth; delay may increase the risk.

Intestinal obstruction may occur in the infant for a variety of reasons: atresia, stenosis, congenital aganglionosis, meconium ileus, or malrotation. Lesions characterized by complete obliteration of intestinal lumen are classified as atresia. Those that produce a narrowing or partial obliteration of the lumen are classified as stenosis.

Procedural considerations. The major instrument set and pediatric intestinal instruments are required, plus culture tubes, syringes, and a 25-gauge needle.

Usual prepping is done.

Operative procedure

1. The abdomen is opened through an incision appropriate to the exposure of the particular form of obstruction.
2. Exploration and displacement of the intestines to the abdominal wall help determine the obstructive lesion. With atresia or stenosis, the entire bowel must be examined to rule out multiple areas of involvement.
3. Detorsion or reduction of bowel decompression or resection is performed when indicated.

Reduction of intussusception

Intussusception is relieved by reduction of invaginated bowel by the hydrostatic pressure of a barium enema or by laparotomy and manual manipulation. Intussusception is the telescopic invagination of a portion of intestine into an adjacent part with mechanical and vascular impairment. Intussusception is the most common cause of intestinal obstruction in the 2-month to 3-year-old age group. A frequent site for intussusception is the ileocecal junction. Intussusception in children is most often idiopathic; other causes may include Meckel's diverticulum, polyps, or hematoma of the bowel. Early diagnosis and reduction are essential to bowel viability.

Procedural considerations. The child is prepped for surgery as described previously. Reduction by barium enema should be attempted only with the full cognizance of the radiologist, surgeon, and pediatrician, with the operating room team on standby. Should reduction not be accomplished, a laparotomy must be done. The major instrument set is used with the addition of pediatric intestinal instruments.

Operative procedure

1. A transverse or right paramedian incision is made, and the peritoneum is entered (Fig. 29-10, *A*).
2. The cecum and ileum are identified; the intussusception is located and elevated with fingers (Fig. 29-10, *B* and *C*).
3. If there is no evidence of bowel compromise, the bowel immediately distal to the intussusception is occluded with one hand and stripped proximally with the other.
4. The abdomen is closed in layers, and the wound is dressed.

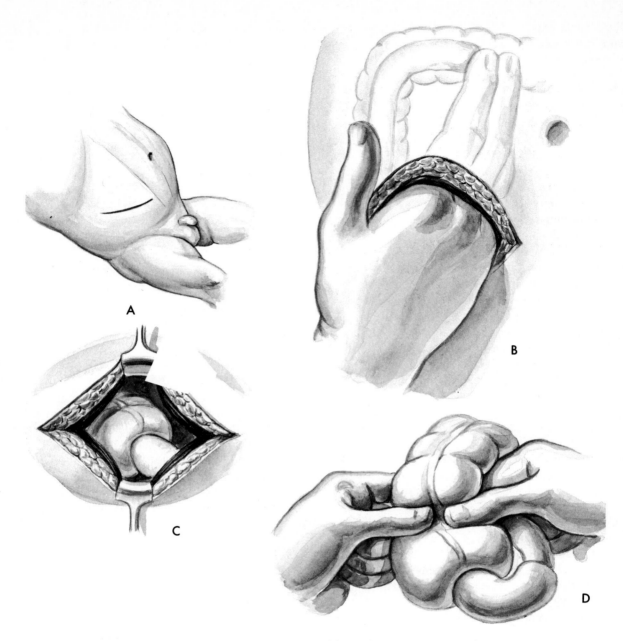

Fig. 29-10. Reduction of intussusception. **A,** Transverse abdominal incision. **B,** Location of intussusception. **C,** Mass delivered into incision. **D,** "Milking" reduction. (From Lewis, J.E.: Atlas of infant surgery, St. Louis, 1967, The C.V. Mosby Co.)

Colostomy

Colostomy is the surgical construction of an artificial excretory opening from the colon. Most congenital anomalies that result in colonic obstruction require a temporary colostomy. These include imperforate anus and Hirschsprung's disease. Both conditions ultimately require further pelvic operative procedures, and proper construction of a colostomy is important. In Hirschsprung's disease, the colostomy must be placed in a section of bowel containing ganglia.

Procedural considerations. A major instrument set and pediatric intestinal clamps are used.

The child is prepped as described previously.

Operative procedure

1. A transverse incision usually is preferred, and the abdomen is entered in the right upper quadrant for a transverse colostomy or the left lower quadrant for a sigmoid colostomy.

2. The loop of colon is freed of peritoneal attachments until it can be brought easily through the abdominal wall without tension.

3. The edges of the mesentery are then sutured to the parietal peritoneum, and the serosa of the colonic loop is sutured with fine absorbable suture materials to the peritoneum and fascia as well as the skin.
4. The colostomy may be sutured immediately. Some surgeons prefer to close the skin under a colostomy loop; others prefer to suture mucosa directly to skin edges. This decision may depend on the location of the colostomy. An important point is that each layer must be securely attached to the serosa of the colon to prevent evisceration and prolapse. The posterior wall of a loop colostomy may be divided by electrosurgery several days after surgery.

Hepatic portoenterostomy (Kasai procedure)

The Kasai procedure is the construction of a bile drainage system by utilizing an intestinal conduit. Biliary atresia is a disease that results from nonpatent extrahepatic bile ducts that prevent the drainage of bile from the liver and lead to eventual cirrhosis. The Kasai procedure re-creates a drainage system using a limb of intestine. This procedure is indicated in patients with extrahepatic biliary atresia who are under 3 months of age. All atretic segments of the existing bile ducts are removed. An operative cholangiogram and frozen section biopsy of the hepatic duct remnant are prerequisites to the actual procedure.

Procedural considerations. The infant is positioned supine over an x-ray plate. Both a major instrument set and transplant instruments are required, with the addition of the following:

3-way stopcock
Syringes
 3 TB
 1 3 cc
 1 6 cc
 1 12 cc
Injectable saline
Hypaque dye (mix half dye, half saline)
Foley catheter and urimeter
Petri dishes
Ligaclips
Umbilical tape
Mineral oil
Jelco catheters, 18 and 20 gauge
Light handles
Sterile specimen cup
Taut cholangiogram catheter

Have available

Deaver retractors
Kittner or Cherry dissectors
Carmalt hemostats
Kocher forceps
Bowel clamps
Head light
Drain
Malecot catheter
Tru-cut biopsy needle

Operative procedure

1. A right upper quadrant incision is made and the gall bladder is identified.
2. A small catheter is placed into the gallbladder and secured with a purse-string suture. Radiopaque dye is instilled into the gallbladder, and an x-ray film is taken. The surgeon notes free flow of bile through the ducts and the duodenum. Occasionally, free flow of bile will be seen. These patients are then categorized as having correctable biliary atresia. In such situations a liver biopsy is performed, and the incision is closed. The majority of patients with correctable biliary atresia demonstrate progressive improvement. More commonly, though, there is a very small amount of flow or none at all. In these cases of noncorrectable biliary atresia, the Kasai procedure is performed.
3. Because of the high incidence of associated anomalies, a thorough inspection of the intraabdominal organs is then performed.
4. The hepaticoduodenal ligament is explored and all drainage structures are ligated (Fig. 29-11, *A*).
5. The hepatic duct remnant is identified and traced to the liver hilum. The remnant is transected as high as possible, using frozen section biopsies as a guide. Frozen section biopsies are also obtained at the portahepatis to denote the presence of ductules. Precise identification of this location is essential (Fig. 29-11, *B*).
6. The proximal jejunum is usually used as the intestinal conduit. A meticulous anastomosis is performed at the portahepatis as previously identified, using a single running layer of absorbable sutures (Fig. 29-11, *C*).
7. The conduit is exteriorized with a double-barreled Roux-en-Y approach (Fig. 29-11, *D*).
8. A liver biopsy is then performed.
9. A drain is placed, and the incision closed in layers.

The procedure described above is one approach of many. Others include exteriorization of the jejunal conduit as a cutaneous jejunostomy or use of double Roux-en-Y loops, avoiding any need for an enterostomy.

Resection of tumors

Nearly two thirds of childhood cancer occurs as solid malignancies. As is always the case, the therapy administered depends on the type of tumor. Examination and judicious investigation of all unusual masses are imperative. Thorough diagnostic workup and prompt definitive treatment may result in cure, even if the tumor is proved malignant. Chemotherapy and radiation therapy are adjuncts to surgical excision of tumors.

Wilms' tumor

Wilms' tumor, also known as nephroblastoma, is the most common intraabdominal childhood tumor. It presents as a painless mass whose enlargement may laterally distend the abdomen.

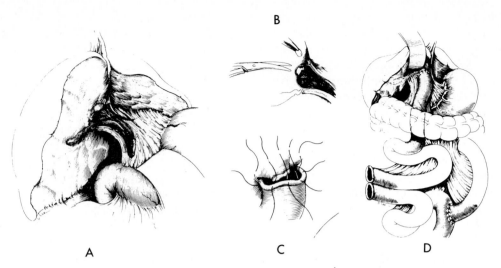

Fig. 29-11. The Kasai procedure. **A,** Exploration of hepaticoduodenal ligament and ligation of drainage structures. **B,** Transection of hepatic duct remnant using frozen section biopsies as a guide. **C,** Anastomosis of jejunal conduit at portahepatis. **D,** Exteriorization of conduit using double-barreled Roux-en-Y approach. (Reprinted with permission from Coran A.G., and others: Surgery of the neonate, Boston, 1978, Little, Brown and Co.)

Procedural considerations. The patient is positioned supine with a roll under the affected side. Both chest and abdomen are prepped. Infrequently, the tumor extends into the inferior vena cava as well as the atrium, and in such cases cardiopulmonary bypass should be readily available. Because of the possible need to clamp the inferior vena cava, lines are placed in the arms and neck. Clean gloves and instruments should be available for inspection of the contralateral kidney. Careful attention should be given when handling tumor and lymph nodes to avoid tumor spillage.

Operative procedure. If the tumor is operable, the following aspects are important:

1. The transabdominal approach, which may be extended to a combined transabdominal-transthoracic approach, is used to inspect abdominal contents and clamp the vessels of the renal pedicle before tumor dissection.
2. All suspicious lymph nodes are removed, placed in separate containers, and labeled. If no suspicious nodes are present, biopsies are obtained of those in adjacent areas.
3. The opposite kidney is explored before dissection of the tumor.
4. The extent of the tumor can be marked with hemostatic clips to facilitate radiation therapy.
5. The entire primary tumor is removed if doing so does not place the patient in jeopardy.
6. Any residual tumor is marked with clips.
7. Due to its close proximity to the kidney, the adrenal gland is usually removed.
8. The abdominal cavity and viscera are thoroughly inspected for evidence of tumor extension or metastases.

Extensive surgery may include partial colectomy or partial resection of the diaphragm.

Neuroblastoma

Neuroblastoma, one of the most common solid tumors of childhood, is a highly malignant tumor. It arises from neural crest tissue and can develop along any sympathetic ganglion chain, with the most common sites the retroperitoneum and adrenal medulla. The mass is usually firm, irregular, and nontender. It is a silent tumor in its early stages and metastasizes rapidly. Treatment includes an operation to ligate the tumor's blood supply and remove as much of the tumor as possible, as well as chemotherapy and radiation.

Sacrococcygeal teratoma

A sacrococcygeal teratoma is a tumor that originates early in embryonic cell division. The sacrococcygeal area is the most common extragonadal site of teratoma. The tumor presents as a large protuberance rising from the sacrococcygeal area. It may be irregular or symmetrical, varies in size, and may be pedunculated.

A sacrococcygeal teratoma is usually resectable in the newborn but may undergo malignant changes if not removed early in life. Tumors resected in the newborn period show microscopic evidence of malignant cells, but surgical cures have been achieved. Early surgical resection is important because these tumors are not sensitive to irradiation and are only temporarily responsive to chemotherapy.

The tumor is in the area of the sacrum and coccyx but may extend into the pelvis or abdomen. Resection is usually feasible by placing the patient in the Kraske's (jack-

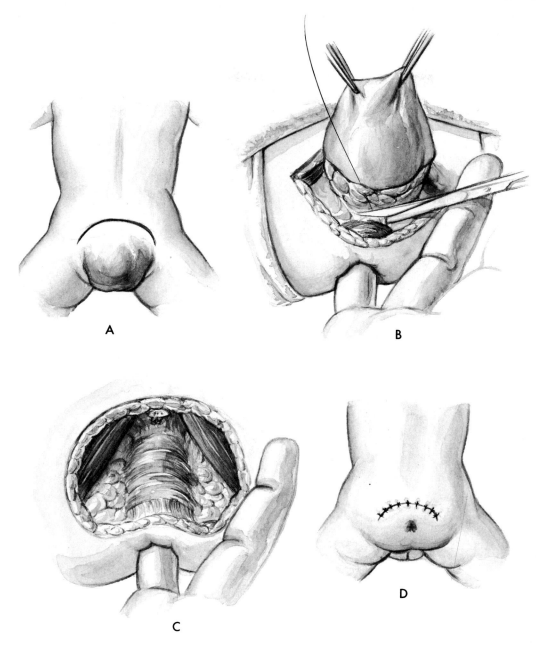

Fig. 29-12. Excision of sacrococcygeal teratoma. **A,** U-shaped incision. **B,** Dissection of teratoma. **C,** Tumor excised while rectum remains intact. **D,** Closed incisional line. (From Lewis, J.E.: Atlas of infant surgery, St. Louis, 1967, The C.V. Mosby Co.)

knife) position and excising the tumor mass and coccyx en bloc (Fig. 29-12).

Infrequently, in cases where the tumor extends high into the pelvis, an abdominal incision may be required in addition to the perineal approach.

Other surgical procedures

The following procedures require emergent colostomy at the time of presentation. Definitive repair of the anomaly usually occurs at about 1 year of age.

Resection and pullthrough for Hirschsprung's disease

Resection and pullthrough for Hirschsprung's disease, the definitive surgical procedure, consists of the removal of the aganglionic portion of the bowel and anastomosis of the normal colon to the anus. Hirschsprung's disease is characterized by the absence of ganglion cells in a distal portion of the bowel. The distal colon is more frequently involved, but the disease may encompass the entire colon, with a less favorable prognosis. The absence of ganglion cells results in a lack of peristalsis. The normal proximal colon becomes dilated, and abdominal contents do not pass through the involved segment. The child presents with an abnormally distended abdomen. On barium enema, proximal distention of the colon is seen, then a transition zone where the bowel appears funnel shaped, followed by the distal aganglionic segment, which is narrowed. The child is taken to the operating room for a "leveling" colostomy. Multiple frozen section biopsies of the muscularis of the proximal colon are done to determine the presence of ganglion cells. The colostomy is performed at the most distal portion of the colon that contains ganglion cells. Some surgeons prefer a routine right transverse colostomy at this time and delay frozen section biopsies until the time of the definitive procedure. The child is returned to the operating room for definitive repair at 1 year of age, if clinical and nutritional status permit.

Several surgical techniques have been devised. Soave's procedure of endorectal pullthrough employs internal bypass of the involved segment. The internal sphincter muscle of the anus is kept intact for continence.

Procedural considerations. The patient is prepped and draped from the nipples to and including the buttocks, genitals, perineal area, and upper thighs to permit positioning for the perineal stage without redraping. (Before preparation, the rectum may be irrigated with warm saline solution.)

A folded towel is placed under the buttocks. The patient is placed in the supine position with knees bent and legs in a modified "ski" position (hips and knees flexed) to facilitate abdominal and perineal approaches without redraping. An indwelling catheter is inserted to keep the bladder empty during the operation. The major instrument set, extra towels and gloves, as well as the following are required:

> Foley catheter (check size) and urimeter
> Kitners (30-60)
> Small Kocher forceps
> Medium Kocher forceps
> 2 Syringes, 3 cc
> 1 Syringe, 5 cc
> Needle, 25 G
> Injectable saline
> Penrose, ¼ inch
> Sterile safety pins
> Large rakes (dull)
> 3 Small tonsil suction tubes
> Hegar dilators

> *On second Mayo:*
> Minor set
> 6 extra curved mosquitos
> Small needle pad
> 2 Tonsil hemostats
> Penrose, ¼ inch
> Sterile safety pins
> Electrosurgical pencil, hand controlled
> Suction

Have available

Deaver retractors
Long instruments
GIA
Ligaclips
Extra #15 blades
Salem sump
K-Y Jelly
Red rubber catheter (22 to 24 Fr)
Mineral oil

Operative procedure

1. A left paramedian incision that includes the sigmoid colonic stoma, if present, is made.
2. The stoma is freed from the abdominal wall, and the left colon is mobilized. (If there is no sigmoid colonic stoma, the extent of aganglionic intestine is established by biopsy and frozen section, and all involved colon excised. If a stoma is present and the area has already been established as normal, the colon above it consititutes the proximal end of the resection.)
3. The mesocolon and the vessels of the intestine to be resected are divided close to the intestine, with care taken to preserve the blood supply to the rectum (Fig. 29-13, *A*).
4. The mucosal tube is freed from the outer muscular layers by sharp and blunt dissection with Metzenbaum scissors and a gauze-tipped instrument (Fig. 29-13, *B*).
5. A muscular sleeve is transected, and traction sutures of silk no. 4-0 are placed on the distal edge (Fig. 29-13, *C*). The mucosa is stripped down to the anus. The depth of the dissection may be checked by inserting a finger in the anus (Fig. 29-13, *D*).
6. When the mucosa is adequately freed, the perineal phase is started, and the perineal instrument table is used.
7. The anus is dilated and retracted with Allis forceps. A circumferential incision is made, and the mucosal stripping is completed (Fig. 29-13, *E*).
8. The proximal portion of the intestine is pulled through the rectal muscular sleeve and out the anus (Fig. 29-13, *F*). If the portion of colon to be resected is large, it is excised abdominally before the proximal portion of the intestine is pulled through the anus.
9. Absorbable sutures are used to secure the seromuscular layers of the intussuscepted colon to the rectal muscular cuff. The colon is divided into axial or longitudinal quadrants, and an anastomosis is performed with no. 3-0 absorbable sutures (Fig. 29-13, *G*).
10. Gowns and gloves are changed, and abdominal instruments are used. The abdominal phase of the operation is completed by approximating the proximal edge of the muscular cuff to the seromuscular layer of the colon with silk no. 4-0 sutures (Fig. 29-13, *H*). The abdomen is closed in the routine manner, without the use of drains.

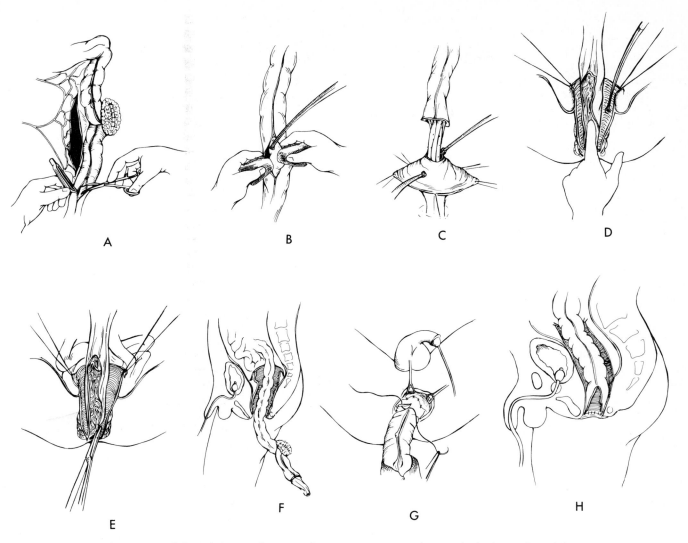

Fig. 29-13. Pull through for Hirschsprung's disease. **A,** Dissection of mucosal tube begun through longitudinal incision. **B,** Gauze-tipped dissecting instrument used to dissect entire circumference of tube. **C,** Muscular sleeve transected. **D,** Depth of dissection determined by inserting finger in anus. **E,** Circumferential incision made. **F,** Mucosal tube and proximal portion of colon and stoma pulled through rectal muscular cuff. **G,** Anastomosis performed between all layers of colon and anal mucosa. **H,** Anastomosis completed. (Modified from Boley, S.J.: An endorectal pull-through operation with primary anastomosis for Hirschsprung's disease, Surg. Gynecol. Obstet. 127(2):353, Aug. 1968. By permission of *Surgery, Gynecology, and Obstetrics*.)

Repair of imperforate anus

An imperforate anus is repaired by establishing colorectoanal continuity through the external anal sphincter and closure of fistulas, if present. Imperforate anus presents in a variety of forms classified as low, intermediate, or high lesions. Females commonly present with low lesions, and males primarily exhibit high lesions. A covered anus and anovulvar fistula is an example of a low lesion. A high lesion consists of a blind rectal pouch, a "flat bottom," and a posterior urethral fistula or fistula to the bladder. This type is the most prevalent and the most difficult to repair.

Repair of low imperforate anus in a female: anal transposition

Procedural considerations. The infant is placed in the lithotomy position with the legs extended on skis. A Foley catheter is inserted, and the perineum is prepped and draped. The major instrument set is required, with the addition of the following:

Extra towels
Needle-point electrosurgical tip
Suction
Nasal speculums
Small tonsil suction tube

Senn retractors
Foley catheter (check size) and urimeter
Kittner dissectors
Penrose, ½ inch
Sterile rubber bands with small brass safety pins
K-Y jelly
Hegar dilators
Vaseline gauze
Nerve stimulator

Operative procedure

1. An electrical stimulator is applied to define the center of the true anus.
2. Stay sutures are placed in the fistula, and it is excised using an oval incision (Fig. 29-14, *A*).
3. The bowel is dissected free from surrounding struc-

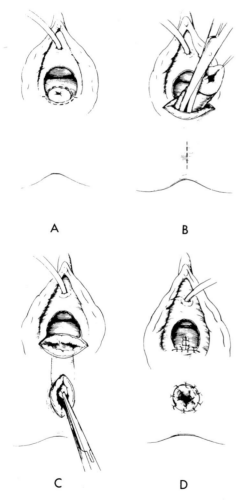

Fig. 29-14. Anal transposition. **A,** Fistula excised using oval incision. **B,** Dissection of bowel from surrounding structures. **C,** Vertical midline incision at site of true anus; identification of external sphincter fibers; mobilized rectum pulled down through subcutaneous tissue to new location. **D,** External sphincter sutured to rectal mucosa; new anus constructed with interrupted sutures through all layers. (Reprinted with permission from Coran, A.G., and others: Surgery of the neonate, Boston, 1978, Little, Brown and Co.)

tures, with care taken not to damage the vagina (Fig. 29-14, *B*).
4. When the dissection is complete, a vertical midline incision is performed at the opening of the true anus, and the fibers of the external sphincter are identified (Fig. 29-14, *C*).
5. The mobilized rectum is pulled down through the subcutaneous tissue to its new location.
6. The end of the fistula is amputated. With interrupted sutures of 4-0 silk, the external sphincter is sutured to the rectal serosa.
7. Using 4-0 Dexon, a new anus is constructed with interrupted sutures through all layers (Fig. 29-14, *D*).
8. A drain may or may not be placed in the anterior incision before it is closed in layers with interrupted 4-0 Dexon sutures. A Hegar dilator is used to calibrate the size of the new anus after closure.

Repair of high imperforate anus: the posterior sagittal anorectoplasty

When a high imperforate anal anomaly presents, surgical intervention is indicated within 24 to 48 hours of life. A transverse or sigmoid colostomy is performed to irrigate the hiatal lumen and to remove meconium plugs while allowing proximal colon function. After the colostomy, further diagnostic studies, such as cystogram and vaginograms are done. The posterior sagittal anorectoplasty (PSARP) is the definitive surgical procedure and is performed when the condition and size of the child permits, usually around 1 year of age.

The PSARP is a highly technical procedure that utilizes electrostimulation throughout and may require position changes (Fig. 29-15).

Procedural considerations. The child is placed in a prone jackknife position with the hips flexed. Adequate padding must be placed under the hips to avoid compression injury to the femoral nerves. The major instrument set is required with the addition of the following:

Foley catheter (check size) and urimeter
Catheter tray (disposable)
Muscle stimulator and probe
Needle-point electrosurgical tip
Feeding tubes, 5 Fr and 8 Fr
Mastoid retractors
Senn retractors
Stevens tenotomy scissors
Marking pen
Hegar dilators
K-Y jelly

Operative procedure

1. The electrostimulator is used to locate the true anus, and a midsagittal incision is made through the skin from the midsacrum to the anterior border of the anal site.
2. Dissection continues through subcutaneous tissue until the external sphincter muscle layers are identified.

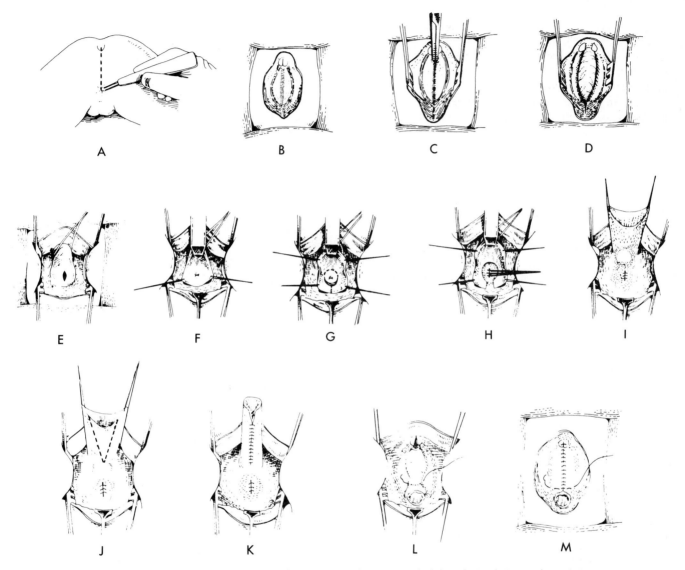

Fig. 29-15. Posterior sagittal anorectoplasty. **A,** Line of incision and electrical stimulation to determine appropriate anal site. **B,** Midsagittal incision through the coccyx and the external sphincter fibers of the anus, showing the striated muscle complex deep to the anal site; subcutaneous external sphincter extending about halfway to the coccyx; superficial external sphincter inserting on the coccyx; levator deeper in midline. **C,** Right-angled forceps beneath levator ani. **D,** All layers of striated muscle partially retracted laterally exposing visceral endopelvic fascia. **E,** Sagittal incision in terminal bowel after proximal dissection around rectum and placement of a tape around the rectum proximally. **F,** Retracted rectotomy showing fistula site. **G,** Hemicircumferential incision through mucosa-submucosa for placement of first sutures to close fistula. **H,** Completed closure of the fistula orifice. **I,** Stippled area where muscular bowel wall is left in place and clear area above where periotoneum may be encountered. **J** (dotted line), The extent of anterior wedge resection for tapered repair of rectum. **K,** Approximation of the tapered edges of rectum. **L,** First and deepest suture for approximation of the levators to establish the beginning of the canal. **M,** After reapproximation of the levator ani to the coccyx, interrupted sutures are placed in the edges of the superficial external sphincter muscle. (From de Vries, P.A.: Posterior sagittal anorectoplasty. In Holmann v. Kap-herr, S., editor: Anorektale Fehlbildungen. Stuttgart, Gustav Fischer Verlag, 1984. Reprinted with permission.)

3. With electrostimulation, these fibers are dissected midsagittally, exactly in the midline.

4. A midsagittal split of the coccyx is performed, and the striated muscle complex found beneath the coccyx is incised sagittally along with the visceral endopelvic fascia. Electrostimulation is used to aid in identifying muscle complexes.

5. Next the rectal pouch and urethra are identified, and the bowel is incised vertically to expose the fistula.

6. The fistula is closed in layers, first the mucosa with interrupted absorbable sutures and then the muscle layer with 5-0 Prolene.

7. The rectum is then mobilized and tapered to allow its placement within the muscle complexes. Tapering consists of excising a wedge of bowel from either the ventral or dorsal surface. The edges are approximated and the mucosal layer closed with 5-0 absorbable interrupted sutures. The muscularis layer is closed with interrupted 5-0 Prolene sutures.

8. Again using electrostimulation, the tapered rectum is placed deep within the muscle complex. Then 5-0 Prolene sutures are used to reconstruct the muscles. The seromuscular layer of the bowel is incorporated into these sutures to keep it securely positioned within the muscle complex.

9. The external sphincter muscles and coccyx are reapproximated.

10. Excess bowel is trimmed before securing it to the skin edges of the anus.

11. Running absorbable subcuticular sutures are used to close the skin.

In cases of very high rectal pouches and fistulas, an abdominal approach may be required. At this point, after the midsagittal incisions and dissections are completed, a rubber tube is placed through the pelvis with one end in the peritoneal cavity and the other through the center of the anus to the skin, where it is temporarily sutured. The child is turned supine, and an abdominal incision is performed. The rectal pouch is mobilized and the fistula closed. The bowel is tapered as described previously, and the terminal portion is attached to the rubber tube, which then is used to pull the rectum through the anal orifice. The bowel is sutured to the muscle complex, and reapproximation of the coccyx and external sphincter muscle is done as described earlier.

BIBLIOGRAPHY

Alagille, D.: Extrahepatic biliary atresia, Hepatology 4:7S, 1984.

Altman, R.P., and Stolar, C.J.: Pediatric hepatobiliary disease, Surg. Clin. North Am. 65:1245, 1985.

Anderson, K.D.: Congenital diaphragmatic hernia. In Welsh, K.J., and others, editors: Pediatric surgery, ed. 4, Chicago, 1986, Year Book Medical Publishers.

Anderson, K.D.: Esophageal replacement. In Welsh, K.J., and others, editors: Pediatric surgery, ed. 4, Chicago, 1986, Year Book Medical Publishers.

Atkinson, L.J., and Kohn, M.L.: Berry and Kohn's introduction to operating room technique, ed. 6, New York, 1986, McGraw-Hill.

Bates, T.A., and Broome, M.: Preparation of children for hospitalization and surgery: a review of the literature, J. Pediatr. Nurs. 1:230, 1986.

Benson, C.D.: Infantile hypertrophic pyloric stenosis. In Welsh, K.J., and others, editors: Pediatric surgery, ed. 4, Chicago 1986, Year Book Medical Publishers.

Bishop, H.C.: Ileostomy and colostomy. In Welsh, K.J., and others, editors: Pediatric surgery, ed. 4, Chicago, 1986, Year Book Medical Publishers.

Boix-Ochoa, J.: Gastroesophageal reflux. In Welsh, K.J., and others, editors: Pediatric surgery, ed. 4, Chicago, 1986, Year Book Medical Publishers.

Coran, A.G., Behrendt, D.M., Weintraub, W.H., and Lee, D.C.: Surgery of the neonate, Boston, 1978, Little, Brown and Co.

Cox, J.A.: Inguinal hernia of childhood, Surg. Clin. North Am. 65:1331, 1985.

Cullen, M.L., Klein, M.D., and Philippart, A.I.: Congenital diaphragmatic hernia, Surg. Clin. North Am. 66:1115, 1985.

deVries, P.A., and Cox, K.L.: Surgery of anorectal anomalies, Surg. Clin. North Am. 65:1139, 1985.

deVries, P.A., and Pena, A.: Anorectal malformations—posterior sagittal anorectoplasty for intermediate and high imperforate anus anomalies. In Welsh, K.J., and others, editors: Pediatric surgery, ed. 4, Chicago, 1986, Year Book Medical Publishers.

deVries, P.A., and Pena, A.: Posterior sagittal anorectoplasty, J. Pediatr. Surg. 17:638, 1982.

Donovan, E.F.: Perioperative care of the surgical neonate, Surg. Clin. North Am. 65:1061, 1985.

Frentner, S.: Abdominal wall defects: omphalocele and gastroschisis, Neonatal Network, Dec. 29, 1987.

Grosfield, J.L.: Neuroblastoma. In Welsh, K.J., and others, editors: Pediatric surgery, ed. 4, Chicago, 1986, Year Book Medical Publishers.

Hatch, E.I., and Baxter, R.: Surgical options in the management of large omphaloceles, Am. J. Surg. 153:449, 1987.

Hersh, S.P.: Psychological implications of operations in children. In Welsh, K.J., and others, editors: Pediatric surgery, ed. 4, Chicago, 1986, Year Book Medical Publishers.

Johnson, D.G.: Current thinking on the role of surgery in gastroesophageal reflux, Pediatr. Clin. North Am. 32:1165,1985.

Kneedler, J.A., and Dodge, G.H.: Perioperative patient care, ed. 2, Boston, 1987, Blackwell Scientific Publications.

Lampkin, B.C., and others: Solid malignancies in children and adolescents, Surg. Clin. North Am. 65:1351, 1985.

Lilly, J.R.: Biliary atresia: the jaundiced infant. In Welsh, K.J., and others, editors: Pediatric surgery, ed. 4, Chicago, 1986, Year Book Medical Publishers.

McConnell, E.A.: Clinical considerations in perioperative nursing, Philadelphia, 1987, J.B. Lippincott Co.

Mackie, R., Peddie, R., and Pendleton, R.: Perioperative care plan guides, AORN J., 40:192, 1984.

Martin, L.W., and Alexander, F.: Esophageal atresia, Surg. Clin. North Am. 65:1099, 1985.

Martin, L.W., and Torres, A.M.: Omphalocle and gastroschisis, Surg. Clin. North Am. 65:1235, 1985.

Martin, L.W., and Torres, A.M.: Hirschsprung's disease, Surg. Clin. North Am. 65:1171, 1985.

Othersen, H.B.: Wilms' tumor. In Welsh, K.J., and others, editors: Pediatric surgery, ed. 4, Chicago, 1986, Year Book Medical Publishers.

Pena, A.: Surgical management of anorectal malformations: a unified concept, Pediatr. Surg. Int. 3:82, 1988.

Randolph, J.G.: Esophageal atresia and congenital stenosis. In Welsh, K.J., and others, editors: Pediatric surgery, ed. 4, Chicago, 1986, Year Book Medical Publishers.

Randolph, J.G.: Experience with the Nissen fundoplication for correction of gasteoesophageal reflux in infants, Ann. Surg. 198:579, 1983.

Ravitch, M.M.: Intussusception. In Welsh, K.J., and others, editors: Pediatric surgery, ed. 4, Chicago, 1986, Year Book Medical Publishers.

Rodgers, B.M.: Gastrostomy: indications and technique. In Welsh, K.J., and others, editors: Pediatric surgery, ed. 4, Chicago, 1986, Year Book Medical Publishers.

Rushton, C.H.: The surgical neonate: principles of nursing management, Pediatr. Nurs. 14:141, 1988.

Schuster, S.R.: Omphalocele and gastroschisis. In Welsh, and others, editors: Pediatric surgery, ed. 4, Chicago, 1986, Year Book Medical Publishers.

Shaw, A.: Disorders of the umbilicus. In Welsh, K.J., and others, editors: Pediatric surgery, ed. 4, Chicago, 1986, Year Book Medical Publishers.

Sickler, W.K.: Hirschsprung's disease. In Welsh, K.J., and others, editors: Pediatric surgery, ed. 4, Chicago, 1986, Year Book Medical Publishers.

Stevenson, R.J.: Non-neonatal intestinal obstruction, Surg. Clin. North Am. 65:1217, 1985.

Templeton, J.A., and O'Neill, J.A.: Anorectal malformations. In Welsh, K.J., and others, editors: Pediatric surgery, ed. 4, Chicago, 1986, Year Book Medical Publishers.

Tiche, S., Dobson, J., and Otker, L.: Pediatric teaching, AORN J., 39:793, 1984.

Vane, D.W., West, K.W., and Grosfield, J.L.: Hirschsprung's disease: current management, Perinatology-Neonatology, Nov/Dec 1987, p. 26.

Ward, H.C., and Brereton, R.J.: Cervical repair of esophageal atresia, J. Pediatr. Surg. 23:802, 1988.

Whaley, L.F., and Wong, D.J.: Nursing care of infants and children, ed. 4, St. Louis, 1990, The C.V. Mosby Co.

Wilkins, S., and Pena, A.: The role of colostomy in anorectal malformations, Pediatr. Surg. Int. 3:105, 1988.

Woolley, M.M.: Teratoma. In Welsh, K.J., and others, editors: Pediatric surgery, ed. 4, Chicago, 1986, Year Book Medical Publishers.

30 Geriatric surgery

PATRICIA FELICE MECKES

As a biologic process, aging has changed little in the last 300 years. We age neither faster nor slower than we did in Colonial America, and our maximum life span has not changed substantially. Essentially, we will enjoy a period of sustained but undramatic growth in the elderly population for the next 20 years. Beginning in the year 2010, however, with the aging of the baby boom, the gerontology boom will emerge, whether we're prepared for it or not.

The older population, which includes those 65 and older, numbered 28.5 million in 1985 and represented 12% of the U.S. population. The number of older Americans increased by 2.8 million or 11% since 1980, compared with an increase of 4% for the under-65 population. By 2030 there will be about 65 million older persons, which represents 2½ times their number in 1980. If current fertility and immigration levels remain stable, the only age groups to experience significant growth in the next century will be those past 55 (AARP, 1986).

Another important trend is the estimated 25,000 centenarians in the United States, a number that is rapidly increasing. Now surpassing the 80 to 85 age group, the 100+ elderly are the fastest-growing age group among the over-65 United States population. The Census Bureau, generally conservative in its estimates of the aged population thus far, now predicts an astonishing 1 million American centenarians by the year 2050 and close to 2 million of them by 2080. Advances in health care and the treatment and prevention of disease may mean that the average percentage of centenarians within each generation—currently about 1%—could increase to 2% or more in future years (Brandt, 1988).

Translating these demographics into health care trends produces even more startling implications for perioperative care. As a result of the "graying" of America, the health care business will never be the same. Adults over 65 currently account for 41% of all hospital bed days, but by 2000 the figure will rise to 58%. Older Americans will become health care's primary consumers (Dychtwald and Zitter, 1987).

Of all persons age 60 and over, 50% will require surgery before they die, and those over 75 will require one-third more surgery than all other age groups. Prior to discharge, older adults in acute hospitals will require surgical intervention 40% more often than any other age group.

This dramatic growth in elderly (over 65) and aged (over 85) surgical patients necessitates an astute awareness by the perioperative nurse in recognizing the special needs of these patients. Understanding how normal aging changes and chronic disease impact the successful outcome of any surgical procedure is of utmost importance and will therefore be the major emphasis of this chapter.

PERIOPERATIVE NURSING CONSIDERATIONS
Preliminary evaluation

Before an elderly patient actually arrives in the operating room for surgery, many preliminary decisions are made by the physician to determine whether the benefit of surgery outweighs potential risks. In the not too distant past, the attitude of some surgeons was to avoid surgery in geriatric patients until all nonsurgical modalities were exhausted. Because surgical morbidity and mortality increase with age, the surgeon's reluctance is understandable. Most surgeons now tend to agree, however, that age alone is not a contraindication to surgery. More recently attitudes have changed toward a more aggressive approach and a belief that surgical risk can be substantially reduced by careful evaluation preoperatively.

The decision for surgery is within the purview of the physician, but nurses should be aware of its implications. Important factors that need to be evaluated are: (1) life expectancy versus the natural course of the disease; (2) comfort versus complications; (3) motivation versus chronic morbidity; and (4) risk of nonoperative management versus hazards of surgical failure (Ferris, 1976).

1. *Life expectancy versus natural course of disease.* If the patient has surpassed the expected norm for number of years of survival (persons reaching age 65 in 1985 had a life expectancy of 18.6 years for females and 14.6 years for males), surgical intervention may not be appropriate if the prognosis of the disease is poor. Conversely, if the patient has several years of life expectancy left and the prognosis is good, surgical treatment may be the treatment of choice.

2. *Comfort versus complications.* The need for independence is of utmost importance to elderly persons,

and they are far more interested in maintaining health than longevity. Complications of surgery are not well tolerated by the elderly and can quickly develop into life-threatening situations. If surgical intervention will further incapacitate an already debilitated individual, alternative treatment should be considered. However, if surgery will help to alleviate debilitating conditions and improve independence, it should be considered an appropriate modality of care.

3. *Motivation versus chronic mortality.* Many elderly patients are reluctant to undergo surgery. They are concerned that the surgery will not improve their quality of life and that it will make them more dependent on others or destine them to a life in a care facility. In addition, they do not want to withstand the pain, discomfort, and rigors of surgery and the recuperative period necessary to treat a condition that does not really bother them all that much anyway. This lack of motivation will have a negative impact on the results of the surgery. The decision then becomes whether the chronic morbidity of the disease or the mortality risk of surgery on an unmotivated patient is less detrimental to the patient. Patients who show a strong sense of determination in doing all that is necessary to get well and stay well will be more likely candidates for surgery than those who believe illness is a prelude to death. Obviously the outcome of surgery is enhanced if the patient is motivated to have a positive result.

4. *Risk of nonoperative management versus hazards of surgical failure.* Mortality rates for emergency surgery in elderly patients is double that of elective surgery. When an acute emergency condition taxes an already overburdened physiologic state, the chances of survival are less likely. The elderly patient's family can take no consolation in knowing that the surgical procedure was successful even though their loved one died. In order to increase the chances of survival from a surgical procedure, the elderly person must be in optimum condition, and adequate preoperative assessment and preparation must precede an elective procedure.

Another important consideration relates to the extent of surgical treatment. Should it be radical, modified, or staged (Vowles, 1979)? The decision for the extent of surgery relies heavily on the patient's physical status at the time of surgery and how extensively the disease has progressed. The surgeon may justify a radical procedure if it will enhance the elderly person's life.

Assessment

In elderly persons a preoperative medical assessment is conducted mainly to determine present physiologic functioning so that operative risk will be identified and post-

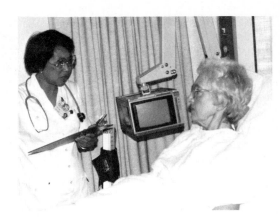

Fig. 30-1. Allowing the elderly person to respond to questions independently, without prompting from family members, helps maintain the patient's dignity and control.

operative complications minimized and to establish the presence and status of any concomitant disease process that could negatively affect the outcome of the surgery. The preoperative nursing assessment is conducted to establish presurgical baseline data so that health status changes, primarily during the intraoperative and postoperative periods, will be more readily recognized.

Using chronologic age as a valid predictor of a patient's response to surgery is not advisable. A person of 75 can be in better physiologic and psychologic condition for surgery than a much younger person. Using biologic age as a measurement criterion is much more reliable. Establishing biologic age, however, becomes the greatest challenge. Chronic conditions may interfere with the elderly person's ability to distinguish between recent and long-standing ailments. Therefore, the preoperative interview, especially in elderly persons, should be conducted in a quiet, relaxed environment with as few distractions as possible. The elderly person should be allowed to respond to each question independently without prompting from a spouse or other family members unless absolutely necessary (Fig. 30-1). This helps to maintain the patient's dignity, independence, and control, which are extremely important to the older adult.

Normal age-related changes

In general, the aging process imposes a decline in organ functions, altered responses to pain and temperature, alterations in pharmacokinetics, and atypical signs and symptoms of disease, all of which may vary from one elderly person to the next. Having a clear understanding of normal age changes helps to establish appropriate nursing diagnoses and care plan development. The following review of systems focuses on age-specific changes of particular importance to perioperative care planning.

Physiologic changes

Integumentary system. The skin loses elasticity and subcutaneous fat and becomes more prone to shear force and pressure injury. Because of the thinness of the skin and small vessel fragility, hemorrhaging is quite common. The skin tends to be dry and lack turgor, which may or may not be attributed to dehydration.

Respiratory system. Lungs lose elasticity, which contributes to an increase in functional residual capacity, residual volume, and dead space. Calcification of costal cartilages, dorsal kyphosis, and osteoporosis results in a rigid chest wall. Muscles responsible for inhalation and exhalation may be weakened, resulting in a diminished ability to increase and decrease the size of the thoracic cavity. All these changes contribute to a minimal tidal exchange that makes the elderly patient more susceptible to pulmonary complications.

Cardiovascular system. A 35% decrease in coronary artery blood flow is more likely in elderly persons. Because of a shift in blood flow, there is a greater decrease in circulation to the kidneys and liver than to the brain and heart. Blood pressure rises as a result of increased arterial resistance. When the elderly person is at rest, the heart rate remains approximately the same as that of a younger person. However, the older heart requires a longer recovery time after each beat, which means that it reacts poorly to stress and anxiety-produced tachycardia. In general, the capacity of the cardiovascular system to tolerate and buffer insults is limited.

Digestive system. The secretion of salivary and digestive glands decreases, mucus becomes thicker, and saliva becomes more alkaline. Decrease in peristalsis and a reduction of gastric motility—results of muscle tone loss—cause a delay in stomach emptying. The absorption of drugs is affected because of a reduction of blood flow to abdominal viscera, hydrochloric acid, and delayed gastric emptying. Decrease of total body water and plasma volume results in a smaller volume of distribution for water-soluble drugs. Lean body mass decreases and the percentage of body fat increases, which increases the volume of distribution and storage of lipophilic drugs such as diazepam and lidocaine (Galazka, 1988). These factors are of particular importance for assessing the patient's response to preoperative, anesthetic, and postoperative medications.

Urinary system. Nephrons decrease in function with age so that by age 75 a person has probably lost a third to a half of original nephron function. Elasticity and tone are lost in the ureters, bladder, and urethra, which leads to incomplete emptying of the bladder. Benign prostatic hypertrophy is almost universal, as it is found in 70% of elderly male patients. Total bladder capacity also declines, so that elderly persons experience a more frequent and urgent need to urinate. Because blood flow to the kidneys is decreased, elimination of drugs through these organs is affected. The danger lies in the possible cumulative and adverse effects of drugs. Close observation and consideration of the impact of age-related changes on the kidneys are extremely important during the perioperative period. During this period of the patient's hospital stay, the greatest number and variety of drugs are given, increasing the chances for adverse and consequential results.

Musculoskeletal system. A significant change in the elderly person's skeleton is the loss of bone mass, which contributes to skeletal instability and makes fractures of the hip and vertebrae very common in aged persons. Curvature of the spine and arthritis of the joints are also commonplace. Back pain is related to dehydration and decreased flexibility of the vertebral disks. Poor posture tends to be proportional to the degree of back pain experienced and may greatly compromise internal organ function.

Nervous system. Although not functionally significant, a steady loss of neurons begins at about age 25. Inappropriate or slow response to stimuli is primarily a result of a decrease in some organ systems of the ability to send reliable messages to the brain and spinal cord. Nerve cells are particularly sensitive to lack of oxygen. Because elderly persons may have, in varying degrees, cerebral arteriosclerosis and atherosclerosis, decreased blood flow and nervous system deficits such as insomnia, irritability, visual motor deficits, and memory loss are not uncommon. Other neurologic changes significant to perioperative care include a loss of position sense in the toes, decreased tactile sense, and an increased tolerance to pain. In addition, benign hypothermia (temperature below 98.6° F) is a common problem in the elderly. In the operating room, thermoregulatory balance between heat gain (metabolic production, muscular contraction, and hot ambient temperature) and heat loss (radiation, convection, evaporation, ventilation, cold fluid infusion, blood loss, antithermoregulatory drugs, and impaired heat production) is difficult at best to maintain in older surgical patients (Biddle and Biddle, 1985).

Sensory changes. Sensory changes in vision, hearing, and cognition may have an impact on the patient's response to care. Farsightedness or presbyopia is a result of the lens becoming more rigid and less pliable. Consequently, visual acuity and accommodation are decreased. Color perception changes, due to a yellowing of the lens, make distinguishing blue, green, and purple more difficult for the elderly person. Of particular importance in the operating room is an awareness of the older person's difficulty in adapting to changes in light. Moving patients from a dimly lit holding area to the bright lights of the operating room can cause momentary "blindness."

Presbycusis, or loss of hearing sensitivity, is irreversible, bilateral, and primarily sensorineural, although metabolic and mechanical causes are also possible. It is the most frequent cause of hearing loss in the geriatric patient. Hearing loss, which appears to be greater in men than women, is mostly within the higher frequencies (above

1000 Hz). In addition, cerumen thickens and the eardrum becomes less pliable, which also contribute to diminished hearing. Often geriatric patients are labeled confused or senile because they respond inappropriately to questions they did not hear or describe what they see inaccurately because of poor vision.

Psychologic changes

Physiologic and psychologic stress may result in confusion in the geriatric patient, which is analogous to convulsions in the pediatric patient. In the elderly, mental change is more significant than a rise of temperature or blood pressure and can be a warning of some underlying problem. Confusion should therefore not be dismissed as an expected behavior of the geriatric patient who is, after all, just "senile." The most important assessment factor is to determine whether the confusion is chronic or acute. Chronic conditions such as depression and Alzheimer's disease can make communication with the patient difficult. Depending on the stage of disease, patients may or may not be able to understand explanations. Family members are the best resource in determining the patient's ability to comprehend and respond to questions and/or instructions. Behavioral changes such as aggressiveness, agitation, and paranoia are not uncommon. Restraints may be necessary in the operating room to assure patient safety. Taking the time to talk slowly, being deliberate in movements, getting to know the patient, and developing a trusting relationship prior to surgery can help to lessen the patient's anxiety and control the combative outbursts that occur in some Alzheimer patients.

Acute confusional states in the elderly can be precipitated by any number of conditions (Charatan, 1976). Some of the most common causes of acute confusion that might be seen in the geriatric surgical patient are: embolus or thrombosis, cardiac arrhythmia, diabetes, anemia, hemorrhage, B_{12} deficiency, infection, tranquilizers, sedatives, cardiovascular drugs, (diuretics, antihypertensives, and digitalis), fecal impaction, urinary bladder distention, dehydration, and electrolyte imbalance. Even the disruption of relocation into the hospital, which brings the patient into an unfamiliar environment, can cause acute confusion, particularly during the postoperative period. Validation of the patient's previous mental state with a relative or significant other can help to determine if the onset occurred since hospitalization.

Routine laboratory and diagnostic tests

The physiologic changes of aging do not significantly alter the diagnostic values of CBC, urinalysis, and blood chemistries; therefore, abnormalities should be evaluated. The chest x-ray may reveal increased AP diameter, osteopenia, and degenerative joint disease. The heart size should appear normal, even in the elderly. Cardiomegaly can contribute to postoperative complications and should be eval-

uated (Seymour and others, 1982). The ECG may show P-wave notching, ST depression, and T-wave flattening or inversion. An increase in bundle branch block, hemiblock, and first-degree block may also be noted, largely as a result of degenerative disease of the conduction system. Other diagnostic tests that are considered important for elderly surgical patients are hemoglobin or hematocrit, BUN, glucose, and arterial blood gases. Serum electrolytes should be evaluated when patients are on diuretics because muscle relaxants, mechanical ventilation, and IV fluids can exacerbate an electrolyte disturbance (Katz, 1985).

Because most elderly patients are on several medications, assessing their drug history is important. Ordinarily digoxin and nitroglycerin are stopped during the perioperative period, whereas diuretics and antihypertensives may be taken as needed but not used routinely during the postoperative period. Any patient who had been receiving steroids within the previous 12 months should receive parenteral steroids starting the evening before surgery and continuing through the initial postoperative course.

Control of diabetes is often difficult during the perioperative period. For patients on oral hypoglycemics, the medication is stopped and serum glucose and urinary sugar closely monitored. Long-acting parenteral insulin is discontinued, and regular insulin is given during the preoperative period. Patients who are fasting the morning of surgery should have an IV inserted with 5% dextrose and water and receive half their usual morning dose of insulin. Thereafter, until the patient assumes a normal diet, serum glucose levels and urine fractionals are covered as necessary with insulin.

Additional assessment data

Another very important but often overlooked area of assessment is dental evaluation. The condition of the patient's temporomandibular joint and the presence of mouth pathology can make the difference between a smooth and safe anesthetic and a disaster. Mouth pathology, like any number of physiologic, psychologic, or social factors, can affect the nutritional condition of the patient. Many elderly persons simply do not care to eat because of ill-fitting dentures or poor dentition.

Life changes can also affect the nutritional state. Of particular importance are the losses endured with aging such as the loss of one's spouse, family, or friends through death or relocation; loss of a prior standard of living through retirement; or loss of physical or mental well-being. These changes can affect older persons to the point that they either cannot afford to buy nutritious foods or lose the ability or interest to prepare food. The ultimate effect, among other things, is a nutritionally debilitated patient. Therefore, any nutritional deficits should be corrected prior to surgery because the success of the operative procedure, the rate of wound healing, and the length of hospital stay are directly related to the nutritional state.

Determination of operative risk

After assessment of the patient occurs, any number of medical conditions may be identified which can add to the patient's operative risk (see the box below). Whenever possible, these conditions are treated medically before surgery. Sometimes correction is not possible, and the risk of forestalling surgery outweighs any other medical prob-

---

RISK FACTORS FOR SURGERY IN ELDERLY PATIENTS

General
Dehydration
Anemia
Malignancy
Recent stroke
Acute confusion, depression, dementia, pseudodementia

Cardiovascular
Recent myocardial infarction
Unstable arrhythmias
Decompensated congestive heart failure
Unstable angina
Uncontrolled hypertension

Pulmonary
Infection
Decompensated chronic obstructive lung disease
Smoking

Gastrointestinal/nutritional
Active peptic ulcer disease
Hepatic insufficiency
Severe malnutrition

Endocrine
Adrenal insufficiency
Hypothyroidism or hyperthyroidism
Uncontrolled diabetes

Genitourinary
Infection
Obstruction

From Barry, P.P.: Primary care evaluation of the elderly for elective surgery, Geriatrics 42:77, 1987. Copyright © 1987 by Geriatrics. Reprinted by permission.

---

lem. The determination of operative risk of the patient is generally based on the physical status scale of the American Society of Anesthesiologists (Dripps and others, 1988). Although the actual classification of the patient is done by the anesthesiologist or anesthetist, noting the parameters from which a decision is made is important.

Class 1: No evidence of physiologic, biochemical, or psychiatric disturbance; the condition necessitating surgery is not systemic
Class 2: Mild to moderate systemic disturbance from the condition requiring surgery or other processes
Class 3: Severe systemic disturbances
Class 4: Severe systemic disturbances of a life-threatening nature that may or may not be correctable with surgery
Class 5: The patient is in serious condition with little chance of survival

In general, patients 80 years old and older are classified as Class 2 and are considered at higher risk based solely on their age (Galazka, 1988).

Preoperative education

The preoperative interview is also an opportune time to evaluate the patient's psychosocial status and educational needs. As previously mentioned, the motivation of the patient can have an effect on operative risk and successful surgical outcomes. Being astutely aware of the patient's emotional status is on a par with evaluation of physiologic status. Many times the patient's concerns are focused on spouse or other family members rather than on the impending surgery. An unexpected hospitalization can be very disruptive to an elderly patient who perhaps was the sole caretaker of an ill spouse, a parent, or even a pet. The worry of how that individual or pet will be cared for can have an effect on the surgical outcome. In addition, the concern for quality of life and the fear of institutionalization after surgery can be extremely upsetting. Utilizing the assistance of the social worker to arrange for resources may help to allay the patient's concerns.

Family members who are present should be included in the preoperative educational session for teaching the patient about perioperative routines. Assuring that postoperative routines such as turning, coughing, deep breathing, and leg exercises are understood and performed correctly is especially important. Having backup support from a family member helps to assure successful outcomes.

Education should be conducted at a time when the patient is at rest rather than during preoperative preparations. Too much stimuli from outside sources can interfere with the patient's ability to concentrate and motivation to learn. Giving the patient postoperative instructions in written form also helps to assure successful outcomes. The written instructions, used as an immediate reference, allow elderly persons to maintain some control over their own care without continually having to ask for help from others. Patients should, however, be made aware that assistance is available when needed.

Nursing diagnoses for geriatric surgical patients

In evaluating, synthesizing, and prioritizing the data collected during the preoperative assessment, the perioperative nurse can formulate nursing diagnoses that will form the basis of the plan of care.

Examples of nursing diagnoses that pertain to many geriatric surgical patients include:

- Potential for infection
- Potential fluid volume deficit
- Ineffective thermoregulation
- Potential for impaired skin integrity
- Sensory/perceptual alterations (visual and/or auditory)

Planning

As a result of anatomic and physiologic effects of aging, geriatric patients have, in varying degrees, general decline in organ function and an altered ability to recover from stressful events. In addition to normal age changes, many older adults suffer from one or more chronic conditions that influence the risk of surgery. Successful surgical outcomes in the geriatric patient depend upon elective versus emergency surgical procedures, optimum physical condition of the patient, thorough preoperative assessment, close intraoperative and postoperative monitoring, and preventive measures to decrease the likelihood of complications.

An example of a geriatric surgical patient Sample Care Plan is shown on pp. 1010-1011.

Implementation

Perioperative geriatric patient care is very similar to the care provided to younger adults. However, modifications are made that consider age-specific differences between the two groups. The perioperative nurse who recognizes the special needs of the elderly patient during this, the most critical period of the patient's hospitalization, helps to enhance the course of surgical intervention and postoperative recovery.

Remember that sensory deficits occurring either as a result of age-related changes or merely because eyeglasses and hearing aids are removed can make communication with geriatric patients more difficult. In addition, if preoperative medications have not been adjusted in smaller dosages for the older adult, cognitive impairment may result, thus giving the nurse the impression that the patient is "senile." Unresponsive or uncooperative behavior is therefore expected and ignored. As discussed earlier, acute

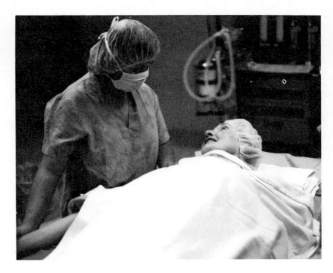

Fig. 30-2. The perioperative nurse's presence and reassuring touch help to allay patient's anxiety prior to anesthesia induction.

confusion in the elderly is the most important indicator of possible underlying conditions that could seriously and adversely affect surgical intervention and outcomes.

The nurse should take advantage of the time spent in preoperative holding or the surgical corridor to introduce herself or himself and explain events to follow. Because a surgical mask is generally not required in these areas, this time is opportune for talking with the older adult and thus facilitating better communication. Once the patient is taken into the operating room, reassuring touch and remaining close to the patient, particularly during anesthesia induction, can help to allay anxiety (Fig. 30-2).

The choice of anesthesia in the elderly patient depends upon physiologic status, length of the operative procedure, and preference of the anesthesiologist or anesthetist. Accurate predictions of how the elderly patient will respond to drugs or anesthesia are difficult to make because of decrease in system function. The nurse should be prepared to respond quickly in assisting the anesthesiologist or anesthetist to stabilize the patient when adverse reactions occur.

Protection of skin integrity is of utmost importance. Loss of subcutaneous fat, poor skin turgor, and tissue fragility can all potentiate a postoperative skin problem. Aging changes in the skin accentuate bony prominences and make positioning one of the most important considerations of care. Elderly patients should be lifted into position, rather than slid or dragged, to prevent shearing injuries.

Often, because of musculoskeletal deformity, elderly patients cannot fully extend the spine, neck, or upper and lower extremities. Using pillows or padding devices to compensate for these skeletal changes not only makes the patient more comfortable during the procedure but also

Sample Care Plan

NURSING DIAGNOSIS:
Potential for wound infection related to intraoperative procedures and length of surgery secondary to age-associated reduction in efficiency of the antigen-antibody reaction and endocrine function

GOAL:
Patient will be free from infection throughout the postoperative period.

INTERVENTIONS:
Monitor for breaks in aseptic technique throughout the procedure.

Take corrective action for breaks in techniques immediately.

Perform preoperative skin preparation using appropriate technique as defined by AORN recommended practices and hospital policy.

Restrict traffic within the operating room.

Keep doors closed during surgical procedures.

Check equipment and assemble all supplies prior to surgery to prevent intraoperative delays.

Confine and contain contaminants.

Assure availability of antibiotics as needed.

NURSING DIAGNOSIS:
Potential fluid volume deficit related to NPO status and intraoperative blood and body fluid losses secondary to age-associated decreases in total body water and plasma volume

GOAL:
Patient will maintain adequate fluid volume levels intraoperatively and postoperatively.

INTERVENTIONS:
Monitor and record intraoperative intake and output.

Provide visualization of sponges and suction canister.

Closely monitor blood versus irrigation fluid amounts in suction bottle.

Assure visualization of the urine drainage bag.

Assure availability of blood replacement as needed.

Assure availability of IV fluids as needed.

Report intake and output to PACU nurse.

NURSING DIAGNOSIS:
Ineffective thermoregulation related to poikilothermy secondary to age-associated physiologic decompensation

GOAL:
Patient will maintain normothermia ± 1° F throughout the perioperative period.

INTERVENTIONS:
Use warm blankets during transport to operating room and replenish as needed throughout the perioperative period.

Place warmed blanket on operating room bed prior to patient transfer.

Use hyperthermia blanket beneath patient for lengthy procedures; begin warming prior to patient's arrival in operating room.

Maintain room temperature at comfortable levels.

Monitor patient for fluctuations in temperature.

Provide additional head covering (cloth or plastic) during surgical procedure.

Prevent overexposure of patient.

---

prevents residual pain or injury postoperatively (Fig. 30-3). Depending on the situation, positioning the patient prior to anesthesia may be best so that the patient can direct positioning efforts in regard to comfort.

Temperature fluctuations are common in the elderly due to changes in thermoregulation. Warming devices are highly recommended, particularly when a lengthy surgical procedure is expected. Prepping solutions should be carefully chosen to prevent skin irritation and warmed to help decrease hypothermic effects. Assuring that the patient is not lying in prep solution or on wet linens also helps to reduce skin injury and inadvertent lowering of body temperature.

As the body is exposed to cold temperatures, blood is shunted away from peripheral body parts to the head. Because the head lacks fat depots and vasoconstriction capabilities, heat loss from the head can be as much as 25% to 60% of total body heat loss (Biddle and Biddle, 1985). Elderly patients should therefore have some form of head covering to prevent the ill effects of hypothermia.

Age-related decline in the immune system and some age-associated diseases have a detrimental effect on the

Sample Care Plan—cont'd

Use warmed prep solutions.

Administer warmed blood and blood products and IV fluids at room temperature.

Administer warmed irrigation fluids.

Remove wet linens prior to transport to PACU.

NURSING DIAGNOSIS:

Potential impairment of integrity related to surgical positioning secondary to alterations in skin turgor, sensation, peripheral tissue perfusion, and skeletal prominence

GOAL:

Patient will maintain skin integrity intraoperatively.

INTERVENTIONS:

Assess potential pressure areas prior to anesthesia and positioning.

Avoid shearing forces by utilizing a four-person lift when transferring patient to or from the operating room bed.

Place safety strap above the knees; prevent undue pressure on the popliteal space and heels.

Provide pillows and other padding devices during positioning to protect potential pressure areas.

Maintain body alignment within restrictions imposed by musculoskeletal age-related changes.

Prevent wrinkling of linen under the patient or positioning devices.

Place electrosurgical dispersive pad in the most appropriate area while avoiding bony prominences.

Avoid pooling of solutions under the patient.

Apply tape sparingly to prevent skin injury during removal.

NURSING DIAGNOSIS:

Sensory/perceptual alterations: visual and/or auditory related to removal of eyeglasses and/or hearing aid in the operating room secondary to age-associated changes in sensory organs

GOAL:

Patient will accurately perceive and interpret environmental and sensory stimuli throughout the perioperative period.

INTERVENTIONS:

Remove operating room mask to introduce self and explain procedures prior to surgery.

Ask the patient to state his or her name and continue to call the patient by stated name.

Attract the patient's attention prior to speaking.

Face the patient directly when speaking.

Speak slowly and distinctly in a low-pitched, clear voice.

Use gestures to supplement words.

Write instructions as needed to clarify information.

Allow ample time for patient to ask questions.

Prepare patient for changes in light intensity.

Assist patient with transfers and mobility.

Inform patient prior to positioning or procedures done prior to anesthesia.

---

aging body's ability to appropriately respond to infectious agents. In the lungs, the cough reflex and ciliary action weaken specialized defense mechanisms against foreign body invasion. Incomplete emptying of the bladder can cause urinary tract infection. Immobility and drug therapy can alter flora in the intestines and make the body more vulnerable to infectious organisms. Because infection and delayed healing of wounds are poorly tolerated and often fatal in the debilitated elderly patient, strict adherence to aseptic technique is extremely important. Because length of surgical procedure is related to incidence of infection,

assuring that needed supplies and equipment are readily available is important. This practice prevents unnecessary waiting for retrieval during the procedure and decreases exposure of the surgical site and also the length of time the elderly patient is under anesthesia.

Fluctuations in fluid volume are common in the geriatric patient. Volume deficits occur as a natural course of aging, whereas volume excess can occur from intraoperative fluid replacement. Careful measurement of intake and output is essential. Assuring that sponges, suction bottle contents, and urinary drainage are closely monitored also helps to prevent potentially fatal complications.

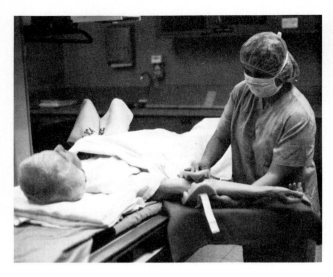

Fig. 30-3. Pillows or padding devices aid patient comfort and prevent residual pain or injury postoperatively.

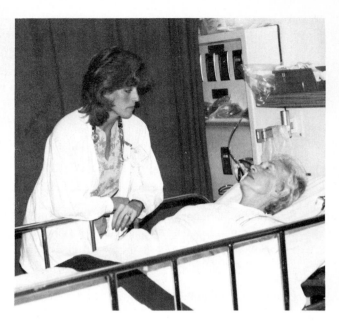

Fig. 30-4. Explanations to the elderly patient prior to any procedure will enhance cooperation.

Evaluation

Before transporting the patient to the PACU, the perioperative nurse should assess the care provided intraoperatively by evaluating expected versus actual outcomes. Specific outcome criteria and goals established for each nursing diagnosis provide the basis for evaluation of care.

The skin is examined for signs of injury, particularly over bony prominences and under the electrosurgical dispersive pad. To prevent skin injury postoperatively, wet linens from beneath the patient are removed, and the patient is carefully lifted from the OR bed to the PACU stretcher. Anticipated frequency of dressing change, such as in a draining wound, should govern the method used to secure the dressing. A minimal amount of tape should be used because its removal can cause additional skin trauma. Depending on the wound site, rolled gauze over the primary dressing may be better so that tape does not have to be applied directly to the skin. Another alternative is Montgomery straps. For smaller wounds the least possible amount of hypoallergenic tape should be used. Because infection is poorly tolerated, the choice of dressing should maximize wound protection while being the least irritating to the skin.

In collaboration with the anesthesiologist or anesthetist, an assessment of intake and output is completed and recorded. Because of the consequences of postoperative dehydration or fluid volume overload in the elderly patient, fluids are increased or decreased accordingly. Blood loss is carefully evaluated, recorded, and reported. The wound is closely observed for bleeding prior to dressing application and postoperatively as the elderly person's ability to recover from hemorrhage and shock is extremely poor.

Evaluation of body temperature is extremely important in the elderly because postoperative hypothermia is quite common and can precipitate agitation and confusion. To prevent any adverse response, the patient should be covered with warmed blankets throughout the recovery period.

As previously discussed, the elderly patient responds poorly to infectious agents. Monitoring the patient frequently for potential infectious complications is extremely important because physical reserves following surgery are greatly reduced. Special attention to sterile and/or clean procedures and frequent handwashing can make the difference between an uneventful surgical outcome and one fraught with complications.

Depending on the patient's level of consciousness, explanation should be given about the impending transfer to PACU as a form of reality orientation. As appropriate, the patient should be introduced to the PACU nurse and told what to expect in the unit. Explanations should always precede any procedure. Often the elderly person is reluctant to cooperate simply because no one has taken the time to explain what is going to happen (Fig. 30-4).

Because of the relatively fine line between stability and the development of postoperative complications, the elderly patient's response to surgery must be closely evaluated. Verbal communication between the perioperative and PACU nurses should include any pertinent preoperative and intraoperative information that could affect postoperative care outcomes, including intake and output; allergies; type and location of catheters, drains, packing, and implantable devices; anesthesia and medications received; and any unusual occurrences that could affect the patient's recovery (Fig. 30-5).

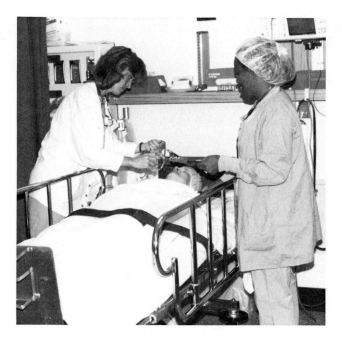

Fig. 30-5. Pertinent information that could affect postoperative care outcomes is communicated to the PACU nurse.

Documentation of goal evaluation can be phrased as outcome statements:

- The patient's skin integrity was maintained, free of redness, bruises, and abrasions; patient will report no pain or impairment of the skin or joint mobility.
- The patient's fluid balance was maintained; urinary output was within normal limits; patient's skin had good turgor, and vital signs were stable.
- The patient's temperature was ± 1° F of normal range; skin was warm to touch, and patient verbalized comfort.
- The patient will exhibit no signs of infection on post-operative evaluation; wound will be free of redness and swelling; lab values and vital signs will be within normal limits.
- The patient accurately perceived and interpreted environmental stimuli, expressed and demonstrated understanding of procedures, and responded appropriately to auditory and verbal stimuli.

SURGICAL INTERVENTIONS

Unlike the pediatric patient, surgery in the elderly does not include special instruments, equipment, or drapes that are made for the geriatric patient exclusively. Surgical procedures that can be considered classically geriatric are governed more by pathology than by anatomy because the spectrum of diseases in the geriatric population is quite different than in younger adults.

Throughout the remainder of this chapter, surgical procedures that are commonly seen in geriatric patients are discussed briefly. Reference is made to other sections of

the text for a more in-depth description of the technical aspects of the procedures.

Common surgical procedures in geriatric patients

A survey of the top 25 most frequently performed surgeries in the United States (1986) included all age groups; 56% of those surgeries were performed on patients 60 years of age and over (Table 30-1). Of the 14 surgeries performed most often in the 60+ age group, the most common was transurethral prostatectomy at 91%, followed by knee replacement (86%), open reduction and internal fixation of fractured femur (84%), bone marrow biopsy (65%), unilateral simple mastectomy (63%), contrast cerebral arteriogram (59%), cystoscopy (56%), combined right and left heart catheterization (55%), venous catheter (54%), balloon angioplasty (53%), left cardiac catheterization (51%), inguinal hernia repair (46%), wound debridement (45%), and total cholecystectomy (39%). An update (1988) reveals similar results (Healthweek, 1989).

Looking at procedures done only in geriatric patients, Keating (1987) reported on surgical diseases and procedures most commonly affecting patients 65 years and older (see the box on p. 1015). His additions to the list previously reported include cataract with intraocular lens, pacemaker implants, above and below-knee amputations and amputations of the toes, thoracentesis, transuretheral resection of bladder lesion, laparotomy for gastrointestinal and genitourinary conditions, sympathectomy, permanent tracheostomy, total hip replacement, and repair and plastic operations on bones except facial.

Abdominal surgery

Surgery on the biliary tract constitutes the majority of abdominal procedures and surgical mortality in the aged. One third of emergency abdominal surgeries in patients over 70 are for biliary disease (Goldman and others, 1983). Most often, operations are performed for complications of calculous disease and less often for malignant obstruction of the bile ducts.

Acute cholecystitis should be treated by cholecystectomy. Conservative treatment of an acute condition followed by interval cholecystectomy is not advisable because elderly men are prone to perforation of an acutely inflamed gallbladder, and the mortality rate is 15% to 25%. All biliary surgery in patients 70 and older should be done with antibiotic prophylaxis (Halter, 1985). See Chapter 12 for an in-depth description of operations of the biliary tract.

Upper gastrointestinal bleeding corresponds with higher mortality in geriatric patients particularly if the bleeding is from a gastric ulcer. The incidence of gastric ulcer increases with age. Diagnosis is established in more than 90% of cases by gastroscopic biopsy (Keating, 1987). Some ulcers get very large and quickly extend outside the stomach into the liver and pancreas. Bleeding gastric ulcers are best treated by gastric resection. In poor-risk patients,

Table 30-1. Top 25 most frequently performed surgeries*

Rank	Procedure	Total	By age group				Payment		Average stay (days)	Percent mortality
			0-17	18-39	40-50	60 +	Medicare and Medicaid	Other		
1	Cervical cesarean section	820,960	27,807	782,140	11,012	0	135,009	685,951	5.0	<0.1
2	Total cholecystectomy (gall bladder removal)	534,767	4,267	155,523	168,423	206,555	194,638	340,129	7.9	1.2
3	Abdominal hysterectomy	468,022	483	192,806	226,139	48,594	64,155	403,868	5.9	0.1
4	Left cardiac catheterization	426,031	697	19,649	186,415	219,270	170,494	255,537	4.1	0.7
5	Transurethral prostatectomy	374,882	265	518	31,892	342,208	288,544	86,339	6.9	0.7
6	Appendectomy	271,901	90,365	122,583	37,858	21,093	33,650	238,251	4.8	0.2
7	Repair of obstetric laceration	266,211	9,331	253,501	3,380	0	46,465	219,748	2.7	<0.1
8	Contrast myelogram	256,816	1,404	100,634	101,586	53,193	47,324	209,493	NA	0.5
9	Intervertebral disk excision	237,227	792	90,871	103,160	42,404	34,732	202,496	8.9	0.1
10	Forceps delivery w/episiotomy	231,015	13,391	215,896	1,728	0	31,277	199,739	2.6	<0.1
11	Wound debridement (removal of foreign material)	178,360	15,342	48,594	34,989	79,436	90,662	87,699	NA	5.7
12	Cystoscopy (examination of bladder w/cystoscope)	166,580	3,956	29,910	39,478	93,236	89,640	76,941	NA	1.3
13	Open reduction of fracture w/ internal fixation (femur)	163,458	3,286	10,632	12,557	136,983	130,450	33,007	9.8	4.5
14	Combined right/left heart catheterization	156,951	9,705	8,661	52,008	86,577	74,528	82,423	4.1	1.6
15	Vaginal hysterectomy	154,950	0	70,267	54,747	29,936	30,989	123,962	5.9	<0.1
16	Balloon angioplasty	148,122	90	5,392	63,804	78,837	57,625	90,497	NA	1.1
17	Unilateral simple mastectomy	122,605	78	7,703	37,963	76,862	61,620	60,986	NA	0.1
18	Venous catheter	122,487	6,459	19,615	30,009	66,408	69,766	52,719	NA	22.3
19	Dilation & curettage, postdelivery	119,660	6,532	108,654	4,474	0	17,017	102,644	2.2	<0.1
20	Tonsillectomy/adenoidectomy	119,294	112,598	6,377	172	148	14,513	104,782	1.4	<0.1
21	Bone marrow biopsy	110,653	6,180	13,260	18,646	72,566	71,545	39,107	NA	7.7
22	Repair of inguinal hernia	109,087	9,112	24,023	25,788	50,164	41,975	67,112	3.1	0.1
23	Knee replacement	98,575	80	895	12,315	85,285	74,016	24,559	NA	.6
24	Contrast cerebral arteriogram	94,200	1,508	12,285	25,193	55,214	48,413	45,787	NA	1.7
25	Open reduction of fracture w/ internal fixation (tibia/fibula)	93,511	8,794	35,395	26,904	22,419	19,972	73,539	NA	0.1

*Surgeries performed in United States short-term, general, nonfederal hospitals, 1986.

NA = figures not available.

suture plication with vagotomy and pyloroplasty can lessen the operative risk (Rossman, 1986). See Chapter 11 for an in-depth description of ulcer surgery.

Hernia

The elective repair of inguinal and femoral hernias can be performed under local anesthesia. General or spinal

---

SURGICAL PROCEDURES PREDOMINANTLY AFFECTING PATIENTS AGED 65 YEARS AND OLDER

Frequency at Least Four Times That of the Population Aged 45 to 64 Years
Lens surgery on the eye
Pacemaker implantation
Arthroplasty and reconstruction of the hip
Above-knee amputation

Frequency at Least Twice That of Population Aged 45 to 64 Years
Thoracentesis
Transurethral prostatectomy
Open reduction of fractures except maxillo-facial
Below-knee amputation

Additional Surgical Procedures
Ileostomy, colostomy, other ostomy
Operations on biliary tract and gallbladder, other than cholecystectomy
Gastrostomy and miscellaneous procedures on stomach
Miscellaneous bladder procedures
Miscellaneous procedures on prostate
Colectomy
Small intestine resection
Ventricular shunts in adults
Repair and plastic operations on bones except facial
Total hip replacement
Arthrocentesis
Cystoscopy
Urethroscopy
Amputation of toes
Sympathectomy
Permanent tracheostomy
Complete mastectomy

anesthesia is not believed to be necessary and may predispose the elderly patient to significant cardiopulmonary and urologic complications (Rossman, 1986). Decisions for local versus spinal or general anesthesia are made based on the patient's overall physiologic status and surgical risk.

In elderly men, the coexistence of inguinal hernia and prostatism is fairly common. Depending on the size of the prostate, the hernioplasty should be postponed until after the prostate surgery.

Progressive pulmonary insufficiency in an elderly patient with symptomatic inguinal hernia can cause postoperative problems. Therefore, hernia repair is advisable only when incarcerated and under local anesthesia. As with other emergency procedures in the elderly, mortality from emergency inguinal hernia repair in the aged is between 7% and 22%, whereas elective hernia repair has a 1.2% to 2% mortality (Nehme, 1983).

Not unusual in the aged are large neglected scrotal hernias. The repair of these hernias is not routine in that the abdominal wall defect may be so large that primary repair cannot take place without tension. Synthetic abdominal wall replacements are helpful in management of such large hernias. The repair of huge scrotal hernias can have a tremendous impact on the personality of the geriatric patient who is much relieved after removal of what can be considered an accessory appendage that is offensive, difficult to clean, and often an impedence to daily activities. See Chapter 13 for an in-depth description of herniorrhaphy.

Genitourinary surgery

The predominant reason for urologic surgery in elderly men is prostatism. Indications for prostatectomy are obstructive signs and symptoms that are persistent and progressive. Prostatism may be silent or have minimal symptoms in the presence of severe bladder decompensation. Prostate surgery, especially transurethral resection of the prostate (TURP), is relatively safe and generally well tolerated. TURP is indicated if the surgeon feels that total resection can be accomplished in 1 hour and there is no bladder disease or impairment to urethral access. Suprapubic prostatectomy, a transvesical adenoma enucleation, is the preferred method when the adenoma weighs over 60 gm or when a stone, diverticulum, or other bladder condition must be treated concurrently (Wheatley, 1988).

Other indications for suprapubic resection are unsuitability of the patient for lithotomy position, a severe stricture of the posterior urethra, or a small bladder capacity. Complications can include pulmonary embolism, but this potential can be minimized by early postoperative ambulation. Sudden dilution of blood from bladder irrigation may occur after TURP and cause hyponatremia and hypotension requiring prompt reversal (Keating, 1987). See Chapter 15 for an in-depth description of prostate surgery.

Ophthalmic surgery

Most ophthalmic procedures are minimally invasive and have a high success rate. Because elderly patients may have concurrent systemic disease, however, even a low-stress procedure should not be treated lightly.

Cataract surgery is among the most common and successful of all surgical procedures. Nearly a million cataract operations are performed in the United States each year, and more than 90% of patients regain the potential for full visual acuity (Kozarsky and Cavanagh, 1988). Intraocular lenses can be safely implanted in the majority of patients. Microsurgical wound closure assures a secure incision that allows immediate ambulation. The procedure is brief and can be done on an outpatient basis and under local anesthesia. The surgical stress is considered so low and visual rehabilitation so rapid that severe visual impairment is considered a reasonable indication to perform surgery even if the elderly patient is debilitated. See Chapter 18 for an in-depth description of cataract surgery.

Orthopedic surgery

Osteoporosis is the most obvious skeletal change that occurs with advancing age. It leads to susceptibility to fracture. An approximate loss of 40% of the mineral content of the bone must be present before detectable change is evident on x-ray. To some degree osteoporosis is related to a lessening of physical activity, but it is also related to lessened hormonal secretion. Thus, postmenopausal women are more prone to develop the condition and therefore more likely to sustain a hip fracture.

Age-related changes in bone increase the incidence of displaced femoral and intertrochanteric fractures of the upper femur. Because the usual cause of death in patients with upper femur fracture is pulmonary embolus, surgery is designed to relieve the severe pain, allow movement in and out of bed, and return the patient to his or her former environment as quickly as possible with minimal debilitation.

A displaced femoral neck fracture must be surgically repaired or healing will not occur. In elderly patients, 70 and older, prosthetic replacement is usually done because it allows for early ambulation and will last throughout the remaining years of the patient's life. Intertrochanteric and subtrochanteric fractures are best treated with internal fixation. These methods also allow for early mobility (Whitesides, 1988).

Degenerative joint disease (osteoarthritis) and inflammatory polyarticular disease (rheumatoid arthritis) are the primary indications for total joint replacement in the hip and knee (DeAndrade, 1988). See Chapter 22 for an in-depth description of hip and knee surgery.

Cardiovascular surgery

Cardiovascular disease remains the number one cause of death in the elderly. Of 753,800 persons dying of heart disease, about 404,000 were 75 years or older. Of this group 58% of deaths were females; however, in those 55 to 74, 64% of deaths were men. Women tended to have cerebrovascular disease, whereas men had more aneurysmal disease of the aorta (Rossman, 1986).

Coronary bypass surgery is performed in increasing numbers in patients over 65 with an operative mortality of 3% to 6%. Elective peripheral vascular reconstructive procedures are also encouraged in the geriatric patient. Patients older than 80 are reported to have had as little as 5.5% hospital mortality and a 13.8% complication rate in various vascular procedures including cerebrovascular reconstruction, aortic aneurysms, grafts of upper and lower extremity vessels, and embolectomy in acute arterial occlusion (Edwards and others, 1982).

In another group of 80-year-olds undergoing elective aortic aneurysmectomy, the patients' mortality rate was reported to be only 4.7%, and 86% of the patients were reported to have quality of life equal to or better than preoperative status (O'Donnell and others, 1976). The facts that 25% of abdominal aortic aneurysms 4 to 7 cm in diameter do rupture and that the operative mortality rate for ruptured aneurysm is about 40% provide a strong argument for elective surgery in carefully screened and prepared elderly patients. See Chapters 26 and 27 for a more in-depth description of vascular and cardiac surgery.

Additional considerations

Every surgical procedure carries with it a certain amount of risk no matter what the age of the patient. As discussed previously, the physiologic deficits of aging increase surgical risk in the aged patient. Procedures that are performed in the thorax or the peritoneal cavity are considered of high mortality risk. Procedures of moderate risk include vascular and hip procedures, and low-risk procedures include prostatectomy and mastectomy. However, any procedure, even those considered low risk, can have poor outcomes, depending on the patient's overall condition.

No particular surgical technique is applicable to elderly patients. As described by Vowles (1979), careful assessment, good preoperative preparation, skillful anesthesia, gentle handling of tissues, and the necessary care to get it right the first time and so avoid complications and the need for secondary operations are the steps most likely to lead to success.

REFERENCES

American Association of Retired Persons: A profile of older Americans, Washington, DC, 1986, the Association.

Barry, P.P.: Primary care evaluation of the elderly for elective surgery, Geriatrics 42:77, 1987.

Biddle, C.J., and Biddle, W.L.: A plastic head cover to reduce surgical heat loss, Geriatric Nurse Jan./Feb. 1985, p. 39.

Brandt, E.: To cherish life, Parade Magazine Oct. 1988, p. 4.

Charatan, F.B.: Acute confusion and the elderly, Hosp. Phys. 12:8, 1976.

DeAndrade, J.R.: Total hip joint replacement. In Lubin, M.F., Walker, H.K., and Smith, R.B.: Medical management of the surgical patient, ed. 2, Boston, 1988, Butterworths.

Dripps, R.D., Eckenhoff, J.E., and Vandam, L.D.: Introduction to anesthesia: the principles of safe practice, ed. 7, Philadelphia, 1988, W.B. Saunders Co.

Dychtwald, K., and Zitter, M.: The elderly as healthcare consumers, Healthcare Exec. 2:28, 1987.

Edwards, W.H., Mulherin, J.L., and Rogers, D.M.: Vascular reconstruction in the octogenarian, South. Med. J. 75:648, 1982.

Ferris, P.: Surgical management of the elderly, Hosp. Prac. 11:65, 1976.

Galazka, S.S.: Preoperative evaluation of the elderly surgical patient, J. Fam. Prac. 27:622, 1988.

Goldman, L.D., Steer, M.L., and Silea, W.: Recurrent cholangitis after biliary surgery, Am. J. Surg. 145:450, 1983.

Halter, J.B.: Alterations of autonomic nervous system function. In Andres, R., Bierman, E.L., and Hazzard, W.R.: Principles of geriatric medicine, New York, 1985, McGraw-Hill.

Katz, J.D.: Anesthetic considerations for geriatric patients, Conn. Med., July 1985, p.424.

Keating, H.J.: Preoperative considerations in the geriatric patient, Med. Clin. North Am. 71:569, 1987.

Kozarsky, A.M., and Cavanagh, H.D.: Cataract surgery. In Lubin, M.F., Walker, H.K., and Smith, R.B.: Medical management of the surgical patient, ed. 2, Boston, 1988, Butterworths.

Nehme, A.E.: Groin hernia in elderly patients, Am. J. Surg. 146:257, 1983.

O'Donnell, T.F., Darling, C., and Linton, R.R.: Is 80 years too old for aneurysmectomy? Arch. Surg. 111:1250, 1976.

Rossman, I.: Clinical geriatrics, ed. 3, Philadelphia, 1986, J.B. Lippincott Co.

Seymour, D.G., Pringle, R., and Shaw, J.W.: The role of the routine preoperative chest x-ray in the elderly general surgical patient, Post Grad. Med. J. 58:741, 1982.

Top 25 most frequently performed surgeries, Healthweek, May 1989, p. 38.

Top 25 most frequently performed surgeries, Healthweek, Nov. 1989, p. 59.

Vowles, K.D.J.: Surgical problems in the aged, Bristol, 1979, John Wright and Sons Ltd.

Wheatley, J.K.: Transurethral resection of the prostate. In Lubin, M.F., Walker, H.K., and Smith, R.B.: Medical management of the surgical patient, ed. 2, Boston, 1988, Butterworths.

Whitesides, T.E.: Surgery for hip fractures. In Lubin, M.F., Walker, H.K., and Smith, R.B.: Medical management of the surgical patient, ed. 2, Boston, 1988, Butterworths.

BIBLIOGRAPHY

Burden, N.: Preoperative assessment of the ambulatory surgical patient, J. Postanesthesia Nurs. 1(1):48, 1986.

Carrick, L.: Considerations for the elderly surgical patient, Geriatric Nursing, Jan./Feb. 1982, p. 43.

Crawford, F.J.: Ambulatory surgery: the elderly patient, AORN J. 41:356, 1985.

Dean, A.F.: The aging surgical patient: historical overview, implications and nursing care, Perioperative Nurs. Quart. 3(1):1, 1987.

Elderly 21 percent of population by 2040. Hospitals Mar. 1985, p. 41.

Jackson, M.F.: High risk surgical patients, J. Gerontological Nurs. 14(1):8, 1988.

Latz, P.A., and Wyble, S.J.: Elderly patients: perioperative nursing implications, AORN J. 46:238, 1987.

Meckes, P.F.: Perioperative care of the elderly surgical patient, Today's OR Nurse 6:8, 1984.

Omerod, B.H.: Perioperative nursing care of the elderly outpatient, Perioperative Nurs. Quart. 3(2):22, 1987.

Walker, M.L.: Growing old: increased surgical risks in the elderly, AORN J. 43:887, 1986.

Waugaman, W.R.: Surgery and the patient with Alzheimer's disease, Geriatric Nurs. July/Aug. 1988, p. 227.

INDEX

A

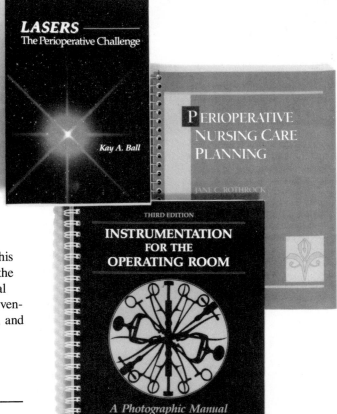
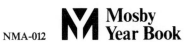